HANDBUCH DER NEUROLOGIE

HERAUSGEGEBEN

VON

O. BUMKE UND O. FOERSTER
MÜNCHEN BRESLAU

SIEBZEHNTER BAND

SPEZIELLE NEUROLOGIE IX

ERKRANKUNGEN DES RÜCKENMARKS UND GEHIRNS VII

EPILEPSIE · NARKOLEPSIE · SPASMOPHILIE · MIGRÄNE
VASOMOTORISCH-TROPHISCHE ERKRANKUNGEN
NEURASTHENISCHE REAKTION · ORGANNEUROSEN

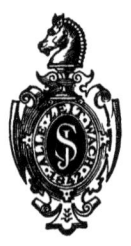

SPRINGER-VERLAG BERLIN HEIDELBERG GMBH
1935

EPILEPSIE · NARKOLEPSIE SPASMOPHILIE · MIGRÄNE VASOMOTORISCH-TROPHISCHE ERKRANKUNGEN NEURASTHENISCHE REAKTION ORGANNEUROSEN

BEARBEITET VON

E. BRAUN · R. CASSIRER † · R. HIRSCHFELD · J. HUSLER
W. JAHRREISS · H. RICHTER · J. WILDER
S. A. KINNIER WILSON

MIT 24 ABBILDUNGEN

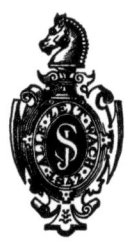

SPRINGER-VERLAG BERLIN HEIDELBERG GMBH
1935

ALLE RECHTE INSBESONDERE DAS DER ÜBERSETZUNG
IN FREMDE SPRACHEN, VORBEHALTEN.
COPYRIGHT 1935 BY SPRINGER-VERLAG BERLIN HEIDELBERG
URSPRÜNGLICH ERSCHIENEN JULIUS SPRINGER IN BERLIN 1935
SOFTCOVER REPRINT OF THE HARDCOVER 1ST EDITION 1935

ISBN 978-3-662-27285-5   ISBN 978-3-662-28772-9 (eBook)
DOI 10.1007/978-3-662-28772-9

Inhaltsverzeichnis.

Seite

Epilepsie und verwandte Krankheiten 1
  The Epilepsies. By Dr. S. A. KINNIER WILSON-London 1
    Introduction 1
    Definition and Classification 4
    Symptomatology 6
    Individual epileptic Symptoms 22
    Clinical Types 26
    Clinical variants 31
      Motor variants S. 31. — Sensory variants S. 38. — Psychical variants S. 40. — Visceral variants S. 41.
    Semeiology apart from fits 44
    Clinical pathology 45
    Morbid anatomy 49
    Pathological states accompanying epilepsy 52
    Experimental convulsions 52
    Pathogenesis of epileptic fits 55
    Neural mechanisms of discharge 58
    Physiological theories of discharge 59
    General etiological considerations 61
    Diagnosis 67
    Course and prognosis 70
    Treatment 73
    Literature 84

Narkolepsie. Von Primararzt Dr. J. WILDER-Wien 87
    Vorwort S. 87. — Definition S. 87. — Geschichte S. 88. — Symptomatologie S. 88. — Beziehungen der Schlafanfälle zum affektiven Tonusverlust S. 102. — Atypische Zustände S. 102. — Der Nachtschlaf der Narkoleptiker S. 106. — Der neurologische Befund bei der Narkolepsie S. 107. — Vegetatives System S. 107. — Andere Laboratoriumsbefunde S. 110. — Der äußere Habitus S. 110. — Das psychische Bild S. 110. — Ätiologische Faktoren S. 111. — Beziehungen zur Epilepsie S. 120. — Verlauf, Prognose S. 122. — Häufigkeit S. 124. — Alter S. 126. — Geschlecht S. 126. — Beruf S. 126. — Pathologische Anatomie, Lokalisation S. 127. — Pathogenese S. 128. — Nomenklatur S. 135. — Differentialdiagnose S. 136. — Therapie S. 138. — Forensische und soziale Bedeutung S. 139.
  Literatur 140

Spasmophilie. Von Professor Dr. J. HUSLER-München. (Mit 6 Abbildungen) . . 141
  I. Tetanoide Spasmophilie (Spasmophilie im engeren Sinne) 141
  II. Spasmophilie im weiteren Sinne 159
  Literatur 164

Die Migräne. Von Privatdozent Dr. H. RICHTER-Budapest 166
  I. Symptomatologie des Migräneanfalles 167
    1. Allgemeines über das Auftreten, Periodizität, Dauer und Verlauf des Migräneanfalles 167
    2. Der gewöhnliche (vulgäre) Migräneanfall 169
    3. Die Augenmigräne (Migraine ophthalmique) 175
    4. Die ophthalmoplegische Migräne 180
        Schwindel und Gleichgewichtsstörungen 187
    5. Die mit Epilepsie kombinierte Migräne 189
    6. Psychische Störungen bei Migräne 194
    7. Hysterische Reaktionen bei Migräne 197
    8. Interparoxysmale Erscheinungen bei Migräne 198

		Seite

II. Pathogenese der Migräne 198
    1. Pathomechanismus des Migräneanfalles 199
    2. Ätiologie der Migräne 217
    Anhang. Symptomatische Migräne 229
III. Zur Differentialdiagnose 231
IV. Prognose 232
V. Therapie der Migräne 233
Literatur 242

Vasomotorisch-trophische Erkrankungen. Von Professor Dr. R. Cassirer † und Dr. R. Hirschfeld-Berlin. (Mit 16 Abbildungen) 246
  I. Die Raynaudsche Krankheit 246
    Ätiologie S. 246. — Symptomatologie S. 249. — Verlauf S. 264. — Pathologische Anatomie und Pathologie S. 266. — Diagnose S. 272. — Therapie S. 276.
  II. Die Akroasphyxia chronica (Akrocyanose) 281
  III. Die Erythromelalgie 286
    Ätiologie S. 287. — Symptomatologie S. 288. — Pathologische Anatomie und Pathogenese S. 294. — Diagnose S. 296. — Verlauf und Prognose S. 298. — Therapie S. 298.
  IV. Die Akroparästhesien 299
    Ätiologie S. 300. — Symptomatologie S. 300. — Verlauf S. 301. — Pathologie S. 301. — Diagnose S. 304. — Therapie S. 305.
  V. Die multiple neurotische Hautgangrän 306
  VI. Die Sklerodermie 312
    Ätiologie S. 312. — Symptomatologie S. 316. — Hemiatrophia faciei progressiva S. 330. — Verlauf und Prognose S. 343. — Pathologische Anatomie S. 344. — Pathogenese S. 349. — Diagnose S. 357. — Therapie S. 361.
  VII. Das akute umschriebene Ödem (Quinckesches Ödem) 366
    Ätiologie S. 367. — Symptomatologie S. 373. — Prognose S. 388. — Pathogenese S. 389. — Diagnose S. 392. — Therapie S. 397.
Literatur 400

Die neurasthenische Reaktion. Von Professor Dr. E. Braun-Kiel. (Mit 2 Abbildungen) 426
  I. Pathogenese 426
    Einleitung S. 426. — Konstitutionelle Nervosität S. 426. — Neurasthenische Reaktion S. 427. — Erschöpfung und Übermüdung S. 429. — Krankhafte Überempfindlichkeit S. 431. — Reizbare Schwäche S. 432. — Das Funktionssubstrat S. 434.
  II. Klinische Stellung und Ätiologie 440
    Die reine neurasthenische Reaktion S. 440. — Grenzen zur konstitutionellen Nervosität S. 441. — Körperliche Krankheiten und Schädigungen als Ursachen S. 444. — Pseudoneurasthenische Erscheinungen S. 446. — Die psychischen Ursachen S. 448. — Neurasthenische Reaktion ein vitales Syndrom S. 453. — Biologische und soziale Hilfsursachen S. 453. — Die Krankheit unserer Zeit S. 455.
  III. Symptomatologie. Ausgänge und Behandlung 456
    Randsymptome S. 456. — Die vegetativ-nervöse Regulationsstörung S. 457. — Körperliche Symptome S. 458. — Prognose S. 466. — Psychogene Entwicklungen S. 467. — Therapie S. 468.
Literatur 471

Die sog. Organneurosen. Von Privatdozent Dr. W. Jahrreiss-Köln 477
  I. Psychophysische Korrelationen 477
    1. Begriffe und Begrenzungen 477
    2. Die seelische Beeinflussung des vegetativen Nervensystems in der Norm und im Experiment 480

Physiologische Vorbemerkungen S. 480. — Einfluß seelischer Vorgänge auf vegetative Funktionen S. 485. — Die Wirkungsweise seelischer Beeinflussung vegetativer Funktionen S. 489. — Begriff des Organismus S. 491. — Psychovegetative Korrelationen und Leib-Seele-Problem S. 492.

II. Die organneurotischen Betriebsstörungen 494
   1. Allgemeiner Teil 494
      Verursachung und Entstehung S. 494. — Erkennen und Verlauf S. 502. — Behandlung S. 506.
   2. Besonderer Teil 509
      Kreislaufsystem S. 509. — Funktionelle Störungen der Atmung S. 514. — Urogenitalsystem S. 520. — Haut S. 522.

Anhang: Die sog. „Koordinationsneurosen" 523
   1. Allgemeiner Teil 523
   2. Besonderer Teil 527
      a) Koordinatorische Beschäftigungsneurosen (Bewegungsneurosen) 527
      b) Stottern 529

Literatur 531

Namenverzeichnis 541

Sachverzeichnis 561

Epilepsie und verwandte Krankheiten.

The Epilepsies.

By

S. A. KINNIER WILSON.

London.

The common nervous affection known everywhere as "epilepsy", still described with equal frequency and inaccuracy as a "disease" whose cardinal symptom is the recurrent fit, is familiar to laity and medical profession alike. An ancient malady, theories propounded at different epochs to explain its phenomena have till recent times only mirrored the prejudices of the minds devising them; and it has been claimed as a therapeutic reserve by each successive brand of healer, from the priest to the psychoanalyst. That knowledge of its intimate nature is at length being gained, however, can scarcely be doubted; but the complexity of its problems, banal though the condition is, still hinders full insight into its mystery. Despite the glaring prominence of its major clinical features they shed at best but a feeble light on epileptic genesis, while by reason of their brevity the chance for objective investigation is often rendered unavailing. Modern research, in consequence, is concerning itself with the induction of fits experimentally, with discovery of the physicochemical changes accompanying them, and with their control by other methods than the purely medicinal. The result is that time-worn theories are undergoing revision and the way is being cleared to a better understanding of epileptic manifestations.

Introduction.

At the outset some exposition of what the term should convey is indispensable.

1. The traditional view is based on the contention that a disease called "epilepsy" exists, its salient symptom being the occasional fit. This "disease" is alleged to be progressive, rather intractable, and prone to result in mental deterioration. Its cause being unknown, it is labelled "idiopathic", in contrast with other well-recognised morbid states often disclosed by similar fits, e. g. cerebral vascular disease, brain tumour, encephalitis, and so on. But the epithet is obsolete, serving merely to cloud the issue. It is curious that the patently symptomatic nature of so many epilepsies has not yet sufficed to convince everyone of the untenable character of the hypothesis constituting this "idiopathic" variety a self-contained and circumscribed entity. No less confusion has been engendered by resort to such terms as "genuine" or "essential" to characterise the "disease", as though fits of a symptomatic kind were merely casual or in some way "false". The best present-day opinion declines to accept the implication underlying the "idiopathic" doctrine, viz. that of "epilepsia sine materie," affirming on the contrary that all epilepsy is symptomatic, whether its basis is discoverable or not; as we shall see, many causes of fits are well substantiated, and warrant the belief that further research will eventually

reveal the origin of those whose source still escapes inquiry. Yet so stereotyped has this view of epilepsy as a "disease" become that the conception is still often transferred to *any* case of fits, with the innuendo that there lurks something forbidding or sinister in its aspect and prognosis, an implication altogether at variance with the facts.

The truth is no class of nervous symptom has suffered more from nosological artificialities than that termed "epileptic". Even if we imagine a patient displaying occasional fits to be the subject of a "disease" which might as well be called "epilepsy" as anything else we are unable to demarcate its boundaries. As every clinician can vouch, a person may have one fit only in the course of his life, or a few, at the widest intervals, witness the case of a lady who had a seizure at the age of 14, when her period of reproductive activity commenced, and another at 44, at its close. To pronounce such cases epileptic in the traditional sense is inequitable, yet the nature of the attacks may not permit description by any other name if the word is to retain its value. Convulsions in infancy, again, do not authorise a diagnosis of epilepsy with the ominous meaning attached thereto that some still suppose is proper to the term; but when fits appear first in middle life or later, partisans of the "disease" theory admit the possibility of an "organic" basis distinct from any conceivably underlying the "idiopathic" form. Such inconsistencies vanish if the view of epilepsy as a disease per se is abandoned. Instead of "the epilepsies" it might be preferable to employ alternatives of more non-committal nature, e. g. "paroxysmal disorders" or "convulsive states," a series of diverse conditions distinguished by the occasional occurrence of "fits," but at the risk of perpetuating notions inherited from a less well-informed era the word will doubtless continue in vogue. For didactic purposes, too, it may be expedient to differentiate epilepsy "of unknown origin" in some terminological way, however undesirable from the standpoint of physiology and pathogenesis.

2. Should nosological and connotative difficulties be provisionally settled by considering all varieties symptoms or syndromes only, we are at once faced by the cognate problem of defining what constitutes a fit. This interpretative question becomes almost impossible to answer in any completely satisfactory manner. The physician may think he knows a fit at sight, but might be somewhat embarrassed in specifying the criteria on which he depends. Facts compel the admission that the property of uncontrolled discharge is probably common to all cell-groups on occasion whatever their particular function, even though a distinction is drawn between permanent instability in a diseased tissue and temporary instability in a healthy tissue; and if this generalisation is acceptable allowance must be made for the greatest diversity and heterogeneousness in the phenomena. It is open to the clinician to claim any transient, paroxysmal, disorderly, uncontrolled, and recurrent manifestation of any neural process as in essence a "fit", and this on any physiological plane. In its ordinary acceptation the word designates conditions as wide apart as convulsive twitches restricted to a segment of a limb and highly coordinated acts of the whole person, sometimes of long duration, comprised under the term "hysterical." Although often considered to embody unvaryingly the idea of malregulated movement, it cannot be confined to attacks of a hyperkinetic class, being used legitimately for certain others of which motionlessness is the cardinal feature. That is to say, "fit" and "convulsion" are not synonymous, nor is the expression "convulsive fit" tautological. Again, common parlance allows such phrases as "a fit of laughter", "a fit of sneezing", "a fit of temper", and so forth, occurrences seeming to differ toto caelo from those usually placed in the class of epileptic symptoms but nevertheless sharing some or all of the characters mentioned above as ordinarily

connoted by the term. A major attack ranges from a disturbance on the highest level (the conscious aura) to disorders of sensory, motor, and visceral nature; other forms may be confined almost entirely to affection of one of these systems. Once initiated, the epileptic process spreads far and wide through the neuraxis, or remains strictly confined; the aura, occurring by itself, may constitute a larval fit; loss of consciousness, as in various examples of petit mal, can supervene almost monosymptomatically. A faint, a cry, a laugh, may be as definitely epileptic as a flicker of finger and thumb, cyanosis, or defaecation. The possibilities in truth are legion; no rigid semeiological framework can be fashioned to embrace them all. Some clinical types may appear remote from epilepsy as currently understood and the objection be raised that they would thus be made equivalent to other orders of phenomena never thought epileptic. Clinical traits such as rapidity of onset, paroxysmal character, failure of control, crudity, disorderliness, transience, interruption of the stream of consciousness, and recurrence are probably foremost in the mind whenever we think of "attacks" or "fits" of any sort, but none is pathognomonic, while from a given case one or several may be lacking and others seemingly foreign to usual conceptions be in evidence. For instance, the aura of a major fit is often a hallucination of one or other sense, as a rule neither ill-regulated nor excessive in intensity or other quality; yet when it occurs it must be assigned an integral share in the whole process of the fit. Further, some movements of certain attacks are quasi-purposive and coordinated, devoid of all convulsive element; those of petit mal and of limited JACKSONian seizures may be conspicuously slight, displaying none of the violence or exaggeration suggested by "fit" and hardly distinguishable in some aspects from tic or myoclonus. Recent years have brought to the fore curious cases of postencephalitic tonic or tonico-clonic movement, and of respiratory spasm, whose respective classification with tic or epilepsy appears to depend more on personal choice and predilection than on any canons of nosology — distinction is difficult when the above-mentioned characters are not plainly present or prove ambiguous. Generally recognised with ease, uncertainty sometimes besets the diagnosis of petit mal, and is opportunely cloaked by employment of the colourless word "faint". Vagueness may also be thought inseparable from fits implicating visceral centres, chiefly or exclusively, for in the absence of skeletal muscle involvement, interference with consciousness, and other banal signs, divergence from ordinary epileptic notions is sometimes extreme. Yet of the reality of such visceral attacks no doubt can be entertained, aside from the fact that accompaniments of an identical kind are accepted without cavil in any major case. It appears neither inconceivable nor absurd that some bouts of tachycardia, diarrhoea, polyuria, etc., even of neuralgia, might be registered in the class.

Thoughtful contemplation of the epileptic field can thus scarcely fail to discount in some degree the value of conventional fit characteristics forming its landmarks. Of these, perhaps the least mutable comprise suddenness in onset, brevity of duration, and habit of recurrence. Without doubt such features are customary in the average case, yet some varieties (notably epilepsia partialis continua) are protracted in their manifestations, repetitions may be extraordinarily infrequent, and even initial abruptness loses significance when the aura is long drawn out. Clouding of consciousness is not a cardinal element; with greater reason disorder of motility might be claimed to be of the essence of epilepsy, and if the term be taken in its widest sense, to cover visceromotility, the assertion may perhaps stand. However this may be, the specificity of all such characters is further diminished by consideration of the epileptic borderland, with its migraine, vertiginous attacks, narcolepsy and other states whose clinical expression comprises features of similar or identical kinds. Hence to institute standards even in regard to the main types of epileptic fit becomes an almost Sisyphean task. Their phenomena edge off by gradations from the motor convulsive seizure to psychical, sensory, or visceral symptoms of a highly disparate sort, yet refuse to be divorced for any physiological reason. Ignorance of the exact nature of the epileptic discharge accounts indubitably for hesitation over the epileptic character of this or that symptom; but if the same processes can reasonably be postulated in action behind these diverse syndromes selection becomes arbitrary and unwarrantable. For the present it is wise to eschew schematic definition and allow elasticity in respect of epileptic symptoms; however general the agreement on the habitual manifestations of the affection, any endeavour to circumscribe it by a series of Procrustean slices transgresses modern views on the nature of disease.

History and Literature. The antiquity of the condition is exemplified by the Hippocratic use of the word to denote a malady "seizing" the patient ($\dot{\epsilon}\pi\iota\lambda\alpha\mu\beta\acute{a}\nu\omega$, $\dot{\epsilon}\pi\iota\lambda\eta\psi\iota\alpha$, a taking hold of) and considered of divine origin (hence also termed $\dot{\iota}\epsilon\varrho\acute{a}$ $\nu\acute{o}\sigma o\varsigma$, the "sacred disease"). Latin writers spoke of morbus sacer, morbus deificus (because it increased the priest's reputation for sanctity), morbus caducus (the "falling disease"), morbus sideratus ("star-struck") or morbus comitialis, since its unpropitious occurrence in an assembly or comitia sufficed to stop the proceedings. In England records of "falling sickness" date back at least as far as the manual for nuns entitled "Ancren Riule" (circa 1210), whose author refers to the "disease commonly so called". In its long course epilepsy has probably altered less than any other affection known to medicine, as the lines of LUCRETIUS show.

GALEN recognised different varieties, including perhaps the JACKSONian, to judge by the following excerpt:

"There is another form of epilepsy which is more rare; this begins in any part of the body, and mounts to the head in such a manner that the patient is sensible of it himself." He refers to cases commencing in the leg, but whether it was a march of convulsive movement that he observed, or merely an ascending aura (in one, a kind of cold vapour, '$\alpha\check{\delta}\varrho\alpha$ $\tau\iota\varsigma$ $\psi\upsilon\chi\varrho\acute{a}$') is not very clear.

The course of epilepsy through the centuries has been sketched by HERPIN, whose personal contributions are conspicuous amid others heralding a new era of scientific interest in the first half of the nineteenth; before, and later, to enumerate but a few, came the works of PORTAL, ESQUIROL, TROUSSEAU, RUSSELL REYNOLDS, HUGHLINGS JACKSON, and GOWERS. Other studies comprise those of ALDREN TURNER, FÉRÉ, BINSWANGER, CESTON, PAGNIEZ, CROUZON, MUSKENS, LENNOX and COBB. As may be imagined, the literature of the subject has reached huge dimensions; the Index Catalogue of the U.S. Surgeon-General's Office (1925) contains about 3000 titles, and GRUHLE's review for the years 1910 to 1920 deals with some 1000 articles.

Speciesal studies of the history of epilepsy have been written by JOSAT and by BES DE BERC.

Definition and Classification.

From the introductory paragraphs the difficulties encountered at the very onset can be realised; they explain the vexed state of contemporary knowledge, evident to all who scan monographs and treatises on the subject, and vitiate to no little extent theoretical discussions and practical conclusions based on statistics. If there is no agreement on what constitutes epilepsy, how is it possible to decide who are epileptics? The prevalence of uncertainty lays open to criticism various efforts at *definition* and *classification*.

1. According to TURNER, the only entirely characteristic symptom of epilepsy is the periodic recurrence of attacks of loss, or impairment, of consciousness, sometimes accompanied by convulsion; yet that authority qualifies his own assertion by admitting the genuineness of epileptic phenomena without such impairment or loss, and its development in states outside the category. Others, e. g. GOWERS and MUSKENS, prefer not to essay the task, being content to specify more or less fundamental traits without their formal embodiment in a definition. The clinical polymorphism of the affection defeats the best attempts of the

schematists at codification based on *symptoms*. Apart from protean aspects of the fit itself, diverse features of pre- and post-convulsive states must not be overlooked; the latter include the most varied sets of opposites, from sleep to fugues, stupor to combativeness, speedy recovery to prolonged headache, fatigue and malaise. Some of these are indistinguishable from accompaniments of seizures signalizing hysteria. As will be noticed later, not a few conventional clinical differences between hysterical and epileptic fits do not retain the diagnostic value ascribed to them.

2. Approaching the problem from another direction, some observers have essayed definition on *etiological* lines. In the opinion of Rows and Bond emotional disorder underlies every case; hence, relegating symptoms to a minor position, and accounting them negligible from either biological or psychological standpoint, these writers affirm that however heterogeneous the clinical types "some emotional state involving a disturbance of consciousness, and some reaction to express the emotion," compose the essence of epilepsy, which they define as a "functional mental illness" whose somatic manifestations are preceded by "complex mental activities". True though the assertion may be, so far as *some* epilepsies are concerned, and significant as may be, on occasion, the participation of a psychical factor, this view of the question at issue scarcely commends itself to the neurologist familiar with the "organic" basis of many attacks. Nor is his scepticism weakened by evidential claims for the influencing of neural processes by emotional agencies.

3. We owe the soundest attempts at *physiological* definition to the genius of HUGHLINGS JACKSON, whose thoughtful exposition must appeal to many minds: "Epilepsy is not one particular grouping of symptoms occuring occasionally from local discharge; whether it puts muscles in movement or not, that is, whether there be a convulsion or not, matters nothing for the definition." And again, "it does not matter for the definition whether there be loss of consciousness or not." In his view epilepsy "is the name for occasional, sudden, excessive, rapid, and local discharges of grey matter". The formal statement can hardly be bettered; it has the advantage of comprehending the multiplicity of symptoms on any physiological level, from highest to lowest, and of being etiologically independent. By laying stress on both suddenness and rapidity of evolution JACKSON seeks to limit the conception of discharge so as to exclude other processes of similar nature differing in these particulars. Apparently some such restriction is also favoured by GOWERS, who affirms that symptoms of "a truly epileptic nature endure only for a few minutes, and often only for a few seconds."

Notwithstanding such pronouncements, it is impracticable to define what is epileptic and what not by reference to the time factor, which cannot be specified with exactitude, nor does brevity allow for various pre- and post-convulsive conditions that are certainly far from short. Some may bridge the difficulty by dismissing both of these as indirect manifestations and not an integral part of the whole process, although this amounts almost to a petitio principii. Besides, as already remarked, the definition will not serve for the accepted variety distinguished by the term "epilepsia partialis continua". A second objection concerns the technical word "discharge," since there are types (admitted by both JACKSON and GOWERS) consisting mainly of inhibitory phenomena without any trace of excessive discharge. Loss of consciousness itself, in JACKSONian phraseology a "negative" symptom, plainly indicates cellular arrest rather than activity. Perhaps the principal feature of the average case of petit mal is cessation of function in one or other form, while the initial stage of major attacks not infrequently illustrates action of the same inhibitory process, e. g. loss of sight or of speech. Under circumstances yet obscure stimuli inaugurating a fit may be followed by restraint of motor discharges, a variety which may be termed "inhibitory epilepsy" (see below). Thirdly, the involuntary flexor spasms of paraplegia, caricaturing movements of tic douloureux, contortions of athetosis and dystonia lenticularis, and other spasmodic syndromes, represent local discharges of grey matter that are also intermittent, excessive, and sometimes individually brief; their differentiation from epileptic symptoms, however facile, depends rather on extrinsic than intrinsic characters. Phenomena of these different kinds impair the validity of the JACKSONian definition and exemplify afresh the intricacies of the epileptic state.

Fluidity in conception and haziness of clinical outlines account no less readily for disagreement in regard to *classification*.

1. Some observers choose an arrangement based on the *time of life* at which the affection develops, thus: infantile convulsions, adolescent, menstrual, climacteric, and senile types. It is, however, too simplistic to possess any merit.

2. A much more useful division depends on *symptomatic* forms, distinguishing JACKSONian (or partial) epilepsy, grand mal, petit mal, myoclonus epilepticus, and numerous variants (to be specified later).

3. Tabulation in accordance with *etiology* is preferable, and were more data to hand the advantages it offers would doubtless lead to its adoption. The subject is discussed on a later page, but it is well to note now that actual exciting causes of fits must be disengaged from morbid conditions with which their appearance may be associated.

4. Classification founded on *pathology* might have something to recommend it, for many known toxic, humoral, vascular, neoplastic and other disease-states favour epileptic development. Here again, however, a proviso is needful to obviate misunderstanding; the pathology of epilepsy should consist of such tissue-changes as can be shown to accompany the affection unvaryingly and whose presence is responsible for the symptoms; but whether any of this nature exist is problematical. The fit represents the liberation of energy, yet very little of it can be due to the discharge of abnormally nourished neural units, the greater part being produced by consecutive discharges of *normal* cells. Temporary instability of healthy mechanisms, whose activity is revealed by "positive" symptoms, is not likely to yield evidence of cytological change, for after the attack a restitutio ad integrum takes place; hence modifications of neural and other tissues found in chronic cases post mortem are almost certainly the exhausting *effect* of repeated discharge and not their instrument. Thus the various diseased states in whose presence fits have been remarked do not properly constitute the specific pathology of epilepsy, though their analytic study aids in penetrating the mystery of pathogenesis; and since "vascular epilepsy" does not differ clinically from "toxic" or any other epilepsy a pathological arrangement is of value only in so far as etiological research is thereby facilitated.

Even if factors in fit production have been determined on a fairly wide scale the circumstances under which they give rise in a particular case to one clinical variety rather than another are so obscure as to prove really enigmatical; hence much more study is requisite ere a scientific scheme of classification on an etiological basis can be devised.

Symptomatology.

The cardinal feature of all epilepsies being constituted by the fit, it is natural to give first consideration thereto. In their observed clinical characters, however, epileptic attacks vary enormously, and descriptive arrangements once thought adequate need to be revised. The time-honoured division into grand and petit mal has its value, but each must be interpreted in a very elastic fashion if it is to embrace all the types not definitely belonging to the other; and, as will be shown, varieties are being recorded for which a fresh terminology is desirable. A general sketch of the components and stages of epileptic fits may serve as introduction to their examination in detail.

It is customary to distinguish three phases in the epileptic paroxysm, viz. 1. The aura or warning, 2. the developed convulsion, and 3. a post-convulsive state with diverse sequelae. Of these, the aura is for present purposes understood to refer solely to a feeling or sensation of one or other modality immediately preceding the stage of unconsciousness (which may or may not eventuate), and must be clearly separated from prodromata or precursory symptoms, signals of an on-coming fit in existence possibly for hours or even days before. These antecedents are sometimes known only to the patient himself, sometimes obvious to relatives or friends. In the great majority of cases the aura or instant warning is identical for each of the attacks of a given epileptic, announcing the imminence of the dreaded fit. Its isolated development, however, is not seldom remarked. The stage of actual seizure, when the patient lies in the throes of his convulsion, endures for two or three minutes, perhaps, much exceeding the time occupied by the aura, which is usually a matter of seconds. Sometimes this phase fails to evolve according to rule, the warning being succeeded by partial or otherwise modified manifestations, "fragments" of the fullblown convulsion in one or other of its aspects. The process becomes arrested at some point, for reasons difficult to fathom. In the intervals between typical major attacks such fragments are fairly often noted; they were claimed long ago by HERPIN to represent complete seizures curtailed to their initial symptoms, but this view scarcely accords with the facts of observation or at least embodies only a partial truth, for it is not invariably the opening symptoms that are reproduced. As for the third phase, that of sequelae, their range is amazingly wide and nature correspondingly diverse; further, in severity and duration they cannot be considered by any means regularly proportional to the intensity of the second.

This description according to phases is applicable to the generality of epileptic fits though subject to much modification; whatever the clinical type, simple or complex, brief or protracted, an endeavour should always be made to ascertain its prelude, content, and after-effects.

The common division into two main classes, major or severe, and minor or slight, is sanctioned by the experience of generations. Of these, the first (grand or haut mal) is composed essentially of loss of consciousness (often profound and sometimes lengthy) with violent generalised muscular spasms; a very brief period of unconsciousness, without the latter, or with insignificant twitches, characterises the second (petit mal). Occasionally trivial movement takes place of which the subject is aware throughout. Both forms may be ushered in by a fall from the erect position, the severe, invariably so. The relation of loss of senses to onset of convulsion is inconstant; in those of maximum degree the two are simultaneous, whereas other fits often begin with muscular spasm (e.g. turning of head and eyes, twisting of trunk) registered in the patient's sensorium ere oblivion supervenes. Preliminary to both comes, of course, the afferent warning in most instances.

We may now examine more closely the several features of (classical) attacks, major and minor, reserving for later discussion epileptic variants and certain individual symptoms. In accordance with custom these components will be taken in the following order:

1. Prodromes. — 2. Auras. — 3. Contents. — 4. Sequelae.

1. Prodromes. By the term are to be understood such preliminary symptoms and signs as may be noted to occur at a varying period of hours or possibly days before the culminating paroxysm; foreshadowing more or less infallibly the near approach of an attack, they must be distinguished (as already pointed out) from the immediate aura, which is the first stage in the development of the epileptic process proper.

To ascertain what percentage of cases is thus preceded is no easy task, largely because of their coming under the cognisance of laymen only, as a rule, who, failing to connect prodromes with the subsequent fit, may tend to overlook them. Intelligent patients and relatives, however, are duly impressed thereby and soon grasp their import. A division into temporary and continuous varieties, favoured by some, is not so suitable as one of a systematic kind irrespective of duration.

a) Motor system. The most common of all are myoclonic twitches, sudden starts affecting one or other limb, on either or both sides, upper and lower, and occasionally the trunk. An object is jerked from the patient's hand, his arm will inflict an unintentional blow on himself or his neighbour, a convulsive shudder will endanger equilibrium or throw him to the ground. This motor jactitation appears preeminently during his early waking hours, in bed, when rising, or at breakfast; hence the more usual happenings include upset of a teacup, toss of comb or brush across the room and so forth. They are rarer during the day or in the evening, and occasionally mark the process of falling asleep. It has always struck me as curious how seldom patient or friend alludes to "the jumps" of his own accord and how frequently their occurrence is substantiated in answer to enquiry.

Myoclonic epilepsy not merely tends to precede major fits but often remains interparoxysmally as a feature of many cases, occurs by itself as a variant, or persists alone for months or years ere a generalised seizure takes place. Further reference to it will be found below (p. 33).

Other precursors in the class are a general fidgetiness, restlessness by day or night, and, conversely, reduction of motor activity. Occasional bouts of yawning or sneezing belong rather to the visceromotor group. Patients suffering from minor epilepsy sometimes manifest similar disorders for a day or two before a more typical fit.

b) Sensory system. Sensory prodromes of a *subjective* nature include headache or other cephalic discomfort, vertigo, paraesthesiae referred to some part of body or limbs or of a migratory kind, visual and auditory phenomena such as recurrent flashes of light or noises in the ears, or of a complex character and more highly specialised. These may undoubtedly in most instances be taken to constitute larval or incomplete auras, as though the epileptic process were momentarily obtruding itself into consciousness. Vertiginous attacks are occasionally rather severe, but brief, probably a petit mal variant.

Objective change in sensibility affecting certain segmental areas was found by MUSKENS in a series of hospital cases and by a few subsequent observers (MAES and CLAUDE, BAUGH, DE CRINIS, etc.). The zones revealing hypalgesia (it is the sensation of pain which is commonly involved) are those from about C 7 or C 8 to D 5 or D 6, rarely at lower levels (lumbosacral). Once or twice it has seemed possible to demonstrate the change in personal cases but opportunities come more freely to those resident in institutions. MUSKENS avers that the field of diminished appreciation of painful stimuli tends to increase up to the time of discharge.

c) Visceral, sympathetic and vasomotor systems. A varied assortment of transient or rather continuous symptoms is comprised under this heading, among which may be noted anorexia or its reverse, a ravenous appetite; coated tongue, constipation, flatulence, dyspepsia, bouts of polyuria and pollakiuria; cutaneous eruptions and erythemas, urticaria, pruritus and other vasomotor troubles (to which FÉRÉ in particular devoted attention); also vague sensations of a visceral kind, malaise, sense of oppression, tightness at chest and heart, and so on. Sleepiness or lethargy sometimes develops prior to a major attack.

d) Psychical system. Alterations in mood and emotional expressions are not infrequent as signs of the approaching climax; these include irritability of temper, apathy, sullenness, depression, "fits" of silence or reserve, desire to be "left alone", apprehension, etc. The epileptic is sometimes "insufferable" until relieved by the discharge. Other premonitory indications are more subtle, and evident only to the entourage; there is a change in aspect, a look in the patient's eyes, an expression on his face, defying closer analysis but declared unmistakable.

Of no little interest is a sense of physical and mental well-being, a pre-convulsive euphoria and eutonia, remarked by some epileptics. Its subject feels particularly well and becomes exceptionally cheerful with unusual flow of spirits, a gaiety of mood no less foreboding because spontaneous. The Russian novelist DOSTOIEVSKY has told of his experiencing supreme ecstasy just before his attacks, contrasting with the painful mental depression that succeeded them. A patient under the care of SPRATLING was "transported" with marvellous delight only a short while before succumbing to a major seizure. On the whole, physical exaltation predominates over psychical in such cases as have come under personal notice. Others complain of a recurrent feeling of unreality and strangeness in regard to their environment, a "dreamy state" identical with that of uncinate epilepsy (see below) and providing a further example of the reproduction of auras, complete or modified, as a prodrome.

Sometimes attacks are ushered by a temporary psychotic condition with delusions and perhaps hallucinations. Fainting fits analogous to some kinds of petit mal may occur. Two instances of epistaxis preceding a major fit have come under personal observation, and a similar case is quoted by MUSKENS. Other possibilities need not be listed, for the variety is endless.

Broadly speaking, the prominence and frequency of definite precursors appear to vary directly with the interval elapsing between fits; when the latter are numerous, or come on each other's heels, prodromes vanish. In the course of a given case mutation of types is sometimes observed, but usually they are as specific as the auras.

Consideration of objective changes in body fluids and excretions discovered in the pre-convulsive period and of their possible bearing on etiological and pathogenic questions is conveniently deferred to a later point.

2. Auras. So far, the assumption has been that prodromata can be differentiated from auras by including under the latter term only such symptoms as instantly announce the coming attack, forming in fact the first recognisable signals of the commencing process in the brain. Yet distinction may not prove a simple matter, for some of the former continue practically to the moment of onset, while others are placed by different observers in different categories. The rare *preconvulsive* automatisms, as an example, are taken for prodromes by GOWERS, but for auras by MUSKENS. A patient may run a short instance ere falling in a fit, start to undress himself, exhibit automatic reactions betokening fear, or become aggressive or excited; sometimes a scream as of anguish (not the characteristic and unmistakable epileptic cry) precedes by a mere second or two the act of convulsive seizure. In one sense the point is more academic than practical, since both series of phenomena are epileptic and both intimate the advent of the storm; but experience teaches the propriety of confining the aura strictly to a sensation or feeling spontaneously arising in consciousness, of one or other mode, or to some more elaborate presentation, describable at the time or later recalled. Though belonging to the psychical series, it is nothing else than the first conscious indication of the commencement of a process that is about to manifest signs of the physical series. The aura, thus defined, either precedes or accompanies visible spasm, but must be kept distinct from the latter, which belongs to the content of the fit.

This view is opposed to that of GOWERS, who, taking the word to connote "subjective commencement", includes thereunder consciousness of motion or of sensation, or a mental state. As will be seen later, I accept and exemplify the occurrence of muscular sense hallucinations as a genuine aura, but GOWERS seems to me mistaken in arguing that the patient's consciousness of the beginning spasm constitutes a "motor aura" because it can be regarded as a "motor sensation". Moreover, he says explicitly that unilateral auras include "a motion or sensation" in one side of the tongue, etc., and that attacks commence with "a sensation or motion" which "may be referred to almost any part of the body". Apart from the anomaly of "referring" a motion anywhere, this manner of regarding the phenomena is calculated to mislead, since loss of senses is taken as the dividing line between aura and fit, whereas in many with a definite aura (e. g. JACKSONian attacks) consciousness may be spared.

The word itself is a relic of antiquated conceptions and etymologically pointless, but enshrines the idea of a wind or vapour moving, a "sensation" so likened by the sufferer. A fine historical study of the aura and its vicissitudes was written by HERPIN eighty years ago. Since the days of HUGHLINGS JACKSON and of advance in doctrines of cerebral localisation it has engaged particular attention as an index to the position of the "storm centre"; but while many do in fact provide a clue to locality others are too complex for the purpose.

As is the case with prodromes, auras occur in multitudinous variety. A number of different classifications have been proposed, but it is not easy to fix groups that are mutually exclusive, and a topical arrangement obviates the difficulty only in part; preference should be assigned to one based on psychophysiological divisions, as follows:

a) Auras of somatic sensibility. — *b) Auras of visceral sensibility.* — *c) Complex auras, inclusive of mental states.* — *d) Special-sense auras.*

The uni- or bilaterality of the warning has to be taken into consideration for practical purposes, but should not be made a distinctive criterion. Views differ on the relative frequencies of auras as a whole, and of particular varieties; some are common and others rare, but reliable figures must always be troublesome to procure and will probably under-represent the facts, since something may be experienced that afterwards escapes the memory, or if noted at the moment proves beyond recall. In his large collection of 2013 cases GOWERS obtained a history of aura in 60 per cent., but other observers have recorded a much smaller proportion (HERPIN 27 per cent., BINSWANGER 31 per cent.). From personal notes during twenty-five years' hospital and private experience I find 50 per cent. represents the average.

It is hardly necessary to point out the erroneousness of the old view ascribing a prime rôle in fit causation to the aura, which was taken to be of peripheral origin, though the cerebral process can undoubtedly be modified by manipulation of the limb in which it starts (as will be shown in due course). The specificity of the warning for a given case is subject to few exceptions, but variability characterises JACKSONian auras on occasion; in one patient tingling usually began in the hand but sometimes in the foot, while another felt numbness in either fingers or face, more or less indifferently. If the aura is complex its components do not always appear in the same sequence or identically. In the course of a long case it may slowly alter, ordinarily becoming less pronounced. Combinations of more than one distinctive type are known.

a) Auras of somatic sensibility. Among the most banal in this common class may be enumerated sensations of numbness, tingling, pricking, "pins and needles," cramplike feelings, and other analogous subjective experiences. Often something is declared to creep or run over the body, pass up the spine, rush from limb to head, and so on. A sensation of "stiffness" is not infrequent. Thermal paraesthesiae are seldom remarked; in one case they consisted of a feeling of icy coldness down the whole of the left side, including the face and left half of the tongue. Whether pure pain ever occurs is a point of importance for cortical physiology; intensity of pricking is closely allied to it, and GOWERS refers to a patient who felt "as if a knife were being plunged into the arm." An aura of "cutting pain" in the ear is mentioned by PÖTZL. One of my own described "painful pricks, like stabs" in the region of the heart, though in this instance, as in another recorded by FOERSTER (pains in bladder and rectum) the symptom probably comes within the visceral class. None the less such subjective realisation of pain must presumably have a *cortical* origin in JACKSONian cases and by analogy in the others.

The aura in a JACKSONian variety reported by COLLIER consisted of "horrible pain" in the right hand; but his assertion that it could not have arisen in any higher structure than the optic thalamus is open to criticism.

So far as concerns generalised fits these diverse derangements of sensibility are often bilateral in the limbs, or involve the body and its members simultaneously or in rapid succession; sensations may seize both arms and pass up to the head, or affect trunk and arms, or commence in legs and move headward; sometimes their course ascends or descends irregularly, or passes across from one side to the other.

When, however, such paraesthesiae form the prelude to a JACKSONian or unilateral attack their "march" is often highly informative. In the first place, it is much more usual for the aura to commence in the periphery of arm or leg than elsewhere; when the former is the part affected, the sensation often singles out thumb and forefinger, or those on the ulnar side or all together. Palm, dorsum, or wrist is also a site of election, but no example of commencement by the middle finger alone has come under personal notice (since there is reason to believe a pre- and postaxial representation of sensibility exists at the cortical level that finger ought perhaps to escape). In the case of the lower limb, the great toe or all the toes, sole, instep, and the foot as a whole, constitute the usual places, especially the first. By comparison, onset at upper segments of either leg or arm is rare.

The sequence thereafter, as a general rule, corresponds to the topical arrangements of sensory centres in the post-rolandic cortex. Thus should the toes be earliest engaged, spread by continuity next implicates ankle, leg, and thigh in ascending series, passing by the side of the trunk to shoulder, face and head. At this point, however, consciousness is frequently lost, descent to arm, wrist and fingers being seldom described. When the last-named segment is the initial point, a reverse pattern of march occurs, the sequence being fingers, forearm, upper arm, shoulder, face and head; in this case it is not exceptional for the aura to advance further by passing down the side of the trunk, sometimes into the leg itself. These two modes do not represent the only occurrences, for the arm may be involved secondarily to the leg by a fresh start in the fingers and ascending participation; the sequence therefore becomes toes, leg, trunk, fingers, arm, face. Several cases of the kind have been personally observed; it was wellknown to GOWERS, and has been fully substantiated by SITTIG. The supposition in such instances is that the march corresponds to some physiological "schema" of somatic segments rather than to juxtaposition of cortical points.

On occasion the aura begins in the face, usually round the lips and corner of the mouth, after which neck, shoulder, arm, and fingers become consecutively its seat. The tongue may share in the sensation. Not infrequently, in facial cases, paraesthesiae are felt round both sides of mouth and lips. Among other combinations allusion must be made to spread from fingers (usually forefinger and thumb) to the ipsilateral angle of mouth and cheek, a sequence of which I have seen examples repeatedly; also to a preaxial or postaxial passage of the aura in upper or lower limb, e. g. along radial or ulnar aspect of the arm, or homologous sides of the leg (SITTIG, VAN VALKENBURG). The finger-mouth extension is readily accounted for by the propinquity of corresponding centres on the cortical surface.

At what moment in the course of these somatic intimations unconsciousness supervenes is a question to which no uniform answer can be given; as a general though not invariable rule once face and head are reached from below spasm sets in and awareness comes to an abrupt stop; on the other hand, as is well recognised, the epileptic process often fails to advance beyond the stage of paraesthesiae. Again, auras commencing in face and head are sometimes immediately followed by insensibility. From one or two curious cases mentioned by GOWERS it would appear that the abnormal sensation may first ascend and then descend a limb (or vice versa) ere consciousness is submerged in the epileptic flood (cf. also POPPER, SITTIG).

Hitherto reference has been made solely to cutaneous modes, but certain remarkable cases distinguished by an *aura of the muscular sense* must not be overlooked. In these, the patient feels as though his limb, or some part of his body, were moving, before any visible displacement can be detected by himself or others. Several instances of this peculiarity have come under personal observation.

One was that of a soldier wounded in the right parietal lobe during the Boer war, who subsequently developed JACKSONIAN fits. The aura consisted of a feeling that the left arm was being steadily and irresistibly elevated from his side to a position above his head, impelling him to direct his gaze to the limb preparatory to seizing it; yet there was no corresponding movement whatever.

A recent example concerns a youth with left infantile cerebral hemiplegia and homonymous hemianopia, whose aura takes the form of seemingly powerful flexion of fingers and contraction of wrist and forearm, giving the impression that his hand is rising to his mouth; all the while the limb lies motionless on his lap.

Other variants of the same phenomenon are on record; it is not altogether rare, doubtless being sometimes missed owing to faults of enquiry. Properly regarded as a hallucination of the muscular sense, its occurrence mainly if not solely in unilateral cases, with involvement of the parietal cortex, suggests that the site of the mechanisms concerned may some day be determined with exactitude.

b) Auras of visceral sensibility. Foremost place in the group must be assigned to the familar *epigastric sensation,* possibly the most frequent of all; it is habitually referred to the pit of the stomach in the midline, sometimes nearer the umbilicus, sometimes behind the sternum. An apparent localisation to right or left must be considered unusual. Intelligent epileptics may be able to convey some idea of its nature by resort to such terms as a "sinking feeling", a cramp, pain, spasm, a "gripping" sensation, flutter, trembling, "rumbling" and what not; it may be likened to some more definite movement, "as if the stomach were turning over," shifting, or becoming contracted. But more often, perhaps, the patient feels incapable of describing a sensation unlike anything within the range of his experience and falls back on similes that cannot be taken literally — "it feels as if there was a hole in my stomach," "it's a funny feeling as if my inside was emptied of everything." An "intense feeling of hunger" can be better understood. In a considerable number the epigastric component of the aura is instantly followed by an impression of something rising within the chest; a sensation of choking, of difficulty in breathing, a clutch or grip at the throat, are common accompaniments, while palpitation is rare. The speed with which these occur and unconsciousness sets in often makes it impossible for the subject to recall details afterwards, or to say more than that there is a "rush from stomach to head" that overwhelms him.

The constituents of the fully developed aura can be traced with greater facility in vasovagal types (see below).

For some reason warnings referred to other viscera in the same pneumogastric distribution come under notice far less often, e. g. cardiac or respiratory commencements (pain at the heart, palpitation, dyspnoea, sense of strangulation, tightness in the chest, etc.) though, as has just been shown, they may succeed those originating in the abdominal division.

It is also convenient to include under the same general caption sundry vague conditions of malaise, faintness, weakness, powerlessness, and others difficult for the patient to describe and the physician to locate.

Allusion can here be made suitably to the variety of *cephalic* sensations initiating fits. Of moderate frequency, they comprise simple types such as headache, neuralgic pains, pressure, heaviness, sense of fullness, numbness, throbbing, etc.; an allegation that "the blood rushes to the head" or brain is quite common. But in other cases the experience is more elusive, or baffles description, and some picturesque but metaphorical image is chosen to express the inexpressible, "I feel as if my brain is being stirred about," "as if my brains are boiling over." One patient averred that the right side of his head seemed to be fixed while the left half was rotating. Sometimes he is conscious of a blow, a snap, "something seems to burst within my brain, at the back," and has difficulty in deciding whether he hears or feels it.

Generally speaking, warnings referred to the head itself are instantly followed by abolition of consciousness, and have to be distinguished from the complex states discussed in the succeeding paragraphs; they may, however, form the ultimate stage in a rapidly advancing epigastric aura, or occur in combination with one or other of the special sense types.

c) Complex auras, inclusive of mental states. Some previous writers have employed the term "psychical auras" for this particular category, but since in accordance with the definition given above all auras are psychical it has no differentiating value and should be abandoned. In the class the most interesting is that now universally known as the *uncinate aura* or syndrome, to which HUGHLINGS JACKSON directed attention on a number of occasions, and which consists essentially of what he described as a "dreamy state" coupled, usually, with a sensation of smell or taste. The latter may precede, accompany, or succeed the other; sometimes awanting, it can occur by itself. As for the dreamy state, it can be extremely brief, or prolonged into the space of a few minutes. Comprised thereunder are conditions for which a variety of phrases have been coined by those with experience of it; "a feeling of having been there before", "feeling of being somewhere else", "reverie", "double consciousness", "recurrence of an old dream", "memories of thing that happened in childhood", "feeling of strangeness and unreality". Sometimes the sensation is so peculiar and evanescent as to elude depiction; it so transcends reality that the subject feels he is quivering on the brink of the unknown; sometimes there are "terrible thoughts" that cannot be expressed.

The combination creates a particular type shown by JACKSON to occur in association with lesions of the uncinate region of the temporal lobe, and often made the subject of research since his first contributions (ANDERSON, BUZZARD,

CLARKE, CRICHTON-BROWNE, MILLS, GOWERS, FOSTER KENNEDY, and many more). To its detailed study in cases of epilepsy (without gross lesion) a chapter is devoted elsewhere [1]. With the hope of clarifying conceptions and of introducing some order into a rather involved topic a provisional classification was there attempted, and is here reproduced. Four main types can be distinguished:
  A. The "Familiarity" or "Déjà vu" type. — B. "Strangeness" or "Unreality" type. — C. "Panoramic memory" type. — D. Abortive type.

In given cases one or more of the first three may blend with another, and to either of the first two visual or auditory hallucinations be added; the latter sometimes occur with the third. From a large selection one of each type may be chosen.

Type A. "It seems to take me to a set of circumstances in which I have found myself before, or to a place where I have been before. I feel that certain things are happening as they have happened previously, or that people are coming together as at some former time."

Type B. "All of a sudden everything around me seems strange and different. I've been at the table talking to people, and I've said to myself, I know you, and you, and you, and at the same time they have been unreal and different. They have never noticed anything and yet the feeling has been there."

Type C. "I go into a curious state in which I suddenly remember all sorts of things that happened when I was a child. They are stupid, old-fashioned things of my childhood, things that I have done in days gone by, in other places. I remember silly things like swinging, playing with toys with other girls, and then I go off."

Type D. "I call it a vision, but I never can get at it. It is a funny sensation which lasts only a minute; it is always the same, and if only I could get at the root of it I should tell you. I keep puzzling over it."

The rather common feeling of "being somewhere else" need not be set in a class by itself, for it exists or is implicit in more than one of the above types.

As already remarked, to these peculiar mental experiences is united in general a hallucination referable to olfactory or gustatory system, illustrated by the case of a patient who complained of a pungent smell, as if he were inhaling gas, and of another into whose mouth came with the dreamy state a bitter taste of lemons.

However heterogeneous these clinical instances, they are identical in constituting the aura of typical epileptic fits; elaborate, simple, or elusive, each is a portent of the coming crisis. Dreamy states clearly belong to a different order of mental experience from tastes or smells, and according to HUGHLINGS JACKSON ought not be regarded as epileptic because not the result of discharge; they are produced, he argued, by overactivity of centres as yet untouched thereby. His distinction between discharging and release phenomena (the olfactory-gustatory sensation being assigned to the former and the dreamy state to the latter), however, seems to furnish an example of the artificialities into which a rigid definition drives the analyst. In one sense it matters little from the viewpoint of epilepsy as a whole whether a particular symptom is derived from excitation or from escape, being none the less a part of the total process though arising from the activity of centres that are not being discharged crudely, violently, or excessively. Moreover, the dreamy state does not stand alone; it is linked, by a host of transitional forms, with minor intellectual or emotional warnings, recurring fragments of psychical experience identical in all essential aspects with auras on other levels in the psyche. Here fall to be included ill-defined fears, a sense of something impending, something miserable or terrifying, which may or may not be united with a clear conception of its cause; words, sentences, ideas keep echoing in the head for a moment or two, sometimes known, sometimes incapable of recall later. One patient described "a feeling

---

[1] Modern Problems in Neurology, 1928. Chap. IV.

of dread, as if someone were going to strike me," an unchanging aura the explanation of which eluded discovery. In another case it took the form of repetition in the patient's brain of the last chance words, whatever they were, that reached her ears from without. The experience may be more intricate, compounded of elements from more than one system; thus an epileptic's aura consisted in his taking the terminal position of a row of twelve men in military formation; a superior in rank stepped forward and boxed the ears of each in turn, knocking him down, while the subject stood in fearfulness awaiting the inevitable end; as his ears were boxed he became insensible. It is unnecessary to annotate further these infinitely varied mental intimations, many of which are scarcely separable from those discussed in the next group, viz. the auras of the special senses.

Allusion has just been made to the occurrence of emotional constituents in the warning, the great majority being characterised by a feeling of apprehension, fear, or even terror. But to another affective aspect of epileptic consciousness little attention has been paid. Now and again cases are encountered where the subject declares that his attacks have been associated with some of a distinctly *pleasurable* kind. In my MORISON Lectures[1] (1930) the point was examined, and two cases described; one was that of an intelligent lady of 32, suffering from uncinate epilepsy, whose aura ("I feel as if my mind and my body are coming apart") was accompanied by a delectable feeling, so much so that at first she used to welcome the sensation as a "dream of delight," though never able to specify wherein the pleasure consisted. Another patient, whose fits seem to have been little more than a prolonged petit mal, noted their highly agreeable content; "I felt that I had been away somewhere in a pleasing dream which I was enjoying to the full." In a third example the statement was made: "I felt as if my brain were leaving my body for the moment, and used rather to welcome it, as a not unpleasant feeling."

Perhaps it is not a coincidence that in each the pleasurable sensation occurred in connexion with dreamy states, though in one of them, when the fits became more severe, the much commoner feeling of ill-defined anxiety supplanted it. Two instances of epilepsy with apparently motiveless but compulsive and unrestrained laughter as an aura have come under personal notice, while others of epileptic fits having been induced by that act, itself resulting from tickling the soles of the feet, are on record (FÉRÉ quotes those of VAN SWIETEN, ESQUIROL, and REYNOLDS). Under what precise circumstances agreeable emotion becomes the precursor of fits, affording an impressive contrast with the doubtless more natural feeling of apprehension or even anguish, is difficult to ascertain.

For further analysis of these complex uncinate and allied auras, and their bearing on tempting problems of double consciousness, paramnesia, phenomena occurring in drowning and other states of semisuffocation, etc., the reader is referred to the chapter already mentioned.

d) Special-sense auras. Some idea of the relative frequency of the class can be gathered from figures published by GOWERS; among 1145 cases special sense auras were present in 274 as follows: visual 175, auditory 68, gustatory 18, olfactory 12.

The last two have been dealt with apropos the uncinate syndrome and need not be particularised again, except to say that they sometimes occur by themselves and trouble may be experienced in recollecting their precise quality. One may blend with the other to produce a flavour (an olfactory "taste"). Mostly unpleasant, linkened to something "rotten", "metallic", "bitter", and so on, the presence of a sensation of taste can sometimes be inferred from concomitant smacking movements of labial muscles, or of the tongue, as though to moisten

---
[1] Brit. med. J. **11** (1930).

the lips. Smells also are described by such epithets as "vile", "horrid", "putrid", "chemical", "rubbery", etc. or resemble something gaseous (like "strong smelling-salts", "ether", "fumes of an acid"), rarely embodying a pleasant sensation ("like passing a perfume shop"). MILLER mentions a case in which an overpowering scent of the most cloying variety made his patient's limbs tremble with a feeling of passion.

Auras referable to the *visual* system range widely from a low to a high degree of specialisation. Commencing with the former, we note among the simplest varieties sensations of light, sparks, stars, flashes, twinkles, and of colour in the mass, reds, blues, greens, yellows, etc., appearing in blotches, or as a mist tingeing all objects, a "coloured vision". The tints may change from moment to moment, reds and blues predominating. Sometimes either or both (lights and colours) assume a definite shape, balls, whirling circles, wheels, spirals whose outlines alter as they move to and fro, or cross the field, or pursue a complicated course, coming nearer or retreating to a distance. Such kaleidoscopic spectra are not as a rule comparable to the teichopsia of migraine in their exact characters.

For a minute analysis of many details consult the BOWMAN Lecture by GOWERS, and the HUGHLINGS JACKSON Lecture by the same authority.

In a higher class come the visual hallucinations of objects, faces, figures, scenes, in endless variety, sometimes arising out of the former group but generally independent of it, and similar to those of the uncinate class. For example, one patient constantly saw a human shape clad in white which appeared far out in the right visual field and crossed to the left, always with back turned and going away from him. Another described in faithful detail the figure of a little old man in a black overcoat and hard hat; on his back was a knapsack hung over his shoulders by a strap, half of canvas, half of string. This image was perceived vividly for about two seconds ere the onset of unconsciousness. The particular type may vary from one fit to another, as in the case of an epileptic who sometimes saw a silk-hatted and frook-coated man pass through railings and go down steps; at others it was a procession of vehicles coming from the right and moving to the left. OBANIO's patient saw his own mirror image (with an accompanying olfactory hallucination of methyl salicylate). Some alleged "ghost" apparitions may conceivable have had a basis in visual phenomena antecedent to an epileptic fit.

Apparent increase or decrease in the *size* of objects forms another variety-Macropsia is exemplified by the case of a woman who finds objects in front of her enlarging and coming very close, as though about to graze her face; after a few seconds they become misty, then she "goes blind" and falls unconscious. Just before his fits a patient saw everything greatly magnified, three times its normal size (VERAGUTH). Micropsia is perhaps less rare; in one case everything seemed tiny and far off, while the patient had a simultaneous feeling of being transported to a mountain top though still conscious of remaining in her room. Sometimes the content of visual hallucinations itself undergoes magnification or reduction; the lilliputian variety is well known though rare as an aura; conversely, in a personal case visions occurred of people passing who seemed to be unusually large and unpleasantly near.

For closer discussion of dysmetropsias and their pathogenesis see an article of mine published elsewhere [1].

Mutations and combinations of visual elements are observed from time to time, and are well exemplified by the case of a young female epileptic who first

---

Trans. Ophthalm. Soc. **36** (1916).

sees three bright shimmering circles to the right; then objects become twice as large as normal, and next are blotted out by a bright red patch spreading from centre to periphery of the field; its completion coincides with loss of consciousness.

Apparent *movement* of objects, an occasional variety, was a feature in the complex aura of a medical man who, after a confused recollection of past events accompanied by a smell (incapable of definition) and a general pleasurable feeling, suddenly would notice the ornaments on the mantlepiece shimmering in an up-and-down motion and then rotating from right to left; twitching of muscles and unconsciousness ensued.

Double vision is mentioned by GOWERS though no case has come under personal notice. The rare hemianopia belongs to the "inhibitory" class referred to later.

Elements derived from other sensory systems may be combined with those of a visual order, as has been noted en passant, e. g. paraesthesiae, visceral sensations (epigastric), smell or taste, and also those of the auditory group; this latter combination is exemplified by the aura of a woman who suddenly heard the penetrating voice of a girl she used to know in her school-days, and immediately saw a crowd of schoolmates dancing in front of her in their nightgowns.

Auditory warnings, like those of vision, can be subdivided into low and high grades, comprising on the one hand such crudities an "hissing", "buzzing", "drumming", a "snap", "bang", "explosion"; thence passing by as intermediate type, such as "bells", or "whistles", to specialised varieties including voices, music, or singing on the other. Like those of a visual nature, also, they sometimes manifest a crescendo or diminuendo homologous with macropsia and its converse. In one case the aura took the form of a voice at a distance singing "Roses in Picardy," distinct though faint; gradually coming nearer, the last notes seemed loudest of all; thereafter came a sense of terror, loss of speech, and unconsciousness. Auditory warnings generally involve both sides but may be unilateral, as with a patient who invariably heard a peculiarly worded advertisement (once seen in a shop-window) audibly repeating itself in his left ear; anomalously, they may appear located in the back of the head, or round it, or far above; local signature occasionally fails altogether. In some cases the experiences are confused or ill-differentiated, a mere "noise" or "hubbub of talk", or not to be understood literally, as when a patient remarked, "I seem to hear everything that has ever been said to me in all my life." There may be recognition of the general character of the aura but inability to specify the particulars; a patient said it was as if she had been sharing in a long conversation, but she never could recall it, although always feeling just on the point of remembering what had been heard and said.

Except in complex (e. g. uncinate) auras, it is uncommon for those of hearing to occur with other types, or be coupled with cruder phenomena such as vertigo.

A final question concerns what may be termed *auras of inhibition.* In the course of positive manifestations (chiefly, perhaps, visual or auditory) a negative phase may supervene, or, seemingly, the two processes may coexist; blindness succeeds the vision, "everything goes dark", or silence the sounds, a sudden sense of absolute quiet. In one case of combined visual and auditory type voices clearly heard at the outset ceased abruptly, though the lips of the figures from which they had come continued to move. Initial loss of sight (hemianopic, total) or hearing may form an inhibitory aura; inability to speak, also, may be regarded as a similar negative phenomenon, whether primary or secondary to some other constituent of the whole, as in the case of a youth who after intense buzzing in the head was deprived of all power to say what he had clearly in his mind to utter; a few minutes later he was unconscious. If under such circumstances inhibition is considered to overcome discharge it may be taken in reality for the opening phase of the developing fit as opposed to the warning, an "inhibitory epilepsy" rather than an "inhibitory aura". The point is difficult to decide; some variety of paraphasia is not exceptionally rare before loss of senses, and a striking instance of paragraphia is on record (GORDON); the patient was writing to dictation and for several seconds continued to make errors ere he fell off his chair convulsed. If we abide by our definition both of these symptoms ought rather to be included in the content of the fit than classed as an aura, though doubtless they are indicative of disorder on the "sensory" side of speech. But the sudden "blank" in conscious appreciation of sights and sounds, like numbness or deadness of the skin, or loss of smell or taste (were this to be observed), must be considered a "negative" warning due to a process of inhibition.

The importance of auras taken as a whole does not reside in their variety, multiplicity, or individual features so much as in the light their types and combinations shed on "schemata" of cerebral function and on paths followed by irradiating impulses.

3. Content of the Fit. After prodromes and auras (both of which, as has been remarked, may fail), the symptoms and signs of the developed fit come under notice. A description will first be given of the complete epileptic seizure.

Major attack. With the onset of unconsciousness the patient, if erect, falls to the ground, or if sitting, slides off his chair, to the accompaniment, perhaps, of a characteristic cry. His whole musculature is seized in a powerful tonic spasm, turning the head strongly to one or other side, or back, while the trunk is slowly twisted round en suite. The arms, in extreme tonic rigidity, mostly flexed and adducted, fists clenched and thumbs driven into palms, adopt and hold for a time their attitudes, while lower limbs extend and stiffen with some inward rotation, inversion of feet, and bending of toes. Gripped in the universal spasm, chest and abdomen become temporarily fixed, the immediate consequence being seen in flushed and livid features, whose grimacing and often asymmetrical contortion accentuates the realism of the "seizure". The eyes, generally deviated, with lids open, are insensitive to touch; their pupils dilate in accord with the cyanosis. After perhaps some twenty or thirty seconds of such tetanic contraction, during which slow changes in posture may follow local modifications of its intensity, its place is taken by slight muscular vibrations, felt rather than seen, which rapidly assume a visibly clonic character; abrupt and forcible jerks convulse the segments of the body in a series of violent shocks, more or less identical and synchronous on the two sides, that seem about to rend the helpless frame or dislocate its joints. With remission of thoracic fixity apnoea gives way to stertorous breathing, during which frothy saliva exudes, tinged with blood if tongue or cheek has been nipped by the teeth at the tonic phase, or in a clonic snap of the jaws. Simultaneously lividity yields to increasing aeration, but convulsive movements persist though lessening in frequency; evacuation of contents of bladder, bowel, or seminal vesicles may now be remarked. Finally, with a last jerk often as severe as any of its predecessors, the muscular torment ends in relaxation; emptied of tone, body and limbs subside into positions impressed on them by gravity, and the patient lies prostrate, passing insensibly to the recuperative stage of deep slumber and quiet breathing, or, less often, emerging soon to awareness of his surroundings. A minute or two cover the duration of the clonic period, an indefinite time the third or terminal.

This sketch of the common type of major fit gives its general outline and detail requires filling in; further, departures therefrom are both numerous and diverse. Their consideration may be postponed to a later point, when individual symptoms come to be discussed.

Minor attack. Often described indifferently by the patient as a "faint", "turn", "sensation", etc., (words in reality embodying some conception of its nature, a "faint" corresponding to loss of senses, a "turn" to a feeling of rotation or imbalance, a "sensation" to some affective element therein), the petit mal attack varies as widely in its characters as does the major, more so, indeed, because of its relative formlessness. Sometimes it consists purely in trifling loss of senses, a momentary arrest of the conscious stream, a "blank" or "absence" (the "absence épileptique" of the French), betrayed to the onlooker by a vacant look or fixed expression, pallor of facies, cessation of talk or failure to answer, or other negative signs; often unaware of his lapse, the patient "comes to" to find surprise or concern depicted on the faces of those about him. Throughout its moments he may have kept his feet, but may, or may not, have relaxed his grasp of any object held in the hand. In addition to suspension of such activities as are engaging him, slight twitches are sometimes observed, flickers round the mouth, rolling up of eyes, blinking, little quasi-purposive motions of lips and tongue. Perhaps more noticeable phenomena are in evidence, such as anteroflexion of head, which sinks in nodding movement on the chest, or of the head and body, or outstretching of arms in tonic fashion; a limb or part of a limb may be mildly convulsed; swaying of the body may precede an abrupt fall; or head and eyes may twist round and an arm be elevated, etc. In many cases such transient motor disturbances are coordinated rather than convulsive or myoclonic, and pass by easy gradations to fits of a somewhat more intricate kind that yet cannot be plainly classed with the ordinary major seizure.

Other examples of these epileptic brevities are unaccompanied by loss of senses, the patient experiencing merely a temporary mental confusion, or indeed little else than an aura of one or other kind, yet proving unable subsequently either to specify or to recall the incident. Any of the different types of warning already described may form the prelude to an abortive attack of such insignificance as to escape the notice of all but the practised eye, and perhaps revealed solely by some post-epileptic manifestation (as recounted below). Another common variant consists merely of a vertiginous sensation, a "turn" in the literal sense, during which the subject is dazed, feels about to fall, and may be conscious of some rotation of himself or his environment. There may be no more than a sudden loss of power in the legs, an inhibitory phenomenon akin to those already mentioned, resulting in a fall; in one or two personally observed instances the patient sank more gradually, on to his hands and knees, yet was up again in a moment, without even a fleeting indication of unconsciousness being discerned. Despite the transience of all average petit mal fits urine is sometimes passed involuntarily, furnishing on one occasion a definite clue to its nature that could not be derived from the parents' description.

In most attacks the return to full awareness is as immediate as its loss is sudden; the thread of conversation is resumed, the activity of the moment is continued, without a falter. On the other hand, symptoms may ensue whose complexity or duration is altogether disproportionate to the preceding functional disorder. The importance of this fact of observation cannot be stressed too much, for the true character of minor fits is often not realised until a major attack takes place or unless recurring peculiarities of behaviour on the patient's part compel attention.

As will be seen later, some types of coordinated, visceral, and other epilepsies might fairly be considered little else than variants of this minor class, whose limits are as indefinite as its clinical forms are multitudinous.

The content of fits other than grand and petit mal is described under their respective headings, in a later section.

4. **Sequelae.** For clearness of exposition the manifold after-states of the fit may be subdivided into those of a *physical* and a *psychical* character respectively. Among unsolved epileptic problems is that of the relations subsisting between type of attack and type of sequela, which has not yet progressed towards a reasonable solution. Some patients are positively ill after their fit, others feel much better than before; the return to normality may be speedy, or delayed; post-epileptic conduct is often at once rational, yet sometimes ugly, antisocial, even criminal; stupor may ensue, or hypomanic excitement; a confusional period elapses, or one of flawless automatism, during which the patient wanders far without ever betraying to the casual witness that he is "not himself".

a) On the *physical* side, it is possibly most usual for sleep to set in, sometimes after a brief time of wakefulness when the senses are regained. Its depth may be so profound as to constitute a danger should the sufferer, alone or unobserved, have fallen beside a fire, or turned his face into the pillows at the end of his convulsions.

A tragic instance was that of a youth who after an encouraging prognosis in consultation went off by train the same night to a distant town; on arrival he was found asphyxiated, his face buried in the cushions of the compartment he occupied alone. This curious tendency to turn over ("epileptic pronation") deserves note.

Headache, severe and generalised, follows sleep or develops without it and may last for hours or all day. *Vomiting,* not rare, occurs in similar circumstances and also may be attended by risk, viz. of food entering the glottis. *Myalgia,* another frequent after-effect, testifies to the muscular strains of powerful contraction, but ere long passes off. Interest has centred round the question of *postepileptic paralysis* (the "epileptic hemiplegia" of BRAVAIS and TODD), differing opinions being expressed in regard to its frequency, nature, and importance. The problem concerns *postconvulsive* palsy, be it noted, and not that constituting a form of inhibitory or akinetic epilepsy (described below), for some writers have confused the two. Apart from weakness consecutive to concentrated and exhausting discharges of neuromuscular units, a debility of varying degree, often both slight and evanescent, personal experience has brought no case of *enduring* residual palsy except among local epilepsies having their origin in definite pathological states (tumour, vascular disease, etc.). Even in serial types and status epilepticus rapid recovery is the rule. Should paralysis disproportionate to the fit's severity be in evidence the possibility of underlying structural change ought to be considered. To other sequels such as aphasia, ageusia, anosmia, hemianopia, etc., the same remark applies; when not fleeting and negligible they persist only if local conditions have modified the usual after-effects of the paroxysm itself.

Among those discussing the subject are HUGHLINGS JACKSON, CHARCOT, DUTIL, CLARK, CLARK and PROUT, MUSKENS, FÉRÉ, TURNER, COLLIER.

As regards cutaneous and deep *reflexes,* during the terminal period of complete atony and powerlessness the knee-jerk is sometimes abolished, personal researches on the point fully corroborating the result of old studies conducted by BEEVOR and repeated by GOWERS. More generally, dependent no doubt on a minor degree of coma and of tonus reduction, the negative phase fails to develop, exaggeration being observed, together with ankle clonus and extensor plantar response. The latter can frequently be obtained on both sides for a few minutes after moderately severe bilateral convulsions, attesting temporary change of function in the pyramidal system. Its continuance thereafter must arouse suspicion of an existing basis distinct from motor discharges. The state of the abdominal reflex usually corresponds.

Post-paroxysmal symptoms and signs connected with sympathetic and biochemical functions, the blood, urine, and other body fluids, etc., are considered together in a subsequent section.

Among various physical *accidents* contingent on violence of convulsion, ecchymoses round eyes or under conjunctiva are sometimes seen; of the bitten tongue the patient is only too painfully aware; broken teeth, scalp and facial cuts, burns and scars disfigure the chronic epileptic; an occasional fracture results from the crash of falling, or dislocation (commonly of the shoulder, and apt to recur) during the fit; a similar accident may involve the lower jaw.

b) Temporary *psychical* derangements often characterise the recuperative stage. Conspicuous among these is a state of *postepileptic automatism*, varying in extent and duration within wide limits. It may consist of no more than simple automatic repetition of everyday actions such as undressing, rearranging the bedclothes, hunting for objects, fumbling in pockets, and so on; however natural, circumstances can render it inconvenient or even compromising. This is particularly apt to be the case when such involuntary behaviour follows in the train of a minor attack (as happens with greater frequency than after grand mal) whose evolution has been almost too brief for notice or of whose true nature the bystander is ignorant. The awkwardness of the situation is exemplified by the case of a youth who unbuttoned his trousers to micturate in the street (analogous instances are reported by TROUSSEAU, GOWERS, COLMAN and others), and that of a boy at hospital who purloined what he could find in his neighbours' lockers. "Kleptomania" of this sort is not rare; one of COLMAN's patients, after a petit mal in an ironmonger's shop, placed a large coal-scuttle on each arm and walked out with them. Less equivocal if equally irresponsible was the action of another boy in seizing the nearest cake of soap to hurl it through the ward windows. Other automatic conduct includes attempts at climbing, or sometimes a quick run. A little boy used to race out of the ward and hide under a grand piano in the day-room; this so-called "epilepsia procursiva," trivial in itself, was changed to tragedy when (as subsequently transpired) during a similar postepileptic state he ran along a country road and stumbled into a deep pool where he was drowned. Often the automatism assumes the form merely of rambling talk, incoherent, repetitive, or paraphasic; a woman patient always said "Oh Robert, Robert, Robert" a dozen times or more; another, entering a baker's shop for threepennyworth of rolls, after an almost unrecognisable "absence" asked for a pound of plaice.

Sometimes the acts are coloured by emotion and violent in character, especially, perhaps, in the case of patients who are under restraint. The epileptic becomes aggressive, insolent, combative, hypomanic, dangerous to himself and others, even homicidal, as forensic cases have frequently revealed; a patient suffering from fits after a frontal injury threw his infant daughter out of the window on to a stone-flagged yard, where she fractured her skull and was killed. He was arrested on the capital charge, but I was able to certify his irresponsibility in view of the incident having demonstrably occurred during a postepileptic confusional state. COLMAN alludes to another in which under analogous circumstances a youth nearly succeeded in mutilating the external genitalia of his small brother.

In various respects postconvulsive phases can be identified with *somnambulism*, particularly as regards nocturnal fits; the patient may emerge from his house in night attire, or dress and return to bed, or walk about aimlessly; a little boy of whom I know always went downstairs to the kitchen to fall asleep again in the same chair. Diurnal fits may be followed by similar automatisms partaking of the character of *fugues* ("poriomania"), of which numerous instances might be quoted. On two occasions a patient resident in south London made his way on foot in postepileptic vacuity to the Hampstead police station in north London, to which he had no apparent object in going, and of the route taken no conscious memory was retained. Another, similarly affected, walked from south-east London to Paddington railway station, bought a ticket to Penzance in Cornwall, and only awoke to reality when in the Cornish express far to the west. In my MORISON Lectures (1930) reference is made to a sufferer from petit mal who during the war fell into difficulties by his transgressing military regulations when in a condition of seeming normality but really of epileptic amnesia.

Postepileptic fugues differ in no essential from those succeding hysterical states or occurring in non-epileptic persons who develop a double personality, of which some reported cases have become classical. As a rule, however, the former are of relatively short duration.

It is unnecessary to designate any of these mental sequelae "hysterical" or "hysteroid," though resembling in emotional content the commoner manifestations of that affection. All are explicable on the view (often urged by HUGHLINGS JACKSON) that temporary impairment of highest (psychical) level control follows discharge of its centres, with consequent release of others, equally complex but of a functionally lower psychical grade. Anticipating for the moment, however, what is afterwards discussed, we must point out that mere removal of control will not altogether explain the positive activity of lower levels, otherwise the phenomena of epileptic fits should occur much more readily than they do when states of unconsciousness are induced in any fashion. Acts of the kinds enumerated above may be so purposive to all outward appearance as to deceive the unskilled observer and raise questions of grave forensic importance should the patient come in conflict with laws regulating society; but the impelling motives are not accounted for by simple release.

Whether automatic actions ever replace fits in the sense of being "equivalent" to them (so-called "masked epilepsy" or "epilepsia larvata") is a subject provocative of much debate. It constitutes in reality part of the larger theme of "psychical equivalents" in general, i. e. the occurrence of interparoxysmal "attacks" of a different order, regarded as substitutes for fits. In view of the fact that antecedent minor seizures may be so trivial as to be quite overlooked, the allocation of such psychical outbursts to a primary class is natural, though often erroneous; but in other cases no record of actual epileptic phenomena of either major or minor type may be obtainable. To deny the genuineness of "equivalents" is perhaps therefore unwarranted. At a later point we will revert to the subject.

Individual epileptic Symptoms.

After analysis of the successive phases of epileptic fits of the more ordinary kinds it is convenient to review some individual symptoms, together with certain aspects of semeiology bearing on problems of localisation and pathogenesis.

1. The epileptic cry. More often absent than present, the cry uttered by the patient as he falls in the initial phase of his convulsion is sometimes shrill, sometimes lower in pitch, resembling a moan or a groan rather than a scream. In most cases it is definitely inspiratory and not, as the usual statement affirms, caused by expulsion of air through the spasmodically closing glottis, but by its inward suction during diaphragmatic descent. Once heard, it is not likely to be forgotten, though whether its comparison (by RUSSELL REYNOLDS) to the "cry of a distracted peacock" is just may be decided by those who have had experience of both.

2. Loss of consciousness. All severe general fits are attended by loss of consciousness; others may not be. In minor attacks it is also habitual, yet some show no more than clouding of the senses, which, in others still, may be retained. Unconsciousness may supervene at the onset, without a trace of warning, or ensue later; it may be extremely brief, even momentary, or endure for some time after the seizure is ended. By itself it forms no gauge of epileptic severity; a JACKSONian attack may evolve from first to last without loss of senses, and a minor fit consist of nothing else than a fleeting conscious "blank" or "epileptic absence." Motor convulsion frequently begins before insensibility develops, the subject being aware of his head and eyes turning or his arm moving, but that this succession of events is more likely to distinguish the so-called "organic" variety (alleged by GOWERS and MUSKENS) does not accord with personal experience.

3. **Types of movement.** Minute observation of the types of movement seen in ordinary fits of a major kind aids in the solution of interpretative problems concerning the sites and mechanisms of discharging phenomena. It is customary to subdivide convulsions into a tonic and a clonic phase, the former preceding the latter as a general rule; JACKSONian attacks are mainly clonic; a special variety occurs in circumstances corresponding more or less intimately to physiological decerebration and is known as the "tonic fit" (see below), clonic accompaniments being absent.

The *tonic stage* is one of practically universal immobility; a number of movements, mutually cancelling each other, are developed with abruptness and force; the result is a state of rigidity, a "single big useless movement", in JACKSON's words. Transient postures thus assumed vary considerably from case to case; symmetrical or asymmetrical on the two sides, affecting trunk more than limbs or vice versa, or all equally, they constitute a maximum of movement in a minimum of time. In most, the eyes turn conjugately to one side, and with them the head, a moment later; it is exceptional for the latter to move in an opposite direction. Sometimes the head twists slowly from one side to the other, becoming stationary in its second position. Forced as far as it will go, the trunk follows it, through an angle of perhaps 90 degrees or more; on rare occasions this tonic motion is not arrested, but continues till the patient has rotated in a circle round his longitudinal axis, or rolls off the bed. Ordinarily, arms are flexed and legs extended, in harmony with the most frequent forms of muscular action of the respective limbs; elbows are flexed to aright angle or less, forearms pronated, wrists strongly flexed, fingers straightened at metacarpophalangeal joints and thumb pressed firmly against the first two, or grasped in the clenched fist; finger flexion may be more pronounced on ulnar than on radial side. For the legs, extension is the habitual posture, at all joints, with inversion of feet and plantar flexion of toes.

Modifications are often remarked; sometimes flexion prevails, the body being curved forward while knees and elbows almost meet, or with powerful anteroflexion of trunk all four limbs may be outstretched; sometimes arm and leg flex on one side, extend and abduct on the other; not infrequently one arm extends to the other's flexion, trunk and legs being in extension.

Facial contraction, mainly bilateral, is commonly greater on the side to which the head turns, affecting cheek and mouth more than periocular and frontal groups; the eyes are usually open. The lower jaw is fixed, very seldom deviating, with mouth shut or partly so; thoracic and abdominal muscles are equally rigid.

No uniformity is to be expected in the phenomena of the tonic phase, nor are clinical possibilities exhausted by the various descriptions that have just been given.

The tetanizing innervations of the first part of the fit give place after a period of seconds or perhaps a minute to the *clonic stage,* which does not commence abruptly but by a palpable and then visible series of vibratory contractions in one or other division of the rigid musculature. These speedily develop into clonic spasms, which become more and more separable and distinct, the muscles relaxing in their fractional intervals and being again seized by violent jerking movement. When finally spaced out, a second or more may elapse between each, until the last supervenes. Rarely, however, the body as a whole appears to shake all over in a coarse tremor, the individual excursions of which are much narrower in range and succeed each other more quickly than in the usual variety. Clonic convulsions affect such segments as have been most involved in tonic contraction, so that postures are to a considerable extent maintained; but with gradually increasing flaccidity between successive twitches the limbs tend to fall away till at length gravity alone decides their position. For a time the arms continue to be jerked in strong flexion, while the originally extended legs, now relaxed in some degree, are agitated by short, sharp, kicklike movements, of limited excursion, bilaterally synchronous and symmetrical; rarely a sort of crude alternation is seen, imagined by some to resemble walking reflexes of the decerebrate animal. The jolts communicated to the unconscious body are responsible for some of the accidents already mentioned; intermittent thoracic spasm ejects saliva and causes the "foaming at the mouth" which never fails to impress the lay mind.

These exaggerated and caricatured movements of the general convulsion compose a medley in which the individuality of each is lost. Their types are capable of much variation, and no even approximate uniformity can be claimed for them. Alternatives range from fits which are all tonic to others yielding only phasic movements, through intermediate grades; under recent care has been a little girl whose attacks throw the left limbs and face into clonic convulsions, with head and eyes deviated to the left, but right arm and leg continue tonically extended, and abdominal muscles are "boarded" in strong bilateral tonic spasm, without twitches. When in JACKSONian cases the "second side" becomes involved its contractions are often tonic rather than phasic, seizing the whole half much more quickly than in the first instance (an example of clonic spasms preceding tonic). Long observation of the changing motor phenomena, sometimes "explosive," sometimes inhibitory, does not warrant the ascription to them of any identifiable "meaning"; they cannot reasonably be likened to reflex automatisms escaping into activity by removal of higher control. In FOERSTER's graphic metaphor, the fit does not resemble a horse the breaking of whose bridle frees him, but one which suddenly rears because the spurs are jabbed into his flanks. Speculations indulged in by some (e. g. PIERCE CLARK), to the effect that convulsed movements are similar to those of the foetus in utero and denote an attempt (an "unconscious wish") on the part of the epileptic to retreat for shelter from an unsympathetic environment into the stillness of the amniotic fluid, cannot be taken seriously, as they run counter to the facts of clinical observation and are plainly based on insufficient and ex parte study of available data.

It is however equally important to note the occurrence, at one or other phase, of more or less normal *coordinated* movement. For example, the patient may during the fit make champing movements of the jaws, may smack his lips, spit, clutch at his throat; in the course of petit mal quasipurposive actions of such a kind are often seen. To the routine question whether he bit his tongue the parents of a little boy answered "no, but he bit the lady next door". Postconvulsive (as already illustrated) and occasionally also preconvulsive periods are distinguished by similar phenomena bearing the stamp of cortical activity yet beyond voluntary control; moreover, some fits (described below) seem to consist solely of analogous "deliberate" acts. Since, then, individuality of movement may be preserved before, during, or after the phase of actual convulsion and since a special type is composed of a coordinated series, any artificial symptomatic barrier between "hysterical" and other kinds of fit tends to break down; differences of form and degree only, not of intrinsic nature, separate hystero-epilepsy from other epilepsies.

This consideration leads to the interesting question of the relation of the *time factor* to the particular mould in which epileptic disorders of motility are cast. If the motor elements of a convulsive fit could be extended, or lengthened in time, would they not possibly show more coordination than they actually do? The swiftness of the average major fit seems to determine the manifestation of movements "all at once", productive of universal contention and tonic rigidity. Were the fit more drawn out its features might well appear less convulsive and more deliberate. Variability in duration of aura, convulsion, and postconvulsive automatism is determined by factors of which we have little or no knowledge, and accounts for phenomena so diverse as to render individual fits hardly comparable one with another, yet the differences are not radical.

4. **Reflexes.** During the attack itself examination of tendon reflexes is difficult or impossible on account of spasm; their subsequent condition has already been discussed. The *corneal reflex* is abolished in conformity with the degree of unconsciousness, and the *pupils* do not react to light at the same stage; in less severe cases their response may be maintained throughout. At the onset of a fit pupillary contraction may be observed, but dilatation is usual, from the tonic phase onward till consciousness returns. A connexion between iris and vascular system is suggested by a record of RUSSELL REYNOLDS in the case of a child in convulsions, with dilated pupils and extremely weak pulse; his finger on the latter, and watching the eye, the observer noted sudden and simultaneous contraction of the pupil and filling of the radial artery. Involuntary *sphincter* action has already been mentioned, micturition being common and defaecation rare; as a general rule, it is a characteristic of nocturnal rather than diurnal fits, though exceptions are found. Passage of urine cannot well be correlated with either depth of unconsciousness or violence of convulsion, for it distinguishes, as has been shown, some instances of petit mal; further, as has also been stated, it constitutes one of the prodromes, and I have seen a case in which the aura ceased promptly if the patient was able to micturate. Facts of these kinds point to the conclusion (reached also on other grounds) that urination may be part of the epileptic process and not an incidental and indirect sequel; its occurrence in association with visceral types of epilepsy will be reverted to later. *Lachrymation* and *salivation,* occasionally rather obvious, seem more the mechanical result of spasmodic action than due to the enhanced activity of corresponding reflexes. I do not recall having seen any instances of *erection* or *emission,* though noted by older writers, the former at the tonic and the latter at the clonic stage.

5. **Vascular symptoms.** Many direct observations have been made of the vascular state on the threshold of an attack, and some of the exposed brain during it. Consensus of opinion holds that cerebral and general pallor or anaemia is often visible just as the seizure commences. This circulatory change is confirmed by the frequent record of failure of the peripheral *pulse* at the outset, and the rarer one of retinal arterial constriction at the same moment (MOXON, TROUSSEAU, JACKSON, FAGGE, BROADBENT, etc.). Some cases reported by RUSSELL are very convincing and, together with older and newer instances, rather discount GOWERS' generalisation that such failure is "certainly exceptional". In this connection

it is pertinent to recall the fact that cessation of the heart-beat in the STOKES-ADAMS syndrome is accompanied by transient unconsciousness, with or without convulsions. The condition of the pulse during the successive stages of the fit is rather variable; often small and slow at the tonic period, it accelerates thereafter, but sometimes no material change is remarked. Doubtless its vagaries depend on depth of coma and particular type of fit; it is much disturbed in some visceral forms of attack.

Initial *pallor* of face and skin is commoner in petit mal than in grand mal, but if not at first evident it becomes noticeable during the tonic stage, at the end of which it is nearly always replaced by *cyanosis*; the patient is "black round the lips," or a dusky and livid hue tinges the whole complexion, until the blood is better aerated by increasing freedom of respiratory movement. The aspect of the epileptic in the cyanotic phase is alarming, and occasionally he seems (to unaccustomed eyes) in articulo mortis. Yet at the end of the convulsive period, when everything is over, twice or thrice I have noticed such absolute pallor and total arrest of pulse and breathing as to mislead me into imagining for appreciable moments that exitus had occurred; during the tonic phase no such semblance of death has been personally observed.

Body temperature is little influenced even by severe attacks, though often rising several degrees in the course of status epilepticus. According to SPRATLING an elevation to 100° F. has been observed in single major seizures. It is less likely to be disturbed by extensive muscular contraction than by direct involvement of regulatory centres as a visceral component; patients suffering from vasovagal attacks often complain of icy coldness followed by flushing and perspiration, but whether objective change in temperature occurs does not appear to be known. Of some interest are cases (in children) distinguished by the development of fits in association with fever, of which a few examples have come under personal notice (see below).

Clinical Types.

To aid description epileptic syndromes are often grouped in accordance with 1. the clinical character of the seizures, 2. their frequency and periodicity, and 3. the time of their occurrence. Such an arrangement however applies almost exclusively to fits of unknown origin (cryptogenic fits), especially in institutional cases, which are more likely to belong to that category than those of identified causation and capable, it may be, of radical treatment. On the other hand, advances in therapeutics make it increasingly difficult to ascertain what might be called the "natural course" pursued by epilepsy. Statistical compilations dealing with frequencies, intervals between paroxysms, recurrences, and so forth, tend to become obsolete, for they seldom if ever incorporate figures derived from other epilepsies than the cryptogenic variety, and provide no information as to the relative percentages of major and minor fits of all kinds (e. g. in cerebral tumour, vascular disease, eclampsia etc.). So far as I am aware no endeavour has been made to ascertain whether any specific types of epileptic reaction are allied with particular processes of disease, or to compare clinical variants numerically on an etiological basis. There can be little doubt that conventional tabular studies are apt to convey wrong impressions in regard to the syndrome considered as a whole.

On purely empirical grounds it has long been the custom to distinguish epileptic classes according as the attacks are restricted to 1. major and 2. minor types, or 3. occur in a combined way. The appended table furnishes data affording some idea of the comparative frequency of these three general divisions among epilepsies of unknown origin.

Even in this "common or genuine" epilepsy (as MUSKENS seeks to term it) types are met with which are neither major, minor, nor combined. The same writer introduces another

Author	Number of cases	Percentage		
		Major	Minor	Combined
SPRATLING .	1325	60,0	5,5	32,0
TURNER . .	280	58,2	3,8	38,2

category, "primary myoclonic epilepsy," alleging it to be the most frequent of all; among more than 2000 cases he found less than 20 per cent. in which major fits were the sole mode of discharge. An analysis by GOWERS of petit mal cases showed 30 per cent. to occur alone and 70 per cent. in combination with major epilepsy.

To harmonise these divergencies, extreme as they are, would perhaps not be impossible, but the point they illustrate is the uselessness of figures in the absence of classificatory agreement and presence of epileptic variants.

1. The *major type* (so far as concerns cryptogenic epilepsy) begins either by a single severe fit with no recurrence for months or longer, or by comparatively quick repetition after a few days or weeks. From a series of cases investigated by GOWERS the second fit was ascertained to have occurred within a week in 14 per cent., within a month in 25 per cent., within six months in 28 per cent., and within a year in 10 per cent. Once the affection becomes confirmed, intervals between attacks vary greatly, and can hardly perhaps be reduced to a formula. All such broad generalisations, moreover, ignore the effects of treatment. Major fits come singly, or in little runs of two or three; their incidence is seldom characterised by any regularity, except perhaps in the case of socalled menstrual epilepsy (see below). Evidence suggesting a relative numerical constancy of attacks for a measured period of, say, a year at a time has sometimes been obtained, but many examples of the type do not conform to any rule. If, in some, frequency increases with the chronicity of the affection, in others the exact converse is the case.

Uncomplicated instances of the *minor type*, less abundant than the preceding, are subject to similar variation as regards numerical form. Generally, attacks are very frequent in their recurrence, a daily incidence being quite common, not merely of one or two fits but of many; yet, per contra, varieties are known in which they are spaced out to weeks or even longer, in the latter case, however, being often associated with major seizures. The minor type sometimes persists for many months, or years, ere severer convulsions develop. Seldom is any alternation or other interconnexion to be traced between the two; and if the major attacks sometimes yield to treatment minor seizures may continue relatively uninfluenced.

The *combined type*, to which numerous cases of petit mal eventually pass, is moderately common; minor fits are generally found to outnumber the others, though by no means invariably. What may perhaps be termed the "worst" specimens of the affection belong mostly to this combined category, if quantity of seizures is taken as the criterion. Sometimes a series of petit mal attacks precedes a severe fit; sometimes recurrence of the latter seems as it were to blot out daily repetition of the other for a time; the mild variety may be largely diurnal, the severe, nocturnal.

2. Another clinical grouping has reference mainly to *periodicity*. The term *serial epilepsy* is employed to designate the occurrence of a succession of major (sometimes of minor) fits at brief intervals over a limited period. No standard exists whereby to estimate whether a batch of seizures should thus be described or not; little runs of three, four, five or more attacks may come within some hours, or perhaps a day and a night, but sometimes their number exceeds a

dozen in a corresponding period and thereafter an indefinite stage of relief sets in. An occasional patient may always have his seizures in pairs. Short serial outbursts often seem to be introduced by a gradual numerical increase in isolated attacks, or by quick recurrences of the minor form; they constitute a kind of subacute epilepsy developing irrespective of any night or day rhythms that may have been evident.

Distinguished chiefly by the fact that consciousness is not regained between individual fits of the series, *status epilepticus* (état de mal) exemplifies the affection at its maximum. In the severest form, the postconvulsive sleep of one attack is cut short by development of the next, and so on without respite till eventually exhaustion is piled on exhaustion, coma sets in and deepens, pulse and respiration are accelerated, temperature rises and the immediate prognosis becomes ominous. A considerable proportion of chronic demented epileptics die in status; but if the convulsions are less continuous and less weakening recovery ensues once an after-stage of collapse or delirium is safely passed. The condition seems independent of sex, age, and time of onset of the original epilepsy. Computation of the average interval elapsing between initial paroxysm and first status period is impracticable, for the data are conspicuously diverse; generally speaking the type of case must be well-established, its course unfavourable, and predisposition evident, ere the likelihood of status supervening need be feared. Reduction of sedative treatment on too drastic a scale sometimes operates as a factor in its causation. The number of attacks during its continuance varies within wide limits, occasionally touching almost incredible figures; one of LEROY's patients had 488 major fits in 24 hours, and one of CLARK and PROUT's 542 in 48. Development is as a rule preceded by augmentation in fit frequency either by way of short serial phases or a gradual rise over a given period; rarely has it been fulminant. At the outset intervals of perhaps an hour, or half an hour, elapse between successive fits, but soon they are so curtailed as to render the convulsions almost unceasing; interparoxysmal rest may vanish altogether, one or other part of the body remaining in continuous spasm. Duration ranges from perhaps a few hours to as much as several days; overlapping of tonic and clonic phases, noticed at the climax, disappears with a change for the better; the end is marked by local twitching only, or slight general tremors. In a given case the number of status periods is subject to wide variation; one generally paves the way for another, rarely proving unique. Two or three sometimes suffice to lead to death in the last, but as many as seven have been noted.

Should the attacks be of moderate severity, however numerous, the prognosis need not alarm; in the case of a girl of 13, reported by MCDOUGALL, a group of 3,231 separate major fits occurred in 17 days; of these, 2,258 were observed in 6 consecutive days, being at the rate of 1 every 3,8 minutes. Despite this well-nigh unbelievable record the case ended in perfect recovery.

Like other features of epilepsy, status has never been given precise definition. Embodying the element of continuity in convulsions over a certain time, it can hardly be restricted to the cryptogenic type with predominance of grand mal seizures. Not only are so-called symptomatic varieties prone to issue in status as the underlying disease advances, but JACKSONian cases also may culminate in the same condition. Phases of the variant known as pyknolepsy (q. v. infra) may amount practically to status, while epilepsia partialis continua (as its name implies) constitutes in essence the same phenomenon; and the term need not be refused to series of "absences épileptiques," illustrated by a case in which 769 such attacks occurred in 12 hours (CLARK and PROUT). At least, variants and equivalents must be allowed if, broadly considered, incessant repetition without intervals of adequate recovery is taken to compose the integral feature of the state.

Not known, apparently to the ancients, its first description was given by CALMEIL. Among the best studies are those of BOURNEVILLE, LORENZ, CLARK and PROUT, TOULOUSE and MARCHAND, and (in particular) BOUTTIER.

3. Another clinical arrangement depends on the *time-relations* of fits, having regard either to their appearance by day or night on the one hand, or to the life-period at which they first manifest themselves or to which they are mainly confined on the other. Any value the method possesses concerns less the facts of observation justifying it than possible reasons for such variables, and this is a matter to be dealt with preferably under the heading of Pathogenesis (see below), since it entails discussion of both endogenous and exogenous factors. For centuries patients have sought to connect the recurring attacks of their malady with particular cosmic influences (seasonal, lunar, atmospheric, etc.), or with special periods of life; still now and then is the belief cherished that on attainment of his fourteenth or twenty-first year the patient will experience a change for the better or his fits will leave him. In no case does an alleged relationship of epilepsy to one or other division of time warrant the establishment of a corresponding clinical type except perhaps as regards the following varieties.

a) Study of epileptic recurrences with suffucent material and over an adequate period has long since led to the conclusion that *diurnal* and *nocturnal* types can be distinguished. To these, a third must be added, viz. one in which fits occur indifferently during sleep or the waking hours. For the better part of a century statistical analyses have been published at intervals showing with some unanimity that attacks take place in greater numbers by night, or by both night and day, than by the latter alone. They have also proved the existence of two nocturnal maxima, viz. one in the early hours of rest and a second towards four or five o'clock in the morning. The chief diurnal "peak" is found within an hour of two of the patient's getting up. Members of the nocturnal and diurnal groups react in antithetically opposite ways to factors influencing the development of convulsions (whatever they turn out to be), for fit-incidence is falling to its lowest in the case of the former at the very time it is rising in the case of the latter. Further, if nocturnal epileptics are made to sleep by day their seizures increase during that period (witness the proclivity to convulsion if they 'take a nap'), but the converse distinguishes the diurnal class; their nights however wakeful are comparatively or entirely free. Nocturnal epilepsy sometimes persists unrecognised for months or years, until a fit in the day reveals the truth. As already mentioned, the significance of such variations will be examined later.

For numerical details and analyses see articles by ECHEVERRIA, FÉRÉ, RODIET, PICK, IAMHANZI, HARTENBERG, LANGDON-BROWN and BRAIN, PATRY, and MARCHAND. Though practically all of these refer solely to epilepsies of unknown causation five among the 66 patients studied by LANGDON-BROWN and BRAIN suffered from "organic" lesions, but the time-incidence of their fits did not differ from that of the rest.

b) The relation of convulsions to the catamenial flow in female subjects is well authenticated. This so-called *menstrual epilepsy* seldom occurs in pure form, so to say, yet when it does it cannot fail to impress both patient and observer. In the majority the attacks take place just before the monthly period, or during its course, being rarer after its cessation. Should fit-incidence be more frequent than menstrual, it may increase at such times. Facts of observation lend no support to lingering belief in or hope for disappearance of seizures (if already in being) with establishment of the menses; indeed, fits sometimes then begin. Etiological relationships between the two states will be noticed subsequently.

c) The term *infantile convulsions* is based on a time subdivision and though sanctioned by long usage possesses no advantage except that of being noncommittal. Fits during the first three years of life differ in no material respect from those of later years, and their relegation to a separate category continues, perhaps, in deference to an attitude of mind loading the word "epilepsy" with sinister import. A history of convulsions in infancy, in the course of teething and other episodes, was obtained in 18,7 per cent. of 1000 epileptics (TURNER), in 34 per cent. of 100 (FÉRÉ), 19,6 per cent. of 500 (PATRICK and LEVY), 27,5 per cent. of 200 (MUSKENS), 29 per cent. of 1365 (SCHLAPP), 31,6 per cent. of 1000 (SHANAHAN). Of the last-mentioned collection only 200 (20 per cent.) continued to suffer from fits uninterruptedly into later life; only 15 of 111 children with infantile attacks were found to have shown no remission eight years later (THOM).

Wide differences of opinion exist as to the significance of these early manifestations, some maintaining they are only of passing moment, others insisting that they portend a subsequent epilepsy. Unnecessary confusion has been caused by attempts to discriminate between different kinds of infantile convulsions; MUSKENS, for example, seeks to separate "occasional convulsions" (in children with febrile disorders), encephalitic fits, infantile eclampsia (spasmophilic phenomena, mainly of rickets), "emotional or anger convulsions", and others still, from "common or genuine" epilepsy of childhood, though admitting the impossibility of drawing a hard-and-fast line between epilepsy and eclampsia. According to the views here adopted such endeavours are beside the point; it is irrational to hold that infantile convulsions are "antecedents" of the adult malady, and still worse (as some do) to make them "causes" of the latter, for they are nothing else than epileptic themselves, constituting a variant solely in respect of incidence on early years. The opinion expressed many years ago by FÉRÉ, that the convulsions of infancy are etiologically and symptomatically identical with epilepsy, must receive endorsement if that term is employed in a wide and inclusive sense. That some factors are operative in early years rather than later, that immature nervous systems may be more susceptible than those of the adult, that clinical forms of one or other sort should be more frequent in the case of children, are considerations which in no way invalidate the main proposition. And if there is trouble in differentiating what is "epileptic" and what not in regard to infantile spasmodic symptoms, precisely the same difficulty must be faced in respect of adult syndromes. Further, if a child has a solitary convulsion of any kind the problem of whether "epilepsy" is going to develop presents no features distinguishing it from the identical problem in the case of an adult's first attack. The real importance of the matter consists in the urgency of scrutinising every case of infantile fits for immediate or remote causes and dealing with them promptly; neglect of such precautions must be partly responsible for the not very uncommon reappearance of epileptic attacks after a long remission in the years of childhood.

To others (already mentioned) who have dealt with the subject the names of HOCHSINGER, FORD and SCHAFFER, BOSSERT, BURR, VOGT, BIEULAC, GÖTT, MORSE, LUCAS and SOUTHARD, CRAMER, and COOKSON may be added.

d) Such terms as *adolescent, climacteric* and *senile* epilepsy have little to recommend them. The first of these no doubt denotes one of the principal types, in the sense that attacks often commence at that time of life; menopausal instability occasionally acts as a precipitating, more regularly as an aggravating factor; senile epilepsy, incapable of precise definition, merits brief comment. Its association with the period of involution leads the observer to suspect an arteriopathic basis for the phenomena, and this is often evident (cf. SCHUPFER). Of 40 cases beginning after the fourth decennium a family history of epilepsy was found by Turner in 10 per cent., but delayed hereditary influence is of less import as a determinant than coexisting "organic" change of one or other kind. When middle life sees the first appearance of fits attention should be directed to the vascular system, intracranial pressure, evidence of syphilis and, in general, to the probability of structural disease. Such etiological factors apart, however, the senile form offers no features distinguishing it from any other.

Clinical variants.

In addition to ordinary major and minor varieties, of everyday occurrence, cases come under notice presenting similarities to the phenomena of epilepsy as generally understood, but may not seem to resemble each other, at least in outward appearance. To such conditions the term *epileptic variants* may conveniently be applied; some are of course quite well-known and far from rare, others are unusual and their epileptic nature not at first sight evident. Commencing with clinical types characterised by modifications of a motor kind, we may usefully adopt the appended classification.

1. Motor variants.

1. Jacksonian (partial) epilepsy. — 2. Myoclonic or regional epilepsy. — 3. Tonic epilepsy. — 4. Coordinated epilepsy. — 5. Epilepsia partialis continua. — 6. Pyknolepsy. — 7. Inhibitory or akinetic epilepsy.

1. Jacksonian Epilepsy. In this term the name of the English master, Hughlings Jackson, is commemorated, though the particular variety it denotes (to which alone the expression "epileptiform" was first applied and should be confined) was, as he well knew, familiar to Prichard, Bravais and Todd before him, even possibly to Galen (see p. 4). It is taken, after Jackson, to signify local or partial attacks of epilepsy, unilateral in the first instance, without loss of consciousness, pursuing a "march" in accordance with the disposition of motor centres in the rolandic cortex.

Unilateral convulsions commence in any part of face, trunk, or limbs, habitually though not invariably assuming a clonic form throughout. Sometimes initial spasms are tonic rather than clonic, at others the former mode affects the "second" limb (e. g. the arm if the leg is first involved), or the "second" side (if spasm spreads across the body). Practical experience recognises three places where fits of this group mostly begin, viz. 1. hand, 2. face or tongue, or both, and 3. foot. Jackson's physiological explanation of these clinical facts was that the spasm selects segments having the greatest number of "voluntary uses"; and the order given above, in accordance with this view, also specifies the relative frequency of the three, the hand coming first. Whether the explanation suffices must however be considered open to question, for a large number of Jacksonian seizures start with a sensation instead of a motion; and though sensory centres for the hand are more highly developed than those for, say, the shoulder, both sensory and motor initial symptoms not infrequently affect other divisions of the former segment than thumb and forefinger, which are the parts employed in the most varied ways. Sometimes, too, the aura is referred not to the most sensitive regions of the hand, the finger-tips, but to palm or wrist.

On a previous page detailed description has been furnished of the Jacksonian aura, its classical forms and occasional variants. To a large extent the motor phenomena follow identical lines, with or without antecedent sensations. As regards the hand, clonic flexor spasm seizes forefinger and thumb principally, less often the ulnar digits, sometimes all together; it never seems to commence in the middle finger, or invade the extensors primarily. In the face, the lower division may be affected unilaterally, upper groups bilaterally;

should the tongue first be caught it deviates away from the side of the lesion. Orbicularis oris may contract on one or, more usually, both sides. Fits beginning in the foot nearly always cause strong dorsiflexion of the great toe, but now and then all the toes flex, with inversion at ankle and drawing up of heel. Local commencement otherwise is distinctly uncommon; spasm may start in the larger muscles of shoulder, upper arm, hip or thigh, and rarely in those of the abdomen on one side only.

The march of the convulsions obeys the same physiological laws as have been illustrated in the case of sensory spread, most often extending rapidly over the whole of one half of the body; they may be localised in one limb only or part of a limb, or confined to face and neck; in numerous instances they pass over to the other (second) side ere abandoning the first, affecting the former identically but more commonly not; for example, intermittent spasm may be found on the first side and tonic spasm on the second, or both varieties may (in either of the two orders, tonic-clonic or vice versa) traverse the first in succession and only one the second. This is shown by the case of a woman where tonic extension of the right leg was followed by clonic twitches advancing from ankle, knee, and hip to the right arm and face; immediately after, the whole left side became involved together in tonic spasm. Another variation is provided by a case in which twitching commenced in the ball of the right thumb, rapidly affecting the right arm as far as the shoulder; then both legs were suddenly relaxed and the patient fell without losing consciousness; the movements died out in the right arm just as intermittent spasm appeared on the right side of the face, and when it, too, ceased, he began to "talk nonsense". Crossing to the second side is generally coincident with deviation of head and eyes away from that first affected to the other. As a rule convulsion dies out quickest in the segment originally concerned and from other parts in the order of their invasion. Sometimes the march is peculiarly deliberate, the discharges anomalous.

In a case closely watched throughout, the fit commenced by flickering contractions of the right abdominal muscles for a few seconds; spasm then started afresh, a moment later, in the toes of the right foot, passing up the limb in clonic convulsions to the groin, where it ceased entirely. After an interval of two minutes it began once more, in the right side of the abdomen, traversing trunk to shoulder and travelling down arm to fingers; in this limb, however, the spasm was of tonic type, impressing on it a rigid attitude of semi-flexion; the right lower face was the seat of clonic twitches during the tonic phase of the arm. Ten minutes was the average total duration of an observed series.

Only muscles accustomed to act individually are implicated in JACKSONian fits of mild degree; if more severe, bilateral couples (e. g. muscular pairs of thorax and abdomen, of upper face, throat, etc.) are mostly affected together, though the hemispheric discharge is unilateral. But to this rule there are frequent exceptions, running contrary to the doctrine embodied in BROADBENT's law, according to which bilateral groups have a representation in each half of the brain. For instance, I have seen several cases of strictly one-sided clonic spasm of recti and obliqui abdominis (as have other clinical observes, e. g. HARRIS) a condition incapable of "voluntary" imitation.

Despite the universally received view that the cortex "knows nothing of muscles" and that only movements are represented therein, the phenomena of JACKSONian epilepsy compel its reconsideration. In addition to prolonged unilateral abdominal clonus, a combination of twitching of right forefinger and thumb with isolated simultaneous flickers confined to right depressor labii inferioris has come under notice. The latter point illustrates the argument, for such contractions seem to prove that an individual muscle can be innervated from the cortex. Both cases also show dissociation of normal physiological pairs by cortical motor disorder.

Whether the discharging process continues strictly hemispheric in site as both halves of the body become involved in a severe JACKSONian seizure is doubtful; probably spread to the opposite hemisphere takes place at least in some cases, for observed data warrant the conclusion. Moreover, none other is permissible when, as occasionally happens, unilateral fits become generalised, with loss of senses. Instantaneous transmission of nervous impulses brings anatomically separate centres into the closest physiological rapport, for sometimes the whole of one side is simultaneously seized by spasm; differing rapidities of invasion doubtless account for (or are at least one of the factors in) the ranging of clinical modes from tonic rigidity to phasic movement.

It is sometimes possible to modify the contractions of a slow attack by external manipulation; for example, when biceps brachii is in tonic spasm forcible hyperflexion at the elbow, approximating the two ends of the muscle, may cause the spasm to leave it and appear in an antagonistic group (cf. HOLMES). Deliberate prevention of movement, either by strong and urgent exercise on the patient's part or by the observer's hold on the limb, frequently proves effectual (the latter procedure, known to ARETAEUS, has been rediscovered empirically by generations of epileptics); another time-honoured method consists in the application of a ligature to the part concerned. Such modes of interference with the action of discharging centres can be explained by afferent influence thereon and are considered in connexion with the variant known as reflex epilepsy (q.v. infra), where also comment on the excitation of JACKSONian and other types of fit by external stimuli will be found.

Motor paresis of fluctuating degree often follows a unilateral attack, and is discussed above in connexion with sequelae (p. 20).

A question once hotly debated concerns the occurence of genuine JACKSONian seizures in hysteria; today it must be answered in the negative, for, as has been shown, physiological dissociations take place in the former that are beyond volitional reproduction. On the other hand, hysterical convulsions sometimes are of local or unilateral distribution and so, in a sense, "JACKSONian"; careful study of their phenomena will, however, confirm their origin on a higher level than that of the precentral gyrus. Discussion has also centred on the problem of "idiopathic" JACKSONian fits, that is, of local convulsions observing a march from an initial focus but unaccompanied by evidence, early or late, of coexisting structural disease. COLLIER goes so far as to assert that "the commonest cause of JACKSONian epilepsy is idiopathic epilepsy," but few in my belief will support the opinion from personal experience. Despite occasional cases seemingly innocent of any local lesion, the fact that in the great majority some or other form of recognisable tissue change can be either found or reasonably postulated (in only 8,4 per cent. of 130 JACKSONian cases reported by FINCHER and DOWMAN did the etiology remain undetermined) must lead to an opposite conclusion. One or two JACKSONian patients in whom unilateral convulsions were the sole residuum of an infantile encephalitic hemiparesis, discoverable in their history yet completely in abeyance otherwise, have been personally observed.

The frequency of partial fits varies enormously, being generally greater in inverse ratio to the range covered; in one case, 900 attacks occurred in 24 hours, but were restricted to left face, tongue, and side of the neck. When thus confined, they may become almost continuous on occasion, and scarcely to be distinguished from the corresponding type mentioned on a later page.

From a vast literature reference can be made here only to a few papers of historical or other interest, e. g. those by PITRES, BÄUMLER, MCKENDRICK, ROLLAND, MILLS, MÜLLER, REDLICH.

2. Myoclonic Epilepsy. This variant is more common than is generally imagined. It takes the shape of irregular twitches of one or other part of the body in multimuscular groups, and colloquially is often termed "the jumps".

Fully described by RUSSELL REYNOLDS in the middle of last century, the frequency of such jerking movements without loss of consciousness still seems to be underestimated. Of modern writers only MUSKENS has devoted particular attention thereto, one of his statistical studies [1] having established their presence at one or other period in no fewer than 185 out of 300 epileptics. Not much complained of spontaneously, regarded with unconcern or even ignored, careful enquiry often elicits a history of their existence for a longer or shorter time prior to the first paroxysmal fit, while continuance during intervals between major attacks is also frequent (see under Prodromes, p. 8 above). Myoclonus may form the sole epileptic indication, as in the case of a girl of 18 (in whose family a brother suffered from fits and three other members had had convulsions in infancy) who for four years had noticed, practically every morning, sudden and violent jerks of the arms, sufficient to throw things out of her hands. Up to the time of observation no other epileptic phenomenon had ever occured.

Either uni- or bilateral, myoclonic symptoms affect some definite region of the body (whence the synonym "regional epilepsy"); one or both arms are shot suddenly forwards or out (in one case always preceded by tickling in the palms of the hands) the head jerkily flexed or extended, the trunk curved or straightened. A frequent incident during the process of dressing consists in the patient's being thrown to the floor. Facial involvement is exceptional. Occasionally the briefest of conscious "blanks" appears to accompany the condition, which, though liable to develop at any moment, generally selects night or morning as favourite hours.

Myoclonus, as a term, denotes abrupt muscular contractions of varying intensity, and is known to depend on other processes besides those of an epileptic nature. Among the myoclonias are some producing movement and displacement at one or other joint by simultaneous implication of several muscles, a tic-like feature, and these (rather than such as consist in flickering contraction of isolated muscles) belong to the class under review. None the less it may be difficult at the bedside to effect discrimination; and whether the distinction constitutes a basic difference is more than doubtful, for both can occur in the same subject, and at the same time. In some epileptics myoclonic phenomena are widespread and almost continuous, supplying a link with the epilepsia partialis continua discussed below; they may, or may not, exhibit a familial incidence.

The *familial myoclonus epilepsy* of UNVERRICHT represents clinically a combination of two syndromes, yet each may vary profoundly in degree and extent, while sporadic occurrence has been reported. Though the myoclonia is sometimes more pronounced, persistent, and progressive than in ordinary cases, neither that nor its hereditary character suffices to make the condition a nosological entity, as some would maintain (cf. CLARK). The UNVERRICHT syndrome is by no means rare, and does not differ in any essential feature from the clinical commonplace of fits combined with "jerks".

For descriptions see UNVERRICHT's original article and the monograph by LUNDBORG; also reviews or cases by CLARK and PROUT, REYNOLDS, DIDE, MANNINI, CROUZON and BOUTTIER, SICARD and LERMOYEZ, CATALANO, etc.

Similar criticism applies to the intermittent or sporadic type of RABOT, which would appear to be nothing else than a stage in the evolution of the more progressive variety, or merely an example of the usual syndrome.

3. Tonic Epilepsy. Fits characterised by tonic contractions only, to the exclusion of the clonic or phasic element, have long been known. Many so-called "cerebellar" fits belong to this group; their physiological localisation chiefly

---
[1] Epilepsia Vol 1. 1909.

concerns postural mechanisms of the mesencephalon. From the pathological standpoint, generalised attacks distinguished by assumption of tonic attitudes and occurrence of tonic muscular contractions, often superimposed one on the other, are most likely to develop in consequence of lesions functionally dissociating cerebral hemispheres from cerebello-mesencephalo-pontine levels. Such tonic fits consist essentially of bilateral extension and inversion of all four limbs, with arching of back and head; frequently, however, the arms are flexed at elbows, adducted at shoulders, wrists flexed and hands closed. One or both sides of the face may be involved; the eyes may be directed to one side, and the head turn with them, or the latter may from the first be strongly contracted. In some instances the fit begins by slow flexion of one arm and extension of the ipsilateral leg; then the former extends while trunk and opposite limbs are seized in turn. A further variety takes the shape of tonic adduction of arm and leg with abduction of the contralateral limbs, followed by rotation of head and trunk away from the side primarily affected. Other possibilities include fragmentary manifestations of tonicity, confined to head and body.

In general, two main forms can be distinguished, one consisting of immediate bilateral and symmetrical tonic spasms of the whole musculature, throwing the body into the posture assumed in decerebrate rigidity; the other commences locally and pursues a deliberate march or course till all segments are implicated, evolving slowly and asymmetrically through successive phases of tonic contraction and often combined with complete rotation round the patient's long axis. A number of such fits, either personally observed or culled from the literature, were described in extenso in a paper[1] dealing with decerebrate rigidity. The fully developed type is not seldom ushered in by rapid, deep, grunting respiration or other change in the rhythm of breathing, accompanied by less noticeable affection of the pulse and, frequently, by abundant sweating.

A remarkable case (asphyxial in origin) was that of a suicide who hanged himself and was cut down when in extremis. Tetanic convulsions soon began, increasing in intensity and affecting the whole body. Arms were rigidly extended, hands clenched, thumbs pressed into palm, legs stretched out, jaws tightened, head drawn back, with extreme opisthotonus; during the fits (which continued for ten hours) breathing was almost entirely suspended; between them the patient was bathed in perspiration.

The majority of such tonic attacks doubtless proceed from a basis of structural disease, and have often been given description (HUGHLINGS JACKSON, STEWART and HOLMES, FIRTH, FOERSTER, MARTIN, REYNOLDS etc.); but brief tonic fits, constituting not much more than a rather elaborate petit mal seizure, also occur, and deserve mention for their unusual features. A case in point is that of a young woman whose so-called "menstrual epilepsy" is as follows; a sudden inspiratory cry is succeeded by outstretching of rigid arms, strong opisthotonus, and a backward crash to the floor, with legs extended and stiff; cyanosis at once sets in, and micturition occurs; then as suddenly muscular relaxation appears, no trace of intermittent movement being seen, and violent vomiting brings the fit to a close. Tonic phases and local tonic convulsion form a portion of many major and minor epilepsies, of JACKSONian and notably of numerous hysterical attacks. Elsewhere[1] is narrated the case of a boy whose tonic seizures rolled him off the bed or caused the adoption of slowly changing postures reminiscent of decerebrate rigidity; no lesion could be discovered, but whether hysterical or not they belonged to an exclusively tonic variety and were coupled with loss of senses stertorous breathing, and slight "foaming at the mouth."

Within recent years the term *striatal epilepsy* seems to have come into vogue for somewhat heterogeneous cases of tonic spasm, of a partial, unilateral, or

---

[1] Brain **43** (1920).

generalized kind, imagined (on the analogy of PARKINSONian and other involuntary movements) to have its substratum in lesions of the basal ganglia (WIMMER). Known also as "spastic epilepsy" (KNAPP), "extrapyramidal" (STERLING) or "subcortical epilepsy" (SPILLER), this plausible attribution of tonic contractions to the corpus striatum must be received with very considerable reserve. Not a few of the examples cited by these observers can be reasonably assigned either to tetany or to painful cramps, and it seems inadvisable to widen the horizon of the epilepsies by inclusion of categories of such distinctiveness. Further there is no novelty except its proposed name in the conception, for cases of the kind have long been known; one under personal care is that of a youth with symptoms of postencephalitis, in whose unilateral and purely tonic attacks the left foot extends and becomes inverted, the left leg is in extension, head bent over to the left and trunk slightly arched, with concavity to that side; the arm is flexed at elbow, abducted at shoulder, and fingers generally flexed; some spasm of the left orbicularis oris is noticed but the mouth does not deviate; consciousness is preserved. Discovery of striatal lesions post-mortem (STERTZ) in a case of this nature (showing also torsion-spasm, however, as did WIMMER's) is of course no proof of the striatal origin of the fits; on the contrary, they most likely had an extra-striatal source since these ganglia were the seat of destructive processes. Besides, as has been illustrated already, tonic phases and seizures occur much too frequently in generalised, JACKSONian, petit mal and hysterical cases to justify reference of the tonic component exclusively to the striatal system (see also below, in the section on Pathophysiology).

4. **Coordinated Epilepsy.** By this term, possibly not the most appropriate that might be devised, is denoted a type composed of coordinated and quasi-purposive movements, like many of those distinguishing hysterical attacks. Considered by TROUSSEAU intermediate between epilepsy and hysteria and assigned by GOWERS preferably to one or the other "disease", such phenomena break down artificial symptomatic barriers between "functional" and other kinds of fit (*all* fits are nothing else than temporary disorders of function) and exemplify the occurrence of epileptic processes on the highest levels of activity. We have already seen how both before and after the paroxysm movements of a coordinate class are observable, and during its course as well (page 24). In one case a patient waved his right arm in circles ere falling unconscious and convulsed, and in another (GOWERS) the fit began with his hopping round the room on one leg. Sometimes the whole motor content is not convulsive in any feature, but purely coordinate. This is admittedly true of various instances of petit mal, and is shown by the case of a patient (with epileptic ancestry) who turns pale, loses touch with his surroundings, raises his closed fist and shakes it, blinks his eyes, then looks sideways as though peering round the corner. In this connexion it is of interest to recall JACKSON's view that the anatomical substratum of minor epilepsy has a frontal site. Be that as it may, development of epileptic symptoms of this highest-level quality must on clinical grounds be conceded, and their acceptance possesses the supreme merit of bringing heterogeneous fit manifestations within a uniform physiological scheme.

5. **Epilepsia partialis continua.** Another motor variant, doubtless somewhat rare, has received but scant attention despite its physiological interest. It differs from the general myoclonic type in that the twitching is limited to one segment of the body (hence the term "monoepilepsy"), nearly always peripheral, such as wrist and fingers, is practically continuous between infrequent paroxysmal JACKSONian or generalised fits, and on the whole consists less in formed movements than in irregular, individual muscular contractions. Known also as "polyclonia epileptoides continua", most though not all of the reported cases have

had a background of structural disease of the cortex. Among several personally observed is that of a young man of 30, an epileptic since childhood, who for 15 years has noticed more or less continuous jerky and abrupt twitches of the right upper limb, usually causing flexion but sometimes also extension of the fingers, and either of wrist. His major fits commence in this part, becoming generalised with great rapidity.

The interest of the condition resides in the apparently ceaseless character of the phenomena, as though due to persistent excitation of the cortical reflex arc, and in the absence of any trace of the exhaustion paresis or paralysis often characterising JACKSONian epilepsy; the latter observation is probably explicable on the ground of relative mildness of discharge.

Further information can be gained from articles by KOSHEWNIKOW, ORLOWSKI, CHOROSKO, SPILLER, KRUMHHOLZ, SCHMIERGELD, LONG-LANDRY and QUERCY, POLLOSSON and COLLET, D'HOLLANDER, etc.

6. Pyknolepsy. The word pyknolepsy ($\pi v \varkappa v \acute{o} \varsigma$, crowded, frequent) was coined by MEYER for a subvariety principally affecting children between the ages of perhaps four and twelve years and distinguished by amazingly numerous repetitions of extremely brief mental "blanks", a complete momentary arrest of the mental stream, during which the child looks vacant or stares, his eyeballs may roll and his eyelids flicker, and in a few seconds he is himself again. Tonic and clonic elements of any obstrusive kind are conspicuous by their absence. If seated, his limbs may relax, but a fall from the erect position does not occur. The most impressive feature of the state is the frequency of the attacks, sometimes running into hundreds daily, hence the graphic American expression "myriad spells".

Their sudden onset in most examples is paralleled by an equally sudden disappearance after weeks, months, or years, never to return; this happened in the case of a most intelligent little boy who used to have dozens as he sat on a chair in the outpatient clinic, and who has fulfilled the promise of his youth. Yet occasionally the prognosis turns out to be unfavourable, for major fits sometimes develop later. No unique and unmistakable clinical trait divides pyknolepsy from petit mal, of which it is obviously a mere variant; hence its formulation as a nosological entity or "disease" cannot be justified. That the little fits subside spontaneously can hardly be taken to constitute a differentiating criterion, in view of the exceptions that occur, however rare they be; nor is it reasonable to exclude from the category cases otherwise typical if they manifest symptoms suggestive of ordinary petit mal, e. g. clonic movements, pallor, subsequent mental confusion or automatism, and so forth. The monotonously unvarying character of the pyknoleptic seizures perhaps forms a distinctive feature, yet a similar remark is applicable to numerous cases of minor epilepsy; I recall that of a little child whose head used to sink in a nodding movement on his chest scores of times every day, in precisely the same fashion at each recurrence. Clinical interest and weight attach rather to the circumstance that for this particular type a gratifying outcome can be predicted with some confidence even though the explanation is still to seek.

The literature includes studies by FRIEDMANN, HEILBRONNER, STIER, ADIE.

Under the nondescript title of "lightning spasms" (Blitzkrämpfe) attention has been directed to the occurrence in infants and young children of sudden contractions tending to curl the patient into a ball, as it were; the head is bent forward on the chest and the knees are doubled up on the abdomen so as to meet it. By some these "lightning convulsions" have been compared to movements accompanying the act of sneezing. As has long been known, however, not only do some examples of petit mal consist essentially of a general emprosthotonic series of contractions, but "salaam" tics or spasms must also be borne in mind. LEHMKUHL, on the other hand, uncritically allots the type to the "striate" category (q. v. supra), with a basis in structural brain disease.

7. Inhibitory or Akinetic Epilepsy. Many epileptic phenomena are inhibitory and not excitomotor in nature. Arrest of function distinguishes one or other phase, initial or later, in both major and minor fits, while some postconvulsive symptoms generally attributed to exhaustion might be better regarded as exemplifying inhibition. Both GOWERS and JACKSON refer to the possibility of sensory excitation being succeeded not by motion but by its opposite (see above, page 5), and one or two cases were reported by the former in which an aura of acute paraesthesiae in the arm was followed by powerlessness of the same member. For these and analogous instances illustrating inhibition of motor centres by epileptic sensory discharges the term proposed at the head of this paragraph may find acceptance. A personally studied case of the kind has been published in detail elsewhere [1], and others alluded to briefly by HOLMES and COLLIER.

A further case in point is that of a man of 52 suffering from "attacks of trance"; the aura, an intense and peculiar smell like that of "burning fat", is at once succeeded by his falling into a trance-like state during which he turns pale, loses touch with his environment, and is utterly incapable of moving a finger.

The fact that strong stimulation sometimes leads to arrest of function finds expression in popular phrases such as being "thunderstruck", or "struck all of a heap", which include the idea of temporary "paralysis". This sequence of immobility after a sensory discharge offers a certain resemblance to the negative or refractory phase of a reflex arc following overexcitation. Attacks distinguished by powerlessness constitute a heterogeneous group, yet among them are cases providing links between epilepsy, catalepsy, narcolepsy and cataplexy; for example, a patient who suffered from infrequent major convulsive fits to the age of 14 thereafter developed another kind, precipitated by hearty laughter and having as components pallor, clouding of consciousness, and absolute arrest of voluntary movements. A transition of this kind from convulsive to inhibitory epilepsy (or cataplexy, perhaps) shows that no impassable symptomatic boundary divides affections for which separate nomenclature sometimes proves misleading.

2. Sensory variants.

1. Sensory epilepsy. — 2. Reflex epilepsy. — 3. Affective epilepsy.

1. Sensory Epilepsy. That paroxysmal manifestations should be confined to afferent mechanisms is more than a theoretical possibility. Not only do the sensations of the JACKSONian aura march along physiological lines like a corresponding motor fit but they may be followed by transient loss of sensibility, together constituting the whole of the disturbance. The numbness that had started round the lips and involved the right face arm and leg (in a case personally studied) was found to be accompanied by loss in recognition of tactile stimuli, which gradually receded from the proximal zones of each limb; the last segments to recover were the hand and foot. Analogous observations have been made by HOLMES (who also noted interference with painful and thermal impulses) and seem to indicate some departure from the rule governing cases of local convulsive phenomena, for the segment first becoming insensitive does not always lead in recovery.

Perhaps some paroxysmal neuralgias may eventually prove to be classifiable with the epilepsies.

2. Reflex Epilepsy. The term is in usage to signalise cases where one or other kind of fit follows on the heels of some extrinsic stimulus, but has never been defined with precision. Formerly employed in a general way to connote fit development in consequence of peripheral "irritation", older writers enumerate as

---

[1] J. of Neur. 8 (1928).

examples those "reflexly" induced by adenoids, errors of refraction, carious teeth, dyspepsia, helminthiasis, tight prepuce, and what not. The expression "secondary epilepsy" was proposed by NOTHNAGEL for rare instances of peripheral nerve injury succeeded after an interval by major attacks, with or without a corresponding aura; curiously enough, the aftermath of the war does not appear to have brought such conditions with it. "BROWN-SÉQUARD's epilepsy", also regarded as "reflex", consisted in the production of convulsions (in guinea-pigs) by excitation of a cutaneous epileptogenous zone over face and neck after previous section of the sciatic nerve, or of half the cord (cf. BRAMWELL and GRAHAM BROWN).

In a specific sense, reflex epilepsy should be reserved for the occurrence of fits as an instant sequel to external stimuli, impulses reaching the brain by any sense avenue. Cases of the kind are not very unusual; a boy of seven went off into an attack whenever his head or face was touched, but if forewarned none took place (HUGHLINGS JACKSON). It closely resembles an earlier one reported by DUNSMURE, in which, however, immediate "loss of power" resulted. Another (WOODCOCK) is that of a little boy whose sister remarked that whenever she drew his right stocking off he had a fit. In a personal instance the hat-elastic under a little girl's chin slipped up and hit her nose, a convulsion ensuing; this incident led to the discovery that flicking or tapping the nose invariably precipitated a seizure consisting in widened pupils, tonic spasm of arms and thorax, respiratory arrest, cyanosis, and slight salivation (this case was also seen by KENNEDY). Instances of *reflex Jacksonian epilepsy*[1] are met with; one distinguished by rightsided convulsions beginning in the hand was remarkable in that they were caused not merely by touches or knocks on that member but also by similar stimuli applied to the right leg, and (less often) by unexpected sights or sounds of a disturbing nature. I have also observed tonic unilateral spasm seize the left limbs of a little boy in consequence of any jar or knock, whenever applied. The comparative ease with which local fits can be started reflexly by handling the segment concerned is an old observation. What seems a significant factor in most cases is that the reflex arc should be seized unawares; but the element of the surprise cannot be considered indispensable since fits may develop in its absence.

Another variety may be given the name of *acousticomotor epilepsy* (cf. OPPENHEIM), and is distinguished by the subject's falling to the ground on any abrupt auditory stimulus, not always either loud or alarming; a girl of 19 had suffered in this way since the age of seven, any noise for which she was unprepared causing collapse on her knees, which had often sustained minor injuries (cf. PUTNAM and WATERMANN). Another case of the same kind was complicated subsequently by major fits.

As regards this reflex class similar duplication of epileptic processes is traceable; an external stimulus either excites or inhibits discharge. The acousticomotor type exemplifies action of the latter mechanism, as does the case of DUNSMURE (quoted above). Another known to me concerns an old lady whose nurse discovered by accident that if a stream of water from a sponge was directed on the head during her bath insensibility supervened, all limbs were relaxed, and she sank motionless to its foot. The only satisfactory way of interpreting arrest of JACKSONian convulsions by ligature of the segment immediately affected is on the assumption of reinforcement thereby of some restraining influence exercised by sensory on motor centres. Many epileptics discover for themselves that a powerful and sharp stimulus of one or other kind may so impress the sensorium as to check incipient discharge (see under Treatment, p. 80).

---

[1] See my MORISON Lectures, Brit. med. J. 2 (1930).

3. Affective Epilepsy. Proposals have frequently been made for separation of certain fits claimed to be neither epileptic nor hysterical, not in respect of their content, which is identical with that of major attacks, but because of their alleged etiology. They belong to the "reflex" category in the sense of being provoked from without but by excitants invariably of an affective kind, hence the suggested title "affective epilepsy". Stated to occur mainly or solely in psychopaths, they have also been termed "psychasthenic fits".

The subdivision, however, is based on the erroneous conception of epilepsy as a "disease" with pathognomonic characters, a "genuine" malady capable of being "simulated" by other conditions, and on the equally mistaken idea that its attacks develop spontaneously, without any precipitant. Arguing from these faulty premises, several observers (BRATZ, OPPENHEIM, BONHOEFFER, STALLMANN, SPILLER, FRINK, etc.) affirm that the seizures merely "simulate" epilepsy, representing the maximal type of a series whose mildest grade consists of giddiness, faintness, and other neurotic trifles; some allege that the patients never become mentally deteriorated or suffer from petit mal. These latter features, however, cannot be relied on for differentiation from ordinary epilepsy (of unknown origin); moreover in the course of time cases once labelled "affective" are often found to belong to the cryptogenic or, alternatively, the "organic" class (GUTTMANN). Segregation only adds to existing confusion. Affective stimuli form but a small group amid the vastly larger number of determinants all of which are alike in acting simply as a spark to ignite convulsible material; besides, in a given case excitants of different orders may be in action at different times. Subdivision is carried much too far if quality of stimulus is to be employed for differentiation. The most that can be said for "affective" epilepsy is that it denotes the occurrence, in psychopathic and hysterical subjects, not of hysteroepilepsy (as might have been expected from emotional incitements), but of major epileptic fits. But this merely proves that hysterical and other epilepsies are much more closely related than is commonly allowed.

For criticism see also articles by STEFFENS, APELT, ALZHEIMER, NOTKIN, and others.

A number of characteristic examples have come under personal observation and one or two recorded elsewhere [1], but their total is relatively insignificant, though the war brought cases of the kind in some abundance. The view of ROWS and BOND (see above, p. 5) that every epileptic fit represents a reaction to express emotion is too exaggerated a claim to be seriously considered.

3. Psychical Variants.

The term "psychical equivalents of epilepsy" is objectionable for more than one reason; if behind psychical symptoms processes of stimulation and inhibition identical with those underlying epileptic symptoms in other systems can rationally be postulated, then these psychical syndromes are not "equivalent" to epilepsy but are in fact epileptic. Defined by TURNER as comprising the mental symptoms of pre- and postconvulsive states occurring without convulsion, this view of their character is tantamount to an admission of identity, not equivalence, with the affection itself. Thus conceived, the phrase incorporates diverse psychical disorders accompanying grand and petit mal and any of the variants, inclusive of dreamy states (for which the word "psycholepsy" was coined by JANET), epileptic mania, fugues, automatisms and analogous features mentioned passim in our descriptions and thereby is bereft of any specific usefulness.

---

[1] Brit. med. J. **1** (1927); J. of Neur. **8** (1928).

Admittedly, however, a tendency exists to regard any sudden irresponsible and uncontrolled outburst of erratic conduct (transient it must be, and perhaps accompanied by diminution of conscious awareness) as an "equivalent" of an epileptic seizure, even in the absence of any personal or family history of the condition. No doubt in at least some cases the mental derangement follows a minor "lapse" so mild and fleeting as to be overlooked, but whether this is true of all must be left an open question. Rare instances of fits being *preceded* by acts of impulse are on record, and so far as facts of observation allow there is no difficulty in accepting incidents of violence or of misdemeanour as having their origin in processes identical with those known to distinguish some epileptic cases; but it would be a mistake to assign all such outbreaks to an epileptic category.

On the other hand, evidence has accumulated proving the occasional occurrence of bouts of bad temper in members of epileptic families and the fact has been utilised to support the hypothesis of genuine equivalents. In a number collected by DAVENPORT the patient was a sufferer from both, while among his relations they appeared either separately or together. The "epileptic temper" is well-known and has often been described (RIBOT, BINSWANGER, RAECKE), but whether its substitution for epileptic fits renders it a true equivalent is uncertain, in view of its appearing also in families with insanity as a feature, but without epilepsy. One known to me is remarkable for the prominence of all three traits; bad temper is shown in three members none of whom has ever had a fit; the familial insanity, however, rather complicates the point at issue. DAVENPORT's conclusion is against acceptance of bad temper as an equivalent, for it may occur without either of the others; it is best regarded as due to an undetermined factor having its greatest effect when acting on a nervous system that is specially liable to the major affection.

4. Visceral variants.

Obscurities arise with approach to the question of epileptic syndromes of viscerosensory and visceromotor origin, and the observer must proceed warily, content to record if he cannot yet explain. On general grounds participation of visceral centres in epileptic displays must of course be conceded. As the discharge sweeps over different levels it can scarcely be supposed to exercise selectivity; it is "brutal," as JACKSON said, and does not spare mechanisms belonging to the sympathetic system. Here are included circulatory, respiratory, vasomotor, vesical, rectal, renal, vagal, salivary, sudatory, pupillary, and other phenomena. It is however undoubtedly possible for variants to occur that are confined to discharges in sympathetic centres, sensorimotor symptoms of somatic type being absent. That by far the greater number of the ganglionic collections concerned with affective and vegetative life fringe the fourth and third ventricles cannot be without significance, it is therefore permissible to speak in general terms of *periventricular epilepsy*[1], by which may be designated types with localisation of the disorder in neurosympathetic centres round the ventricular system.

The actual nucleus or focus of the "nerve-storm" cannot always be determined with any nicety, although consideration of the clinical phenomena will frequently provide an index thereto; at all events an open route must be postulated between the discharging focus and the percipient cortex, since in few of the seizures to be described is consciousness ever lost. On the contrary, the subject is only too acutely aware of some paroxysmal disturbance referred to his viscera, and equally incapable of restraining it. The assumption is that abnormal impulses

---

[1] Modern Problems in Neurology, 1928. p. 38.

ascend to the cortex and are there interpreted as accurately or (for most instances) as imperfectly as may be, in accordance with previous experience or with lack of it.

1. Prominent in the general category of visceral epilepsies come the fits known (after GOWERS) as *vasovagal attacks,* also designed "pseudoangina", and popularly if non-committally, "nerve-storms"; in their physical concomitants they are akin to what is nowadays termed by the psychiatrist "anxiety neurosis".

FREUDian doctrine teaches that any syndrome of which anxiety (Angst) is a pronounced feature has to do with the psychosexual system of activities, and that the mental and physical symptoms are the inevitable accompaniment of conflict within the personality; but this simple explanation will not cover all cases, and ignores the well-established principle that a given syndrome may be of diverse etiology and varying localisation.

A typical example is characterised by palpitation, difficulty in breathing, suffocating sensation in the throat, nausea, hot flushes or icy coldness, pallor, sweating, shivering and tremors; and often, also, by an indescribably distressing sentiment of fear, impending trouble, even of imminent dissolution. Slowing of pulse-rate and change in respiratory rhythm (sometimes tachypnoea) are common. The symptoms point in a general way to derangement of function mainly referred to viscera supplied by the pneumogastric nerve, presumable started in vagal nuclei on the floor of the fourth ventricle and the adjacent vasomotor centres; but radiation therefrom by neurosympathetic paths to analogous ganglia of the floor and sides of the third is common enough; in particular, polyuria and pollakiuria are very frequent at the close. Cases of the kind, presenting numerous variations of the generic picture, have engaged my attention for many years and have been reported [1] from time to time; only one or two need here be selected.

A male patient has attacks in series, four to six a day for five or six days, with an interval of weeks between them. Lasting for about 30 seconds, they begin with a sudden "jump" at the heart, and to this succeed pallor, giddiness, icy coldness, trembling, tachypnoea, and inability to speak. As the attack finishes an overpowering "nightmare" of depression seizes him, making him feel frankly suicidal. Every hour (for hours in succession) in the course of the serial fits, he voids clear limpid urine in large quantities.

It is impossible not to recognise in this case a sequence of visceral and affective or emotional disorders whose locus is precisely that of ganglionic centres round the fourth and third ventricles, inclusive of palaeothalamus. Especially worthy of note is the fact that the fits (which have continued for 12 years) were at first preceded by an unpleasant "rotten" taste in the mouth, bringing with it a strong feeling of familiarity and a peculiar dreamy sensation compared to that of "going under gas". Association of the uncinate aura with periventricular epilepsy is of singular significance, for the fact that a viscero-affective seizure follows stamps the latter with the epileptic seal and justifies its acceptance as an epileptic variant; further, spread from temporal to ventricular grey matter exemplifies an unusual line taken by physiological excitation (or release), and suggests the possibility of still others that are not generally known.

As for the angor animi characteristically present, words of the patients are far more graphic than a laboured description: "Oh my God! I'm going! I'm going!"; "I feel, is this it? Is this death at last?" We also note retention of consciousness, though frequently a sense of unreality, closely allied to that of the uncinate syndrome. Sometimes, again, the senses are preternaturally acute. Particular attention is drawn to the fact that on occasion the patient is conscious of a sensation of being unable to move, as if in a trance; one said, "I struggle inwardly, but nothing happens; I try to call out, but I say nothing;" and another, "I hear everything they say to me but I cannot utter a single sound." Such

---

[1] Brit. med. J. 1 (1913); 2 (1930); Lancet 2 (1913); J. of Neur. 8 (1928).

occurrences clearly link the condition to narcoleptic and cataplectic fits, because of their feature of inability to move or innervate, and constitute a phenomenon of inhibition accompanying those of escape or excitation, precisely as in other epileptic variants already discussed.

The connexion is illustrated also by the case of a youth of 23, who has suffered from peculiar attacks for six years, at irregular intervals. These commence by a sensation at the heart ("as if it were moving in a circle" to the accompaniment of "painful pricks") and in the stomach (which seems to "turn right over"); and the customary sequence of giddiness, trembling, "hot waves", laboured breathing, etc. is experienced in severe form. Thereafter he feels extremely drowsy and sometimes falls fast asleep. He has often observed that the fits are induced by unrestrained laughter, and occasionally, too, by his being tickled; at such a moment the syndrome unrolls itself forthwith.

Provocation of the vasovagal attack by a pleasurable emotion is remarkable, but the case also shows the affinity of laughing with sleep; and the production of a periventricular fit by a stimulus which in other circumstances gives rise to the cataplectic attack undoubtedly narrows the gap between narcolepsy and epilepsy.

Vasovagal fits are often seen in persons with a family history of epilepsy, migraine, or insanity. The hypothesis that they can in many instances be considered epileptic variants does no violence to the facts and is consonant with what is known of epileptic phenomena otherwise.

Reactions of visceral centres cannot be expected to be identical with those of somatic centres; allowance must be made for differences, histological and physiological, in the ganglionic collections being discharged. The extended nature of the average attack cannot of itself form an insuperable objection to acceptance of the theory, for some are quite brief; just as a faint may be a type of bulbar inhibitory fit, so may a vasovagal seizure be one of a less rapid, less "brutal", more coordinated and more far-ranging kind.

Widely differing etiological circumstances may throw into action the same mechanism. On the physical side, anaphylaxis, commotio cerebralis, disorder of intracranial circulation, toxicosis, encephalitis, tumour, disseminated sclerosis, etc. are conditions in whose course the vasovagal symptom-complex may appear episodically; it is known, also, to be derived secondarily from disease of the viscera concerned. From the psychical aspect, concomitants of anxiety neurosis and of nightmare find expression through the same channels. The cardinal features of the condition undoubtedly conform to the general sense in which the term "fit" is understood, and do in fact constitute a periventricular variety; psychogenic or physiogenic in origin, the syndrome seems in reality to be localised and its pathogenesis more readily discoverable than is the case with the major affection.

2. Less definite in constituent features but equally suggestive of neurosympathetic impairment, transient in nature if somewhat extended in time, are peculiar attacks distinguished by continual *yawning* with constant voiding of urine, and followed by violent giddiness, headache, and occasional vomiting. Such cases possibly indicate derangement of visceral centres (of the third ventricle) regulating sleep and fluid interchange, with subsequent spread to others on the floor of the fourth. They belong, at least, to the epileptic borderland, part of their symptomatology having affinities with that of migraine.

3. Another unusual visceral association is provided by cases of ordinary epilepsy appearing to exhibit *rise of temperature* as a regular accompaniment. Doubtless some are feasibly explained by a temporary state accountable for both fit and fever, a toxaemia of microbial or metabolic origin, for example. There are children who react to any febrile disturbance, e. g. recurrent bronchitis, with a fit. But in others the question arises whether the fever may not be of neural

derivation. In the case of a schoolboy of 15, who for two years had an occasional epileptic seizure, all associated with muscular effort (wrestling, swimming, running, in the gymnasium, etc.), on each occasion the temperature rose immediately to $103°$ or $104°$ F., falling again within a few hours. The fit itself consisted of pallor, unconsciousness, and micturition; its constituents were solely visceral; and possibly the fever can be ascribed to transient involvement of heat-regulating centres by the same process.

4. Some other varieties consist of little else than isolated neurosympathetic disorder. Cases whose description as "faint" or "fit" seems almost a matter of choice belong here; syncopal attacks are in essence visceral, and termed "faints" if of circulatory origin, but "fits" if considered neural, though whether this constitutes a distinction without a difference is debatable. Opportunity was afforded to observe a peculiar form in an elderly man who had also suffered from occasional major fits for many years; the attack in question consisted in his sitting motionless, unconscious, and turning a greyish colour, immediately his respiration accelerated in a rapidly rising series of ever shorter and quicker breaths, becoming slower again in about half a minute and the arrhythmia ending with a deep sigh. The symptom-complex was seemingly limited to visceral ganglia of the medulla and floor of fourth ventricle, a disturbance that is frequently accompanied by transient clouding of the senses. Petit mal, of course, is merely a descriptive epithet; and when its phenomena are analysed they are sometimes found to consist of no more than such isolated visceral discharges or escapes.

The connexion of fever with epilepsy has been studied by MUSKENS; GOWERS' *Borderland* deals with a variety of visceral types; cf. also contributions by BONNIER, NOTHNAGEL, LÉVI, RYLE, VINNING, RUSSELL, etc. Under the title "diencephalic autonomic epilepsy" a visceral form (of organic derivation) has been reported by PENFIELD, but his claim to its being a "new conception" in neurology is unfounded.

Semeiology apart from fits.

When the question of fits is left aside and the epileptic examined objectively, there may be little or nothing to engage attention. Many patients during interparoxysmal periods enjoy perfect health and their nervous systems are demonstrably intact. Others, less well, utter complaints referable to heart, circulation, stomach, or bowel for which long use of sedatives may be largely to blame. Vasomotor instability or paresis is moderately common, especially in the confirmed epileptic, whose extremities are often cold and bluish — here also protracted medication may be partly responsible. "Stigmata" on which stress was wont to be laid by older writers are of dubious value, for none can be considered pathognomonic except, paradoxically, such as are incidental. Oliver WENDELL HOLMES said of the obsolete silver nitrate treatment that it "turned epileptics into Ethiopians"; the dusky hue (which I have once seen) was unmistakable, but fortuitous. Identical comment applies to the *facies epileptica*, defined by SPRATLING as resulting from a combination of dementia, facial scars, and bromide acne. No doubt a visitor to an institution for chronic and deteriorated cases will see (or used to see) examples of the "epileptic face", but not so the physician in out-patient practice; at most there is a dull or heavy look, coupled perhaps with poor emotional expression, which, added to a somewhat greasy skin, may be taken for what it is worth as an epileptic sign. Former observers, also, were much occupied with the presence of "stigmata of degeneration", comprising deformities of teeth, jaws, palate, ears, face, etc.; but in the absence of agreement on what constitutes a physical stigma, and their occurrence in many subjects of mental defect without epilepsy, endeavours to correlate them with the clinical symptoms of prognosis are useless.

More interest attaches to the *epileptic temperament* or character, on which inordinate stress has been laid by a number of writers, especially those claiming for the affection an origin in the psychical sphere. We are asked to believe that some form of mental obliquity distinguishes the great majority of epileptics, who are also egocentric, volatile, or rapt in religious fervour; of irritable temper and feeble judgement, suspicious or credulous, dreamy or impulsive, hesitant or hasty, timorous or fanatic, the "character" of the epileptic can be made to comprise almost anything. If some alleged traits are exceptional and others less so, none is distinctive. Divergencies of opinion as regards frequency and degree of prominence are partly accounted for by differences in the class of material studied. The neurologist no doubt generally sees early and uncomplicated cases, yet were the temperament pre-existing as a foundation for convulsive development it would have been much more manifest in personal experience than it has proved. Many epileptics have a normal mental endowment, intellectual and emotional, unimpaired by the progress of their malady.

Among the class (if tradition does not deceive) have been men famous in different walks of life, Julius Caesar, Mahomet, Peter the Great, Napoleon, Swedenborg, etc.

Should the patient start life with exiguous mental equipment, handicapped by heredity or retarded by early disease, psychical deterioration may set in as his ailment advances; but whether repetition of exhausting discharges by itself entails the likelihood of later mental involution, in persons normally gifted at the outset, must be considered doubtful. In no discussion of this vexed question can the cognate problem of the harmfulness of long-continued drug-taking be ignored. On the whole, neither length of illness nor frequency of fits is calculated to induce mental failure; nor do observed data warrant the conclusion that one type of attack rather than another in the end acts prejudicially.

To disentangle the essential from the incidental in respect of epileptic personality demands a wide purview of the subject. Life is very difficult for these patients, and much that is confidently attributed to underlying temperament can with greater reason be assigned to chronic invalidism and unfortunate circumstance. Mental sluggishness may be the outcome of bromide and a narrowed horizon of activity, emotional imbalance a consequence of unrealisable aims. No view of the problems can avoid being one-sided if it overlooks the fact that many patients rise superior to their infirmity, do their work in the world, never enter institutions, and betray no sign of either affective instability or intellectual deficit.

Among those dealing with various aspects of epileptic psychology may be mentioned CLARK, KENNEDY, KRETSCHMER, NINDE, Rows and BOND, WIERSMA.

Clinical pathology.

In addition to a purely clinical approach, the secrets of epilepsy have been explored from the side of chemistry and metabolism; body fluids and excretions have been analysed both before and after the discharge in the hope thereby of winning knowledge of what actually takes place in the tissues during fits, as well as of any enduring processes behind the liability to recurrence. Despite numberless researches the results are in part disappointing, because contradictory; but various facts have emerged that augur well for the success of further investigations by the same methods.

The best critical reviews on the whole subject are those of PAGNIEZ and of LENNOX and COBB.

1. Blood. So far as concerns *cytology*, neither reds nor whites show deviation in the course of the affection except of an incidental kind, but it is otherwise at the time of the paroxysm. According to DI GASPERO and DE CRINIS, leucopenia precedes, and leucocytosis follows some six hours after; the latter, together with eosinophilia, was found by WUTH during the attack, yet decrease has been noted in the same circumstances (TARGOWLA). Absence of concord probably means that leucocytic count and formula are of little weight. *Serum albumen* generally does not exceed normal limits, and any irregularities of content do not appear to be related to fits (MEYER and BRÜHL), though some consider they are (FRISCH, DE THURZÓ). Measurements of *fibrin* were conducted by LENNOX and ALLEN in 100 epileptics, of whom 34 for some obscure reason exhibited abnormally high concentration; in the whole series a figure 19 per cent. above the average ascertained for healthy subjects by POSTER was noted, but whether this is connected with the convulsive phenomena remains to be determined. An unmodified *coagulation time* is the rule (THOM, WUTH). Other *physical properties* (sedimentation, viscosity, flocculation) are not radically changed, except for an occasional augmented rate of the first of these (GEORGI, WUTH, LÖWENBERG).

2. Cerebrospinal fluid. The *cytology* is unaffected interparoxysmally, although an amount above 5 cells per c.mm. may sometimes be found (PATTERSON and LEVI, LENNOX and COBB, DE THURZÓ). Increase during status has been reported (PAPPENHEIM, BAYLAC et al.). Its *pressure* may be higher than is customary aside from obvious causes such as intracranial lesions and the inevitable rise in relation to the fit itself, and is subject to irregular fluctuations (DALMA, CLAUDE et al., DIELMANN, REDLICH and PÖTZL). *Total protein* passes the accepted limit of 50 mgm. in a few cases (OSNATO et al.); its significance for epilepsy is not evident, in view of its occurrence also in states of an "organic" kind. No particular change in *physical properties* takes place. An increase of the "interferometric rate" was remarked by JACOBI. The LANGE goldsol reaction was normal in 91 per cent. of 200 fluids (LENNOX and COBB), and in 287 of 300 (DE THURZÓ); a mild change may be seen in the luetic zone (KULKOW).

Some think the mastic reaction more sensitive than any of the other colloid methods for epileptic fluids, and recently a China ink test has been devided by DE THURZÓ, which in his hands gave a positive reaction in no less than 87 per cent., a rather astonishing result.

The *Wassermann test* in blood and fluid yields a positive response very seldom, but its etiological value is then of course unmistakable.

3. Protein Metabolism. In view of the alleged harmfulness of meat diets it is imperative to ascertain whether abnormal metabolism of protein or pathological susceptibility to it distinguishes the epileptic. Broadly speaking, any unusual concentration of protein products in the blood follows seizures but does not cause them. This is true of blood urea (HARTENBERG), creatinine (BRÜHL), non-protein nitrogenous substances (WUTH, LENNOX et al.); similar comment is applicable to the question of urea, etc., in the fluid. The concentration of various *antiproteolytic ferments* in the blood has been examined repeatedly (PFEIFFER et al., FRISCH and WALTER, SACKS and ZANDER), a minority of cases exhibiting increase. As for *protein sensitiveness*, observations are rather conflicting and clinical results indeterminate. Skin tests were performed by WALLIS and his colleagues upon 122 epileptics, of whom 28 were "positive" in regard to peptone, while 37 per cent. in all gave reactions to one or other food material. This allergic factor was also present in other series (e. g. that of WARD and PATTERSON), but some workers have not succeeded in procuring evidence of its activity. In the opinion of LENNOX and COBB the patient betraying such sensitiveness is exceptional, and this accords with personal experience; reaction to milk in one case was striking, and the consequence of its elimination impressive, but with a number of others search proved negative.

Further remark on the question of protein-feeding is postponed to the section on treatment, where also reference to protein injections will be found.

4. Carbohydrate Metabolism. A study of 267 epileptics conducted by LENNOX and BELLINGER failed to disclose any abnormality of *blood sugar* or any direct relation between its level and the oncoming of fits. Its increase during convulsions can be ascribed to utilisation of available glycogen in the body. In another series of researches the same workers [1] found that after glucose ingestion 10 per cent. of 140 epileptics had high sugar curves not explicable by coexisting disease-conditions and presumably indicative of potential diabetes. A subnormal glucose tolerance curve was noticed in a large number of institutional cases by MACKAY and BARBASH, who however were not able to establish any connexion between fit frequency and sugar level. Fluctuations and variations are influenced by so many factors as to have no specific bearing on the problem. During interparoxysmal periods normal curves in blood, urine, and spinal fluid have repeatedly been recorded (HOLMSTRÖM, NIELSON, WEEKS, LENNOX and ALLEN, OSNATO et al., etc.).

The fact is now well established that either convulsions or coma, or both, may coincide with deprivation of blood sugar whether spontaneous or due to insulin. These *hypoglycaemic fits*, easily producible by experiment in animals (MACLEOD, FOSHAY, etc.) are rare in man, and though occurring in severe form with a low sugar content are often independent of its level. Other factors must undoubtedly be incriminated (MILLER and TRESCHER, MÜLLER and PETERSON, SJÖGREN and TILLGREN, JOHN). Whatever the precise mechanism of the reactions, hypoglycaemia alone is not responsible.

See also articles by RUSSELL BRAIN, FRANK, WILDER, NIELSEN and EGGLESTON, WALTHER, CANEO.

5. Fat Metabolism. Less is known of fat metabolism in epileptics, though studies of blood cholesterol are concordant in proving reduction of that substance with the occurrence of fits (POPEA and VICOL, ROBINSON et al., GLEN DUNCAN, PEZZALI); but there is disagreement on the precise connexion, for while some workers have observed diminution prior to paroxysmal discharge others have not. The subject none the less is likely to prove of importance in view of the frequent success of a fat dietary (see below).

6. Basal Metabolism and Endocrine Disorder. Measurements of the rate of oxygen consumption in 130 epileptics revealed an average for the group of 3 per cent. below the norm (LENNOX and WRIGHT); reduction has also been found by others (BOOTHBY and SANDIFORD, NIELSON, BOWMAN and FRY), but denied as well (FRISCH, TALBOT et al.). Doubtless variations of non-pathogenic significance occur in interparoxysmal periods; in some cases low rates are accompanied by clinical evidence of glandular underfunction. Decreased consumption may precede attacks, and relative anoxaemia precipitate them in susceptible subjects. The question has other aspects bearing on the mechanism of fit production and is alluded to at a later point.

The endocrine features of epileptic cases, objectively considered, are scarcely capable of formulation. Only a minority exhibit low metabolic rates conceivably due to *thyroid* deficiency, yet this can hardly ever be verified by ordinary clinical tests. Evidence concerning *parathyroids* depends inter alia on the calcium content of blood and spinal fluid, which is commonly within normal range (see below) and on possible connexions between epilepsy and tetany. Though general opinion rightly judges the two conditions distinct and separable, some factors tending to produce contractions in the subjects of tetany are identical with those calculated to cause fits in epileptics; according to COLLIP these are tissue anoxaemia, disturbance of ionic equilibrium, and of p_H ratio. The matter is again referred to at a subsequent stage. No convincing

---

[1] Arch. of Neur. 18 (1927).

clinical argument for implication of the *adrenals* has been advanced; increased secretion before fits should cause changes in pulse rate, blood-pressure and blood sugar, which have not in point of fact been observed. The output of the gland must be increased with the muscular efforts of the convulsion, but injection of adrenalin does not precipitate fits (LENNOX and COBB, BERTOLANI), as some have alleged. So far as the *pituitary* is concerned, only in very few cases does it appear to be diseased: and such a state must be regarded as accidental in respect of epilepsy. Mild degrees of altered function are perhaps rather less uncommon (cf. TUCKER and McKENNAN), but the evidence therefor is never impressive. On the other hand, the amount of hypophyseal secretion in the spinal fluid can be estimated by SAWASAKI's method; in 71 out of 80 non-epileptic fluids it was present in measurable quantity, and absent in 40 of 79 epileptic (ALTENBURGER and STERN). Pursuing a similar line of research in regard to epileptic serum, ALTENBURGER and GUTTMANN failed to obtain rhythmic contractions in the isolated guinea-pig uterus by its employment; these data point to underfunction of the posterior lobe, the significance of which is not plain. Of the *gonads* in the male little is known bearing on the question under discussion; their relation in the female to the menstrual type of fits has been the subject of previous comment (p. 29). From a distant period a host of observers have busied themselves with connexions between ovario-uterine function and fit development, which is often held to be aggravated by the catamenia and relieved by pregnancy. There is no evidence of persisting ovarian malfunction in epileptic women. Increased capillary permeability accompanying menstruation may be one of the factors called into play during that physiological phase.

In addition to textual references, aspects of endocrine-epilepsy relationships have been discussed by MARCHAND, TOULOUSE and MARCHAND, REBATTU, EVERKE, WINTER, LIND.

7. Acid-base Equilibrium. General opinion agrees that the core of the convulsion problem must be sought in the reactive capacity of nerve-cells, which is intimately dependent on physicochemical processes largely concerned with the circulation. Experimental evidence, added to that of the clinical laboratory, has been steadily accumulating in favour of the view that changes in oxygen content of the blood, in equilibrium of electrolytes and acid-base ratios, in permeability of cell-membranes and state of fluids in the tissues, directly or indirectly affect the liability to fits.

By definition, the hydrogen-ion concentration of a fluid is the ratio between its acid and basic elements, and is known as p_H; for blood plasma a normal figure ranging from 7.33 to 7.39 obtains, and a shift in a direction less than the first of these constitutes a state of acidosis, beyond that of the second a state of alkalosis. The chief basic elements of the serum include sodium, potassium, calcium and magnesium, with traces of ammonia. All of these have been repeatedly measured in epileptics (spinal fluid as well as blood) and found during interparoxysmal periods to remain within normal limits, though sometimes exhibiting fluctuations that tend towards greater alkalinity (LENNOX and ALLEN, HAMILTON, FRISCH and FRIED, BISGAARD and NORVIG, etc.). The acid constituents (mainly carbonate and chloride, with phosphate of minor importance) are also normally concentrated in epileptic plasma and spinal fluid (LENNOX and ALLEN, OSNATO et al., etc.).

At the time of seizures, however, alterations take place whose significance can best be gauged by reference to experimental epilepsy (see later). A large increase in acid excretion occurs during fits (GAMBLE and HAMILTON); it is decreased before and augmented after (VOLLMER). According to DI RENZO convulsions are preceded for 24 to 48 hours by addition to the alkaline reserve of the blood, a maximum being reached in the last hour; the alkaline content is then quickly depleted just before convulsion, which coincides with a rapid liberation of acid. Whether such changes in p_H ratio are adequate to account for the phenomena must however be left over for later consideration. The p_H of brain tissues may not be identical with that of the plasma, while asphyxia and muscular contractions are responsible to some, perhaps a large, extent for the temporary acidosis.

It is convenient to incorporate with the present section certain data derived from x-ray technique or observable should the brain be exposed during life, in respect of chronic epilepsy.

Encephalography. When the spinal fluid above the foramen magnum is replaced by air radiography often discloses abnormal meningeal spaces over frontal and parietal regions and along the vertex; shrunken frontal poles, deepened sulci, retrocession of cortex from dura; also dilatation of lateral and sometimes of mesial ventricles. Subarachnoid spaces elsewhere (occipital, basal, temporal) are by contrast rarely if ever distended. These changes unquestionably signify accumulation of fluid in pools where normally little is to be found; and this "water-logged" condition is without doubt a contributory factor in epileptogenesis. Frequent though it is in confirmed epilepsy, it does not occur with unfailing regularity by any means.

Among those who have obtained encephalograms of the kind are PANCOAST and FAY, FAY, FOERSTER, DANDY, WARTENBERG, BINGEL, CARPENTER.

Direct Operative Observations. The exposed brain surface has repeatedly been studied not only at rest but during the whole course of a major fit (HORSLEY, LERICHE, KENNEDY, MIXTER, FOERSTER, GUTTMANN, HORRAX, etc.); the appearances in traumatic cases are naturally somewhat different but bear on the general question (FOERSTER and PENFIELD, PENFIELD, etc.). In chronic cases greatly distended subarachnoid spaces are commonly found over the frontoparietal area, with a milky, semitranslucent leptomeninx; pial hyperplasia is evident along the larger veins, and minute whitish granulations about the size of a millet seed may be seen in the same positions. The gyri are often soft on palpation.

This was precisely the condition in a case personally observed; the patient was 28 years old and had suffered from major fits since infancy, their local commencement (left hand) furnishing a clue to the focus of initial discharge.

FAY's description of the phenomena during the attack is informative: a tonic movement on the patient's part was associated with immediate pallor of the cortex, followed, a few moments later, by a fan-like suffusion of reddish congestion over the exposed region, so intense and rapid as to simulate a subarachnoid haemorrhage. This was coincident with the clonic phase, which was violent; incision of the arachnoid allowed about one ounce of clear fluid to escape and the attack immediately subsided. In that observed by KENNEDY sudden whitening of the brain was succeeded by venous engorgement so severe as to cause it to protrude beyond the level of the operative wound.

The bearing of these facts on the mechanism of fit production will be examined presently.

Morbid anatomy.

As explained in the Introduction, a cardinal distinction must be drawn between lesions of the central nervous system that are frequently *accompanied* by convulsions and any which may be considered to *cause* them. The fit is the symptom whose recurrence has to be accounted for pathologically, and since it is often preceded by a definite aura, localisable and unvarying, or commences by a local spasm, no diffuse and unsystematised morbid condition is capable of being regarded as its specific cause. However originated, the processes of a fit spread through normal physiological mechanisms with extreme rapidity; hence for a large part of epileptic symptomatology it is irrational to expect any recognisable morbid anatomy. In the case of focal commencement a focal lesion may perhaps be discoverable; but even under such circumstances no particular histological change can reasonably be looked for, since cells must be living in order to be discharged, and recuperation is the rule.

It thus becomes clear that the recurrent dynamic phenomena of convulsions may leave no trace of structural derangement behind them and that in the strict sense the fit, the fundamental symptom of epilepsy, has *no* histopathology. This inference, based on physiological considerations, is amply confirmed by the findings of morbid anatomy, for no connexion has ever been established between clinical types and cerebral changes. In their search for the anatomical basis of "idiopathic epilepsy" THOM and SOUTHARD submitted 205 brains of institutional epileptics to study, finding those of patients with a minimum number of convulsions (fewer than one a month) to be actually *less* "normal-looking" than those from cases of frequent daily fits.

The *gross lesions* often found associated with chronic epilepsy depend largely on the clinical class examined, and are useless for purposes of comparison. Most of the published reports concern demented institutional cases, often with congenital nervous defects, and thus the matter of purely epileptic pathology is seriously complicated. Statistics on the weight of epileptic brains are consequently valueless; moreover, they seldom if ever include cases of better social class, uninfluenced by either mental or somatic deterioration. Up to the age of 25 the brains of epileptics were stated by MUNSON to be much lighter than normal, and after that age approximately the same; yet this conclusion is at once refuted by instances of macrocephalic epilepsy, in which they greatly exceed the average (WIGGLESWORTH and WATSON). We are much in need of accurate information on the cerebral condition of "pure" cases of the affection.

When autopsy records in chronic examples (most of which, it will be understood, have complicating elements) are scrutinized, no special type of *macroscopic* lesion is found to predominate. Among the commoner features may be enumerated abnormal amounts of cerebrospinal fluid beneath the arachnoid, and sometimes above it (the "wet brain" of the postmortem room); thickening of dura, of pia and arachnoid, with or without intermeningeal adhesions; ventricular distension; ependymal granulations: convolutional atrophy and lobar shrinkage; and, sometimes, abnormalities of brain pattern (cf. LIND, and the annual reports of the Craig Colony for Epileptics, New York). Which of these changes may be a cause of recurrent convulsions, and which a consequence, will be difficult to decide; some observers take the parenchymatous atrophy to result from long-continued fluid pressure, the latter forming a distinctly pathogenic agent in the epileptic process. But cases are seen presenting no such involutional changes. No pathological standards of what constitutes meningeal thickening, ventricular dilatation, or cortical sclerosis are in existence.

The condition of the *Pacchionian bodies* has been studied by FAY and WINKELMAN, who in 80 per cent. of epileptic brains examined were able to detect evidence of hypo- or hyperplasia, of fibrosis or infiltrative change in these structures and the neighbouring arachnoid. According to WEED the villi have a normal cycle of evolution and involution, active growth not commencing till about the tenth year of life. Since they constitute the chief outlets for cerebrospinal fluid, failure to develop properly at an early period (aplasia or hypoplasia), hypertrophy consecutive to some infective or toxic process, or premature degeneration as a result of trauma or for other reasons, must result in temporary or permanent collections of subarachnoid fluid over the vertex and elsewhere. This pathological condition merits attention because of its bearing on problems of pathogenesis.

Noteworthy alterations have also been seen in the *choroid plexuses*, consisting of reduction in number and size of their villosities ("microplexia") and of sclerosis and atrophy affecting both glandular parenchyma and perivascular mesoderm (ALLENDE-NAVARRO). This line of study also deserves further prosecution, pointing as it does to the importance of the "ecto-mesodermic barrier" in epileptic causation.

Histopathology has failed to make any contribution of significance, speaking generally, so far as the cerebral cortex is concerned; on a priori grounds the fact occasions no surprise. To older descriptions of chromatolysis, nuclear vacuolation, changes in cellular network and so forth (MOTT, ANDRIEZEN, CLARK and PROUT etc.) no specificity can be assigned, nor to marginal and other types of gliosis (BLEULER, TURNER). For more than half a century attention has been focussed on *sclerosis of the cornu Ammonis*, found by JELGERSMA in many chronic cases, and also by FISCHER, WORCESTER and others. Turner observed the condition in considerably more than 50 per cent. of 115 brains coming from "idiopathic" cases. Later observers (PRATZ, KOGERER, WEIMANN, SPIELMEYER) have corroborated the finding; it consists of an ischaemic change (patchily distributed), whereby nerve-cells shrink and degenerate, lipoids appear, and gliosis supervenes. Noted by the last-named observer in no less than 80 per cent. of 126 epileptic brains, it is ascribed by him to the effects of frequently repeated angiospasm (without visible vascular disease); analogous alterations involve many PURKINJE cells and adjoining molecular layers of the cerebellum. A study by TAFT of 50 cases of general paralysis led to his discovery of sclerosis of AMMON's horn in 18 out of the 19 associated clinically with fits. Thus it would be a mistake to dismiss the lesions as of minor interest, but at the same time their relation to the affection may be quite incidental. This is suggested by the experimental work of ORR, who, introducing bacteria into the general circulation, found resultant lesions of ischaemic character involving definite anatomical sites in the brain; among these were invariably the cornu Ammonis and fornix, in which situations the bloodvessels are terminal. Moreover, similar lesions have been seen in carbon monoxide poisoning. So far as concerns convulsions per se, therefore, they can have neither etiological nor symptomatic value.

Considerable discussion has ranged round the question of certain *cell-inclusions*, originally discovered by LAFORA in two cases of myoclonus-epilepsy and regarded by him as composed of amyloid or hyaline substance; their histochemical reactions sometimes point to an intermediate constitution. Presumably due to metabolic disturbance of cytoplasm, LAFORA does not attribute their presence to myoclonic fatigue but believes they determine the occurrence of myoclonic phenomena. The corpora amylacea are scattered diffusely or localised to some neuronic system or systems.

They were found in a similar case by WESTPHAL and SIOLI, but their precise significance remains to be determined (cf. SPIELMEYER, BIELSCHOWSKY, PILOTTI, WEIMANN) for they are not confined to epileptic types, and were not seen in myoclonus-epilepsy by PARHON.

Nothing seems to be known of the state of *periventricular ganglia* in confirmed epilepsy, despite the frequency with which they must be involved in many types of fit. It is curious, too, how little attention has been allotted to the *sympathetic system*; in a long search no record of its systematic examination among epileptic autopsy material has come under notice. Comparative neglect, also, has been the fate of the *endocrines*; they were studied by PRIOR and JONES in 14 cases (8 male and 6 female), without any constant changes being discovered except perhaps in respect of the adrenals; but since most of their patients died in status the affection of its cortex was probably secondary to exhaustion. Signs of unusual activity characterised the pituitary in 4 instances; active thymus tissue was present in 3 males and 1 female. A persistant thymus was found by VOLLAND in 20 per cent. of 100 epileptic autopsies, in 9 of their 14 cases by PRIOR and JONES, but in only 0,7 per cent. of 423 at the Craig Colony. Among 396 thyroids examined by BUSCAINO 71 per cent. of those from epileptics contained crystals taken to represent an abnormal protein. A selective action on chromophil cells of adrenals and pituitary was noticed by SCHOU and SUSMAN; the researches of CLAUDE and SCHMIERGELD were inconclusive.

Pathological states accompanying epilepsy.

The paucity of the findings of morbid anatomy need occasion no comment, for the clue must be sought elsewhere. With this end in view, persistent effort has been made to categorize the types of lesion, structural or nutritional, found in practice to be associated with epileptic attacks. Their number and variety, however, are almost bewildering; and it is no less unfortunate that they often fail to supply any hint of the exact way in which the cellular reaction concerned is facilitated.

A. Humoral and Vascular Cerebral States. These may be summarised as follows:

1. Disease or disorder of cerebral blood-vessels: thrombosis, embolism, haemorrhage, arteriosclerosis, endarteritis obliterans, endarteritis calcificans (GEYELIN and PENFIELD).
2. Disorder of cerebral circulation: morbus cordis (cf. MOON), heart-block, anaemia, asphyxia of various origins, interference with carotid and vertebral streams, anomalies of venous sinuses, any condition causing venous obstruction or delay.
3. Disorder of cerebrospinal fluid regulation and flow: hydrocephalus, internal or external, fluid stasis, cerebral oedema, rise in fluid pressure, etc.

This catalogue of morbid states with which convulsions may occur does not exhaust the possibilities yet is sufficiently comprehensive to illustrate their multiplicity.

B. Cerebral Disease-conditions. Conditions affecting cerebral parenchyma and interstitial tissues and liable to be associated with fits are equally heterogeneous; their tabulation is appended.

1. Cerebral tumours, of varying site and histopathological texture.
2. Infections and toxi-infections, encephalitis, syphilis, tuberculosis, abscess; toxins of many specific fevers and exanthems, of common or rare meningitic affections, etc.
3. Toxidegenerations and scleroses, disseminated sclerosis, tuberous sclerosis, diffuse sclerosis, WESTPHAL's pseudosclerosis, PICK's cortical atrophy, ALZHEIMER's disease; plumbism, alcoholism, and other toxicoses.
4. Cerebral trauma.
5. Some forms of congenital and heredofamilial disease.

Amid all this pathological diversity one or two points stand out clearly. Fits are not the invariable accompaniment of each and every affection that has been enumerated; in some, they are few and far between; with others (e. g. fevers and exanthems) they often occur solely at the onset. Almost any cerebral lesion, whatever its nature, may be found in union with epilepsy under circumstances which it is the task of the investigator to discover and specify. If this entails acceptance of an unknown, a "functional instability" or "convulsive tendency", at any rate the problem is simplified by narrowing of the field.

Experimental convulsions.

A preliminary point of importance that emerges from a vast amount of research, old and new, is the ease and certainty with which normal animals can be made to develop convulsions. In their case no question of inheritance arises. But the fundamental problem of recurrence (as in human cases) has not as yet been solved by experimentation.

Study of methods reveals two chief technical procedures for induction of the convulsive state, viz. 1. the neural, and 2. the humoral, respectively.

It is of some relevance to note at once that these may act separately or together. This has been demonstrated by DANDY and ELMAN, who provoked convulsions in cats by oral administrations of absinthe in sufficient quantity. They next made pre-rolandic lesions by either cortical or subcortical extirpation or introduction of a foreign body, and within from 1 to 5 months their animals became much more sensitive to the effect of absinthe, $^1/_3$ to $^1/_7$ of the original dose now proving epileptogenic. The addition of a pathological cerebral factor increased the facility and aggravated the degree of action of the convulsant; in other words, cerebral injury lowered the convulsion threshold.

A. Taking the **humoral factor** first, we may define it comprehensively as that component in the production of experimental epilepsy (animal and human) which consists in disturbance of body fluids and biochemical constitutents either mechanically or consecutive to the action of exogenous or endogenous noxae.

A convenient tabulation of humoral factors follows.

1. Mechanical. a) *Increased intracranial pressure.* — b) *Increased permeability of cell-membranes.* — c) *Alteration of water balance; oedema.* — d) *Pressure on or ligation of carotids and vertebrals.*

2. Exogenous. a) *Convulsants (alcohol, lead, acid fuchsin, camphor, absinthe, thujone, cocaine, picrotoxin, santonin, etc.).* — b) *Hypoglycaemia produced by insulin.* — c) *Foreign proteins.* — d) *Anoxaemia (variously induced).* — e) *Change of acid-base equilibrium; alkalosis (variously induced).*

3. Endogenous. *Toxic derivatives in blood, urine, or spinal fluid, or of endocrine source.*

1. In the *mechanical* group of epileptogenic factors attention may first be turned to *rise of intracranial pressure* which exerts an influence definitely predisposing to fits. When it is decreased by the use of hypertonic solutions a higher dosage of absinthe than usual is necessary, and conversely if it is raised (ELSBERG and PIKE). A convulsant acts most readily when pressure is high.

Incidental to the convulsion itself, an initial fall in fluid pressure is succeeded by pronounced rise during the seizure (MACDONALD and COBB).

The effect of *increased permeability of membranes* has been studied by SYZ, who after a variety of mechanical injuries to the brain (in frogs) found (by injection of acid fuchsin as a convulsant) that tonic and clonic attacks were induced with ease and that the dye was diffusely absorbed throughout the brain and cord to a definitely greater degree than in controls. Despite the complexity of the processes the conclusion would appear to be that augmented permeability adds to the effectiveness of the convulsing agent. The question of oedema will be discussed presently in connexion with other factors. *Pressure on the large bloodvessels* supplying the brain, or their ligature, has been known since the days of ASTLEY COOPER to be provocative of spasms, in both normal and epileptic subjects, as well as in animals (KUSSMAUL and TENNER, STEWART et al., FLESCH, TSIMINAKIS, and many more). SCHIFF and, later, HILL induced epileptiform clonic spasm in themselves by compression of one carotid artery; effects no doubt vary in different persons owing to free anastomosis, but the inference that deficient blood-supply is apt to be accompanied by fits, unilateral or general, must be regarded as established.

2. In the *exogenous* class the precise mode of action of various convulsants has not been verified, though there is evidence to suggest that some (e. g. absinthe, and its active principle thujone) directly stimulate the motor cortex in the intact animal (GOTCH and HORSLEY, BOYCE, HORSLEY, UYEMATSU and COBB, KEITH, etc.). The mechanism of the action of others requires elucidation, a comment applying with no less force to the germane question of anticonvulsants, viz. bromide, luminal, etc., in respect of which only meagre experimental and pathological data are at hand. Fits secondary to *insulin hypoglycaemia* have already been mentioned (p. 47) and the difficulties connected with their exact causation pointed out. Abnormal *sensitiveness to proteins* has also been discussed, but direct clinical experiments are scanty and not very illuminating. Much more impressive are the data relating to acid-base equilibrium, oxygen tension, and water balance; the work of many observers, added to and summarised by LENNOX and COBB, justifies the following general conclusions.

a) Acidosis tends to inhibit seizures, and alkalosis to cause them. Acidosis may be induced experimentally by resort to fasting, by the use of a diet rich in fat and poor in carbohydrate (ketogenic diet), or by making the subject rebreathe expired air or inhale a mixture containing a high percentage of carbon dioxide. Conversely, if the latter acid is "blown off" by forced voluntary respiration, the blood quickly becomes more alkaline, and a fit may ensue. This *hyperventilation* or hyperpnoea was minutely studied by ROSETT, and his results confirmed by FOERSTER and a number of others (GUTTMANN, HENDRIKSEN, WOLFF and LENNOX, FOG and SCHMIDT, etc.). Alkalosis can also be brought about by the ingestion of alkali in sufficient amount to derange normal acid-base equilibrium, and acidosis in a correspondingly opposite way.

b) Increased tension of oxygen in the tissues tends to delay seizures, and decrease to induce them. Simple hyperventilation causes not only a relative alkalosis due to disappearance of carbon dioxide but also a reduction of free oxygen in peripheral vessels and tissues owing to its being more firmly bound to haemoglobin under these circumstances. If, however, the procedure is accompanied by inhalation of carbonic acid gas fits do not appear, for its presence helps to liberate oxygen from the haemoglobin and O_2 tension in the tissues is thus increased. Since cellular deficiency in oxygen is one of the factors causing convulsions, the "purpose" of the latter may be to counteract this effect (CAMPBELL). Alkalosis and anoxaemia are mutually supplementary in producing attacks, acidosis and oxygenation in preventing them. So far as concerns experimental fits, lack of oxygen may be largely compensated for by increase in carbon dioxide content.

In 27 of 33 cases a fall in blood-pressure was noted by FOG and SCHMIDT to accompany hyperpnoea, but they do not accept it as one of the agents in artificial fit production since no parallelism exists between it and the seizures.

c) Oedema of the brain tends to bring on attacks, and dehydration to diminish them. Dehydration can be rapidly effected by intravenous injection of 50 per cent. sucrose, and thereby susceptibility to experimental convulsions is diminished (KEITH); reduction of fluid intake is not so potent. The factor of oedema cannot be rigidly separated from those mentioned above, for anoxaemia and alkalosis both cause passage of fluid through capillary walls, while acidosis acts conversely. Control or modification of major fits can be regulated in some degree by measures leading to diminution of fluid in and over the brain (FAY), and there is evidence that ketogenic diet and acidosis produce their results in part by removal of surplus extracellular fluid (BRIDGE and IOB). On the other hand, anticonvulsants such as acetone, ethyl aceto-acetate and diacetone alcohol do not cause dehydration of brain tissue (KEITH).

d) For years experimenters have sought for some specific *endogenous* toxin, to be obtained from blood, urine, or spinal fluid. In most instances blood has been taken from epileptics and injected into animals (CENI, MEYER, HELD, PAGNIEZ, CUNEO, PFEIFFER et al., and others), but the results are unconvincing, because not free from ambiguity. Combinations of epileptic blood and fluid were utilised by TREVISANELLO, who stated that the effect on guinea-pigs was different from that produced by similar material from normal persons, anaphylactic reactions occurring in the former instance but not in the latter. In some ways seizures resemble anaphylactic crises, and the point deservers further study. No satisfactory evidence is forthcoming in favour of the view that endocrine derangement leads to the production of toxins responsible for fits. It is true that in parathyroidectomised animals the same agents induce tetany as in man are causative of convulsions, yet not only is the calcium content of body fluids normal in epileptics (as noted above) but treatment with that substance or with parathyroid extract is also ineffectual in diminishing attacks. Again, susceptibility to fits is apparently increased by experimental thyroidectomy but, as has been shown, there is little proof of hypothyroidism in epileptic subjects, or of their seizures being ameliorated by thyroid extract.

For experimental and clinical data see papers by FISCHER and LEYSER, UYEMATSU and COBB, BISGAARD, MASSAGLIA, ELSBERG and STOOKEY, REDLICH, etc., and the review by LENNOX and COBB.

B. Neural factor. When in these days so much attention is being directed to humoral constituents the importance of the *neural factor* must not be underestimated. Direct excitation of motor centres may result in the development of unilateral or generalised attacks. The observation is old, as far as concerns the laboratory (cf. SHERRINGTON), but has of late been amply confirmed in human patients on the operating table. According to FOERSTER, in man certain definite epileptogenic areas can be traced on the cerebral cortex (precentral, postcentral, frontal adversive field, parietal adversive field, etc.), where quantitative electrical stimulation induces an aura (this depends on the region excited) and initial clonic or tonico-clonic movements which may spread unilaterally or even become general. Many of the cases he observed were of traumatic origin, with cicatricial contraction of tissues at the site of the wound, gentle pull on the adherent dura also sometimes being followed by convulsions; assuming that this procedure must inevitably cause a drag on vessels caught by the scar or on vascular growth therein subsequent to injury, FOERSTER believes that a vasomotor reflex thus evoked is responsible for the onset of the fit. Despite this plausible theorising, the direct excitation of convulsions by the electric stimulus must not be overlooked, nor the part played by the strength of the current.

Pathogenesis of epileptic fits.

If now the information garnered in preceding sections is carefully sifted, it can be summarized as implying the existence of three or four determinants, at most, for the production of epileptic phenomena. A fit is a disturbance of nervous tissue without question, not of any specific and unvarying mechanism, but simply of the subject's neural network in one or other of its parts. The disorder exteriorizes itself mostly via pyramidal systems, but it may commence anywhere, so to say; witness the manifold and polymorphic auras. Concisely put, the crux of the pathogenic problems is to ascertain whether discharge is initiated neurally or is preceded and effected by humoral or vascular change; or whether, conceivably, simultaneous action is requisite. At the present time no direct solution can be offered. What evidence has accumulated is indirect and collateral, and may be set down as follows.

1. The mechanical determinant consists of delay in absorption of spinal fluid by the usual channels, its collection in pools under (and sometimes over) the arachnoid, back pressure, and consequent supracortical oedema. Yet the problem still presents itself, to explain the occurrence of fits, given such pathological conditions. Perhaps oedema in some way augments cellular excitability; but, ex hypothesi, it is a permanent state, whereas the fits are intermittent.

2. Vascular determinant. Abundant material supports the contention that the *vascular determinant* is of significance. Many years ago the presumptive circulatory phases were thus epitomised by FRANCIS HARE:

a) Vasoconstriction, causing rapid rise in general blood-pressure. — b) Cardiac inhibition (vagal) to counteract the effects of the above, inducing a sudden fall in pressure. — c) Immediate cerebral anaemia, productive of unconsciousness and tonic spasm. — d) Improvement of heart-beat, causing rise of pressure, returning cerebral circulation, relaxation of tonic spasm, and clonic convulsions. — e) Reestablishment of blood pressure and cerebral circulation; arrest of convulsions; sleep recuperative of exhaustion.

It is possible to harmonise the facts of clinical and experimental epilepsy with this sketch of pathogenic sequences, at least to some extent; but there are more than a few obscurities. Though HUGHLINGS JACKSON himself favoured the possibility of the paroxysm's being caused by local vascular contraction, and imagined that series of different movements are developed by successive involvement of cerebral arterioles, neither the proximate cause of the sudden initial angiospasm nor its starting-point is known. Whether cerebral vasomotor change commences in the corresponding bulbar centre or locally as a sympathetic reflex from vessel walls remains undetermined; and even if assigned pathogenic significance, by itself it seems insufficient to evoke the attack. Many local cerebral anaemias are unaccompanied by discharging phenomena (there is often no convulsion with the flaccid palsies of embolism and thrombosis); on the other hand, were anaemia the cause per se, numerous conditions of which unconsciousness is a feature should be followed by fits, but in fact are not. Nor can so integral an epileptic phenomenon as the aura be thus explained, for it often has the character of a normal sensation or sensory presentation; and to suppose that neural activity is combined with anaemia in the brain of the normal subject is absurd. If, however, the aura is considered to arise in consciousness before vasoconstriction, we are faced with the enigma of its own causation and how it is responsible for the succeeding angiospasm. Circulatory changes are admitted to accompany the march of events in the paroxysm, but the association may not be causal. Sudden loss of senses may not be of vascular origin though occurring in union with vascular reaction; the same stimulus might influence both the bulbar vasomotor centre and neural tissues themselves, or the observed circulatory phenomena might conceivably be due to neurogenic disorder of function at the level of the medulla.

On the other hand, cerebral arteries are now known to be under vasomotor control, and evidence is adduced later (p. 83) which shows how fit production can be affected by periarterial sympathectomy of carotids and vertebrals. Though firm proof of the initiation of the whole series of events by vasoconstriction alone is lacking, it has become impossible to withhold from the sympathetic system of the brain some part in favouring, if not in starting, cellular discharge.

3. Of the **humoral determinant** much has already been said. Its hypothetical action has been sketched along the following lines by LENNOX and COBB. Contraction of cerebral vessels will cause deficiency of oxygen supply to brain tissues, and the anoxaemia will dilate capillaries, with outward passage of fluid through their walls. Lowered oxygen tension, oedema, or rise of intracranial pressure, singly or together, may then so interfere with neuronic function as to precipitate a fit. The convulsion will lead to accumulation of carbon dioxide and relative acidosis; in consequence oxygen will be utilised by the tissues, fluid will pass back into capillaries and normal intracranial circulation be restored.

Such a series of physicochemical interchanges may well attend a *major* fit, but the postulated vasoconstriction beginning the process is still unexplained, as is its relation to the aura on the other hand, and to neural activity on the other. The beneficial effect of induced acidosis is not derived from alteration of p_H ratio alone, but from the above mentioned accompanying fluid changes, which combine to decrease in some as yet not fully understood way the irritability of nerve-cells. These lacunae in knowledge lead the advocates of the humoral theory to admit that its several component factors may be effective only in such persons as have a "tendency" to seizures and in whom some pathological circumstance in brain, body, or emotional life alrady exists.

4. Neural determinant. This leads back to the question of the *neural determinant*, in connexion with which the following considerations are opposite.

a) A "susceptibility" or "tendency" can scarcely be ruled out in cases of direct heredity and of epilepsy in homologous (uniovular) twins; and this can be expressed at least as easily in terms of neural instability as of extraneural abnormality. b) The phenomena of reflex epilepsy strongly suggest neural causation and reactions, independent of vascular and humoral interposition. c) To a number of epileptic variants (limited JACKSONian fits, epilepsia partialis continua, petit mal, epileptic "absences", etc.) the relatively diffuse physicochemical processes of vasculo-humoral class seem inapplicable. It is difficult to imagine anoxaemia, oedema, and alkalosis strictly confined to a constellation of cells producing twitches of a corner of the mouth. Yet it would be unreasonable to deny the possible intervention of a vascular component for some forms of petit mal, especially in view of accompanying pallor. d) The occurrence of epilepsy in some structural nervous diseases (tuberous sclerosis, pseudosclerosis, etc.) pleads in favour of a neural factor. e) Certain phenomena of the epileptic fit, e. g. inhibition and radiation, are more readily explicable by neural than by extraneural activities. f) So far as is known to me, mechanical, vascular, or humoral precipitants are never postulated for hysterical fits, which in a number of material respects do not differ integrally from those of epilepsy.

When, finally, the pathogenic problem is surveyed from every angle, it seems illogical to expect one single and unique common factor for the totality of epileptic symptoms. Their immense diversity precludes the likelihood of an identical basis for all; the major seizure differs widely from petit mal, and both from vasovagal attacks, hence theories applicable to it can hardly apply to the others. Neither mechanical, vascular, nor humoral excitant is potentially so pathogenic as the neural, for the three former can scarcely act without the latter, which however, seems capable of inducing a paroxysm by itself. Changes in fluids and non-parenchymatous tissues are contributory rather than provocative, since the most they can do, seemingly, is to augment the irritability of neural mechanisms; the question whether general vasoconstriction, oedema, or alkalosis might arouse a local aura is not only unsolved but probably misconceived. And as the epileptic process commences by this conscious signal, of presumptive nervous origin, its continuation along neural pathways is unquestioned even if the units involved are prepared for abnormal reaction by extraneural influences. This view, indeed, accords best with the data of clinical and experimental study; the convulsive capacity of neurones is facilitated and heightened by preliminary action on the part of surrounding tissues and fluids, and when it is being discharged in the fit concomitant change in these elements takes place. The significance of physiochemical alterations preceding and attending the paroxysm is not undervalued by the assertion that they are of importance chiefly in relation to the major seizure; perhaps, indeed, they account for its severity and excess; but so far as concerns minor, local, myoclonic, reflex, and other epilepsies they are much less in evidence if not absent entirely, the neural factor then predominating, or working alone.

Because of this, the existence of some special proclivity to discharge has often been assumed; whether it be a property of nerve-cells is at present beyond analysis; but the general conclusion does not conflict with the facts of observation. The tendency, however, may not be innate or congenital; perhaps it seldom is; the possibility of acquisition must be borne in mind. An inherent tendency is never postulated for incidental fits characterising tumour, general paralysis, encephalitis, or cerebrovascular cases, and heredity plays a negligible rôle in the common JACKSONian variety, for whose occurrence local cerebral conditions are deemed sufficient. The inference may then be warranted, or is at least feasible, that "susceptibility" may signify little else than a state induced by repetition and the continuing effect of precipitants, whatever their class. The chronic epileptic (without family history of fits) may be constituted not so much by his possessing an obscure congenital reactive capacity of nerve-cells as by his acquiring the facility from simple failure on the observer's part to discover precisely which of the known determinants is causing his malady to perpetuate itself, and to deal with it. If the determinant, however, is one as yet unknown, it need not on that account be congenital.

On the other hand, in cases of direct inheritance and for some of the types already discussed it seems unreasonable to negative the reality of a disposition or proneness to react abnormally in the presence of exciting factors. But though the process of epileptogenesis has been shown to be much more complex than was formerly believed, the number of epilepsies for which no cause other than that of inherent irritability can be discovered is being steadily reduced.

Neural mechanismus of discharge.

We may now seek to ascertain if possible the neural sites of epileptic seizures and the mechanism implicated in their different phases.

1. Probably the assumption is general that ordinary *major attacks* are the outcome of discharges involving cortical nerve-cells throughout the middle (rolandic) level of both hemispheres; whether they commence, as JACKSON affirmed, in the frontal lobes (highest level) is very difficult to decide, unless the common turning of head and eyes is accepted as a frontal symptom, which it may well be. When limbs and trunk are convulsed, simultaneous excitation of motor-cell groups in bilateral rolandic areas is taking place, the first result being contention of movement and consequent rigid immobility, tetanic contractions like those obtained by faradic stimulation of cortical motor points. As intensity diminishes they become phasic or clonic, but this signifies discontinuity of innervation and not change in physiological level. Formal dissociation of tonic from clonic elements introduces much too schematic a conception, for one runs into the other in accord with relative severity and simultaneity of the discharges. Many JACKSONian fits are partly tonic, or pass from one type to the other, without any indication of change in site; both local and general seizures take the kinetic paths of the pyramidal system. The major fit, however, is to be distinguished from the tonic postural fit, not succeeded by phasic movements, which is the outcome of epileptic processes affecting postural mechanisms of the midbrain.

But the phenomena are not confined to the motor regions of the middle level; on the contrary, they range widely and immediately through the neuraxis, involving somatic and sympathetic centres alike and perhaps also those of the cord. Moreover, fits can be induced after decerebration (ROTHMANN, OLMSTED and LOGAN), and convulsions have been seen in the hind limbs of spinal animals (FOERSTER, MUSKENS, UYEMATSU and COBB); in those whose cortical motor areas have been extirpated tonic and clonic spasms are still possible (ROTHMANN, PIKE and ELSBERG). Evidently, then, various divisions of the neuraxis are capable of becoming epileptogenous, and of manifesting both of the usual types of movement; hence exclusive ascription of tonic contractions to the extrapyramidal and of clonic to the pyramidal system is based on ignorance of experimental data and the facts of clinical research.

In decerebrate or decorticate animals, however, a much larger dose of convulsant is necessary for the induction of fits than in the case of intact animals, so that the supposition of greater excitability on the part of cortical motor cells seems justified. Whether under the former circumstances the convulsions evoked are identical in all respects with those of the unoperated animal is a point on which information is regrettably meagre; JACKSON held that it would be "marvellous" if discharges of centres lowest in rank were the same as those from more highly involved centres. But the fact that under artificial conditions neural mechanisms of infracortical site can become epileptogenous in no way invalidates the conclusion that the origin of major convulsions in intact man is cortical.

2. For the elusive *petit mal attack* a specific anatomical locus can scarcely be excepted. It may conceivable result from transient stoppage of hemispheric circulation without invasion of postural centres (for the patient often remains on his feet), possibly originating in vasomotor nuclei of the bulb; or the whole may be of neurogenic nature, a generalised cortical inhibition with escape, perhaps, of a few flickering movements. Its basis is obscure out of all proportion to the trifling character of the symptoms, for the physical substratum of consciousness has still to be discovered.

Some evidence is adduced by MUSKENS appearing to link the latter with integrity of the formatio reticularis of pons and medulla.

3. The site of *myoclonic epilepsy* is less uncertain, since its phenomena are nearly always manifested via pyramidal tracts and have therefore a cortical source. Experiments have however shown the possibility of their occurrence after pyramidal section, whence a secondary spinal or pontobulbar origin must be assumed. Muskens affirms the existence of myoclonic "convulsive centres" at the junction of pons and medulla, controlling the ipsilateral cord by descending (extrapyramidal) paths.

Physiological theories of discharge.

Considerations advanced in the foregoing paragraphs are germane to the much discussed problem of the nature of the functional disorder in epilepsy, for which several theories have been advanced.

1. The Theory of Irritation. Phenomena of JACKSONian epilepsy on the one hand, and of experimental cortical stimulation on the other, favour the view attributing convulsions to irritation of motor centres, begun by a sensory impulse (manifested as the aura) and continued as a kind of avalanche spreading to and overwhelming adjoining and lower centres in succession, these in their turn being compelled to discharge. Various isolated epileptic symptoms are equally suggestive of local excitation at some point or points in reflex arcs passing through the cortex.

2. The Theory of Release. According to another view the phenomena are the consequence not so much of direct stimulation passing from higher to lower levels as of removal of control by the former over the latter; the epileptic process checks the prevailing inhibitory function of cortical centres, and those of lower grade escape into action. Some symptoms, undoubtedly, are best explained in this way; peculiar states of epileptic consciousness, automatisms, coordinated movements, and other pre- and postconvulsive features imply activity unhampered by transcortical inhibition, and to that extent substantiate the theory. Some form of decontrol seems feasible in certain cases of epileptic attack (visceral, periventricular) unattended by loss of senses. But in spite of its attractiveness the conception raises as many difficulties as some may think it appears to dispel. We have to account for the tremendous violence of the discharges, which are in this respect altogether unlike the motor phenomena of spinal mechanisms liberated from prespinal control, e. g. those of spastic paraplegia. The great disorderliness and irregularity of the paroxysmal movements, also, are characters foreign to the systematised and relatively unvarying types of isolated intracortical reactions. More significantly still, this temporary release is followed by convulsions while more permanent release is not; and, conversely, many transient decontrols never have fits for a sequel. It is impossible to avoid the conclusion that another factor than a mere fleeting break in cortical restraint presides over epileptic discharges; were it otherwise, convulsive syndromes should occur vastly more often than they do.

From the standpoint of neurophysiology, excitation and inhibition appear together and are mutually interactive at the cortical level; from that of clinical research, many though not all paroxysmal symptoms are best regarded as excitatory, while some belong to the other class. The aura must surely be placed in the first group when it has the character of a crude sensory experience (a sudden stench in the nostrils, a "sinking" in the stomach, a "rush to the head"), but those of more extended and elaborate type (a feeling of "being somewhere else", with the complex mental state accompanying it) should probably be categorized with the latter, in view of the occurrence of similar hallucinatory forms in persons who are half-drowned or half-suffocated.

But the *negative* symptoms of the epileptic fit cannot be interpreted in terms of either theory, for they are neither excited nor released into action. Auras of blindness, deafness, etc., are purely inhibitory in nature. Loss of senses, again, is a pure negation, and no parallelism can be traced between it and motor accompaniments. Consciousness is absent in negative cerebral states such as concussion and coma, but also during positive, excessive cerebral states, e. g. the period of convulsions. Many clinical instances of the former are free from discharging phenomena; conversely, a JACKSONian patient may exhibit severe paroxysmal movements ere becoming insensible. It seems impossible to elucidate both negative and positive symptoms by reference to the same process, whether that be one of release or otherwise.

If the neurogenic theory be abandoned, similar obscurities face those who rely on disorder of cerebral blood-flow. Cerebral anaemia may result in unconsciousness, but it also diminishes cortical excitability; and absence, not excess, of movement should ensue. Were a cortical anaemia to be postulated inducing loss of senses, with retention of blood-flow at inferior levels, allowing activity of released infracortical systems, such a hypothesis might conceivably provide an explanation of the phenomena of the major seizure, yet it fails to account for those of the JACKSONian variety.

Difficulty in deciding whether a given epileptic symptom is derived from escape or from excitation perhaps arises from a merely verbal use of undefined terms. Of the intimate nature of inhibition we are still ignorant, and have no knowledge of the process whereby sensory function is accompanied in consciousness by sensation. Hence we are not in a position to ascribe the aura either to release of a sensory mechanism from some hypothetical control or to activation by some usual or unusual stimulus. Even if inhibition is first to be removed by a process of de-inhibition, excitation might still be needed to "touch off" the prepared neural unit or system. For these reasons much of the controversy over theories of discharge is academic rather than genuinely physiological, and must await further study on the latter lines.

3. **The Short Circuit Theory.** A modified release theory assumes "simplification" of reflex arcs through the cortex in consequence of cortical "disease" (traumatic, developmental, or whatever it may be), with the result that impulses reaching the brain are not as it were diluted by spread through association systems but compelled to take shorter and abnormal routes; this is imagined to induce discharge. As "long-circuiting" through cortical arcs is considered to delay response, so "short-circuiting" by simplified arcs may precipitate it. The theory is not without plausibility and has been given support on both physiological and pathological grounds (FULTON, SOUTHARD). Yet its application to the multitudinous symptoms of epilepsy is limited, for if it can be utilised to account for convulsions in children and the feeble-minded these form but a small part of the epileptic fraternity.

None of the hypotheses furnishes an adequate explanation of epilepsy in all its aspects; the explosiveness of the major attack cannot be compared with other syndromes in clinical neurology and in this respect is unlike any reasonably set down to either excitation or escape. Perhaps, as already hinted, its violence may be due in part to concurrent metabolic or physiochemical derangement on a widespread scale, acute and sudden, obliterating normal physiological relationships between neural levels.

General etiological considerations.

1. **General Prevalence.** Statistics on the racial and geographical distribution of epilepsy, and its prevalence in different classes of the community, are largely vitiated by the fact that fits may be either unrecognised or concealed, while infantile convulsions are frequently ignored; especially, also, by disagreement on what constitutes the affection. Figures derived from cases resident in institutions or under the care of legal authorities are misleading as regards the total numbers in the population. From a series collated by TURNER the ratio per mille of the general public in certain selected countries is found to range between 2.9 and 0.4. In none of the reports (so far as I have noticed) is attention paid to the occurrence of any other epilepsy than the cryptogenic, an additional reason for discounting their value. Epilepsy manifests no partiality for white or coloured races, for social grades or types of occupation.

Further data will be found in a paper on epileptic oecology by DAVENPORT; consult also the monographs of SPRATLING, TURNER, BINSWANGER, FÉRÉ, MORSELLI. Evidence suggesting that epilepsy is on the decline is adduced by POLLOCK and FURBUSH.

2. **Relative Sex Frequency.** Similar criticism is pertinent to tables of sex incidence; some reveal preponderance of male cases, others the opposite. GOWERS' belief in excess of female epileptics during early years and in a reversed proportion later is refuted by TURNER's figures, showing no pronounced variation at any decennial period. Conclusions, however, depend to such a degree on the material examined as to possess no absolute value.

3. **Age Incidence.** No age is exempt from fits, though some are more likely than others to witness their onset. Ignoring the practical difficulties of the subject (such as failure to recognise nocturnal epilepsy or petit mal, and omission

to remark or recall infantile convulsions) we note the consensus of opinion in respect of diminishing tendency as the years pass. A Table drawn up by TURNER, based on 1000 personally observed examples, is here reproduced.

Table 1. Age at onset of 1000 cases in quinquennial periods from birth to 70.

Age	Males	Females	Total	Percentage
Birth—5 years	104	66	170	17,0
6—10	76	67	143	14,3
11—15	150	131	281	28,1
16—20	106	80	186	18,6
21—25	31	38	69	6,9
26—30	37	16	53	5,3
31—35	20	14	34	3,4
36—40	12	12	24	2,4
41—45	9	9	18	1,8
46—50	7	1	8	0,8
51—55	2	3	5	0,5
56—60	2	3	5	0,5
61—70	3	1	4	0,4
Totals	559	441	1000	100,0

By subdividing age incidence into three periods corresponding to infancy and childhood, youth and adolescence, and adult and late life, the same writer obtains equally instructive numerical ratios, as follows:

Age period at onset	Number of cases	Percentage
Birth—9 years	272	27,2
10—23	557	55,7
24—70	171	17,1

From 11 to 15 is the "dangerous age", coincident with the development of puberty; during infancy and childhood the first 12 months, and the age of 7, more or less, appear to be favourite periods for a start; thereafter no special year or years would seem to be selected. In the female the climacteric is without influence on epileptic genesis. The mean age at onset of TURNER's 1000 cases was 14,8; of the males, 13,7, and of the females, 15,5, figures differing from those of other observers (REYNOLDS, GOWERS, DORAN, etc.).

4. Heredity. Diversities of opinion and discrepancies between clinical records complicate the subject of the relation of epilepsy to inheritance. The reasons are self-evident — dissimilarities in material studied, absence of uniformity in the collection of data, preponderance of institutional and comparative neglect of private cases, obstacles in the way of getting exact information, differences in the genealogical ground covered by search, lack of agreement on what constitutes heredity taint. Enquiry is sometimes restricted to the preceding generation, sometimes extended much more widely, without any definition of what is to be taken as inheritance being fixed. Hence published figures diverge to a degree incompatible with belief in their general accuracy, and are at variance with other conclusions to be discussed presently. The appended Table, compiled from a number of sources, illustrates the point at issue.

Table 2. Percentage of Epileptics with family history of the affection.

Author	Number of cases	Percentage
FINCKH	250	33
MOREAU	364	32
DEJERINE	350	69
GOWERS	2400	40
KNEIDEL	1859	22
SARBÓ	913	42
MARBURG	41	28
RUSSELL BRAIN	200	28
SPRATLING	1070	56
DAVENPORT and WEEKS	372	19
TURNER	676	37

Many others have been collected by STÜBER and merely add to the confusion. Arbitrarily defining direct heredity as epilepsy occurring in parents, grandparents, brothers or sisters, or children; and indirect, its appearance in uncles, aunts, nephews, nieces or cousins, MUSKENS obtained evidence of one or other in 31,1 per cent. males, and 33,6 per cent. females, out of 2000 cases in all. If an approximate mean is taken for a number of statistics less open to objection than others, a figure of between 25 and 30 per cent. results.

Though personal experience compels me to affirm that this is too high, it would still leave from 70 to 75 per cent. for which no hereditary factor can be blamed.

But the problem must be approached from another angle. Were inheritance of much import as a determinant, out-patient practice should have brought me numerous instances of the condition among siblings, yet in point of fact this is distinctly rare. MYERSON cites information furnished (1925) by the superintendent of the Massachusetts State Hospital for Epileptics to the effect that among 1500 inmates only 4 families of 11 persons in all were to be found. At the same institution THOM ascertained that 138 marriages of epileptics resulted in 553 offspring, among whom a history of fits was obtainable in only 10 (1,8 per cent.). PILCZ traced 161 children of 144 epileptic mothers, only three turning out to be affected, while MUSKENS (who almost appears to refute his own deductions) states specifically that "so far not one of the offspring of marriages of my former patients has become an epileptic"! When every allowance is made for premature decision, and the fact that a hereditary history distinguished a fair number commencing in later life is also borne in mind, we are still justified in concluding that the influence of the factor is persistently overrated. MYERSON goes so far as to deny its genuineness, arguing that the personal or constitutional determinant may arise de novo in the liefetime of the subject concerned, from his uterine existence onward; a study of 1449 cases convinces BURR that "congenital instability" is all that can ever be transmitted, the disease-state of epilepsy being dependent on external causes. My own experience, as has been indicated, warrants a somewhat similar conclusion; in only about one-fifth of my material has evidence of inheritance been forthcoming, and, at most, what can be thus handed on from one generation to the next is an obscure cellular tendency to excessive reaction demonstrable only if circumstances calculated to evoke it should arise.

5. Trauma. Another highly controversial topic is that of the relation of head injury to subsequent fits. The readiness with which epilepsy is attributed to knocks or blows on the head testifies more to prevailing etiological ignorance than to proven cause and effect, and far exceeds that which the diseases of internal medicine are ascribed to corresponding accidents. Why this should be so offers a tempting line of thought that cannot here be prosecuted. Nearly every epileptic child has fallen out of a perambulator, if credence be given to parental assertions; but how many of the general population have not at one time or another been the recipients of "shocks to the system"?

In 1920 a survey by the Ministry of Pensions of 18,000 patients with gunshot wounds of the head disclosed the existence of nearly 800, or 4,5 per cent., that had become epileptic. BEHAGUE's analysis of 3523 similar French cases revealed the occurrence of the affection in 439, or 12,1 per cent.

With these statistics may be compared those of other wars, scanty though they are; according to ALLEN among 167 American civil war cases of head injury 13,7 per cent., and of 571 Franco-Prussian war cases 4,3 per cent., were ascertained to have developed epilepsy later.

The appended Table comprises figures of civilian origin.

However rigorously elimination of dubious examples is carried out the incontrovertible fact remains, that trauma capitis appears responsible for subsequent epilepsy in a *small* proportion of both civilian and war cases. The difficulty of deciding whether in a given instance a blow or fall on the head has produced

Table 3. Traumatic epilepsy.

Author	Number of cases	Percentage of traumatic causation
WILDERMUTH	210	3,8
TURNER ..	388	7,2
FINCKH ..	250	17,6
BIRO	306	21,0
GOWERS .	3000	3,6
MUSKENS ..	2000	7,4

actual intracranial injury is often extreme, especially in the absence of tangible signs; each case has to be judged on its own merits. Relative severity does not count for much in respect of youthful heads, as is well appreciated; while even in the case of adults failure to procure evidence of visible injury is no guarantee of normality within the skull. Obvious wounds will, if recent, cause contusions, haemorrhages, and oedema, and may be followed by infection and meningeal sepsis or cerebral abscess; at a later period cicatrices may be found to have pulled brain and membranes towards the site of injury and "anchored" the cranial contents (SARGENT, FOERSTER, PENFIELD, GUTTMANN, etc.), with vascular new-formation within the scar. In such circumstances the way is opened for epileptic development as a sequel to the action of mechanical or humoro-vascular determinants; and the fact that cicatrisation and "pull" are of tardy appearance lengthens the interval between injury and epilepsy to one of years, in not a few cases, effectually countering the view that the traumatic variety, to be genuine, must arise within a few months. Often enough, however, no lesion of skull or brain is apparent at the time, and fits arising after a long period may be devoid of local aura, yet exploration over the site of injury sometimes reveals pathological states of arachnitis, adhesions, or oedema that may been have instrumental in causing the affection. By resort to x-rays and encephalography occult lesions of the kind are not seldom discovered. No rule of thumb exists to aid diagnosis; the violence of a blow may be exaggerated, and its alleged intracranial effects apocryphal, but nothing is gained by minimising or ignoring the trauma; the best policy is to search with an accuracy that omits no detail.

Whether JACKSONian or general seizures will follow head injury cannot be predicted merely by reference to its position; of 439 cases analysed by BEHAGUE 35,5 per cent. belonged to the former and 54,4 per cent. to the latter class, but topographical allotment was as follows, viz. parietal, 55 per cent.; frontal 25,9; occipital, 10,5; and temporal 8,3. That is to say, a number of parietal cases developed general and not local convulsions. In the series no instances of epilepsy after cerebellar wounding occurred.

To what extent evolution of traumatic epilepsy is favoured by preexisting factors of a hereditary or personal kind cannot easily be ascertained; although the proportion of cases of definite head injury subsequently becoming epileptic is but a fraction of the totality it is probably incorrect to refer them all to "predisposition". With greater likelihood it may be affirmed that only in some do optimum conditions of mechanical or humoro-vascular change arise, and that if these are in being the neural factor becomes more potent. Antecedent epilepsy not infrequently is aggravated by trauma.

To the inquiring mind it must always seem curious how seldom petit mal or any of the numerous epileptic variants either are ascribed to injury or as matter of observation are evoked by it. The fact may rightly be taken to plead in favour of the view outlined above, viz. that the pathogenesis of the major seizure does not apply in all its features to other epileptic types.

Of *other predisposing causes* listed in the section on pathological states accompanying epilepsy (p. 52) nothing further need be said; heterogeneous though they are, and of differing frequency and moment, their specific effect is to intensify the pathogenic action of one or more of the determinants. But comment on the apparent etiological bearing of some *physical, physiological,* and *psychical* states is desirable.

1. **Cosmic Influences.** A search for causative factors in the physical environment of those who suffer from fits may savour of astrology and the middle

ages to some modernist minds but is none the less worth prosecuting. The belief that epilepsy is worse in spring than at any other *season* dates back to the Hippocratic era; according to LEURET winter is the unfavourable period, but DELASIAUVE could find no support for either view. Studies conducted over three years by TOULOUSE and PIÉRON concerning from 70 to 100 epileptics, showed the existence of two annual curves of rise and fall, with "peaks" in May and October respectively. The same observers found diminution of nocturnal attacks in spring and summer, but increase in autumn and winter, presumably in consequence of shorter or longer nights. Some evidence has accumulated seeming to point to reduction in paroxysmal frequency at times of high *external temperature* (TOULOUSE and PIÉRON, MARCHAND), with which perhaps may be linked the statement of HARTENBERG that lowering of body temperature precipitates fits. The influence of *atmospheric pressure* has been a subject of repeated search, without any clear issue emerging (LOVNER, BELLAVITIS, REICH, MARIE and NACHMAN, DANNHAUSER); residence in high altitudes has sometimes been considered to exercise a favourable effect, sometimes the reverse (cf. BUSCAINO).

2. Sleep. On p. 29 above some description of nocturnal and diurnal types has been given, with their contrasting difference in hours of maximum and minimum response. At the time of awakening and getting up the convulsive tendency of the nocturnal group sinks to a low level, just when it is rising to a high level in the other. Of course, the moment also coincides with a change from recumbent to erect posture, and from rest to activity; which, if either, of these two factors plays a rôle in exciting or, conversely, checking the tendency it is difficult to say. GOWERS decided against the influence of alteration in position, alleging that persons who are as a rule seized after rising do not escape by merely staying in bed. It is tempting to assume an action on the part of physiological mechanisms underlying the presence of sleep, to which the two types (termed by TOULOUSE and PIÉRON the "hypnique" and the "vigile") respond in diametrically opposed fashion. Something may depend on the depth of sleep in the two, as to which no data have been collected; it may inhibit the convulsive tendency of the one because it is itself the expression of an inhibitory function, but as regards the other no explanation except that of insufficient arrest seems feasible. Possibly, however, we should look no less to the physicochemical concomitants of sleep than to its neural basis for a solution of these obscurities. The theory of cerebral anaemia, relied on by PICK, does not harmonise with the facts.

LANGDON-BROWN and RUSSELL BRAIN made the interesting observation that the temporal distribution of the fits of the two classes is not altered by previous treatment with either bromide or luminal; these drugs suppress a proportion of attacks but do not defer them.

3. The Reproductive Functions. Of so-called *menstrual epilepsy* some account has been given in dealing with symptomatology (p. 29), but the etiological connexion is far from being well understood. It is strikingly exemplified by the case of a girl who for one or two years prior to normal menstruation showed a vicarious form (epistaxis), and who noticed that if her nose failed to bleed at one of these monthly recurrences she invariably had a severe epileptic fit instead. The catamenia per se are blameless, as is self-evident; but whether a passing toxaemia of endocrine origin, or increase of capillary permeability comparable to that of the uterine mucosa, is the noxious factor, remains in the realm of speculation. However regular in time and normal in character, the onset of the menses, or some day or two previous, may see the appearance of a major fit in certain cases, making it plain that a dysmenorrhoea is not responsible.

I have knowledge of a remarkable case in which a girl had attacks of petit mal while her mother was menstruating, no doubt a pure coincidence; a somewhat analogous but less obscure instance reported by FILIA concerns a breast-fed infant who had fits under the same circumstances.

Simple ascription to the hereditary factor (often, for that matter, absent) will not, of course, explain the association with the monthly period. Similarly, the menopause exerts occasional influence in conducing to attacks, or in aggravating their number and severity. The personal case quoted in the Introduction, of a solitary fit at puberty (aet. 14) and at the climacteric (aet. 44) is paralleled by one of ELLIOTSON's, where a woman suffered from epilepsy until menstruation was established and thereafter was free until the menopause. Impressive though such clinical data are, vaguenes invests their etiology.

Pregnancy seems occasionally related to epileptic incidence, and in opposite ways, i. e. either by starting the affection or inducing relapse and augmenting frequency, or, conversely, by an arresting or mitigating effect. Examples of the former have been reported by CURSCHMANN, WESTPHAL, GOWERS, etc., and of the latter by EUSIÈRE and DELMAS, REDLICH, BECHTEREW, and others. NERRLINGER collected the statistics of 157 pregnancies in 92 women, finding cessation of fits in 28 per cent. and increase in 35 per cent. The facts supply yet another instance of the disconcerting occurrence in epilepsy of "corresponding opposites", whose explanation is to seek. More curious still, a case is on record (DE LA MOTTE) of fits during pregnancies with sons but not with daughters, and another of identical nature we owe to MUSKENS. What the eventual solution of these epileptic mysteries will turn out to be we can scarcely even imagine.

Acute renal "inflammation" with albuminuria was formerly considered a sufficient reason for the development of "puerperal convulsions", commonly described as *eclampsia*. Occurring about once in 500 labours, and more usual in primiparae, the fact that it seldom recurs and is definitely known without nephritis militates against the renal theory. In the opinion of FÉRÉ, TURNER and others the condition is nothing else than serial epilepsy in acute form, precipitated by an unknown factor independent of heredity, the circumstances of the puerperium, and kidney disorder. Defective renal action often occurs without fits; and these sometimes persist after the incidents of childbirth are over. Eclamptic seizures may constitute a mere episode in the course of a confirmed case. The foetus sometimes perishes during severe attacks, while pregnancy is rarely interrupted by "ordinary" fits, but this distinction does not justify separation of the two conditions.

Experiments conducted on pregnant animals seem to warrant the conclusion that convulsants act more readily in them than in non-pregnant controls (MUSKENS, BLUMREICH and ZUNTZ, EDEL, CHIRÉE, etc.).

4. Psychical States. From the earliest days there have been claims for the production of epilepsy by agencies of a non-physical and non-physiological kind. That it should have been ascribed to divine or satanic influence is of historical interest alone; a present-day analogue is belief in what has been termed "emotional possession". Dismissing the evidence for visceral, metabolic, humoral or other physical causation, some allege that relief from the intolerable pressure of unconscious conflicts is sought in, and accomplished by, the epileptic "flight" into a fit [1], without stopping to inquire whether a "flight" that lands the luckless sufferer in a fireplace or breaks his head open is as convincing a proof of the validity of the theory as might be wished. Since in the course of our discussion numerous considerations have been advanced against the view of a self-contained nosological entity termed "epilepsy" they must throw no less doubt on the existence of any such person as an "essential epileptic"; the arguments of the psychoanalytical school assigning to him an oral- and anal-erotic character, an egocentric and narcissistic personality, can therefore hardly

---

[1] Cf. MENNINGER: Psychoanalytic Rev. **13** (1926), CLARK: J. nerv. Dis. **63** (1926).

apply, aside from the fact the conceptions are much too general to be of any specific value in the matter of paroxysmal etiology.

To say that a given fit is "psychogenic" leaves untouched the physiological problem of the convulsion itself, for which clearly something more is requisite than a mere affective stimulus. The nervous system concerned must be in a state of preparedness; as has been well said, emotion is only the trigger that fires the shot. Buried complexes and unconscious motivation may or may not be discoverable, but they are inert without the other state, and no psychological explanation of the physical phenomena of the convulsion can be anything else than verbal.

No doubt, of course, can be entertained that incidental circumstances of a psychical kind, fright, grief, anxiety, and other affective elements, frequently act as precipitants, and are potent in the immediate causation of fits. Nor can it be questioned, either, that a nervous system congenitally inferior or rendered unstable by incidents of early life may react to the bombardment of emotional stimuli in a fashion different from that of the stable and well-balanced individual. But it is quite another thing to assert that the pathology of the fit is determined by psychical mechanisms; of this, indeed, no even plausible evidence has been offered.

Examples of major epilepsy activated by stimuli of the affective series have often been reported (see p. 40); of various instances within personal knowledge one may here be cited.

It is that of a youth, age 21, who has had grand mal seizures about once a week for two years; his sister, age 30, suffers in the same way. On one occasion she fell convulsed in a corner of the room, and he, overcome with emotion and solicitous on her behalf, knelt down to assist; with words of endearment on his lips he suddenly lost consciousness and had an equally severe fit beside her.

In the experience of GOWERS about one-third of his cases were immediately preceded by inciting factors of the kind, but other writers record a much lower percentage; none except ROWS and BOND (so far as I am aware) claim that in every instance some emotional state can be found. With this latter assertion I am in radical disagreement.

5. Miscellaneous Causes. To specify and illustrate all the other causes, probable and improbable, to which paroxysms have been ascribed would be a task of supererogation. It stands to reason that the presence of any possible source of irritants should be sought for and dealt with; the literature contains many reports of "marvellous" results consecutive to removal of bad teeth, septic tonsils, refractive errors, phimosis, intestinal worms, nasal polypi and what not. In the presence of so distressing a complaint as epilepsy it is wise to hunt systematically for inciting or aggravating factors, and these often turn out to be either comparatively trifling or altogether unsuspected. But it is equally unwise to believe that they account for the convulsive tendency.

Diagnosis.

The epileptic state is recognisable by the symptoms, which consist in one or other variety of fit. No reliance can be placed on any alleged stigmata of mind or body, on any mental attributes or somatic habitus. If the chronic epileptic can be diagnosed by scars on his head or face, or by his emotional or intellectual traits, these are incidental or secondary, and devoid of pathognomonic significance. Hence the physician's first duty is to ascertain as best he may the precise nature of the patient's attacks, which is not always a simple affair. Those who have been resident in hospitals or institutions with abundant opportunity for observing fits, soon learn to appreciate signs of value in reaching a decision; others, as constantly happens, are compelled to judge from description furnished by inexpert witnesses. Even for one familiar with epilepsy in all its aspects the perplexity occasionally felt in listening to verbal narratives is considerable.

1. Occurrence of attacks. In the first place, the *occurrence of attacks* may have to be inferred from evidence of an indirect kind. If nocturnal, with the patient sleeping alone or not within hearing of others, all the phenomena of the major fit may pass unperceived and no knowledge of them be retained in consciousness. Reasonable deductions may then be drawn from morning headache, soreness of limbs or tongue (if it was bitten), presence of blood on the pillow, bed-wetting, and also from ecchymoses round eyes or extravasation beneath the conjunctive. None of these may be noted, however, the earliest proof coming from observation of a diurnal fit.

Again, suspicion should be aroused when complaint is made of involuntary "jumps" or "jerks", especially in the morning; and if for any reason it seems desirable to verify the point no hesitation should be felt in asking "leading questions"; under these circumstances they do not, in my experience, mislead.

In the case of minor fits the difficulty may be greater. It is very common for the patient, whose symptoms have at length come under medical notice, to remark spontaneously that he has long been aware of curious "sensations" or "feelings" or "day-dreams", sometimes not unpleasant, to which no particular attention was paid and which escaped observation; conversely, they may have been unknown to him but visible to the bystander, ignorant of their import. If the possibility of petit mal arises, questions should be directed to the occurrence of any momentary "blank", "lapse", "giddiness" or similar incident, however trifling and evanescent. The epileptic significance of vertigo is always increased when attended by transient mental confusion.

2. Recognition of the generalised fit can never prove troublesome, for its phenomena are too glaring to be misunderstood. When inference from description is required, information should be sought in respect of the epileptic cry, falls and hurts, loss of senses, convulsive movements, cyanosis, tongue-biting, involuntary micturition, frothing at the mouth; especial note should be made of sequelae, their presence or absence, their exact nature and approximate duration. As regards the minor variety, personal observation usually suffices; attention should be focussed on pallor, fixity of expression, flickering movements of eyelids or corners of mouth, staring or rolling up of eyes, and so on; and these should be matters of enquiry when the fit is not seen.

For epileptic variants of a motor kind diagnosis is aided by the characteristic march of the JACKSONian type, and by the distinctive twitches of myoclonic forms. The attacks of pyknolepsy, when well established, occur with such repetitive frequency as to provide chances for personal study in practically every case, and their nature is so like that of a petit mal variety as to involve no diagnostic embarrassment. Tonic epilepsy is often found accompanied by recognisable intracranial disease, but, if not, its salient characters are in any case self-evident. Differentiation from the tonic fits of hysteria will be discussed presently. The rare akinetic variant, practically always JACKSONian, is preceded by a local aura that can hardly be mistaken.

Sensory epilepsies have features of their own which should obviate confusion, a remark applicable also to visceral types. In regard to so-called psychical variants and equivalents each case must be considered on its merits. The problem is beset with difficulties less of a clinical than of an etiological kind; whether a given mental syndrome is classed as epileptic or not will depend to some extent on the personal views of the investigator.

3. Distinction from other paroxysmal syndromes often calls for minute care in observation and faithful weighing of probabilities.

a) Among the commonest of the questions to arise in this connexion is that of ordinary *syncopal attacks*. Transient insensibility, with loss of colour and sinking to the ground, is characteristic equally of faints and petit mal seizures; as a good working rule stress should be laid on the general absence of exciting factors in the latter and their presence in the former. That is to say, states of emotion, physical pain, over-exertion, and conditions involving crowded environment or impure atmosphere are calculated to induce syncope in weakly persons, whereas petit mal is largely independent of such circumstances and its subjects generally have no organ defects. Faints, too, are usually introduced by a sinking feeling, sweating or nausea, a sense of oppression and of heaviness of the limbs; only a few visceral and minor epileptic attacks are ushered in by any aura comparable to part of these. The duration of unconsciousness is briefer in the latter groups, which may be accompanied by micturition and succeeded by mental confusion or automatisms, features foreign to any type of faint. Immediate or quick recovery distinguishes the epileptic patient, a degree of lingering physical disability the other.

b) Severe attacks of *aural vertigo*, the MENIÈRE syndrome, consist of giddiness so fulminant and intense as to throw the patient down, as if he had been struck, and are associated with violent vomiting; these features, together with retention of consciousness, relatively long duration, slow return to the normal, and the coexistence of nerve-deafness and tinnitus, compose an unmistakable picture. But mild bouts of labyrinthine vertigo, sudden and brief, embracing also a transient sense of confusion, with or without a fall and forced movements, offer a much more close resemblance to epilepsy; they are, indeed, on the borderland. Distinction is facilitated by the presence of enduring labyrinthine symptoms and signs, as well as by absence of postparoxysmal confusion or automatism. Rare cases of major epilepsy commence with an aura of vestibulo-auditory type, but are of course at once recognised by the convulsions.

c) Perhaps not so frequently as in other days the observer may have to differentiate epileptic from *hysterical seizures*. Diagnosis rests on a) the intrinsic features of the attack, and b) the circumstances under which it occurs. As regards the first of these, the grande crise hystérique, now seldom if ever witnessed, embodies prolonged and fluctuating tonic spasms of extension and opisthotonus (arc de cercle) or of anteroflexion, alternating or mingling with wild quasipurposive movements expressive of emotion (attitudes passionelles), or representing and reproducing some prior experience laden with affective tone. Her limbs quivering and breast heaving, with tremulous eyelids and flushed face, the hysteric gives vent to cries, or talks and mutters, resisting any effort to compose her and often needing restraint owing to the violence and impulsiveness of her actions. When the eyes are forcibly opened (for orbiculares are held in tense contraction) the eyeballs roll up and in till only the whites remain visible. Milder and briefer fits generally exhibit some or other of the same characters; though she lies limp and "lifeless" on the floor, resistance to opening of the eyes, or the blepharospasm of the lids, and a cutaneous analgesia disproportionate to the degree of conscious impairment, generally reveal the true nature of the case.

From the negative side, it suffices to remark the absence of cyanosis and of tongue-biting (yet the latter may occur) or profound unconsciousness and (usually) of sphincteric decontrol. Rarely, however, the hysteric wets herself at one stage or another of the performance. The corneal reflex, commonly, retained, is sometimes reported to have been abolished, and the pupils inactive to light. A BABINSKI sign is not obtainable at any stage, though often no plantar response can be elicited.

Attention, however, should also be given to the circumstances of the fit. Many years ago CHARCOT insisted on the diagnostic value of the fact that hysterical seizures seldom or never take place when the patient is alone, or in a water-closet, whereas the reverse is not infrequently the case with the epileptic. Hysterical subjects never hurt themselves seriously, and often show informative foresight in avoiding the risk.

A friend of mine was eye-witness of a scene during the darker days of the war, when at a convalescent hospital Army Council orders were read out to a circle of shell-shocked soldiers standing on a gravel court. Five or six became hysterical and promptly developed fits, but all without exception first made their way to a grassy lawn before succumbing.

Both intrinsic and extrinsic features obviate any diagnostic difficulty, except perhaps in the case of brief and abortive attacks, or when a fleeting petit mal seizure passes unnoticed and only a postepileptic "hysteria" is observed. Some tonic fits are rather difficult to categorize, evolving without clonic spasms and introducing at one or other phase an opistotonic movement reminiscent of that neurosis; an example of the kind is fully described elsewhere[1]. GOWERS states they are specially apt to occur in boys, and my experience is similar. Non-hysterical cases are differentiated by depth of unconsciousness, suddenness of fall, pallor or cyanosis, occurrence of aura and time occupied. Nor should the question of motivation be overlooked.

Hysteria of this somatic kind appear to be a vanishing quantity, and if distinctions between the two states are still thought necessary the fact that each is a syndrome and not a disease tends to impair the value of clinical contrasts. On the borderland of the two occur fits whose classification with one, to the exclusion of the other, is almost impossible; nomenclature makes an artificial separation hardly corresponding to reality.

d) Clinicians of other times were much occupied with criteria serving as they believed, to distinguish *organic* from *idiopathic* epilepsy. Much of the trouble expended was beside the point, according to present-day views. The convulsions of alcoholism, uraemia, lead poisoning, general paralysis, cerebral tumour, and so forth, cannot be recognised at the bedside by any specific and intrinsic marks; they are identical with those of so-called cryptogenic origin. In my experience none of the alleged distinctions is of any worth, unless myoclonus be excepted; diagnosis, as always, rests on detection of their cause, which in the case of the maladies enumerated is generally simple, It is naturally of the utmost importance to recognise local and active brain disease, and equally desirable to discover the presence of quiescent lesions; but so far as concerns their epileptic manifestations, neither a precise aura nor a local commencement may accompany either of these two cerebral conditions, whose existence not infrequently has to be inferred by other means. Conversely, some, to all appearance "idiopathic", cases begin in a local fashion.

I have had but little experience of *simulated* epilepsy, formerly considered part of the stock-in-trade of professional beggars, criminals, and soldiers. One fit of the kind that came under personal notice was a very poor imitation of the real thing. The art is now probably lost, like many another.

Course and prognosis.

No comprehensive formulas can be devised whose application to a given case will cover the possibilities, while questions on the outlook and prospects of cure have always to be met. Even after but one fit expression of opinion on the future is often sought forthwith. For guidance on the problem several considerations have to be borne in mind.

---

[1] Brain **43** (1929) (case 7).

1. Of these, by far the most significant is whether a cause can be discovered, or not. This will entail patient scrutiny of every system of the body, by present-day technique, and may, of course, prove negative. Should, however, some positive symptom or sign be found its lead must be followed up. Recognition of an exciting as opposed to a determining cause is not to be neglected, because of the desirability of avoiding or controlling the cirumstances that may have brought it into action.

2. Should somatic examination furnish no evidence, the attacks are, for the time being, relegated to the cryptogenic group. Under these conditions prognosis is influenced by a series of factors, as follows. a) The *age at onset* must be duly noted; cases commencing before 20 perhaps do less well than those beginning later. On a previous page facts concerning the prospects of children suffering from infantile convulsions have been adverted to; the proportion developing epilepsy thereafter is small. In adult and senile epilepsies can nearly always be traced underlying lesions of an identifiable kind, prognosis depending on ability to deal with these. b) Importance also attaches to the *physical and mental endowment* of the person concerned. A physical weakling or mental defective stands less chance of repelling his infirmity than an otherwise healthy and normal subject. c) The *influence of heredity* has to be assessed; patients weighed down by a wretched neuropathic or psychopathic diathesis will be handicapped to a material degree. But here, as elsewhere, the quality of that inheritance must be examined; and arrest of fits can be, and often is, secured in cases from which the hereditary factor is not absent, provided other predisposing elements do not aggravate its effect. 4. Of significance, too, are the *frequency, character*, and *times* of the attack, and the *duration* before treatment is begun. Constantly recurring and severe generalised fits are less amenable to therapeutic measures than mild cases with long intervals of freedom; on the other hand, minor epilepsy is undoubtedly more apt to prove intractable than the major variety, except as regards pyknolepsy, which seems to cure itself. If fits occur by night and day indifferently, or observe no particular periodicity and in each recurring instance are unexpected, they will not yield so readily as in other cases characterised by a certain uniformity. A possible reason for this is the sureness with which reappearance can be guarded against, in the latter, by preliminary medication. The longer the affection has been in existence the less effectively can its sinister course be controlled. But, even so, we need not dispair of the chronic epileptic, in view of recent accretions to knowledge discussed already, especially as regards mechanical and humoral determinants.

3. The prognosis of epileptic variants depends on their course, as does that of all cases originating in known structural or nutritional disorder. Once the "habit" of epileptic reaction is set up removal of the cause may not have the beneficial result imagined on theoretical grounds likely to ensue, but this consideration should not influence decision, e. g. to operate when the evidence points to a local lesion capable of surgical remedy. For the epilepsies of the numerous pathological states catalogued on p. 52 no prognostic rule can be laid down other than this, that appropriate treatment of the underlying condition is bound to affect favourably the subsequent course of the case, though care and judgment should be exercised ere an actual cure is guaranteed.

4. When the cause remains hidden, some time should be allowed to elapse before a confident expression of opinion is offered; the response of the patient to treatment has to be added to painstaking estimation of the relative values of the different factors mentioned in paragraph 2 above. In a majority of cases, my personal conviction is that the type can be regarded as benign and the outlook reassuring; those of malignant nature form by contrast a rather small minority.

Spontaneous cessation seems to be an ever-present object of hope on the part of parents and friends, but the event is too rare to be relied on, yet not so much so as to be ignored. I have seen several thus distinguished, and observed for a sufficiently long period to justify the assertion. But the paroxysmal state is peculiarly deceptive; intervals of freedom, e. g. after infantile convulsions or fits at puberty, may extend to a number of years, only to be succeeded at another time of physiological stress by their reappearance. Expectation of relief or of arrest at one or other of the outstanding periods of life is unjustified by facts; yet now and again a case is encountered whose record discloses steady improvement with the passing of time and complete epileptic abeyance in later life. And I have no hesitation in affirming that successful treatment can often be accomplished by simple methods and is, as a fact, so accomplished to a much greater extent than is generally imagined.

5. Another question is frequently asked; is there any danger to life in a major attack, or during a state of postconvulsive automatism? In the course of the seizure itself death is practically unknown, imminent as it may seem to the uninformed eye. Risk of fatal respiratory arrest or interference with cardiac action at the stage of tonic spasm is more apparent than real. But danger of a serious kind attends the various accidents of the convulsion, alluded to already, among which that of "epileptic pronation" is not one of the least. The possibility of choking must be remembered if the fit occurs at table or of passage of food into the lungs if vomiting takes place in the period of unconsciousness. On another page is cited the case of a little boy who was drowned in a pool of water during a postepileptic confusional state; this form of accidental death is perhaps most to be feared, though all are rare and the likelihood of any remote.

The dangers of status epilepticus must be considered apart, for in the first place few patients pass into it, and in the second the accompanying circumstances are more responsible than the fits themselves. This is shown by the records (p. 28) of cases of a severe kind from which recovery has been complete.

As regards the cognate question of *epileptic mortality* disagreement is rife and misconceptions abound. At the National Hospital from the years 1902 to 1925 inclusive 1898 patients were admitted with the diagnosis of "idiopathic epilepsy", of whom 15 died. In spite of the fact that admission is restricted to the more serious types the death-rate was a mere 1,07 per cent. The majority of the fatalities occurred in status and only two were the result of accident, i. e. less than half of 1 per cent. But if we are to judge by the figures of the Registrar-General's Review for England and Wales (the year selected being 1925) epilepsy is a surprising second on the list of killing (nervous) diseases, as the appended Table shows.

Table 4. Deaths attributed to Nervous Diseases (England and Wales), 1925.

Disease	Number of deaths (male and female)
Cerebral apoplexy	27031
Epilepsy	2123
Paralysis	2098
Meningitis	1814
General paralysis of the insane	1539
Ear and mastoid	1183
Cerebral tumour	1035 etc.

The mixed character of these descriptive terms for "diseases", however, is so absurd as to deprive them of any precise significance; and no information can be gleaned from the figures on the all-important matter of the pathological basis of the "epilepsy" that is declared to be only less fatal than "apoplexy". But the Review shows also that of these 2123 epileptic deaths as many occurred between the ages of 70 and 75 as between 10 and 15; and that more patients live to over 60, eventually to die of their affection, than succumb below the age of 20. Though the numerical data are rendered suspect by failure to differentiate the "epilepsy" to which they refer, at their face value they assuredly do not support traditional views still obtaining currency, and might be taken to suggest that the subjects of the affection may live as long as any one else.

A closer analysis of the fallacies underlying statistics on the mean age at death of epileptics, and of mortality tables dealing with the condition generally, will be found in my article[1] on epilepsy and life assurance.

6. A final question merits passing notice, since to it also an answer is sometimes demanded; what is the chance of epilepsy developing in a member of a family marked by epileptic ancestry? This possibility is contingent on a number of factors and no ready reply can in fairness be expected; but since some 75 per cent. of "idiopathic" cases have already developed symptoms by the age of 21 the prospect thereafter is distinctly in favour of freedom and increases with the years. That is to say, the chances are greatly against its appearance later (as much perhaps as 50 to 1) if the person concerned has been immune to the age mentioned.

Treatment.

A humiliating chapter in the history of medicine might be written on the vicissitudes of epileptic treatment from the earliest times, when CELSUS saw patients drinking the blood of wounded and dying gladiators, to the present era of enlightenment, when "cures" as empirical and irrational are still being vended in the medical market place. There is scarcely a substance in the world, as SIEVEKING declared, capable of passing through the gullet of man, that has not at one time or another enjoyed the reputation of being antiepileptic. In HENNING's bibliography of 1798 no less than 152 pages quarto are filled with reference to treatment alone; by 1852 HERPIN could say discouragingly that epilepsy is "une affection pour laquelle on a tout essayé, tout vanté, tout dénigré." The unbelievable variety of therapeutic agents experimented with testifies much more to human ingenuity than intelligence; nail-parings of hands and feet were recommended to the eighteenth century patient for their efficacy in the falling sickness[2], yet only a few years ago there came into my hands a pamphlet extolling the magical properties of a bot-fly infusion.

But the source of therapeutic failure is clear enough; the epileptic fit is the expression of normal nervous activity increased to a morbid degree, self-perpetuating by repetition; and since discharge is followed by return to a normal cellular state the core of the problem is to reduce excitability without at the same time injuring normal function. Hence little surprise need be felt at the monotonous regularity with which curative efforts have been defeated, though now at length the future has become more promising.

1. Prophylaxis. Contributory factors rendered active by trauma at birth might be made less prevalent by better obstetrical practice, and others tending to initiate convulsions in the predisposed can be neutralised by suitable hygiene, including removal of manifest causes of irritation such as have already been mentioned. Perhaps some day eugenics will enact a more imposing rôle in preventive medicine by reduction or suppression of congenital nervous defects. The hygiene of the mind, too, must not be overlooked when there is reason to suppose a potential cause of mischief lurks within.

Whether transmission of epileptic tendencies should be controlled by forbidding *marriage* to members of epileptic stocks is an extraordinarily complicated question incapable of any stereotyped solution. In themselves, marital

---

[1] Brit. med. J. 1 (1927).
[2] Ana of Medical Literature, Vol. 3, p. 120 (1825).

relations are without influence on the development of fits; as we have seen, pregnancy may or may not modify their course, if already occurring, and may or may not precipitate them in a predisposed subject. As regards the matter of children, however, a number of considerations have to be reviewed. Briefly, when there is evidence of cryptogenic epilepsy in direct or indirect line of descent the possibility of its reappearing cannot be ignored. Although due emphasis has already been laid (p. 62) on collected data refuting common and exaggerated views of epileptic heredity too little known of human inheritance for an accurate forecast in any given case. My practice is to ascertain all the germane familial facts and to express an opinion in frankness; if the evidence points to transmission of nervous or mental disease in general, or of epilepsy in particular, the problem solves itself, and the proposed marriage is stated to be inadvisable; if the hereditary factors appear of minor potency, and the previous history of the individuals concerned is unimpeachable, then the decision can be left to them (as indeed it must always be) but the chances are declared to be in their favour. The physician is often compelled to adopt an agnostic attitude and to leave the situation at that. He is aware that hereditable conditions sometimes seem to arise de novo in embryonic tissues, without proof of actual inheritance, in which case risk of epileptic development may be involved, yet none, so far as can be seen, of epileptic transmission.

It is scarcely needful to point out that the discussion applies solely to cryptogenic epilepsy — as would appear, a slowly diminishing class. For all types whose causation is obvious or presumptive no anxiety on the score of possible transmission should be entertained. Acquired characters (to which those of known epilepsy belong) do not reappear in a succeeding generation.

2. Immunity. Epileptic manifestations are sometimes controlled by nature's own methods. This feature has engaged surprisingly little attention, though the Father of medicine oberved two thousand years ago that intermittent fever replaced or mitigated epilepsy, whence the adage "Quartana epilepsiae vindex appellatur". More than a century ago ESQUIROL commented on diminution or disappearance of fits in the course of "accidents fébriles"; this was noticed during an epidemic of measles at Bicêtre (BOURNEVILLE and BONNAIRE), at the Salpêtrière (SÉGLAS), in the course of a typhoid epidemic (BOURNEVILLE); GOWERS quotes the case of a child ("with strong inheritance") who suffered from fits to the age of seven, when they ceased during an attack of typhoid and did not recur till 27. Scarlatina is mentioned by TURNER as having a similar effect. In my own experience measles and chickenpox have sometimes produced noteworthy amelioration continuing long after the illness.

Older authors, also struck with the favourable influence exerted by febrile diseases, had advocated the establishment of malaria or erysipelas to cure epilepsy long before the idea was applied to general paralysis (cf. HAMMOND, LENOIR).

No attempt at explanation seems to have been made, however except by HARE, who believed the pyrexia dilates the bloodvessels generally, thus inducing a beneficial effect; he also quoted a case of GARROD's in which recurrent epilepsy of 30 years' duration ceased entirely after the development of attacks of acute articular gout. This remarkable circumstance can be properly accounted for on humoral lines, but that pyrexial vasodilatation represents the mechanism of exanthematous arrest does not appear probable. The subject deserves further study from both clinical and experimental sides.

3. General Hygiene. Common sense will lead to painstaking scrutiny of the patient's mode of life, with a view to correcting irregularities or faults. On the physical side, he should be allowed to take his share in games and recreations even at some little risk, unless clear evidence of deleterious effect is forthcoming. The salutary and bracing effect of being considered a normal person must be balanced against the danger (should it be present) of aggravating attacks by undue muscular exertion. He should not be denied the pleasures and indulgences of youth except when the nature of his case makes it imperative to forego them; he should then substitute regular exercise under supervision or in the quiet of home. Even swimming, riding, cycling, etc., need not be vetoed if practised in moderation with some companion. Skin, kidneys, and bowels must be kept in order with unfailing attention; a good physique must be promoted in every possible way, faulty postures adjusted, deep breathing enjoined, and the circulation prevented from becoming sluggish. In a word, to secure a healthy body and actively functioning systems is one of the prime aims of epileptic hygiene.

On the *mental* side nothing should be done that is likely to sow, in a sensitive mind, the seed of inferiority. Wherever possible, the patient should be retained a useful member of society; discouragement must be eschewed and optimism fostered. The necessity of avoiding emotional stress or excitement is self-evident. Such aptitudes as he possesses for any intellectual pursuit are to be utilised, and an atmosphere of normality sedulously cultivated. His thoughts should be diverted from the apprehensiveness fatal to improvement; on the other hand, if frank discussion of the nature of his case is believed desirable, or if experience of an affective kind are found to have been instrumental in its onset, no hesitation should keep the physician from taking the patient into confidence and explaining in what way or ways the latter can help himself.

As a preliminary to this regimen of physical and mental hygiene it will always be essential to ascertain (1) whether any particular abnormality of mind or body is acting as a precipitating cause, and (2) whether any combination of circumstances seems responsible for individual fits. A search for the first of these will entail complete physical examination and suitable psychological questioning, nor should any stone be left unturned in the hunt. The chance should be seized at the onset, before a neural habit is formed. Universal experience condemns the attitude of mind that is satisfied with the euphemism of "nerve faints" and a statement that the patient "will grow out of them". The golden opportunity for correction of contributory elements comes at the beginning; airy promises of arrest on completion of some physiological period ignore the fact, as has been truly said, that one of these may be death itself. Of equal value is careful enquiry with a view to detecting any immediate excitant, or excitants acting in unison. Not infrequently patient or parents have already observed something that "seems to bring the fit on"; it may be injudicious feeding, violent exercise, constipation, physical fatigue and the keeping of unusual hours, or recurring anxiety, emotional strain and so forth. Whatever the tale, it should be attentively listened to, and if credence be justified a line for future treatment may be indicated. In numerous examples, however, no hint of a possible immediate cause can be gleaned.

The question of *education* and avocation is often brought before the practitioner in the hope of guidance on a difficult matter demanding no little thought. Many points have to be considered; the patient's age and sex, mental capacity, tastes and inclinations have to be borne in mind, together with the type of case, the stage it has reached, and some estimate of its probable course. Broadly speaking, mental exercise is as wholesome as physical, and any idea of its "injuring the brain" can be brushed aside. Indeed, neglect of ordinary education will only serve to impress the patient (if of normal endowment) with the suspicion of his being in some way "different" from others, a harmful conception, to be studiously avoided. Moreover, it is only right that he should be fitted for his station in life as far as is practicable, since his future may be prejudiced owing to such neglect if the infirmity should turn out to be not merely moderate but actually curable. Some epileptics are ineducable and unemployable from the beginning; for many more, the comparative ease of an epileptic colony, with its graded occupations and opportunities of self-expression, at different levels, is welcome; but the great majority are not so handicapped as to require this seclusion, and choice of some suitable life-work may be perplexing. General principles must influence decision. Practical wisdom suggests preference for an out-door employment, one not calculated to involve risk or danger, or some sedentary calling to which the same remark applies. In-door occupations have a disadvantage owing to the possible absence of fresh air. A successful living can often be made on the land, chicken- or bee-farming, fruit-growing, gardening, etc., being among the pursuits chosen.

4. Diet. The dietary of the epileptic has been a happy hunting-ground for empirics and charlatans ever since the Hippocratic era, but evidential proof of its influence on fit production is as a general rule conspicuously absent, with one or two exceptions, to be noted presently.

A bland, simple, easily assimilated diet, sufficient for the requirements of the person concerned, neither excessive in quantity for any one meal nor hurriedly eaten, summarises the food question. Exclusion of meat, however, is widely ordered, and of animal food as a whole, without either clinical or experimental justification. Researches by WEEKS et al. on the comparative effect of high and low protein diets were inconclusive, like those of GOWERS long ago. Allusion has been made (p. 46) to the lack of evidence for abnormal protein metabolism in persons subject to fits, and to the equivocal results of protein sensitisation tests. Only an occasional patient is benefited by meat restriction, or by omission of some food article capable of inducing allergic phenomena; in a few cases (as has also been mentioned) increase of anti-proteolytic ferments can be demonstrated. Despite the paucity of pertinent data, empiricism has resorted to injections of peptone (MILLER, AULD, EDGEWORTH, etc.) and of milk (WEIDNER, SCHWARTZ, and others) without any unambiguous results being gained. Another form of protein injection, antirabic vaccine, employed by OSSOKIN and OCHSENHANDLER, HOROSHKO, MILIZYN, is claimed to have been beneficial.

Of none of these have I had personal experience, nor of another foreign protein, viz. rattlesnake venom (crotalin) vaunted by SPANGLER and FACKENHEIM, but condemned by THOM, RUSSELL, JENKIN and PENDLETON.

A dietary for which plausible claims have been made is one from which *common salt* is excluded (TOULOUSE and RICHET, BALINT, TURNER, etc). Its rationale is based on the theory that chloride increases nerve-cell irritability, though clinical experimentation has proved rather unconvincing (WEEKS et al., SHERRILL, LENNOX and ALLEN). A salt-free diet lowers chloride concentration in the blood and sometimes appears to diminish fits (FREUDENBERG, VOLLMER). During interparoxysmal periods chloride (inter alia) keeps within normal limits (see p. 48), but aggravation of the epileptic tendency by its increase ought not perhaps to be denied, especially since intravenous injection may cause tetany in animals (LENNOX and COBB).

Fasting as a method for treating epilepsy has often proved of striking if temporary value (GEYELIN, GOLDBLOOM, GAMBLE et al., MORIARTY, SCHOU and TEGLBJOERG, LENNOX et al., LENNOX and COBB, KARGER, and others). Its disadvantages are manifest, viz. the discomfort it entails and the limited period for which it can be indulged. The procedure is accompanied by decrease of protein and basal metabolism, retention of uric acid, low blood sugar, absence of salt, removal of water from the tissues, and presence of acidosis. To decide which of these several factors may be chiefly responsible for the beneficial results has provoked much discussion, owing to the number and complexity of the processes. In the opinion of some, the action of fasting is really a triple effect of high fat diet (from the patient's own tissues), salt starvation, and acidosis (owing to reduction of plasma bicarbonate); others lay stress on the attendant dehydration and drainage of water from extra- and intracellular sites. Whatever be the exact mechanism (probably more than one is involved) the clinical usefulness of the method cannot be gainsaid, but its applicability must always be rather restricted.

Closely related to the question of fasting is that of the merits of a *ketogenic diet*. If the value of starvation as a check to epileptic development can be attained by a less uncomfortable method, based on similar metabolic changes, the advantage must at once be apparent. Fasting corresponds in reality to a highfat and low carbohydrate diet, and this is known as a ketosis-producing combination.

Ketosis is a form of acidosis. The ketones are β-oxybutyric acid, diacetic acid, and acetone; these acid substances, produced in a number of ways, appear in excess when fats are insufficiently "burned" owing to lack of carbohydrate available for the purpose. Fat is largely ketogenic, carbohydrate the reverse. Ingestion of the latter soon reduces and stops formation of ketones. (The word is merely shortened from acetone, which is one of the ketone bodies.)

A large number of clinical experiments have been conducted on ketogenic lines, especially in children (WILDER, PETERMAN, HELMHOLZ, TALBOT et al., BRIDGE and IOB, VOLLMER, MCQUARRIE and KEITH, TALBOT and MORIARTY, etc.). The chief reason why the diet has hitherto proved more satisfactory in young people than in adults is that ketosis can be produced with greater readiness in the former on a low ratio between ketogenic (fat) and antiketogenic (carbohydrate and protein) foodstuffs. A 3 : 1 or 4 : 1 ratio causes sufficient ketosis for the desired effect.

As with fasting, the manner in which the dietary acts favourably on epileptogenesis has not yet been fully elucidated. Some observers attach most importance to the acidosis, others to removal of surplus extracellular fluid from the tissues. The superiority of ketosis over starvation resides in the length of time it may be practised; its disadvantage is that the body eventually becomes adjusted thereto, plasma bicarbonate returns to a normal level, and seizures reappear even with ketone bodies recoverable in the urine. A combination of the two procedures has its value, fasting for some days, or a week, being followed by resort to a ketogenic diet. As an emergency method, the former can be recommended, e. g. to tide the patient over a difficult time, when status may appear imminent.

TALBOT's book contains all necessary information on caloric requirements in the matter of ketogenic-antiketogenic balance, with numerous menus suitable for children; others are supplied by BRAIN and STRAUSS.

5. Medication. Sedative treatment by means of drugs is an obvious method for controlling epilepsy, purely symptomatic though it be.

a) First place must be assigned to *bromide*, introduced by LOCOCK in 1857.

It is not mentioned by HERPIN (1852), whose favourite medicaments were oxide of zinc, ammoniacal sulphate of copper, and zinc valerianate. Early records were published by WILKS, ROGERS, RAMSKILL, HUGHLINGS JACKSON, MCDONNELL and especially by DUCKWORTH WILLIAMS (1865). After that date references are abundant.

The medicinal value of salts of bromine in reducing or abolishing the tendency to seizures needs no exposition; they were for years the sheet-anchor on which everyone relied, and if today their use has perhaps become less constant the sterling properties of the drug have in no wise altered.

Little enough is known of the precise way in which bromide acts on nerve-cells, or indeed, whether it may not produce its effects by rendering the walls of cerebral capillaries more permeable. According to GÄRTNER, in experimental poisoning by sodium bromide its localisation in glial cytoplasm can be detected. Many years ago HUGHLINGS JACKSON surmised that the efficacy of the bromides might be due to their replacing the more common chlorides of the body. Proof of his theory has been long in coming, but evidence that decrease of chloride intake enhances the usefulness of bromide medication has frequently been obtained in recent times (cf. ULRICH and see p. 76 above).

The chemical serves in the great majority of cases to diminish the frequency and mitigate the severity of epileptic seizures of all kinds; for a smaller number it seems to achieve a cure, in the sense that eventual omission is not followed by a relapse; at the other end of the scale are those which remain uninfluenced. Choice of salt matters little, nor does any advantage accrue by a mixture of bases, to which numerous prescribers seem partial. If good results depend solely on the amount of bromide present lithium and ammonium salts should be found most efficacious, for their percentage of the halogen is 92 and 81 respectively, that of potassium bromide being 67, and of sodium bromide 57. But clinical observation confirms the superior merits of the last two, though on occasion one salt or another appears to answer best in a particular instance without reference either to its base or its bromide content.

The dosage selected varies with the nature of the case in regard to severity and frequency of attacks, and the age of the patient. Rarely if ever is a daily administration of more than 60 grs. desirable; satisfactory results generally follow a morning and evening dose of 25 grs., which is usually well borne. On the whole, there is a tendency to overdo the necessary amount, but the effect should not be dissipated by inadequate quantity for a single dose; in other words, 15 grs. twice a day may well be preferable to 10 grs. thrice. Further, common sense suggests the advisability of seeking to concentrate on that period of the twenty-four hours (if such there be) which is most likely to witness attacks; hence for nocturnal cases a single dose on retiring often proves efficacious, for morning cases a dose at night and another on waking but before rising. The principle is manifestly capable of extension; in respect of fits at the catamenial flow the daily dosage should be increased or if necessary doubled for some days beforehand. In all such matters each patient must be considered individually, and a careful record kept of the response to treatment. Systematic administration is imperative, and this can often best be secured by restricting it to twice, or once, a day; neglect of so simple an undertaking is fatal. Every out-patient physician knows the old story of relapse from failure to continue regular treatment. Once a good result is obtained, the paroxysmal "habit" counteracted and intervals of freedom lengthened, or actual arrest seemingly effected, the amount can be lessened by degrees; the safest way at first is to reduce total but not separate dosage, e. g. ordering the medicine twice a day instead of three times, then once, then on alternate days, and so forth. Decision on the exact point in the course of a case at which diminution should started must rest with the observer and no hard-and-fast rules can be laid down; it is always preferable to err on the side of delayed reduction, for premature curtailment of a medicinal regime not only invites relapse but in some peculiar way often impairs the efficacy of the original dosage when it is again adopted. I have for a very long time made it a practice not to begin graded withdrawal until two years have passed in security, and have sometimes been impressed by the unwillingness of the patient to accept a proposal for even moderate decrease.

Undoubtedly those cases respond best to bromide that best tolerate its long-continued use. If judiciously administered, no complication need be feared; but when the total amount is too high symptoms of bromism may develop, in the shape of mental dullness and apathy, loss of memory, and general sluggishness of the functions of the body — in particular, a stagnant circulation with cold and blue extremities. Bromide acne sometimes covers face and back, its apparition being attributable more to drug impurities and personal idiosyncrasy than actual dosage. It can be obviated to a large extent by the use of arsenic in the bromide mixture; if rather inveterate, it should be treated with sulphur ointments or by resort to vaccine methods [1]. In a comparatively small number of cases bromide is badly tolerated from the outset and becomes harmful when pushed; the patient's well-being is upset mentally and physically, without compensatory improvement in respect of control of attacks. Under such circumstances other methods must be chosen. The confirmed epileptic, too, does badly with the drug; its effects are then procured only at the expense of serious toxic and other untoward symptoms. But if a "bromide life", as it may be termed, has been lived for years, unwise reduction with a view to bettering the patient's general condition may only serve to incite development of status.

Although major epilepsy responds well in average examples to bromide administration, greater difficulty is often experienced with the minor variety, for which, accordingly, other medicaments may have to be tried.

Combinations of the drug with other sedatives are much in vogue; some of the latter will be mentioned presently.

There are many preparations (secret or otherwise) on the market whose staple ingredient is simply one or other salt of bromide. They include bromocarpine (potassium bromide and pilocarpine), bromipin or brominol (bromide and sesame oil), bromalin (hexamin ethyl bromide), GÉLINEAU's dragées (potassium bromide, antimony arsenate, and picrotoxin), sedobrol (sodium bromide and sodium chloride), "ozerine" (potassium bromide and ammonium carbonate), "TRENCH's remedy" (potassium and ammonium bromide), etc. Of all those (not "secret") which I have tried the dragées of GÉLINEAU have seemed the best; they are in solid form and convenient for use, while the total dosage can be suitably modified by taking more or fewer.

b) *Luminal* (phenyl-ethyl-barbituric acid), introduced in 1912 (its French equivalent is gardenal) was at first thought likely to supplant bromide as a remedy of choice, though it is not its equal in general applicability; luminal sodium is soluble and has proved in personal experience as efficacious as the original. The same principles should be observed as in the case of bromide; an endeavour should be made to concentrate on the times when fits may appear, and the effect should not be weakened by too small and too frequent doses. In general, it is best to commence with say half a grain of the sodium salt morning and evening, increasing to three-quarters or one grain if desirable; three or four grains in the 24 hours should represent a maximum. On the whole, major epilepsy responds better to luminal than the minor form; other types and variants also do well with it, especially perhaps those of the epileptic borderland and cases with mental symptoms. The drug is often serviceable, also, in conjunction with bromide (luminal sodium is incompatible with the ammonium salt), or borax, or other sedatives used for epileptic treatment.

Its advantages (apart from tablet form and convenient bulk) are comprised in the absence of mental depression and lowering of somatic function when exhibited for a long period; disadvantages include the comparative ease with which tolerance is established. Its effective dose, also, is not far removed from the toxic dose, since scarlatiniform and other rashes appear with some readiness; vertigo, ataxia, and either restlessness or torpor and stupor may develop if the

---

[1] Cf. Taylor, Brit. med. J. **2** (1913).

drug is pushed too far. The risk of sudden stoppage is the same as with bromide, viz. abrupt increase of fits.

According to personal experience luminal acts best in mild and moderate epilepsies, given alone; for more severe or semi-chronic cases its combination with bromide or other sedative is advisable; and it appears to have least value in serial types recurring at longish intervals.

The literature on the subject is lengthy; a few selected papers are those of FUCHS, DERCUM, SANDS, GOLLA, TYLOR, FOX, DARLING, RUSSELL BRAIN, JOHNSON, FRANKHAUSER, DIVRY, VAN DER LOEFF and BARNHOORN.

c) Other valuable if somewhat uncertain medicaments include *borax* (introduced by GOWERS) and some of its compounds. Sodium biborate in doses of 5—15 grs. twice a day or of 10 grs. thrice often proves very satisfactory for both major and minor varieties either by itself or coupled with bromide or luminal. In 1920 PIERRE MARIE advocated treatment with the double tartrate of borax and potassium; a dosage of 45 grs. in the 24 hours was recommended. Borax serves well in traumatic and "organic" cases also and no particular disadvantages attach to its use. *Belladonna* in union with bromide also merits favourable mention; to secure the best results not less than from 5 to 15 minims of the tincture should be taken two or three times a day. At the National Hospital it has long enjoyed a reputation in regard especially to petit mal; five grains of sodium bromide and five minims of belladonna twice daily or oftener, have frequently justified the confidence reposed in the combination. Many other medicines have been given trials and some on occasion seem to benefit the patient e.g. zinc oxide, iron, digitalis or strophanthus, calcium; opiates and hypnotics generally fail to exert any particular influence. *Dialacetin*, however, praised by CUSHNY as superior to luminal, occasionally procures relief (HALL, WORSTER-DROUGHT); representing a combination of dial with allylparacetaminophenol, it has been given with advantage in cases of nocturnal epilepsy. Little attention has been paid to *nitroglycerine*, whose effect is commonly dismissed as inappreciable; but I have been impressed with its usefulness in selected cases, notably those for which bromide has been taken over a number of years. On theoretical grounds it should prove of value for minor attacks resembling faints, and I have found it so in practice; in visceral fits, too, it is remarkably helpful, being in point of fact almost a specific; given in the form of liquor trinitrini, combined with liquor strychninae and a small dose of sodium bromide, it can be strongly recommended.

No useful purpose would be served by further comment on the list of drugs vaunted at one time or another; all must stand the test of experience, and if those which have successfully done so can be numbered on the fingers of one hand we should always be prepared to institute empirical treatment (in the absence of etiological knowledge) with any alleged remedy until failure compels us to discard it.

6. Symptomatic Treatment. *During an actual seizure* of major type nothing can be done except to loosen the clothes at the neck for freedom of respiration, to obviate accident by a quick consideration of the circumstances and the use of common sense, to prevent tongue-biting by insertion between the teeth of any suitable object at hand, cork or indiarubber being preferable to harder materials. The patient should be allowed to sleep his attack out, nor is any stimulant requisite. In the case of fits preceded by an aura of measurable duration the possibility of arrest always presents itself. JACKSONian convulsions can sometimes be curbed, and their onset checked, by gripping the part involved, by a ligature tied firmly round the segment in which they begin, or by forcible extension of a limb that is flexing; in the former instance a piece of tape can be left in situ, ready for an emergency. Blistering in a circle round the segment first affected has had its advocates, as a kind of "permanent" control, but this can be more rationally effected by ascertaining the cause of the JACKSONian fits and dealing with it. When aura and convulsions are of a more general kind a powerful or violent stimulus may so influence the sensorium as to inhibit the commencing discharge; smelling salts may be applied to the nostrils, or amyl nitrite inhaled; GOWERS mentions chewing a piece of ginger, and NOTHNAGEL advised swallowing a mouthful of common salt. No allusion to the merits of *alcohol* in this connexion has come under my notice; considered taboo for all epilepsies, it has within my knowledge proved a valuable means of warding off a fit in more than one case. A patient whose attack seemed to "work about him" before its actual evolution was always able to arrest it by a glass of beer, and another, by a tablespoonful of whisky; the influence of alcohol in dilating capillaries and stimulating cardiac action deserves bearing in mind. Epileptic subjects occasionally discover some or other precedure for themselves; in one instance an epigastric aura was never followed by an attack if eructation could be brought about; in another, immediate getting out of doors sufficed.

The treatment of *status epilepticus* depends to some extent on the particular circumstances inducing it. Should it have followed omission of bromide or other sedatives the natural remedy is to institute such measures without delay; but if it develops in spite of appropriate medication little benefit will be derived from massive increase.

When status is threatened, it may sometimes be averted by the use of bromide and opiates in combination; the prescription of CLARK and PROUT can be recommended for the purpose, composed of tinct. opii m. 5, potass. bromid. grs. 25, chloral hydrat. grs. 20, and liq. morph. sulph. m. 60. It is administered by mouth or rectum and repeated in two hours. Should the condition have supervened because of premature abandonment of sedation, large doses of bromide and choral must be tried; 60 grs. of the former may be combined with 20 or 30 grs. of the latter for rectal administration every four or six hours. Other means of controlling the convulsions should however be sought; hypodermic injection of luminal sodium (grs. 1—3) in a freshly prepared solution can be approved (cf. KIMBER), and bromide (10 per cent.) may be utilised in the same way. Repeated drainage of spinal fluid by lumbar puncture is also serviceable, and instillation of bromide solutions by the same route has sometimes appeared to assist. Hypodermics of hyoscine hydrobromide (gr. 1/75 or 1/50) repeated within an hour or two, are a useful adjunct on occasion; paraldehyde [1] in doses up to 8 dr., mixed with an equal quantity of olive oil and given per rectum, is another sedative worthy of trial. Chloroform inhalation is of course only a temporary expedient, but may be resorted to at an early stage, not later; oxygen inhalation, too, may be applied with advantage. Venesection and injection of saline can be performed in the robust.

In all cases, undue depressant effects must be combated by the utmost support to the strength of the heart and body generally, for which strychnine, digitalis, and alcohol may be required, and by careful attention to food and drink, nor must diuretics and cathartics he overlooked. Plain nourishing liquids should be given by nasal tube from the outset.

7. Surgical Treatment. Any surgical treatment applicable to the epilepsies has hitherto concerned mainly, though not solely, the collateral pathological states found from time to time in connexion therewith. When fits constitute the incidental accompaniment of such varieties of cerebral lesion as may be

---

[1] Cf. Collier. Lancet **1928 I**.

amenable to surgical skill it is proper to deal with these accordingly in the expectation of effecting a cure, or at least relief. But for those of cryptogenic character the question of operative interference, if it is to be raised from the level of sheer empiricism, must be decided by reference to the mechanism of production of fits, and only after knowledge of their precise determinants has been gained. Whether that stage has yet been reached can hardly be stated positively, though we must allow that at the present time we are better aware both of what goes on during a fit and of what pathological conditions result from or are combined with frequent attacks than were those of an older generation.

a) Trephining, an ancient remedy, can have no justification if it is proposed with a view to relief of intracranial pressure, for, as is recognised, epilepsy of unknown origin is not accompanied by such a state in any permanent fashion. On the other hand, as we have seen, oedematous conditions of meninges and brain not infrequently are associated with chronic epilepsy, and if these can be removed, or at least alleviated, by opening the skull and incising the membranes the operation may be thought to possess a modicum of virtue. In 1911 a series of 20 cases of the kind, in which craniotomy was performed and "fenestration" produced were reported by ALEXANDER and encouraging results claimed. He chose otherwise intractable cases and in every instance noted oedema of the pia-arachnoid. Analogous measures have been adopted by others before and after him, notably KOCHER and DANDY, but the method, however palliative, has never been viewed with much favour.

Dehydration, however, can be accomplished by resort to a simpler and different technique. TEMPLE FAY has published his findings in a series of 22 patients in whom active dehydration was effected by magnesium sulphate, intravenous glucose, spinal drainage, and restriction of fluid intake. So far as concerns the last of these, liquid allowed in the 24 hours ranged from a minimum of six ounces to a maximum of 18. His cases were observed for a period of two and a half years, and favourable results accrued. The procedure is based on a sound theory but in practice it is not a little unpleasant and requires faithful cooperation on the part of the epileptic. Further clinical research along the same lines is desirable, for in other hands control of the water-balance factor by similar means has not apparently been beneficial.

The question of trephining in *traumatic epilepsy* should be influenced by two considerations; firstly whether there is clinical or clinico-pathological evidence of a focal origin for the fits and secondly whether the lesion consequent on operation is likely to prove less of an irritant than the original one. Vague histories of a blow or fall on the head are insufficient for practical purposes unless substantiated by clinical proof of local abnormality in the shape of aura or commencing spasm; but when the type of fit manifestly belongs to the JACKSONian class, or though generalised reveals by its initial phenomena the cortical site of the discharging lesion, the matter of exploratory operation should be seriously discussed. Researches alluded to in a previous section have shown conclusively how meningo-cortical cicatrices slowly contract and exercise a "pull" on cerebral tissues; but since a clean excision of brain substance is not followed by much glial hyperplasia and cicatricial "pull" it is evident that the sequelae of injury and of operation are not identical. In other word, the knife will not leave behind it an irritant scar comparable to that of the trauma. There can be little doubt that removal of the actual point from which convulsions start and radiate, small though it be, has in a large number of cases been succeeded by enduring freedom from attacks. Similar considerations should guide decision in cases of chronic infantile hemiplegia distinguished by persistent fits with local commencement;

if they do not respond to accepted medical treatment the possibility of their being caused by cystic arachnoid accumulations of fluid and being relieved by operation should be entertained.

b) Excision of the cervical sympathetic ganglia, practised a number of years ago, was based on the conception that vasodilatation of cerebral vessels would follow thereby, so counteracting the anaemia inducing fits. Comparatively encouraging results were reported by JONNESCO and WINTER, the latter of whom obtained arrest or improvement in 44 cases out of 122, a success just as great as that of various other methods of treatment. In other hands they have been disappointing, more or less (e. g. WAGNER), yet the effect of periarterial sympathectomy of the carotid has definitely been beneficial (TINEL, BOJOVITCH, HIRSCH et al.). There can be no doubt that vasomotor control of cerebral arteries is a physiological fact, or that alterations in vessel calibre accompany the phenomena of the epileptic fit. Such circumstances throw new light on old ideas of epileptic causation, and study of vascular-cellular relationships may yet prove fruitful for treatment.

A suggestive experiment made by PENFIELD also becomes of interest in this connexion. His case was that of a boy who suffered from generalised attacks and in whom periarterial sympathectomy of the right carotid and vertebral arteries was performed, with the result that convulsive movements thereafter were strictly confined to the right side of the body, the left being free. Further investigation along similar lines may prove very informative.

8. Psychotherapeutic Treatment. That psychoanalysis and psychotherapy in general should have left epilepsy severely alone was hardly to be expected. Attention has already been given to resemblances between some epileptic and some hysterical fits, to induction of the former by affective stimuli such as commonly introduce the latter, to "equivalents" of a psychical kind, and to polymorphic auras and other symptoms belonging to the psychical series. Involvement of the mental level in epilepsy, at one phase or another, is apparent to every observer. But whether such data justify the view assigning to the condition a psychogenic origin, and one amenable to psychological treatment, is more than dubious. Throughout these pages the evidence for the physiological basis of epilepsy has accumulated to such a degree as to render suspect any other hypothesis. It is impossible to regard with patience the assumption of STEKEL that the tongue-biting of the convulsed epileptic is not accidental but the expression of his unconscious longing to bite and to see blood, or any of the numerous other "meanings" attached to the crude phenomena of the major seizure.

To me at present it seems that the proper attitude to adopt is to accept psychical factors initiating fits as only one among several classes, and to deal with them as with any other inciting causes, i. e. by removal where possible. Should such removal be accomplished by psychological methods it will be a gain to the patient, and eminently justifiable; but the physiological problems of the fit are untouched by psychotherapy.

Among those claiming good results by methods of the kind are Rows and BOND, STEKEL, PIERCE CLARK, GRAVES, WITTELS, HEBERER. Others are cited in REDLICH's article submitting the psychological theory to keen criticism.

If, in conclusion, a summary of present-day knowledge in respect of epileptic causation and treatment may be attempted, it will embrace the general statements that acidosis, dehydration, and oxygenation should be promoted; that alkalosis, oedema, and lowering of oxygen tension should be avoided; that recognisable excitants should be withdrawn or rendered harmless; and that the irritability of the "charged" nervous system should be reduced by sedatives.

Literature.

ADIE: Brain **47** (1924). — ALEXANDER: Lancet **1911 II**. — ALLEN: (a) Boston med. J. **174** (1906). (b) Arch. of Neur. **20** (1928). — ALLENDE-NAVARRO: Schweiz. Arch. Neur. **18** (1926). — ALTENBURGER u. GUTTMANN: Z. Neur. **112** (1928). — ALTENBURGER u. STERN: Z. Neur. **112** (1928). — ALZHEIMER: Z. Neur. **1** (1910). — ANDERSON: Brain **9** (1886). — ANDRIEZEN: Brit. med. J. **1897 I**, Nr 1896. — APELT: Epilepsia, Bd. 1. 1909. — ARETAEUS: Extant Works (New Sydenham Society), 1856. — AULD: Brit. med. J. **1920 II**.

BARBASH: J. ment. Sci. **77** (1931). — BAUGH: J. ment. Sci. **56** (1914). — BÄUMLER: Dtsch. Z. Nervenheilk. **39** (1910). — BAYLAC: Bull. Soc. méd. Hôp. Paris **47** (1923). — BECHTEREW: Arch. f. Psychiatr. **19** (1880). — BEEVOR: Brain **5** (1882). — BEHAGUE: C. r. Congr. Luxembourg 1921. — BELLAVITIS: Note Psichiatr. **18** (1930). — BERO, BES DE: Thèse de Montpellier 1871. — BERTOLANI: Riv. sper. Freniatr. **49** (1926). — BALINT: Neur. Zbl. **22** (1903). — BIELSCHOWSKY: Z. Neur. **18** (1912). — BIEULAC: Thèse de Paris **1920**. — BINGEL: Klin.Wschr. 1 (1922). — BINSWANGER: Nothnagels Handbuch, Bd.12. 1899.— BIRO: Dtsch. Z. Nervenheilk. **23** (1903). — BISGAARD: Acta med. scand. (Stockh.) **61** (1925). — BLEULER: Münch. med. Wschr. **42** (1895). — BOJOVITCH: Rev. de Chir. **63** (1925). — BONHOEFFER: Allg. Z. Psychiatr. **42** (1918). — BONNIER: Le vertige, 1904. — BOOTHBY and SANDIFORD: J. of biol. Chem. **54** (1922). — BOSSERT: Z. Neur. **67** (1921). — BOURNEVILLE: (a) Gaz. méd. Paris **4** (1874). (b) Progrès méd. **27** (1899). — BOURNEVILLE et BONNAIRE: Progrès méd. **10** (1882). — BOUTTIER: Questions neurologiques d'actualité, 1922. — BOWMAN and FRY: Arch. of Neur. **14** (1925). — BOYCE: Brit. med. J. **1893 II**, Nr 1716. — BRAIN, RUSSELL: (a) Quart. J. exper. Physiol. **16** (1926). (b) Quart. J. Med. **19** (1926). (c) Lancet **1929 I**; **1929 II**. — BRAIN and STRAUSS: Recent Advances in Neurology, 1930. — BRAMWELL and GRAHAM BROWN: Rev. of Neur. **3** (1905). — BRATZ: (a) Allg. Z. Psychiatr. **63** (1906); Mschr. Psychiatr. **29** (1911). (b) Mschr. Psychiatr. **47** (1920). — BRAVAIS: L'hémiplégie épileptique, 1827. — BRIDGE and IOB: Amer. J. Psychiatr. **10** (1931). — BROADBENT: Lancet **1887 I**. — BROWN-SÉQUARD: C. r. Soc. Biol. Paris **2** (1851). — BRÜHL: Z. Neur. **84** (1923). — BUSCAINO: (a) Schweiz. Arch. Neur. **11** (1922). (b) Riv. Pat. nerv. **30** (1925). — BURR: (a) Arch. of Neur. **7** (1922). (b) Arch. of Pediatr. **39** (1922). — BUZZARD: Lancet **1906 I**.

CALMEIL: De la paralysie considérée chez les aliénés, 1826. — CAMPBELL: J. of Physiol. **60** (1925). — CANEO: Riv. sper. Freniatr. **49** (1925). — CARPENTER: Amer. J. med. Sci. **173** (1927). — CATALANO: Riv. sper. Freniatr. **49** (1925). — CELSUS: See Van Wageningen. Nederl. Tijdschr. Geneesk. **72** (1923). — CENI: Riv. sper. Freniatr. **32** (1906). — CESTAN: Les épilepsies, 1922. — CHARCOT: Oeuvres complètes, Tome 2. 1894. — CHIRÉE: Ann. de Gynéc. **5** (1908). — CHOROSKO: Neur. Zbl. **27** (1908). — CLARK: (a) Arch. Neur. a. Psychopath. (N. Y.) **2** (1899). (b) J. nerv. Dis. **63** (1926). (c) Amer. J. med. Sci. **172** (1926). — CLARK, PIERCE: Brain **43** (1920). — CLARK and PROUT: Amer. J. Insan. **59** (1902); **60** (1903—04). — CLARKE: Lancet **1900 I**. — CLAUDE: C. r. Soc. Biol. Paris **97** (1927). — CLAUDE et SCHMIERGELD: Encéphale **4** (1909). — COBB: Epilepsy, 1928. — COLLIER: Lancet **1928 I**. — COLMAN: Lancet **1890 II**. — COOKSON: Arch. Dis. Childh. **11** (1927). — COOPER, ASTLEY: Guy's Hosp. Rep. **1** (1836). — CRAMER: See BRUNS and ZIEHEN: Handbuch der Nervenkrankheiten im Kindesalter, 1912. — CRICHTON-BROWNE: Lancet **1895 II**. — CRINIS, DE: (a) Die Beteiligung der humoralen Lebensvorgänge am epileptischen Anfall, 1920. (b) Spezielle Pathologie und Therapie der inneren Krankheiten von KRAUS u. BRUGSCH, 1922. — CROUZON: Le syndrome épilepsie, 1929. — CROUZON et BOUTTIER: Bull. Soc. méd. Hôp. Paris **45** (1921). — CUNEO: Riv. sper. Freniatr. **49** (1925). — CURSCHMANN: Dtsch. Z. Nervenheilk. **75** (1922). — CUSHNY: Textbook of Pharmacology, 1928.

DALMA: Riv. sper. Freniatr. **49** (1925). — DANDRY: (a) Ann. Surg. **70** (1919). (b) Amer. J. Psychiatr. **6** (1927). — DANDY and ELMAN: Bull. Hopkins Hosp. **36** (1925). — DANNHAUSER: Z. Neur. **96** (1925). — DARLING: Arch. of Neur. **9** (1923). — DAVENPORT: (a) J. nerv. Dis. **42** (1915). (b) Arch. of Neur. **9** (1923). — DAVENPORT and WEEKS: J. nerv. Dis. **38** (1911). — DEJERINE: Hérédité dans les maladies du système nerveux, 1886. — DELASIAUVE: Traité de épilepsie, 1854. — DERCUM: Ther. Gaz. **35** (1919). — D'HOLLANDER: Arch. méd. belges **72** (1919). — DIDE: Ann. méd.-psychol. **10** (1899). — DIELLMANN: Münch. med. Wschr. **74** (1927). — DIVRY: Encéphale **17** (1922). — DORAN: Amer. J. Insan. **60** (1903). — DUNCAN, GLEN: J. ment. Sci. **76** (1930). — DUNSMURE: Edinburgh med. J. **20** (1874). — DUTIL: Rev. Méd. **3** (1883).

EDEL: Allg. Z. Psychiatr. **65** (1908). — EDGEWORTH: Brit. med. J. **1920 II**, Nr 3125. — ELLIOTSON: Quoted by Féré (v. i.). — ELSBERG and PIKE: Amer. J. Physiol. **81** (1926). — ELSBERG and STOOKEY: Arch. of Neur. **9** (1923). — ESQUIROL: (a) Traité des maladies mentales, Tome 1. 1838. (b) Quoted by LENOIR (v. i.). — EUSIÈRE et DELMAS: Montpellier méd. **30** (1910). — EVERKE: Mschr. Geburtsh. **61** (1923).

FACKENHEIM: Zbl. Neur. **49** (1926). — FAGGE: Textbook of Medicine, Vol. 1. 1886. — FAY: (a) Amer. J. Psychiatr. **8** (1929). (b) J. nerv. Dis. **71** (1930). — FAY and WINKELMAN:

Arch. of Neur. **23** (1930). — FÉRÉ: (a) Épilepsies et épileptiques, 1897. (b) C. r. Soc. Biol. Paris **40** (1888). — FILIA: Rev. Hyg. et Méd. infant. **2** (1903). — FINCHER and DOWMAN: J. amer. med. Assoc. **97** (1931). — FINCKH: Arch. f. Psychiatr. **39** (1905). — FIRTH: J. of Neur. **1** (1920). — FISCHER: Neur. Zbl. **12** (1893). — FLESCH: Wien. klin. Wschr. **28** (1915). — FOERSTER: (a) Z. Neur. **94** (1924—25). (b) Zbl. Neur. **44** (1926). (c) Verh. Ges. deutsch. Nervenärzte, 1926. (d) Dtsch. Z. Nervenheilk. **94** (1926). (e) Die Leitungsbahnen des Schmerzgefühls, 1927. (f) Brain **53** (1930). — FOERSTER and PENFIELD: Brain **53** (1930). — FOG and SCHMIDT: J. of Neur. **12** (1931). — FORD and SCHAFFER: Arch. of Neur. **18** (1927). — FOSHAY: Amer. J. Physiol. **73** (1925). — FOSTER: Arch. int. Med. **34** (1924). — FOX, TAYLOR: Lancet **1927 II**. — FRANK: Verh. Ges. inn. Med. **36** (1924). — FRANKHAUSER: Z. Neur. **17** (1913). — FREUDENBERG: Z. Kinderheilk. **41** (1926). — FRIEDMANN: Dtsch. Z. Nervenheilk. **30** (1906). — FRINK: N. Y. med. J. **93** (1911). — FRISCH: (a) Z. exper. Med. **56** (1927). (b) Wien. klin. Wschr. **41** (1928). — FRISCH and FRIED: Z. exper. Med. **49** (1926). — FRISCH and WALTER: Z. Neur. **79** (1922). — FUCHS: Münch. med. Wschr. **61** (1914). — FULTON: Muscular Contraction, 1926.

GAMBLE: J. of biol. Chem. **57** (1923). — GAMBLE and HAMILTON: Hopkins Hosp. Bull. **41** (1927). — GÄRTNER: Z. exper. Med. **51** (1926). — GASPERO: See Lewandowskys Handbuch der Neurologie, Bd. 5. 1912. — GEORGI: Dtsch. Z. Nervenheilk. **83** (1924—25). — GEYELIN: Med. Rec. **99** (1921). — GEYELIN and PENFIELD: Arch. of Neur. **21** (1929). — GOLDBLOOM: Canad. med. Assoc. J. **12** (1922). — GOLLA: Brit. med. J. **1921 II**, Nr 3165. — GORDON: J. of Neur. **8** (1928). — GOTCH and HORSLEY: Philos. trans. roy. Soc. Lond. **182** (1892). — GÖTT: See Pfaundlers und Schlossmanns Handbuch der Kinderheilkunde, Bd. 4. 1924. — GOWERS: (a) Lancet **1879 I**. (b) Trans. ophthalm. Soc. **15** (1895). (c) Epilepsy, 1901. (d) The Borderland of Epilepsy, 1907. (e) Brain **32** (1909). — GRAVES: Cited by REDLICH (v. i.). — GRUHLE: Zbl. Neur. **34** (1923). — GUTTMANN: (a) Z. Neur. **119** (1929). (b) Z. Neur. **136** (1931).

HALL: Lancet **1924 II**. — HAMILTON: J. of biol. Chem. **65** (1925). — HAMMOND: Medical Annual, 1901. — HARE, FRANCIS: Austral. med. Gaz. **22** (1903). — HARRIS: Lancet **1896 I**. — HARTENBERG: (a) Encéphale **19** (1924). (b) Presse méd. **32** (1924). — HEBERER: Cited by REDLICH (v. i.). — HEILBRONNER: Dtsch. Z. Nervenheilk. **31** (1907). — HELD: Berl. klin. Wschr. **57** (1920). — HELMHOLTZ: J. amer. med. Assoc. **88** (1927). — HENDRIKSEN: Acta psychiatr. (København) **5** (1930). — HENNING: Analecta litteraria epilepsiam spectantia, 1798. — HERPIN: L'Épilepsie, 1852. — HILL: Allbutts System of Med., Vol. 8. 1910. — HIRSCH: J. amer. med. Assoc. **80** (1927). — HOCHSINGER: Dtsch. Klin. **7** (1912). — HOLMES: Lancet **1927 I**. — HOLSTRÖM: Uppsala Läk.för. Förh. **29** (1924). — HOROSHKO: Z. Neur. **98** (1925). — HORRAX: See COBB and MACDONALD: J. of Neur. **4** (1923). — HORSLEY: (a) Brit. med. J. **1892 I**, Nr 1622, Nr 1623, Nr 1631, Nr 1638, Nr 1639. (b) Brain **29** (1906).

JACKSON: (a) A study of convulsions 1870. (b) Brit. med. J. **1890 I**, Nr 1523. — JACKSON, HUGHLINGS: (a) Med. Tim. Gaz. **1864**, 1. (b) Ophthalm. Hosp. Rep. **5** (1866). (c) Lancet **1878 II**; **1881 I**; **1895 I**. (d) Brain **11** (1888); **22** (1899); **29** (1906); **32** (1909). (e) Selected Writings, Vol. 1. 1931. — JACOBI: Z. Neur. **85** (1923). — JAMHANZI: Boll. manicom. Ferrara **1** (1909). — JANET: Les obsessions et la psychasthénie, 1903. — JELGERSMA: Nederl. Tijdschr. Geneesk. **24** (1888). — JENKIN and PENDLETON: J. amer. med. Assoc. **68** (1914). — JOB: Amer. J. Psychiatr. **10** (1931). — JOHN: Arch. int. Med. **39** (1927). — JONNESCO: Zbl. Chir. **24** (1897); **26** (1899). — JOHNSON: Lancet **1922 II**. — JOSAT: Recherches historiques sur l'épilepsie, 1856.

KARGER: Klin. Wschr. **5** (1926). — KEITH: Amer. J. Dis. Childr. **41** (1931). — KENNEDY: Arch. of Neur. **9** (1923). — KENNEDY, FOSTER: Arch. int. Med. **8** (1911). — KIMBER: Brit. med. J. **1906 I**. — KNAPP: Mschr. Psychiatr. **46** (1919). — KNEIDEL: Cited by STÜBER (v. i.). — KNOWLEDGE: Brit. med. J. **1927 I**. — KOCHER: Dtsch. Z. Chir. **36** (1893); Korresp.bl. Schweiz. Ärzte **28** (1898). — KOGERER: Z. Neur. **86** (1923). — KOSHEWNIKOW: Neur. Zbl. **14** (1895). — KRETSCHMER: Zbl. Neur. **35** (1924). — KRUMBHOLZ: J. nerv. Dis. **40** (1913). — KULKOW: Arch. f. Psychiatr. **88** (1929). — KUSSMAUL u. TENNER: Molesch' Untersuchungen, Bd. 3. 1857.

LAFORA: Revue neur. **30** (1923). — LANGDON-BROWN and BRAIN: Lancet **1929 I**. — LEHMKUHL: Mschr. Kinderheilk. **36** (1927). — LENNOX: (a) Arch. int. Med. **38** (1926). (b) Arch. of Neur. **17** (1927). — LENNOX and ALLEN: (a) Arch. of Neur. **23**, **24** (1930). (b) Quoted by LENNOX and COBB, l. c. — LENNOX and COBB: (a) Arch. of Neur. **18** (1927). — (b) Arch. of Neur. **20** (1928). (c) Epilepsy, 1928. — LENNOX and WRIGHT: Arch. of Neur. **20** (1928). — LENOIR: Thèse de Paris **1901**. — LERICHE: Presse méd. **28** (1920). — LEROY: Thèse de Paris 1880. — LEURET: Arch. gén. Méd. **2** (1843). — LÉVI: (a) Presse méd. **13** (1905). (b) Arch. of Neur. **15** (1926). — LEYSER: Mschr. Psychiatr. **52** (1922). — LIND: Med. J. Austral. **2** (1926). — LOCOCK: Lancet **1857 I**. — LOEFF, VAN DER and BARNHOORN: Neurotherapie, Juli/Okt. 1926. — LONG-LANDRY and QUEROY: Revue neur. **26** (1913). — LORENZ: Inaug.-Diss. Kiel 1890. — LOVNER: Arch. f. Psychiatr. **41** (1906). — LÖWENBERG: Z. Neur. **87** (1923). — LUCAS and SOUTHARD: Boston med. J. **166** (1912). — LUCRETIUS: De rerum natura. — LUNDBORG: Die progressive Myoklonus-Epilepsie, 1903.

MACDONALD and COBB: J. of Neur. 4 (1923). — MCDONNELL: Dublin med. J. 37 (1864). — MCDOUGALL: J. ment. Sci. 65 (1919). — MCKENDRICK: Brain 22 (1899). — MACKENNAN: Arch. of Neur. 4 (1920). — MACLEOD: Carbohydrate Metabolism and Insulin. 1926. — MCQUARRIE and KEITH: Amer. J. Dis. Childr. 34 (1927). — MAES and CLAUDE: Ann. Électrobiol. 10 (1907). — MANNINI: Gazz. Osp. 21 (1900). — MARBURG: Wien. klin. Wschr. 32 (1919). — MARCHAND: (a) Revue neur. 38 (1922). (b) L'hygiène ment. 26 (1931). — MARIE, PIERRE: Presse méd. 28 (1920). — MARIE e NACHMAN: Arch. di Antrop. crimin. 5 (1913). — MARTIN: J. of Neur. 5 (1925). — MASSAGLIA: J. Lancet 44 (1924). — MEYER: (a) Mschr. Psychiatr. 31 (1912). (b) See SACHS and HAUSMAN: Nervous and Mental Disorders, 1926. — MEYER and BRÜHL: Z. Neur. 75 (1922). — MILIZYN: Mschr. Psychiatr. 61 (1926). — MILLER: (a) Amer. J. med. Sci. 168 (1924). (b) J. of Neur. 8 (1927). — MILLER and TRESCHER: Amer. J. med. Sci. 174 (1927). — MILLS: (a) Boston med. J. 94 (1906). (b) J. amer. med. Assoc. 51 (1908). — MIXTER: Arch. of Neur. 9 (1923). — MOON: Lancet 1926 II. — MOREAU: See BINSWANGER, l. c. — MORIARTY: Amer. J. Dis. Childr. 28 (1924). — MORSE: J. amer. med. Assoc. 78 (1922). — MORSELLI: Eulenbergs Realenzyklopädie, Bd. 7. 1895. — MOTT: Croonian Lectures, 1900. — MOTTE, LA: Quoted by MUSKENS (v. i.). — MOXON: Lancet 1881 I. — MÜLLER: Dtsch. Z. Nervenheilk. 28 (1905). — MÜLLER and PETERSON: Klin. Wschr. 5 (1926). — MUNSON: Annual Rep. Craig Colony 1918. — MUSKENS: (a) Arch. f. Psychiatr. 36 (1903). (b) Die Epilepsie, 1928. — MYERSON: The Inheritance of Mental Diseases, 1925.

NERRLINGER: Inaug.-Diss. Straßburg 1889. — NIELSEN and EGGLESTON: J. amer. med. Assoc. 94 (1930). — NIELSON: Med. J. Rec. 122 (1925). — NINDE: Auditory Memory Test in Institutional Epileptics, 1924. — NOTHNAGEL: Dtsch. Arch. klin. Med. 3 (1867). — NOTKIN: J. nerv. Dis. 72 (1930).

OBANIO: Quoted by MILLER (v. supra). — OCHSENHANDLER: Schweiz. Arch. Neur. 15 (1924). — OLMSTEDT and LOGAN: Amer. J. Physiol. 66 (1923). — OPPENHEIM: (a) Mschr. Psychiatr. 9 (1903). (b) Z. Neur. 42 (1918). — ORLOWSKI: Neur. Zbl. 15 (1896). — ORR: J. of Neur. 11 (1930). — OSNATO: Brain 50 (1927).

PAGNIEZ: (a) Presse méd. 32 (1924). (b) L'Épilepsie, 1929. — PANCOAST and FAY: Amer. J. Roentgenol. 21 (1929). — PAPPENHEIM: Neur. Zbl. 36 (1917). — PARHON: Bull. Soc. rom. Neur. 3 (1926). — PATRICK and LEVY: J. amer. med. Assoc. 82 (1924). — PATRY: Amer. J. Psychiatr. 10 (1931). — PENFIELD: (a) Arch. of Neur. 21 (1929). (b) Canad. med. Assoc. J. 23 (1930). — PETERMANN: J. amer. med. Assoc. 90 (1928). — PEZZALI: Riforma med. 39 (1923). — PFEIFFER: (a) Klin. Wschr. 4 (1925). (b) Z. Neur. 103 (1926). — PICK: Wien. med. Wschr. 49 (1899). — PIÉRON: Unpublished records, quoted by MARCHAND (v. supra). — PIKE and ELSBERG: Amer. J. Physiol. 72 (1925). — PILCZ: Jb. Psychiatr. 46 (1928). — PILOTTI: Riv. sper. Freniatr. 14 (1922). — PITRES: Revue neur. 8 (1888). — POLLOCK and FURBUSH: Ment. Hyg. 11 (1927). — POLLOSON and COLLET: Revue neur. 28 (1914—15). — POPEA and VICOL: C. r. Soc. Biol. Paris 93 (1925). — PORTAL: Sur la nature de l'épilepsie, 1827. — PÖTZL: Med. Klin. 19 (1923). — PRICHARD: Diseases of the Nervous System, 1822. — PRIOR and JONES: J. ment. Sci. 64 (1918). — PROUT: Amer. J. Insan. 60 (1903); 61 (1904). — PUTNAM and WATERMAN: Boston med. J. 153 (1905). Case 2.

RABOT: Thèse de Paris 1899. — RAECKE: Transitorische Bewußtseinstörungen der Epileptiker, 1903. — RAMSKILL: Med. Tim. Gaz. 1863, 2. — REBATTU: Lyon méd. 131 (1922). — REDLICH: (a) Mschr. Psychiatr. 30 (1911). (b) Z. Neur. 48 (1919). (c) Nervenarzt 2 (1929). — REDLICH and PÖTZL: Z. Neur. 3 (1910). — REICH: Zbl. Nervenheilk. 14 (1903). — RENZO, DI: Riv. Pat. nerv. 36 (1930). — REYNOLDS: (a) Rev. of Neur. 4 (1906). (b) Brit. med. J. 1921 II, Nr 3159. — REYNOLDS, RUSSEL: Epilepsy, 1861. — RIBOT: The Psychology of the Emotions, 1896. — RISGAARD u. NORVIG: Z. Neur. 83 (1923). — ROBINSON: Lancet 1927 II. — RODIET: Arch. de Neur. 32 (1910). — ROGERS: Lancet 1862 II. — ROLLAND: De l'épilepsie Jacksonienne, 1888. — ROSETT: Brain 47 (1924). — ROTHMANN: (a) Z. klin. Med. 44 (1902). (b) Dtsch. Z. Nervenheilk. 45 (1912). — ROWS and BOND: Epilepsy, 1926. — RUSSELL: (a) Proc. roy. Soc. Med. 1 (1907). (b) Clin. J. 34 (1909). (c) S. afric. med. Rec. 20 (1922). — RYLE: Guy's Hosp. Rep. 78 (1928).

SACKS u. ZANDER: Biochem. Z. 188 (1927). — SANDS: Arch. of Neur. 5 (1921). — SARBÓ: Der heutige Stand der Epilepsie, 1905. — SARGENT: Brain 44 (1921). — SAWASAKI: Pflügers Arch. 209 (1925). — SCHIFF: Lehrbuch der Physiologie, 1858. — SCHLAPP: Quoted by SHANAHAN (v. i.). — SCHMIERGELD: Presse méd. 16 (1908). — SCHOU and SUSMAN: Brain 50 (1927). — SCHOU and TEGLBJOERG: Hosp. tid. (dän.) 68 (1925). — SCHUPFER: Mschr. Psychiatr. 7 (1900). — SCHWARTZ: Allg. Z. Psychiatr. 82 (1925). — SÉGLAS: Thèse de Paris 1880. — SHANAHAN: Amer. J. Psychiatr. 7 (1928). — SHERRILL: J. metabol. Res. 5 (1924). — SHERRINGTON: Proc. roy. Soc. B. 97 (1924—25). — SICARD and LERMOYEZ: Bull. Soc. méd. Hôp. Paris 46 (1922). — SIEVEKING: Epilepsy, 1861. — SITTIG: Brain 48 (1925). — SJÖGREN u. TILLGREN: Acta med. scand. (Stockh.) 65 (1927). — SOUTHARD: Amer. J. Insan. 64 (1907—08). — SPANGLER: Med. J. Rec. 122 (1925). — SPIELMEYER: (a) Histopathologie

des Nervensystems, 1922. (b) Z. Neur. **119** (1927). — SPILLER: (a) J. abnorm. a. soc. Psychol. **1** (1907). (b) J. amer. med. Assoc. **52** (1909). (c) Brain **50** (1927). — SPRATLING: Epilepsy, 1904. — STALLMANN: Allg. Z. Psychiatr. **88** (1911). — STEFFENS: Arch. f. Psychiatr. **39** (1904). — STECKEL: Cited by REDLICH (v. supra). — STERLING: Revue neur. **2** (1924). — STERTZ: Der extrapyramidale Symptomenkomplex, 1921. — STEWART: J. of exper. Med. **8** (1906). — STEWART and HOLMES: Brain **27** (1904). — STIER: Z. Neur. **80** (1922—23). — STÜBER: Zbl. Neur. **25** (1921). — SYZ: Amer. J. Psychiatr. **7** (1927).
TAFT: J. of Neur. **2** (1921). — TALBOT: (a) Amer. J. Dis. Childr. **28** (1924). (b) Boston med. J. **196** (1927). (c) Treatment of Epilepsy, 1931. — TALBOT and MORIARTY: Amer. J. Dis. Childr. **33** (1927). — TARGOWLA: C. r. Soc. Biol. Paris **93** (1925). — THOM: (a) Epilepsia **5** (1915). (b) Boston med. J. **175** (1916). (c) Arch. of Neur. **10** (1924). — THOM and SOUTHARD: Rev. of Neur. **13** (1915). — THOM: Illinois med. J. **26** (1914). — THURZÓ, DE: J. of Neur. **11** (1930). — TINEL: Revue neur. **41** (1925). — TODD: Clinical Lectures, 1861. — TOHEVERRIA: Ann. med.-psychol. **1** (1879). — TOULOUSE and MARCHAND: (a) Rev. de Psychiatr. **17** (1913). (b) Presse méd. **30** (1922). — TOULOUSE and RICHET: Quoted by TURNER (v. i.). — TREVISANELLO: Zbl. Bakter. **69** (1913). — TROUSSEAU: (a) Clin. med. **1** (1867—1868). — TSIMINAKIS: Wien. klin. Wschr. **28** (1915). — TUCKER: Arch. of Neur. **2** (1919). — TURNER: (a) Rev. of Neur. **2** (1904). (b) Epilepsy, 1907.
ULRICH: Med. J. Rec. **126** (1927). — UNVERRICHT: Dtsch. Z. Nervenheilk. **7** (1895). — UYEMATSU and COBB: Arch. of Neur. **7** (1922).
VALKENBURG, VAN: Zbl. Neur. **24** (1914). — VERAGUTH: Dtsch. Z. Nervenheilk. **24** (1903). — VINNING: Lancet **1922 I**. — VOGT: Epilepsie im Kindesalter, 1910. — VOLLAND: Z. Neur. **3** (1910). — VOLLMER: (a) Klin. Wschr. **4** (1925). (b) Z. Kinderheilk. **41** (1926). (c) Fortschr. Ther. **4** (1928).
WAGNER: Zbl. Chir. **52** (1925). — WALLIS: Lancet **1923 I**. — WALTHER: Klin. Wschr. **4** (1925). — WARD and PATTERSON: Arch. of Neur. **17** (1927). — WARTENBERG: Z. Neur. **94** (1924—25). — WEED: Amer. J. Physiol. **58** (1921). — WEEKS: J. metabol. Res. **8** (1923). — WEIDNER: Dtsch. med. Wschr. **50** (1924). — WEIMANN: (a) Mschr. Psychiatr. **51** (1922). (b) Z. Neur. **90** (1924). — WESTPHAL: Dtsch. med. Wschr. **45** (1919). — WESTPHAL and SIOLI: Arch. f. Psychiatr. **63** (1920). — WIERSMA: Fol. neurobiol. **3** (1910). — WIGGLESWORTH and WATSON: Brain **36** (1914). — WILDER: (a) Mayo Clin. Bull. **2** (1921). (b) Arch. int. Med. **38** (1926). — WILDERMUTH: Neur. Zbl. **16** (1897). — WILKS: Med. Tim. Gaz. **1861**, 2. — WILLIAMS, DUCKWORTH: On the Efficacy of the Bromide of Potassium, 1865. — WIMMER: Revue neur. **2** (1925). — WINTER: (a) Dtsch. Arch. klin. Med. **67** (1902). (b) Münch. med. Wschr. **70** (1923). — WITTELS: Cited by REDLICH (v. supra). — WOLFF and LENNOX: Arch. of Neur. **23** (1930). — WOODCOCK: Lancet **1919 II**. — WORCESTER: J. nerv. Dis. **24** (1897). — WORSTER-DROUGHT: Lancet **1925 II**. — WUTH: (a) Untersuchungen über die körperlichen Störungen bei Geisteskrankheiten, 1922. (b) Z. Neur. **101** (1926). (c) Bull. Hopkins Hosp. **38** (1926).
ZUNTZ: Zbl. Gynäk. **26** (1902).

Narkolepsie.
Mit Benützung der nachgelassenen Schriften EMIL REDLICHs †.

Von JOSEF WILDER-Wien.

Vorwort. Die Bearbeitung dieses Kapitels war dem besten Kenner dieses Gebietes, Prof. EMIL REDLICH, zugedacht. Eine Reihe von wichtigen Vorarbeiten hat REDLICH bereits geleistet, als ihn am 7. 6. 30 vorzeitig der Tod hinwegraffte. Das gesamte in seinem Nachlaß vorgefundene Material zu dieser Frage wurde von mir unter dem Titel „Epilegomena zur Narkolepsiefrage" im Jahre 1931 publiziert. Im Aufbau und Auffassung folgt dieses Kapitel hier dem Plane REDLICHs, die textliche Fassung und insbesondere die Erweiterung durch Berücksichtigung der großen Anzahl der in den Jahren 1930—1934 publizierten Fälle stammen von mir.

Definition. Unter Narkolepsie wollen wir hier verstehen eine chronische Erkrankung, charakterisiert in der Regel durch zwei Reihen von Erscheinungen: 1. Anfälle von mehrmals täglich auftretendem kurzen unbezwinglichen Schlaf (Schlafanfälle) und 2. eine eigenartige Reaktion auf freudige oder traurige Emotionen, bestehend in plötzlicher, meist mehrere Sekunden dauernder Erschlaffung der gesamten Skeletmuskulatur und Unmöglichkeit einer aktiven Bewegung, wodurch der Kranke unter Umständen zu Boden stürzt und bewegungslos liegen bleibt bei voll erhaltenem Bewußtsein.

Diese Definition soll nur zur vorläufigen Orientierung dienen. Sie hat dieselben Schwächen, wie jede Krankheitsdefinition. Die Narkolepsiefrage befindet sich gerade im Stadium einer lebhaften Diskussion, so daß es wenige Punkte dieser Definition gibt („Krankheit", „Schlaf" usw.), die nicht bei dem einen oder anderen Autor auf Widerspruch stoßen würden. Doch entspricht diese REDLICHsche Fassung der Meinung der überwiegenden Mehrheit der Kenner dieser Frage. Allerdings wird in folgendem (wie bei jeder anderen Krankheit) auf die notwendigen Einschränkungen und Erweiterungen dieser Definition hingewiesen, ebenso wie auf die Ausnahms- und auf die Grenzfälle.

Geschichte. Obwohl sich die Alten mit dem Problem des Schlafes lebhaft befaßten — GALEN, ARETAEUS, hinterließen Bücher über Lethargie —, wissen wir nicht, ob ihnen auch das Krankheitsbild der Narkolepsie bekannt war. Als der eigentliche Entdecker der Narkolepsie gilt GÉLINEAU (1880), welcher das Krankheitsbild mit seinen beiden Haupterscheinungen beschrieben und als eigene Krankheitseinheit erkannt hat. GÉLINEAU selbst zitiert allerdings auch einen Fall von CARRÉ aus dem Jahre 1862, der aber vom Autor nicht richtig gewürdigt wurde. GÉLINEAU hatte jedoch in Deutschland Vorläufer. WESTPHAL hat im Jahre 1877, F. FISCHER im Jahre 1878 je einen typischen Fall genau beschrieben. FISCHER faßt die Krankheit als epileptoid auf, WESTPHAL ebenfalls, jedoch mit Betonung, daß damit die Eigenart des Krankheitsbildes nicht voll gewürdigt ist. So ist es begreiflich, daß manche Autoren von der GÉLINEAUschen Krankheit, andere vom Morbus WESTPHAL-GÉLINEAU sprechen. Die Kenntnis der Krankheit war aber nicht sehr weit gedrungen, zum Teil wurde das Krankheitsbild auch durch die Arbeiten LHERMITTES und seiner Mitarbeiter, welche auf dem Standpunkt stehen, daß es fließende Übergänge zwischen den verschiedenen Arten von Schlafsucht gibt, und von „den Narkolepsien" sprechen, wieder verwischt, ebenso wie durch die Arbeiten FRIEDMANNs über Pyknolepsie. Eine wichtige Etappe in der weiteren Heraussonderung und Erforschung der Frage bilden insbesondere die Arbeiten von GOWERS und von LÖWENFELD. Dann kamen jedoch zwei Umstände, welche das Interesse an der Frage wieder in den Vordergrund rückten: 1. wurde man im Weltkriege auf viele, bisher ärztlich nicht beobachtete Fälle aufmerksam dadurch, daß die Soldaten auf Horchposten, bei militärischen Übungen usw. einschliefen und 2. kamen die Encephalitisepidemien mit ihrem Heer verschiedenartigster Schlafstörungen, bei denen man immer häufiger auch narkolepsieartige Bilder bemerken konnte. Es war vor allem EMIL REDLICH, der seit dem Jahre 1914 in verschiedenen Arbeiten und Vorträgen, gestützt auf eine wachsende Zahl eigener Fälle, die Aufmerksamkeit auf diese Krankheit immer wieder gelenkt hat und sich um die Erforschung ihres Wesens, ihrer Symptomatologie und Therapie bemühte. Eine immer wachsende Zahl von Publikationen zeugt davon, daß es ihm gelungen ist, das Interesse für diese Krankheit, die in früheren Lehrbüchern gar nicht oder nur mit ein paar Worten erwähnt wurde, so zu wecken, daß sie wohl nicht mehr vom Terrain der medizinischen Forschung verschwinden wird. Und so scheint es begreiflich, daß manche Forscher (JANZEN, VILLAVERDE) sogar von einer GÉLINEAU-REDLICHschen Narkolepsie sprechen. Um einen Begriff von dem steigenden Interesse an den Problemen der Narkolepsie zu geben, genügt die Erwähnung des Umstandes, daß in den 2 Jahren seit REDLICHs Tod weitaus mehr Fälle von Narkolepsie publiziert wurden als in den 50 Jahren seit GÉLINEAU.

Symptomatologie. Bei der Besprechung der Symptomatologie wollen wir zuerst schildern, wie ein typischer Fall aussieht, und zwar in seinen Hauptsymptomen. Selbstverständlich gibt es zahlreiche in verschiedener Hinsicht atypische Fälle, mit atypischem Verlauf, atypischen Symptomen usw. und es gibt auch Fälle, deren Einreihung Schwierigkeiten macht. Doch ist dies auch bei anderen Krankheiten nicht anders. In der überwiegenden Majorität der Fälle spielt sich aber die Krankheit so ab, daß in der Pubertät oder um das 20. Lebensjahr herum meist ohne erkennbare Ursache sich zu verschiedenen Tageszeiten ein imperatives Schlafbedürfnis einstellt, dem der Kranke nicht widerstehen kann. Es kann so stark sein, daß man von einem *plötzlichen* Einschlafen sprechen kann, meist aber versucht der Kranke einige Sekunden oder Minuten gegen den Schlaf anzukämpfen — vergeblich. Der Schlaf übermannt ihn überall, wo er gerade ist, beim Arbeiten, beim Essen, beim Kartenspielen, im Gespräch mit Freunden, selbst bei politischen Diskussionen, beim Stehen und Gehen, beim Chauffieren, Radfahren, im Kino, in der Kirche, auf der Toilette (THIELE und BERNHARDT), intra coitum (B. FISCHER, SINGER, HOFF und STENGEL), nach dem Urinieren (SCHILDER), den Soldaten beim Marschieren, auf Posten, im Gespräch mit dem Vorgesetzten, beim Reiten, den Arzt beim Ordinieren und Auskultieren (GRÜN), den Studenten bei der schriftlichen Prüfung usw. Es ist ein wahrer Dornröschenschlaf, wie er in dem Märchen geschildert wird, bloß daß er nicht Jahre, sondern Minuten dauert. Es werden Fälle erwähnt, wo der Patient mit zum Mund erhobenem Glas ,,zwischen Lipp- und Kelchesrand" wie WILSON sagt, einschläft, oft beim Füllen eines Glases mit Wasser. Ein Kranker CAVEs, ein Gärtner, wurde zum erstenmal vom Schlaf übermannt, gerade als er kniend am Gartenbeet arbeitete; plötzlich fiel er hin und blieb schlafend liegen. *Hiermit ist das erste und das zweite Merkmal charakterisiert, welches den narkoleptischen Schlaf vom physiologischen Schlaf unterscheidet: 1. sein besonders imperativer Charakter und 2. das Auftreten unter unphysiologischen Umständen.*

Allerdings ist hier schon eine kleine Einschränkung zu machen. Wohl sind es unphysiologische Umstände, unter denen dieser Schlaf eintritt, doch muß man hinzufügen, daß Umstände, unter denen auch normalerweise eine Schläfrigkeit oder ein Schlaf einzutreten pflegt, das Auftreten des Schlafes so außerordentlich begünstigen, daß sich wohl die *Mehrzahl* aller Schlafanfälle eher durch ihren imperativen Charakter und ihre Häufigkeit als durch die Merkwürdigkeit der *äußeren Umstände* auszeichnet. Denn auch unter den aufgezählten, besonders sonderbaren Umständen sind viele, die bei näherer Betrachtung weniger sonderbar erscheinen, vor allem *monotone Tätigkeiten:* es ist sicher krankhaft, daß eine so große Anzahl der Patienten am Volant des Autos so vom Schlaf übermannt wird, daß sie das Auto in einen Straßengraben fahren und in größter Lebensgefahr schweben. Aber die Mehrzahl der Automobilisten kennt die starke Schläfrigkeit bei langer, monotoner Fahrt und erst kürzlich hat KAPLINSKI über das häufige Einschlafen bei Chauffeuren und Straßenbahnführern berichtet. Das Einschlafen im Marschieren war bei übermüdeten Soldaten eine bekannte Erscheinung im Krieg (,,corticaler Übermüdungsschlaf" nach PFISTER) usw. Es soll aber noch besonders betont werden, daß sich der Schlafanfall einstellt mit Vorliebe nach dem Essen, ferner in Ruhe, beim Sitzen oder Liegen, in Wärme, bei Musik (ZADOR, THIELE-BERNHARDT), bei mechanischer, monotoner Tätigkeit, bei Ermüdung, nach schlecht durchschlafenen Nächten usw. Ein Patient von CAVE schlief besonders im Frühjahr ein, ein anderer fühlte sich besser im Winter, ein Kranker GRÜNs fühlte sich besser im Gebirge — Umstände, die an manche physiologische Erscheinungen erinnern.

Doch gibt es auch hier immer wieder Ausnahmen, die an das Pathologische des Zustandes gemahnen. Wir würden es verstehen, wenn die Patienten bei *Aufregungen* weniger oft einschlafen würden, doch wird dies nur in einem Fall von CAVE gemeldet, hingegen finden wir in den Fällen von GÉLINEAU, WESTPHAL, KAHLER, STRANSKY, TSIMINAKIS usw. Einschlafen gerade bei Aufregungen. Ist allerdings diese Erscheinung in einem geringeren Grade nicht auch bei Normalen nach Aufregungen zu beobachten? Wir sagten, daß in den meisten Fällen *Ruhe* ,,einschläfernd" wirkt. Und doch gibt es Fälle (GOLDFLAM, CAVE), wo sich bei Ruhe die Anfälle bessern und es ist eine bekannte Erscheinung, daß die Schlafanfälle sich beim Eintritt ins Spital in der Regel so rapid verringern, daß ihre Beobachtung auf Schwierigkeiten stößt (ein Umstand, der von manchen Autoren bei Beurteilung von evtl. therapeutischen Effekten übersehen wird). Der Widerspruch ist aber vielleicht nur ein scheinbarer: wohl wirkt Ruhe ,,einschläfernd", aber auch die *Ermüdung* und diese fällt mit dem Eintritt ins Spital weg. Und doch scheint es wiederum Fälle zu geben (CAVE, THIELE und BERNHARDT), bei denen die Anstrengung bestimmter Art, z. B. der Beruf eines Laufburschen die Anfälle eher verringert. Wir haben also hier ein Charakteristikum vor uns, das die Schlafanfälle mit dem physiologischen Schlaf *gemeinsam* haben: *die Umstände, welche den physiologischen Schlaf begünstigen, pflegen in der Regel auch den narkoleptischen Schlaf zu begünstigen.*

Wie sieht nun ein solcher *Schlafanfall* aus? Es ist sehr wichtig zu betonen, daß er sich in seinem Aussehen *in nichts vom physiologischen Schlaf* unterscheidet. Nur wenige Autoren bestreiten dies (ADIE, STRAUSS, WILSON). Doch sind alle Argumente, welche angeführt werden, um den Unterschied hervorzuheben, nicht stichhaltig, denn sie basieren auf der Nichtberücksichtigung der zahllosen Varietäten, welche der normale Schlaf darbietet und welche besonders jene Autoren genau kennen, welche sich speziell mit dem Verhalten des Menschen im normalen Schlaf befassen. Verzeichnen wir bloß einige Charakteristika des normalen Schlafes und vergleichen wir sie mit dem, was wir vom narkoleptischen Schlaf wissen. Das Gefühl der Müdigkeit, der Schläfrigkeit, der Augenschwere geht auch dem narkoleptischen Schlaf voraus, wenn es auch in manchen Fällen sehr kurz dauert; doch kommt es auch beim normalen Schlaf hier und da vor, daß man ,,hinfällt und schläft wie ein Toter". Auch Gähnen kommt vor, wenn auch nicht häufig. Im narkoleptischen sowie im normalen Schlaf sind die Muskeln in der Regel erschlafft, das Gesicht oft etwas gerötet, die Atmung verlangsamt und vertieft, hier und da sogar schnarchend, öfters besteht ein Schwitzen, die Tränensekretion ist gehemmt (THIELE-BERNHARDT), die Pupillen sind verengt, sie reagieren jedoch und erweitern sich beim Erwachen trotz Lichteinfall (STRAUSS, SEREJSKI fanden übrigens die Pupillen reaktionslos). Manchmal gehen dem Schlafe typische hypnagoge Halluzinationen voraus (B. FISCHER, DOYLE und DANIELS). Im Schlafe selbst kommt es häufig zu Träumen, welche die Patienten nachher wiedergeben können und die sich in nichts von den gewöhnlichen Träumen unterscheiden. ROTHFELD erwähnt Erektion im Schlaf (und bei Unterdrückung desselben), LEVIN Secessus urinae. Wir sprachen davon, daß der Schlaf nicht unterdrückbar ist. Gerade das könnte man als Argument gegen die Schlafnatur der Anfälle benützen, denn der normale Schlaf ist auch bei sehr großer Müdigkeit nur in der Minderzahl der Fälle nicht irgendwie unterdrückbar. Daher ist es wichtig zu betonen, daß man das Wort ,,nicht unterdrückbar" nicht wörtlich nehmen darf. In der Mehrzahl der Fälle ist es wohl möglich, den narkoleptischen Schlaf zu coupieren, jedoch mit sehr großer Mühe und mit Beschwerden (besonders Kopfschmerzen, was ja ebenfalls beim Normalen vorkommt), so daß die meisten Kranken es später gar nicht versuchen, den Anfall zu unterdrücken, insbesondere, da sie die Erfahrung machen, daß bei Coupierung eines Schlafanfalles der nächste um so eher und um so heftiger auftritt. Ein Fall ROSENTHALS z. B. konnte den Anfall bis zu 2 Stunden unterdrücken. Die Art, wie die Kranken aber den Schlaf coupieren, ist ein weiteres Argument für die Schlafnatur der Anfälle, denn wir begegnen da lauter vom Normalen her bekannten Mannövern: Rauchen einer Zigarette (LHERMITTE und PEYRE), Waschen mit kaltem Wasser, Hinausgehen in frische Luft, Herumgehen, Anstrengung, Schwimmen, eine Schale Kaffee, Kneifen der Haut. Beim Fall LHERMITTE-PEYRE hatte auch interessante Arbeit einen unterdrückenden Einfluß. Hingegen kann das Fixieren eines Gegenstandes, bekannt von der Technik der Hypnose, bei manchen Fällen (nicht bei allen) einen Schlafanfall provozieren. Wir sehen hier also eine weitere Reihe von Umständen, welche auf den narkoleptischen Schlaf provozierend oder hemmend wirken und die sich wiederum mit analogen Einflüssen auf den normalen menschlichen Schlaf decken. Selten wird der Schlaf durch einen Gähnanfall ersetzt (REDLICH, MÜNZER).

Es dürfen aber nicht verschiedene Erscheinungen unerwähnt bleiben, die — wenn sie auch nur in einer kleinen Minderzahl der Fälle vorkommen — von jenen in den Vordergrund geschoben werden, welche daran zweifeln, ob es sich beim narkoleptischen Anfall um einen wirklichen Schlaf handelt. Es sind dies vor allem gewisse *motorische Reizerscheinungen*, welche bei verschiedenen Fällen, sei es unmittelbar vor dem Einschlafen, sei es im Schlaf, beobachtet wurden, Zuckungen oder Zittern besonders im Gesicht, weniger oft in den Extremitäten, sogar einzelne einfache koordinierte Bewegungen (CAVE), in einem Fall von RIZATTI (postencephalitisch!) sogar eine stärkere motorische Unruhe (wie sie ja aber auch sonst im Schlaf der Postencephalitiker häufig ist). Wir erwähnen noch Zucken der Augenlider, Verschieben des Unterkiefers, leichte Streckbewegungen. Obwohl diese Erscheinungen sicher zum Denken Anlaß geben und unser besonderes Interesse verdienen, darf man nicht vergessen, wieviele dieser Erscheinungen im normalen Schlaf vorkommen, wenn man bloß die Schläfer etwas genauer beobachtet. Denjenigen, die im Kriege Gelegenheit hatten, mitten unter einer großen Anzahl Schlafender die Nacht zu verbringen, ist dies am besten bekannt. Wir erwähnen auch als Beispiel die Arbeit DE LISIS über die Myoklonien des Normalschlafes. Eine zweite Reihe von Erscheinungen, die nicht ganz in den Rahmen des Schlafes hineinzupassen scheinen, betrifft schon große Ausnahmen: Es sind dies subjektive Symptome, die an eine *Aura* des epileptischen Anfalles erinnern, wie Blitz vor den Augen und optische Halluzinationen (FRÖDERBERG), befehlende Stimmen (MÜNZER), „träumerische Zerstreutheit" (THIELE und BERNHARDT), Licht im Kopf (PASKIND, WILSON), Schwindel (PASKIND, SOLOMON), Druck in der Stirne und in den Augen (URECHIA und BUNTBACESCU), Sensationen im Epigastrium oder im Herzen, Mikropsie, Parästhesien, Doppelbilder (WOHLFAHRT, JANZEN). Für diese Erscheinungen gilt ebenfalls das oben Gesagte: Die Akten darüber sind wohl noch nicht abgeschlossen, doch darf man nicht an die ungeheure Mannigfaltigkeit verschiedener Sensationen vergessen, die sich auch beim Normalen einstellen bei Schlafeintritt, Schlafunterdrückung, Übermüdung. Speziell bei Ermüdung und Erschöpfung sind ja Störungen auf somatischem und psychischem Gebiete beobachtet worden, die über den Rahmen der soeben besprochenen Anomalien weit hinausgehen.

Wir wollen jetzt eine andere Eigentümlichkeit des narkoleptischen Schlafes hervorheben, die ebenfalls zu Diskussionen Anlaß gegeben hat. Wir haben schon erwähnt, daß die Patienten bei der Arbeit, beim Stehen, Gehen usw. vom Schlafe überfallen werden. Und hier gibt es zwei Typen von Verhaltungsweisen. Der eine Typus, bei dem der Schlaf vielleicht nicht mit der äußersten Heftigkeit und Plötzlichkeit eintritt und der dem Schlaf keinen großen Widerstand entgegensetzt, wohl aus der Erfahrung heraus, daß es nicht viel nützt, sucht sich rasch einen Sitz- oder Liegeplatz und schläft dort ein, ein Lehrer geht in ein leeres Nebenzimmer, ein Chauffeur hält den Wagen an und legt sich am Wegesrand usw. Bei einer anderen Gruppe von Fällen jedoch, die mitten in einer Tätigkeit vom Schlaf befallen werden und die diese Tätigkeit entweder nicht unterbrechen wollen oder infolge der relativen Plötzlichkeit des Schlafeintrittes nicht unterbrechen können, geschieht es nicht allzu selten, daß sie in der begonnenen Tätigkeit fortfahren, bloß daß diese dann irgendwie verkehrt ausfällt: Der Gärtner flicht den Kranz weiter, aber so falsch, daß die Arbeit unbrauchbar ist, der Schreibende produziert ein mehr oder weniger unverständliches Gekritzel, ein Patient WOHLFAHRTs aß das Ei mit der Schale, ein Patient REDLICHs klopfte sich mit dem Hammer auf die Finger, ein Gehender geht weiter bis er stolpert, ein Sprechender murmelt noch ein paar unverständliche Worte usw. Es kommt auch zu Unfällen dabei (NOACKs Kranker wurde überfahren, ein Fall von THIELE-BERNHARDT durchbrach die Bahnsperre, ein anderer fiel mit dem Kopf in ein Schaufenster). Dies sind übrigens alles Erscheinungen, die auch beim normalen Schlaf bzw. bei Ermüdung hier und da vorkommen und eher geeignet sind, ein Argument für als wider die Schlafnatur der narkoleptischen Anfälle zu liefern. Wenn ein Patient im Stehen vom Schlaf übermannt wird, so kann es geschehen, daß er langsam zusammensinkt, ja, auch daß er umfällt. Interessanter sind aber die Fälle, wo dies nicht der Fall ist, wo der Kranke stehenbleibt (CAVE), wo der Muskeltonus normal ist (CURSCHMANN, PRANGE). Denn die Weiterbetätigung im Schlaf und die letzten erwähnten Erscheinungen sprechen gegen die Identifizierung der Schlafanfälle mit den später zu besprechenden Anfällen von Tonusverlust (STRAUSS). Im Schlafanfall sieht man eben öfters das Fehlen der innervatorischen Hemmung, sowie das Fehlen des Tonusverlustes. Daß auch Sprechen aus dem Schlaf vorkommt, versteht sich von selbst. Somit wäre eine weitere Reihe von Symptomen bei den Schlafanfällen besprochen, welche von manchen Autoren (wie wir meinen, zu Unrecht) gegen die Identifizierung mit dem normalen Schlaf angeführt werden.

Und nun kommen wir zu einer Eigenschaft der narkoleptischen Anfälle, welche die führende und wichtigste Gemeinsamkeit mit dem normalen Schlaf bildet. Es ist, wie die Literatur zeigt, außerordentlich schwierig, heutzutage eine Definition des Schlafes zu geben, welche ihn genügend deutlich von anderen Zuständen von Bewußtlosigkeit unterscheidet. Eine Eigenschaft wird aber von allen als wesentlich und prinzipiell wichtig genannt, die mehr oder weniger prompte *Reversibilität* des Zustandes, die Eigenschaft, daß man die Bewußtseinsveränderung im Schlafe durch relativ geringfügige äußere Reize wieder vollständig aufheben kann. Und diese ganz charakteristische Eigenschaft hat auch der Schlaf des narkoleptischen Anfalls. Man kann einen schlafenden Narkoleptiker ohne weiteres durch die ganz gewöhnlichen taktilen und akustischen Reize sofort *aufwecken*. Manchmal geht es etwas schwieriger, manchmal leichter, genau wie bei gewöhnlichem Schlaf. Nach dem Aufwachen benimmt sich der Narkoleptiker genau wie der normale Schläfer, er blickt evtl. etwas überrascht um sich, er reibt sich die Augen, streckt sich evtl. Manchmal bleibt noch kurze Zeit eine gewisse Schläfrigkeit und Dösigkeit, auffallend häufig jedoch (häufiger meines Erachtens als beim normalen, künstlich unterbrochenen Schlaf) ist er sofort ganz frisch und munter. Diese prompte Erweckbarkeit steht in einem seltsamen, fast grotesken Kontrast zu der Unwiderstehlichkeit des Schlafanfalles, in einem Kontrast, der meines Erachtens ein ungeheures theoretisches Interesse hat und der bisher noch gar nicht gewürdigt wurde. Es gibt genug Fälle, wo nichts in der Welt einen Narkoleptiker am Einschlafen hindern kann, wenn man ihn aber eine Minute später wecken will, so gelingt schon eine leise Berührung dazu, und er ist sofort munter und frisch, hat auch gar kein Schlafbedürfnis mehr. Es sieht also fast so aus, als ob es nicht um den Schlaf, sondern um das Einschlafen ginge, als ob es sich nicht um eine Schlaf-, sondern um eine *Einschlafstörung*, nicht um einen Schlaf-, sondern um einen *Einschlafanfall* handeln würde. Von diesem Gesichtspunkt aus ist aber leider das Narkolepsieproblem bisher noch nicht behandelt worden. Daran muß man aber streng festhalten: das *Kriterium der Reversibilität, der Erweckbarkeit ist ein wesentliches Kriterium des narkoleptischen Anfalls* und man darf nicht, wie es hier und da geschieht, auch Fälle, die nicht erweckbar sind, zur Narkolepsie zählen. Durch dieses Kriterium hauptsächlich unterscheidet sich der narkoleptische Anfall von anderen Zuständen von Bewußtlosigkeit, insbesondere von den epileptischen und komatösen (mit Ausnahme vielleicht gewisser hysterischer Zustände).

Fragen wir uns nun, was geschieht, wenn man den Narkoleptiker nicht weckt, so ist das identisch mit der Frage nach der *Dauer des narkoleptischen Anfalles*. Dies ist jedoch schon eine Frage, die mit gewisser Vorsicht gestellt werden muß, weil sie an heikle Punkte des Narkolepsieproblems rührt. Die überwiegende Mehrzahl der Schlafanfälle, bei der überwiegenden Mehrzahl der Narkoleptiker dauert einige Minuten, durchschnittlich 5—15 Minuten. Selten weniger (wie z. B. 30—45 Sekunden in einem Fall von CAVE), selten mehr, $^1/_2$ Stunde und darüber. Allerdings kommt es öfters vor, wenn ein Narkoleptiker *unter günstigen Umständen* einschläft, im Bett liegend, bei äußerer Ruhe, daß er auch 1—2 Stunden, selten drüber schläft. Doch ist es vielleicht hier gestattet, von einem ,,Übergang des narkoleptischen Anfalls in einen physiologischen Schlaf'' zu sprechen. Manche Autoren allerdings, welche die ,,Narkolepsien'' weiter fassen, zählen auch die Fälle von ständiger Somnolenz, von tagelang dauerndem Schlaf zur Narkolepsie, sehr zum Schaden der Sache. Vereinzelte Grenzfälle allerdings gibt es, die bei der strengen Trennung, wie sie mit LÖWENFELD, REDLICH die überwiegende Mehrzahl der Autoren will, nicht leicht zu rubrizieren sind, wie etwa Fälle, die neben Schlafsucht oder Dauerschlaf auch narkoleptisch aussehende Anfälle haben oder Fälle, wo Schlafsucht und Narkolepsie in einer und derselben Familie vorkommen, doch gibt es solche Fälle bei jeder Krankheit und sie sind kein Grund das Krankheitsbild zu verwischen, dessen scharfe Heraushebung uns schon manche neue Erkenntnisse gebracht hat und noch neue zu bringen verspricht. REDLICH schlägt für diese Fälle von Schlafsucht z. B. bei Hirntumoren den GOWERSschen Ausdruck ,,Somnosie'' vor.

Die Frage nach der *Häufigkeit* des Auftretens der Schlafanfälle ist so zu beantworten, daß bei der Mehrzahl der Kranken auf der Höhe des Krankheitsbildes 3—6 Anfälle täglich aufzutreten pflegen, doch sind auch Fälle mit 10—20 Anfällen keine extreme Rarität. Die Zahl der Anfälle ist übrigens begreiflicherweise nicht jeden Tag dieselbe, da diese ja von verschiedenen äußeren Momenten zum Teil abhängig sind. Ein Extrem sind die Fälle, wo der Schlafanfall nur einige Male im Jahr auftritt, obwohl dies zu Beginn der Erkrankung weniger selten ist und auf der anderen Seite stehen diejenigen Fälle, wo bis zu 100 (JELIFFE), ja, bis zu 200 Anfälle im Tag (GÉLINEAU) vorkommen. Es ist fast selbstverständlich, daß bei solchen Fällen die Anfälle kürzer, oft etwa 1 Minute zu dauern pflegen.

Betrachten wir schließlich noch einige Momente, durch welche Schlafanfälle künstlich *provoziert* werden können, da dies mit Rücksicht auf die späteren Erörterungen wichtig erscheint. *Alkohol* hat keinen provozierenden Einfluß auf die Anfälle, obwohl sich unter den Narkoleptikern auch einzelne alkoholintolerante befinden. Durch *Calcium* gelang es ZADOR Schlafanfälle hervorzurufen (intravenöse Injektion von 10 ccm Afenil, destilliertes Wasser war unwirksam), doch ist sein Fall nicht ganz sicher; dasselbe sah jedoch auch BASSOE, ferner in einem Fall REDLICH und in einem ich selbst; es gibt jedoch auch negative Fälle, wie ich mich selbst überzeugen konnte. Durch *Hyperventilation* gelang es STRAUSS, ferner SEREJSKI und FRUMKIN Schlafanfälle hervorzubringen, allerdings bei postencephalitischen Fällen, die sich, wie wir sehen werden, in mancher Hinsicht etwas anders verhalten. Bei 2 anderen postencephalitischen Fällen, ferner bei Fällen echter Narkolepsie konnten WOHLFAHRT, STRAUSS, BEYERMANN, REDLICH und auch ich keinen Schlaf provozieren. Auch THIELE und BERNHARDT konnten durch Hyperventilation nur leichte tetanoide Erscheinungen, aber keinen Schlaf provozieren.

Zusammenfassend kann man also sagen, *daß bei den Einschlafanfällen der Narkolepsie mit imperativer Gewalt mehrmals täglich ein mehrere Minuten dauernder kurzer physiologischer Schlaf eintritt, in welchem der Kranke alle Merkmale des Schlafenden hat, öfters auch träumt, leicht erweckbar ist oder auch spontan nach kurzer Zeit, zumeist erfrischt, aufwacht.*

Affektiver Tonusverlust. Die zweite Erscheinung, welche für die typische Narkolepsie charakteristisch ist, steht in der neurologischen Symptomatologie so einzig da, daß es begreiflich ist, wenn sie — besonders seit den Hinweisen REDLICHS — allgemeines Interesse erweckt hat. Eröffnet doch jedes neue neurologische Symptom neue Einblicke in pathologische und physiologische Vorgänge. Dieses Symptom, welches bereits GÉLINEAU gut bekannt war, hat verschiedene Namen bekommen. GÉLINEAU nannte es Astasie oder Chûte, KELLER „Sturzanfälle", LÖWENFELD „kataleptische Starre", HENNEBERG „kataplektische Hemmung", TRÖMNER „Affektatonie", STRAUSS „reaktiver Anfall", ROSENTHAL „Adynamic" (für die leichteren Anfälle) usw. Am populärsten (auch in fremden Sprachen) wurde jedoch die Bennung REDLICHS „affektiver Tonusverlust", weil sie die wesentlichsten Momente des Zustandes in sich enthält [1]. Es handelt sich darum, daß unsere Kranken bei gewissen Emotionen, oft schon leichter Art, bei *Freude, beim Lachen, bei Ärger, Zorn, Schreck, Überraschung*, von eigenartigen Schwächezuständen befallen werden. Meist blitzartig, jedenfalls aber sehr schnell, tritt ein Nachlaß jener physiologischen Innervation ein, welcher die menschliche Muskulatur auch im Ruhezustand unterliegt, und die wir *in der Klinik* als Tonus der Muskulatur bezeichnen, obwohl sie mit der sog. tonischen Innervation des Tierexperimentes nichts gemeinsam hat. Die ganze Skeletmuskulatur wird schlaff, atonisch, der Körper sinkt plötzlich machtlos in sich zusammen und da zugleich auch eine vollständige Unmöglichkeit einer willkürlichen oder reflektorischen Innervation vorhanden ist. klappt der ganze Mensch, wie ein willenloses Bündel toter Muskeln, in sich zusammen, stürzt evtl. je nach der Situation, wie vom Blitz getroffen zu Boden, unfähig sich auch nur ein wenig zu bewegen, unfähig zu sprechen, zu lachen (!), dabei aber bei vollkommen klarem Sensorium, sich seines Zustandes vollständig bewußt, mit erhaltenem Willensantrieb zur Bewegung, der sich bloß nicht in Handlung umsetzen kann. Und dieser schwerste Zustand einer vollkommenen Paralyse der Willkürmuskulatur (denn man muß ja auch von dieser sprechen und nicht bloß vom Tonusverlust) dauert in der Regel nur wenige Sekunden, der Kranke fühlt dann, wie sehr rasch, evtl. auch ganz plötzlich seine Muskeln ihre Kraft wiedergewinnen und der Mann, der soeben noch wie tot umgefallen war, fühlt sich vollkommen frisch und munter. Dieser Zustand: bei vollem Bewußtsein zu sein und sich nicht rühren, keinen Laut hervorbringen zu können, wird nur in seltenen Fällen allzu tragisch genommen, dazu dauert er zu kurz, wiederholt sich zu oft, der Zusammenhang mit der Emotion ist viel zu deutlich, nur in seltenen Fällen haben die Patienten dabei das Gefühl des Vergehens, das gehört nicht zu den typischen Erscheinungen des affektiven Tonusverlustes. Sonst wäre es auch schwer erklärlich, daß die meisten dieser Kranken überhaupt erst nach Jahren einen Arzt konsultieren oder auch gar nicht. Verletzungen im Anfall sind nicht häufig, kommen aber vor.

---

[1] Die noch immer manchmal gebrauchte Bezeichnung Geloplegie (Lachschlag) ist hier ganz falsch (s. u.).

So verhält es sich zumindest in den Fällen von typischem schweren Tonusverlust. Doch ist die Symptomatologie des affektiven Tonusverlustes viel mannigfaltiger, die Abweichungen sehr viel zahlreicher als bei den im Vergleich dazu einförmigen Schlafanfällen. So gibt es seltene Fälle, wo der Tonusverlust mehrere Minuten dauert, evtl. von seltsamen Kopfsensationen, einmal sogar von Gehörstäuschungen begleitet war (FRÖDERBERG). Die vereinzelten Fälle, wo von einem tagelang dauernden Tonusverlust die Rede ist, wo z. B. ein Patient, der später eine Narkolepsie bekam, nach einer Explosion tagelang eine Schwäche in den Beinen verspürte (STRAUSS), sind derzeit bezüglich ihrer Zugehörigkeit zum Tonusverlust noch sehr fraglich. Schon REDLICH u. a. betonten, daß der Tonusverlust etwas in sich hat, das an gewisse Affektreaktionen beim Normalen erinnert. Und tatsächlich sind die Fälle, wo der Normale beim starken Lachen Gegenstände aus der Hand fallen läßt oder sich anhalten muß, ebenso wie bei einer plötzlichen Trauernachricht usw. außerordentlich häufig; daß jemandem vor Zorn die Sprache versagt, daß jemand vor Staunen mit offenem Mund stehenbleibt, daß jemandem vor Schreck die Beine erstarren, ist nichts Seltenes und Sprachwendungen im Volksmund aller Länder geben Zeugnis davon. So drückt z. B. der Wiener den höchsten Grad der Überraschung, so aus: „Ah, da legst Di(ch) nieder und stehst net auf!" Auch das Nachlassen des Blasensphincters bei Frauen bei starkem Lachen ist bekannt. Mancher „Feigling" ist es nur deshalb, weil er schon bei einem geringen Angstaffekt „wie gelähmt ist" und weder sich verteidigen, noch davonlaufen kann. Auch in der dichterischen Darstellung der starken Affekte, in der Darstellung der bildenden, der darstellenden Kunst findet man auf Schritt und Tritt irgendwelche Grade von affektivem Tonusverlust beschrieben und nachgebildet. Ob der affektive Tonusverlust der Narkolepsie jedoch wirklich eine bloße Steigerung des normalen Verhaltens ist, wie etwa manche Schlafanfälle oder ob die Analogie nur eine äußere ist und es sich in Wirklichkeit um etwas qualitativ ganz anderes handelt, ist bis jetzt noch nicht entschieden, ja, nicht einmal untersucht worden.

Wir haben schon erwähnt, daß es charakteristisch ist für diese Anfälle, daß sie ausschließlich im Anschluß an gewisse Affekte auftreten, niemals ohne diese (auf gewisse Ausnahmen werden wir noch weiter unten eingehen). Man darf sich aber nicht der falschen Ansicht hingeben, daß es sich um affektiv außerordentlich ansprechbare sensitive Individuen handelt. Davon ist gar keine Rede. Die Narkoleptiker zeichnen sich in der überwiegenden Mehrzahl der Fälle gar nicht durch ein besonders gesteigertes Affektleben aus, mehrmals werden darunter sogar träge, affektiv etwas stumpfe Individuen erwähnt. *Nicht ihr Affektleben ist gestört, sondern die Reaktion ihres Muskelapparates auf die gewöhnlichen, ja, oft sogar auf ganz schwache Affekte* (s. unten). STRAUSS drückt das sehr gut so aus: es handelt sich dabei nicht um Affektlabile, sondern um Reaktivlabile. Und tatsächlich ist man erstaunt zu sehen, wie häufig man unter den auslösenden Situationen solche findet, die man sich als stürmisch wirkende Emotionen nur schwer vorstellen kann. Ein Kranker WESTPHALs fiel zusammen, als er zwei sich balgende Knaben sah und für einen derselben Partei ergreifen wollte, ein Kranker SOMERs fiel zusammen, als er von einem affektiven Tonusverlust erzählen wollte, ein Kranker WILSONs beim Erzählen eines aufregenden Traumes. Wir finden ferner Tonusverlust beim Öffnen eines Briefes, beim Anrufen eines im Auto vorüberfahrenden Freundes, bei Lob, bei Drohung mit Kitzeln, bei einem Befehl des Chefs, beim Begrüßen eines vorgesetzten Offiziers, beim Eintritt des Chefarztes, bei einem herzlichen Händedruck, beim Dankenwollen für eine Zigarette, beim überraschenden Begegnen eines Reptils, einer Schnecke, eines Hundes, eines Wachmanns, wenn ein Auto von hinten kommt, die Schnur eines Pakets reißt. Wir finden mehrere Fälle, wo das Angeln unmöglich war, weil jedesmal, wenn ein Fisch anzubeißen schien, der Tonusverlust kam, so daß Patient alles fallen ließ und einer sogar dabei vom Boot ins Wasser fiel; bei mehreren Fällen passierte es auf der Jagd, daß die Abgabe eines Schusses dadurch unmöglich wurde. Man könnte eine ganze Psychologie der Affekte bzw. ihrer körperlichen Auswirkung am Menschen auf dem Studium dieser Anfälle aufbauen. Wäre es so, daß nicht die Qualität der Affekte, sondern eben ihre Intensität eine Rolle spielen würde, so begegneten wir manchen Überraschungen. Sicher machen wir uns von der Intensität der Affekte eine ganz falsche Vorstellung, wenn man die Affekte nur nach ihrem „Inhalt", d. h. nach der auslösenden Ursache beurteilt. Diesem Eindruck kann man sich insbesondere dann nicht entziehen, wenn man sich etwa mit Neurotikern in psychoanalytischer Art befaßt. Wir werden also vielleicht nicht überrascht sein, wenn ein Mann bei CAVE etwas Blinkendes auf der Straße erblickt, sich danach bückt, bemerkt, daß es eine goldene Uhr ist und in diesem Momente schon macht- und kraftlos auf der Straße daliegt. Sonderbar ist jedoch, daß sich der affektive Tonusverlust so häufig findet bei Tätigkeiten, die eine gewisse Aggression beinhalten — also nicht bloß auffallend oft bei verschiedenen Sportarten und hier wiederum bei Angeln, Jagd, Ringen, sondern auch beim Schlagen der Kinder, der Tiere; z. B. WENDEROWIČ und CAVE beschreiben je einen Fall, wo ein Landmann ein Pferd, eine Kuh schlagen wollte, in diesem Momente kraftlos wurde, sich an das Tier stützen mußte und erst nach einigen Sekunden fähig war sich aufzurichten und die beabsichtigte Handlung durchzuführen. Auch THIELE und BERNHARDT sahen Ähnliches. (Sollte es ein Zufall sein, daß der Kranke WENDEROWIČ ein Sodomit war und seine Narkolepsie kurze Zeit nach Verlust eines Pferdes, der ihn sehr kränkte, bekam?) ROSENTHAL beschreibt dasselbe beim Schlagen eines Hundes. Viele Autoren erwähnen Ähnliches beim Züchtigen eines Kindes. Man hat aber sicher den individuellen psychologischen Faktoren bei den einzelnen Fällen vorläufig zu wenig Beachtung geschenkt. Und vorläufig mit Recht. Denn zuerst interessiert uns, bei dieser neuen Gelegenheit die Psychologie der Affekte an einem neuen objektiven Symptom studieren zu können, das Gemeinsame. Das Individuelle, das wir ja auch auf andere Weise genügend studieren können, kommt erst in zweiter Linie als unbedingt notwendige Ergänzung und als Kontrolle hinzu. Jedenfalls soll aber an dieser Stelle betont werden, daß eine individuelle psychologische Durchforschung eines Narkolepsiefalles bisher noch nicht in genügender Weise erfolgt ist, wenn wir nicht den Fall MISSRIEGLERs erwähnen. Ich selbst konnte bei einem oberflächlichen Eingehen auf psychogene Faktoren in 2 Fällen in mehreren Sitzungen nichts von besonderem Interesse erheben. Wenn wir nun bei den aggressiven Handlungen verbleiben, so haben wir wiederum auffallend häufig den affektiven Tonusverlust beim Versuch der Kranken, ihre Kinder zu züchtigen. Dann möchten wir noch eine Gruppe von Auslösungsursachen erwähnen, die vielleicht ein wenig überraschend, aber bei näherer Überlegung verständlich sind: So wird bei 2 Fällen erwähnt, daß sie beim Kartenspiel nur dann den Tonusverlust haben, wenn sie ein besonders gutes Blatt bekommen und nie, wenn sie ein schlechtes Blatt haben, bei 2 Fällen, daß sie beim Tennisspielen dann zusammenklappen, wenn sie einen besonders guten Ball gegeben haben und nicht bei einem schlechten. THIELE-BERNHARDT, ROSENTHAL erwähnen Ähnliches beim Billardspiel, THIELE und BERNHARDT beim Schachspiel. Ein Patient ZEHRERs bekam den Zustand bei Musik, jedoch nur, wenn ein flotter Marsch gespielt wurde. Das wird uns weniger wundern, wenn wir erfahren (s. unten), daß freudige Emotionen als Auslöser des Tonusverlustes überhaupt überwiegen (auch Schadenfreude, THIELE-BERNHARDT). Aber regt es nicht zu psychologischen Studien über den Witz und die Witzbolde an, wenn wir erfahren, daß ein Patient CAVEs nur den Zustand bekam, wenn er selbst einen Witz erzählte, niemals, wenn er über den Witz eines anderen lachen mußte (Ähnliches bei THIELE-BERNHARDT). Und wenn wir auch wissen, daß die Überraschung oft eine auslösende Rolle spielt, werden wir verstehen, daß ein Patient LEVINs den Tonusverlust beim Lesen schon bekam, wenn sich der Sinn eines gelesenen Inhaltes plötzlich änderte? Oder beim bloßen Versuch zu lesen? Es entspricht auch vielleicht nicht ganz unseren Erwartungen, daß der affektive Tonusverlust beim Coitus bzw. Orgasmus relativ selten ist (ROTHFELD, LOPEZ und SEMON, LEVIN). P. LOEWY beschreibt Tonusverlust beim Urinlassen. Man muß hier ausdrücklich betonen, daß die häufigste und kräftigste Ursache von Tonusverlust das Lachen ist[1]. Es bestand im Anfang ein gewisser Zweifel darüber, ob es der Akt des Lachens selbst ist oder der heitere Affekt, welcher den Tonusverlust bewirkt. Für ersteres schien eine gewisse Ähnlichkeit mit dem sog. Lachschlag OPPENHEIMs zu sprechen (s. unten), der nur durch starkes Lachen ausgelöst wurde und die Tatsache, daß viele Patienten behaupten, sie könnten den Tonusverlust unterdrücken, wenn sie sich bemühen nicht stark zu lachen. Letzteres scheint jedoch darauf zu beruhen, daß nicht das Motorische des Lachens, sondern auf dem Wege der Unterdrückung des Affektausdrucks der Affekt selbst abgeschwächt wird, wofür wir ja auch Analogien beim Normalen leicht finden können. Denn viele Patienten geben ausdrücklich an, daß es eben nicht der Akt des Lachens ist, sondern der heitere Affekt, der den Tonusverlust auslöst (REDLICH, LEVIN u. a.). Kranke von PASKIND, WOHLFAHRT z. B. geben ausdrücklich an, daß schon ein Lächeln genügt. Ein Patient WILSONs ging sogar so weit, daß er sich eine Art absichtlich gekünstelten Lachens zurechtlegte, weil bei diesem Lachen der Tonusverlust nicht eintrat. Während wir in einem Falle sehen, daß Drohung mit Kitzeln den Tonusverlust auslöst, geben z. B. ROTHFELD, THIELE-BERNHARDT ausdrücklich an, daß Kitzeln selbst ohne Einfluß ist und auch ich konnte mich davon überzeugen. Schreck spielt wohl oft eine Rolle, aber doch keine so ausgedehnte, als wir nach Analogien mit dem Normalen annehmen würden. Wohl fällt z. B. ein Patient SEREJSKIS und FRUMKINS schon bei plötzlicher Annäherung des Reflektors wie vom Blitz getroffen um, aber es finden sich auch Fälle, wie z. B. der von CAVE, wo ein Kranker bei Gefahr 1 Stunde laufen konnte. Es drängt sich der Eindruck auf, daß nicht so sehr der Schreck wie das Moment der Überraschung ausschlaggebend ist, das Unerwartete. Das kann man an den früher gegebenen Beispielen deutlich verfolgen und dies ist ja nach den älteren Psychologen der Komik auch das Ausschlaggebende beim Witz und bei der Komik, während neuere Psychologen (FREUD) wiederum eher geneigt sind, dem Aggressionstrieb dabei eine Rolle zuzubilligen. Und es haben ja sicherlich beide Schulen recht, die eine erfaßt mehr die Technik, die andere die unbewußten Motive des Witzes. Von sonstigen Affekten fällt uns die relativ häufige Rolle von Zorn und Ärger auf, die ja in uns ebenfalls aggressive Tendenzen wecken.

Nun beginnen sich aber in der letzten Zeit Beobachtungen zu mehren, welche bei diesen Fällen auch Tonusverlust angeben bei Gelegenheiten, bei denen ein zugehöriger Affekt nicht ohne weiteres ersichtlich ist. Es sind vorläufig noch vereinzelte Beobachtungen, aber sie haben alle etwas Gemeinsames, so daß es sich schon verlohnt, sie näher zu betrachten. Es sind dies Angaben über Tonusverlust beim Versuch zu laufen, beim Laufen, nach langem Laufen, bei plötzlichem Wenden, beim Versuch etwas zu werfen, beim Nageleinschlagen, beim Holzhacken, ferner bei Tisch im Momente des Hinüberreichens von Gegenständen. Man muß bei der Beurteilung dieser Fälle natürlich vorsichtig sein,

---

[1] So fanden THIELE und BERNHARDT unter 25 Fällen Lachen als Ursache 15, Freude 5mal, Schreck usw. nur 5mal.

es kann dabei in manchen Fällen auch ein Affekt mitspielen, der nur für uns nicht sofort einfühlbar ist. Dafür scheint besonders eine Angabe eines WILSONschen Kranken zu sprechen, der aussagte, daß ihm beim Servieren eines Tennisballes plötzlich der Gedanke aufschießt, ob er es wohl gut machen wird und der in diesem Momente eben den Tonusverlust bekommt. Sicher jedoch ist es nicht in allen Fällen so. Man muß in Hinkunft besser auf solche Auslösungsursachen achten, die ja etwas Gemeinsames zu haben scheinen insoferne, als dazu eine *plötzliche Innervation* notwendig ist; vielleicht spielt auch dabei das Unerwartete eine Rolle; daraufhin ist noch nicht untersucht worden, aber es gibt Kranke, die angeben, daß sie überhaupt den Tonusverlust nicht bekommen, wenn sie einen Witz u. dgl. schon erwarten.

Jedenfalls kann man vielleicht schon heute die zahlreichen vorliegenden Beobachtungen zusammenfassen und feststellen: *Von allen Auslösungsursachen des affektiven Tonusverlustes spielt die Gruppe der heiteren, der freudigen Affekte eine Hauptrolle und darunter das Lachen eine führende Rolle. Bei genauerer Betrachtung der Inhalte (Auslösungsursachen) der Affekte finden wir gewisse Gemeinsamkeiten. Es überwiegen Momente, bei denen der Aggressionstrieb eine Rolle spielt und die etwas Plötzliches, Unerwartetes, Überraschendes beinhalten.* So könnte man in hypothetischer Weise weitergehen und sagen: die Anomalie des affektiven Tonusverlustes besteht nicht in einer Anomalie der Affekte, sondern in einer Anomalie der motorischen Reaktion auf diese Affekte. Man könnte sagen, diese Reaktion ist *paradox*; denn es handelt sich hier um äußere Umstände und um Affekte, die eine plötzliche Anspannung der Muskulatur erfordern, eine plötzliche Innervation, eine plötzliche Hemmung bzw. Gegeninnervation oder zumindest eine plötzliche Umstellung zu einer erhöhten Innervationsbereitschaft. Das Gegenteil tritt jedoch ein. Dies scheint der Punkt, wo die eigentliche Störung liegt. Ich habe darauf hingewiesen, daß es eine große Reihe von Affekten gibt, bei denen Tonusverlust noch niemals beobachtet wurde, z. B. Schmerz, Trauer, Kummer, Liebe, Begeisterung, Angst (im Gegensatz zu Schreck), Hunger usw., Erwartung (diese coupiert sogar den Tonusverlust), Sehnsucht, Haß, Neid, Scham, Stolz, Reue, Ekel, Unrast, Demut, Sympathie, Verachtung, Heiterkeit (im Gegensatz zu Freude und Lachen) usw. Man könnte also im affektiven Tonusverlust ein Beispiel jener zahlreichen paradoxen Reaktionen vermuten, welche wir besonders im Bereiche des vegetativen Systems kennen, die jedoch auch dem animalen Nervensystem nicht fremd sind. Ich konnte für das Gebiet des vegetativen Systems zeigen, daß die Ursache solcher Paradoxien sehr oft im Zustande der *peripheren* Organe liegt und gewissen Gesetzmäßigkeiten folgt („Ausgangswertgesetz"). Es könnte aber auch so sein, wie es mit REDLICH die meisten Autoren annehmen, daß die z. B. im Thalamus zweifellos vorhandenen anatomischen Beziehungen zwischen Affekten und der Körpermuskulatur irgendwie gestört sind (s. Zwangslachen, mimische Facialisparese bei Thalamuserkrankungen usw.). Für die Annahme, daß die Plötzlichkeit der Einwirkung der Affektsache (bzw. nach mir die Notwendigkeit einer plötzlichen motorischen Umstellung) eine Rolle spielt, sprechen wiederholte Angaben von Patienten, daß dieselbe Ursache gar keinen Effekt hat, wenn sie schon erwartet wird (besonders bei CAVE), spricht ferner der Umstand, daß sich der affektive Tonusverlust bei Lachen z. B. bei Wiederholung der Ursache erschöpft (SOLOMON u. a.).

Hier liegt also das erste Charakteristikum der Tonusanfälle und gleichzeitig ihr Unterschied von den Schlafanfällen: das ist *ihr Zusammenhang mit Affekten*. Auf einzelne Ausnahmen, sowohl beim Schlaf wie beim Tonusverlust, haben wir bereits hingewiesen und wollen hier noch einen, allerdings postencephalitischen Fall von CAVE hinzufügen, der anscheinend ohne besonderen Anlaß einfach beim Gehen den Tonusverlust bekam (man muß sich hier jedoch auch an die von SCHILDER und GERSTMANN beschriebenen „Bewegungslücken" bei Encephalitikern erinnern).

Ein weiterer Unterschied gegenüber den Schlafanfällen ist, daß der Tonusverlust ein viel weniger einförmiges und stereotypes Bild bietet, als es in der Regel mit den Schlafanfällen der Fall ist. Hier kommen gegenüber dem Typus des plötzlichen Nachlassens der Innervation am ganzen Körper viel mehr atypische Formen vor. Wohl ist die Plötzlichkeit die Regel und jene Fälle, wo sich der Tonusverlust in rascher, aber doch deutlich merkbarer Reihenfolge auf die einzelnen Körperpartien, etwa vom Gesicht zu den Füßen absteigend, ausbreitet, die Ausnahme. Hingegen gibt es vom Betroffensein des ganzen Körpers so viel Ausnahmen, daß man von einer Regel kaum mehr sprechen kann. So häufig sind die Fälle von sog. *partiellem Tonusverlust*, bei dem nur ein gewisser Körperteil vom Tonusverlust betroffen wird: ein Einknicken in den Knien, die zum Schlag erhobene Hand sinkt kraftlos herunter, der Unterkiefer, der Kopf, die Augenlider sinken herab usw. Ob auch gelegentlicher Secessus urinae dazu gehört, steht noch nicht fest. In der Mehrzahl der Fälle betrifft dieser Tonusverlust jenen Körperteil, der gerade innerviert werden sollte, es gibt jedoch auch Fälle, wo er in Körperpartien auftritt, die mit der beabsichtigten Innervation nichts zu tun haben. Dieser partielle Tonusverlust ist bisher ein Rätsel, doch will es mir scheinen, daß er sich am ehesten mit meiner Hypothese der paradoxen Innervationswirkung bei Affekten in Einklang bringen ließe. Es ist meistens so, daß ein einzelner Kranker den partiellen Tonusverlust immer wieder in derselben Art bekommt oder daß er bei schwächeren Affekten bzw. im Beginn der Krankheit einen lokalisierten, später oder bei stärkeren Affekten einen generalisierten Anfall bekommt.

Der Tonusverlust ist mit Willen noch viel weniger unterdrückbar als der Schlaf; nur vereinzelte Ausnahmen sind bekannt, so 2 Fälle von CAVE, bei denen der Tonusverlust eher zu unterdrücken war als der Schlaf. Die dazu notwendige Willensanstrengung scheint eine sehr große zu sein und man muß sich außerdem bei der Selbstschilderung solcher Kranken vor Täuschungen hüten, denn der Tonusverlust dauert ja ohnehin sehr kurz. Die Ermüdung scheint keine besondere Rolle zu spielen, nur in einem einzelnen, wiederum postencephalitischen Fall von CAVE wird das Gegenteil angegeben.

Wir erwähnten den kompletten und den partiellen Tonusverlust. Damit ist jedoch die Reichhaltigkeit der Symptomatologie des Tonusverlustes noch nicht erschöpft. Es gibt noch recht häufig einen *abortiven Tonusverlust*, eine Art von *Äquivalent des Tonusverlustes*. Selten sind die Fälle, die bei Aufregung nur diesen abortiven Tonusverlust haben, aber recht häufig jene Fälle, wo er neben ausgeprägten Anfällen auftritt. Und hier wird wiederum von den Kranken angegeben, daß es bei leichteren Affekten der Fall ist. Es handelt sich dabei um subjektive Sensationen mehr als um objektiv wahrnehmbare Erscheinungen, subjektive Sensationen allerdings, die ihre Zugehörigkeit zum Tonusverlust dadurch manifestieren, daß sie bei denselben Affekten auftreten wie dieser und weiters dadurch, daß sie oft *auch bei dem vollentwickelten Anfall*, sei es vorher, sei es während des Anfalls, vorhanden sind. Also eine Analogie mit der Anfallsaura des Epileptikers, die ja bekanntlich auch isoliert als ein kleiner Anfall auftreten kann. Es sind dies zumeist verschiedene Parästhesien, oft ein Gefühl der Schwäche, z. B. in den Gesichtsmuskeln, ohne daß eine solche Schwäche wirklich nachweisbar wäre, manchmal dazu eine gewisse Vernebelung des Sehens oder auch ein Tremor, ein Schütteltremor, eine Myokymie im Gesicht oder in den Extremitäten, welche bei Affekten auftreten, Zittern oder Zuckungen der Lippen, der Augen, der Gesichtsmuskulatur, Grimassieren, torquierende, choreiforme Bewegungen der Extremitäten, des Rumpfes, Zungenkrampf — Erscheinungen also, die, zum Teil wenigstens, besonders bei nervösen Individuen, bekannt sind und bei unseren Kranken subjektiv vielleicht bloß dadurch eine besondere Note bekommen, daß bei ihrem Auftreten der Kranke befürchten muß, einen echten Tonusverlust zu bekommen.

Wir haben also hier eine Reihe von Erscheinungen erwähnt, die hier und da neben dem Tonusverlust auftreten, die Symptomatologie eines solchen Anfalls bereichern können. Es gibt aber Fälle, wo noch mehr dieser Symptome *zum Anfall* dazugehören, sei es in Form einer Aura — ein Umstand, der von jenen in den Vordergrund gestellt wird, die eine Verwandtschaft zur Epilepsie behaupten —, sei es auf der Höhe des Anfalls. Wir finden Angaben über Parästhesien, besonders im Gesicht, Steifigkeitsgefühl, über Nebelsehen vor oder im Anfall, über motorische Unruhe und Parästhesien vorher (ROSENTHAL), öfters Hitzegefühl oder Kongestion, Licht oder Blitz im Kopf (PASKIND, WILSON usw.), seltsame Kopfsensationen und Gehörstäuschungen (ein Fall von FRÖDERBERG), ferner Zuckungen, Verziehen des Gesichtes, ticartige Kopfbewegungen, Vorstrecken der Zunge, Zittern besonders im Gesicht, Schütteltremor, Würgen im Hals, Druck auf der Brust usw. B. FISCHER spricht direkt von Krämpfen im Anfall. Es soll hier betont werden, daß am häufigsten und am stärksten diese Erscheinungen bei postencephalitischen Fällen entwickelt sind. So finden wir in einem Fall CAVEs Schütteltremor, leichte Bewußtseinstrübung, undeutliches Sprechen, in einem anderen Blässe, Schwitzen, Zittern und Doppelbilder, im Fall von VADASZ Blickkrämpfe. Es handelt sich um wahre „subcorticale Anfälle", ein Terminus, den ROTHFELD für eine Gruppe von Anfällen vorschlägt, zu denen er auch die Narkolepsie, den Tonusverlust usw. zählen möchte. Und tatsächlich fällt eine gewisse Analogie zu den Blickkrämpfen der Postencephalitiker auf, die in vielen Fällen von einer reichhaltigen pyramidalen, extrapyramidalen oder vegetativen Symptomatologie begleitet sind (s. WILDER und SILBERMANN, Beiträge zum Ticproblem. Berlin: S. Karger 1927).

Durch diese Erscheinungen wird das Problem des affektiven Tonusverlustes ein wenig kompliziert, doch darf man nicht vergessen, daß es sich doch eher um Ausnahmen handelt, und man darf nicht vergessen, das in einzelnen Fällen die Affekte eben auch noch andere Wirkungen als die auf die Muskulatur haben können. Anderseits muß man hier nochmals vermerken, daß ähnliche Erscheinungen auch schon bei den Schlafanfällen Erwähnung fanden, wo also von einer Affektauswirkung keine Rede ist.

Ein wichtiger, vielleicht der wichtigste prinzipielle Unterschied zwischen den Einschlaf- und Tonusanfällen besteht jedoch in der Reversibilität: *die Anfälle von Tonusverlust kann man nicht coupieren!* Man kann einen Kranken aus einem solchen Anfall nicht „erwecken". Nur in einem einzigen und hier wiederum postencephalitischen Fall von STRAUSS gelang es, durch Schütteln angeblich den Anfall zu coupieren und auch hier gilt dieselbe Vorsichtsmaßregel, die schon oben erwähnt wurde, die ohnehin kurze Dauer des Anfalls ist zu berücksichtigen. Einzelne scheinbare weitere Ausnahmen gehören, wie ich weiter unten zeigen werde, nicht zum echten affektiven Tonusverlust.

Was ergibt die objektive Untersuchung des Patienten im Anfall, die wohl leichter durchzuführen ist als die im Schlafanfall, wo der Patient sofort erweckt wird, aber anderseits durch die sehr kurze Dauer dieses Anfalls sehr erschwert wird? Die Reflexe im Anfall werden von manchen erloschen gefunden (WILSON, GOZZANO, CAVE, CURSCHMANN-PRANGE), von anderen herabgesetzt (WAGNER, VILLAVERDE), beides nur ganz vorübergehend, während die dritten sie ganz normal finden (FRÖDERBERG, BROMBERG, REDLICH). Es scheint mir nicht angebracht, daraus weitgehende Schlußfolgerungen ziehen zu wollen, wissen wir doch, daß ein Nachlaß des Muskeltonus auf die Sehnenreflexe einen herabsetzenden Einfluß ausüben kann (daher die Kunstgriffe von Negro, von Sträussler bei Prüfung der Patellarreflexe), ebenso wie eine stärkere Anspannung der Muskulatur (daher Kunstgriff von Jendrassik); es gibt hier eben bekanntlich ein gewisses Optimum der Muskelspannung und dieses ist im Tonusverlust unterschritten. Damit soll aber nicht gesagt sein, daß dieses fallweise Fehlen der Sehnenreflexe schon ein geklärtes Problem ist. Denn wir finden z. B. im Gegensatz zu der Mehrzahl der Autoren, welche normale Pupillen, welche Plantarbeugung der Großzehe beim Babinskischen Versuch finden, auch vereinzelte Angaben über unausgiebige Pupillenreaktion (Cave, Wilson) und über positiven Babinski (Wilson). Einzelne Autoren (z. B. Gozzano) glauben ferner im affektiven Tonusverlust auch Zeichen von Vagotonie beobachtet zu haben.

Es wäre schließlich noch zu vermerken, daß ebenso wie beim Schlafanfall es Wagner bei einem Kranken gelang, durch Afenilinjektion den affektiven Tonusverlust zu provozieren, bei einem anderen nicht. Eine gewisse Bedeutung könnte dabei der Befund Wagners haben, nach welchem bei dem positiven Fall der Blutkalk nach 5 Minuten von 11 mg-% auf 16 mg-% gestiegen war, während sich im anderen, negativen Fall nach 6 Minuten ein normaler Blutkalk fand, so daß Wagner geneigt ist, den affektiven Tonusverlust auf plötzliche Calciumschwankungen nach oben im Blute zurückzuführen. Leider ist sein Material zu gering.

Schließlich ist noch ein sehr wesentlicher Unterschied zwischen dem Schlafanfall und dem Tonusanfall hervorzuheben: das ist die *Dauer* des Anfalls. Im Gegensatz zum Schlafanfall, welcher 5—15 Minuten und noch länger dauert, dauert der affektive Tonusverlust nur wenige Sekunden, selten bis 1—2 Minuten. Ausnahmen sind selten, wie z. B. der auch sonst nicht ganz typische Fall von Fröderberg, bei welchem der Anfall 5—10 Minuten anhielt. Nach Redlich hält der affektive Tonusverlust selten mehr wie 2—3 Minuten an.

Die *Häufigkeit* der Anfälle von affektivem Tonusverlust ist eine sehr verschiedene, auch bei ein und demselben Kranken. Das ist begreiflich, da sie doch auch vom Vorhandensein entsprechender Affekte, also von äußeren Umständen abhängig ist. So gibt es also Kranke, welche in ihrem ganzen Leben nur ein- oder zweimal einen solchen Anfall hatten und daneben andere, welche ihn mehrmals täglich haben, ja imstande sind, an einem lustigen Abend 20mal hintereinander den Tonusverlust zu bekommen oder 30mal täglich (Thiele und Bernhardt). Der Fall von Vadasz erzählt von 100 Anfällen pro Tag. Das hängt nicht nur von dem Grade der Disposition des Kranken ab, sondern auch von seiner ganzen Einstellung zu diesen Anfällen. Viele, aber durchaus nicht alle Kranke, werden von den Anfällen so stark beunruhigt, daß sie jeden Anlaß zu einem Affekt meiden, daß sie sich ganze Kunstgriffe zurechtlegen, um z. B. nicht zu lachen, welche einen ganz ängstlichen Gesichtsausdruck bekommen, wenn irgendwo gelacht wird (Redlich), ja nicht allzu selten sind Kranke, welche durch diese Anfälle ganz asozial werden, die Menschen meiden, in kein Theater, kein Kino gehen usw. Was nun den Grad der Häufigkeit der beiden Reihen von Anfällen im Verhältnis zueinander betrifft, so gibt es da sehr verschiedene Kombinationen. Neben den zwei Extremen, die noch zu besprechen sind, d. h. den Fällen, die isoliert nur Schlafanfälle oder nur den Tonusverlust haben (Ausnahmen!), stehen die schon etwas zahlreicheren Fälle, bei denen die eine oder die andere Erscheinung so stark im Vordergrund ist, daß die Patienten, die z. B. sehr häufig, mehrmals täglich einen Schlafanfall, einen Tonusverlust haben, die andere Erscheinung äußerst selten, vielleicht nur ein oder das andere Mal in ihrem Leben hatten. Und davon gibt es alle Übergänge zum Haupttypus, der mehrmals täglich in relativ regelmäßigen Zwischenräumen seinen Schlafanfall hat und daneben etwas seltener und in ganz unregelmäßigen Intervallen, nicht jeden Tag, den Tonusverlust bekommt.

Beziehungen der Schlafanfälle zum affektiven Tonusverlust. Wir haben uns bemüht, die wichtigen prinzipiellen Unterschiede zwischen den zwei Reihen von Anfällen hervorzuheben. Doch darf man nicht glauben, daß es sich hier immer um zwei rein koordinierte, nebeneinander einhergehende Erscheinungen handelt. Es werden vielmehr Fälle berichtet, die, wenn sie auch nur Ausnahmen darstellen, dafür zu sprechen scheinen, daß es gewisse Beziehungen zwischen diesen zwei Erscheinungen geben muß. Diese Beziehungen scheinen sogar verschiedener Art zu sein. So sind die Fälle nicht allzu selten, wo ein Affekt *statt des Tonusverlustes Schlaf* auslösen kann (WESTPHAL, GÉLINEAU, KAHLER, B. FISCHER, SOMER, REDLICH). Ja wir finden sogar wiederholt die Angabe, daß solche affektive Schlafanfälle den spontanen Schlafanfällen vorausgingen. Ferner gibt es Fälle, wo *bei Unterdrückung von Schlaf Tonusverlust* eintritt (z. B. 2 Fälle von CAVE), weiters Fälle, wo der *Tonusverlust spontan* ohne Affekt einzutreten scheint (REDLICH, MATZDORFF, BONHOEFFER, GRUSZECKA, WILSON, WENDEROWIČ, ZEHRER, LEVIN u. a.). Allerdings bin ich der Meinung, daß es sich bei der Mehrzahl dieser Fälle um etwas anderes handelt als um affektiven Tonusverlust ohne Affekt (s. unten). Wir haben weiters Fälle, wo der *Tonusverlust in Schlaf übergeht* (GÉLINEAU, KAHLER, MILLER, DANIELS und DOYLE) und dann noch die sog. *Wachanfälle* ROSENTHALs (s. unten), wo nach dem Erwachen Tonusverlust zu bestehen scheint. Wir sehen also alle möglichen Arten von Beziehungen, welche dafür sprechen, daß hier engere Zusammenhänge bestehen könnten, auf die wir theoretisch später eingehen werden.

Atypische Zustände. Wir haben gesagt, daß die Narkolepsie durch die zwei Reihen von Anfällen, die Schlafanfälle und die Anfälle von affektivem Tonusverlust ausreichend charakterisiert ist. Damit ist aber nicht gesagt, daß ihre Symptomatologie mit diesen Anfällen erschöpft ist. Vielmehr kommen dabei in einem unvergleichlich weniger obligaten Ausmaß auch verschiedene andere Zustände vor, die wir im letzten Abschnitt zum Teil bereits angedeutet haben und die wir hier als atypische Zustände zusammenfassen wollen. Es handelt sich dabei hauptsächlich um Zustände, die bezeichnenderweise nicht leicht einzureihen sind, weil sie einerseits mit dem Schlaf, andererseits mit dem affektiven Tonusverlust etwas zu tun haben und deren Wesen daher sehr umstritten ist. Zwei davon haben wir bereits erwähnt; es sind dies die Anfälle von spontanem Tonusverlust und die Anfälle von Tonusverlust beim Erwachen. Wir wollen von vornherein bemerken, daß wir uns nicht jenen Autoren anschließen können, welche überhaupt den Schlafanfall mit dem Tonusverlust fast identifizieren und im affektiven Tonusverlust auch einen Schlaf sehen, und zwar einen Körperschlaf ohne Hirnschlaf, einen Körperschlaf bei erhaltenem Bewußtsein also. Und auch nicht jenen Autoren, die (STRAUSS) den Unterschied nur darin sehen, daß einmal der Affekt eine Rolle spielt und ein andermal nicht und von „spontanen" und „reaktiven Anfällen" sprechen. Dazu sind die Unterschiede, die wir hervorgehoben haben und die nicht bloß in der affektiven Bedingtheit, sondern auch in der Reversibilität, in der Dauer usw. bestehen, viel zu groß. Aber daß Beziehungen vorhanden sind, läßt sich nicht leugnen und man sieht sie am besten gerade in den so schwer einzureihenden atypischen Formen.

a) Anfälle von nichtaffektivem, spontanen Tonusverlust. Je mehr man sich in das Studium der Literatur vertieft, desto mehr sieht man, daß die hier und da vorkommenden Anfälle dieser Art manche Besonderheiten gegenüber den Anfällen von affektivem Tonusverlust bieten, Besonderheiten, welche von den Autoren gar nicht oder nur wenig beachtet werden. Nehmen wir hier als Beispiel eine der Krankengeschichten WILSONs und zwar seinen Fall T. T. Es handelt sich um einen 41jährigen Mann, der seit 20 Jahren typische narkoleptische Schlafanfälle hat, fast täglich, nicht selten mehrmals täglich. Sie kommen sehr plötzlich, dauern 4—5 Minuten und Patient erwacht aus ihnen spontan oder kann mit Leichtigkeit erweckt werden. Er ist nachher vollkommen frisch. Er schläft sogar im Gehen ein und erwacht, wenn er an einen Laternenpfosten anrennt. Außerdem hat er seit derselben Zeit auch bei Aufregungen eine sonderbare Schwäche in den Gliedern, so daß er in den Knien einknickt oder sogar fällt. Diese Anfälle dauern außerordentlich kurz, fast momentan und sind verbunden mit Parästhesien im Kopf und im Körper, sowie starkem Herzklopfen. Er bekommt sie bei Lachen, Ärger, Zorn, wenn er seine Kinder schlagen will usw. Insofern haben wir eine ganz typische Krankengeschichte eines Narkoleptikers vor uns. Aber dieser Kranke hat auch noch eine dritte Art von Anfällen. Diese bekommt er zu jeder Zeit, aber *gewöhnlich, wenn er ruhig in einem Sessel sitzt oder auf dem Sofa liegt*, gegen eine Mauer lehnt u. dgl. Es ist ein Lähmungsgefühl, das ihn überkommt, *die Augen sind geschlossen* und er ist absolut außerstande, seinen Finger auch nur um einen Bruchteil eines Zentimeters zu bewegen, dabei weiß er jedoch ganz scharf, was um ihn vorgeht und hört alles, wiederholt ließ er dabei die Zigarette zwischen seinen Fingern weiterbrennen und hat sich so arg verbrannt, ohne imstande gewesen zu sein, etwas dagegen zu tun; er sagt „jemand könnte mich ermorden und ich könnte mich nicht rühren". Er macht innerlich die größten Willensanstrengungen dagegen ohne Erfolg und jemand, der ihn sieht, wird nichts davon merken. Manchmal gelingt es ihm, einen unartikulierten Laut hervorzubringen, um die Aufmerksamkeit auf sich zu lenken. Der Anfall dauert *gewöhnlich 3—5 Minuten. Eine bloße Berührung oder Schütteln genügt, um den Anfall zu unterbrechen,* „den Bann zu brechen". Diese Anfälle kommen dann, *wenn er versucht, den Schlafanfall zu unterdrücken.*

Es ist meine Meinung, daß gerade die Anfälle von diesem Typus (von WILSON zu den Übergängen und Äquivalenten gezählt) und nicht der typische Anfall von Tonusverlust das darstellt, was man den „Körperschlaf" ohne „Hirnschlaf" oder kurz den „*Schlafanfall ohne Schlaf*" nennen könnte. Beachten wir, daß er wohl mit dem affektiven Tonusverlust die Gemeinsamkeit der Innervationsunfähigkeit bei voll erhaltenem Bewußtsein hat; um wieviel mehr hat er jedoch gemeinsam mit dem Schlafanfall: das Auftreten bei Ruhe, im Sitzen oder Liegen, die Dauer (der Tonusverlust „momentan", der Schlafanfall und dieser Anfall etwa 5 Minuten), die prompte Reversibilität durch Berührung usw., was im affektiven Tonusverlust nicht vorkommt und schließlich das Auftreten im Moment, wo Patient mit seinem Willen einen Schlafanfall unterdrücken will. Es ist so, als ob es ihm gelungen wäre, sein Bewußtsein, aber nicht seinen Körper wach zu erhalten. Er schläft, er muß geweckt werden, aber nur körperlich. Diese Zustände erinnern an manche Zustände beim Normalen, die ins Gebiet des Alpdrucks, des Pavor nocturnus usw. fallen. Es sind dies nicht bloß jene Träume, in denen alles mögliche Schreckliche geschieht, während wir uns absolut nicht bewegen können. Es führen davon Übergänge zu jenen, ebenfalls fast allen Normalen bekannten Schreckträumen, in denen wir wissen, daß es nur ein Traum ist und vergeblich alle Bemühungen machen, um zu erwachen, bis schließlich zu jenen schon ans Pathologische grenzenden Zuständen, wo man aus einem solchen Schrecktraum erwacht, aber noch immer eine Weile unter seinem Bann steht, sei es, daß man nicht imstande ist, die Schrecksituation mit voller Klarheit als nur traumhaft zur Kenntnis zu nehmen, sei es, daß man noch immer sich nicht bewegen kann. Wir werden später darauf hinweisen, wie häufig und wie hochgradig gerade solche nächtliche Erlebnisse bei Narkoleptikern sein können. Hier wollen wir nur noch kurz auf das Gegenstück dieses Zustandes des Körperschlafes hinweisen, auf den Somnambulismus, den man den Hirnschlaf ohne Körperschlaf nennen könnte oder als Pendant zum „Schlafanfall ohne Schlaf" den „Wachanfall ohne Wachsein". Der Fall WILSONs steht nicht vereinzelt da und wir können unter jenen Fällen, die als Tonusverlust ohne Affekt beschrieben wurden, immer wieder solche finden, bei denen in puncto Dauer, Reversibilität usw. viel mehr Gemeinsamkeiten mit dem Schlafanfall als mit dem Tonusanfall bestehen. Wir finden das auch unter den oben erwähnten Fällen von affektivem Tonusverlust bei Unterdrückung des Schlafes und es finden sich unter den Fällen von CAVE z. B. solche, welche diesen von WILSON so treffend beschriebenen Zustand im Bett vor dem Einschlafen zu bekommen pflegen und durch eine Berührung „geweckt" werden müssen. Wir fassen also zusammen: Es gibt bei der Narkolepsie eine ganze Reihe von Erscheinungen, die sich am besten unter dem Namen *Dissoziationserscheinungen* zusammenfassen lassen. Es sind dies Fälle von Dissoziation zwischen Hirnschlaf und Körperschlaf, die in verschiedener Form auftreten können (s. unter Nachtschlaf der Narkoleptiker) und die man im Gegensatz zu den Schlafanfällen auch mit ROSENTHAL als Wachanfälle bezeichnen kann (ROSENTHAL selbst jedoch versteht darunter eine bestimmte eng umschriebene Gruppe dieser Zustände). Die Übergänge zu den wirklichen Schlafanfällen sind fließend, denn auch bei diesen ist der Schlaf oft nur sehr oberflächlich und öfters berichtet der Kranke, er habe gehört, was um ihn vorging.

b) Zu diesen Anfällen von Körperschlaf gehören auch vereinzelte vom beschriebenen Typus abweichende Anfälle. So beschreibt z. B. ROSENTHAL Zustände, bei denen Patient im Anfall *nicht nur alles wahrnimmt, sondern auch gehen kann*, so lange, bis er auf ein Hindernis stößt. WILSON beschreibt Zustände, die er „*rêverie*" nennt, in denen der Patient den Eindruck des Schlafenden macht, aber alles merkt, sich an alles erinnert und anscheinend das Gefühl hat, den Zustand jederzeit abbrechen zu können. PENTA erwähnt Tagträume. Dann gibt es eigentümliche Zustände von „*Zerstreutheit*", man könnte sie vielleicht auch „*Schlaftrunkenheit*" nennen, in denen die Patienten plötzlich alles verkehrt machen; sie sind dabei eigentlich nicht bewußtlos, sie sind eher das, was man im gewöhnlichen Sprachgebrauch „geistesabwesend" nennt: Ein Koch macht z. B. statt der bestellten Eier eine andere Speise, ein Kartenspieler nimmt plötzlich die Karten vom Tisch und reicht sie seinem Nachbar (CAVE). Die Kranken merken den Fehler sofort oder sehr bald und korrigieren ihn womöglich, eine eigentliche Amnesie besteht nicht. Die Verwandtschaft aller dieser Zustände mit Zuständen von Schlaftrunkenheit, von Erscheinungen bei starker Übermüdung, bei Schlafunterdrückung, bei jähem Aufwecken des Normalen ist offenkundig. Allerdings gibt es auch hier, aber besonders bei postencephalitischen Fällen, deren Schlaf ja überhaupt Dissoziationserscheinungen bietet (z. B. die „Pseudoschlafzustände" MARINESCOs) Zustände, deren Zuteilung schon nicht so ganz klar ist, aber immerhin noch im Rahmen des soeben Ausgeführten liegen kann; so z. B., wenn ein Patient CAVEs im Schlafanfall *sinnlose Handlungen begeht* und unverständliche Worte murmelt. Ein möglicherweise encephalitischer Fall CAVEs hatte vor Auftreten einer typischen Narkolepsie von Jugend auf Anfälle von *Tonusverlust (spontan?) mit Dyspnoe, Flimmern vor den Augen, Zittern der Arme, Zuckungen im Gesicht und in den Extremitäten*, Anfälle, die besonders im Sitzen oder Liegen kamen, ein paar Sekunden bis 1 Minute dauerten und evtl. durch eine tiefe Inspiration coupiert werden konnten. Hier zu erwähnen sind z. B. 2 nicht ganz typische Fälle von ROTHFELD, bei denen teils im Schlafanfall, teils beim Versuch, den Schlaf zu überwinden, *Erektionen* auftraten.

ROTHFELD betont gewisse Beziehungen zwischen Schlaf, sexuellen Vorgängen und Lachen, welche auch bei der Narkolepsie größere Beachtung verdienen: sexuelle Erregungen rufen Schlaf und Lachen hervor, das Lachen kann Schlaf erzeugen (beim Normalen Schlaf nach Orgasmus), Schlafzustände verbinden sich mit sexuellen Erregungen. Hier wäre ein Fall von mir zu zitieren, der jahrelang Anfälle von Zwangslachen verbunden mit Erektion hatte, die dann zur Aura eines epileptischen Anfalls wurden; ein Bruder des Patienten hatte Epilepsie, ein anderer Anfälle von Zwangslachen. Nehmen wir einen Fall von FELIX FRISCH hinzu, eine Frau, die an Anfällen von Zwangslachen litt, welche in der Pubertät schwanden, um im Klimakterium wiederzukehren, ähnlich wie es sich in einer Narkoleptikerfamilie von HOFF und STENGEL mit den Schlafanfällen verhielt (Mutter hat Schlafanfälle bis zur Pubertät und im Klimakterium, zwei Söhne in der Pubertät, eine Tochter bis zm Klimakterium). Ich selbst sah einen Patienten, der Schlafanfälle mit Pollutionen hatte, doch erwies sich die Sache als hysterisch und schwand sofort unter Psychotherapie, bei einem anderen Neurotiker, der am Morgen Zustände von ,,Trance", wie er es nannte, hatte, in denen er einen schweren Alpdruck hatte mit Unmöglichkeit, sich zu bewegen, waren diese Zustände regelmäßig mit Erektionen verbunden. Wenn man also auch hier manches mit Vorsicht aufnehmen muß, so hat ROTHFELD sicher Recht, wenn er meint, daß es zwischen Schlaf, Lachen, Sexualität und, fügen wir hinzu, Tonusverlust Zusammenhänge gibt, sowohl bei Normalen als auch bei der Narkolepsie, die eines näheren Studiums wert sind.

c) Eine Gruppe von Anfällen hat besonders ROSENTHAL hervorgehoben und ihnen den Namen ,,*Wachanfälle*" gegeben, sie finden sich schon in der älteren Literatur hier und da erwähnt und werden auch bei WILSON, WEIR MITCHELL, STRANSKY, CAVE beschrieben. THIELE und BERNHARDT fanden sie in 4 von 25 Fällen. Sie werden von ROSENTHAL mit PFISTERS ,,verzögertem psychomotorischen Erwachen" bei Normalen in Beziehung gebracht und bestehen darin, daß der Patient aus seinem Nachtschlaf erwacht, ganz bei Bewußtsein ist, jedoch nicht imstande ist sich zu bewegen, meist auch nicht imstande ist zu sprechen. Der Zustand vergeht entweder spontan oder bei irgendeiner äußeren Einwirkung. Eine meiner Patientinnen z. B. konnte erst ,,ganz erwachen", d. h. sich bewegen und aufstehen, wenn man sie im Bette umdrehte. Wir haben hier wieder Dissoziation zwischen Hirnschlaf und Körperschlaf und sehen gleich Analogien zu manchen oben beschriebenen Zuständen. Bei den Wachanfällen ROSENTHALS erwacht gewissermaßen das Gehirn viel früher als der Körper, bei den analogen Störungen, die dem nächtlichen Schlaf *vorausgehen*, schläft sozusagen der Körper früher ein als das Gehirn, bei den ,,Schlafanfällen ohne Schlaf", die untertags zustande kommen, wie bei dem näher beschriebenen Fall WILSONS, gelingt die Unterdrückung des Hirnschlafes, aber nicht die des Körperschlafes. Während also beim normalen Menschen der Hirn- und der Körperschlaf eng assoziiert sind, das Gehirn, der Wille imstande ist, nur beides zusammen zuzulassen oder zu unterdrücken, das Gehirn einschläft, wenn der Körper es verlangt, der Körper einschläft, wenn das Gehirn in Schlaf verfällt, so sehen wir hier Dissoziationserscheinungen dieser beiden Komponenten des Schlafes, wie sie beim Normalen nur in viel geringerem Grade und unter ganz besonderen Umständen auftreten.

Man könnte also diese ganze Gruppe von Anfällen — nicht aber die Anfälle von affektivem Tonusverlust — auch *Dissoziationszustände* nennen oder auch *Dysgrypnien* und ihnen noch anfügen die in vielen Fällen, besonders bei CAVE, THIELE-BERNHARDT u. a. beschriebenen Zustände von Alpdruck, von *Pavor nocturnus* mit Unbeweglichkeit. Mit monotoner Einförmigkeit erleben diese Patienten hier und da nachts dasselbe: Sie erwachen entweder aus einem Angsttraum oder aber mit dem Gefühl, jemand sei im Zimmer oder jemand steige durchs Fenster, sie erleben alle Phasen von Angst und Verzweiflung, sind aber außerstande, sich zu rühren oder auch nur um Hilfe zu rufen. Doch gehören diese Zustände bereits in ein anderes Kapitel, bei welchem man noch reichlich Schlafdissoziationserscheinungen finden kann, in das Kapitel des *Nachtschlafes* bei der Narkolepsie. Hier wollen wir nur noch zum Abschluß erwähnen, daß auch ein Fall erwähnt wird, wo der morgendliche Wachanfall mit Desorientierung einherging, also vielleicht auch das Gehirn nur *partiell* erwacht war. Interessant ist ein Fall von BROCK, wo Wachanfälle nur im Anschluß an narkoleptischen Schlaf auftraten.

Der Nachtschlaf der Narkoleptiker. REDLICH war es, der darauf hingewiesen hat, daß der Nachtschlaf bei den Narkoleptikern viel häufiger gestört ist, als man bei oberflächlicher Betrachtung annehmen würde. Häufig geben die Kranken an, sie schliefen gut, während die Umgebung berichtet, daß sie durch das *Herumwälzen*, das *Sprechen aus dem Schlaf*, durch *somnambule Zustände* dieser Patienten gestört wird. Diese Störung geht sogar öfters so weit, daß niemand mit ihnen im selben Raum schlafen kann. Diese Beobachtung, die man ursprünglich nur so aufzufassen geneigt schien, daß der gestörte Nachtschlaf irgendeine Rolle bei der Schlafsucht untertags spielen könnte, erweist sich immer mehr als von tieferer Bedeutung für die narkoleptische Schlafstörung, als Ausdruck derselben Störung wie die Schlafanfälle und andere Erscheinungen, als Fundgrube der verschiedenartigsten Dissoziationserscheinungen des Schlafes. Man darf allerdings nicht glauben, daß alle Narkoleptiker an nächtlichen Schlafstörungen leiden. Ganz normaler Schlaf ist gar nicht selten, auch tiefer Schlaf kommt vor, aber auch abnorm langer Nachtschlaf ist nicht selten, manche Patienten können auch 10, 12 Stunden in einem Zug schlafen, allerdings ist dieser lange Schlaf oft kein ruhiger Schlaf. Sehr häufig ist der Schlaf unruhig, oftmals unterbrochen, die Schlaftiefe scheint sehr zu schwanken, die Kranken wälzen sich im Schlaf herum, sie sprechen aus dem Schlaf, ja sie stehen auf und gehen herum, wobei sie verschiedene, oft unsinnige Hantierungen vornehmen; lautes Aufschreien aus dem Schlaf ist nicht selten, ebenso wie ausgesprochener Pavor nocturnus. Grelle, lebhafte, angsterfüllte Träume werden immer wieder berichtet. Schon REDLICH wies darauf hin, daß zwischen diesem schlechten Schlaf und der Narkolepsie eigentümliche Beziehungen zu bestehen scheinen. Oft tritt diese Schlafstörung *zugleich* mit der Narkolepsie auf, manchmal geht sie ihr voraus, manchmal besteht sie seit Jugend oder seit 10, seit 20 Jahren vor dem Auftreten der Narkolepsie (CAVE). REDLICH wies ferner darauf hin (und seither wurden auch noch weitere Fälle beschrieben), daß der Narkolepsie manchmal eine Zeit vorausgeht, wo der Schlaf aus äußeren Gründen gestört ist (Nachtarbeit usw.). Manchmal berichtet der Patient, daß sein Schlaf in der Kindheit, in der Pubertät gestört war, sei es im Sinne einer Schlaflosigkeit, sei es — und dies häufiger — Schlafsucht. Fälle, wie der von PASKIND, bei denen berichtet wird, daß Patient nach der Geburt durch 5 Monate ohne Unterbrechung geschlafen hat, werden eher den Verdacht auf encephalitische oder traumatische Genese lenken. In seltenen Fällen besteht eine ständige Schlafsucht bei Tage (CAVE) oder eine dauernde Müdigkeit (BEYERMANN, nach ROSENTHAL sogar in einem Viertel der Fälle), eine Mattigkeit am Morgen nach dem Erwachen (GRÜN). Manchmal bildet sich der Typus der Schlafumkehr heraus, wie er bei den Postencephalitikern bekannt ist, d. h. Schlaflosigkeit in der Nacht, Schlafsucht bei Tage (KAMMANN, CAVE, PASKIND, PENTA u. a.), allerdings auch hier wiederum vorwiegend bei postencephalitischen Fällen. Ein schläfriges Aussehen haben viele der Kranken ständig. — Diese Dissoziationserscheinungen des Schlafes bieten viel Bemerkenswertes. So ist z. B. bei solchen Fällen Somnambulismus in der Kindheit oder in der Familie beobachtet worden.

Fragen wir uns, ob die Dauer des Nachtschlafes einen Einfluß hat auf die Zahl der Schlafanfälle bei Tag, wie es naheliegend wäre anzunehmen, so müssen wir vorerst feststellen, daß nur ganz ausnahmsweise ein verlängerter Nachtschlaf zu einer Abnahme der narkoleptischen Anfälle führt, wie in einem (encephalitischen!) Falle CAVEs. Es kommt übrigens auch das Gegenteil vor (SOLOMON), daß langer Nachtschlaf eher zur Vermehrung solcher Anfälle führt, etwas, was sich auch beim Normalen mitunter angedeutet findet. In der überwiegenden Majorität der Fälle hat die Dauer des Nachtschlafes oder, besser gesagt, der verlängerte Nachtschlaf keinen besonderen Einfluß auf die Zahl der Anfälle, vielmehr ist es so wie Cave sagt, daß Verlängerung ohne Einfluß ist, Verkürzung des Nachtschlafes jedoch zu einer Vermehrung der narkoleptischen Anfälle führt.

Es liegt nahe, daß so manche Patienten versuchen, durch einen ausgiebigen Nachmittagsschlaf die Zahl der Anfälle zu vermindern und die Arbeitsfähigkeit zu steigern. Manchmal gelingt dies auch, und zwar nicht allzu selten (z. B. Jeliffe, Solomon, Wagner, Cave u. a.). Meistens sind dann die Patienten etwa 2—3 Stunden frei von Schlafanfällen; aber es fehlt auch nicht an Fällen, wo dieser Nachmittagsschlaf ganz ohne jeden Einfluß ist.

Der neurologische Befund bei der Narkolepsie ist *in der Regel ganz negativ*, wenn wir von den Fällen symptomatischer, besonders postencephalitischer Narkolepsie absehen. Dort, wo sich kleine Abweichungen von der Norm finden, haben sie öfters eine besondere Erklärung. So finden wir leichte Differenzen der Sehnenreflexe in Fällen von Redlich, Kahler, Stransky, Levin, Ratner, die in einem Teil der Fälle von den Autoren auf die im Röntgenbild nachweisbare Drucksteigerung im Schädel zurückgeführt werden. In einem Fall Rosenthals findet sich Babinski und Oppenheim angedeutet. Ein Fall von Goldflam mit Zungenkrämpfen nach links bot ein Abweichen der Zunge nach links, Wilson erwähnt Doppelbilder ohne Lähmung, also wahrscheinlich Konvergenzschwäche und diese findet sich auch bei Rothfeld und in den meisten (familiären) Fällen von Hoff und Stengel. Brock und Zehrer erwähnen sympathische Ophthalmoplegie, Kennedy Doppelbilder und Zuckungen bei plötzlichen Geräuschen, Redlich ticartige Zuckungen im Platysma und Migräne, Wohlfahrt verschiedene Zuckungen, 2 wahrscheinlich symptomatische Fälle von Cave hatten Kopfschmerzen, einer davon Konvergenzschwäche. 3 Fälle von Redlich, ferner je 1 Fall von Levin, von Serejski und Frumkin und von Cave hatten leichten Nystagmus. Bei zahlreichen Fällen mit schläfrigem Aussehen, die ich selbst sehen konnte, kann man von einer leichten habituellen Ptosis sprechen, die für die Lokalisation der Störung von einer gewissen Bedeutung sein kann (s. unten). Der Muskeltonus wird öfters herabgesetzt gefunden (Rosenthal, Thiele u. a.). Fügen wir noch dazu, daß sich in ganz vereinzelten Fällen (Thiele, Beyermann) positiver Chwostek fand und daß neben Fällen mit normaler elektrischer Erregbarkeit (Redlich, Beyermann), in einzelnen Fällen auch erhöhte Erregbarkeit gefunden wurde (Thiele, Mankowsky, Beyermann). Bei Beyermann sank diese erhöhte Erregbarkeit nach erfolgreicher Behandlung in einem Fall herab. Marinesco, Sager und Kreindler behaupten Zunahme der Erregbarkeit im physiologischen Schlaf. C. P. Richter fand dabei den Hautwiderstand erhöht; diesen Befund hat der Narkoleptiker angeblich auch im Wachen.

Damit erschöpfen sich die dürftigen und wenig charakteristischen Befunde am animalen Nervensystem. Reichhaltiger sind die Abweichungen von der Norm, die wir am vegetativen Nervensystem finden.

Vegetatives System. Einige Befunde kehren hier so häufig wieder, daß wir ihnen eine Bedeutung kaum absprechen können. Es sind dies vor allem *Fettsucht, Herabsetzung des Grundumsatzes* und *Lymphocytose*. Schon Redlich betont die relative Häufigkeit einer ausgesprochenen Fettsucht, die er unter 100 Fällen in 17 Fällen findet, manchmal zugleich mit der Narkolepsie entwickelt und bis zu 20 kg reichend, und zwar auch bei nicht postencephalitischen Fällen. In der neueren Literatur hat sich der Prozentsatz von Fällen, die entweder ausgesprochene Fettsucht oder deutliche Gewichtszunahme während oder vor der Narkolepsie zeigten, beträchtlich vermehrt, sei es, daß man jetzt auf dieses Symptom mehr achtet, sei es, daß unter den Fällen mehr postencephalitische Fälle mitlaufen. Wilson, der den Begriff der Narkolepsie weiter faßt, findet noch mehr Fälle mit Fettsucht. THIELE und BERNHARDT fanden in allen ihren 25 Fällen eine Gewichtszunahme, besonders zu Beginn der Erkrankungen und parallele Schwankungen der Fettsucht und der Narkolepsie, CAVE fand unter seinen 42 Fällen 18 mit ausgesprochener Gewichtszunahme, meist zugleich mit der Erkrankung, mit einem durchschnittlichen Gewichtszuwachs von 12 kg. Ein Fall, der aus einer fettsüchtigen Familie stammte, nahm in 3 Jahren 45 kg zu. Außerdem fand er die meisten Fälle ihrem Wuchs nach stark übergewichtig, und zwar betrug das durchschnittliche Übergewicht bei den Männern 11 kg, bei den Frauen 20 kg. MÜNZER fand bei 79 encephalitischen Fällen Fettsucht 34mal, hingegen ausgesprochenen Parkinsonismus nur 7mal. Ich finde auch einen allerdings symptomatischen (hypophysären) Fall von PFANNER mit Magersucht, Senium praecox und akromegaloiden Zügen. REDLICH, LHERMITTE u. a. weisen übrigens auch auf die bekannte Erscheinung der Schlafsucht bei Fettleibigkeit hin (der „fette Joy" in den Pickwickiern usw.). Solche Fälle, die übrigens oft so eng an der Grenze der Narkolepsie liegen, daß REDLICH ausdrücklich eine „symptomatische Narkolepsie bei Fettsucht" unterscheidet, beschrieben z. B. SAINTON, GOLDFLAM, LHERMITTE, REDLICH. SAINTON spricht da von einer Autointoxikation der Fettleibigen. Allerdings entsteht da immer auch die Frage, ob die Fettsucht selbst nicht wiederum symptomatisch ist, wie die folgenden 2 Fälle REDLICHS zeigen.

Fall 1. 43jähriger Mann aus fettleibiger Familie. Patient, seit vielen Jahren fettleibig, wiegt jetzt 140 kg. Vor 14 Jahren Lues (!), mehrmals behandelt, zuletzt vor 9 Jahren. Seit 4 Jahren schläft er untertags wiederholt für mehrere Minuten ein, erwacht spontan. Niemals affektiver Tonusverlust. Nachtschlaf gut, spricht aber aus dem Schlaf und hat gelegentlich Secessus urinae. Zeitweise Durst. Grundumsatz — 26,4%, spezifisch-dynamische Eiweißwirkung normal, 20% Lymphocyten. Auf Thyreoideapräparate angeblich Besserung der Schlafanfälle. — Fall 2. 50jähriger Mann aus fettleibiger Familie, derzeit 130 kg schwer, schläft untertags öfters ein, besonders wenn es warm ist. Nachtschlaf in letzter Zeit unterbrochen. Sella erweitert, Dorsum dünn. Niemals affektiver Tonusverlust.

Diese Fälle sollen als Beispiel dienen, daß die Narkolepsie bei Fettsucht zu der oben beschriebenen echten Narkolepsie oft nur sehr lose, aber theoretisch dennoch interessante Beziehungen hat.

Der *Grundumsatz* bei den Narkoleptikern zeigt sehr oft Anomalien, wenn auch selten hochgradige, und zwar bewegen sich diese Anomalien, wie man eigentlich schon aus der Häufigkeit der Fettsucht erwarten sollte, fast ausschließlich im Sinne einer Herabsetzung. So konnte REDLICH 17 Fälle zusammenstellen, darunter 7 eigene, von denen nur einer eine Erhöhung zeigte, und das war eine gravide Frau, 3 waren normal und 13 zeigten eine Herabsetzung verschiedenen Grades (4 weniger als —10%, 2 mehr als 30%). In der späteren Literatur finde ich weitere 26 Fälle, von denen 5 geringe Erhöhung, 4 normalen Befund, 3 eine Herabsetzung unter —10%, 15 eine höhergradige Herabsetzung zeigen. Weiteres fanden THIELE und BERNHARDT in ihren 28 Fällen in 64% normalen Befund, in 21% Verminderung über —10%, in 15% Vermehrung über +10%; diese Autoren finden aber eine herabgesetzte spezifisch-dynamische Eiweißwirkung, während REDLICH in seiner Zusammenstellung gerade in der spezifisch-dynamischen Eiweißwirkung keine eindeutige Veränderung finden konnte. Wir sehen also, daß die Befunde derzeit noch sehr divergent sind, was zum Teil vielleicht mit Verschiedenheiten der Technik zu erklären ist. Den Arbeitsstoffwechsel fanden THIELE und BERNHARDT normal.

Blutbefund. REDLICH hat zuerst die Aufmerksamkeit auf eine oft beträchtliche Lymphocytose gelenkt, welche sich bei der Narkolepsie findet. Er fand sie in 7 eigenen Fällen (von 19) und sie findet sich auch in zahlreichen Fällen der Literatur, bei denen danach gefahndet wurde. Es fehlt allerdings nicht an Fällen, bei denen die Lymphocytenzahlen normal waren. THIELE und BERN-

HARDT fanden in ihren 25 Fällen fast stets eine Lymphocytose, in den Fällen CAVES finden sich ebenfalls Fälle mit Lymphocytose. Die Lymphocytenzahlen übersteigen 30, 40, ja 50%. Auch ein von mir publizierter Fall von Narkolepsie nach Kastration hatte über 40% Lymphocyten und ich sah sie fast in allen persönlich untersuchten Fällen. Die Bedeutung dieser Lymphocytose ist unklar. Etwaige Zeichen von Hyperthyreoidismus finden sich bei diesen Fällen nicht (s. auch Grundumsatz). REDLICH ist geneigt, sie als konstitutionell zu betrachten, als Ausdruck eines Status lymphaticus, KAHLER als Zeichen hypoplastischer Konstitution, BAUER als Infantilismus. Ich selbst konnte darauf hinweisen, daß ich im Jahre 1919 bei mir und mehreren anderen eine eigentümliche Schlafsucht, verbunden mit beträchtlicher Lymphocytose konstatieren konnte. Ich führte dies auf die damals in Wien ganz abnormen Ernährungsverhältnisse zurück (erste Nachkriegszeit). Was den sonstigen Blutbefund betrifft, so hatten nur einzelne Fälle (REDLICH, MAKAROV, LEVIN) eine Eosinophilie. Auf die Fälle von Narkolepsie bei Polycythämie werden wir noch beim Kapitel symptomatische Narkolepsie zurückkommen.

Auch im Bereich des *vegetativen Nervensystems* finden sich außer den bereits erwähnten Anomalien noch so oft Abweichungen von der Norm, daß es sich wohl um einen wesentlichen Zusammenhang mit der Narkolepsie handelt. Leider lassen unsere Untersuchungsmethoden des vegetativen Nervensystems ja bekanntlich noch viel zu wünschen übrig und in vielen Fällen von Narkolepsie wurde darauf überhaupt nicht geachtet. Immerhin finden wir manches Bemerkenswerte. Man kann die Anomalien, die sich hier finden, mehr oder weniger im Sinne einer erhöhten Vagusansprechbarkeit deuten, wie es ja auch viele Autoren tun; in erster Linie THIELE und BERNHARDT. Der Puls zeigt keine besonderen Anomalien, in den Fällen von THIELE-BERNHARDT hatte er meist Frequenz 60—70, der Blutdruck ist öfters erniedrigt (REDLICH u. a.). Herabgesetzte oder paradoxe (vagotone) Adrenalinreaktion, verstärkte Pilocarpinreaktion sah REDLICH in seinen Fällen, ferner KAHLER, ROTHFELD, SPERLING und WIMMER, THIELE, WOHLFAHRT. Doch finden sich auch seltene Fälle mit umgekehrtem Verhalten (LEVIN, RATHNER?). THIELE und BERNHARDT sahen in ihren 25 Fällen fast immer eine vegetative Labilität mit Tendenz nach der vagotonen Seite hin. Sichtbare vasomotorische Störungen vermerken STRAUSS, ZEHRER, ZADOR, REDLICH, RAYNAUDsche Krankheit DOYLE-DANIELS. Das Capillarbild bietet nichts Charakteristisches (eigene Fälle, THIELE-BERNHARDT). Auf diese Störungen legt STRAUSS besonderes Gewicht. Auch andere subjektive und objektive Symptome, welche sich allerdings bloß gelegentlich finden und nach denen auch nicht systematisch gefahndet wurde, sprechen mehr im Sinne einer erhöhten Vagusansprechbarkeit. So erwähnt REDLICH verstärkte respiratorische Arhythmie, positiven okulo-cardialen Reflex von ASCHNER, auffallende Bulimie, Speichelfluß, Schwitzen, Neigung zu Stuhlverstopfung. Es findet sich öfters verstärkter, elevierter, weißer Dermographismus (PFANNER); vielleicht gehören auch die Parästhesien hierher. Die Temperatur zeigt in der Regel keine Anomalien. Der Wasserhaushalt wurde nur wenig beachtet; REDLICH allerdings hat ihm sein Interesse zugewendet, er sah in einem Falle Polyurie und Polydipsie, ebenso LEVIN, BAILAY und FULTON. In 2 Fällen sah er Pollakisurie. Verschiedenartige Störungen sahen auch THIELE und BERNHARDT öfters, aber keine Gesetzmäßigkeit. Das Verhältnis von Wasseraufnahme und -ausscheidung ist oft normal, aber wir sehen auch hier und da eine leicht herabgesetzte oder noch öfters eine leicht überschießende Wasserausscheidung (REDLICH, MÜNZER). Der VOLHARDsche Wasserversuch ergab REDLICH, ebenso wie mir selbst, sehr verschiedene Resultate. Der Versuch, den VOLHARDschen Wasserstoß durch Pituitrin zu hemmen (nach HOFF und WERMER), ergab normale

Hemmung (REDLICH, eigene Fälle). REDLICH versuchte auch einmal den Einfluß von Präphyson, einmal von Thyroxin auf den VOLHARDschen Versuch, beides ohne deutlichen Effekt.

Gehen wir zum *Stoffwechsel* über, so haben sich bisher keine eindeutigen Störungen erwiesen. Der *Nüchternblutzucker* wurde in der letzten Zeit vielfach untersucht und normal befunden, doch heben THIELE und BERNHARDT mit Recht hervor, daß sich oft Werte an der unteren Grenze der Norm finden; in ihrer Arbeit finde ich auch ausgesprochen subnormale Werte (67, 68, 70 mg-%). Die ausgesprochenen Fälle von Hypoglykämie von HARRIS, sowie von MARINESCO, FAÇON und Mitarbeiter werden jedoch meines Erachtens zu Unrecht zu der Narkolepsie gezählt. Auch der *Liquorzucker* ist normal (TSIMINAKIS, THIELE-BERNHARDT). LEVIN, MÜNZER, PASKIND, WOHLFAHRT, ich u. a. prüften auch die *alimentäre Blutzuckerkurve* und fanden sie normal, nur bei WOHLFAHRT war sie herabgesetzt, bei SCHILDER erhöht. In meinen Fällen war auch die hypoglykämische Phase in der 2. und 3. Stunde normal. Die Dextrose- und Galaktosetoleranz an der Zuckerausscheidung gemessen, ist nicht erniedrigt (REDLICH, ich, THIELE und BERNHARDT u. a.). WOHLFAHRT fand in einem Fall den *Insulineffekt* auf den Blutzucker verstärkt, die *Adrenalinhyperglykämie* war normal oder erniedrigt.

Der *Blutkalk* war in meinen eigenen Fällen, sowie in denen von BASSOE, von THIELE-BERNHARDT normal. Letztere finden manchmal auch im *Kochsalz-Stoffwechsel* deutliche Störungen.

Andere Stoffwechseluntersuchungen liegen nicht vor, und das ist bedauerlich, denn meines Erachtens sind gerade auf diesem Gebiete weitere Aufklärungen über die Narkolepsie zu erwarten. Besonders fehlen vergleichende Untersuchungen im Anfall und außerhalb desselben.

Andere Laboratoriumsbefunde. Der *Liquor cerebro-spinalis* wurde in einer ganzen Reihe von Fällen untersucht und stets normal befunden, selbstverständlich mit Ausnahme einiger „symptomatischer" Fälle. Kochsalzgehalt im Liquor ist normal (THIELE-BERNHARDT). STRANSKY ließ auch den *Pituitringehalt des Liquors* untersuchen, der Befund war spurweise positiv (biologische Probe). Die *Senkungsgeschwindigkeit* des Blutes war in den Fällen von THIELE und BERNHARDT herabgesetzt, bei LHERMITTE und PEYRE normal. Das *Encephalogramm* nach Lufteinblasung war in 4 Fällen von THIELE und BERNHARDT normal, in 2 Fällen Erweiterung, in einem (traumatischen) Asymmetrie der Ventrikel, einmal atypische Lage des Aquädukts. Die Wa.R. im Blut ist negativ, mit Ausnahme der luischen Fälle.

Eine gewisse Bedeutung wird von manchen Autoren den *Röntgenbefunden der Sella* zugeschrieben, die wir weiter unten beim Kapitel Hypophyse erwähnen.

Der *internistische Befund* ist immer normal.

Der äußere Habitus bietet außer der schon erwähnten Fettsucht manchmal auch andere Anomalien. So fand REDLICH in mehreren Fällen das typische Bild der lymphatischen Konstitution. THIELE und BERNHARDT fanden in ihren Fällen das Vorwiegen des untersetzten, evtl. auch athletischen Körperbaues. In manchen Fällen werden akromegaloide Züge erwähnt. SCHILDER beschreibt eunuchoiden Hochwuchs.

Das psychische Bild bietet in den meisten Fällen nichts Abnormes, doch sind neurasthenische Beschwerden nach REDLICH nicht selten und auch psychopathische Züge werden in einer ganzen Anzahl von Fällen vermerkt. Leichte Imbezillität notieren REDLICH, NOAK, BOAS, B. FISCHER, JANZEN, JAKOBSOHN, THIELE-BERNHARDT (evtl. ist nur von geringer Intelligenz die Rede). Eine Patientin von REDLICH, eine von SEREJSKI und FRUMKIN hatte in der Jugend ein eigentümliches, scheues Wesen, machte als Kind einen Selbstmordversuch.

Der Patient HENNEBERGs war deutlich dement. Der Kranke VILLAVERDEs war „phantasiereich". Ein Kranker REDLICHs, ebenso wie einer von NOAK und mein Kastrat zeigten Neigung zu Gewalttätigkeiten. Ein Patient REDLICHs wollte ein Perpetuum mobile erfinden. Eine Patientin von B. FISCHER hatte gelegentliche Halluzinationen und epileptische Anfälle. Ein Fall von LEVIN hatte vorübergehende amnestische Zustände. Ein Kranker EDELs, einer von THIELE-BERNHARDT waren schizophren, ein Fall FRÖDERBERGs paranoid, ebenso ein Fall SCHILDERs. Eine Kranke JELIFFEs litt an zirkulärem Irresein. Ein Patient REDLICHs, der nur intermittierend an Schlafanfällen litt, hatte periodische Depressionszustände und ein Patient CAVEs, ein Cycloider, hatte die Narkolepsie nur in den depressiven Phasen (vielleicht encephalitisch). THIELE-BERNHARDT finden nicht bloß bei den encephalitischen Fällen die typische Psyche der Encephalitiker sehr häufig, sondern gelegentlich auch bei genuinen Fällen. Stottern finden wir in je 2 Fällen bei REDLICH und bei WOHLFAHRT; manchmal Enuresis in der Kindheit. Ein Fall STRANSKYs hatte als Kind Augenzuckungen, ein anderer hatte Myoklonien (encephalitisch?). Bei DENYER lag Hysterie vor. Ein Fall CAVEs (encephalitisch?) wurde erst 10 Jahre nach Beginn der Narkolepsie nervös. THIELE und BERNHARDT, DOYLE und DANIELS betonen die Initiativarmut und Langsamkeit der Reaktionen. Meines Erachtens sind dies Anomalien, wie sie an einem größeren Material zum Teil unvermeidlich sind. Ein engerer Zusammenhang zwischen diesen Anomalien und der Erkrankung bzw. den einzelnen Anfällen wurde nicht festgestellt, womit jedoch nicht gesagt ist, daß das Zusammentreffen unbedingt rein zufällig sein muß. Speziell die Frage einer evtl. gemeinsamen Anlage gelangt im nächsten Abschnitt (Heredität) nochmals zur Sprache. Auch die „Encephalitis-Psyche" verdient Beachtung.

Ätiologische Faktoren. *1. Heredität, Konstitution.* Ein hereditär-familiäres Auftreten ist unleugbar in einer kleinen Gruppe von Fällen vorhanden. Es ist nicht bloß an und für sich wichtig, sondern es zeigt auch verschiedene Eigentümlichkeiten, die lehrreich sind. Bei WESTPHAL hatte die Mutter des Patienten nach einem Schädeltrauma (!) vorübergehend ähnliche Anfälle, bei F. FISCHER hatte eine Schwester vorübergehend Schlafanfälle. Bei BALLET war der Großvater ein „großer Schläfer", bei NEWMARK hatte der Großvater ebenfalls Narkolepsie. Bei REDLICH waren Großvater und Vater, bei JAKOBSOHN der Vater große Schläfer. Bei BAUER, bei THIELE und BERNHARDT hatte der Vater ähnliche Schlafanfälle, bei ROSENTHAL zwei Brüder (gleichzeitig erkrankt; Wa.R. verdächtig). REDLICH wies seinerzeit darauf hin, daß es sich bei einem Teil der Fälle somit nicht um richtige Narkolepsie, sondern um Schlafsucht handelt und daß kein Fall auch den affektiven Tonusverlust zeigte. Seit REDLICHs Tod hat sich das Material noch weiter vermehrt. Es kamen noch hinzu: die kurz erwähnten Fälle von THIELE und BERNHARDT (Neffe, Tante, Cousin), SCHILDER (Vater und Sohn), CAVE (Vater und Tochter, beide nur Schlafanfälle), DOYLE und DANIELS (Mutter, Tochter und Sohn) und dann die Fälle von HOFF und STENGEL: 1. Vater Narkolepsie ohne Tonusverlust, Sohn postencephalitische Narkolepsie und Tonusverlust; 2. Großvater und Enkel nur Schlafanfälle; 3. Vater nur affektiver Tonusverlust, ein Sohn nach psychischem Trauma Narkolepsie ohne Tonusverlust, der zweite Sohn Psychoneurose mit Schlafsucht, alle haben eine Konvergenzschwäche; 4. Mutter in der Pubertät und im Klimakterium Schlafanfälle, zwei Brüder von ihr dasselbe in der Pubertät, eine Schwester menstruell und die Tochter seit der Pubertät (ist 15 Jahre alt), bei allen fiel auf, daß sie bei fieberhaften Erkrankungen viel schliefen; die zwei untersuchten Mitglieder der Familie hatten Konvergenzparese. Es waren dies im Jahre 1931 bereits 15 Familien, also etwa 6% der publizierten Fälle. Interessant ist, daß in einer Familie von

Hoff und Stengel auch isolierter affektiver Tonusverlust ohne Anfälle von Schlaf aufscheint. Aber es existiert nur eine Familie (Thiele), in der zwei Mitglieder (Tante und Nichte) eine voll entwickelte Narkolepsie mit beiden Arten von Anfällen hatten; ferner sah Rolandi, daß zwei Brüder, deren Mutter, vier Geschwister (darunter eine Zwillingsschwester) und ein Brudersohn Narkolepsie hatten. Diese Tatsachen wollen wir uns vorläufig vermerken, sie sind sehr wichtig und wir kommen auf sie bei der Besprechung der Pathogenese und der Abgrenzung der Krankheit noch einmal zurück. Hier wollen wir noch vermerken, daß z. B. Strauss genaue Nachforschungen in der Familie eines Falles gepflogen hat, ohne auf irgendwelche Schlafanomalien zu stoßen und daß auch ein Zwillingspaar existiert (ob eineiig nicht bekannt), wo nur einer der Zwillinge Narkolepsie hatte. Hier möchte ich auch einen Fall erwähnen, den ich im Wiener psychiatrischen Verein 1933 demonstriert habe: Seit Jugend Somnambulismus, später Narkolepsie und Fettsucht, in der Familie Fettsucht, Diabetes und Somnambulismus.

Man kann immerhin aus diesen Daten einen Schluß ziehen, der sich auch sonst manchmal aufdrängt, nämlich, daß bei der Narkolepsie *eine gewisse angeborene Disposition* eine wichtige Rolle spielt. Das nahm auch Redlich an, auch Kahler, der von einer „narkoleptischen Reaktionsfähigkeit" spricht, ebenso wie J. Bauer, der von einer Vererbung des „Narkolepsiesubstrates" (in Anlehnung an Kehrers Choreasubstrat) spricht. Man kann aber auch direkt daran denken, daß sich eine abnorme Anatomie, Chemie, Gefäßversorgung usw. der betreffenden Zentren vererbt (s. unten) oder eine abnorme Funktion jener komplexen Faktoren, die außer den Zentren für den Schlaf in Frage kommen.

Wir finden in der Aszendenz und bei den Geschwistern der Narkoleptiker (die Deszendenz wird in der Literatur ein wenig stiefmütterlich behandelt) noch andere Momente, die zu vermerken sind: Alkoholismus (Redlich, Noak, Kahler, Hilpert, Thiele, Wenderowič, Stiefler, Pfanner). Redlich ist jedoch (offenbar auf Grund seiner Studien über den Unterschied zwischen dem Material des Spitales und dem der Privatpraxis) nicht geneigt, diesem Umstand eine nennenswerte Rolle beizumessen. In 2 Fällen fand ich Lues, in 3 Fällen Fettsucht in der Familie. Nervosität in der Familie wird nur hier und da vermerkt, ebenso psychopathische Züge (Curschmann, Prange, Levi, Gélineau, Rathner?, Kennedy). Psychosen verschiedener Art werden erwähnt, sowohl aus dem manisch-depressiven Formenkreis als auch aus dem schizophrenen (Löwenfeld, Wenderowič, Rosenthal, Edel, Redlich, Wilder). Organische Nervenkrankheiten spielen keine große Rolle (Tabes und multiple Sklerose bei Henneberg). Nicht ohne Bedeutung scheint Epistaxis in der Familie zu sein (s. unten), wie z. B. bei Paskind, wo sie mit periodischem Kopfschmerz verbunden war. Migräne erwähnt Lopez und Semon, Thiele und Bernhardt sahen bei ihrem großen Material keinen einzigen Fall. Die Frage der Epilepsie wird gesondert besprochen (s. unten). Es ist schließlich vielleicht nicht überflüssig, zu erwähnen, daß keine von den ausgesprochenen hereditären Erkrankungen in irgendeiner nennenswerten Häufigkeit bei der Narkolepsiefamilie auftritt.

Fassen wir das Gesagte zusammen, so muß man sich den Ansichten von Kahler, Redlich, J. Bauer u. a. anschließen, daß die Fälle von familiärer Narkolepsie, wenn sie auch nicht zahlreich sind, doch — neben manchen anderen Argumenten — dafür sprechen, daß irgendein konstitutioneller Faktor dabei eine Rolle spielen muß. Von einer familiären oder hereditären Erkrankung kann man natürlich nicht sprechen. Wenn wir aber die Gesetzmäßigkeiten der Konstitutionslehre betrachten, so werden wir auch hier von vornherein erwarten, daß dieser konstitutionelle Faktor bei der Entstehung des Krankheitsbildes der Narkolepsie gegenüber anderen Faktoren einmal eine große, einmal eine geringe Rolle spielen wird. Daher darf man vielleicht vorschlagen, eine Gruppe abzusondern, bei welcher der konstitutionelle Faktor eine besonders große Rolle zu spielen scheint und die, wie wir gesehen haben, auch sonst einige wichtige Eigentümlichkeiten bietet und sie *die Gruppe der familiären Narkolepsie* nennen, wobei wir gerade hier mit der Auffassung des Terminus Narkolepsie nicht allzu streng sein wollen.

2. *Encephalitis.* Abgesehen von einem unsicheren Fall von W. M. KRAUSE aus dem Jahre 1921 war REDLICH der erste, welcher Fälle von Narkolepsie nach Encephalitis beobachten konnte und welcher die grundlegende Bedeutung dieser Tatsachen für das ganze Narkolepsieproblem sofort erfaßt hat; waren es ja gerade diese Fälle, welche ihn zu seiner Auffassung und zu seiner Lokalisation der Narkolepsie geführt haben. Seither ist die Zahl der Fälle nach Encephalitis epidemica im ständigen Wachstum begriffen und viele sind schon geneigt, die Narkolepsie überhaupt als eine Art von Encephalitis aufzufassen oder zumindest von einem starken Anwachsen der Narkolepsie seit den Encephalitisepidemien zu sprechen (s. unten). Betrachtet man die neuere Literatur, so merkt man ferner eine gewisse Tendenz die verschiedenartigsten fieberhaften Erkrankungen aus der Anamnese der Kranken, speziell solche von der Art der Grippe und Influenza, auch wenn sie weit zurückliegen, mit der Narkolepsie in Beziehung zu bringen und es muß zugegeben werden, daß die Argumente dafür in so manchem Falle sehr gewichtig sind. In den folgenden Ausführungen befassen wir uns mit der Encephalitis epidemica ECONOMO und werden die anderen selteneren Arten von Encephalitis anschließend gesondert betrachten. REDLICH hat bis zum Jahre 1930 7 eigene und 21 Literaturfälle sammeln können (STIEFLER, PERRIER, SPILLER, MANKOWSKY, GRUSZECKA, HERMANN, RIZATTI, SYMONDS, FROCASSI, PAPASTRATIGAKIS, LHERMITTE und NICOLA, ADIE, WILSON, WENDEROWIČ, STRAUSS, MINZA, BONHOEFFER, ROSENTHAL, STOCKERT u. a.). Seit dem Jahre 1930 konnte ich noch mindestens 20 sichere Fälle zusammenstellen neben einer großen Reihe von nicht ganz sicher postencephalitischen Fällen. Bis 1932 zählte MÜNZER schon 79 Fälle. Man kann also die Zahl der postencephalitischen Narkolepsiefälle auf etwa 20% aller Fälle schätzen, also eine große Gruppe, die um so mehr eine Besprechung verdient als sie manche für die Auffassung der Narkolepsie wichtige Besonderheiten bietet. Gerade auf diese Besonderheiten wollen wir hier Gewicht legen. Geschlecht: Kein Unterschied gegenüber der echten Narkolepsie, d. h. starkes Übergewicht der Männer. Alter: Trotzdem die Encephalitis ebenso wie die Narkolepsie eine Erkrankung des jugendlichen Alters ist, scheint sich der Beginn der Narkolepsie bei den postencephalitischen Fällen öfter nach dem 20. Lebensjahr abzuspielen als bei der echten Narkolepsie. Symptomatologie: Im großen und ganzen besteht kein prinzipieller Unterschied zwischen den Symptomen der echten und der postencephalitischen Narkolepsie. Hier wie dort sehen wir in rascher oder langsamer Entwicklung dieselben Anfälle auftreten, die typischen Schlafanfälle einerseits, den typischen affektiven Tonusverlust andererseits. Sicherlich, die Erwartung, daß man hier neben der Narkolepsie auch Zeichen der gewöhnlichen postencephalitischen Schädigungen finden wird, erweist sich als berechtigt, aber *nur in einem geringen Teil der Fälle und in einem auffallend geringen Grade.* So fand MÜNZER in 49 von 79 Fällen keinen Parkinsonismus, aber in 50% Fettsucht. THIELE-BERNHARDT fanden unter 7 Fällen nur 1 psychisch normalen, bei den anderen die typische Encephalitikerpsyche. Wir können hier auch eine Vorliebe für gewisse Symptome erblicken, die sich für die Lokalisation der Narkolepsie als wichtig erweisen werden. Es sei noch deutlicher gesagt: Wir haben eine ganze Reihe von Fällen nach Encephalitis, die außer den Erscheinungen der Narkolepsie

absolut gar nichts Neurologisches bieten und die dennoch ihrem Verlauf nach keinen Zweifel übriglassen, daß sie tatsächlich encephalitischer Genese sind. Ferner finden wir in der Gruppe der encephalitischen Fälle besonders viel *atypische* Fälle und besonders viel *atypische Erscheinungen*, was uns ja bei einem verstreuten entzündlichen Prozeß kaum wundern wird. Gerade aber diese Abweichungen vom Typus haben hier, wo kein Zweifel daran besteht, daß es sich um anatomische Veränderungen handelt, eine besondere Bedeutung für die Frage der Pathogenese und Lokalisation der Krankheit, wenn sie auch in dieser Hinsicht noch recht wenig ausgenützt sind. Was das Intervall zwischen der akuten Erkrankung und der Narkolepsie betrifft, so schließen sich die Erscheinungen letzterer entweder unmittelbar an das akut-encephalitische Stadium an oder es entsteht ein Intervall zumeist bis zu 6 Monaten (REDLICH). Doch sind auch größere Intervalle bekannt, so z. B. 2 Jahre (STRAUSS, BONHOEFFER, TSIMINAKIS), 3 Jahre (HOFF und STENGEL, 4 (REDLICH), 5 (LHERMITTE), ja sogar 10 Jahre (ein nicht ganz sicherer Fall von WOHLFAHRT). Die Encephalitis bei diesen Fällen ist nach REDLICH zumeist eine *leichte*. Hervorzuheben ist *das Überwiegen der somnolentophthalmoplegischen (lethargischen) Form* und man muß schon hier erinnern, daß REDLICH die Narkolepsie gerade dorthin lokalisiert, wo ECONOMO die Herde bei dieser Form fand, d. h. in die Gegend des hinteren Anteils des 3. Ventrikels und des vorderen Anteils des Aquaeductus Sylvii. Hervorzuheben ist ferner das Vorkommen *symptomarmer oder abortiver Encephalitisformen* in der Vorgeschichte dieser Fälle, offenbar von ähnlicher Lokalisation; so erwähnen WAGNER, KAMMAN, CAVE eine rein somnolente Form, WOHLFAHRT nur Augenkrämpfe, in einem anderen Fall bloß Doppelbilder bei Lachen und bei Müdigkeit. In 2 Fällen CAVES war es eine delirante Form. In einem Fall von TSIMINAKIS begann die Encephalitis mit Pavor nocturnus, welcher dann auch als Dauersymptom bestehen blieb. Was die neurologischen Erscheinungen der Postencephalitis betrifft, so fand sie REDLICH unter seinen Fällen 7mal fehlend, 8mal nur andeutungsweise vorhanden, und nur 5mal ausgesprochen. Öfters findet man so oligosymptomatische Formen, wie bei WOHLFAHRT (nur Doppelbilder, Zittern der Zunge, Nystagmus und Seborrhoe), bloß leichte Gesichtsfeldeinschränkung (CAVE), bloß Hypomimie (CAVE, HOFF und STENGEL), bloß eine etwas monotone und verlangsamte Sprache und Speichelfluß nachts (RIZZATI) oder nur ganz leichten Parkinsonismus (WAGNER, KAMMAN). Bei diesen dürftigen neurologischen Bildern muß die relative Häufigkeit oft nur leichter *Augensymptome* auffallen, auf die schon REDLICH hingewiesen hat (s. auch STIEFLER, MANKOWSKY, BONHOEFFER, SYMONDS, STRAUSS, PENTA, WAGNER, WOHLFAHRT, RATNER, KAMMAN, RIZZATTI, HOFF und STENGEL). Es handelt sich dabei um Ptosis, leichte Pupillenstörungen verschiedenster Art, Akkommodationsparese, Konvergenzschwäche, Doppelbilder, Nystagmus usw. Neben den Augenmuskelstörungen sind vegetative Erscheinungen bei diesen Fällen auffallend häufig. Fettsucht haben wir schon erwähnt. Potenzstörungen erwähnen WOHLFAHRT, HOFF und STENGEL. Auch die Seborrhoe kann man dazu zählen, Polyurie (REDLICH, RIZZATTI), exzessiven Hunger und Durst (REDLICH, SEREJSKI und FRUMKIN, RIZZATI, CAVE). REDLICH findet, daß der Nachtschlaf besonders schlecht ist in jenen Fällen, bei denen sich die Narkolepsie unmittelbar an die akute Phase anschloß; hier erinnern die Verhältnisse an die bekannte Umkehr der Schlafperiode, wie sie bei Postencephalitikern auch sonst häufig ist (Schläfrigkeit bei Tag, Munterkeit bei Nacht); manchmal wird direkt von einer solchen Umkehr gesprochen (PENTA). CAVE erwähnt ständige Somnolenz. In einem anderen Falle dieses Autors ging dem Auftreten der Narkolepsie zuerst durch 4 Jahre eine dauernde Müdigkeit voraus. Im Schlaf selbst finden wir dieselben Erscheinungen wie bei der echten Narkolepsie, d. h. Unruhe im Schlaf, Sprechen aus dem Schlaf, Somnambulismus und wir müssen uns daran erinnern, daß ja diese Erscheinungen bei Postencephalitikern überhaupt sicht selten sind, ja, daß hier oft der Schlaf auf die bei Tage extrapyramidal gehemmte Motilität einen enthemmenden Einfluß hat; fast anarthrische Kranke sprechen im Schlafe klar und deutlich, Kranke, die sich kaum mehr bewegen, können im Schlaf flott nachtwandeln. Die bekannten typischen postencephalitischen Charakterveränderungen der Jugend beschrieben auch STRAUSS, WAGNER, WOHLFAHRT, CAVE, RIZZATI. Aus alledem geht wohl mit großer Wahrscheinlichkeit hervor, daß diejenigen Encephalitisherde, welche zur Narkolepsie — sagen wir es zuerst vorsichtig — disponieren, nicht dort liegen, wo die choreatisch-hyperkinetische Form lokalisiert wird (Striatum), auch nicht dort, wohin der Parkinsonismus lokalisiert wird (Substantia nigra), sondern dort, wohin die somnolent-ophthalmoplegische Form lokalisiert wird, sowie dort, wohin die vegetativen Störungen lokalisiert werden, und das ist der hintere Teil des 3. Ventrikels mit den angrenzenden Partien. Ob auch das häufigere Vorkommen der Charakterveränderung, die ja bisher nirgends lokalisiert wurde, im Zusammenhang damit eine Bedeutung hat, läßt sich derzeit nicht sagen. Sonstige Befunde: In 6 Fällen ist Lymphocytose verzeichnet (REDLICH, STIEFLER, MÜNZER, MANKOWSKY, STRAUSS), doch gibt es auch hier Fälle mit normalen Lymphocytenzahlen (WAGNER, KAMMAN, CAVE). Der Grundumsatz ist auch hier öfters nicht unbeträchtlich erniedrigt (ROSENTHAL, WOHLFAHRT). Das Encephalogramm war bei WAGNER normal. Der Liquor in der Regel ohne Besonderheiten: RATNER erwähnt erhöhten Druck. Die Zuckertoleranz im Falle WAGNERs war normal. Ein Fall von THIELE hatte niedrigen Blutzucker (68 mg-%). Der von STRAUSS erwähnte Nüchternblutzucker von 38 mg-% beruht auf einem Druckfehler (schriftliche Mitteilung des Autors an mich). Hyperventilation rief bei STRAUSS, bei SEREJSKI Schlaf hervor, bei WOHLFAHRT und einem zweiten Fall von STRAUSS nicht. Blutcalcium in einem Fall (WAGNER) normal. RIZZATI fand auch hier Vagotonie, wobei zu bemerken ist, daß die Vagotonie sich bei den Postencephalitikern überhaupt in etwa 80% der Fälle findet (MARINESCO). Die Adrenalinwirkung bei dieser Gruppe von Narkolepsien wurde teils schwach (WOHLFAHRT, MÜNZER), teils normal befunden (STRAUSS). Auf die nicht unbeträchtlichen Unterschiede in der Prognose und Therapie der postencephalitischen Narkolepsie gegenüber der idiopathischen werden wir bei den betreffenden Abschnitten eingehen. REDLICH hebt hervor, daß bei der postencephalitischen Narkolepsie der affektive Tonusverlust seltener ist als bei der echten. Es gibt also eine größere Anzahl von Fällen, die bloß Schlafanfälle haben. Wir konnten in der neueren Literatur noch 3 sichere und 4 fragliche postencephalitische Fälle dieser Art finden. Andererseits gibt es hier auch Fälle, wo nur affektiver Tonusverlust ohne Schlafanfälle vorhanden war (MÜNZER, ROSENTHAL, TSIMINAKIS, WAGNER). Man muß also die Behauptung REDLICHs erweitern und sagen: bei der encephalitischen Narkolepsie kommt viel öfter als bei der idiopathischen eine forme fruste vor, bei der entweder nur Schlafanfälle oder nur affektiver Tonusverlust auftreten. Auf die theoretische Bedeutung dieser Spaltung der Symptome werden wir noch eingehen. Wachanfälle beschreiben ROSENTHAL, BONHOEFFER usw. Jedenfalls wird es sich empfehlen, bei jedem Fall von Narkolepsie nicht bloß eine genaue Anamnese bezüglich evtl. abortiver Encephalitis zu erheben, sondern auch auf die verschiedenen kleinen Zeichen von Postencephalitis zu achten (Ptosis, Pupillendifferenzen, paradoxer Argyll-Robertson, Konvergenzschwäche, Hypomimie, Monotonie der Sprache, Seborhoe, Fehlen des Armpendelns, Lagebeharrungsversuch von SCHILDER-HOFF, Reflex von PUUSSEP usw.).

Narkolepsie wird nicht bloß mit der Encephalitis epidemica in Zusammenhang gebracht, sondern es scheint so gut wie sicher, daß sie auch nach anderen Encephalitisformen hier und da auftreten kann, nach Grippe (SIEBERT), Recurrens (ESLEVIČ), nach einer fieberhaften disseminierten cerebrospinalen Affektion (REDLICH), nach anderen unklaren fieberhaften Affektionen (WAGNER), nach Denguefieber (TSIMINAKIS), nach Masern mit Delir (CAVE, LUST?), Pneumonie mit Delir (CAVE), Parotitis (CAVE), Scharlach (CAVE, COHEN), Ptomainvergiftung (CAVE), Typhus abdominalis + exanthematicus + Recurrens (SEREJSKI und FRUMKIN), 3 Tage nach einer Vaccination (COHEN). Wir haben also hier unter dem Sammelbegriff Encephalitis alle möglichen Infektionskrankheiten zusammengestellt, allerdings mit der in vielen Fällen unbewiesenen Voraussetzung, daß die Narkolepsie dabei auf dem Umweg über eine Hirnschädigung encephalitischer Art entstanden sein mag, obwohl auch der Zusammenhang mit diesen Infektionen nicht in allen Fällen bewiesen und in manchen gar nicht beweisbar war. Es finden sich außerdem bloß in der neueren Literatur mehr als 20 Fälle, besonders bei CAVE, bei welchen eine „Influenza" in der Anamnese angegeben wird, in einem verschieden langen Zeitraum vor dem Auftreten der Narkolepsie, bei manchen Fällen knapp vorher, bei anderen in einem Abstand bis zu 10 Jahren. Auch unter diesen Fällen dürfte sich manche Grippe- oder epidemische Encephalitis verbergen.

3. Endokrine Drüsen. Schon bei der Erwähnung der häufigen Anomalien des Fettstoffwechsels, des Grundumsatzes usw. mußte die Frage auftauchen, ob bei der Narkolepsie nicht auch die endokrinen Drüsen irgendwie im Spiele sind. Auch die so häufigen vegetativen Anomalien verschiedener Art legen ja diese Vermutung nahe, wissen wir doch, daß die endokrinen Drüsen mit dem vegetativen Nervensystem in vielfacher Weise verknüpft sind und daß ihre Anomalien zu den häufigsten Ursachen vegetativer Dysfunktionen gehören. Und tatsächlich ist es bald aufgefallen, daß sich bei den Narkoleptikern recht häufig endokrine Stigmen finden.

Hypophyse. REDLICH war der erste, der die Aufmerksamkeit auf diese Drüse gelenkt hat, und zwar hauptsächlich deshalb, weil bei Erkrankungen der Hypophyse sehr häufig Schlafsucht und manchmal auch ausgesprochene narkoleptische Zustände beschrieben werden. REDLICH selbst hat einen Fall von Hypophysentumor beschrieben, bei dem in zwei längeren Zeitperioden typische narkoleptische Anfälle bestanden, die sich zugleich mit den anderen Erscheinungen des Tumors auf Jod gebessert haben. Ich selbst sah bei 2 Fällen von hypophysärer Kachexie Zustände, die ganz an affektiven Tonusverlust erinnerten, aber spontan ohne Affekt entstanden waren und mit einem ganzen vegetativen Anfallssyndrom einhergingen. Umgekehrt werden in manchen Fällen von Narkolepsie Syndrome beschrieben, die an eine Erkrankung der Hypophyse denken lassen, ohne daß man eine solche sicher beweisen könnte, so z. B. Bilder von hypophysärem Infantilismus oder sogar Zwergwuchs (PFANNER), von Dystrophia adiposo-genitalis, akromegale Züge (THRASH und MASSEE), eunuchoider Hochwuchs (SCHILDER) usw. Besonders BEYERMANN trat in der letzten Zeit dafür ein, der Hypophyse eine größere Rolle bei der Narkolepsie zuzuschreiben und stützt sich u. a. auf die Erfolge der entsprechenden Organotherapie (s. unter Therapie). Bei der Diskussion dieser Frage spielen die nicht seltenen sonderbaren Röntgenbefunde der Sella turcica eine Rolle, welche sich gelegentlich auch bei encephalitischen und traumatischen Fällen zeigen (THIELE-BERNHARDT). In erster Linie wird da über eine abnorme Kleinheit der Sella berichtet (4 Fälle von REDLICH, ferner KAHLER, JANZEN, COHEN, VILLAVERDE, ROSENTHAL, RATHNER, BEYERMANN, ROTHFELD u. a.). Aber auch andere abnorme Sellabefunde werden mitgeteilt: erweiterte Sella (DERCUM,

ESLEVIČ, THIELE und BERNHARDT), Sellabrücken (BEYERMANN, THIELE-BERNHARDT), ein Befund, der von vielen als nicht pathologisch angesehen wird, Kalkschatten im Sellabereich (BEYERMANN) usw. Übrigens sei hier erwähnt, daß auch andere pathologische Befunde in der Nähe der Sella angeführt werden, so z. B. von BEYERMANN (Verkalkungen der Glandula pinealis) oder von FRÖDERBERG (Usuren am Clivus, Verkalkungen an der Hirnbasis und am Plexus chorioideus) usw. In zahlreichen Fällen jedoch, z. B. in 10 von 19 Fällen von THIELE und BERNHARDT war der Röntgenbefund normal. Auf die Schlafhypothese SALMONs, welcher der Hypophyse beim Schlaf überhaupt eine große Rolle zuschreibt, wird weiter unten hingewiesen.

Daß es Fälle gibt, bei welchen sehr viele Symptome auf die Hypophyse hinweisen, die aber (zumindest im Beginne) schwer zu rubrizieren sind, möge folgender Fall meiner Beobachtung beweisen. I. H., ein etwa 40jähriger Bühnenarbeiter, war bis vor 3 Jahren gesund. Vor 3 Jahren wurde er wegen einer linksseitigen eitrigen Otitis media operiert, nach 1 Jahr Rezidiv und Radikaloperation. *Seit dieser Zeit* begann eine rasch zunehmende Fettsucht trotz starker Nahrungseinschränkung, welche zu einer Gewichtszunahme von 20 kg in einem Jahre führte, ferner eine Abnahme der Libido und der Potenz, stärkerer Durst (trinkt angeblich um 2 Liter Wasser mehr als früher), Obstipation, ferner wird er stundenlang von einem intensiven Geruch („Leichengeruch") verfolgt, so daß er öfters die Quelle dieses Geruches vergeblich sucht. 8 Monate nach der Operation begann er überall einzuschlafen, 4—5mal täglich, sogar beim Stehen; er ist sehr leicht erweckbar, schläft aber manchmal unter günstigen Umständen 4 und 5 Stunden. Zugleich wurde der Nachtschlaf schlechter, unruhig, er setzt sich auf die Bettkante, fällt auch manchmal vom Bett herunter, spricht aus dem Schlaf (vom Theater usw.), träumt sehr lebhaft, besonders vom Krieg. Auch beim Tagschlaf hat er ähnliche Träume. Wenn er gehindert wird am Einschlafen, ist er benommen und schläfrig, aber auch nach dem Schlafanfall fühlt er sich matt und schwach. 4 Monate nach Beginn der Schlafanfälle stellten sich auch Anfälle von typischem affektiven Tonusverlust ein nach Aufregungen und beim Lachen und besonders bei einem plötzlichen Befehl oder scharfen Tadel seitens eines Vorgesetzten. Post coitum sehr matt. Er hat eigentümliche Wachanfälle, die man als partielle Wachanfälle bezeichnen könnte, er kann in der Nacht beim Erwachen manchmal irgendeine Extremität nicht bewegen und das dauert etwa 20 Minuten. Seit der Erkrankung ist er ganz alkoholintolerant. Arbeit oder Ruhe haben keinen Einfluß auf die Anfälle, aber Hitze vermehrt sie. Objektiv findet sich folgendes: Starke Adipositas, bei den Mammae ist möglicherweise auch das Drüsenparenchym vergrößert, aber kein Colostrum, die größte Fettansammlung abdominal. Die Körperbehaarung gering, die Axillarhaare äußerst reduziert, die Crines pubis schütter, horizontal begrenzt; hingegen ist seit der Erkrankung dem Patienten ein sehr verstärkter Haarwuchs im Gesicht aufgefallen. Die Hoden sind klein, der Penis ganz auffallend klein. Neurologisch ist der Befund gering: keine Geruchsstörung, Fundus, Gesichtsfeld normal, aber auffallend starkes Schwitzen auf der linken Stirne und den angrenzenden Kopfpartien und (vorübergehend) eine Hypästhesie im linken Trigeminus für alle Qualitäten inklusive Schleimhäute. Sonst nur geringfügige Reflexdifferenzen. Wa.R. war negativ, ebenso Schädelröntgen. Wichtig ist, daß einige Monate nach Beginn der Erkrankung Glykosurie festgestellt wurde, und zwar 4%, welche mit ganz geringfügigen diätetischen Maßnahmen verschwunden war, um nach $^1/_2$ Jahr wiederzukommen. Ich verfolgte den Fall noch etwa $^3/_4$ Jahre, dann ist er aus meinen Augen entschwunden. Ich erfuhr aber, daß die auf meine Veranlassung halbjährlich vorgenommenen Röntgenaufnahmen schließlich doch einen Befund ergab, der für einen suprasellaren Tumor sprach.

Auch für *Thyreoidea* liegt einiges Material vor. Man sieht hier und da Strumen (REDLICH, DERCUM, KAHLER, BAUER, STRAUSS). Ein Fall von REDLICH entstand nach Thyreoidektomie. Hypothyreose erwähnen STRAUSS, ESLEVIČ, LEVIN, BEYERMANN, SCHILDER, THIELE-BERNHARDT. Letztere sahen aber auch einen Fall von Basedow. Wir erinnern uns an die Schläfrigkeit, ja, manchmal Schlafsucht der Myxödematösen. Doch ist das Material hier zu gering, um ein zufälliges Zusammentreffen auszuschließen. Wir verweisen ferner auf die manchmal beschriebenen Erfolge der Thyreoideabehandlung, aber auch auf ihre Mißerfolge bei manchen Fällen, wo der erniedrigte Grundumsatz verschwunden war, ja, in Fällen, in denen bereits die Erscheinungen einer Thyreotoxikose erzielt wurden.

Genitaldrüsen. Hier sind abnorme Befunde so häufig, daß man sie nicht übersehen kann. Allerdings muß man sich sowohl hier als auch bei der

Thyreoidea und besonders bei der Hypophyse vor Augen halten, daß heutzutage die meisten Symptome auch bei Erkrankung der vegetativen Zentren im Zwischenhirn entstehen können, daß ferner Störungen z. B. der Genitaldrüsen auf einer Erkrankung der Thyreoidea, besonders aber der Hypophyse beruhen können. Es ist sehr oft nicht möglich, dies bei einem Fall sicher zu entscheiden und unsere Gruppierung bedeutet also bloß eine rein äußerliche, nach oberflächlichen, landläufigen Gesichtspunkten vorgenommene Einteilung. Bei dieser Unsicherheit ist es beim Kapitel Genitaldrüsen vielleicht gut, einen von mir publizierten Fall voranzustellen, wo es bei einem nach Kriegstrauma operativ kastrierten Mann vorübergehend zu Erscheinungen von Narkolepsie und Tonusverlust kam, welche später spontan schwanden; bei dem Mann, der aus einer psychotischen Familie stammte und ein Psychopath war, ergaben die genauen Untersuchungen des vegetativen Nervensystems verschiedene Anomalien (Vagotonie, Lymphocytose usw.), welche nach operativer Affenhodentransplantation zum Teil verschwunden sind. Ein Fall von ZADOR bei einer Frau mit Ovarialoperation ist leider als Narkolepsie nicht vollkommen sicher. Wir haben schon bei der Besprechung der postencephalitischen Narkolepsie erwähnt, daß dabei Potenzstörungen öfters vermerkt werden. Das ist aber auch bei der genuinen Narkolepsie der Fall (STRANKY, HOFF und STENGEL, SEREJSKI und FRUMKIN u. a.). Daß aber die Beziehungen auch hier nicht allzu einfache sein dürften, dafür spricht ein Fall WOHLFAHRTs, bei welchem Potenzverminderung bestand; im Frühjahr wurde bei diesem Kranken die Narkolepsie ärger, hingegen traten da morgendliche Erektionen wieder auf (neben Polyurie). Erstes Auftreten nach erzwungener sexueller Abstinenz finden wir bei SEREJSKI und bei CAVE. Viel häufiger sind verschiedene objektive kleine Zeichen, die wir auf Hypogenitalismus zu beziehen pflegen, mangelhafte oder verspätete Entwicklung der Genitalien, der sekundären Geschlechtsmerkmale, besonders der Behaarung, infantiles Aussehen usw. (JOLLY, DERCUM, MOELLENHOFF, KAHLER, STIEFLER, JANZEN, ESLAVIČ, BAUER, ZEHRER, ROSENTHAL, SEREJSKI und FRUMKIN, BEYERMANN, WOHLFAHRT u. a.). Auch THIELE und BERNHARDT fanden bei ihren Fällen öfters Zeichen von Hypogenitalismus. Auch hier sind die Beziehungen nicht eindeutig; so berichtet REDLICH über einen Fall, bei dem sich im weiteren Verlauf die Entwicklung nachholte (also bloß eine verspätete Entwicklung) und der dann über vermehrte Libido und erhöhte sexuelle Erregbarkeit klagte. Obwohl das Frauenmaterial bedeutend kleiner ist, finden sich auch hier ähnliche Zeichen von Hypogenitalismus, besonders Menstruationsstörungen. Im Gegensatz zur Epilepsie muß man aber hervorheben, daß Zusammenhänge der Anfälle mit der Menstruation fast fehlen (z. B. HOFF und STENGEL berichten über einen solchen Fall). E. FISCHER, BALLET, KAHLER sahen menstruelle Häufung der Anfälle. Beginn der Erkrankung in der Pubertät ist jedoch sowohl bei Männern wie bei Frauen häufig. Hingegen scheinen gewisse Zusammenhänge mit dem Klimakterium (HOFF und STENGEL) und besonders mit der Gravidität zu bestehen. So meldet BALOGH Auftreten der Narkolepsie während zweier Graviditäten (encephalitisch ?), KOLLEWIJE während einer Gravidität (fraglicher Fall), ebenso NEVERMANN und SZATMARY (auch intra partum), ROSENTHAL Auftreten von Wachanfällen während zweier Graviditäten (encephalitisch ?), GRUSZECKA Häufung von Tonusverlust dabei usw. Hier wäre auch nochmals an die Familie von HOFF und STENGEL zu erinnern, in welcher eine Frau in der Pubertät und im Klimakterium, eine andere umgekehrt, bloß menstruell und bis zum Klimakterium, Schlafanfälle hatte, um zu zeigen, daß die Zusammenhänge hier oft komplizierter Natur sind.

Für andere endokrine Drüsen ergeben sich keine sicheren Anhaltspunkte. Zusammenfassend kann man heute nur so viel sagen, daß es bei der Narkolepsie in vielen, aber bestimmt nicht in allen Fällen Anhaltspunkte dafür gibt, daß auch die endokrinen Drüsen irgendeine Rolle dabei spielen, und zwar kommen in Frage in erster Linie die Hypophyse, in zweiter die Keimdrüsen, in dritter die Schilddrüse.

REDLICH hat trotz der auch von ihm selbst betonten Problematik der Methode mehrere Fälle auch nach ABDERHALDEN-PREGL untersuchen lassen. Es bauten ab: Fall 1. Thyreoidea ++, Hypophyse +. Fall 2. Thyreoidea ++. Fall 3. Thyreoidea +, Hypophyse ++, Thymus +. Fall 4. Thyreoidea +, Hypophysenhinterlappen +, Thymus +, Stammganglien +. Fall 5. Thyreoidea angedeutet, Ovar angedeutet (Frau). Fall 6. Hypophysenvorderlappen angedeutet, -hinterlappen schwach, Parathyreoidea +, Nebennieren +. Fall 7. Thyreoidea +, Placenta +, Stammganglien + (gravid). Fall 8. Alles negativ. Bei ROAK waren Hypophyse und Hoden negativ, bei WIMMER und SPERLING Hypophysenvorderlappen angedeutet, bei ZEHRER Thyreoidea, Hypophyse und Hirnrinde angedeutet. Schlüsse lassen sich daraus kaum ziehen. Auch THIELE und BERNHARDT sahen keine charakteristischen Befunde.

Kann man wie bei einigen anderen ätiologischen Faktoren von einer *endokrinen Gruppe von Narkolepsien* sprechen? Dafür ist das sichere Material (z. B. Fall WILDER) doch zu gering.

4. Schädeltraumen. Es kann nicht ohne Bedeutung sein, daß in einer ganzen Reihe von Fällen Schädeltraumen in der Anamnese angegeben werden, Traumen verschiedener Art und Lokalisation, öfters jedoch in auffallendem zeitlichen Zusammenhang mit dem Auftreten der Narkolepsie. Solche Fälle publizierten GÉLINEAU, GOWERS, NOAK, STIEFLER, SINGER, GOLDFLAM, SOMER, KAHLER, GILLESPIE, BONHOEFFER, WILSON, REDLICH, ROSENTHAL, THIELE und BERNHARDT, URECHIA und BUMBACESCU. In der neueren Literatur fand ich noch weitere 7 Fälle, davon 3 bei THIELE und BERNHARDT, also etwa 8% aller Fälle. Darunter sind allerdings auch Fälle mit einem weit zurückliegenden Trauma oder geringfügigen Trauma enthalten, aber auch Fälle, bei denen ein schweres Schädeltrauma der Narkolepsie kurz vorausging, wie bei REDLICH, GOLDFLAM und HAENEL.

Man kann also meines Erachtens von einer *posttraumatischen Gruppe* sprechen, und sie gesondert studieren, um so mehr, als es mir scheint, daß sich auch bei diesen Fällen, ebenso wie bei den encephalitischen auffallend viele nicht vollkommen typische Fälle finden, die wohl hier wie dort zum Teil durch Nachbarschaftssymptome bedingt sind.

5. Lues. In einigen Fällen finden wir Lues in der Anamnese oder positiven Wassermann (SOMER, REDLICH, THIELE und BERNHARDT, ROSENTHAL, CAVE u. a.), in anderen Fällen handelt es sich um Lues der Hypophyse (REDLICH, MARKOW), oder um eine basale Meningoencephalitis luetica (GUILLAIN, MOLLARET und THOYER). Allerdings sind fast alle diese Fälle nicht sicher als Narkolepsie zu bezeichnen. Da wir schließlich auch Lues der Eltern finden, ist es vielleicht nicht unberechtigt, auch an die Möglichkeit einer *luischen Untergruppe* zu denken.

6. Andere Faktoren. Polycythämie. In der letzten Zeit scheint sich auch eine Narkolepsie bei Polycythämie abzuzeichnen. Wir haben hier die Fälle von GÜNTHER (mit Fettsucht, vasomotorischen und respiratorischen Störungen), einen ganz typischen Fall von LHERMITTE und PEYRE, der außer Fettsucht sonst überhaupt kein klinisches Symptom hat, encephalitische und genuine Fälle von SALUS, Fälle von NEISSER, MÜNZER, KRAUS, von GUILLAIN, LECHELLE und GARCIN, von Moreau, einen fraglichen Fall von WILMAERS, ein Fall von LHERMITTE, VALERY-RADOT usw. Aber auch im Material von THIELE und BERNHARDT finde ich 5 Fälle mit etwa 6 Millionen Erythrocyten und erhöhtem Hämoglobingehalt, davon allerdings nur 1 genuiner Fall, 2 encephalitisch, 1 luisch, 1 encephalitisch und luisch. Hier muß man allerdings erwähnen, daß manche Internisten (LICHTWITZ) ein hämatopoetisches Zentrum im Zwischenhirn annehmen, daß Polycythämie bei Akromegalie keine ungewöhnliche Erscheinung ist usw. Ein anderer eigentümlicher ätiologischer Faktor scheint *Nasenbluten* zu sein; nicht bloß, daß Fälle bekannt sind, wo es dem Auftreten der Narkolepsie lang (STRANSKY) oder kurz vorausging (MENDEL, WEECH), wo die Narkolepsie damit endete (MCNAMARA) oder sich besserte (HILPERT), wo es periodisch oder in Verbindung mit Kopfschmerzen auftrat (WOHLFAHRT, WILSON), auch in der Familie des Narkoleptikers wurde familiärer periodischer Kopfschmerz mit Epistaxis beschrieben (PASKIND). Hierher gehört vielleicht auch ein Fall von THIELE-BERNHARDT (Encephalitis mit Nasenbluten). Eine Erklärung dafür steht allerdings aus; es sind mir keine Fälle bekannt, wo andere Blutungen, z. B. Hämorrhoidalblutungen eine Rolle spielen würden. — *Erschöpfung, Überanstrengung*, besonders wenn sie auch mit Nachtwachen verbunden war, scheint eine Rolle zu spielen (GOWERS, REDLICH, JOLLY, HENNEBERG, KAHLER, CURSCHMANN-PRANGE, SPERLING und WIMMER, THIELE u. a.). Es ist auch möglich, daß es auch *arteriosklerotische* Fälle gibt (GRÜN, ERMAKOV, POPOVA und SKVORCOV). Ich habe mit URBACH einen Fall von allergischem MENIÈRE publiziert, bei welchem im Verlauf der Erkrankung durch ein paar Tage typische Einschlaf- und Tonusverlustanfälle auftraten. Damit ist alles erschöpft, was sich an möglichen ätiologischen Faktoren erheben läßt und man kann daraus vorläufig bloß diesen sicheren Schluß ziehen (REDLICH), daß man von einer klaren eindeutigen Ätiologie bei der Narkolepsie derzeit nicht sprechen kann.

Beziehungen zur Epilepsie. Diese viel diskutierte und auch heute noch sehr umstrittene Frage muß gesondert besprochen werden, wenn man einigermaßen klar sehen will. Die ersten Autoren, FISCHER, WESTPHAL, dachten an etwas Epileptoides, aber schon GÉLINEAU sprach sich für die scharfe Trennung der beiden Krankheiten aus. Denselben Standpunkt nahm auch REDLICH ein. OPPENHEIM dachte an die Möglichkeit gewisser Übergänge, WILSON hielt von seinem Standpunkt die ganze Diskussion für müßig, aber noch bis in die letzte Zeit meldeten sich Stimmen, die für engere Beziehungen zwischen diesen beiden Krankheiten plädieren (KLEINE, LEWY, ZADOR, RATHNER, SEREJSKI und FRUMKIN). Als Argumente wurden angeführt vorerst gewisse *Ähnlichkeiten in den Manifestationen* beider Krankheiten, Aura (die aber meist nicht vorhanden ist), Bewußtseinstrübung, anfallsweises Auftreten, kurze Dauer usw., aber mit Recht betont WILSON, daß dies Kriterien sind, welche fast für alle „Anfälle", welcher Art immer, gelten und man müßte auf diese Weise fast alle Anfälle zur Epilepsie rechnen; allerdings weist das anfallsartige Auftreten bei verschiedenen Krankheiten, also auch bei der Epilepsie, auf irgendeinen gemeinsamen Mechanismus hin, aber worin dieser Mechanismus besteht, wissen wir nicht. Daß die Unterschiede überwiegen, liegt klar zutage: das Fehlen der Aura in den meisten Fällen, die für den Schlaf charakteristische Art der Bewußtseinstrübung, mit Träumen, ohne Amnesie, mit leichter Erweckbarkeit, ohne Secessus urinae, ohne Konvulsionen usw. Was den *affektiven Tonusverlust* betrifft, so sind die Ähnlichkeiten schon größer, denn das Argument jener, welche die affektive Auslösung als Unterscheidungsmerkmal anführen, ist sicher, wie WILSON und REDLICH an einer Reihe von Fällen von Epilepsie mit affektiver Auslösung zeigen, nicht stichhaltig. Man darf allerdings dabei nicht vergessen, daß, während beim Tonusverlust die affektive Auslösung wesentlich ist, sie bei der Epilepsie eben nur in Ausnahmefällen vorkommt, die bei der großen Masse der Epileptiker überhaupt nicht ins Gewicht fallen. Man darf schließlich nicht an die Hauptsache vergessen, an die bei der Epilepsie vorhandene, beim Tonusverlust fehlende Bewußtseinsstörung (einzelne Ausnahmen auf beiden Seiten sind eben atypische Zustände). Bedenken wir ferner die fehlende Charakter- und Intelligenzveränderung bei der Narkolepsie (auf vereinzelte Ausnahmen haben wir bereits hingewiesen). Die Mittel zur Provokation der epileptischen Anfälle (Alkohol, Carotidenkompression nach TSIMINAKIS, in der Regel auch Hyperventilation) versagen bei der Narkolepsie, ebenso wie die Mittel zur Coupierung epileptischer Anfälle, Brom, Luminal usw. So bleibt schließlich nicht viel anderes Gemeinsames übrig als dies, daß es sich bei beiden Krankheiten eben um *anfallsweises* Auftreten der Erscheinungen handelt.

Und doch sprachen auch so vorsichtige Forscher wie OPPENHEIM und REDLICH von „Übergängen", von gewissen „Beziehungen" und doch gibt es eine Reihe von Autoren, die auch heute noch von einer strengen Trennung beider Krankheiten nichts wissen wollen (s. o.). Worauf stützen sich diese Meinungen? Es gibt wirklich ein gewisses nicht allzu großes Tatsachenmaterial, welches zum Nachdenken Anlaß gibt. So kommt in der Familie der Narkoleptiker hier und da Epilepsie vor (ein Bruder der Mutter bei HILPERT, vielleicht ein Bruder bei WILSON, die Mutter in einem unsicheren Fall von ZADOR, eine Nichte bei GRÜN, der Vater bei HOFF und STENGEL). Mit Recht sagt REDLICH, daß angesichts des häufigen familiären Vorkommens der Epilepsie man sich eher wundern muß, daß man nicht mehr solcher Beispiele findet, denn die hier aufgezählten, zum Teil sogar unsicheren Fälle umfassen nicht mehr als 2% des Materials, also kaum eine in Betracht kommende Ziffer. — Auch Linkshändigkeit, die sich in den Familien von Epileptikern häufig findet (REDLICH), sieht man bei Narkoleptikern und bei ihren Familien selten (2 Fälle von REDLICH, 1 von THIELE-BERNHARDT) und auch die Migräne spielt hier keine nennenswerte Rolle. Die Bedeutung der elterlichen Trunksucht für die Epilepsie wurde ja früher sehr überschätzt; immerhin erinnern wir daran, daß auch diese in den Narkoleptikerfamilien nicht auffallend häufig vertreten ist. Die zweite Frage, die zu erörtern ist, ist diese: kommen bei Fällen von Narkolepsie epileptische Anfälle vor? Kommen bei der Epilepsie narkoleptische Zustände vor? Das hier von den Autoren zitierte Material hält sehr oft genauerer Kritik nicht stand, so ist z. B. in den Fällen von HAENEL und von LAFORA die Epilepsie, im Fall von BRAILOWSKY die Narkolepsie nicht sicher usw. Die Fälle, die von WILSON zitiert werden, entsprechen seiner weiten Auffassung von den „Narkolepsien", aber nicht der Narkolepsie in unserem Sinne. Es bleiben aber doch einige Fälle, die beachtet werden müssen. In einem Falle von GOWERS bestand typische Epilepsie und außerdem Schlafanfälle; auf Brom verschwanden die epileptischen, nicht aber die Schlafanfälle. In einem Falle von WORSTER-DROUGHT bestanden („wahrscheinlich") epileptische Anfälle und daneben Schlafzustände. In einem Falle von GOLDFLAM bestanden zuerst Schlafzustände, später epileptische Anfälle; GOLDFLAM selbst glaubt, daß es sich nicht um echte Narkolepsie gehandelt hat. Ein Fall von THIELE-BERNHARDT bekam später Epilepsie. In keinem dieser Fälle ist affektiver Tonusverlust beschrieben, nur EDEL beschreibt einen Fall, bei dem nach Schädelschuß epileptische Anfälle auftraten, später beim Lachen Tonusverlust, auch Einschlafen, die epileptischen Anfälle wurden manchmal durch Affekte ausgelöst; man darf nicht vergessen, daß es sich um einen traumatischen Fall handelt. Etwas häufiger sind Schlafanfälle bei der echten Epilepsie, die sich von den narkoleptischen, soviel auch ich gesehen habe, anscheinend in gar nichts unterscheiden; vielleicht dauern sie im Durchschnitt etwas länger. Solche Fälle beschrieben OPPENHEIM, FÉRÉ, ZIEHEN, REDLICH). REDLICH beschreibt auch einen Fall, bei welchem die Schlafanfälle vielleicht epileptische Äquivalente darstellen (vielleicht ist es auch beim Fall GOLDFLAMS so).

Eine 52jährige Frau, seit 10 Jahren amenorrhoisch, bekommt seit 1^1/$_2$ Jahren Anfälle von Übelkeit, Erbrechen und starkem Schlafbedürfnis, seit ^{1}/$_2$ Jahr Anfälle von Bewußtlosigkeit mit nachfolgendem Schlaf; nach dem Anfall öfters leicht desorientiert. Die Anfälle kommen besonders zur Zeit der ausbleibenden Menstruation. Kein Tonusverlust. Epileptoide psychische Veränderung. Durst und Polyurie. Im Liquor bloß leichte Eiweißvermehrung, Neurologisch und intern o. B. ABDERHALDEN: Parathyreoidea +++ (eine Reaktion, die sich besonders häufig bei Epilepsie findet), Hypophysenvorderlappen +, Ovar +.

Man kann also wohl mit REDLICH daran festhalten, *daß Narkolepsie und Epilepsie zwei voneinander scharf zu trennende Krankheiten sind.* Besonders ist hervorzuheben, daß auch Jahrzehnte dauernde Narkolepsie nie in Epilepsie übergeht. Die gewissen nicht allzu häufigen motorischen Reizerscheinungen beim narkoleptischen Schlaf und Tonusverlust haben eine eigene Note und auf ihre Erklärung werden wir noch eingehen. Bei der Epilepsie gibt es zweifellos hier und da Schlafanfälle vom Charakter der narkoleptischen Anfälle (Tonusverlust kommt dabei anscheinend nicht vor). Und schließlich könnte es ja auch eine Kombination beider Krankheiten in seltenen Fällen geben, obwohl bisher ein wirklich sicherer Fall dieser Art, speziell auch mit affektivem Tonusverlust, nicht bekannt ist. Da es sich bei beiden Krankheiten um Anfälle handelt, die vielleicht einzelne Erscheinungen gemeinsam haben, so denkt REDLICH auch an gewisse Beziehungen pathogenetisch-lokalisatorischer Art und meint schließlich: „Man kann, wenn man will, beide zusammenfassen in eine große Gruppe, man kann Übergänge herstellen, aber das kann man schließlich auch sonst bei vielen Erkrankungen, die trotzdem ihre Selbständigkeit behaupten können." Solche Zusammenfassungsversuche haben manche Autoren unternommen. So faßt KLEINE Epilepsie, Hypnolepsie, Pyknolepsie, episodische Dämmerzustände, Verstimmungszustände, Dipsomanie und Migräne in eine Gruppe zusammen. RATNER zählt zu der von ihm aufgestellten Gruppe der „Diencephalosen" Pyknolepsie, Narkolepsie, Geloplegie, Affektepilepsie, manche Formen von manisch-depressivem Irresein, Hysterie.

Verlauf, Prognose. In den typischen Fällen beginnen die narkoleptischen Schlafanfälle in oder nach der Pubertät, zugleich mit ihnen oder etwas später die Anfälle von affektivem Tonusverlust, beide in verschieden starker Ausprägung und gegenseitiger Mischung, und die Krankheit erreicht sehr bald ihren Höhepunkt, um in der Regel auf diesem Jahre und Jahrzehnte hindurch zu verbleiben. Ob bis ans Lebensende, wissen wir nicht, merkwürdigerweise fehlt darüber jedes Material in der Literatur, woraus mir ersichtlich erscheint, daß die Narkolepsie wahrscheinlich die Lebensdauer nicht verkürzt. DOYLE und DANIELS erwähnen ganz kurz einen Exitus nach Röntgenbestrahlungen des Schädels. Hingegen sind Fälle bekannt, die ohne Hinzukommen irgendwelcher weiterer Symptome ihre Krankheit 11 Jahre (SPERLING und WIMMER), 12 (BOAS, REDLICH), 13 (JANZEN), 15 (SINGER, ADIE, REDLICH), 16 (GOLDFLAM, REDLICH), ja, sogar mehr als 20, mehr als 30 Jahre behielten (STIEFLER, WILSON, ZEHRER, GOLDFLAM, REDLICH, JAKOBSOHN, FREUND, BALLET, CAVE, ROTHFELD, THIELE-BERNHARDT, DOYLE-DANIELS u. a.). Man kann also wohl von einem *chronischen,* man kann wohl (derzeit zumindestens) von einem *unheilbaren* Leiden sprechen. Was die Progredienz betrifft, so haben wir bereits angedeutet, daß eine *Progredienz im Beginn* wohl nicht obligat, aber häufig ist, daß aber dann die meisten Fälle Jahrzehnte hindurch nicht weiter progredient bleiben und auch sonst körperlich und psychisch intakt.

Von diesem Typus nun, dem die Mehrzahl der Fälle angehört, gibt es selbstverständlich auch verschiedene Abweichungen im Verlauf. Die Abweichungen, die das Alter des Krankheitsbeginns betreffen, werden weiter unten besprochen. Es wurde schon erwähnt, daß die beiden Arten von Anfällen meist zugleich oder knapp hintereinander entstehen. Wenn dies nicht der Fall ist, so gehen in den meisten Fällen die Schlafanfälle voraus, meist nur ein wenig, aber manchmal dauert es auch sehr lange, bis zu den Schlafanfällen auch der affektive

Tonusverlust hinzukommt. Das ist sehr wichtig zu wissen, denn es gemahnt natürlich zu besonderer Vorsicht, bei der Beurteilung jener Fälle, die uns als reine Schlafanfälle ohne Tonusverlust präsentiert werden. Hier heißt es oft abwarten, denn wir kennen Fälle, wo sich der affektive Tonusverlust erst nach ein paar Monaten (KENNEDY, PASKIND, BROMBERG, ROSENTHAL), nach 1 Jahr (ADIE, ROSENTHAL, LEVIN, CAVE), nach 2 Jahren (BROCK, LEVIN, THIELE-BERNHARDT, CAVE), nach 4 Jahren (THIELE, CAVE), nach 6 Jahren (CAVE), ja, sogar nach 8 Jahren (SEREJSKI und FRUMKIN) und nach 10 Jahren (SPERLING und WIMMER), nach 16 Jahren (DOYLE und DANIELS) einstellte. Seltener sind die Fälle, wo der affektive Tonusverlust den Schlafanfällen vorausgeht (LEVIN, STRANSKY, THIELE und BERNHARDT, CAVE, RATNER) und dann ist das Intervall gewöhnlich nur einige Monate oder sogar nur Wochen (VADASZ, THIELE-BERNHARDT); aber GIESEN sah auch ein Intervall von 1 Jahr und von 12 Jahren, so daß Fälle mit isoliertem Tonusverlust eher als eine Sondergruppe zu betrachten wären, als die viel häufigeren Fälle mit isolierten Schlafanfällen. An solchen Fällen ist nämlich kein Mangel, viele von ihnen sind allerdings nicht lange genug beobachtet, um ein späteres Auftreten der zweiten Art von Anfällen auszuschließen. In REDLICHs Statistik über 100 Fälle waren in 72% beide Arten von Anfällen vorhanden, in 2% waren die Angaben unsicher, in 12% fehlten verwertbare Angaben und in 12% waren bloß Schlafanfälle vorhanden. Ich konnte dann noch 25 Fälle ohne Tonusverlust sammeln, es ist aber zu bemerken, daß sich unter diesen 25 Fällen 9 Fälle von symptomatischer Narkolepsie befanden (Encephalitis, Lues, Hypophysenaffektion), es dürfte also der Prozentsatz nicht viel größer sein als bei REDLICH. DOYLE und DANIELS hatten unter 67 Patienten 8, d. h. ebenfalls in 12% keinen Tonusverlust. Unter diesen Fällen ist auch ein 11 Jahre beobachteter Fall von CAVE. Seltener sind die Fälle, wo nur affektiver Tonusverlust ohne Schlafanfälle vorkommt (MÜNZER, WILSON, VILLAVERDE, der MÜNZERsche Fall sicher encephalitisch), aber die Mitteilungen über diese Fälle mehren sich in der letzten Zeit. Wir erwähnen die Fälle von FOUCHÉ (Tonusverlust und Wachanfälle, traumatisch), TSIMINAKIS (encephalitisch), ROTHFELD, HOFF und STENGEL. Der Fall von ROTHFELD ist 9 Jahre, der von MÜNZER 10 Jahre beobachtet. Man sieht also auch bei dieser atypischen Verlaufsart eine besondere Häufigkeit von symptomatischer Narkolepsie, so daß man sogar sagen kann: Fälle, welche durch viele Jahre bloß *eine* Reihe von Anfällen bieten, sind verdächtig auf symptomatische Narkolepsie, ausgenommen vielleicht die Fälle von familiärer Narkolepsie.

Zwischen diesen beiden Extremen aber, zwischen den ganz typischen Fällen, bei denen mehrmals täglich Schlafanfälle und öfters, gewöhnlich mehrmals wöchentlich Anfälle von affektivem Tonusverlust vorhanden sind (letztere begreiflicherweise viel unregelmäßiger und inkonstanter, da sie ja durch Ausweichen vor den spezifisch wirksamen Affekten stark reduziert werden können), gibt es Übergänge, das sind Fälle, bei denen das Krankheitsbild ganz von *einer* Art der Anfälle beherrscht wird, während die andere Art nur sehr selten, ein paar Mal im Jahre oder sogar nur einige Male im Leben auftritt, ja, es gibt sogar Fälle, bei denen z. B. nur ein einziger affektiver Tonusverlust (ROTHFELD) oder nur einige wenige Schlafanfälle bekannt sind (CAVE, GIESEN) und diese Fälle sind wichtig, da sie ja zusammen mit den Fällen, bei denen es nur *eine* Art von Anfällen gibt, dafür sprechen, daß die beiden Arten wohl nicht der Ausdruck eines und desselben Mechanismus sein dürften. Gleichzeitig aber sprechen diese Fälle doch ziemlich eindeutig für die Auffassung jener Autoren, welche, wie REDLICH, ADIE, SEREJSKI und FRUMKIN, keine Bedenken tragen, auch diese Fälle von isoliertem Auftreten, z. B. des affektiven Tonusverlustes, zur Narkolepsie zu zählen.

Weitere Abweichungen vom typischen Verlauf ergeben sich in einzelnen (!) Fällen dadurch, daß es zu *spontanen Besserungen* in der Zahl und Schwere der Anfälle kommt, Besserungen, die vorübergehend oder auch bleibend sein können, so in 2 Fällen von GOLDFLAM nach 10 und nach 16 Jahren, in 3 Fällen von THIELE und BERNHARDT (1 traumatisch), in 1 Fall von LHERMITTE und PEYRE, in 3 Fällen von CAVE (in 1 nach 9 Jahren, beide fraglich encephalitisch). DOYLE und DANIELS sahen in 30 von 67 nicht näher beschriebenen Fällen Besserungen verschiedenen Grades, besonders bei Fällen mit Tonusverlust. Überhaupt haben die metencephalitischen Fälle, wie REDLICH und MÜNZER betonen, eine relativ viel bessere Prognose, obwohl es auch hier Fälle gibt, die durch viele Jahre beobachtet wurden (WAGNER 11 Jahre, THIELE-BERNHARDT 13, CAVE 16 Jahre). Dies gilt nach REDLICH speziell für jene Fälle, bei denen sich die Schlafanfälle unmittelbar an das akute Stadium der Encephalitis anschließen. Darum muß man mit der Beurteilung derjenigen postencephalitischen Fälle, bei denen therapeutische Erfolge berichtet werden (und sie werden hier am häufigsten berichtet), sehr vorsichtig sein. Die Besserung bezieht sich evtl. auch auf den affektiven Tonusverlust (PASKIND). Seltener ist ein vollständiges Verschwinden der Anfälle (zumindest für die Beobachtungsdauer). So berichtet z. B. ROSENTHAL über einen postencephalitischen Fall mit isoliertem affektiven Tonusverlust, der sich spontan verlor, in der Folgezeit traten aber in zwei Graviditäten Wachanfälle auf. SYMONDS berichtet über einen postencephalitischen Fall, bei welchem nur die Schlafanfälle verschwanden, nicht aber der schlechte Nachtschlaf und der affektive Tonusverlust. Einen Fall von *echter* Narkolepsie, der spontan ganz ausheilte, scheint es nicht zu geben. Hingegen scheint es eine besondere Gruppe von *Pubertätsnarkolepsie* zu geben, welche nach der Pubertät verschwindet; solche Fälle wurden in einer Narkoleptikerfamilie von HOFF und STENGEL beschrieben, auch von ROSENTHAL; bisher lauter Fälle ohne affektiven Tonusverlust. Auch *Verschlechterungen* im Laufe der Narkolepsie kommen plötzlich vor, auch nach jahrelangem Bestehen, so z. B. bei einem Fall von CAVE nach Influenza. Der *Beginn* der Narkolepsie geht manchmal mit einer Schlafsucht oder mit einer Schlaflosigkeit einher, diese Fälle sind begreiflicherweise auf eine larvierte Encephalitis verdächtig und werden von den Autoren verschieden rubriziert. Selten kommen andere Symptome im Beginne der Erkrankung vor, deren Zusammenhang mit dem Leiden noch nicht ganz feststeht, so z. B. in einem Falle von STRAUSS Zuckungen im Musculus temporalis, bei WOHLFAHRT Zuckungen im Gesicht und in den Extremitäten.

Diese Prognose, gut quoad vitam, schlecht quoad sanationem gilt also vor allem für die echte Narkolepsie, für die symptomatische ist ja von vornherein anzunehmen, daß dort, wo eine Beseitigung der Ursache möglich ist, auch an die Möglichkeit des Ausheilens der Narkolepsie gedacht werden muß. Unglücks- und sogar Todesfälle im Schlafanfall sind sehr selten, kommen aber vor.

Häufigkeit. Die Narkolepsie gehört zu den seltenen Krankheiten. Aber die außerordentliche progressive Vermehrung der Zahl der Publikationen in den letzten Jahren muß auffallen. Es sind bisher seit WESTPHAL etwa 250 Fälle dieser Krankheit publiziert worden. Von diesen sind etwa 130 in den letzten 2 Jahren veröffentlicht worden. Im Jahre 1924 konnte REDLICH auf 11 eigene Fälle und 14 Fälle der Literatur verweisen. Diese ungeheure Vermehrung der publizierten Fälle ließ manche Autoren als sicher annehmen, daß sich die Zahl der Narkolepsiefälle vermehrt hat und man schrieb diese Vermehrung begreiflicherweise den Encephalitisepidemien zu. Nun kann es wohl keinem Zweifel unterliegen, daß durch die postencephalitischen Fälle, deren Zahl wir ja weiter oben derzeit auf etwa 20% geschätzt haben und die früher, in der Narkolepsiestatistik vor dem Jahre 1917 fast gefehlt haben, tatsächlich eine deutlich wahrnehmbare Vermehrung der Narkolepsiefälle eingetreten ist. Aber es wäre verfehlt, die ganze Vermehrung der letzten Jahre auf diesen Umstand zurückführen zu wollen. Schon REDLICH hat auf Grund seiner Erfahrungen darauf hingewiesen, daß der Weltkrieg es war, welcher ein *scheinbares* Anwachsen der Fälle mit sich gebracht hat. Viele Fälle von Narkolepsie, sehr viele sogar, betrachten ihre Narkolepsie eigentlich nicht als Krankheit, sondern als Eigenheit, als Unbequemlichkeit, die nicht in die Hände des Arztes gehört. Das kommt so recht deutlich zum Vorschein, wenn man in den Krankengeschichten sieht, wie viele Jahre, ja sogar Jahrzehnte es dauert, bis die Narkoleptiker und das oft bloß zufällig, wegen anderer Störungen in die Hände des Arztes kommen. CAVE fand an seinem Material, daß die Männer im Durchschnitt 5, die Frauen 10 Jahre brauchen, bis sie sich zu diesem Schritt entschließen. Darum sind ja auch alle Narkolepsiestatistiken, die sich auf das Datum der erschienenen Arbeiten oder auf das Datum des Spitaleintrittes beziehen, unrichtig; hier muß man zum Unterschied von den meisten anderen Krankheiten ausdrücklich das Datum des *Krankheitsbeginnes* als Grundlage nehmen. So findet z. B. CAVE ein sonderbares Anwachsen der Aufnahmen im Jahre 1927, während dieses Jahr, wenn man das Datum des Krankheitsbeginnes betrachtet, nichts Besonderes bietet. Die Rolle des Weltkrieges in der Geschichte der Narkolepsie war nun diese, daß durch den militärischen Dienst mit seinem Exerzieren, Posten stehen usw., so manche Soldaten als dienstuntauglich, als krank erkannt wurden und zur Begutachtung in die Hände des Neurologen kamen. So erhielt z. B. REDLICH einen Teil seines Materials. Und das war neben der Encephalitis die zweite Ursache der Vermehrung der Narkolepsie. Als dritte Ursache kann man vielleicht die Arbeiten REDLICHs bezeichnen, der es verstanden hat, das Krankheitsbild so weit zu popularisieren, daß viele Fälle, welche bisher unentdeckt waren, erkannt wurden und Interesse erregten. Und mit der Vermehrung der Arbeiten in den verschiedenen Ländern wird diese Wirkung noch vervielfacht. Man darf diese Wirkung vielleicht sogar als die Hauptursache der Vermehrung der Narkolepsiefälle betrachten, denn wir alle haben wohl schon die Erfahrung gemacht, wie durch irgendwelche Arbeiten die Aufmerksamkeit auf ein seltenes Krankheitsbild gelenkt wird und sich plötzlich die Fälle in unglaublicher Weise vermehren.

Wie häufig ist also die Narkolepsie? CAVE fand sie unter den Patienten der Mayoklinik in einem Verhältnis von 1:8 610, also in etwa 0,12 $^0/_{00}$ des Krankenmaterials. Man kann also wohl noch immer von einer sehr seltenen Krankheit sprechen, aber nicht extrem selten, denn ich sehe wohl jedes Jahr 1—2 Fälle (an einem rein neurologischen privaten und Spitalsmaterial).

Ich habe auch, um mir ein Bild zu machen darüber, ob auch nach dem Krankheitsbeginn genommen, ein Anwachsen der Fälle zu konstatieren ist, im Jahre 1931 eine Statistik von willkürlich ausgewählten 100 Fällen zusammengestellt — für eine derartige

Tabelle 1.

1901	1902	1903	1904	1905	1906	1907	1908	1909	1910	1911	1912
1	1	0	0	0	2	0	2	2	2	2	4

Tabelle 1 (Fortsetzung).

1913	1914	1915	1916	1917	1918	1919	1920	1921	1922	1923	1924
2	1	1	0	6	2	2	6	6	5	11	9

Tabelle 1 (Fortsetzung).

1925	1926	1927	1928	1929	1930
11	10	8	1	2	1

Statistik sicher ein zu geringes Material. Es spräche, soweit die Statistik verwertbar ist, gleichfalls im Sinne eines Anwachsens in den Jahren seit dem Krieg bzw. seit der Encephalitisära.

Natürlich darf man angesichts der langen „ärztlichen Latenzzeit" der Narkolepsie aus dieser Statistik nicht etwa auf eine *Abnahme* in den *allerletzten* Jahren schließen. Während in unserer Statistik also der Höhepunkt in den Jahren 1923—1927 liegt, sieht man in 20 Fällen von BERNHARDT-THIELE den Gipfel in 1925—1927 und bei LEVIN (43 Fälle 1926—1928).

Aus der Literatur ergibt sich, daß das Vorkommen der Narkolepsie an kein bestimmtes Land und an keine Rasse gebunden ist. Wir haben Berichte aus Europa, Amerika und Australien, von Weißen und Schwarzen, von Ariern und Semiten, von Schweden und Griechen.

Alter. Wir haben schon erwähnt, *daß der Beginn der Narkolepsie mit Vorliebe ins jugendliche Alter fällt,* daß sich Ausnahmen von dieser Regel besonders häufig unter den symptomatischen Fällen finden. REDLICH hat in einer Statistik von 100 Fällen gefunden: das erste Auftreten vor dem 10. Lebensjahr in 4 Fällen (STIEFLER, JANZEN, JAKOBSOHN, WEECH), im 2. Dezennium in 54 (!), im 3. in 23, im 4. in 18 und jenseits des 40. Jahres in 3 Fällen (in 5 Fällen keine Angaben). THIELE und BERNHARDT hatten in ihren 25 Fällen 9mal, also in 44% den Beginn im 2. Dezennium. Wir fanden bei weiteren 70 Fällen folgende Zahlen: im 1. Dezennium 4%, im 2. 39%, im 3. 28%, im 4. 18% und darüber 9%. Rechnet man jedoch die encephalitischen Fälle ab, so bekommen wir im 2. Dezennium 48%, im 3. 23% — also ähnliche Zahlen wie REDLICH.

Geschlecht. REDLICH fand in seinen 100 Fällen 79% Männer und 21% Frauen. THIELE unter 25 Fällen 7 Frauen, also mehr, jedoch bei genuiner Narkolepsie unter 21 Fällen 5 Frauen. Ich fand Zahlen in der neueren Literatur (nach REDLICHs Tod), welche zwischen jenen von THIELE und von REDLICH stehen: 24 Frauen gegen 72 Männer. Es ist aber wiederum bemerkenswert, wie viele Fälle von symptomatischer Narkolepsie sich bei meinen ersten 19 Frauen befinden: 2 sichere, 5 wahrscheinliche Encephalitiden, 3 luische Fälle, 1 hypophysärer Fall — also 11 symptomatische oder auf symptomatisch verdächtige Fälle. Es ergibt sich daraus, daß *an dem starken Überwiegen der Männer bei der Narkolepsie und besonders bei der genuinen Form nicht zu zweifeln ist.* Wie sollen wir uns das erklären? Meines Erachtens kommen da nicht bloß irgendwelche hereditär-konstitutionellen Gesetzmäßigkeiten in Frage, sondern noch 2 andere, vielleicht wichtigere Faktoren: 1. die endokrinen Drüsen, wobei aber zu bemerken ist, daß sonst die Frauen mit ihrem labilen Endokrinium überall dort, wo es sich um endokrine Krankheitseinflüsse zu handeln pflegt, überwiegen; 2. ein *exogener Faktor,* wahrscheinlich in Form von beruflicher Anstrengung, denn dieser Umstand spielt in den meisten Krankheiten eine Rolle, wo es sich um ein Übergewicht der Männer handelt. Das müßte man sich nicht unbedingt so denken, daß es berufliche Schädigungen spezifischer Art sind, welche eine wesentliche ätiologische Rolle spielen, aber wer es wiederholt beobachtet hat (und die meisten Autoren bestätigen dies), wie unter dem Einfluß von körperlicher und psychischer Ruhe die Anfälle im Spital verschwinden, der wird sich dem Eindruck kaum entziehen, daß durch die männlichen Berufe eine Narkolepsie erst manifest, erst zu einer „Beschwerde" wird. Das wird ja wohl nicht für alle, aber für sehr viele Fälle gelten.

Beruf. Wir finden ziemlich viel *schwerarbeitende* Berufe, ferner Berufe, die eine gewisse *Monotonie* der Arbeit und ein Arbeiten in heißen Räumen mit sich bringen. So gab einer meiner Patienten, welcher in einer Brauerei mit dem Durchsieben der Gerste in einem heißen Raum beschäftigt war, an, daß auch andere Arbeiter dabei öfter einschliefen. Ähnliches berichtet KAPLINSKI über Chauffeure, Straßenbahnführer, Motoristen, die bei Automaten arbeiten. Dies alles kann sich so erklären, daß eben eine Anlage zur Narkolepsie unter solchen Umständen manifest wird (wobei es noch immer unklar ist, wieso es dabei auch zu affektivem Tonusverlust kommen soll). THIELE und BERNHARDT finden unter ihrem Material auffallend viele Monteure und Mechaniker, manche von ihnen hatten jedoch die Narkolepsie schon vor dem Eintritt ins Berufsleben; mir fiel die große Zahl der Chauffeure und Autofahrer auf, wir finden auch Heizer, Führer von Dampfpflügen usw. Man könnte evtl. die Möglichkeit erwägen, ob nicht die verschiedenen Abgase dabei eine Rolle spielen, wobei man sich andererseits die nicht unbeträchtliche Menge von Landarbeitern und Soldaten vor Augen halten muß.

Pathologische Anatomie, Lokalisation. Es liegt bisher kein einziger anatomischer Befund bei Narkolepsie vor[1]. Alle Vermutungen über die Lokalisation oder die Natur des Krankheitsprozesses, welche den Erscheinungen der Narkolepsie zugrunde liegen, müssen daher vorläufig mehr oder weniger hypothetisch bleiben. Manche Autoren zweifeln sogar daran, ob ein positiver anatomischer Befund überhaupt zu erwarten ist, da es sich auch um eine rein funktionelle Störung handeln kann. Nichtsdestoweniger konnte es REDLICH im Jahre 1924 unternehmen, eine Lokalisation des Leidens zu versuchen und er stützte sich dabei auf die Tatsache des Auftretens von typischer Narkolepsie nach Encephalitis epidemica. ECONOMO konnte nämlich zeigen, daß bei der lethargischen oder somnolent-ophthalmoplegischen Form, die Herde der Encephalitis auffallend stark in der Gegend des vorderen Teiles des Aquaeductus Sylvii und den kranial davon gelegenen Partien des 3. Ventrikels lokalisiert sind. Er griff daher die alte MAUTHNERsche Hypothese auf, daß sich in dieser Gegend, welche nach hinten an die vorderen Teile des Oculomotoriuskernes angrenzt (daher die Ptosis bei der lethargischen Form) und vorne an die wichtigsten vegetativen Zentren des Zwischenhirnes (der Schlaf als vegetativer Vorgang) ein Zentrum befinde, welches für den Schlaf bzw. seine Störungen von wesentlicher Bedeutung sein müsse. Gestützt auf sein tiefes biologisches Wissen verfiel jedoch ECONOMO nicht in den Fehler der meisten seiner Vorgänger, einfach ein „Schlafzentrum" zu supponieren, welches in einer ähnlichen Weise funktionieren sollte, wie etwa die motorischen Rindenzentren oder die Sprachzentren. Er verschloß sich nicht der Erkenntnis, daß der Schlaf ein biologischer Vorgang ist, welcher schon bei niedrigen Lebewesen, ja sogar bei den Pflanzen vorkomme, daß er nicht eine bloße Angelegenheit des Gehirnes, sondern eine biologische Angelegenheit des Körpers sei, eine Eigenschaft des Protoplasma. ECONOMO unterschied den „Hirnschlaf", das Auslöschen bzw. die Herabstimmung der psychischen Tätigkeiten vom „Körperschlaf", welcher den ganzen Körper umfaßt, dessen sämtliche Organe im Schlaf Zustandsänderungen erfahren. Er wußte gut, daß der Schlaf ein vegetativer Vorgang ist. Da aber andererseits eine Bedeutung der erwähnten Hirnpartien für den Schlaf ihm sicher schien, so stellte er sich vor, daß es sich hier bloß um ein höheres *Regulierungszentrum* des Schlafes handeln könne, um ein „*Schlafsteuerungszentrum*", wie er es nannte und für diese Annahme schien ihm auch das häufige Vorkommen der Schlafumkehr bei der Encephalitis zu sprechen. Weitere Untersuchungen schienen diese Hypothese ECONOMOS immer mehr zu stützen und heute ist sie so verbreitet, daß man wohl von einer offiziösen Theorie sprechen kann. Eine Reihe von Fällen (LUCKSCH, ADLER, HIRSCH, PETTE, MARINESCO-SAGER-KREINDLER, SCHWAB) von Tumoren, Erweichungen usw. mit genauem anatomischen und klinischen Befund bestätigten eindeutig diese Lokalisation und sehr zur rechten Zeit kam hier auch ein Anencephalus von CAMPER, bei welchem nicht bloß das Großhirn, sondern auch zum größten Teil die Thalami optici fehlten, ein „Mittelhirnwesen" also,

---

[1] LEY, SELS und VAN BOGAERT beschreiben einen fraglichen Fall (65jähriger Mann, Auftreten von Schafanfällen nach Aufregungen, Dauer der Anfälle $1/4$—$1/2$ Stunde, kein Tonusverlust, Übergang in Dauerschlaf und Koma); der Obduktionsbefund war negativ bis auf leichte Atherosklerose, leichte Ependymitis und verstärkte Gefäßfüllung.

welches trotzdem eine Schlaf- und Wachperiodik zeigte. Pötzl war es, welcher alle diese Fälle zusammenfaßte und zu einer noch präziseren Lokalisation des Schlafsteuerungszentrums in überzeugender Weise gekommen ist. Er umgrenzt es auf Grund dieser Fälle folgendermaßen: kranialwärts vom Oculomotoriuskern, die Gegend der hinteren Commissur und die angrenzenden Teile des Thalamus opticus umfassend (dorsalwärts etwa bis zur Höhe der Habenula), hauptsächlich im Gebiete des Nucleus Darkschewitsch (im Falle Gampers fehlten Pulvinar thalami, Habenulae, Meynertsches und Viq d'Azyrsches Bündel). Pötzl meint übrigens, daß auch Thalamusherde für den Schlaf von Bedeutung sein können. Auch die interessanten Versuche von W. R. Hess sprechen für diese Auffassung. Und gerade die Dissoziationen des Schlafes bei der Narkolepsie zeigen deutlich, daß ein Regulierungsapparat gestört ist.

Wie verhält es sich aber mit den anderen Symptomen der Narkolepsie? Hier sind wir noch mehr auf Hypothesen angewiesen, ist uns ja nicht einmal das Wesen aller dieser Begleiterscheinungen der Narkolepsie vollkommen klar. Wir gehen auf diese Details daher lieber im Kapitel „Pathogenese" ein. Nur das wichtige Symptom des affektiven Tonusverlustes und seiner Lokalisation wollen wir hier kurz streifen. Man wird den Tonusverlust verschieden lokalisieren wollen, je nachdem man ihn mehr als dem Schlaf verwandt ansieht oder als eine Erscheinung für sich. Redlich neigte mehr zu der letzten Meinung und war daher geneigt, den Tonusverlust mehr als ein Nachbarschaftssymptom von seiten des Thalamus und des strio-pallidären Systems zu betrachten. In letzter Zeit lernte ich jedoch einen Fall kennen, der fast dafür zu sprechen scheint, daß der affektive Tonusverlust in die unmittelbarste Nähe des Economoschen Schlafzentrums, wenn nicht in dieses selbst zu lokalisieren ist.

Die Krankengeschichte des Falles, der im Wiener Verein für Psychiatrie im Jahre 1932 von Herschmann demonstriert wurde, wurde mir von diesem mittlerweile frühverstorbenen Forscher zur Verfügung gestellt. Ein 27jähriger Mann bekommt seit einigen Jahren bei Freude oder komischen Situationen ein Schwächegefühl, so, daß er zusammenfällt oder sich setzen muß. Dauer einige Sekunden, keine Bewußtseinstrübung, die Anfälle können durch Willensanstrengung manchmal abgekürzt werden. Seit einem Monat klagt er über zunehmende Kopfschmerzen pulsierenden Charakters, die vom Hinterhaupt nach vorne ausstrahlen, und über Erbrechen. Seit einer Woche Doppelbilder. Die Vermutung Herschmanns, es könne sich um eine Affektion in der Gegend der Mauthner-Economoschen Region handeln, wurde unabhängig davon auch vom Okulisten Dr. Kestenbaum ausgesprochen. Die Doppelbilder konnten nämlich nur im Sinne einer äußerst seltenen Störung, nämlich einer Divergenzlähmung gedeutet werden. Der sonstige neurologische Befund war dürftig: feinschlägiger gemischter Nystagmus beim Seitenblick, besonders nach links, der linke Cornealreflex etwas schwächer, leichte Schwäche im 2. und 3. Facialisast links, fragliche Schädigung des linken Cochlearis und des linken Hypoglossus, an den oberen Extremitäten Reflexe vielleicht links Spur stärker, eine Abweichtendenz der Arme nach rechts, die B.D.R. rechts Spur schwächer. Eine beiderseitige Stauungspapille, das Bild eines Hydrocephalus internus im Röntgen bestätigten die Vermutungsdiagnose eines Tumor cerebri. Was jedoch besonders interessant ausfiel, war das Ergebnis der Encephalo- und der Ventrikulographie; der Röntgenbefund nach Lufteinblasung direkt in die Ventrikel lautete nämlich: „Seiten- und 3. Ventrikel erweitert, links mehr wie rechts, ebenso Foramen Monroi, der hintere Teil des Aquaeductus Sylvii und der 4. Ventrikel nicht dargestellt, ein pflaumenkerngroßer unregelmäßiger bogenförmiger Tumor ragt von vorne in das rechte Ventrikeldreieck hinein." Eine Ergänzung erfuhr dieser Befund durch die lumbale Lufteinblasung; diese ergab: „Konvexität und basale Zisternen gefüllt, Ventrikel nicht, die Cisterna chiasmatis in den Sellaeingang hinabgedrängt, Hydrocephalus occlusus." Es wurde occipital trepaniert, wobei nichts Besonderes auffiel, die Dura wurde nicht eröffnet.

Hätten wir mehrere Fälle dieser Art, so wären sie vielleicht geeignet, die fehlenden Obduktionsbefunde zu ersetzen. Vorläufig bleibt jedoch die Lokalisation des affektiven Tonusverlustes noch immer sehr hypothetisch.

Pathogenese. Wenn wir uns über die Pathogenese der *Krankheit* Narkolepsie eine Vorstellung machen wollen, müssen wir einige Überlegungen über ihre *Symptome* anstellen, da es sich ja dabei um in der Neurologie neuartige und daher noch unklare Erscheinungen handelt. Wir wollen dabei die Schlafanfälle als die führende Erscheinung im Krankheitsbilde zuerst besprechen. Da muß man wohl erwähnen, daß es Autoren gibt (WILSON, ADIE, STRAUSS u. a.), welche nicht davon überzeugt sind, daß es sich *um wirklichen Schlaf* handelt und sie verweisen insbesondere auf gewisse durchaus inkonstante und nicht häufige Nebenerscheinungen, welche diesen Schlaf begleiten können, z. B. eine Art von Aura oder die oben erwähnten motorischen Reizerscheinungen, Zuckungen, Tremores, andere Bewegungen. Nun sind wir der Meinung, daß es sich, zumindest bei einem Großteil dieser Erscheinungen um Dinge handelt, welche auch beim normalen Schlaf mindestens ebenso oft vorkommen, wie etwa der Somnambulismus, bei welchem wir dennoch nicht daran zweifeln, daß er im *Schlaf* erfolgt; und wir wissen, daß unsere Patienten eben abnormale Schläfer sind, welche zu einer Dissoziation von Hirn- und Körperschlaf auch in der Nacht neigen. Wollen wir daran zweifeln, daß sie in der Nacht schlafen? Aber immerhin, die Frage dieser motorischen Erscheinungen ist noch nicht so eindeutig geklärt, daß man anderes als vage Hypothesen aufstellen könnte. REDLICH denkt z. B. daran, daß es sich dabei um Irradiationserscheinungen auf die eng benachbarten Stammganglien handeln könnte, um striäre Erscheinungen bei den Hyperkinesen, um thalamische bei den Parästhesien, wie ja die so häufig vorhandenen vegetativen Anomalien dafür sprechen, daß der Prozeß bei der Narkolepsie nicht eng an das Schlafzentrum geknüpft ist, sondern auch die benachbarten vegetativen Zentren im Tuber cinereum betreffen kann.

Wir zweifeln nicht daran, daß es sich bei den sog. Schlafanfällen ebenso um Schlafstörungen handelt, wie bei dem so häufig in eigenartiger Weise gestörten Nachtschlaf der Narkoleptiker. Können wir uns nun über die Art dieser Störung eine Vorstellung machen? Das hängt davon ab, welche Vorstellung wir uns vom Schlaf machen und gerade dieses Kapitel der Physiologie ist auch in den letzten Jahrzehnten ein Gegenstand so lebhafter Diskussion, daß uns in diesem Rahmen kaum etwas übrigbleibt als die wichtigsten dieser Theorien aufzuzählen und ganz einfach ohne jede Begründung uns einer dieser Theorien anzuschließen, allerdings jener, welche gerade in den letzten Jahren besonders viel Anhänger hat.

Sehen wir von den teleologischen Auffassungen ab, die uns hier nicht interessieren, so kommen folgende Theorien in Frage: die vasomotorischen Theorien, welche den Schlaf teils auf eine Hyperämie, teils auf eine Anämie des Gehirnes zurückführen, die Drucktheorien, welche teils den Liquordruck, teils den osmotischen Druck im Nervengewebe zum Gegenstand haben, die chemischen Theorien, von denen jene, die mit Ermüdungsstoffen operieren, die bekanntesten sind, die neueste Theorie ist die Bromausschüttung in die Oblongata von ZONDEK und BIER, die hormonalen Theorien (SALMON, MINGAZZINI und BARBARA), welche in der periodischen Tätigkeit verschiedener Inkretdrüsen in Anlehnung an den Winterschlaf der Tiere eine Erklärung suchen, die psychologischen Theorien (CLAPARÈDE), die psychoanalytischen Theorien (Flucht in einen Urzustand), die schon etwas teleologisch gefärbt sind und schließlich die verschiedenen nervösen Theorien, wie die von PURKINJE, von MARINESCO, TRÖMNER u. a., welche alle das gemeinsam haben, daß sie in einer Leitungsunterbrechung oder in einem Reizmangel eine Erklärung suchen. ECONOMO nun und mit ihm andere neuere Autoren stellen sich aber auf einen Standpunkt, der zu einem Teil schon von BROWN-SÉQUARD vertreten wurde, daß Schlaf eben nicht bloß Hirnschlaf ist, daß der Schlaf auch keine Narkose ist, sondern ein komplexer *biologischer* Vorgang, welcher beim Menschen aktiv reguliert wird, und sehr viele Tatsachen sprechen für diese Auffassung, die wir hier nicht alle anführen können. ECONOMO, der von einem Schlafsteuerungszentrum spricht, denkt auch an die Möglichkeit, daß es neben dem Schlafzentrum noch ein *Wachzentrum* gibt, welches alternierend mit dem ersteren das Übergewicht bekommt und ROSENTHAL nimmt sogar *nur* ein Wachzentrum an. PÖTZL steht ebenfalls auf dem Standpunkt, daß es sich um verschiedene Zustände eines und desselben Zentrums handelt. Wenn man nun den Schlaf, wie es PÖTZL näher ausführt, als einen vegetativen Vorgang par excellence betrachtet, wenn man sich vor Augen hält, wie alle vegetativen Funktionen, jede in ihrer Art jenen periodischen Wechsel mitmachen, welchen wir Schlafen und Wachen nennen, so kann man wohl davon sprechen, daß es sich um ein Zentrum handelt, welches eine Funktion beherrscht, die sich in allen vegetativen Vorgängen äußert und somit, wie PÖTZL es tut, von einem „Zentrum der Zentren" sprechen. Damit ist allerdings noch nicht gesagt, wodurch und auf welche Weise dieser aktive Vorgang ausgelöst wird und schon gar nicht, wodurch er beeinflußt werden kann. Hier kommen so manche der früher aufgezählten Theorien zur Geltung, denn dies kann durch Ermüdungsstoffe, durch vasomotorische Vorgänge, durch Hormone usw. geschehen. W. R. HESS hat durch ingeniös ausgedachte Experimente darzulegen versucht, daß es eine Periodik in der Funktion des *vegetativen Nervensystems* ist, welche hierfür verantwortlich ist und dies ist uns ein willkommener Anlaß, darauf hinzuweisen, daß man ja auch umgekehrt behaupten kann, der Schlaf schaffe erst diese Periodik (wenn sie auch ohne „Hirnschlaf" sich zeigen kann). Auf keinem Gebiete ist diese Fragestellung nach Ursache und Wirkung so heikel, wie gerade auf dem Gebiete des vegetativen Nervensystems. Wenn PÖTZL immer wieder das Prinzip der *Reziprozität* für die Funktion der Hirnzentren vertritt, indem er nachzuweisen versucht, daß z. B. Zentren, welche Erregungen aussenden, auch solche empfangen, „absaugen" können, so gilt dieses Prinzip in höchstem Maße vor allem für das vegetative Nervensystem. Nehmen wir ein Beispiel: Das Adrenalin reizt den Sympathicus (strenggenommen wirkt es wie Sympathicusreizung), aber Sympathicusreizung bringt notwendigerweise auch eine Adrenalinausschüttung mit sich; und dasselbe gilt für Thyreoidea und Sympathicus, für Inselapparat und Vagus usw. Ist hier nicht jede Frage nach dem primum movens praktisch ganz müßig und erinnert sie nicht an die Frage „was früher war, die Henne oder das Ei?" Wir können also bloß sagen, daß der Schlafvorgang, so wie wir ihn im gewöhnlichen Sprachgebrauch verstehen, d. h. der Hirnschlaf, in engster, und zwar reziproker Verbindung mit allen vegetativen Vorgängen, besonders aber den assimilatorischen, den parasympathischen steht und dasselbe gilt sicher auch für die hormonalen, die vasomotorischen, die chemischen Theorien usw. Es ist sicher notwendig und angezeigt, alle diese Theorien auch an dem Fall der Narkolepsie nachzuprüfen, was bisher nicht geschehen ist. Vorläufig müssen wir uns bloß diese enge reziproke Verknüpfung vor Augen halten und den Umstand, daß es eine Stelle im Gehirn gibt, welche wohl nicht für den Schlaf verantwortlich ist, aber für die Koordination der Schlafvorgänge und deren Affektion Störungen im *Ablauf* dieser Vorgänge verursacht.

Und von diesem Standpunkt muß man meines Erachtens die Schlafanfälle der Narkolepsie betrachten. Nicht als Lähmungs-, Hemmungs- oder Reizerscheinungen, nicht das Zuviel oder Zuwenig an Schlaf interessiert uns hier, sondern es handelt sich dabei um nichts anderes Pathologisches als um Störungen in der normalen *Periodik* des Schlafes und um Störungen der *Koordination der einzelnen Schlafkomponenten* (Nachtschlaf, Wachanfälle, Körperschlafanfälle). Die meisten Fälle der Narkolepsie zeigen eigentlich kein besonderes Zuviel oder Zuwenig an Schlaf und es wäre daher meines Erachtens angezeigt, weil fruchtbar, nicht von „Schlafstörungen" zu sprechen, sondern von „Einschlaf- und Erwachstörungen".

Schwieriger ist die zweite Gruppe der Erscheinungen zu deuten, der affektive Tonusverlust; denn hier herrscht über das Wesen der Erscheinung, welche in der Pathologie keine rechten Analoga hat, noch weniger Einigkeit. Nicht bloß in der Nomenklatur (s. unten), sondern in der Definition der Erscheinung selbst. Wir haben schon erwähnt, daß die meisten Autoren die plötzliche Erschlaffung in den Vordergrund stellen, welche beim Stehen allein schon dazu führt, daß das Individuum zusammenfällt (darum nennt auch GÉLINEAU diese ganze Erscheinung *Astasie* oder *Chûte*). Nun ist es ja nach meiner Auffassung wirklich kein Zufall, daß sich die meisten Fälle von Tonusverlust in aufrechter Position ereignen (s. frühere Ausführungen über Aggression), man darf jedoch nicht übersehen, daß dies nicht immer der Fall ist, daß es auch z. B. beim Essen, beim Coitus usw. zum Tonusverlust kommen kann. Nun ist die Erschlaffung der Muskulatur bei diesen Zuständen nicht bloß subjektiv den Patienten sehr stark bewußt, sondern auch objektiv zahllose Male nachgewiesen. Dabei wird aber von den meisten Autoren übersehen, daß sich die Erscheinungen des Anfalls nicht darauf beschränken, daß tatsächlich auch eine *Unmöglichkeit zur aktiven und reflektorischen Innervation der Skeletmuskeln vorhanden ist, also doch eine Art Lähmung*. Das subjektive Gefühl der Kranken dabei entspricht wohl schon dem Gefühl der Lähmung, denn sie machen ja zum Teil heftige Willensanstrengungen, um eine Bewegung zu produzieren. Und doch scheuen sich alle Autoren von einer Lähmung zu sprechen, man spricht höchstens von innervatorischer Hemmung, ohne aber diese Ablehnung des Wortes Lähmung irgendwie zu begründen. Es ist vorläufig leider noch Gefühlssache, wenn sowohl die Patienten als auch die Autoren nicht von einer Lähmung sprechen (auch ich würde es nicht tun) und man kann nur vermuten, daß das Wort hauptsächlich abgelehnt wird, weil es sich um Zustände von so kurzer Dauer handelt; und wir kennen in der Pathologie wohl Reiz-, nicht aber Lähmungserscheinungen von so blitzartig einsetzendem und so rasch und vollkommen vorübergehendem Charakter; eine Lähmung braucht immer einige Zeit zu ihrer Entwicklung und auch zu ihrem Verschwinden. Bleiben wir also dabei, daß es sich um eine *innervatorische Hemmung* handelt, dann kann man allerdings auch den Verlust des Tonus, also der physiologischen Ruheinnervation unter denselben Begriff der innervatorischen Hemmung subsummieren. Worin besteht aber dieser Vorgang? Hier suchen die Autoren in zwei Richtungen. Die einen sehen das Wesentliche in einer gewissen Analogie mit dem Schlaf, in welchem es ja ebenfalls in der Regel zu einer hochgradigen Hypotonie und zu einem Mangel an motorischer Innervation kommt; daß gerade bei den narkoleptischen Schlafanfällen manchmal das Gegenteil zu sehen ist (Schlafen im Stehen und Gehen), beweist vielleicht nicht viel[1], da wir ja hier besonders reichlich Abweichungen von der Norm, Dissoziation der Schlafkomponenten sehen. Auf diesem Standpunkt steht z. B. LHERMITTE und seine Schule, welche direkt von „Schlafäquivalenten" sprechen. Die anderen berufen sich auf das Verhalten des Normalen im Affekt, indem hier ein gewisser Einfluß auf den Muskeltonus zu beobachten ist. Allerdings sind diese normalen Erscheinungen noch sehr schlecht studiert. Während z. B. die einen behaupten, daß es beim normalen Lachen zu einem Tonusverlust, zu einer Innervationserschwerung kommt, welche in Grenzfällen schon stark an den pathologischen Tonusverlust erinnert (kommt es ja bei Frauen nicht so selten dabei sogar zu einem Nachlassen des Sphincter vesicae und zum Secessus urinae), behauptet z. B. ROTHFELD, daß das Lachen den Tonus steigert, traurige Affekte ihn herabsetzen. KELLER ist aber z. B. der Meinung, daß jeder

---

[1] Daß aber Schlaf und Atonie nicht dasselbe sind, sehen wir beim Schlaf mancher Tiere. PÖTZE zitiert z. B. den Klammerreflex der Vogelzehen, der Sichelkrallen der Faultiere, der Zehenhacken der Fledermäuse.

Affekt den Tonus steigere. LÖWENFELD betont den Tonuswechsel im Affekt. Solange man hier noch so sehr im Dunkeln tappt, müssen begreiflicherweise jene Theorien, welche im affektiven Tonusverlust bloß eine Steigerung oder eine Abänderung des normalen Verhaltens im Affekt sehen, auf sehr unsicherer Basis beruhen, was im Interesse der Aufklärung des Problems sehr zu bedauern ist. Vielleicht werden hier Untersuchungen in der Art der Studie von STRAUSS über das Zusammenschrecken oder von AUGUSTE FLACH über die tänzerische Darstellung von Affekten weitere Aufklärung bringen. Es ist interessant, daß STRAUSS dabei (sogar bei einem Narkoleptiker) keinen Tonusverlust beim Zusammenschrecken (nach Schuß) beobachten konnte. Eine dritte Reihe von Autoren, vor allem REDLICH, stützt sich mehr darauf, daß mit dem Tonusverlust allein die Begleiterscheinungen des Affektes beim Narkoleptiker manchmal nicht erschöpft sind, daß man dabei öfters auch *hyperkinetische* Erscheinungen verschiedener Art beobachten kann (s. oben). Diese Autoren suchen eine mehr anatomische und pathologische Erklärung und REDLICH glaubt, daß es sich dabei teils um eine Störung im benachbarten Thalamusgebiet handelt, dessen Bedeutung für die Beziehungen von gewissen Affekten zu der Motilität bekannt ist, teils um Irradiation auf das benachbarte striopallidäre System mit seinen bekannten Beziehungen zum Muskeltonus. Ich selbst deutete schon weiter oben die Hypothese an, daß die Art der Affekte und der von mir hervorgehobenen nicht affektiven Auslösungsmomente des Tonusverlustes etwas Gemeinsames haben, es sich um plötzlich aufschießende und mit plötzlicher Anspannung der Körpermuskulatur einhergehende Affektstöße handelt, welche ferner teils offenkundig, teils im tiefenpsychologischen Sinn (Lachen) eine Aggressionstendenz oder Bremsung einer Aggression beinhalten. Es ist nun von vornherein anzunehmen, daß die von mir zusammengestellten Auslösungsursachen (Schlagen, Jagen, Angeln, Schießen, plötzliches Umwenden, Beginn des Laufens), aber auch Lachen, bei welchem ja nach den älteren psychologischen Anschauungen das Moment der Überraschung, nach den neueren der plötzlichen Lustabfuhr eine Rolle spielt, der Orgasmus usw. die Notwendigkeit einer plötzlichen Innervation beinhalten, ja einer Innervation, welche auch eine gesteigerte Bereitschaft, eine gesteigerte Anspannung aller Kräfte, mit einem Wort eine Steigerung dessen, was wir eben Tonus nennen. Die Störung kann nun hier entweder so zustande kommen, daß statt dieser Anspannung eine paradoxe Innervation erscheint, eine Hemmung (ich habe vorgeschlagen einfach von „paradoxem Tonusverlust" zu sprechen); etwas Ähnliches nimmt z. B. PÖTZL an, indem er von einer „*denervatorischen* Hemmung" infolge einer absaugenden Gegenreaktion der Zentren spricht. Man kann aber auch denken, daß eben diese erforderliche Anspannung einen Zustand von erhöhtem „Tonus" in der Muskulatur schafft, welcher nach meinem „Ausgangswertgesetz" besonders geeignet ist, auf weitere Reize mit einer Reaktionsumkehr zu antworten, also mit einer Erschlaffung. Übrigens unterscheiden sich diese beiden Auffassungen voneinander nur von ihren verschiedenen Gesichtspunkten, indem die eine denselben Zusammenhang mehr von einem zentralen, die andere von einem peripheren Gesichtspunkt betrachtet. Dies alles sind jedoch Hypothesen, ebenso wie STRANSKYs „Schaltschwäche" zwischen kortikofugalen Bahnen und subcorticalen Zentren u. a. Eine sichere Kenntnis vom Wesen und von der Pathogenese des Tonusverlustes haben wir heute noch nicht.

Fassen wir nun diese beiden Haupterscheinungen der Narkolepsie zusammen, um über die Pathogenese des Krankheitsbildes etwas auszusagen, so können wir uns auf den Standpunkt stellen, daß es sich einerseits um Anomalien in der Funktion des Schlafsteuerungszentrums im 3. Ventrikel handelt, andererseits um eine Erscheinung, welche von manchen Autoren auf dieselbe Regulationsstörung zurückgeführt wird, von anderen als eine Nachbarerscheinung, auf eine Störung in der Koordination der Beziehungen von Affekten zur Skeletmuskulatur bzw. ihrem Tonus aufgefaßt wird. Die anderen Erscheinungen der Narkolepsie machen dann keine weiteren Schwierigkeiten. Die anderen Anfälle, die „Wachanfälle", die „Körperschlafanfälle", die Störungen des Nachtschlafes beruhen ebenfalls auf Störungen der Schlafkoordination, die vegetativen Erscheinungen auf Störungen in den so eng benachbarten vegetativen Zentren des Zwischenhirns, die hyperkinetischen Erscheinungen auf Störungen in dem ebenfalls benachbarten striopallidären System.

Wie kommen aber diese Störungen zustande, was für krankhafter Vorgang liegt ihnen zugrunde? Hier müssen wir nun zwei Gruppen von Narkolepsien unterscheiden: eine Gruppe, bei der wir den Prozeß, der für die Erscheinungen verantwortlich ist, mehr oder weniger kennen. Diese Gruppe nennt REDLICH u. a. in Analogie mit der Epilepsie die Gruppe der *symptomatischen Narkolepsien*, hervorgerufen durch Encephalitis, Hirntumoren, Traumen, Lues usw., also cerebrale Störungen von einer Lokalisation, welche der soeben besprochenen Auffassung entspricht. Daneben steht aber eine größere Gruppe, welche keinerlei Anhaltspunkte für eine organische Hirnschädigung bietet, welche in der Gleichförmigkeit ihres Auftretens, Beginn in der Jugend, ungemein chronischer, nicht progredienter Verlauf, evtl. familiäres Auftreten usw. einen anderen Eindruck erweckt und die REDLICH und seine Anhänger als eine Krankheitseinheit, als einen Morbus sui generis betrachten und *echte, idiopathische, genuine Narkolepsie* nennen.

Nichts an dieser Einteilung blieb unbestritten. So bezweifeln einige Autoren, z. B. WILSON, LHERMITTE, SOUGUES, BUMKE, MAKAROFF, ob die Narkolepsie überhaupt eine Krankheit im eigentlichen Sinne des Wortes sei, ob es sich nicht bloß um eine kleine Anomalie, eine Übertreibung des normalen Verhaltens handelt, höchstens aber um ein Symptom. Auch die hier skizzierten Grenzen der Narkolepsie wurden, wie schon erwähnt, von manchen Autoren nicht akzeptiert. Trotz des so scharf umrissenen Krankheitsbildes wollten LHERMITTE und seine Schüler, auch WILSON u. a. von scharfen Grenzen gegenüber verschiedenen anderen Arten von Schlafsucht nichts wissen und sprechen nur von „den Narkolepsien". Auch daß ein eigenartiger Krankheitsprozeß hier zugrunde liegt, wird von vielen bezweifelt, die Narkolepsie sei nur ein Syndrom, welches bei verschiedenen Krankheiten zustande komme, aber nicht eine eigene Krankheit. Wir glauben, daß mit solchen Spitzfindigkeiten, mögen sie sich auch auf ernste Argumente stützen, der Wahrheitssuche nicht gedient ist. Es ist gut und hat bereits Früchte getragen, die typische Narkolepsie von verschiedenen, oft nur oberflächliche Ähnlichkeiten bietenden Grenzgebieten möglich scharf abzutrennen, wenn auch dabei, wie bei fast allen anderen Krankheiten auch, gewisse Grenzfälle übrig bleiben mögen. Es ist notwendig, jene Fälle, bei denen die Narkolepsie nur als Symptom einer wohlbekannten Erkrankung auftritt, abzutrennen von jener großen Gruppe, bei der dies nicht der Fall ist, die auch bei näherer Betrachtung sich als viel mehr typisch, in sich einheitlich erweist und die man — vielleicht nur vorläufig — als genuine Narkolepsie bezeichnen muß.

Betrachten wir nun die symptomatischen Fälle, so bieten sie ja vorläufig keine besonderen Schwierigkeiten. Wir nehmen eben an, daß es sich dabei um Entzündungsvorgänge oder um Druckwirkungen usw. in den oben besprochenen Regionen handelt. Aus unbekannten Gründen entsteht eine Reiz- oder (weniger wahrscheinlich) eine Lähmungswirkung auf das Schlafsteuerungszentrum, aus unbekannten Gründen löst ein Affekt bestimmter Art die motorischen Vorgänge des Tonusverlustes aus.

Bei der echten Narkolepsie ist die Frage schon schwieriger. Hier nehmen REDLICH u. a. eine *konstitutionelle Anomalie* der betreffenden Zentren an; ähnliche Beispiele auf anderen Gebieten kennen wir zur Genüge. Für diese konstitutionelle Schwäche spricht nicht nur die Tatsache des Vorhandenseins familiärer Fälle, sondern auch die Art der Störungen in den betreffenden Familien (s. Fälle von J. BAUER, von HOFF und STENGEL). Der Beginn in der Jugend, die ungemeine Chronizität des Leidens ohne eigentliche Progredienz, die therapeutische Unzulänglichkeit sind weitere Beweise für die Rolle des konstitutionellen Faktors eigener Art, mag man ihn die „narkoleptische Reaktionsfähigkeit" nach KAHLER, mag man ihn das „Narkolepsiesubstrat" nach J. BAUER nennen. Aber wir sehen, daß auch noch andere Faktoren bei der Entstehung der Narkolepsie eine Rolle spielen dürften. Ob sie obligat sind, ist zu bezweifeln. Es sieht so aus, wie bei manchen anderen Erkrankungen, daß es eine Reihe von verschiedenartigen Faktoren geben kann, welche die Krankheit begünstigen, ihr Manifestwerden verursachen, ihre Erscheinungen verstärken können. Da sind in erster Linie die endokrinen Drüsen: es scheint, als ob genitale Hypofunktion, als ob Schilddrüsenhypofunktion die Krankheit öfters begünstigen würde, auch die Hypophyse scheint eine Rolle zu spielen, das ergibt sich nicht etwa bloß aus den nachbarschaftlichen Beziehungen der Hypophyse zu den besagten Zentren usw., sondern einfach aus der Häufung von klinischen Beobachtungen, die in diesem Sinne sprechen. Eine Rolle anderer endokriner Drüsen ist bei der Narkolepsie nicht bekannt. Speziell liegen keine Anhaltspunkte dafür vor, daß das Pankreas, welches im Gegensatz zu der Thyreoidea und Hypophyse den Winterschlaf der Tiere begünstigt, durch seine Hyperfunktion, wie sie in den letzten Jahren unter dem Bilde der spontanen Hypoglykämie bekannt wurde, die Narkolepsie fördern würde. — Neben den endokrinen Drüsen scheint das vegetative Nervensystem eine Rolle zu spielen. Man findet öfters Anomalien im Sinne einer Vagotonie, im Sinne eines Überwiegens der Assimilationsvorgänge über die Dissimilationsvorgänge. Und während der Hinweis auf die Rolle des Endokriniums etwa den Theorien von SALMON, von MINGAZZINI und BARBARA über den Schlaf entsprechen würde, so entspricht dieser Hinweis auf die Rolle des vegetativen Nervensystems etwa den Anschauungen von W. R. HESS. Jedenfalls hat der Vagotoniker im Gegensatz zum unruhigen, Angstparoxysmen unterworfenen Sympathicotoniker eine Neigung zur Depression, Müdigkeit, sogar Schlafsucht, es ist also nicht zu verwundern, wenn es den Anschein erwecken muß, als ob Überwiegen des Vagus die Narkolepsie begünstige, wobei wieder reziproke Beziehungen bestehen: der Schlaf ruft ein Überwiegen des Vagus hervor. — Auch Elektrolytverschiebungen können vielleicht eine Rolle spielen, wie die Tierversuche über die Einspritzung von Calcium ins Infundibulum einerseits, Calciuminjektionen beim Narkoleptiker andererseits ergeben; es würde demnach eine Hypercalcämie die Narkolepsie begünstigen (sicher aber nicht hervorrufen, s. Erfahrungen beim Hyperparathyreoidismus). — Den vasomotorischen Vorgängen wurde von manchen Autoren eine Rolle zugeschrieben und es sieht so aus, als ob eine gewisse Hyperämie, wie sie bei horizontaler Lage, bei Hitze, beim Lachen usw. auftritt, die Narkolepsie begünstigen würde, eine Kongestion wurde ja häufig dabei beobachtet, Blässe fast nie; auch hier wiederum reziproke Beziehungen, Schlaf macht Hyperämie. — Ähnliche reziproke Beziehungen haben wir beim Stoffwechsel: im Schlaf überwiegen die Assimilationsvorgänge, Fettsucht bringt sehr oft Schlafsucht mit sich. Daß Stoffwechselvorgänge überhaupt bei der Narkolepsie eine große Rolle spielen könnten, scheint mir a priori sehr wahrscheinlich; leider liegt aber gerade in dieser Hinsicht fast gar kein positives Material vor. — An meinen allergischen Fall möchte ich hier nochmals erinnern.

Wir haben also eine ganze Reihe von Faktoren, welche, wie die Erfahrung zeigt, bei der Narkolepsie eine Rolle spielen oder spielen können. *Alle* diese Faktoren haben nun außerdem etwas Gemeinsames, sie entsprechen einer Verschiebung im vegetativen System im weiteren Sinne (nach FR. KRAUS) in einer *ganz bestimmten* Richtung. Es ist nur nicht leicht, bei der komplizierten gegenseitigen Verbundenheit des vegetativen Systems diese Richtung eindeutig zu definieren und es ist ein willkürlich gewählter Standpunkt, wenn wir gerade das vegetative *Nervensystem* zum Ausgangspunkt nehmen und sagen: wir bemerken bei der Narkolepsie eine Unterfunktion von Drüsen, welche sonst den Vagus hemmen, ein Überwiegen des Vagus im vegetativen *Nervensystem*, ein Verhalten der Vasomotoren im vagotonischen Sinne, ein Überwiegen der assimilatorischen Vorgänge, welche bekanntlich mit dem Vagus in Verbindung stehen. Alles dies sind Vorgänge, welche zugleich auch mit dem normalen Schlaf Beziehungen haben, und zwar in einem ebensolchen reziproken Sinne.

Wir sehen aber, daß die Narkolepsie auch durch exogene Faktoren begünstigt wird, wie z. B. Anstrengung, Hitze, Schlafmangel, Erschöpfung usw. Es sind dies wohl Faktoren, welche wir auch als schlafbegünstigend kennen, aber es kann ja hier ihr Einfluß auch ein anderer sein.

Die Narkolepsie ist eine Anfallskrankheit und wir müssen uns daher auch die Frage stellen, wie der einzelne Anfall hervorgerufen wird. Auf diese Frage können wir eine Antwort nicht einmal verlangen; wissen wir dies ja nicht einmal bei der bestbekannten Anfallskrankheit, bei der Epilepsie, mit Sicherheit. In Frage kommen hier unbekannte exogene Momente, die für den affektiven Tonusverlust ja sicher sind, ferner Schwankungen im Vasomotorium, im Stoffwechsel, im Liquordruck usw. Diese Frage ist jedoch fast unbearbeitet.

Wollen wir also kurz definieren, so werden wir sagen, daß die symptomatische Narkolepsie durch direkte Einwirkung von bekannten Krankheitsvorgängen auf das Schlafsteuerungszentrum und dessen Umgebung zustande kommt, die genuine Narkolepsie höchstwahrscheinlich auf einer konstitutionellen Minderwertigkeit dieser Zentren beruht und gefördert wird durch Erkrankungen und Anomalien im vegetativen System (Hormone, vegetative Nerven, Elektrolyte, Stoffwechsel usw.) im Sinne einer Verschiebung nach der assimilatorischen, nach der vagotropen Seite hin.

Nomenklatur. Einige Bemerkungen über die Nomenklatur sind angesichts der verschiedenen Vorschläge angebracht. Der Name Narkolepsie stammt von GÉLINEAU; GÉLINEAU zählt die Krankheit zu den Erkrankungen ohne bekannte anatomische Ursache, also nach dem damaligen Brauch zu den Neurosen. Da der Ausdruck Neurose jedoch in den letzten Jahren immer mehr auf die sog. Psychoneurosen, die psychogenen Erkrankungen angewendet wird, zählt sie REDLICH nach seiner Einteilung zu den Neuropathien organischen Gepräges. Der Name Narkolepsie wurde bald beanstandet, denn ναρκεῖν bedeutet mehr „erstarren, gelähmt sein" und nicht schlafen; es würde dieser Ausdruck meines Erachtens eher auf den affektiven Tonusverlust als auf die Schlafanfälle passen. SINGER, TRÖMNER u. a. sind daher für den Namen „Hypnolepsie", aber REDLICH verweist darauf, daß damit ohnehin nur eine Reihe der Symptome, nämlich die Schlafanfälle, bezeichnet werden. CURSCHMANN-PRANGE verdeutscht Narkolepsie mit „Einschlafsucht". Manche Autoren beanstanden übrigens auch die „-lepsie" wegen des damit verbundenen Anklangs an die Epilepsie, gegen welche sie eine möglichst scharfe Grenze gezogen haben wollen. Man versuchte die Schwierigkeit zu umgehen und sprach vom „GÉLINEAUschen Syndrom", aber das entspricht wiederum nicht ganz der historischen Wahrheit, eher wäre der Name „WESTPHAL-GÉLINEAUsches Syndrom" angebracht. Manche Autoren sprechen vom „GÉLINEAU-REDLICHschen Syndrom".

Es ist aber doch wohl am besten, wie ADIE, REDLICH u. a. meinen, den Namen Narkolepsie beizubehalten, ohne diesen Ausdruck wörtlich nehmen zu wollen, was ja auch bei anderen Krankheiten nicht geschieht. Eine andere Meinungsverschiedenheit besteht darin, ob man als Narkolepsie nur das vollausgebildete Syndrom bezeichnen soll, wie es manche (LEVIN z. B.) wollen. Aus dem Inhalt dieses Kapitels ergibt sich wohl ohne weiteres, daß dies nicht angängig ist und REDLICH, MÜNZER u. a. tragen kein Bedenken, nicht bloß Fälle ohne affektiven Tonusverlust, sondern auch Fälle mit bloßem affektiven Tonusverlust zur Narkolepsie zu zählen. Wir sehen ja, daß die eine Reihe von Erscheinungen 10 Jahre und mehr bestehen kann, ehe die andere dazukommt.

Differentialdiagnose. Trotzdem es sich bei der Narkolepsie um ein wohlumschriebenes und kaum zu verkennendes Krankheitsbild handelt, ist es notwendig, die Differentialdiagnose gegenüber einigen Zuständen anderer Art zu besprechen, nicht bloß aus Lehrgründen und nicht bloß wegen der Existenz seltener, nicht leicht zu rubrizierender Grenzfälle, sondern auch deshalb, weil sich in der Literatur verschiedene Vereinheitlichungsbestrebungen geltend machen, welche die sonst ziemlich klare klinische Trennungsgrenze vollends zu verwischen drohen. — In erster Linie wird bei solchen differentialdiagnostischen Erwägungen die FRIEDMANNsche *Pyknolepsie* genannt, weil FRIEDMANN selbst und mit ihm einige andere, wie z. B. GRUHLE, beide als Narkolepsie zusammenfassen und nur von einem Typus I und Typus II sprechen. Die Unterschiede gegenüber der Pyknolepsie sind aber beträchtlich und REDLICH hat sie besonders hervorgehoben: Bei der Pyknolepsie das Auftreten in der Regel mit 5—6 Jahren und Verschwinden in der Pubertät, der Beginn nach einem psychischen Trauma, Anfälle meist nur ein paar Sekunden, aber viel öfter im Tag als bei der Narkolepsie, Bewußtsein dabei meist getrübt, kein affektiver Tonusverlust, psychische Beeinflußbarkeit; sicher gilt das nicht für alle Fälle von Pyknolepsie, aber die Pyknolepsie bildet auch anscheinend (zumindest ätiologisch) keine einheitliche Gruppe, indem mehr epileptoide und mehr psychogene Fälle darunter sind. — Die Beziehungen zur *Epilepsie* wurden schon besprochen und man muß hier nur die Differentialdiagnose gegenüber einer besonderen Art von Epilepsie, den Petitmal-Anfällen, besprechen: die Petitmal-Anfälle kommen auch öfters zur Zeit der Pubertät vor, meistens aber schon früher, sie gehen mit einem Bewußtseinsverlust einher, sie sind nicht reversibel, d. h. die Kranken sind aus ihnen nicht erweckbar, sehr oft Amnesie, sehr oft Blässe im Anfall, öfters Secessus urinae (bei der Narkolepsie eine extreme Seltenheit), meist früher oder später Kombination mit großen epileptischen Anfällen, meist epileptische Veränderung der Psyche, Reaktion auf Luminal u. a. Antiepileptica, wie bei der Epilepsie. — Der *Lachschlag* von OPPENHEIM wird oft mit dem affektiven Tonusverlust beim Lachen verwechselt, es handelt sich aber beim Lachschlag um gelegentliches Auftreten von Bewußtlosigkeit bei starkem Lachen (zumindest starke Bewußtseinstrübung) und ein Fall von OPPENHEIM hatte später auch epileptische Anfälle, wie ja überhaupt Fälle von Epilepsie existieren, bei denen Lachen einen epileptischen Anfall auslöst (WILSON u. a.) oder die Aura eines epileptischen Anfalls bildet (WILDER); bei allen diesen Fällen aber handelt es sich jedoch im Gegensatz zum affektiven Tonusverlust vor allem um eine Bewußtseinsstörung und diese Störung kommt bloß beim lauten Lachen vor (vielleicht durch die damit verbundenen vasomotorischen und respiratorischen Vorgänge im Schädelinnern, also auf mechanische Weise), nicht aber wie beim Tonusverlust durch den bloßen heiteren Affekt. Allerdings sah ich auch einen von REDLICH erwähnten Fall von Hirndrucksteigerung, bei dem es durch lautes Lachen zu einem Zusammenfallen bei vollem Bewußtsein kam, dasselbe kam auch bezeichnenderweise durch starkes Husten zustande, der Fall hatte außer einem beiderseitigen BABINSKI einen negativen neurologischen Befund und blieb durch Jahre hindurch unverändert.

Bei dieser Gelegenheit muß noch erwähnt werden, daß jene nicht allzu seltenen Fälle von Epilepsie, bei welchen eine ausgesprochene Provokation der Anfälle durch Affekte vorkommt, vielleicht Anlaß zu Verwechslungen geben können, die aber näherer Betrachtung kaum standhält.

Außer der Geloplegie OPPENHEIMs unterscheidet ROTHFELD auch eine *Gelolepsie* und neben ihr eine *Orgasmolepsie*. Es sind dies Fälle von lange beobachtetem typischen Tonusverlust beim Lachen und beim Orgasmus ohne Schlafanfälle. Ich glaube, daß kein genügender Grund vorliegt, diese Fälle von den Fällen von isoliertem affektiven Tonusverlust und somit von der Narkolepsie zu trennen; daß dieser Tonusverlust gerade nur beim Lachen vorkommt, ist auch so bei den Fällen von Narkolepsie bekannt. ROTHFELD schlägt übrigens vor, die Narkolepsie, die Orgasmolepsie, Gelolepsie als selbständige Krankheiten, zu den ,,subcorticalen Anfällen" gehörend, zu betrachten.

Die *Hysterie* kann nicht bloß wegen der verschiedenartigen Anfälle bei Affekten Anlaß zu Verwechslungen geben, Anfälle, bei denen auch ein Zusammenfallen vorkommt, sondern auch wegen der bei der Hysterie vorkommenden Schlafanfälle. Nun ist aber die Hysterie eine so polymorphe Krankheit, daß sie, rein äußerlich genommen, der Narkolepsie sehr ähnlich sein kann, obwohl gerade die bei der Narkolepsie typische *Kombination* von Schlafanfällen mit Anfällen von Tonusverlust mir nicht bekannt ist. Es wird sich also bei der Feststellung von Unterschieden zuerst um die allerdings meist nicht sofort zu machende Feststellung des hysterischen Charakters und einer Psychogenie der Erkrankung handeln, daneben wird man bei den hysterischen Schlafanfällen meist eine längere Dauer finden, das Erwecken ist manchmal nicht so leicht möglich, der Schlaf entsteht oft bei anderen Gelegenheiten als den für die Narkolepsie typischen usw., ein Zusammenfallen wird eher bei Unlustgefühlen als beim Lachen stattfinden, nicht so rasch vergehen usw., beide Arten von Anfällen werden eine psychogene Beeinflußbarkeit zeigen, aber immerhin, wie bei den meisten anderen Krankheiten wird die Unterscheidung von der Hysterie oft nicht sofort möglich sein, wenn sie auch bei dem wohlumschriebenen Krankheitsbild der Narkolepsie nicht allzu oft in Betracht kommt.

Ich beobachtete einen Mann, der nach Tisch täglich einen unbezwinglichen Schlaf bekam, aus dem er nur sehr schwer erweckbar war, im Schlaf stets eine Pollution; der Fall erwies sich aber bei näherem Eingehen als typisches hysterisches Konversionssymptom und die Erscheinungen schwanden nach 2—3 Unterredungen.

KLEINE und einige andere von ihm zitierte Autoren beschreiben auch eine periodische *Schlafsucht zur Zeit der Pubertät*; hier dauern aber die Anfälle Stunden bis Tage, der Patient erwacht zum Teil, um seine Notdurft zu verrichten, zu essen usw.; kein affektiver Tonusverlust, manchmal psychische Veränderungen. — Auch bei *Hirndruck* können Anfälle von Einschlafen vorkommen, die an Narkolepsie erinnern, ein solcher Fall ist z. B. von GROSS beschrieben worden; auch hier dauert der Schlaf länger, die Erweckbarkeit ist oft nicht so leicht, es besteht eine ständige Schlafsucht, im Anfall oft Pulsverlangsamung usw. — Auch beim CHEYNE-STOKES sehen wir ein kurzes, reversibles, periodisches Einschlafen, aber in kurzen regelmäßigen Intervallen, man muß aber auf den Atemtypus manchmal achten. — Nach Insulin und bei der spontanen *Hypoglykämie* konnte ich u. a. Anfälle beschreiben, die ganz an Schlaf erinnern, es ist aber ein tiefer, nicht leicht reversibler Schlaf, von längerer Dauer, der auf eine intravenöse oder orale Zuckerzufuhr sofort sistiert. — Die *periodische Extremitätenlähmung* kann mit dem affektiven Tonusverlust oder mit Wachanfällen verwechselt werden; sie ist oft familiär, dauert länger, tritt nicht im Anschluß an Affekte, wohl aber im Anschluß an den Schlaf auf, ohne

Schlafanfälle. — Bei der *Katalepsie* ist die Flexibilitas cerea vorhanden, sie dauert viel länger als der affektive Tonusverlust usw.

Therapie. Hier muß ein Unterschied gemacht werden zwischen der symptomatischen und der genuinen Narkolepsie. Es ist fast selbstverständlich, daß bei der symptomatischen Narkolepsie durch die Beeinflussung der Causa morbi auch die Narkolepsie beeinflußt werden kann. Aber darauf beschränkt sich der Unterschied nicht, sondern es ist sicher, daß viele Fälle von symptomatischer Narkolepsie auch spontan ausheilen können; aber nicht nur dies, sie sind auch einer *symptomatischen* Therapie anscheinend eher zugänglich wie die echte Narkolepsie. Man darf also nicht aus an symptomatischen Fällen erzielten Erfolgen eine Therapie der Narkolepsie überhaupt behaupten. Die echte Narkolepsie kann noch immer als eine *unheilbare Krankheit* gelten, wenn auch einzelne Fälle mit verschiedenen Mitteln und in verschiedenem Maße beeinflußt werden konnten, fast nie dauernd, ein Beweis, daß es sich um eine bloße symptomatische Therapie handelt. — 1. *Genuine Narkolepsie.* Von GOWERS und manchen anderen wird das *Coffein* empfohlen, in vielen Fällen erwies es sich als unwirksam. Relativ viel Erfolge oder teilweise Erfolge, teils mehr auf den Schlaf, teils mehr auf den affektiven Tonusverlust hat man von *Thyreoideapräparaten* gesehen, freilich mangelt es auch nicht an Versagern, auch in Fällen, bei denen der erniedrigte Grundumsatz zur Norm hinaufging oder sogar Erscheinungen von Hyperthyreoidismus auftraten. Manche Autoren hatten mit *Hypophysenpräparaten* Erfolge, in anderen Fällen versagten sie. In der letzten Zeit wurde (JANOTA, DOYLE und DANIELS) über sehr gute Wirkungen von *Ephedrin* berichtet; die Fälle sind zum Teil symptomatische, zum Teil echte Narkolepsie und die Erfolge sind von vielen Autoren bestätigt worden (PENTA, CAVE, COHEN, LAFORA und AYDILLO, VADÁSZ, THIELE und BERNHARDT, COLLINS u. a.). In manchen Fällen wurde auch der Tonusverlust beeinflußt, in den meisten nur die Schlafanfälle. Als Nebenerscheinungen treten manchmal auf: sexuelle Übererregbarkeit, Blasentenesmen, Nervosität, Herzklopfen, Hitze, Schwitzen. Das Ephedrin, welches im Tierversuch Schlaflosigkeit erzeugt, kann auch beim Narkoleptiker, wenn es überdosiert wird, nächtliche Schlaflosigkeit erzeugen und dann nehmen die anfangs verminderten Schlafanfälle wieder zu. DOYLE und DANIELS empfehlen 3mal 0,05 täglich, die letzte Dosis um 5 Uhr nachmittags, bei Schlaflosigkeit letzte Dosis geringer. Widersprechende Resultate, aber sicher auch vereinzelte Erfolge erzielt man mit der Röntgenbestrahlung der Hypophyse, ferner mit Lufteinblasung in die Ventrikel (Encephalographie, BENEDEK und THURZÓ, THIELE und BERNHARDT), angeblich auch mit Bettruhe und Ketodiät. In einem Fall von LHERMITTE und NICOLAS (Lues!) war Lumbalpunktion wirksam, in zahlreichen sonstigen Fällen nicht. Die partielle Pankreasresektion empfiehlt HARRIS, doch war sein Fall (mehrstündige Bewußtlosigkeit) keine Narkolepsie. Vereinzelte Autoren verwenden auch Schlafmittel, in den meisten Fällen haben sie aber keinen oder einen direkt ungünstigen Effekt. Ein Gemisch von Opium, Strychnin und Coffein empfiehlt BOSTOCK, abends Luminal und bei Tag Coffein HILPERT. MISSRIEGLER glaubt in einem Fall mit Psychoanalyse Erfolg gehabt zu haben, VILLAVERDE mit Suggestion, LÖWENFELD mit Hypnose, STRANSKY hatte mit Psychotherapie (SAR-Methode) Erfolg bei einem fraglich hysterischen Fall; demgegenüber stehen zahlreiche Fälle, bei denen die Psychotherapie versagte (SCHILDER, ich u. a.). Verschiedene in der Literatur gemeldete Erfolge (MYERS, MORTON, CARLILL) sind keine Narkolepsien, sondern Hysterien. Ohne Erfolg wurden ferner versucht: Präparate aus Genitaldrüsen, Adrenalin, Natrium salycilicum-Injektionen, Septojod, Atropin, Scopolamin, Opium, Valeriana, Bor, Brom, Calcium, Phosphor, Sauerstoffinhalationen, Strychnin, verschiedene Tonica und Roborantia, Hydro- und Elektrotherapie, Haarseil usw. — 2. *Symptomatische Narkolepsie.* Hier wollen wir vor allem die postencephalitischen Fälle berücksichtigen, da die Therapie bei Tumoren, Lues, Trauma gewissermaßen sich von selbst versteht. Hier wurden Erfolge gemeldet mit PREGLscher Jodlösung, Jodnatrium, Strychnin, Milchinjektionen, Thyreoidea (verschiedene Erfahrungen), zum Teil auch mit Hypophysenbestrahlung, Bettruhe, Kakodylinjektionen. Erfolglos waren Strammonium, Luminal, Diät, Sedativa, Natrium salicylicum, Acriflavin. Bemerkenswert ist, daß in einem Falle von WAGNER mit postencephalitischer Charakterveränderung und isoliertem affektiven Tonusverlust durch Erziehung nur der Charakter, nicht aber der Tonusverlust zu beeinflussen war. — Sämtliche Erfolge beziehen sich sowohl bei der echten wie bei der symptomatischen Narkolepsie zumeist auf die Schlafanfälle, während der Tonusverlust sehr schwer beeinflußbar ist. Nur einzelne Autoren geben, besonders bei Thyreoidea, an, daß sie eher den Tonusverlust beeinflußt haben, demgegenüber stehen viele andere Fälle, wo es sich umgekehrt verhält, ja, wo die Thyreoidea einen direkt ungünstigen Einfluß auf diese Anfälle ausgeübt hat. VADASZ konnte mit Ephedrin die Schlaf-, mit Genohyoscyamin die Tonusanfälle, mit hohen Atropindosen beides beeinflussen. — Zusammenfassend kann man also sagen, daß man bei der Narkolepsie, besonders bei der symptomatischen, einen Versuch mit einem der genannten Mittel machen kann und soll, speziell mit Ephedrin, Thyreoidea, hohen Atropindosen, Lufteinblasung, daß es aber eine kausale oder auch nur eine sicher wirksame symptomatische Therapie bei der genuinen Narkolepsie derzeit noch nicht gibt.

Forensische und soziale Bedeutung. Es kann der Fall eintreten, daß ein Narkoleptiker auf einem entsprechenden Posten sich einer groben Vernachlässigung seiner Pflichten, ja, einer Gefährdung seiner Umgebung schuldig macht, wie dies ja im Kriege bei Soldaten der Fall war. Daß solche Fälle freizusprechen sind, unterliegt wohl keinem Zweifel, falls sie nicht in Kenntnis ihrer Krankheit, gegen besseres Wissen eine solche Aufgabe übernommen haben. Ebensowenig kann bezweifelt werden, daß einem Chauffeur seine Lizenz, einem Maschinisten usw. seine Beschäftigung entzogen werden muß, falls er unter der Arbeit an narkoleptischen Anfällen leidet. Auch Privaten muß das Fahren mit Auto, Motorrad usw. verboten werden. Evtl. kann man Berufe mit starker körperlicher Bewegung empfehlen (THIELE-BERNHARDT). — In einigen Fällen wurde teilweise Kriegsbeschädigung infolge Strapazen anerkannt (GRÜN, THIELE-BERNHARDT), es könnte aber unter Umständen auch ein Kopftrauma [1] Anlaß zu einer solchen gerichtlichen Begutachtung geben. Auch Aufregungen, gestörter Nachtschlaf, seelische Shockwirkungen kommen, allerdings nur als Auslösungsursachen, in Frage. Bei den meisten Fällen ist die allgemeine Erwerbsfähigkeit nicht schwer eingeschränkt, schließlich gehen ja auch die meisten Fälle einem Beruf nach. Aber die engere Erwerbsfähigkeit in bestimmten Berufen kann auch sehr schwer beeinträchtigt sein, z. B. bei einem Chauffeur usw.; hingegen wird sie vielleicht bei einem Bureaubeamten oder einem Kaufmann unter Umständen fast gar nicht eingeschränkt sein. — Gesellschaftlich und sozial sind schwerere Fälle oft sehr geschädigt nicht nur wegen der Schlafanfälle, sondern mehr noch wegen des affektiven Tonusverlustes. Es kommt zu einem Vermeiden von lustiger Gesellschaft, Theater, Kino usw., ja, zu einer vollkommenen Zurückgezogenheit; letzteres nicht sehr häufig. Alle möglichen Triks und Vorsichtsmaßnahmen werden von einzelnen Kranken ersonnen, welche ihnen das soziale Leben ermöglichen, wenn auch mit gewissen, manchmal nur sehr geringen, manchmal aber ziemlich großen Opfern.

---

[1] Hier muß ein zeitlicher Zusammenhang oder sog. Brückensymptome im freien Intervall nachweisbar sein oder auch Nachbarschaftssymptome wie Diabetes insipidus usw.

Literatur.

ADIE: Brain **49**, 257. — ALAJOUANINE et BARUK: Progrès méd. **1926**, 639. BALLET: Rev. Méd. **1882**, 945. — BALOGH: Ref. Zbl. Neur. **39**, 365. — BASSOE: Zit. bei SOLOMON-BAUER: Wien. med. Wschr. **1929 I**, 8. — BENEDEK u. THURZÓ: Ref. Zbl. Neur. **60**, 324. — BEYERMANN: Z. Neur. **128**, 726. — BOAS: Ärztl. Sachverst.ztg **1927**, 262. — BOGAERT: Ann. Méd. **26**, 145. — BONHOEFFER: Wien. klin. Wschr. **1928 I**, 979. — BOSTOCK: Med. J. Austral. **2**, 239. — BRAILOWSKY: Z. Neur. **100**, 272. — BROCK: J. ment. Dis. **68**, 583. — BROMBERG: Arch. of Neur. **24**, 194.

CAMPBELL: Mschr. Psychiatr. **65**, 58. — CARLILL: Lancet **1919 II**, 1128. — CAVE: Arch. of Neur. **26**, 50. — COHEN: Lancet **1932 II**, 335. — COLLINS: Amer. int. Med. **5**, 1289. — CREAK: Lancet **1932 II**, 514. — CURSCHMANN-PRANGE: Dtsch. Z. Nervenheilk. **86**, 97.

DENYER: Brit. med. J. **1930**, Nr 3625, 1172. — DERCUM: J. nerv. Dis. **40**, 185. — DOYLE and DANIELS: J. amer. med. Assoc. **69 II**, 1370; **98**, 542.

ECONOMO: Erg. Physiol. **28**, 312. — Jkurse ärztl. Fortbildg **1929**. — EDEL: Z. Neur. **92**, 160. — ERMAKOV: Ref. Zbl. Neur. **59**, 484. — ESLEWIČ: Ref. Zbl. Neur. **52**, 734.

FISCHER, B.: Z. Neur. **90**, 598. — FISCHER, J.: Arch. f. Psychiatr. **8**, 200. — FOUCHÉ: Proc. roy. Soc. Med. **24**, 313. — FREUND: Ref. Wien. klin. Wschr. **1914 II**, 1618. — FRISCH: Ref. Jb. Psychiatr., Sitzgsber. **1932**. — FROCASSI: Ref. Zbl. Neur. **52**, 331. — FRÖDERBERG: Ref. Zbl. Neur. **59**, 467. — FULTON and BAILEY: J. nerv. Dis. **69**, 1.

GÉLINEAU: Gaz. Hôp. **1880**, 626. — GIESEN: Allg. Z. Psychiatr. **98**, 405. — GILLESPIE: Ref. Zbl. Neur. **48**, 587. — GOLDFLAM: Z. Neur. **82**, 20. — GOZZANO: Zit. bei PFANNER-GRÜN: Z. Neur. **134**, 155. — GRUHLE: Zbl. Neur. **34**, 1. — GRUSZECKA: Ref. Zbl. Neur. **50**, 251. — GUILLAIN, MOLLARET et THOYER: Bull. Soc. méd. Hôp. Paris **46**, 334. — GUILLAIN, LERHELLE et GARCIN: C. r. Soc. Biol. Paris **1931**, 7. — GÜNTHER: Dtsch. Arch. klin. Med. **165**.

HARRIS: J. amer. med. Assoc. **100**, 321. — HERRMANN: Med. Klin. **1928 I**, 22. — HERSCHMANN: Ref. Jb. Psychiatr. Sitzgsber. 1932. — HEVER: Encéphale **1919**, 402. — HEVEROCH: Ref. Zbl. Neur. **40**, 822. — HILPERT: Klin. Wschr. **1925 I**, 32. — HOFF u. STENGEL: Klin. Wschr. **1931 II**, 1300.

JAKOBSOHN: Klin. Wschr. **1927 I**. — JANOTA: Med. Klin. **1931 I**, 272. — JANZEN: Z. Neur. **104**, 800. — JELIFFE: Med. J. a. Rec. **129**, 269.

KAHLER: Jb. Psychiatr. **41**, 1. — KAMMANN: J. amer. med. Assoc. **1929**, 29. — KAPLINSKI: Z. Neur. **147**, 101. — KELLER: Dtsch. Z. Nervenheilk. **112**, 140. — KENNEDY: Brit. med. J. **1929**, Nr 3572, 1112. — KLEINE: Mschr. Psychiatr. **57**, 285. — KLUGE: Z. Neur. **110**, 415. — KOLLEWIJN: Ref. Zbl. Neur. **31**, 352. — KRAUS: Ref. J. nerv. Dis. **53**. — Amer. J. med. Sci. **149**. — KYRIACO u. ROQUES: Ref. Zbl. Neur. **58**, 697.

LAFORA: Ref. Zbl. Neur. **47**, 455. — LAFORA and AYDILLO: Ann. med. int. **1**, 3. — LAMOC: Rev. Méd. **1897**, 699. — LAUDENHEIMER: Ref. Zbl. Neur. **48**, 373. — LEWY: Z. Neur. **110**, 235. — LEY, SELS, VAN BOGAERT: J. de Neur. **32**, 503. — LHERMITTE: Revue neur. **1910 II**, 96, 203. — Ref. Zbl. Neur. **59**, 747. — LHERMITTE et KYRIACO: Gaz. Hôp. **103**, 255. — LHERMITTE et NICOLAS: Gaz. Hôp. **1929 I**, 585. — LHERMITTE et ROQUES: Revue neur. **1928 II**, 729. — LHERMITTE et PEYRE: Revue neur. **37 I**, 286. — LHERMITTE, VALÉRY-RADOT, DELAFONTAINE et MIGET: Revue neur. **39 II**, 565. — LEVIN: Arch. of Neur. **22**, 1172. Ref. Zbl. Neur. **70**, 628. — LISI, DE: Riv. Pat. nerv. **39**, 481. — LÖWENFELD: Münch. med. Wschr. **1902 I**, 1041. — LÖWENSTEIN: Ref. Arch. f. Psychiatr. **85**, 276. — LOEWY: Ref. Jb. Psychiatr. Sitzgsber. 1932. — LOPEZ u. SEMPAN: Ref. Zbl. Neur. **67**, 747. — LUST: Münch. med. Wschr. **1927 I**, 97.

MACNAMARA: Zit. nach WILSON. — MAKAROW: Ref. Zbl. Neur. **52**, 735. — MANKOWSKY: Mschr. Psychiatr. **61**, 340. — MARINESCO: Revue neur. **1921 I**. — MARINESCO, FAÇON, BRUCH, PAUNESCO-PODEANO: Ann. Méd. **33**, 177. — MARKOV: Ref. Zbl. Neur. **43**, 447. — MATZDORF: Dtsch. Z. Nervenheilk. **88**, 1. — MISSRIEGLER: Fortschr. Sex.wiss. **1**, 207. — MÖLLENHOFF: Klin. Wschr. **1925 II**, 2037. — MOREAU: J. de Neur. **32**, 112. — MORTON: J. nerv. Dis. **11**, 615, 884. — MÜNZER: Mschr. Psychiatr. **63**, 97. — Med. Klin. **1928 I**, 10; **1932 II**, 1382. — Z. exper. Path. **5**. — MYERS: Lancet **1920 I**, 491.

NEISSER: Berl. klin. Wschr. **1908 I**, 1206. — NEVERMANN: Dtsch. med. Wschr. **1921 II**, 1164.

PAPASTRATIGAKIS: Encéphale **22**, 354. — PASKIND: Arch. of Neur. **24**, 185. — PENTA: Ref. Zbl. Neur. **61**, 507. — Boll. Soc. Biol. sper. **6**, 1026. — PERRIER: Revue neur. **1925 I**, 1056. — PFANNER: Riv. Pat. nerv. **35**, 80. — POPOVA u. SKWORCOV: Ref. Zbl. Neur. **67**, 186. — PÖTZL: Jkurse ärztl. Fortbildg **1929**, 2. — Med. Klin. **1926**, 1845. — Mschr. Psychiatr. **64**, 1.

RATNER: Mschr. Psychiatr. **64**, 283. — Arch. f. Psychiatr. **86**, 525; **89**, 802. — REDLICH: Mschr. Psychiatr. **37**, 85. — Jb. Psychiatr. **37**, 68. — Handbuch der Neurologie, Erg.-Bd. 1, S. 462. — Z. Neur. **95**, 256; **136**, 128. — Das Grenzgebiet der Epilepsie. Wien 1927. — Med. Welt **1927**, 35. — RICHTER & CIE.: Arch. of Neur. **21**, 363. — ROGER: Les narcolepsies.

Paris: Masson & Co. 1932. — Rolandi: Arch. Pat. e. Clin. med. **13**, 43. — ROSENTHAL: Arch. f. Psychiatr. **96**, 572. — ROTHFELD: Z. Neur. **115**, 516; **138**, 704. — SAINTON: Revue neur. **1901**, 297. — SALMON: Ref. Zbl. Neur. **43**, 25. — SCHILDER: Zit. bei BROMBERG. — Wien. med. Wschr. **1933** I, 326. — SEREJSKI u. FRUMKIN: Z. Neur. **123**, 233. — SIEBERT: Mschr. Psychiatr. **48**, 178. — SOLOMON: Arch. of Neur. **24**, 187. — SOMER: Wien. klin. Wschr. **1921** I, 132. — SOUQUES, BARUK et BERTRAND: Revue neur. **1926**, 532. — SPERLING u. WIMMER: Dtsch. Z. Nervenheilk. **102**, 252. — SPILLER: J. amer. med. Assoc. **86**, 673 (1926). — STIEFLER: Wien. klin. Wschr. **1924** II, 1044. — Wien. med. Wschr. **1926** II, 1110. — Münch. med. Wschr. **1926** I, 981. — STÖCKER: Z. Neur. **18**, 217. — STRANSKY: Wien. klin. Wschr. **1929** I, 18. — STRAUSS: Mschr. Psychiatr. **61**, 265. — Z. Neur. **109**, 401. — SYMONDS: Lancet **1926** II, 1214. — SZATMARY: Zbl. Gynäk. **1931**, 3629. — THRASH and MASSEE: J. amer. med. Assoc. **91** II, 1802. — THIELE: Ref. Zbl. Neur. **46**, 904; **67**, 522. — THIELE u. BERNHARDT: Ref. Zbl. Neur. **61**, 143. — Beiträge zur Kenntnis der Narkolepsie. Berlin: S. Karger 1933. — TRÖMMER: Z. Neur. **101**, 786. — TSIMINAKIS: Wien. klin. Wschr. **1930** II, 1147.
URBACH u. WILDER: Med. Klin. **1934** II, 1420. — URECHIA u. BUMBACESCU: Arch. int. neur. **52** I, 107.
VADASZ: Schweiz. Arch. Neur. **32**, 154. — VILLAVERDA: Arch. f. Psychiatr. **86**, 129.
WAGNER: J. nerv. Dis. **72**, 405. — WEECH: Amer. J. Dis. Childr. **32**, 672. — WEIR-MITCHELL: Zit. nach REDLICH. — WENDEROWIČ: Arch. f. Psychiatr. **72**, 459. — WESTPHAL: Arch. f. Psychiatr. **7**, 631. — WILDER: Z. Neur. **117**, 472. — Nervenarzt **4**, 75. — Dtsch. Z. Nervenheilk. **133**, 280. — WILMAERS: Le Scalpel **1930** II, 1425. — WILSON: Brain **51**, 63. — Proc. roy. Soc. Med. **21**, 1238. — WOHLFAHRT: Acta psychiatr. (København.) **6**, 277. — WORSTER-DROUGHT: Zit. nach WILSON.
ZADOR: Mschr. Psychiatr. **66**, 13. — ZEHRER: Z. Psychiatr. **92**, 263. — ZIEGLER: Ref. Zbl. Neur. **57**, 287. — ZONDEK u. BIER: Klin. Wschr. **1932** I, 760.

Spasmophilie.

Von J. HUSLER-München.

Mit 6 Abbildungen.

Spasmophilie kann als Krankheitsbegriff in sehr verschiedenem Sinne gefaßt werden und wird in praxi auch als Diagnose in wechselndem Sinne gebraucht. Wörtlich genommen müßte man unter *Spasmophilie* (= Krampfbereitschaft) *sämtliche* Krampfzustände überhaupt zusammenfassen, müßte also auch den echt epileptischen mit einbeziehen. Nach pädiatrischem Herkommen aber scheidet von vornherein alles aus, was zur echten genuinen Epilepsie, wie zu den greifbar organischen Prozessen gehört. Es bleiben dann noch zwei Kategorien von Krampfkrankheiten, die Tetanie einerseits und allerhand Krampfzustände funktioneller, im allgemeinen unklarer Herkunft, andererseits. Erstere wird als *tetanoide Spasmophilie*, letztere werden auch als sog. *intermediäre Krampfkrankheiten* — zwischen den Polen Epilepsie und Hysterie liegend — bezeichnet.

I. Tetanoide Spasmophilie (Spasmophilie im engeren Sinne).

Man versteht unter *Tetanie* (infantiler) ein vor allem auf der Basis der Rachitis sich entwickelndes Symptombild, das scharf gekennzeichnet ist durch einen erhöhten Erregbarkeitszustand der peripheren Nerven, dann aber auch der autonomen Apparate und der nervösen Zentralorgane. Diese erhöhte Erregbarkeit ist entweder eine *latente*, die nicht zu deutlichen Spontanmanifestationen führt, oder sie ist eine *manifeste,* d. h. sie gibt sich kund vor allem in motorischen Reizerscheinungen, wie allgemeinen und partiellen Krämpfen, dann in sensiblen Wirkungen, Parästhesien, in besonderen Fällen auch trophischen und Stoffwechselstörungen.

Die ursächliche Verbindung der *infantilen* Tetanie mit der Rachitis, die früher viel umstritten war, steht heute für die ganz überwiegende Mehrzahl der Fälle zweifellos fest, während die in späterer Kindheit auftretende (*puerile Tetanie*) für gewöhnlich nicht auf Rachitis beruht. Wir können in Anbetracht der Seltenheit der Fälle von pueriler Tetanie und der verschwindend geringen Zahl von nichtrachitischen infantilen Fällen mit E. FREUDENBERG *die infantile Tetanie ohne weiteres unter den Oberbegriff Rachitis einreihen. Die Spasmophilie (im engeren Sinne) ist also eine Folge unmittelbar vorausgehender Rachitis.*

Latenzzustand der infantilen Tetanie. Wie oben ausgeführt, besteht eine erhöhte Erregbarkeit mehr minder des ganzen Nervensystems, ohne daß es aber zu äußeren Kundgebungen dieser Erregbarkeit kommt; diese kann aber durch besondere Prüfungsmethodik nachgewiesen werden. Die einfachste Methode hierfür ist die mechanische. Es sind einige Phänomene bekannt, die der näheren Besprechung bedürfen. Am einfachsten und leichtesten zu ermitteln ist das sog. Facialphänomen. Man beklopft den N. facialis etwa zwischen Jochbogen und Mundwinkel mit einem leichten Perkussionshämmerchen. Dieses reizt genügend bei tetanischen Individuen, um deutliche Zuckungen der vom Facialis versorgten Muskulatur auszulösen. Diese Zuckungen äußern sich vor allem an Oberlippe, Unterlippe, am Nasenflügel, um das Auge herum und selbst auf der Stirne. Nicht immer sind diese Teile in gleicher Weise an den Zuckungen beteiligt, am häufigsten sind wohl die Zuckungen um den Mund. Auch die Stärke der Innervierung schwankt sehr stark, in besonders ausgesprochenen Fällen geht die Zuckung wie ein Blitz über die ganze Gesichtsseite, andere Male ist sie nur eben angedeutet. Auch zwischen den beiden Gesichtshälften beobachtet man gelegentlich wesentliche Verschiedenheiten der Reaktion. Vielfach muß man auf der Wange den optimalen Klopfpunkt erst durch einige Schläge suchen. Eine ursprünglich von CHVOSTEK angegebene Reizstelle ist der Punkt unmittelbar vor dem Gehörgang an der Austrittsstelle des N. facialis in den Gesichtsbereich über dem Kieferwinkel. Man spricht bei deutlichem Ausfall der Klopfwirkung vom „CHVOSTEKschen Phänomen". Nach v. FRANKL-HOCHWART können drei Intensitätsgrade unterschieden werden. CHVOSTEK I: Auf Beklopfen der Wange vor dem Gehörgang zucken Augenschließmuskel, Nasenflügel und Mundwinkel; CHVOSTEK II: Bei Beklopfen unterhalb des Jochbogens zuckt Nasenflügel; CHVOSTEK III: Zuckung *nur* am Mundwinkel.

Manchmal ist die Erregbarkeit des Facialisgebietes derart gesteigert, daß es genügt, mit dem Finger vor dem Ohr herunter zu streichen, um enorme Ausschläge in den gereizten Muskelgebieten zu erzeugen (= SCHULTZEsche Variante des Facialphänomens). Allerdings ist nach unseren Erfahrungen dieses Phänomen fast nur bei deutlich manifesten Tetanikern — also solchen *mit* Stimmritzenkrämpfen, Konvulsionen usw. — zu finden.

Nicht in allen Altersstufen kommt dem Facialphänomen eine pathognostische Bedeutung für die Diagnose Tetanie zu. Nur im 1. Lebensjahr dürfte das Zeichen ein absolut verlässiges sein. Mit fortschreitendem Alter verliert es rasch an diagnostischem Wert. Man findet es bei den verschiedensten Abwegigkeiten im Nervenapparat, bei Neuro- und Psychopathen, bei zahlreichen gesunden Schulkindern, die nie tetanisch waren. GÖTT fand das Zeichen häufig im Gefolge von Diphtherie, besonders auch im Vorstadium postdiphtherischer Paresen. Des weiteren wird es bei Epileptikern, aber auch organisch Nervenkranken anderer Art festgestellt, dann bei Phthisikern, bei den verschiedenen Formen der Kachexie, vor allem denen, die mit Exsikkation verbunden sind (CURSCHMANN), aber auch gelegentlich bei anderen Zuständen. Auch bei Frühgeburten ist das Phänomen beobachtet. Wir fanden es wiederholt bei Kindern mit schweren geburtstraumatischen Schädigungen des Gehirns. Andererseits muß betont werden, daß dann und wann auch trotz Fehlens des Zeichens echte Tetanie vorliegen kann.

Es ist klar, daß angesichts der verschiedenwertigen Auslösungspunkte, der Erregung bald am Facialisstamm, bald an Seitenästen, bald vom Muskel aus, das Facialphänomen nichts Einheitliches darstellt. Nur die Auslösung vor dem Gehörgang ist als glatte mechanische Übererregbarkeit des Nerven anzusprechen. Bei der Auslösung von allen anderen Stellen aus handelt es sich mehr um einen Reflex; der von den sensiblen Bahnen des Trigeminus umgeleitet wird. Man hätte es also beim Facialphänomen mit einem gemischten Vorgang zu tun, einer direkt mechanischen und einer reflektorischen Übererregbarkeit.

Ein anderes wertvolles Zeichen der mechanischen Übererregbarkeit ist das *Peroneusphänomen*. Durch Beklopfung des N. peronaeus werden die von ihm versorgten Mm. peronaei zur Kontraktion gebracht. Man sieht die Zuckung der M. peron. nach dem Beklopfen jenes Nervenpunktes. Außerdem wird als Erfolg der Muskelinnervation der laterale Fußrand gehoben. Als Auslösungspunkt gilt die Partie am Unterschenkel unmittelbar unterhalb des Fibulaköpfchens. Man legt zu diesem Zweck den Patienten auf die Seite so, daß der Fußrand hängt. Wie beim Facialphänomen kommt auch hier dem Phänomen pathognostische Bedeutung nur im 1. Lebensjahr zu. In dieser Zeit trifft man das Zeichen nur bei wirklich Tetanischen, später verwischen sich die Grenzen, beim älteren Kind kommt es auch außerhalb dieses Rahmens vor.

Ähnliche und einschlägige Phänomene sind noch folgende: Durch Beklopfung des N. radialis am dorsalen Oberarm kommt es zur Zuckung der Hand. Fingerzuckungen resultieren bei Schlag oder Druck auf den N. ulnaris im Sulc. ulnaris. ESCHERICH bezog ferner die Quadricepszuckung bei Schlag auf diesen Muskel oberhalb des Knies auf mechanische Nervenübererregbarkeit.

Von höherem diagnostischen Werte als die letzteren Phänomene ist das TROUSSEAUsche. Dieses dürfte wohl stets auf Tetanie, sei es auf latente, sei es auf manifeste, zu beziehen sein. Es besteht darin, daß durch Druck auf die Nervenstämme im Sulcus bicipitalis sich eine starke Innervation im Handbereich einstellt. Die Hand tritt in die sog. *Geburtshelferhandstellung* durch Beugung der Finger in den Grundphalangen bei Streckung in den übrigen Gelenken. An Stelle des Druckes auf den Nervenstamm kann man auch mit der Hand oder einer Gummibinde eine Umschnürung der Extremität vornehmen. Dieser tetanische Krampf erklärt sich nicht aus der damit verbundenen Störung der Zirkulation, sondern aus einer wirklich vorhandenen mechanischen Übererregbarkeit. Bei der Bahnung des tonischen Krampfes allerdings müssen wohl sensible Nerven mitsprechen, denn am ungemischten, rein motorischen Nerven läßt sich das Phänomen niemals auslösen (H. SCHLESINGER). Daß es sich um einen tetanischen Krampf handelt, ergibt sich aus der Feststellung von 50 Aktionsstromstößen pro Minute (H. SCHÄFFER).

In ähnlicher Weise kann gelegentlich tetanischer Krampf durch Zug am senkrecht erhobenen Arm ausgelöst werden = PROLsches *Phänomen*. Endlich hat H. SCHLESINGER ein Zeichen zur Darstellung gebracht, welches hier zu registrieren ist. Das Bein wird im Kniegelenk gestreckt und dann im Hüftgelenk stark gebeugt, dies hat einen tonischen Krampf zur Folge mit Supinationsstellung des Fußes und Beugung der Zehen. Der Krampf ist schmerzhaft.

Die Heranziehung der *elektrischen Übererregbarkeit* zur Prüfung auf Tetanie ist für alle Spasmophiliefälle eine unerläßliche Notwendigkeit. Elektrische Übererregbarkeit, vor allem der peripheren motorischen Nerven fehlt in keinem Fall von Tetanie, *sie gilt als führendes Symptom*, und zwar vor allem die Übererregbarkeit durch den galvanischen Strom.

Der Ort der Wahl für die Prüfung dieses sog. ERBschen Phänomens ist die Ellenbeuge. Hier ist der N. medianus leicht mit dem Reiz zu treffen. Die Reizelektrode — zunächst die Kathode — wird in die Ellenbeuge, die indifferente

Elektrode auf die Brust gesetzt, beide nach guter Befeuchtung. Man beginnt die Prüfung mit ganz schwachem Strome und schleicht sich dann in stärkeren ein, und zwar in die Stromstärke, die eben zu einer sichtbaren Zuckung im Erfolgsorgan, dem Daumenballen, führt. Dieser am Ampèremeter abgelesene Wert gilt als Schwellenwert für die Erregbarkeit des Med., und zwar wird dieser Wert sowohl für die Stromschließung wie für die Öffnung bestimmt (KSZ, KÖZ). Dann wird der Stromkreis gewendet und mit der Anode gereizt, wiederum mit Schließungs- und Öffnungsreiz (ASZ, AÖZ). Endlich läßt sich bei Steigerung der Stromstärke Dauerkontraktion im Daumenballen erzeugen: KS-Tetanus. Der weitaus wichtigste Wert ist die KÖZ (s. u.).

Die einzelnen Werte schwanken auch bei vollwertigen gesunden Kindern innerhalb weiter Grenzen. Abgesehen von einer Differenz zwischen rechts- und linksseitiger Erregbarkeit bei gleichen Individuen, stehen die oberen und unteren Grenzwerte bei verschiedenen Individuen in weitem Abstand voneinander. KSZ in der Regel < ASZ, selten KSZ = ASZ. Ungleich wichtiger als die Schließungs- sind die Öffnungszuckungen, vor allem die KÖZ. Die KÖZ liegt beim ganz gesunden Kind ausnahmslos über dem Wert von 5,0 mA. Bei latenter oder manifester Tetanie findet sich gerade dieser Wert besonders stark gesenkt, d. h. also die Erregbarkeit für KÖZ beträchtlich gesteigert. *Alle Senkungen der KÖZ unter 5,0 mA werden seit* Themich *als pathognostisch für Tetanie angesprochen.*

Normalwerte: KSZ am Ulnaris etwa 0,9 mA, ASZ etwa 1,5—2 mA, AÖZ etwa 2,5—3 mA, KS-Tetanus etwa 5 mA, KÖZ = 5,0 mA, meist darüber. Medianus: Am Medianus ergeben sich ähnliche Werte (Husler): KSZ 0,4—2,2, ASZ 1,2—3,0, AÖZ 2,3 bis > als 5,0, KÖZ > 5,0 mA.

Für die AÖZ gelten ähnliche Voraussetzungen wie für die KÖZ. v. Pirquet studierte zuerst eingehend besonders die semiotische Bedeutung der Anodenzuckung beim Säugling. Er führte bei 24 Kindern am N. peronaeus Einzeluntersuchungen in großer Zahl durch, außerdem an spasmophilen Einzelindividuen fortlaufende Prüfungen. Letztere ergaben, daß anodische Übererregbarkeit einer *tetanoiden Spasmophilie* vorausgeht und nachfolgt. Man könnte sagen, sie bildet gewissermaßen das Vor- und Nachstadium einer durch pathognostische KÖZ charakterisierten hochgradigen Erregbarkeit. Zahlenmäßig ausgedrückt: „Das Auftreten der AÖZ unter 5,0 mA ist das Anzeichen einer leichten, aber doch pathologischen Übererregbarkeit". Jenseits des 4. Lebensjahres kann dieser Satz keinesfalls in demselben Ausmaß Geltung haben (Husler). Beim älteren Vollkind ist die Schwankungsbreite sehr groß. Die untere Grenze wurde bei 1,0, die obere bei 5,0 mA für AÖZ gefunden, gemessen allerdings nicht am Peronaeus, sondern am Medianus. Und zwar liegen die Schwellenwerte häufiger unter als über 5,0; das ältere Kind ist demnach anodisch weit erregbarer als der normale Säugling. Übrigens wird auch beim gesunden Säugling die Bedeutung der anodischen Übererregbarkeit in Frage gezogen [1]. Kathodenschließungstetanus tritt bei der Tetanie leichter, also bei geringerer Reizschwelle ein als bei normalem Befinden.

Differentialdiagnostisch ist zu sagen, daß die galvanischen Zuckungswerte bei sicherer *genuiner* Epilepsie sich *nicht* wesentlich von denen der normalen Kinder unterscheiden. Im ganzen scheinen sie ein klein wenig höher zu liegen als die der älteren, was einer leicht verminderten Erregbarkeit entsprechen würde. Die KSZ schwankt bei Epileptikern zwischen 0,7 und 3,3 mA (Norm 0,4—3,0). Das Mittel aus 31 Einzeluntersuchungen ist 1,7 gegenüber 1,4 bei der gleichen Zahl Gesunder (Husler). Praktische Nutzanwendung ist daraus freilich nicht zu ziehen. Die ASZ hatte 0,8—4,3 mA als Grenzwerte (Norm 0,4—3,2). 2,4 war

---

[1] Iwamura: Z. Kinderheilk. 1913.

also das Mittel aus 31 Einzeluntersuchungen gegenüber 1,7 der Norm. Also ähnliche leichte Verschiebung nach oben wie bei der KSZ. Die AÖZ ist so starken Schwankungen unterworfen, daß Grenzen nach dem Pathologischen hin nicht zu ziehen sind, sie dürfte sich aber kaum anders verhalten als bei Gesunden. Auch die KÖZ, der besondere Beachtung geschenkt werden muß, liegt beim Epileptiker in der Regel wie bei Gesunden jenseits von 5,0 mA (HUSLER). Seltene Ausnahmen mit starker Erniedrigung der KÖZ-Werte sind gesondert bei der Besprechung der sog. *Spätklampsie* noch zu berücksichtigen.

Es bedarf wohl keines Hinweises darauf, daß man bei der Feststellung der KÖZ-Werte, wie vor allem auch des Tetanus nicht von höheren zu niederen Reizwerten heruntergeht, sondern umgekehrt sich von niederen Werten in die höheren einschleicht. Letzteres ist wesentlich weniger schmerzhaft und gestattet wesentlich sicherere Feststellungen.

Halten wir also daran fest, daß die Herabminderung des KÖZ-Wertes unter 5,0 mA das wichtigste Zeichen der Tetanie ist, so können wir noch weiter hinzufügen, daß *es keinen echt tetanischen Krampfzustand gibt, bei dem das Zeichen fehlt*, andererseits keinen anderen Zustand, bei dem es gesetzmäßig vorkäme. Nur FALTA und KAHN berichten von einem einzigen Fall chronischer Tetanie, bei dem trotz heftiger Krämpfe das ERBsche Phänomen in den ersten Tagen vermißt und erst nach 2 Wochen als positiv festgestellt wurde. Die Rückkehr zu normalen Werten erfolgte ziemlich synchron mit dem Fortschreiten der Heilung.

Für feinere wissenschaftliche Zwecke haben französische Forscher die Methode der *Chronaxiemessung* begründet. Hierbei wird zuerst die Stromschwelle der Reizbarkeit, die sog. Rheobase bestimmt, dann wird gemessen, wie lange Zeit in eintausendstel-Sekunden ein Strom vom Doppelwert der Rheobase einwirken muß, um eben eine Zuckung auszulösen (Chronaxiewert). Die Rheobase ist bei Tetanie erniedrigt, die Chronaxie verlängert. Die Veränderung hält während des ganzen tetanischen Zustandes an [1].

Eine Prüfung der sensiblen Nerven auf erhöhte Erregbarkeit hat wenig praktische Bedeutung, da schon normalerweise die größten Schwankungen zu beobachten sind. Immerhin hat HOFFMANN festgestellt, daß bei Prüfung am N. ulnaris schon bei niedrigen KSZ-Werten Parästhesien vorkommen, CHVOSTEK fand bei Tetanie Empfindungsreaktionen des N. acusticus bei verhältnismäßig niederen Stromreizungen. Auch Geschmacksempfindungen wurden gelegentlich bei Prüfung der kathodischen Übererregbarkeit im Gesicht ermittelt.

Eine *thermische* Übererregbarkeit wurde nach KASHIDA in Form von Parästhesien und Krämpfen auf thermische Reize hin angegeben. Hierher gehört auch die Registrierung der Auslösung von Krämpfen durch temperatursteigernde Stoffe wie Coffein usw., dann auch durch Heißbäder.

Eine eigentliche Reflexübererregbarkeit besteht bei den verschiedenen tetanischen Zuständen nicht.

Manifeste infantile Tetanie. Das *Symptombild* der manifesten tetanoiden, d. h. echten Spasmophilie ist ein ungemein buntes und abwechslungsreiches. Nicht nur die einzelnen Kundgebungen selbst sind jeweils individuell sehr verschieden, sondern nach Kombination und Intensität der Ausprägung sind alle denkbaren Varianten zu beobachten. Vom einfachsten ein- oder mehrmaligen, leichten, krähenden Inspirium, das sehr leicht übersehen wird, bis zu alarmierenden, schweren Konvulsionen sind alle Zwischenstufen denkbar. Am häufigsten ist bei Säuglingen der *Stimmritzenkrampf* (= Glottiskrampf, = Laryngospasmus). Dieser Zustand äußert sich so, daß plötzlich die bisher ruhige

---

[1] TURPIN: La tétanie infantile. Paris 1925.

und kaum hörbare Inspiration von einem lauten *Ziehen*, d. h. krähenden Ton, begleitet wird. Die Ursache ist eben der Stimmritzenkrampf, der zu einer Stenose oder gar manchmal zu einem vollkommenen, krampfhaften Verschluß der Glottis führt (*apnoische* Form des Laryngospasmus). Sehr häufig ist dieses Krähen von keinerlei weiteren Störungen begleitet, insbesondere auch nicht von einer Cyanose des Kindes oder gar von Erstickungserscheinungen, so daß die gefährliche Lage gar nicht erkannt wird, dies um so mehr, als viele Kinder jeweils zur Auslösung des Stimmritzenkrampfes einer psychischen Erregung bedürfen, wie Erschrecken, Zornausbruch, Schmerz, Hustenanfall (Keuchhustenattacke), Erbrechen u. dgl. Überdies ist dieses krähende Inspirium oft nur ein einmaliges oder nur dann und wann in Stunden sich wiederholendes Ereignis. In schweren Fällen freilich erfolgt der Spasmus nicht in Form einer kurzdauernden Innervation, sondern führt zu einem sekundenlangen, partiellen oder totalen Verschluß des Kehlkopfes. Die Folge davon ist ein Blauwerden des Kindes, ein Erblassen, ein angsterfüllter Gesichtsausdruck, auch eine Innervation der mimischen Muskulatur, die das Ringen nach Luft zur Genüge ausdrückt. Ja, es kann vorkommen, daß in einer ununterbrochenen Kette sich Anfälle an Anfälle reihen, so daß im ersten Augenblick der Gedanke an eine Verlegung der Luftwege durch Fremdkörper oder auch an eine diphtherische Stenose naheliegt. Mit Recht werden die Stimmritzenkrämpfe gefürchtet, denn nicht selten erfolgt rasch und vor voller Erkenntnis der gefährlichen Lage der Erstickungstod. Gar nicht selten spielt sich die Tragödie in der Weise ab, daß laryngospastische Kinder des Nachts oder morgens ohne ersichtliche Ursache tot im Bett gefunden werden. Der laryngospastische Tetanietod des Säuglings und Kleinkindes bildet eines der Hauptkapitel innerhalb der großen Kategorie der *Mors subita infantum*. Übrigens erscheint es uns sehr fraglich, ob es sich wirklich bei diesem tetanischen Tod immer um eine echte Erstickung handelt, also um ein Ausbleiben der Krampflösung am Larynx. Wahrscheinlicher dünkt es, daß über dem Weg anderer Nervenapparate es zu einem Herzstillstand kommt. Vielleicht spielt die Thymus dabei eine Rolle. Wir kennen die reine Erstickungslage sehr gut von der Larynxdiphtherie her und sehen da, wie lange ein schwer stenotisches Kind mit der Erstickungsgefahr ringt, ein Ringen buchstäblich mit jeder Herzfaser! Wir müssen annehmen, daß eine einfache Kohlensäureintoxikation beim Laryngospasmus doch schließlich und endlich diesen Spasmus lösen müßte, wenn nicht andere gefährliche Wirkungen im Spiele wären (vielleicht die des Status cardio-thymicus nach Moro). Viele Umstände, vor allem die obengenannten psychischen, sprechen dafür, daß die Auslösung des Glottiskrampfes eine *zentrale*, d. h. daß die Erregbarkeit des Atemzentrums gesteigert ist, so daß eben unterschwellige Werte zu jenen gefährlichen Impulsen nach der Peripherie führen. Abgesehen von der obengenannten *inspiratorischen Apnoe* wird auch eine *exspiratorische* beobachtet, ein Zustand, bei dem im Exspirium zentralbedingter Atemstillstand eintritt. Diese exspiratorische Apnoe verursacht rasch auftretende Blausucht, dann Leichenblässe, Pulslosigkeit und schließlich bei entsprechender Dauer den Tod.

Genaue Studien über die Atmung der spasmophilen Kinder und ein Versuch, die Respirationserscheinungen für gewisse diagnostische Zwecke heranzuziehen, liegt von Masslow vor. Mit dem Algesimeter von Motschutkowsky werden periphere Reize gesetzt und die entsprechende Reaktion der Atmung studiert, die bei Spasmophilen sehr charakteristisch ist. Es treten infolge der Reizung Krampfreaktionen der Atemmuskeln ein. Diese Krämpfe wiederum drücken sich in den Atmungskurven in Form von Pausen aus, also apnoischen Phasen, sowohl in der Periode der Inspiration wie Exspiration, mit nachfolgendem Weinen und darauffolgender regelmäßiger Atmung. Die Dauer der Apnoe gibt einen gewissen Maßstab für den Grad der Nervenübererregbarkeit beim Kind. Das Schwinden läßt auf Heilung schließen. Dieses MASSLOWsche Respirationssymptom soll beständig und sehr empfindlich sein, dient besonders auch der Diagnose der latenten Tetanie.

Einen weiteren gefährlichen und alarmierenden Ausdruck manifester Tetanie bilden die *allgemeinen Krämpfe* (= tetanische Konvulsionen, = *tetanoide Eklampsie*, auch vielfach kurzweg als Spasmophilie bezeichnet). Diese schweren Krampfattacken unterscheiden sich kaum von echt epileptischen Insulten oder solchen bei schweren organischen Prozessen. Mit aller Heftigkeit treten sie entweder nach oder mit den Glottiskrämpfen oder mit den noch unten zu beschreibenden spastischen Partialkrämpfen auf oder — was vielleicht noch häufiger ist — sie setzen urplötzlich aus scheinbar voller Gesundheit ein. Schon der erste Anfall kann tödlich enden. Wenn er nachts unbemerkt vor sich geht, wird allenfalls das Kind später tot im Bett gefunden. Vielfach erfolgt der tödliche Krampfanfall unmittelbar nach einer Magenfüllung, also nach Leerung einer dargereichten Flasche. Im übrigen findet sich ganz dieselbe Sachlage, wie wir sie vom Glottiskrampf kennen. Auch diese tetanoide Eklampsie stellt ein Hauptkontingent zur sog. „Mors subita infantum". Es kann bei der einmaligen Attacke bleiben, oft stellen sich aber noch weitere eklamptische Paroxysmen ein, manchmal reiht sich Anfall an Anfall. Da nach dem Anfall allgemeine Schlafsucht besteht, kommt das Kind bei diesen Serienattacken aus der Bewußtlosigkeit vielfach durch Stunden nicht heraus *(Status eclampticus)*.

Die diagnostische Sachlage ist nicht immer ganz leicht. Wegen der allgemeinen Konvulsionen, besonders aber, weil auch Manipulationen und Reize am Kind (elektrische Prüfung!) den Insult auszulösen vermögen, ist eine Prüfung der KÖZ und auch eine solche der mechanischen Übererregbarkeits-Phänomene nicht immer möglich oder im Ergebnis nicht eindeutig. Vielfach wird daher auf den Nachweis der tetanischen Grundlagen des Zustandes verzichtet und einfach *bei Krämpfen innerhalb der ersten 3 Lebensjahre ohne weiteres tetanoide Spasmophilie angenommen*. Dieser Standpunkt ist unbedingt zu verwerfen, wir kennen mancherlei Krampfzustände im frühen Kindesalter, die gar nichts mit Tetanie zu tun haben; erinnert sei z. B. nur an die so ungemein häufigen sog. *Gelegenheitskrämpfe*, das sind *initiale Krämpfe* als Einleitung fieberhafter Infekte. Man wird den Krampf zunächst symptomatisch behandeln und dann aber ehestens zum Nachweis der Latenzzeichen der Tetanie übergehen müssen, denn ohne solche ist die Diagnose unbrauchbar und jede Therapie vage und anfechtbar.

Merkwürdigerweise ist das Auftreten einer Eklampsie durchaus nicht vom Grade der Erregbarkeitssteigerung abhängig. Ganz geringe Erniedrigung der Zuckungswerte, kaum nachweisbares Bestehen echter Tetanie reicht aus, um ein plötzliches Auftreten des konvulsivischen Bildes zu begründen. Bei anderen wieder findet man alle Zeichen florider Rachitis, die Latenzsymptome in ausgeprägtester Form, höchste Steigerung der mechanischen und nervösen Erregbarkeit, Glottiskrämpfe, Karpopedalspasmen usw., es kommt aber nicht zu den gefürchteten Konvulsionen. Nach der von GÖTT und HUSLER ausgedrückten Anschauung muß wohl wenigstens für einen Teil der konvulsivischen Formen eine vorbestehende, vielfach erblich bedingte Krampfbereitschaft angenommen werden. Mitunter läßt sich in solchen Familien die Anlage zu Krämpfen bei Geschwistern und anderen Anverwandten nachweisen.

Nach dem Symptom des tetanischen Krampfes hat die Tetanie ihren Namen bekommen, begreiflicherweise, da es im Gefolge der Krankheit zu weiteren, sehr mannigfaltigen Krampfäußerungen kommen kann.

In wesentlich eindeutigerem Sinne als die allgemeinen Konvulsionen sind die spastischen, tetanischen Zustände an Händen und Füßen pathognostisch für Tetanie. Es wurde oben bereits auf das TROUSSEAUsche *Phänomen* der mechanischen Erregbarkeit hingewiesen. Dieselbe Krampfstellung kann sich aber auch ohne besonderen mechanischen Reiz spontan einstellen. Die Finger werden in den Grundphalangen in Starre gebeugt, der Daumen in die Hohlhand eingeschlagen *(Geburtshelferhand,* auch *Pfötchenhand)*. Dabei werden die Arme vielfach bei Beugung im Ellbogengelenk an den Rumpf angepreßt. Ganz ähnlich verhalten sich die Muskelapparate des Fußes: Krampfhafte Supination, Beugung der Zehen in den Grundphalangen bei starker Adduktion und Aneinanderpressung. Diese karpopedalen Spasmen (vielfach sind es nur karpale, die pedalen fehlen), verursachen offenbar Schmerzen, manchmal sogar sehr lebhafte, denn die Kinder dulden keine Manipulationen, zeigen sich in weinerlicher Stimmung, äußern vermehrtes Geschrei.

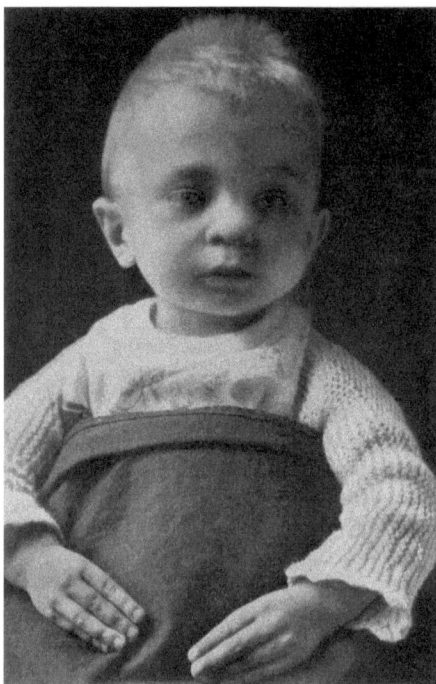

Abb. 1. Manifeste Tetanie bei einem Rachitiker mit Pertussis (Universitäts-Kinderklinik München: v PFAUNDLER.)

Die tonischen Zustände an Händen und Füßen sind wie alle tetanischen Zeichen starker Wandlung unterworfen. Bald sind sie deutlich und unverkennbar, andere Male wieder kaum angedeutet. Beim Erwachsenen wird nicht nur die Pfötchenstellung, sondern Fausthaltung mit gestrecktem Daumen, auch einseitiges Auftreten des Krampfes beobachtet (CURSCHMANN, V. FRANKL-HOCHWART u. a.). An den Zehen trifft man statt der plantaren, gelegentlich auch dorsale Flexion.

Es ergibt sich die Frage, inwieweit auch die übrige quergestreifte Muskulatur sich am tonischen Starrezustand beteiligt? Sehr bekannt ist eine mimische Innervation des Gesichtes in Form von Spitzung des Mundes, Runzelung der Stirne,

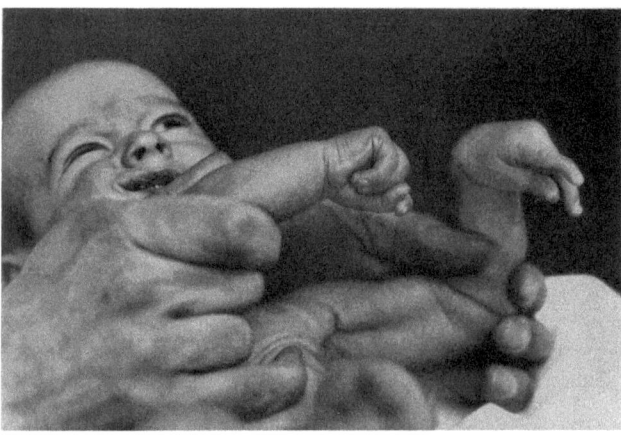

Abb. 2. Tetanie der Hände bei einem 3½ monatigen Säugling. (Universitäts-Kinderklinik München: v. PFAUNDLER.)

Krampfaugen, Verengerung der Lidspalte (= *Tetaniegesicht* nach UFFENHEIMER, Karpfenmund), ein ähnlicher Gesichtsausdruck, wie man ihn vom Tetanus kennt (Risus sardonicus), doch fehlt bei der Tetanie der Trismus. Beim Erwachsenen können zu diesen leichten Gesichtskrämpfen noch allerhand andere Krämpfe kommen, so in den Masseteren, in der Sprachmuskulatur, in den Augenmuskeln. Auch Gähnkrämpfe sind beschrieben, als sehr selten Würgkrämpfe. Wenig praktische Bedeutung und schwer nachweisbar sind die Tonussteigerungen in der Rumpf- und Rückenmuskulatur, immerhin trifft man manchmal Tetaniekinder, die auf der Höhe der Erkrankung eine ganz allgemeine tonische Starre erkennen lassen.

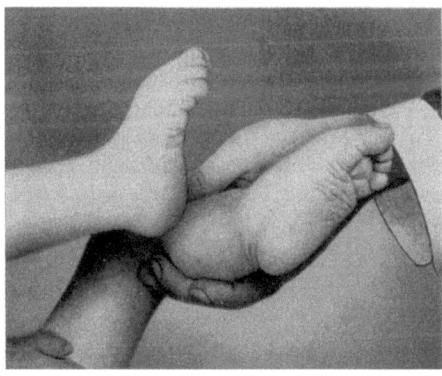

Abb. 3. Typische Tetanie-Stellung der Füße (Univers.-Kinderklinik München: v. PFAUNDLER.)

In der Aufstellung des symptomatischen Inventars der Erkrankung ist man zu immer neuen Funden gekommen. IBRAHIM beobachtete gelegentliche *Sphincteren-Krämpfe*, und zwar sowohl an Blase wie Mastdarm, Krämpfe, die zur vorübergehenden Harn- und Stuhlverhaltung Anlaß geben, wobei die Blasenstörung in Form der Strangurie vielleicht noch häufiger sein dürfte als die Spasmen des Rectums. Des weiteren sind Dickdarmspasmen, ferner solche der Speiseröhre, der Cardia und des Pylorus bekannt geworden. Eine Unzahl von Arbeiten mit zahlreichen Einzelbeobachtungen liegen hier vor.

Innervationsstörungen am Auge sind bereits in Form des vorübergehenden Schielens (FEER) genannt, dazu kommen Pupillenstörungen in Form von Anisokorie, Pupillenstarre, Mydriasis u. a.

Eine fast stets zu Tode führende Krampfinnervation der glatten Muskulatur kommt in den Bronchien vor (= *Bronchotetanie* nach LEDERER), nämlich plötzlich auftretende Atelektase großer Lungenabschnitte unter momentan einsetzender schwerster Dyspnoe. Die Atemfrequenz steigert sich rasch zur höchstmöglichen Höhe, Angst und Erstickungsgefahr, Cyanose prägt sich im Gesicht der Kinder aus. Dazu kommt rasch einsetzendes Fieber, zum Teil mit sehr hohen Graden. Wie bei allen tiefsitzenden Stenosen ist auch hier das Exspirium unvergleichlich stärker betroffen als das Inspirium. LEDERER stellte ein dreieinhalbmal längeres

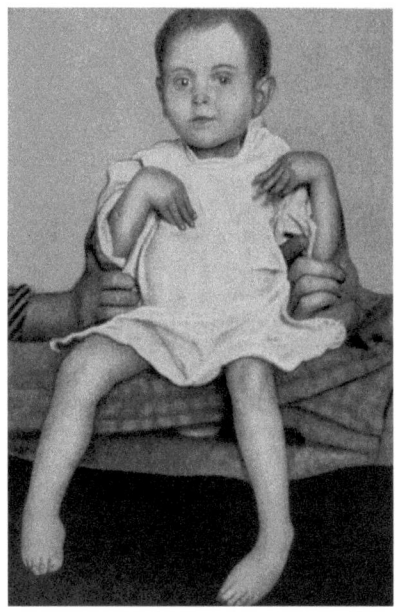

Abb. 4. Tetanische Stellung der Hände und Füße (Universitäts-Kinderklinik München: v. PFAUNDLER).

Exspirium als Inspirium fest. Es können sehr verschiedene Lappen betroffen sein, stets aber läßt sich nach einiger Dauer des Krampfes die atelektatische Verschattung im Röntgenbild in Form eines diffusen Schleiers feststellen. Vielfach wird begreiflicherweise der Zustand mit Asthma bronchiale verwechselt oder eingetretene Atelektase mit Pneumonie (Dämpfung, bronchiales Atmen, feinblasiges Rasseln). Wahrscheinlich ist die Bronchotetanie wesentlich häufiger als vielfach angenommen wird; denn eine Verschleierung der übrigen Tetaniesymptome führt zu leicht zu Fehldiagnosen. An Hand des Röntgenbildes allerdings erscheint die Diagnose nicht gar so schwer. Einige Autoren, wie RIETSCHEL, FINKELSTEIN und GYÖRGY kennen auch eine *spastische asthmatische* Bronchitis auf tetanischer Grundlage, die als leichte Form der Bronchotetanie angesprochen werden könnte.

Wiederholt wurde oben bereits auf die Gefahr des *plötzlichen Todes* bei Tetanie hingewiesen. Nicht nur durch Erstickung infolge Stimmritzenkrampfes, sondern auch infolge unmittelbarer *Herztetanie* (IBRAHIM) kann ein tödlicher Ausgang erfolgen. Diese Herztetanie kann sich in verschiedensten Formen äußern.

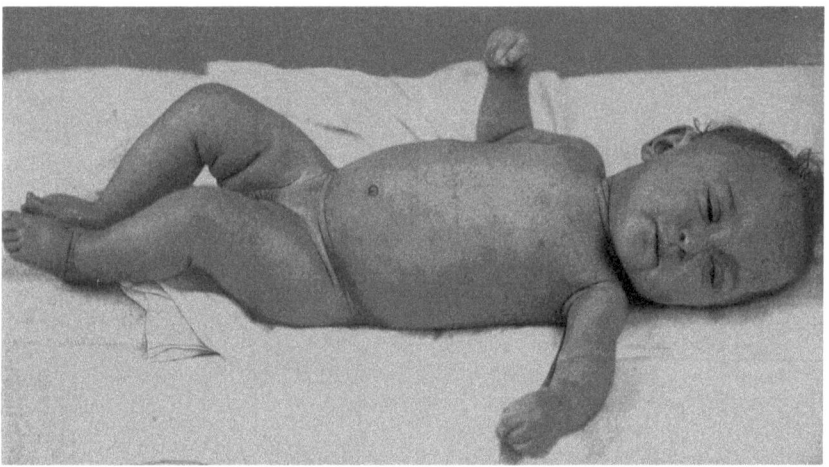

Abb. 5. Karpopedalspasmen bei Tetanie. Ödem der Fußrücken, Karpfenmund. Erschwerte Respiration. 9 Monate alt. Plötzlicher Tod am nächsten Tage.
(Aus der Züricher Kinderklinik, Prof. FEER.) Übernommen aus FEER, Kinderheilkunde. 9. Aufl.

Es sind bradykardische Zustände (KOPLIK) beobachtet, aber auch anfallsweise Tachykardie (FINKELSTEIN). Demnach kann bald eine Sympathicus-, bald eine Vagusreizung sich vordrängen. Im schlimmsten Fall kommt es zum diastolischen Herztod, wie ihn IBRAHIM erstmals beschrieben. Dieser Herztod tritt teils in Verbindung mit anderen, oben genannten spastischen Erscheinungen auf, kann sich aber auch plötzlich ohne andere Begleiterscheinungen einstellen. Als Ursache wurde von E. SCHIFF ein Versagen der autochthonen Herzreize, Kammerflimmern, plötzliche Änderung des Herzgefäßtonus usw. angenommen. Als auslösende Ursachen für Herzstörungen, vor allem aber auch für den Herztod, kommen die verschiedensten seelischen Erregungen in Betracht. FINKELSTEIN berichtet von einer enormen Tachykardie mit 200 Schlägen im Anschluß an eine Magenspülung. Ein anderer Fall ist bekannt, wo ein Kind, zur Nachuntersuchung wiederbestellt, während der elektrischen Prüfung tot umsank. Ähnlich kann ein plötzlicher Schreck wirken. Auch im Anschluß an starke Magenfüllungen (siehe oben) werden immer wieder schwerste Herzstörungen beobachtet. Das Elektrokardiogramm des tetanischen Herzens zeigt eine deutliche Vergrößerung aller Zacken, eine geringe Initial-, vor allem aber eine ansteigende und spitze Finalschwankung (MORGENSTERN). Interessant sind die Untersuchungen von E. SCHIFF bei künstlich erzeugter parathyreopriver Tetanie des Hundes. Die tetanische Übererregbarkeit führte im Experiment nach Wegnahme der Nebenschilddrüsen zu einer Vergrößerung des Herzens im Sinne einer Erweiterung, die offenbar durch Vagusreizung sich erklärt und die nach Heilung der Tetanie sich wieder vollständig zurückbildet. Derselbe Autor und andere stellten übrigens auch im Röntgenbild des tetanischen Kindes eine Vergrößerung des Herzschattens fest („Tetanieherz"). MORO hat in anderem Zusammenhang auf die Verknüpfung von Herzinnervation und Thymus hingewiesen. Möglicherweise spielen solche Innervationen bei einer derartigen Erregbarkeitssteigerung, wie sie die Tetanis mit sich bringt, eine ausschlaggebende Rolle. Häufig beobachtet wurde akuter Tod anläßlich von Ultraviolettbestrahlungen (also Höhensonne bei manifester Tetanie kontraindiziert!), und zwar sogar in den ersten Minuten der Straleneinwirkung!

Man kann zwar nicht behaupten, daß die Tetaniekinder etwa einen ganz bestimmten Typus darstellen, immerhin sind es meistens wohlgenährte, blühend aussehende Geschöpfe; gerade dieser Umstand führt häufig genug verspätet oder gar nicht zum Arzt oder gibt die Veranlassung zu einer Verkennung des Ernstes der Lage. Allenfalls kann eine Habitusveränderung auftreten durch die Entstehung von *Ödemen*. Man findet diese zwar in erster Linie am Hand- und Fußrücken, wo sie nicht selten sofort in die Augen springende, blasse Polster verursachen; sie führen aber auch zu einer Gedunsenheit des Gesichtes. Namentlich bei länger dauernden karpopedalen Spasmen, also bei der sog. „persistenten Tetanie" findet man sie am schwersten ausgeprägt, obwohl sie nach FREUDENBERG nicht als Folge des Muskelkrampfes aufzufassen sind. Es sind vielmehr die ödemerzeugenden Ursachen dieselben Stoffwechselvorgänge, die auch die Krämpfe bedingen. Die genannten Ödeme unterscheiden sich von den üblichen Nieren- oder Herzödemen dadurch, *daß Fingereindrücke nicht beibehalten werden*. Die durch Stoffwechselstörung bedingte erhöhte Wasserbindung zeigt sich auch dadurch an, daß die sog. Quaddelzeit nach v. GROER verkürzt ist. Von anderen vasomotorischen Störungen wären außer gelegentlicher, in fraglichem Zusammenhang mit Tetanie stehende Urticaria zu nennen, sowie eine besondere Neigung zum Schwitzen, wie sie auch dem rachitischen Kind zu eigen ist.

Ein besonders merkwürdiger Befund ist der seit langem bei der Tetanie des Erwachsenen, sowie bei der experimentellen Tetanie nach Entfernung der Nebenschilddrüsen auftretende *Schichtstar*. Ob ein solcher auch beim Kind vorkommt, scheint fraglich, nachdem bisher darüber keine Mitteilung vorliegt, obwohl erfahrene Kenner besonders auch in Nachuntersuchungen dieser Frage besondere Aufmerksamkeit gewidmet haben. Nach PINELES bedarf es einer *chronischen*, durch Jahre hindurch gehenden Krankheit, wie sie nur bei Erwachsenen (oder allenfalls beim älteren Kinde) vorkommt, um derartige organische Veränderungen zu erzeugen. Durch die Literatur mitgeschleift wird bis in die neuere Zeit das Phantom der sog. „*Tetaniezähne*". Man sieht bei jungen Kindern Schmelzdefekte in ungezählten Fällen, bei Kindern, die zwar niemals tetanisch, aber sicher florid rachitisch sind oder waren. Nachdem nunmehr in neuerer Zeit die engeren Beziehungen zwischen Rachitis und Tetanie zweifelsfrei aufgedeckt sind, wird man die genannten Schmelzdefekte auf jene synchrone oder vorbestehende Rachitis und nicht auf die Tetanie beziehen müssen; *Tetaniezähne* sind nichts anderes als Rachitikerzähne. Einen etwaigen sonstigen pathologischen Zahnbefund, der etwa nur für Tetanie charakteristisch wäre, kennen wir nicht.

Verlauf der Tetanie. Das Prädilektionsalter für die spasmophilen Erscheinungen ist die Zeit der ersten 3 Lebensjahre, das ist die Zeit der floriden Rachitis. Allerdings bleiben die ersten 3 Lebensmonate beim normal ausgetragenen Säugling fast stets tetaniefrei, nur bei Frühgeburten sieht man schon nach 6 bis 8 Wochen gelegentlich die eklamptische Form der Tetanie. Nach den Untersuchungen von BENITA WOLF ist die Behauptung, daß das erste Trimenon überhaupt frei von Tetanie bleibe und daß Krämpfe dieser Periode unbedingt eine andere Genese hätten, irrtümlich. Die Diagnose ist freilich nicht immer leicht zu stellen, da mitunter die elektrische und mechanische Übererregbarkeit den eklamptischen Ausbrüchen erst nachfolgt. Im Zweifelsfall ist der Nachweis der Rachitis auf blutchemischem Wege zu erbringen.

Im allgemeinen sind die eklamptischen Formen der Spasmophilie mehr bei jüngeren Säuglingen zu beobachten, die karpopedalspastischen Typen bei den Kleinkindern. Bei der puerilen und Erwachsenentetanie endlich wird fast ausschließlich der Karpopedalspasmus angetroffen.

Die einzelnen Erscheinungen verteilten sich nach einer Zusammenstellung von FREUDENBERG auf 72 Fälle folgendermaßen:

Konvulsionen und Laryngospasmus	23mal
Konvulsionen allein	15 „
Laryngospasmus allein (einschließl. Apnoe)	11 „
Konvulsionen, Laryngo- und Karpopedalspasmus	9 „
Laryngo- und Karpopedalspasmen	3 „
Karpopedalspasmen allein	4 „
Ödeme	14 „

Was die Häufigkeit in der Altersverteilung im einzelnen anbetrifft, so hat man zu erwarten: Im ersten Trimenon nur ganz selten sichere Tetanie; im zweiten Quartal des 1. Lebensjahres nimmt die Zahl bedeutend zu; das Maximum trifft auf das dritte Quartal, im vierten Quartal wieder Abnahme der Frequenz; im 2. und 3. Lebensjahr nimmt die Frequenz weiter bedeutend ab und mit dem vollendeten 4. Jahr ist die obere Grenze der eigentlichen *infantilen Tetanie* erreicht. Die *puerile Tetanie* (ESCHERICH) tritt nur sehr selten auf, erst im Erwachsenenalter wieder ist Tetanie etwas häufiger.

Rezidive der Spasmophilie in früher Kindheit kommen insoweit vor, als Rezidive der Rachitis sich einstellen. Ein Persistieren mehr minder durch die ganze Kindheit hindurch, dürfte nur ganz selten vorkommen; in einem mir bekannten derartigen Falle handelte es sich um Tetanie bei chronischer Cöliakie.

Einer besonderen Erörterung bedarf der Begriff der

sog. Spätekalmpsie oder Spätspasmophilie. THIEMICH, der Schöpfer dieses Begriffes, hat 1906 die Späteklampsie folgendermaßen definiert:

Krämpfe, die auf dem Boden der spasmophilen Diathese entstehen und sich von den gewöhnlichen eklamptischen Anfällen der ersten Kindheit nur durch das höhere Alter der betreffenden Kinder unterscheiden. Sie sind meist, aber nicht immer, die Wiederholung der Säuglingskrämpfe. Sie gleichen der Epilepsie vornehmlich dadurch, daß sie im 5. Lebensjahr (vielleicht auch noch später) auftreten, unterscheiden sich aber von ihr durch das Vorhandensein ausgeprägter tetanoider Symptome und durch die günstige Prognose.

Wegen der möglichen Beziehungen zur Epilepsie oder auch aus differentialdiagnostischen Gründen gegenüber dieser verlangt die Frage *Späteklampsie* genaueste Erwägung. Es ergeben sich vor allem folgende Fragen: Gibt es eine tetanoide Übererregbarkeit in später Kindheit, die zu epileptischen Manifestationen führt? Ist diese Übererregbarkeit in der üblichen Weise in Latenz und Manifestation feststellbar? Welche Bedeutung haben solche tetanoiden Spätkrämpfe? Bilden sie eine eigene Krankheitskategorie für sich, mit feststehendem Verlauf und Ausgang? Oder sind sie einer echten genuinen Epilepsie gleichwertig oder gar mit ihr gleichbedeutend?

Nach THIEMICH hat sich POTPESCHNIGG solchen Fragen gewidmet und kam zur Vermutung, daß Späteklampsie häufiger sei als angenommen wird, daß sie auch noch in späteren Jahren und selbst jenseits der Kindheit auftrete, und daß ihre Träger später „unerkannt in der Schar der Epileptiker verschwinden würden". HUSLER hat dann an der Münchener Kinderklinik bei sehr zahlreichen krampfkranken Kindern die Frage der Spätspasmophilie weiter verfolgt.

Als Kriterien für tetanoide Genese können zunächst in Betracht kommen: Das Facialphänomen, das TROUSSEAUsche Zeichen und vor allem die kathodische Übererregbarkeit. Das Facialphänomen findet sich in der späteren Kindheit derart häufig, daß es für diese Zwecke jeder Bedeutung entbehrt. Das TROUSSEAUsche Zeichen ist ein Attribut der jungen Säuglinge, ebenso wie der Laryngospasmus. Die Karpopedalspasmen sind zwar, wie bereits oben ausgeführt, nach ESCHERICH mit zunehmendem Alter mehr und mehr die Hauptmanifestation einer Tetanie, können aber nur verwertet werden für die wirklich manifest tetanischen Fälle. Das Peronealphänomen kann, wie das Facialphänomen, für das ältere Kind nicht mehr als brauchbarer Hinweis genommen werden. Es bleibt dann nur noch der Nachweis einer galvanischen Übererregbarkeit als Mittel, um einen Krampfzustand als evtl. tetanischen Ursprungs abzugrenzen. Da der Normalwert der KÖZ auch beim älteren Kind jedoch über 5,0 mA liegt, können wir Erniedigungen dieses Wertes als brauchbares Kriterium ansehen. Da nach unseren Untersuchungen das ältere Kind anodisch weit erregbarer ist als der normale Säugling, können wir die anodische Übererregbarkeit nicht im diagnostischen Wert ebenso einschätzen.

Man hat die Bedeutung des Begriffes Späteklampsie darin gesehen, daß damit eine Krankheit sui generis von der Epilepsie abtrennbar ist. Nachuntersuchungen bei sog. Späteklampsie haben aber ergeben, daß es sich durchweg um echte Epilepsie gehandelt hatte. Es zeigte sich, daß gerade die Fälle, die seinerzeit als die typischen Vertreter einer Späteklampsie angesprochen waren, weil bei ihnen die Spasmophilie am längsten und deutlichsten ausgeprägt war, späterhin vollkommen das Verhalten echter Epilepsie boten und der geistigen Destruktion anheimgefallen waren. Das Untersuchungsresultat führte zu folgenden Ergebnissen:

1. Es gibt echte, typische, genuine Epilepsie mit allen epileptischen Folgeerscheinungen, die von ausgesprochenen tetanoiden Symptomen begleitet ist (s. auch die parathyreoprive Tetanie-Epilepsie nach REDLICH, v. FRANKL-HOCHWART u. a.). Die Epilepsie erscheint hierbei von Anbeginn als selbständiges, unabhängiges Leiden.

2. Das Vorhandensein von latenten Zeichen des tetanoiden Zustandes neben konvulsivischen oder ähnlichen Erscheinungen gutartigen Charakters berechtigt ebenfalls durchaus noch nicht ohne weiteres von ,,Späteklampsie'' zu sprechen und eine günstige Prognose zu stellen. Die Krampfkrankheit kann auch hierbei eine selbständige sein, die in keiner Beziehung zur tetanoiden Erregungslage steht (auch sehr niedere KÖZ-Werte [< 5,0 mA] erlauben nur einen Rückschluß auf konkomittierende Tetanie, nicht aber auf die von ihr begleitete oder verursachte Krampfkrankheit.)

3. Wenn auch bei den bisher beobachteten Fällen von Krampfkrankheiten mit tetanoidem Syndrom es sich um eine Kombination zweierlei grundverschiedener Dinge handelte, wäre immer noch denkbar, daß eine Späteklampsie beim älteren Kind vorkommen könnte, bei der der episodische und günstige Verlauf und die Ähnlichkeit mit der Säuglingseklampsie, ferner das *gleichzeitige Bestehen* anderer *manifester tetanischer Stigmata* die Auffassung als echte Späteklampsie berechtigt erscheinen läßt.

Zu 1. Die epileptischen Manifestationen an älteren Tetanoiden unterschieden sich in nichts von denen bei echter genuiner Epilepsie. Alle Einzelheiten des typischen Grand mal waren gegeben. Ferner blieben die Betroffenen keineswegs vom geistigen Verfall verschont. In allen Fällen ergab die Nachforschung, daß der Verlauf der *Tetanie* der denkbar ungünstigste war; die progressive Tendenz im Leiden war sogar eher eine stärkere, als man sonst von der Mehrzahl der Epileptiker gewohnt war. Ein innerer Zusammenhang zwischen Epilepsie und Tetanie ist nicht darzutun. Wohl sind die tetanoiden Zeichen durch Ca und P zum Verschwinden zu bringen, *die Epilepsie aber wird dadurch nicht merklich berührt oder aufgehalten.*

Zu 2. Die latente Tetanie älterer Kinder verknüpft sich, wenn auch selten, gelegentlich mit nichtepileptischen nervösen Störungen — seien es krampfartige oder andere —, so mit neuropathischen oder typisch hysterischen Kundgebungen, dann mit den verschiedenartigsten organischen Erkrankungen (FINKELSTEIN), auch völlig isoliert bei scheinbar ganz Gesunden kommt sie vor. Feststellungen von Übererregbarkeitsphänomen in jedem Alter haben daher zunächst nur symptomatischen, nicht pathognostischen Wert. Keiner der beobachteten „Spätspasmophilien" glich dem von THIEMICH beschriebenen Typus *Späteklampsie.* Bei keinem waren die Anfälle nach Art und Verlauf ähnlich der beim Säugling geläufigen tetanoiden Eklampsie. Zwar ließe sich theoretisch vorstellen, daß gelegentlich die tetanoiden Symptome eine solche akute Steigerung erfahren, daß es zur eklamptischen Explosion kommt: zu *Gelegenheitskrämpfen.* Praktisch konnte aber gerade an solchen Patienten mit Gelegenheits-, Fieberkrämpfen usw., soweit sie außerhalb des eigentlichen Tetaniealters standen, nicht ein einziges Mal eine tetanoide Grundlage ermittelt werden.

Zu 3. Übererregbarkeitsphänomene bei Kindern jenseits des Säuglingsalters weisen somit auch bei gleichzeitigen Krampfäußerungen lediglich auf Spättetanie, nicht aber auf das Wesen der daneben bestehenden Krampfkrankheit. Wohl nur ganz selten ist diese letztere eine echte *Späteklampsie.* Unter 360 klinisch genau beobachteten Krampfkrankheiten der späteren Kindheit fanden *wir* kein Beispiel, wenn auch fünf der Kinder jenseits des 4. Lebensjahres neben den Krämpfen übererregbar im tetanischen Sinne waren.

Nahe verknüpft mit diesen Fragen ist die nach dem *späteren Schicksal ehemals spasmophil gewesener Kinder.* Untersuchungen hierüber liegen vor von THIEMICH und BIRK, sowie POTPESCHNIGG. Die verschiedensten Störungen, und zwar sowohl körperliche Fehler, wie solche des Nervensystems und der Psyche, wurden von den ersteren Autoren festgestellt: Neuropathie in allen ihren Formen, Pavor nocturnus, Somnambulismus, Enuresis, Wutkrämpfe u. a. Epilepsieähnliche Krankheiten oder auch nur das Fortbestehen von Krampfanfällen war in keinem einzigen Fall nachzuweisen. POTPESCHNIGG hatte bei seinen Nachprüfungen ein ähnliches Resultat. Sechs Prüflinge hatten Zeichen von Spätspasmophilie, und zwar teils kathodische, teils anodische Übererregbarkeit. In einem einzigen Fall, wo die Krämpfe bis ins 9. Lebensjahr fortbestanden, hatte die Annahme einer echten Späteklampsie gewisse Berechtigung. Inzwischen sind noch einige weitere kasuistische Mitteilungen letzterer Art dazugekommen, so daß die bisher vorliegenden Beobachtungen nichtepileptischer Späteklampsie äußerst spärlich sind. Auch heute noch gilt mehr minder der ehemals von GÖTT ausgesprochene Satz: „Wir kennen von dieser äußerst interessanten Form bisher eigentlich nicht viel anderes als ihre Existenz."

Die *beim Erwachsenen vorkommende Tetanie* ähnelt im großen und ganzen durchaus der kindlichen Form. Dieselben latent tetanischen Zeichen beobachtet man hier wie dort, wobei die mechanischen Übererregbarkeitszeichen weniger zuverlässig sind als beim Kind oder gar beim Säugling. Maßgebend ist beim Erwachsenen in erster Linie die Erhöhung der elektrischen Reizbarkeit, vor allem die Minderung des KÖZ-Wertes unter 5,0 mA. Die manifesten Symptome ähneln ebenfalls denen der Kinder, allerdings sind die laryngospastischen und allgemeinen Krämpfe viel seltener, das Bild wird vielmehr beherrscht von tonischen Krämpfen an Händen und Füßen *(Arthrogryposis)*, dann sind Parästhesien häufiger oder werden besser und genauer angegeben, wie etwa Kribbeln in den Fingern, Gefühl von „Feuergarben", Ameisenlaufen usw. Hierher gehört auch das HOFFMANNsche Symptom, welches in dem Auftreten von Parästhesien bei Reizung sensibler Nerven gehört. Krampfhafte Innervationen in der Muskulatur des Oesophagus, des Magens, der Blase, des Auges sind festgestellt, endlich auch psychische Störungen depressiver Art oder auch halluzinatorische Verwirrtheit u. dgl. Während wir bei Kindern abgesehen von den Ödemen der distalen Extremitäten kaum organische Erscheinungen wahrnehmen, vermutlich wegen der zu kurzen Dauer der Stoffwechselstörung, sind solche bei der chronischen Erwachsenentetanie zahlreich mitgeteilt: Tetaniestar, vasomotorische Störungen, trophische Störungen der Haut, der Haare und Nägel, Extremitätengangrän. Wie beim Kind an die Rachitis, ist die idiopathische Tetanie des Erwachsenen an die Osteomalacie gebunden, welch letztere ja bekanntlich nichts anderes als die Rachitis des erwachsenen Skeletes ist. Infolge dieser gleichen Abhängigkeit besteht auch Übereinstimmung hinsichtlich der jahreszeitlichen Verteilung. Der Hauptgipfel der Frequenz wird im Winter und Frühjahr angetroffen. Über die Ursache der Osteomalacie besteht Klarheit; sie beruht vor allem auf dem Mangel an D-Vitamin in der Nahrung[1].

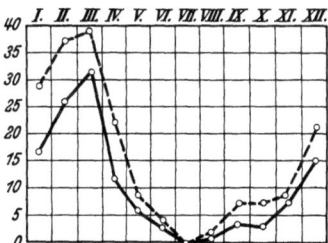

Abb. 6. Die jahreszeitliche Verteilung der manifesten Tetanie auf Grund von 195 in der Heidelberger Kinderklinik zwischen 1911 bis 1918 beobachteten Fällen. Die ausgezogene Kurve entspricht den „spontanen" und die punktierte Kurve der Summe der spontanen und der „symptomatischen" (im Verlaufe anderweitiger Erkrankungen, wie Pertussis, Grippe, Pneumonie, Masern entstandenen) Tetanien. (MORO).

Ob allerdings sämtliche Spontantetanien beim Erwachsenen osteomalacischen Ursprungs sind oder ob einzelne auch andere Ätiologien haben (Epithelkörperchen-Insuffizienzen?), bedarf noch der Feststellung.

Umstritten ist die Frage der *angeborenen Tetanie*. In der Regel dürfte es sich bei solchen Angaben um Irrtümer handeln, denn die Tetanie ist von der Rachitis abhängig, diese hat aber eine gewisse Inkubationszeit der Entwicklung, nämlich etwa 2—3 Monate, so daß schon aus diesem Grunde eine angeborene Tetanie äußerst fragwürdig erscheint. Übrigens wurden wiederholt Neugeborene tetanischer Mütter gesund gefunden, selbst im Blutchemismus.

Interessant ist die *jahreszeitliche Verteilung der Tetaniefälle*. Aus obiger Kurve läßt sich ersehen, daß in den Früh- und Hochsommermonaten die Zahl der Erkrankungen sehr spärlich ist, daß dann im Herbst ein Anstieg erfolgt, der um Februar, März und April seinen höchsten Gipfel erreicht. Diese Beobachtung ist immer wieder übereinstimmend festgestellt worden, so von ESCHERICH, FEER, MORO, auch schon von den alten Autoren. MORO konnte durch weiteres Studium des Frühlingsgipfels der Tetanie ermitteln, daß innerhalb der Haupttetaniemonate wiederum ganz bestimmte Tage und kleine Perioden die Hauptmasse der Erkrankung bringen, während wieder in anderen Wochen die Erkrankungsgefahr gering ist. Diese klimatische und geophysische Häufung hat MORO als Tetaniewetter bezeichnet. Die klimatische Einwirkung sieht MORO in einer Beeinflussung des Hormonapparates des Organismus, die auf eine

---

[1] Ausführliche Bearbeitung des Themas siehe STEPP und GYÖRGY: Avitaminosen, S. 378—402. 1927.

Erhöhung des Erregbarkeitszustandes im gesamten vegetativen Nervensystem hinausläuft. FREUDENBERG und GYÖRGY sprechen von einer *hormonalen Frühjahrskrise*.

Nicht nur die Witterung hat Einfluß auf die Auslösung der Tetanie, sondern vor allem auch Veränderungen in der Stoffwechsellage des Körpers. Nicht selten tritt sie in Erscheinung im Anschluß an Infekte der verschiedensten Art, wie Pneumonie u. dgl. Man hat solche durch Infekte ausgelöste Tetaniezustände auch als *akzidentelle Tetanie* nach FINKELSTEIN bezeichnet.

Pathogenetisch ist in neuerer Zeit die Forschung um ein gutes Stück vorwärts gekommen. Zunächst einmal ist nunmehr einwandfrei festgestellt, daß die Tetanie — wie schon betont — in einen ursächlichen Zusammenhang mit der Rachitis zu bringen ist, wobei aber keineswegs der Grad der Rachitis für die Entstehung des spasmophilen Zustandes ausschlaggebend ist. Ein weiterer für die Pathogenese wichtiger Punkt ist die einwandfreie Feststellung durch FINKELSTEIN u. a., daß bei Brustkindern nur ganz verschwindend wenig Tetaniefälle vorkommen, trotz florider Rachitis, während Flaschenkinder unter sonst gleichen körperlichen Umständen ganz unvergleichlich mehr disponiert sind. FINKELSTEIN hat den Salzen, also der Molke in den artfremden Milchen eine Hauptbedeutung beigelegt. Eine Übersicht über die Mineralzusammenstellung von Frauen- und Kuhmilch ergibt in Äquivalenzberechnung folgende Tabelle nach FREUDENBERG:

Milliäquivalente pro Liter	Na	K	Ca	Mg	P	Cl	Citrat	Anionendefizit
Frauenmilch . .	5,2	1,5	15	0,2	5,0	8,3	10,9	— 2,3
Kuhmilch . . .	15,0	4,0	61	0,5	31,7	23,2	31,2	— 5,5

Der LÖBsche Ionenquotient $\frac{Na + K}{Ca + Mg}$, den FREUDENBERG hieraus errechnet, ist für Frauenmilch 0,44, für Kuhmilch 0,31, d. h. das Milieu der Frauenmilch ist stärker erregbarkeitsfördernd als das der Kuhmilch. Nun bleibt dabei aber der gewaltige Einfluß der Phosphate und der Citrate unberücksichtigt, welch ersterer in der Kuhmilch ein sechsfaches gegenüber dem der Frauenmilch ausmacht. Diese beiden Faktoren gleichen nicht nur die genannte Eigenschaft der Erregbarkeitsförderung völlig aus, sondern wirken an sich durch Entionisierung der zweiwertigen Kationen weit mehr erregbarkeitsfördernd. Nach FREUDENBERG ist demnach der tetanigene Einfluß der Kuhmilch in erster Linie auf ihren hohen Phosphorgehalt zurückzuführen. Während beim Rachitiker bekanntlich Hypophosphatämie besteht, ist umgekehrt beim Tetaniker das Serumphosphat vermehrt (grundlegende Feststellung von FREUDENBERG und GYÖRGY). „Diese Steigerung beantwortet der Organismus des Tetanikers mit einer Senkung des Serumkalkspiegels." Phosphatsteigerung und Kalksenkung im Blut und in den Säften aber begründen die Manifestierung der Tetanie. Unklar bleibt der Grund für jene Phosphatsteigerung. Die MOROsche Schule hat nun diese Phosphatsteigerung mit der hormonalen Frühjahrskrise in Zusammenhang gebracht, ohne angeben zu können, welches Hormon hierbei die entscheidende Rolle spielt. Die genannten Autoren weisen weiter darauf hin, daß neben Ernährung und klimatischen Faktoren noch andere tetaniebegründende Umstände eintreten können, so vor allem die obengenannte Fieberwirkung. Diese führt zur sog. febrilen Hyperventilation, zur Senkung des Kohlensäurespannung des Blutes sowie der Alkalireserve. Diese Umstände wiederum führen zu Veränderungen im organischen Stoffwechsel, besonders im Kohlehydratstoffwechsel. Der spasmophile Zustand tritt in Erscheinung vor allem in dem Moment, wo die Rachitis im Heilgang unterbrochen oder nach anderer Meinung in ein beschleunigtes Tempo übergeführt wird. Bei der Rachitis besteht Azidose, mit dem Eintreten der Tetanie muß es zur Anazidose gekommen sein. Auf diesen Zustand der Anazidose legt FREUDENBERG großes Gewicht, weil die Steigerung des Serumphosphatgehaltes „ebenso wie die Senkung des Kalkspiegels nicht zu tetanoiden Reaktionen führt, wenn eine Azidose vorliegt". „Das Bestehen einer Azidose ist unvereinbar mit tetanoiden Reaktionen, auch wenn der übrige Ionenkonstellation sie begünstigt." (Näheres über diese sehr interessanten Fragen sind in den Originalarbeiten von GYÖRGY und FREUDENBERG nachzulesen, insbesondere siehe auch bei STEPP und GYÖRGY[1]).

Die weit überwiegende Mehrzahl der Tetanieformen rachitogenen Ursprungs wird daher im frühen Kindesalter beobachtet. Es gibt jedoch noch gewisse andere

---

[1] STEPP u. GYÖRGY: Avitaminosen usw. Berlin 1927.

Formen, die mit Rachitis nichts zu tun haben, die deshalb in der Regel an reifere Altersstufen gebunden sind.

Parathyreoprive Tetanie. Nach operativer Entfernung der Epithelkörperchen bei Mensch oder Säugetier tritt zunächst latente, dann plötzlich durch schwere Konvulsionen manifeste Tetanie ein. Man kannte früher namentlich diese Folgeerscheinungen nach Kropfoperationen, wenn die Glandulae parathyreoideae mit der Schilddrüse restlos entfernt wurden. Dasselbe läßt sich experimentell am Tier erzeugen. Die dauernden Krämpfe sind beim Tier verbunden mit allgemeiner Kachexie, mit Tremor und anderem, welche Erscheinungen beim Menschen in der Regel fehlen. Der Verlauf der Erkrankung ist weitgehend durch die Art der Fütterung beeinflußbar: Fleischfütterung beschleunigt den Verfall, Milchfütterung hält ihn auf. Mit der Erkrankung geht Hand in Hand eine Änderung des Chemismus: progrediente Hypocalcämie, Alkalose, Phosphatstauung usw. Im klinischen Verlauf bestehen gewisse Unterschiede zwischen der menschlichen und tierischen Epithelkörperchentetanie.

Ebenfalls zu den experimentellen Tetanien wird die sog. *Guanidin-Tetanie* gerechnet. Guanidin erzeugt im Tierversuch tetanieähnliche Symptome, wie Steigerung der elektrischen Erregbarkeit, Stimmritzenkrämpfe, Konvulsionen. Der Chemismus bei Guanidin-Tetanie ist ein anderer als bei der Epithelkörperchentetanie. Es scheint fraglich, ob überhaupt diese Tetanie mit den echten Tetanien in eine Linie gestellt werden darf.

Die Einführung gewisser Phosphatsalze, vor allem der alkalischen, vermag im Experiment Tetanie zu erzeugen *(sog. Phosphat-Tetanie).* Besonders wenn schon eine latente Tetanie besteht, kann durch *alkalische* Phosphatsalze die Manifestierung erfolgen, während nach ADLERSBERG, PORGES, FREUDENBERG die sauren Phosphatsalze stark antitetanisch wirken. Die Kaliumsalze sind dabei den Natriumsalzen überlegen. Nach FREUDENBERG besteht eine Parallele zur infantilen Tetanie, insofern als die Phosphatzufuhr den Kalkgehalt im Serum vermindert und rein intermediär ihre Wirkungen auslöst.

Bicarbonat-Tetanie stellt eine Sonderform dar, die auch praktisch nicht ganz ohne Belang ist. Übermäßige Zufuhr von Bicarbonat erzeugt einen Zustand von erhöhter Nervenerregbarkeit. Genau so wirkt starker Chlorverlust, beispielsweise durch stark anhaltendes Erbrechen oder durch übermäßig häufige Magenspülungen. Der Chlorverlust führt zu Erhöhung des Bicarbonats im Blut. Solche Fälle sind beim Erwachsenen beschrieben unter der Diagnose „Magentetanie", beim älteren Kind als Folge von chronischem Erbrechen (UFFENHEIMER).

Hyperventilations- oder Atmungstetanie. Von VERNON wurde 1909 zum erstenmal festgestellt, daß übermäßig häufige und tiefe Atemzüge in der Ruhe nervöse Störungen erzeugen. Diese Störungen wurden dann später von GRANT und GOLDMANN als echt tetanische erkannt und von anderen, z. B. FREUDENBERG und GYÖRGY, bestätigt. Der Symptomenkomplex ist völlig identisch dem der kindlichen Tetanie, vom Facialphänomen bis zum Laryngospasmus sind alle Erscheinungen bekannt. Es kommt durch die Hyperventilation zu einer wahren Alkalose bei gleichzeitig unverändertem Gesamtkalk-, niedrigerem Bicarbonat- und Phosphatgehalt (GYÖRGY). Bei der forcierten Atmung verarmt das Blut rasch an Kohlensäure und sekundär an Bicarbonat; die Erniedrigung der freien Kohlensäure kann durch Alkaliausscheidung nicht mehr kompensiert werden, das Säurebasengleichgewicht verschiebt sich gegen die alkalische Seite. GYÖRGY erblickt deshalb in der Alkalose die übergeordnete pathogenetische Ursache dieser Tetanieform.

Prognose. Die allermeisten Fälle von tetanischer Übererregbarkeit bleiben unerkannt und reagieren nach kürzerem oder längerem Bestand spontan wieder ab, wohl nur ein kleiner Teil kommt überhaupt durch die Manifestierung zur Kenntnis. Von diesen wiederum heilt der größte Teil, vor allem bei zweckmäßiger Behandlung rasch ab. Die Prognose der tetanischen Erscheinungen ist also als günstig zu bezeichnen; immerhin besteht die Möglichkeit eines raschen und oft ganz unerwarteten Todes im laryngospastischen Anfall, dann vor allem durch schwere allgemeine Konvulsionen. Diese Frage der Mors subita infantum wurde bereits oben gestreift, eine Gefährdung, die naturgemäß vor allem Säuglinge und Kinder des 2. und 3. Lebensjahres betrifft. Sie kann sich noch bedeutend erhöhen, wenn Komplikationen oder Kombinationen mit anderen Krankheiten vorliegen. Eine ganz besonders gefürchtete, gelegentlich zu enormen spasmophilen Reaktionen führende Kupplung ist die mit Keuchhusten. Des weiteren werden akute Infekte, wie besonders Masern, Grippe u. dgl. spasmophilen Kindern sehr gefährlich. Auch die erste Phase der Behandlung birgt gewisse Gefahren in sich. Vor allem ist das antirachitische Vorgehen — so notwendig es ist — zunächst einmal geeignet, gelegentlich die spasmophile Bereitschaft zu erhöhen. So z. B. ist bekannt, daß Ultraviolettbestrahlungen rachitisch-tetanischer Kinder zu raschen und schwersten, auch tödlichen Krampfexacerbationen führen. Die Aussichten der Tetaniker *für später* werden sehr verschieden beurteilt. In älteren Arbeiten findet sich der Standpunkt vertreten, daß tetanisch gewesene Kinder später zu allerhand schweren Folgezuständen neigen. Geistige, motorische und andere Defekte werden diesen Kindern nachgesagt. Die Grundlage für diese Prognostik bilden die Katamnesen von THIEMICH. Dieser forschte bei Schulkindern, die ehemals tetanisch gewesen waren, nach und fand unter 53 Schulpflichtigen nicht weniger wie 21 Schwachbegabte, aber auch unter den Nichteingeschulten fand sich ein enormer Prozentsatz von Schwachbegabten. Nicht weniger wie zwei Drittel der Kinder war gezeichnet von den verschiedenartigsten neuro- und psychopathischen Abwegigkeiten. Aus diesen THIEMICHschen Feststellungen könnte allenfalls, wie es THIEMICH selbst tat, mit Recht geschlossen werden, daß die schwereren Formen der Tetanie besonders bei solchen vorkommen, die eine Minderwertigkeit des Nervenapparates, sei es im ganzen oder in Teilen von Haus aus besitzen. Schwer konvulsivische Tetanie würde sich demnach vor allem auf dem Boden abwegiger konstitutioneller Anlage entwickeln. Wir können weiter noch aus eigener Erfahrung hinzufügen, daß schwerste Tetanie besonders häufig solche betrifft, die aus miserablem äußeren Milieu kommen, das selbst wieder oft genug seine Wurzeln in anlagemäßigen Minderwertigkeiten hat. Ursache und Wirkung stehen hier noch in einem weiteren Sinne in einer Wechselbeziehung. *Nicht aber darf gefolgert werden aus den durchaus einwandfreien Feststellungen* THIEMICHS, *daß die Tetanie allein etwa die Ursache später hervortretender Unzulänglichkeiten wäre.* Insbesondere muß die Meinung, daß die Tetanie den Boden lege für eine spätere echte Epilepsie, bekämpft werden. Es existieren keinerlei einwandfreie Feststellungen, die einen derartigen Zusammenhang dartun würden. Die elektive Bevorzugung zentral geschädigter oder anlagemäßig minderwertiger Kinder betont neuerdings auch FREUDENBERG; unter 72 tetanischen Säuglingen mit manifesten tetanischen Symptomen (bereits oben zitierte Aufstellung) zeigten nicht weniger wie 9 cerebrale Defekte oder angeborene Mißbildungen. Die Tatsache der erleichterten Manifestierung bei vorbestehenden nervösen Schäden tritt nach demselben Autor sehr deutlich auch dadurch in Erscheinung, daß bei cerebraler Halbseitenlähmung die geschädigte Seite vorzugsweise von der Tetanie betroffen ist. Des weiteren wurde oben schon darauf hingewiesen, daß nach Beobachtungen von GÖTT und HUSLER überhaupt die tetanische Eklampsie von vornherein eine familiäre oder zum mindesten an das Einzelindividuum gebundene, anlagemäßige Krampfbereitschaft voraussetzt. Dieselben Erwägungen erklären auch die allgemein bekannte Tatsache, daß in Schwachsinnigenheimen ein gewaltiger Prozentsatz der Patienten unter Krämpfen in der ersten Kindheit gelitten hat. Zweifellos sind diese Krämpfe zum großen Teil tetanoid-spasmophilen Ursprungs und nur zum kleinen Teil organisch-epileptischen oder echt epileptischer Ätiologie.

Differentialdiagnose. Die Erkennung des latenten Zustandes der Tetanie ist nur durch Prüfung der mechanischen und elektrischen Erregbarkeit möglich. Wo diese Untersuchung bei floridrachitischen Säuglingen und Kleinkindern unterlassen wird, wird dieser Zustand, falls er vorliegt, übersehen. Meist unverkennbar sind dagegen die manifesten Kundgebungen. Die Karpopedalspasmen lassen kaum eine andere Deutung zu. Eine Verwechslung mit spastischen Zuständen cerebralen Ursprungs dürfte kaum vorkommen. Ebenso sicher diagnostizierbar sind die laryngospastischen Funktionsstörungen. Schon anamnestisch sind die Angaben von Krähen oder Ziehen, wenn nicht mit Husten verbunden, höchst verdächtig. Die verschiedenen Formen des Croups wie Diphtheriecroup, Maserncroup usw. lassen sich durch die Begleitumstände wie Atemnot, Fieber usw. in der Regel leicht abtrennen. Auch Verwechslung mit Keuchhusten dürfte angesichts der fehlenden exspiratorischen Hustenstöße nicht in Frage kommen. Die vielen Formen des angeborenen Stridors erledigen sich als Möglichkeiten dadurch, daß ja zum Unterschied von diesen Laryngospasmus im ersten Trimenon kaum zu erwarten ist.

Die eklamptische Form der Tetanie kann weit mehr Schwierigkeiten bereiten, da sie in diagnostische Konkurrenz tritt mit einer größeren Anzahl gerade auch im früheren Kindesalter auftretenden Krampfäußerungen. Wir kommen damit zur Frage der *sog. Spasmophilie im weiteren Sinne,* also der Krampfkrankheiten des Kindes auf *nichttetanoider* Grundlage.

II. Spasmophilie im weiteren Sinne.

Gelegenheits- oder Initialkrämpfe (HOCHSINGER) werden meist singulär auftretende Krampfäußerungen genannt, die namentlich in den ersten 4—5 Jahren bei manchen Kindern auf bestimmte Anlässe, Gelegenheiten hin sich einstellen. Solche Anlässe sind in der Regel Infektionen mit raschem Temperaturanstieg. Die auslösenden Infektionen sind nicht nur ernsterer Art, wie etwa Scharlach oder Diphtherie, sondern oft ganz harmlose wie banale Angina, Grippe oder auch Mumps, Varicellen usw. Des weiteren können belanglose Reize, wie leichte Verletzungen, Harnentleerungsschwierigkeiten u. a., endlich auch starke Erhitzung im Hochsommer gelegentlich Konvulsionen genannter Art erzeugen. Die Krämpfe sind meist durchaus epileptiform, mitunter ungemein schwer, sie setzen wie beim Epileptiker momentan und ohne Vorläufer ein, die Betroffenen zucken in allen Gebieten gleichmäßig klonisch, daneben kann aber auch eine gewisse Starre bestehen. Bewußtlosigkeit, Pupillenstarre, allgemeine Cyanose, Schäumen, Urinabgang können die Anfälle begleiten. Man hat in diesen Gelegenheitskrämpfen ein Äquivalent des Schüttelfrostes erblickt, ein vasomotorisches Phänomen oder auch eine toxische Wirkung auf die Ganglienzellen des Gehirns. Ganz abwegig ist es, in ihnen den Ausdruck einer tetanoiden Spasmophilie oder gar Epilepsie sehen zu wollen. Mit beidem haben die Initialkrämpfe vor und bei Fieber gar nichts zu tun. Allerdings ist zuzugeben, daß bei wirklich Tetanischen eine interkurrente Infektion den ganzen spasmophilen Komplex auszulösen vermag. Hier entscheiden dann diagnostisch die oben ausführlich besprochene Übererregbarkeitsprüfung und allenfalls die Serum-Kalkanalyse. Erfahrungsgemäß machen viele Diagnostiker sich die Aufgabe sehr leicht, indem sie alle nichtorganischen Krämpfe der ersten Kindesjahre einfach und ohne weiteres auf Tetanie beziehen, also auch die Initialkrämpfe. Durch jahrelange Beobachtung solcher Kinder kommen wir zum Ergebnis, daß die Neigung zu Gelegenheitskrämpfen anlagemäßig begründet ist. Die Infektion spielt nur die auslösende Gelegenheitsursache. Es gibt Familien, in denen diese unangenehme Bereitschaft familiär besteht: Mehrere oder gar alle Kinder haben in den ersten Lebensjahren die Neigung, irgendwelche Infektion mit Krampf einzuleiten. Auffallend häufig sind nach unseren Feststellungen die Krampfträger Einzelkinder. Immer sind sie von allgemeiner funktioneller Labilität. Es sind sog. sensible, reizbare Kinder. Sie neigen zu anderen illegalen Äußerungen des Nervensystems, z. B. zu Meningismus bei Fieber, dann zu Hyperreflexien, choreiformer Instabilität, Ängstlichkeit, Labilität der Psyche usw. Auch bei den Eltern dieser Abkömmlinge finden sich die Wurzeln der Konstitutionsanomalie. Wir sind ferner solchen Kindern katamnestisch nachgegangen, um evtl. Beziehungen zur echten Epilepsie festzustellen. Eine solche Feststellung ist in keinem Falle in positivem Sinne gelungen. Diese Tatsache ist besonders wichtig gegenüber der älteren Anschauung, die etwa in einem Satz THIEMICHs gipfelt:

Alle Krämpfe im Säuglingsalter, bei denen die spasmophile Grundlage ausgeschlossen werden kann, auch die ohne Übererregbarkeit auftretenden sog. ,,Fieberkrämpfe" im Sinne HOCHSINGERs[1] sind mit großer Wahrscheinlichkeit als epileptisch zu deuten.

Eine andere zu den sog. Spasmophilen im weiteren Sinne gerechnete Krampfkrankheit des Kindesalters sind die sog. *gehäuften Absenzen*.

Dies sind kleine und kleinste Anfälle von Geistesabwesenheit, die täglich in großer Zahl, entweder immer einzeln oder in gehäuften Serien auftreten. Die eigentliche klonische Krampfkomponente an den Extremitäten fehlt. Durch FRIEDMANN wurden sie 1906 beschrieben, haben aber zunächst wenig Beobachtung gefunden. Auch als 1912 der Autor nochmals sich eingehend mit der Frage befaßte, hatte er nicht viel Erfolg. Merkwürdigerweise ist erst in neuerer Zeit erhöhte Aufmerksamkeit dem an sich häufigen Krankheitsbild gewidmet worden. Im Alter von 4—7 Jahren treten zunächst nach Aufregung, Schreck, Operation od. dgl., oft auch ohne besonderen Anlaß, kurzdauernde und leichte Absenzen auf. Von Anfang an fällt schon die starke Häufung von manchmal bis zu dutzenden, ja bis zu hunderten und mehr Anfällen täglich auf. Die Anfälle sind außerordentlich stereotyp. Es sind ganz kurze Bewußtseinstrübungen von Sekundendauer. Die Kinder empfinden das Kommen und Gehen der Attacken, jedoch ist die Fähigkeit willkürlicher Bewegung, mit Ausnahme der automatisch weiterwirkenden, sowie das Sprachvermögen aufgehoben. Die Anfälle kommen in allen Haltungen und Lagen und unter allen erdenklichen äußeren Umständen. Der Blick ist im Anfall meist starr nach oben gewandt. Wiederholt wurden Attacken auch im Schlaf beobachtet, wobei die Kinder erwachen und sich im Bett aufrichten. Der Verlauf gestaltet sich äußerst langwierig, erstreckt sich stets über viele Jahre, führt aber niemals zu psychischem Verfall. Ergänzend zu den FRIEDMANNschen Beobachtungen können wir hinzufügen, daß nach unserer Erfahrung die betroffenen Kinder zwar im Anfall plötzlich mit starrem Blick in ihrer eben gepflogenen Tätigkeit wie Lesen, Essen, Spielen einhalten, daß sie aber kaum je bei anstrengender Arbeit, beim Laufen, Treppensteigen usw. ihre Absenze bekommen. Im Moment dieser Seelenpause reagieren sie nicht auf Anruf, rasch Vorgesprochenes wird nicht erfaßt und nicht reproduziert, ebensowenig wie vorgezeigte grelle Farben. Auch Schmerzen werden nicht empfunden und rufen keine Abwehr hervor. Ein Teil der Patienten hat keine Spur von Erinnerung an den Anfall, andere geben an, ,,daß etwas los war". Im Anfall beobachtet man keinerlei konvulsivische Zuckungen, auch kein Hin-

---

[1] HOCHSINGER: Deutsche Klinik, Bd. 7.

stürzen. Manchmal sinkt der Kopf nach vorne, gelegentlich auch nach hinten. Eine Auslösung ist im allgemeinen nicht möglich, in der Literatur finden sich allerdings Angaben, daß durch Rückbeugung des Kopfes dann und wann dies möglich sei. Nach dem Anfall fahren die Kinder in der unterbrochenen Tätigkeit fort, ja sie führen sogar begonnene Sätze zu Ende. Hie und da werden vielleicht noch ein paar weitere unzusammenhängende Worte gesprochen. Sichere Prüfungsergebnisse der Pupillen- oder auch anderer Reflexe liegen nicht vor, da der Anfall hierfür zu kurz dauert. In einer ganzen Anzahl von Beobachtungen sind diese Anfälle derart kurz, daß sie überhaupt übersehen werden oder es kann die Aufeinanderfolge so rasch erfolgen, daß das ganze als einfacher Blinzeltic angesprochen wird. Sehr wichtig sind die Beziehungen zu den drei Erkrankungen tetanoide Spasmophilie, Epilepsie, Hysterie. Mit Tetanie hat die Erkrankung wohl niemals etwas zu tun. Sie fällt überdies genau in das Alter, in dem eine echte Tetanie am allerseltensten ist. Schwieriger ist die Abgrenzung gegenüber Epilepsie angesichts der weitgehenden Ähnlichkeit mit dem epileptischen Petit Mal. FRIEDMANN hielt einen Zusammenhang für gelegentlich möglich. In der Tat mögen unter dem Bild der FRIEDMANNschen multiplen Absenzen echte Epilepsien für kürzere oder längere Zeit verlaufen. In typischen Fällen jedoch konnten wir niemals, auch nicht auf Grund katamnestischer Erhebung, eine Indentität mit Epilepsie finden. In der Regel verschwinden die Störungen ebenso spurlos wie sie gekommen sind. Es muß wohl ein prinzipieller Unterschied zwischen der FRIEDMANNschen Krankheit und der echten Epilepsie bestehen. Aber auch mit Hysterie hat die Erkrankung wohl im allgemeinen nichts zu tun. Den Kindern fehlt regelmäßig das sonst gewohnte hysterische Gehaben. Daß sie allerdings auf dem Boden einer neuro-psychopathischen Konstitution entstehen, konnten wir in vielen Fällen durch genaue Anamnestik einwandfrei feststellen.

Bei Erwachsenen ist ein vielleicht damit verwandtes Krankheitsbild beschrieben unter der Bezeichnung *Narkolepsie* (GÉLINEAU). Es sind dies kürzere oder längere Anfälle von Schlafsucht, aus denen der Patient kaum zu erwecken ist. Diese dürften viel mehr hysterische Wurzeln haben als die FRIEDMANNsche Krankheit (s. diesen Band, Kapitel Narkolepsie, S. 87).

Unter dem Namen *orthostatisch-epileptoider Symptomkomplex* wurde von HUSLER eine Kombination von epileptiformen Krampfzuständen mit dem orthostatisch-lordotischen Syndrom beschrieben. Die Betroffenen sind kindliche Individuen, die erstens auf morgendliches Aufstehen aus der Rückenlage oder auf Lordotisierung der Lendenwirbelsäure mit Eiweißausscheidung reagieren und die zweitens nebenher eine wiederholt bekundete Neigung zu Krampfanfällen gerade beim Stehen oder nach Lordotisierung haben. Bei Erkenntnis der besonderen konstitutionellen Grundzüge dieser Kinder kann man einen Augenblick dem Zufall das Zusammentreffen dieser beiden Symptomkomplexe zuschieben. Der scheinbare Zufall entpuppt sich als Notwendigkeit, sobald man einen konkreten solchen Fall genauerer Analyse unterzieht. Die Ohnmacht, die man vom Lorditiker kennt, erreicht bei diesen Kindern einen Grad, der in gleichmäßiger Folge über den Bewußtseinsverlust hinaus bis zu klonischen Krämpfen führt. Im klinischen Typus der betreffenden Kinder dominiert der Vasomotorismus als Leitsymptom. Farbenwechsel, Schwitzen, subjektive vasomotorische Störungen wie Schwindel, Müdigkeitsgefühl, Kopfweh und vor allem der Orthostatismus, Herzklopfen u. a. sind die besonderen Kennzeichen der Kranken. Die Anfälle selbst lösen sich für gewöhnlich in derselben Weise aus wie die orthostatischen Ohnmachten: Bei allen mit Lordotisierung einhergehenden Körperhaltungen, beim längeren Stehen, aber auch bei psychischen Anlässen. Jede progressive Tendenz und die sonst für Epilepsie charakteristischen Veränderungen der psychischen Persönlichkeit fehlen vollkommen. Auch ein Übergang in echte Epilepsie ist nie bekannt geworden.

Unter dem Begriff der Spasmophilie im weiteren Sinne fallen noch zahlreiche andere *epileptoide Krankheitsformen, die auf neuropsychopathischer Grundlage* beruhen, die man deshalb auch als *neuro-* oder *psychopathisches Epileptoid* beim Kind bezeichnet. In allen erdenklichen Varianten bilden Kinder dieser Kategorie häufige Gäste der Kliniken. Die verschiedenartigsten, zumeist den epileptischen besonders ähnlichen Anfälle kommen zur Beobachtung. Bald sind es sehr schwere, bald wieder kleine Attacken, bald mehr singuläre, dann wieder recht zahlreiche, bald kommen die Anfälle ohne jeden Anlaß, dann wieder bilden psychische Traumen eine notwendige Auslösung. Die Abgrenzung gegenüber einer echten Epilepsie ist meist durch Jahre hindurch ungemein schwierig, oft überhaupt nicht möglich, kurzum es handelt sich in der Regel um in ihren Ursachen und Beziehungen gänzlich unklare Zustände. So hat OPPENHEIM den Begriff der sog. *psychasthenischen Krämpfe* formuliert, welch letztere einerseits mit der Hysterie, andererseits mit echter Epilepsie nichts gemein haben. Betroffen sind vorwiegend psychisch schwer belastete und entartete Individuen, bei allen gehen den Anfällen Angstzustände, Phobien oder Tics oder auch vasomotorische Störungen, voraus. Nie erfolgen die Anfälle unvermittelt, sondern stets auf besonderen Anlaß wie Aufregung, Anstrengung u. dgl. Die Anfälle stellen nur eine Episode des Gesamtleidens dar, sind zum Teil typisch epileptiform, zum Teil handelt es sich nur um Bewußtlosigkeiten oder auf einzelne Muskelgebiete beschränkte Konvulsionen. Intelligenz und Gedächtnis bleiben intakt. Die OPPENHEIMschen Kranken sind meistens Erwachsene, und zwar vorwiegend ältere. Identisch oder verwandt mit diesem Typus sind jene Zustände, die ZIEHEN *epilamptische Anfälle* genannt hat. Dann wären hier anzuführen die sog. *affekt-epileptischen Zustände* nach BRATZ, auf dem Boden schwer psychopathischer Konstitution auftretende epileptiforme Zustände, die immer nur nach Gemütserschütterungen, besonders solcher von längerer Dauer, dann aber auch nach akuten Erregungen auftreten. Verwandt mit diesen Zuständen sind wohl die im Kindesalter so häufig beobachteten *respiratorischen Affektkrämpfe* oder das sog. *Wegbleiben* junger Kinder. Hier werden ebenfalls Anfälle beobachtet mit rein affektiver Auslösung. Diese Anfälle sind zwar zunächst nicht epileptiformen Charakters, können sich aber mit epileptischen Komponenten paaren. Bevorzugt sind vor allem die ersten 3—4 Lebensjahre. Später verschwinden die Anfälle. Sicherlich handelt es sich um psychisch nicht ganz einwandfreie Kinder, dazu noch meist um solche mit Erziehungsdefekten, es scheint aber, daß sie sich nicht in der Regel zu dem eigentlichen OPPENHEIMschen psychasthenischen Typus oder zu dem BRATZschen auswachsen. Auch diese Störung hat mit echter Epilepsie sicherlich keine Wesensgleichheit. Die von uns nach Jahren nachuntersuchten Fälle waren bestimmt nicht epileptisch. Dann und wann aber war die Störung familiär. Die Katamnese älterer Individuen ergibt übrigens häufig die Angabe, daß in früher Kindheit Wegbleiben, Atemanhalten, ,,Hinter-den-Atem-kommen" bestanden habe. E. STIER allerdings hat bei 62% der von ihm nachuntersuchten Probanden mit respiratorischen Affektkrämpfen später noch Anfälle gefunden von sehr polymorphem Charakter, Neigung zu Ohnmachten, epileptiforme Attacken usw.

Das Kindesalter neigt prinzipiell ungemein zu Krampfäußerungen. Vor allem besteht wohl die Feststellung zu Recht, daß, da alle neuro- bzw. psychopathischen Konstitutionen gerade im Kindesalter sich deutlich kundgeben, darum auch epileptiforme Krämpfe eine weitverbreitete Erscheinung beim Kinde sein müssen. Die enorme Vielgestaltigkeit der nervösen Konstitutionen, vor allem auch die Tendenz der Konstitutionsanomalien sich zu kuppeln, auf die

die Kinderärzte immer wieder hingewiesen haben, machen es verständlich, daß die mit den Anfällen verbundenen Symptomkomplexe unerschöpflich bunt und variabel sind. Wie schon betont, liegt die Hauptschwierigkeit für den Arzt in der Abtrennung von der echten Epilepsie, welch letzterer die progressive und zerstörende Tendenz innewohnt, während alle genannten spasmophilen Formen epileptoider Art nicht zu einer grundsätzlichen Änderung der Persönlichkeit führen.

Vorstehende differentialdiagnostische Übersicht berücksichtigt nicht die organisch-symptomatische Epilepsie, also die anatomischen oder toxischen Hirnschädigungen. Diese bereiten ja in der Regel keine differentialdiagnostischen Schwierigkeiten, da die ersteren ja mit allerhand Ausfallserscheinungen, vor allem auf motorischem Gebiet, mit Reflexveränderungen, Lähmungen, Spasmen, dann vor allem oft mit Schwachsinn usw. verbunden sind, letztere dagegen in der Regel die infektiös-toxische oder chemische Genese der Krämpfe oder auch etwa eine Stoffwechselvergiftung wie Urämie, Acetonämie, Coma diabeticum usw. ohne weiteres erkennen lassen. Auch die Hysterie hier zu besprechen, die selbstverständlich beim Kind manchmal Krampfäußerungen hervorruft, würde zu weit führen. Über diese ist an anderer Stelle nachzulesen.

Prophylaxe und Therapie der tetanoiden Spasmophilie. Die Verhütung der Tetanie im frühen Kindesalter ist eine Aufgabe, die gleichbedeutend ist mit Verhütung der Rachitis, da die beiden bekanntlich in Abhängigkeit zueinander stehen. Die Rachitisverhütung aber wiederum — heute eine äußerst dankenswerte Aufgabe geworden — ist jedem einfachen Lehrbuch der Pädiatrie zu entnehmen. Ist eine latente oder manifeste Tetanie festgestellt, sind gar laryngospastische oder eklamptische Erscheinungen zur Beobachtung gekommen, so muß eine energische Therapie schon aus Gründen der bestehenden Lebensgefahr eingeleitet werden. Die ältere Methode gipfelte darin, sofort die Milch zu entziehen und die Ernährung ausschließlich mit Kohlehydraten durchzuführen. Eine sofortige Wirkung war dieser therapeutischen Behandlungsmethode nicht abzusprechen. Das wirksame Prinzip war nach HEYMANN und FREUDENBERG die sofort eintretende Phosphatverarmung. Große Nachteile dieser Behandlung bestanden in der durch die Kohlehydrate bedingten Einseitigkeit der Ernährung; auch ist es schwierig, den Kindern quantitativ genügend zuzuführen, sie hungern, des weiteren war mit der Wiederzufuhr von Milch ein Wiederauftreten der Spasmophilie zu befürchten. Es gelingt einfacher mit anderen Mitteln den Phosphorspiegel des Serums zu senken und eine Minderung der Erregbarkeit zu erreichen. Das Mittel der Wahl ist der Kalk. Allerdings sind nach übereinstimmender Erfahrung sehr große Dosen anorganischer Kalksalze notwendig. Kein Zweifel, daß die seit nunmehr bald einem Menschenalter erprobte Therapie sehr verlässig ist. Schwierigkeiten bestehen allerdings darin, daß fast alle Kalksalze ungemein schlecht schmecken und daher in den nötigen Dosen nur sehr schwer beizubringen sind. Vielfach erzeugen sie Erbrechen oder werden überhaupt ohne weiteres vom Patienten abgelehnt. Der Wert der zur Verfügung stehenden einzelnen Salze ist ein sehr verschiedener, die organischen werden den anorganischen vorgezogen. Die Dosierung des Calc. chlorat. sicc. beträgt 4,0—6,0 g pro die, in Milch portionsweise verabreicht. Neuerdings wird vielfach als Injektionspräparat Calc. Sandoz verwendet, das zum Unterschied von anderen Kalkpräparaten nicht die gefürchteten schmerzhaften Nekrosen erzeugt. Doch sind auch hier sehr große Dosen notwendig. Sobald die gewünschte Minderung der Erregbarkeit erreicht ist, meist schon nach Tagen, kann man von hohen Dosen auf niedrige heruntergehen, freilich unter fortgesetzter subtiler Beobachtung des Patienten. Mit Rezidiven muß stets gerechnet werden. Der Zweck der Kalktherapie ist die Erhöhung des Kalkspiegels, Senkung des Phosphorspiegels und Ausübung einer azidotischen Wirkung. Zur Erzielung dieser letzteren sind noch andere Vorschläge gemacht worden: Verabreichung der Salzsäuremilch (SCHEER), von Ammoniumchlorid nach FREUDENBERG und GYÖRGY und endlich von saurem Ammoniumphosphat nach ADLERSBERG-PORGES. Die Verwendung der Salzsäuremilch wird vor allem in Anstalten möglich sein. Im Privathaus sie zu geben, wird sich schon deswegen weniger empfehlen, da die Herstellung nicht ganz einfach ist und manchmal mit Nierenblutung zu rechnen ist, die selbstverständlich eine sorgfältige Nierenüberwachung fordert. Die Verabreichung wird nur für kurze Zeit empfohlen, mit dem Abklingen der Symptome soll auch die Salzsäuremilch sistiert werden. Das Ammonchlorid wirkt dadurch, daß ein Zerfall in Ammoniak und Salzsäure eintritt, welch letzteres sich an Alkalien bindet. Diese Salmiakbehandlung soll sehr prompt wirken, FREUDENBERG gibt an, daß bei 10 Jahre langem Gebrauch er nie erlebt habe, daß ein Tetaniefall nicht prompt angesprochen hätte. Die Dosierung besteht in 0,6 g pro Kilogramm Körpergewicht in 10%iger Lösung zu den Milchportionen gemischt und über den ganzen Tag verteilt (also etwa 3—6 g pro die); das Mittel ist schwer zu nehmen. Bei Überdosierung besteht Gefahr der Cylindrurie, schließlich auch des Kollaps u. a. Man gibt daher die Volldosis zunächst nur für 2 Tage, reduziert dann täglich die jeweils gereichten Mengen um 1 g. Von gleicher Wirksamkeit ist das saure Ammoniumphosphat. Bei Kindern wird dieses wohl selten gegeben wegen stark abführender Wirkung. Die Erwachsenendosis beträgt 15—20 g pro die.

Die antirachitische Therapie muß selbstverständlich mit der antitetanischen in jedem Fall parallel laufen. Von den Hauptmitteln Lebertran, Höhensonne, Vigantol ist folgendes zu sagen. Lebertran wirkt zu langsam, Höhensonnebestrahlungen lösen gelegentlich Krämpfe aus (Todesfall nach eigener Beobachtung!), dagegen ist das Vigantol das Mittel der Wahl. Auf Vigantol haben wir niemals eine gefährliche akute Manifestierung tetanischer Symptome erlebt. Der Satz, daß ,,die Kombination antirachitischer und symptomatischer antitetanischer Behandlung der einzig rationelle Weg sei", wird von niemand bestritten. Die Eklampsien selbst können durch geeignete sedative Mittel coupiert werden. Das Mittel der Wahl ist die rectale Verabreichung von Chloralhydrat in der Dosis von 1 g bei Säuglingen, 1,5 g bei Kleinkindern (10% wäßrige Lösung).

Literatur.

ASCHENHEIM, E.: Über die Beteiligung des vegetativen Nervensystems und über trophische Störungen bei der infantilen Tetanie. Münch. med. Wschr. **1919 II**.
BACHENHEIMER, M.: Über die Kalktherapie bei Spasmophilie. Mschr. Kinderheilk. **14**, 184 (1918). — BEHREND: Die Magnesiumsulfatbehandlung der spasmophilen Krämpfe. Mschr. Kinderheilk. **12** (1913). — BEHREND-FREUDENBERG: Über die Angriffspunkte der tetanigenen Reize. Klin. Wschr. **1923 I**. — BERNHEIM-KARRER: Zur Behandlung der Spasmophilie im Säuglingsalter. Mschr. Kinderheilk. **12**, 453 (1914). — BEUMER-SOECKNICK: Über organische Azidose bei anorganischer Azidose und Alkalose. Z. Kinderheilk. **37** (1924).
ERLANGER, B.: Über die Beziehungen zwischen Spasmophilie und Keuchhusten. Mschr. Kinderheilk. **12**, 473 (1914). — ESCHERICH: Tetanie der Kinder. Wien u. Leipzig 1909.
FREI, MAGDA: Zur Behandlung des Herzstillstandes bei Spasmophilie. Mschr. Kinderheilk. **15**, 376 (1919). — FREUDENBERG: Rachitis und Tetanie. Handbuch von PFAUNDLER-SCHLOSSMANN. — FREUDENBERG-GYÖRGY: Salmiakbehandlung der Kindertetanie. Klin. Wschr. **1922 I**.
GYÖRGY: Die Tetanie der Kinder. STEPP-GYÖRGYs Avitaminosen. Berlin 1927. — GOLLWITZER-MEIER: Tetaniestudien. I. Guanidintetanie. II. Überventilationstetanie. III. Magentetanie. Z. exper. Med. **40** (1924). — GRANT-GOLDMAN: Clinical Tetany by Forced Respiration. Amer. J. Physiol. **52** (1920).
HIRSCH, A. u. SCHNEIDER: Dünndarmgeschwüre als Erscheinungsform der Spasmophilie. Mschr. Kinderheilk. **15**, 181 (1919). — HULDSCHINSKY: Die Beeinflussung der Tetanie durch

Ultraviolettlicht. Z. Kinderheilk. **26** (1920). — HUSLER, J.: Zur Systematik und Klinik epileptiformer Krampfkrankheiten im Kindesalter. Erg. inn. Med. **19**, 624 (1920).

IBRAHIM: Über Tetanie der Sphinkteren, der glatten Muskeln und des Herzens bei Säuglingen. Jb. Kinderheilk. **72** (1910).

JÖRGENSEN: Über die Bedeutung der pathologisch-anatomischen Veränderungen der Gland. parashgr. für den Pathologen durch infantile Tetanie. Mschr. Kinderheilk. **10**, 154 (1912).

LEDERER: Über Bronchotetanie. Z. Kinderheilk. **7** (1913).

MASSLOW: Über Veränderung der Atmungskurven bei Kindern mit spasmophilen Symptomen. Mschr. Kinderheilk. **13** (1914).

RIETSCHEL, H.: Bronchotetanie, Bronchialasthma und asthmatische Bronchitis. Mschr. Kinderheilk. **12**, 261 (1914).

SACHS, F.: Untersuchungen über die Erregbarkeit des vegetativen Nervensystems spasmophiler Kinder. Mschr. Kinderheilk. **15**, 437. — SCHEER: Die Beeinflußbarkeit der Spasmophilie durch Salzsäuremilch. Jb. Kinderheilk. **97** (1922).

THORSPECKEN, O.: Magenuntersuchung bei kindlicher Tetanie. Mschr. Kinderheilk. **10**, 429 (1912).

WERNSTEDT: Beiträge zur Kenntnis der spasmophilen Diathese. Acta paediatr. (København) **1** (1922); **5** (1925).

Die Migräne.

Von HUGO RICHTER-Budapest.

Eine geschichtliche Darstellung über die Entwicklung der Lehre von der Migräne enthalten die Arbeiten von THOMAS (1887) und FLATAU (1912). Letztere enthält auch eine genaue Übersicht über die bis 1912 erschienene Literatur. Von weiteren monographischen Bearbeitungen wären hervorzuheben die Arbeiten von TISSOT (1813), LIVEING (1873), MOEBIUS (1894) und KOVALEWSKY (1902). Neuere Übersichten veröffentlichten CURSCHMANN (1926), HARTMANN (1932) und RILEY (1932).

Die Migräne dürfte, was die Häufigkeit ihres Vorkommens betrifft, unter den nervösen Erkrankungen an erster Stelle stehen. Die Statistiken der Nervenstationen sind in dieser Hinsicht kaum geeignet, über die Häufigkeit dieses Leidens auch nur ein annähernd richtiges Bild zu geben. Dies wird dem Fachmann erst klar, wenn er die genauer erforschten anamnestischen Angaben solcher Krankenabteilungen und Ambulanzen berücksichtigt, wo andere, mit der Migräne in keinerlei Beziehung stehende Erkrankungen behandelt werden. Stichproben, die ich in dieser Richtung machte, zeigten, daß die Zahl jener Migränefälle, die nie ärztlich beobachtet oder behandelt wurden, eine überaus große ist. Es soll hier nur auf die häufigste Art dieser nicht als Krankheit aufgefaßten Migräne hingewiesen werden: auf den einige Stunden lang andauernden „gewöhnlichen" Kopfschmerz der Frauen vor oder während der Periode, den so gewissermaßen als physiologische Begleiterscheinung der Menstruation betrachten. Bei älteren Kranken wird man in der Vorgeschichte oft auf Migräneanfälle stoßen, die vor Jahren oder Jahrzehnten durch längere Zeit bestanden hatten, ohne daß sie ärztlich beobachtet wurden. E. GRIMES fand unter 15 000 Individuen der allgemeinen Praxis 1200 Migränefälle (8%); nur 60% dieser Fälle konsultierten den Arzt wegen ihrer Migräne.

Die Migräne ist eine Anfallskrankheit, sie ist ausschließlich durch den in mehr-weniger regelmäßigen Perioden sich wiederholenden Migräneanfall gekennzeichnet. Der Migräneanfall stellt einen aus subjektiven Beschwerden und objektiven Krankheitserscheinungen zusammengesetzten Symptomenkomplex dar, welcher durch besondere Kombination und Variation dieser Teilsymptome dem ganzen Anfallssyndrom ein spezifisches Gepräge verleiht. Das Leitsymptom des Migräneanfalles ist der Kopfschmerz; die Begleiterscheinungen des Anfalles geben diesem eine besondere Charakteristik und ermöglichen eine Gruppierung der Migräneanfälle in besondere Unterformen. Wir sprechen in diesem Sinne von einer 1. gewöhnlichen Migräne, 2. ophthalmischen Migräne, 3. ophthalmoplegischen Migräne, 4. mit Epilepsie kombinierten Migräne und 5. von einer psychischen Migräne. Das klinische Bild des Migränesyndroms zeigt auch innerhalb der hier erwähnten Anfallsformen eine recht große Abwechslung; durch genauere Beobachtung der Krankheitsfälle haben wir neben den sog. typischen Fällen zahlreiche atypische Erscheinungsformen kennengelernt; hierher gehören die verschiedenen Migräneäquivalente, worunter rudimentäre Anfälle zu verstehen sind, in welchen der Kopfschmerz fehlt und nur eine, oder einige der zum Anfall gehörenden Begleiterscheinungen auftreten. Trotz der großen Verschiedenartigkeit, die sich in den Anfällen kundgibt, muß daran festgehalten werden, daß eine semiologische Sonderung der einzelnen Anfallsformen weder von nosologischem, noch von pathogenetischem Standpunkt aus berechtigt ist, da das Migränesyndrom mit seinen verschiedenen Erscheinungsformen eine einheitliche pathologische Reaktionsform des menschlichen Organismus darstellt. Hierfür spricht vor allem die Erfahrung, daß die verschiedenen

Anfallsformen bei ein und demselben Individuum abwechselnd auftreten können. In pathogenetischer Hinsicht erscheint es notwendig, von der echten Migräne als sog. „symptomatische Migräne" diejenigen Fälle abzusondern, in welchen die Migräneanfälle als Begleitsymptom einer organischen Erkrankung auftreten; sie müssen auch in prognostischer und therapeutischer Hinsicht anders beurteilt werden.

I. Symptomatologie des Migräneanfalles.
1. Allgemeines über das Auftreten, Periodizität, Dauer und Verlauf des Migräneanfalles.

Die Migräne ist die Krankheit des jugendlichen und mittleren Alters. Die gefährlichste Altersperiode für das erste Auftreten des Leidens liegt nach FLATAUS Statistik zwischen 16 und 35 Jahren. Nach anderen Angaben, wie z. B. von HEYERDAHL, GOWERS und MOEBIUS tritt sie in mehr als der Hälfte der Fälle in der Kindheit auf. Die Kindermigräne, mit welcher sich in neuerer Zeit mehrere Autoren (COMBY, HAMBURGER, CURSCHMANN) beschäftigten, offenbart sich gewöhnlich im Alter von 5—6 Jahren. FABRE, BOHNS, E. MENDEL u. a. beobachteten das Auftreten des ersten Anfalles schon im Säuglingsalter. Nach COMBY ist es charakteristisch für die Säuglingsmigräne, daß die Anfälle von kurzer Dauer sind, in 2—3 Stunden verlaufen, während die Anfälle der zweiten Kindheit schon 12—48 Stunden lang andauern. CURSCHMANN und HAMBURGER vermehren die Anzahl der Kindermigränefälle, indem sie das periodische Erbrechen mancher Kinder, bei denen eine erbliche Belastung vorliegt, als Migräneäquivalente einer sich später manifestierenden echten Migräne betrachten. (BALYEAT und RINKEL schätzen die Zahl der an Migräne leidenden Kinder unter 12 Jahren in den Vereinigten Staaten auf 1 Million!) Die Kindermigräne verschwindet nicht selten mit Eintritt der Pubertät und bleibt endgültig aus. In der Mehrzahl der Fälle setzt sie sich aber fort und begleitet den Kranken durch lange Zeit, bei Frauen auch in das postklimakterische Alter. Die mit der Pubertät oder genauer mit der ersten Menstruation einsetzende Migräne ist die häufigste Erscheinungsform der Frauenmigräne. Auch bei Männern ist die Pubertätsperiode entscheidend für das Auftreten der Migräne. Gar nicht selten beobachtet man aber, daß die menstruelle Migräne nicht im Beginn der Pubertät, sondern später, oft nach der Verheiratung, nach der Geburt eines Kindes auftritt und als menstruelle Migräne fortbesteht. Das 40. Lebensjahr wird von den meisten Autoren als die oberste Altersgrenze angegeben, bis zu welcher sich eine echte Migräne manifestieren kann. Ein nach diesem Alter auftretender erster Anfall legt den Verdacht einer symptomatischen Migräne nahe. Bei Frauen bedeutet der Wechsel ein kritisches Alter; bei der Mehrzahl hört in diesem Alter die Migräne auf. Es gibt aber Beobachtungen, laut welchen die ersten Migränefälle erst mit dem Unregelmäßigwerden der Menstruation oder nach Ausbleiben derselben, gewöhnlich in Begleitung von anderen klimakterischen nervösen Erscheinungen auftreten, oder daß die bis dahin mild verlaufende Migräne eine schwerere Form annimmt (RIVIÈRE spricht von einer „migraine tardivement aggravée"). Auch MATHIEU und ROUX beobachteten eine häufige Exacerbation der Migräneanfälle, schon im präklimakterischen Alter. CURSCHMANN erwähnt eine Umwandlung der Migräneanfälle in andere vasomotorische und sekretorische Anfallskrankheiten (Angina pectoris vasomotoria, Asthma, Colica mucosa), die sich im Klimax vollzieht.

Die *häufigere Erkrankung des weiblichen Geschlechtes* ist durch zahlreiche Statistiken älteren und neueren Datums zweifellos festgestellt. GOWERS, MOEBIUS und CURSCHMANN geben als Verhältniszahl 1,5 : 1, FLATAU 2,7 : 1, BING 4 : 1 an; auch ich fand im Krankenmaterial des öffentlichen Ambulatoriums die Verhältniszahl 4 : 1, während bei den Fällen meiner Privatpraxis die Proportion 1,7 : 1 sich ergab. Der Unterschied wird erklärlich, wenn man mit Curschmann annimmt, daß die Migräne in den intellektuellen Berufen entschieden häufiger vorkommt; die Männer des öffentlichen Ambulatoriums gehören durchweg der körperlich arbeitenden Klasse an, während in der Privatpraxis die Kopfarbeiter überwiegen. Nur in diesem Sinne kann man einen Unterschied zwischen den verschiedenen sozialen Schichten annehmen. Bei der Landbevölkerung scheint die Migräne seltener zu sein.

In einer jüngst erschienenen Arbeit behauptet Allan auf Grund erbbiologischer und statistischer Betrachtungen, daß das zahlenmäßige Überwiegen der weiblichen Migräne und die vorherrschende Vererbung von der Mutter auf die Tochter den tatsächlichen Verhältnissen nicht entspricht; wenn man bei der Diagnosenstellung streng kritisch vorgeht, dann findet man nach ihm gleiche Erkrankungszahlen für beide Geschlechter.

Die Periodizität der Anfälle ist eines der wichtigsten Erkennungszeichen der Migräne. Durch die regelmäßige Wiederholung in bestimmten Zeitperioden unterscheidet sich der Migränekopfschmerz deutlich von den übrigen Kopfschmerzarten. Die klassische Form repräsentiert die Migräne des weiblichen Geschlechtes, bei welcher der Anfall mit der ersten Menstruation einsetzt und sich bis zum Wechsel bei jeder Menstruation wiederholt, entweder derselben um 1—2 Tage vorauseilend oder während der Menstruation und seltener nach der Menstruation auftretend. Das Ausbleiben der Menses während der Gravidität und in der ersten Zeit der Lactation bringt in diesen Fällen fast immer auch den Migräneanfall zum Verschwinden. Die Periodizität ist aber nicht immer an die Menstruation gebunden. Die Intervalle können kürzere oder längere sein, nicht selten beobachtet man 7, 10 oder 14tägige Intervalle. Auch bei Männern begegnet man oft einer Wiederholung in regelmäßigen Abständen, wenn dies auch weniger ausgesprochen ist als bei den Frauen. K. Mendel und Church nehmen auch hier eine der weiblichen analoge Wellenbewegung im Ablauf der sexuellen Vorgänge als Ursache der Periodizität an; hierfür scheinen zu sprechen einige Beobachtungen, nach welchen die Migräne der Männer oft nach einem Coitus aufzutreten pflegt. Einer meiner Patienten gab an, sich seit einigen Monaten vom geschlechtlichen Verkehr deshalb zurückgehalten zu haben, weil er nach jedem Coitus einen sich von den üblichen Anfällen durch besondere Intensität auszeichnenden Anfall bekam. Über ähnliche Fälle berichtet Flatau. Ich beobachtete bei einem Beamten seit Jahren eine Sonntagsmigräne, die sich aber auch an anderen Feiertagen, wo er nicht ins Amt ging, wiederholte. Längere Intervalle (3—6 Monate, auch mehrere Jahre) beobachtet man bei der ophthalmischen und ophthalmoplegischen Migräne. Es gibt auch Kranke, die nach ihrer Angabe in ihrem ganzen Leben nur einen oder zwei Migräneanfälle gehabt haben. Die Periodizität der Anfälle ist auch bei ein und demselben Individuum größeren Schwankungen ausgesetzt. Oft wird angegeben, daß die Anfälle früher schwach und selten kamen, später häufiger und intensiver auftraten. Auch kommt es vor, daß die Anfälle zeitweise gehäuft auftreten, namentlich nach größeren Pausen. Bei vielen Migränekranken bringt die kalte Jahreszeit eine Häufung der Anfälle, bei manchen zeichnet sich die Frühjahrsmigräne durch Häufung der Anfälle aus. Bei Verschlimmerung des Migränezustandes werden die Intervalle zwischen den einzelnen Anfällen immer geringer und es kann auch ein solcher Zustand eintreten, daß infolge der dichten Aufeinanderfolge der eine Anfall noch gar nicht abgeklungen ist und schon ein neuer mit erhöhter Intensität einsetzt; diesen Zustand bezeichnete Flatau als Status hemicranicus, Oppenheim als Hemicrania permanens.

Die Dauer des Migräneanfalles ist sowohl im allgemeinen, wie auch im Einzelfall verschieden; sie wechselt mit der Intensität des Anfalles. In der Mehrzahl der Fälle wird über eine eintägige (12stündige) Dauer berichtet; der Anfall beginnt in der Früh beim Erwachen aus dem Schlaf und endet abends mit dem Einschlafen. Manche Kranken erwachen schon mit Kopfschmerz aus dem Nacht- oder Tagesschlaf. Gar nicht selten sind aber Abweichungen nach beiden Richtungen hin. Viele Kranken geben eine halbtägige Dauer ihrer Anfälle an. Ich beobachtete bei einem 30jährigen Mann eine seit 10 Jahren bestehende Migräne, wo der Anfall $1—1^1/_2$ Stunden dauert; auch bei ophthalmischer Migräne habe ich das Abklingen der visuellen Erscheinungen und des nachfolgenden Kopfschmerzes binnen 2 Stunden beobachtet. Nach MOEBIUS gibt es Anfälle, die nur einige Minuten lang dauern. Andererseits wird mitunter über eine längere Anfallsdauer berichtet, die sich auf mehrere Tage oder auch auf 1—2 Wochen erstreckt. Die Intensität des Kopfschmerzes und der übrigen Begleiterscheinungen pflegt gewöhnlich im späteren Verlauf des Anfalles etwas nachzulassen. OPPENHEIM bezeichnete diese Anfälle mit protrahiertem Verlauf als Hemicrania continua.

2. Der gewöhnliche (vulgäre) Migräneanfall.

Der gewöhnliche Migräneanfall ist die häufigste Erscheinungsform der Migräne. In der Mehrzahl der Fälle tritt er ohne vorausgehende Symptome, gewöhnlich in den Morgenstunden beim Erwachen aus dem Schlaf auf. In einer Minderzahl der Fälle wird er durch eigentümliche Vorboten, die sog. *Auraerscheinungen*, eingeleitet, die dem Anfall um einige Stunden, oft auch 1 bis 2 Tage vorauseilen. Die Aurasymptome sind recht abwechslungsreich, wiederholen sich aber im Einzelfall mit einer großen Beständigkeit; bei heftigeren Attacken treten sie deutlicher hervor. Am häufigsten zeigen sie sich auf psychischem Gebiet: Ein unbegründeter Stimmungswechsel mit schlechtem Allgemeinbefinden, Mattigkeit, lästige Müdigkeit, Unfähigkeit zur geistigen Arbeit, Unlust zu jeder aktiven Betätigung kennzeichnen das Herannahen des Anfalles, dabei ist die Gemütsverfassung meist eine deprimierte, viel seltener eine erregte (type de depression und type d'excitation von GRASSET-RAUZIER), bei letzterer innere Unruhe, Ungeduld. Fahle Gesichtszüge, trübe, glanzlose, eingefallene Augen verraten oft auch äußerlich diesen Zustand. Mitunter wird das seelische Unbehagen durch flüchtige, quälende körperliche Sensationen noch mehr gestört. Oppressionsgefühl in der Brust, stichartige Schmerzen in der Herzgegend, Magenschmerzen, Frösteln, Kaltwerden der Finger, häufiger Harndrang, Stuhldrang, lästige Erectionen wechseln im bunten Bild der Auraperiode. Gelegentlich wird Heißhunger oder Durst empfunden. Interessant ist die Beobachtung von SIMON, die er bei einer an Migräne leidenden Mutter und Tochter machte. Beide haben einige Tage vor ihren Anfällen ein unstillbares Verlangen nach salzigen und sauren Flüssigkeiten, ohne daß ein erhöhtes Durstgefühl oder vermehrte Harnsekretion bestünde. LIVEING machte auf schreckhafte Nachtträume aufmerksam, die besonders bei Kindern vor dem Migräneanfall aufzutreten pflegen. Es sind auch von seiten der Sinnesorgane verschiedene Sensationen als Aurasymptome beobachtet worden: Geruchs- und Geschmackshalluzinationen, Schwerhörigkeit, Schwindel und flüchtige Sehstörungen. FLATAU beobachtete in der Aura schwerer Migräneanfälle faszikuläre Zuckungen in verschiedenen Muskelgebieten des Körpers, die oft ihren Platz wechseln. Auch kurz dauernde Aphasien und Parästhesien kommen vor.

Der eigentliche Migräneanfall beginnt mit dem Einsetzen *des Kopfschmerzes* und wird von diesem bis zum Ende beherrscht. Der Kopfschmerz bestimmt die Intensität des Anfalles. Meist beginnt er mit einem leichten Druck an einer bestimmten Kopfstelle, welcher an Stärke und Ausbreitung allmählich zunimmt und auf der Höhe des Anfalles seine schmerzhafte Art gewöhnlich wechselt: doch kommt es nicht immer zu einer vollen Entwicklung dieses intensiven Kopfschmerzes. Es gibt leichte Anfälle, wo der Kopfschmerz über die anfängliche Phase hinaus nicht zunimmt und der Anfall in einigen Stunden abklingt. Die Qualität des Kopfschmerzes wird von den Kranken sehr verschieden gekennzeichnet. LABARRAQUE sagt: »Chacun souffre à sa manière«. Am häufigsten wird er als bohrend, klopfend, schlagend, schneidend, reißend, spannend bezeichnet. In einigen Fällen empfinden die Kranken ein lebhaftes Hitzegefühl im Kopf. PISON kennzeichnete seinen eigenen Kopfschmerz so, als wolle sich die Coronarnaht spalten. Auf der Höhe des Kopfschmerzes klagen viele Kranke über heftige Stiche an einer umschriebenen Stelle, die an Schmerzhaftigkeit den allgemeinen Kopfschmerz noch übertrifft. Der Migränekopfschmerz ist ein ausgesprochener Tiefenkopfschmerz; doch kommt es gar nicht selten vor, daß auf der Höhe des Anfalles sich auch ein oberflächlicher Kopfschmerz hinzugesellt, der sich in den verschiedenen Deckschichten und Nachbargebieten des Schädels bemerkbar macht. Die Intensität des Kopfschmerzes zeigt nicht immer einen allmählichen Auf- und Abstieg, vielmehr beobachtet man wellenartige Schwankungen, zeitweiliges Abflauen mit neuerlicher Verschärfung, die sich öfters wiederholen kann. Bei leichterem Kopfschmerz verrichtet der Kranke noch mechanisch seine Tagesarbeit, der stärkere Anfall zwingt aber die Kranken sich zurückzuziehen, jede körperliche oder geistige Arbeit von sich fernzuhalten. Sie liegen stundenlang bewegungslos in einem abgesonderten, verdunkelten Zimmer, schließen sich von ihrer Umgebung ab und erwarten mit Sehnsucht den Schlaf, der den Anfall zum Schwinden bringt. Jede Bewegung, die geringste körperliche Anstrengung, jeder stärkere Sinnesreiz, sowie die geringste geistige Anstrengung können den Kopfschmerz verstärken. Leichte Kopfschmerzen können durch psychische Einwirkungen günstig beeinflußt werden.

Der Kopfschmerz ist in der Mehrzahl der Fälle halbseitig, doch gehört der beiderseitige Kopfschmerz ebenso zum Anfallsbild der Migräne. Beim Halbseitentypus gibt es Fälle, die immer auf einer Seite ihren Kopfschmerz haben und solche, wo der Kopfschmerz bei den verschiedenen Anfällen die Seite wechselt. Von Kranken dieser letzteren Kategorie hört man oft, daß die Intensität des Kopfschmerzes mit der Seite wechselt, so daß sie schon am Beginn des Anfalles die Intensität desselben voraussagen können. Gar nicht selten kommt es vor, daß halb- und beiderseitiger Kopfschmerz bei ein und demselben Kranken abwechselnd vorkommt oder daß der halbseitige Kopfschmerz auf der Höhe des Anfalles auf die andere Seite übergreift und als beiderseitiger Kopfschmerz weiterbesteht.

Was *den Sitz des Kopfschmerzes* anbelangt, muß man sagen, daß der Migränekopfschmerz sich an allen Schädelsegmenten bemerkbar machen kann; doch gibt es, wenn man die relative Häufigkeit gewisser Stellen berücksichtigt, einige Prädilektionsstellen, deren Kenntnis auch vom differentialdiagnostischen Standpunkt wichtig ist. Die meisten Autoren vermerken hier die Augen-, Stirn- und Schläfengegend an erster Stelle. Es gibt viele Kranke, deren Kopfschmerz sich ständig und fast ausschließlich in diesem Schädelgebiet lokalisiert, wobei die größte Schmerzhaftigkeit abwechselnd in der Augenhöhle selbst, am inneren Knochenrand der Orbita, an der Austrittsstelle des Nervus supraorbitalis, an einer umschriebenen Stelle der Schläfengegend oder in der Stirn angegeben wird. Befragt man aber diese Kranken, ob sie auch anderswo im Kopf Schmerzen haben, so erfährt man in den meisten Fällen, daß sie auch im Hinterhaupt einen Schmerz verspüren, dieser aber mehr ein dumpfer, druckartiger Schmerz ist, der gegen den scharfen, intensiven vorderen Kopfschmerz in Hintergrund tritt.

Intelligentere Kranke, die sich genauer beobachten, geben an, daß der Anfall regelmäßig mit einem dumpfen Hinterhauptschmerz einsetzt und sich erst später nach vorne ausstrahlt. Bei manchen Kranken bleibt der Kopfschmerz bis zum Ende auf das Hinterhaupt lokalisiert. Ich möchte diese Lokalisation des Migränekopfschmerzes deshalb mit Nachdruck betonen, weil der Hinterhauptschmerz von vielen Autoren als ein seltener bezeichnet wird und die Reihenfolge nach der Häufigkeit des Sitzes folgendermaßen angegeben wird: Augen- und Stirngegend, Schläfengegend, Schädeldach, Hinterhaupt. Im Gegensatz zu dieser Feststellung kann ich auf Grund eigener Erfahrungen bei mehr als 2000 Migränekranken behaupten, daß der Hinterhauptkopfschmerz fast in jedem einzelnen Fall vorhanden ist. Die Kranken geben meist die Nackengegend als schmerzhaft an. Die Nackenmuskulatur wird als druckempfindlich bezeichnet, doch ist dieser Nackenmuskelschmerz nur eine Begleiterscheinung des dumpfen, tiefen Kopfschmerzes, der in der hinteren Schädelgrube empfunden wird. Es ist sonderbar, daß der Hinterhauptschmerz des Migräneanfalles, welchen übrigens auch FLATAU und CURSCHMANN als isolierten Anfallskopfschmerz beobachteten, bei den meisten Autoren so wenig Berücksichtigung fand, wo es doch eine Reihe von Migränetheorien gibt, die ausschließlich auf die Schmerzhaftigkeit der Hinterhaupt- und Nackenmuskulatur gegründet sind. Für die Mehrzahl der typischen halbseitigen Migräneanfälle konnte ich folgende Ausbreitungsweise des Kopfschmerzes feststellen: Der Anfall setzt mit einem dumpfen Hinterhauptschmerz ein, welcher von einem Nackenmuskelschmerz begleitet wird. Von hier strahlt der Schmerz in den vorderen Schädelpol derselben Seite aus, wo er eine erhöhte Intensität erlangt. Bei weiterer Irradiation werden Schläfengegend oder Schädeldach ergriffen und die Schmerzhaftigkeit kann sich zum Schluß im Hinterhaupt noch erhöhen. In manchen Fällen erfolgt die Ausbreitung des Kopfschmerzes nicht in dieser Reihenfolge; es kommt vor, daß die Augen-Stirngegend verschont bleibt und nur die Schläfengegend schmerzhaft ist, oder, daß der Schmerz vom Beginn an im Schädeldach am stärksten ist; den Beginn mit einem leichten Hinterhauptschmerz wird man aber in den meisten Fällen nachweisen können. Es kommt vor, daß der Kopfschmerz sich auch auf andere, außerhalb des Schädels liegende Gebiete ausbreitet; am häufigsten auf die Weichteile der hinteren Hals- und oberen Rückengegend, oft auch auf das Gebiet zwischen den Schulterblättern, vorne auf die der schmerzenden Kopfseite entsprechende Gesichtshälfte und seltener in das gleichseitige Armgebiet.

Ein den Migräneanfall regelmäßig begleitendes Symptom besteht in der auffallenden Druckempfindlichkeit der Austrittsstelle des Nervus supraorbitalis auf der Seite des Kopfschmerzes. Ich habe auf dieses Zeichen schon früher aufmerksam gemacht und von mehreren Autoren die Zuverlässigkeit dieses Symptoms bestätigt erhalten. Der Austrittspunkt dieses Nerven ist nicht nur bei solchen Anfällen druckempfindlich, wo der Kopfschmerz in der Stirn- oder Augengegend, also im Gebiet des ersten Trigeminusastes sitzt, sondern in allen Migränefällen. Sein direkter Zusammenhang mit dem Anfallssyndrom erhellt daraus, daß die Druckempfindlichkeit mit dem Ende des Anfalles aufhört.

Unter den Begleitsymptomen des Migräneanfalles stehen Reizerscheinungen von seiten des Magens als *Brechreiz oder Erbrechen* im Vordergrund. Nach den statistischen Erhebungen von LIVEING, MOEBIUS, HENSCHEN u. a. kann man sagen, daß diese in der weitaus größeren Hälfte der Migränefälle vorhanden sind. Der Brechreiz tritt gewöhnlich schon zu Beginn des Kopfschmerzes auf und begleitet diesen oft während des ganzen Anfalles; manchmal tritt er während des Anfalles nur zeitweise auf. Es gibt viele Migränefälle, in welchen es bei bestehendem Brechreiz zu keinem Erbrechen kommt; häufiger ist jedoch die Art, daß der Brechreiz sich allmählich steigert und mit einem

Erbrechen endet. Oft bedeutet das Erbrechen das Ende des Anfalles und wird von den Kranken als ein verläßliches Zeichen des sich lösenden Anfalles betrachtet. Nicht immer ist aber dies der Fall, denn es gibt Fälle, wo das Crescendo Brechreiz-Erbrechen sich während des Anfalles mehrmals wiederholt. Mitunter tritt das Erbrechen schon zu Beginn des Anfalles auf mit einem wässerigen, später galligen Erbrechen aus dem nüchternen Magen. Es gibt auch solche Fälle, wo das Erbrechen während des ganzen Anfalles nicht aufhört und sich später in qualvollen, leeren Brechbewegungen äußert. Erfolgt das Erbrechen im späteren Verlauf des Anfalles, so ist das Erbrochene ein zäher, schlecht verdauter Speisebrei; auch Bluterbrechen wurde beobachtet. Brechreiz und Erbrechen bleiben im Einzelfall beständige Begleitsymptome des Migräneanfalles, doch auch hier gibt es Ausnahmen. Von vielen Kranken werden als leichte Anfälle diejenigen bezeichnet, wo nur Brechreiz besteht, als schwere, die mit Erbrechen einhergehen. Auch kann sich das Bild des Migräneanfalles im Laufe der Jahre so ändern, daß Brechreiz und Erbrechen eine Zeit lang aus dem Anfallsbild verschwinden. Es gibt Kranke, die während ihrer Migräneanfälle überhaupt nie Magenerscheinungen hatten.

Als objektive Magenveränderungen während des Anfalles wurde Erweiterung des Magens (MANGELSDORF) und Pylorospasmus (PEST) beobachtet.

Zahlreiche Beobachtungen bestätigen, daß Magenerscheinungen von den übrigen Anfallssymptomen losgelöst, als Migräneequivalente den Anfall vertreten können. Bei Kindern scheint diese Form häufiger vorzukommen, wie es die Beobachtungen von BUCHANAN, GORDON, DEBRÉ, FABRE, CURSCHMANN, HAMBURGER bestätigen. Es wurden aber solche Magenäquivalente auch bei Erwachsenen beobachtet (BLITZSTEIN und BRAMS, A. SCHMIDT, ROSSBACH). Es handelt sich bei diesen Zuständen entweder um periodisch sich wiederholende Brechanfälle, die bei Kindern aus migränösen Familien ohne jede äußere Ursache und ohne Zeichen einer Magenerkrankung auftreten und später nach dem Einsetzen von typischen Migräneanfällen wieder verschwinden oder um periodische Schmerzattacken in der Magen- oder Nabelgegend, die später in der Pubertät durch Migräneanfälle ersetzt werden. BLITZSTEIN und BRAMS berichten über 32 Fälle von sog. Bauchmigräne, in welchen heftige Schmerzanfälle im Epigastrium 1—4 Tage lang bestanden, bei sonst gesunden Leuten, die aus einer migränösen Familie stammen, unter welchen es auch solche gab, bei denen vor oder nach diesen periodischen Bauchkoliken typische Migräneanfälle sich zeigten. Das intermittierende Auftreten von periodischem Erbrechen und typischen Migräneanfällen wurde auch von anderen Autoren beobachtet.

Eine eigene Beobachtung, die zu diesen Fällen eingereiht werden kann, betrifft einen 26jährigen, von mütterlicher Seite mit Migräne erblich belasteten jungen Mann, der im Alter zwischen 13—19 Jahren einige halbseitige Kopfschmerzanfälle mit Brechreiz und Erbrechen hatte; im Alter von 21 und 26 Jahren hatte er zwei 24stündige Attacken, die aus einem überaus heftigen, sich stündlich wiederholenden und unstillbaren Erbrechen bestanden; Kopfschmerzen sowie die anderen Anfallssymptome fehlten. Das beängstigende Bild der ersten Attacke, wo das später Erbrochene schon blutige Färbung zeigte, veranlaßten den behandelnden Arzt, eine Laparatomie vorzuschlagen, die mit negativem Befund endete. Der zweite Anfall, den ich beobachtete und auf Grund der Anamnese als eine Migräneäquivalente auffaßte, verlief nach 24 Stunden spurlos.

Bei Kranken, die im Anfall an Brechreiz oder Erbrechen leiden, besteht während des Anfalles Appetitlosigkeit, oft ausgesprochene Abscheu gegen das Essen. Migränekranke, deren Anfälle ohne Brechreiz oder Erbrechen verlaufen, zeigen oft auch Appetitlosigkeit, manche dagegen einen ausgesprochenen Drang zum Essen und fühlen nach jeder Nahrungsaufnahme eine gewisse Erleichterung.

Eine weitere charakteristische Begleiterscheinung des gewöhnlichen Migräneanfalls offenbart sich *im psychischen Verhalten* der Kranken. Dieselben Erscheinungen, die man bei manchen Migränekranken unter den Aurasymptomen findet, zeigen sich in den meisten Fällen während des Anfalles, also seelische Verstimmung, Apathie, Abnahme der Willenskraft. Über diese Störungen soll bei der psychischen Migräne ausführlicher berichtet werden. Hier möchte ich nur kurz darauf hinweisen, daß die psychische Alteration, die sich im Migräneanfall einstellt, nicht die Folgeerscheinung des Kopfschmerzes und der übrigen peinlichen Anfallssymptome ist, sondern ein selbständiges Symptom des Anfalles darstellt. Dies beweisen die Fälle, in welchen die psychische Störung als einzige Manifestation in Erscheinung tritt (psychische Migräneäquivalente).

Zu den hier geschilderten Symptomen, die man als regelmäßige Begleiterscheinungen des Kopfschmerzes betrachten kann, gesellen sich dann weitere Symptome, die aber an Beständigkeit weit zurückstehen. Man kann sie nach FLATAU am zweckmäßigsten in drei Gruppen einteilen.

1. Erscheinungen von seiten des Halssympathicus. Sie wurden von DUBOIS, MÖLLENDORF, EULENBURG, MOEBIUS u. a. eingehend dargestellt und als Reiz- und Lähmungserscheinungen des Halssympathicus beschrieben worden. Als Reizerscheinungen sind bekannt: Verengung der Blutgefäße am Gesicht (Gesichtsblässe), kontrahierte, stark pulsierende Schläfenarterie, vermehrter Speichelfluß, Erweiterung der Lidspalte und vor allem eine Erweiterung der Pupille auf der Seite des Kopfschmerzes. Letzteres Symptom, die isoliert erweiterte Pupille mit träger, oder manchmal auch fehlender Reaktion, beobachteten E. MENDEL, PÄSSLER, CURSCHMANN, WESTPHAL und auch ich wiederholt. Als Lähmungserscheinungen von seiten des Halssympathicus wurden Rötung des Gesichts und der Bindehaut, Verengerung der Lidspalte und der Pupille, Tränenfluß und am häufigsten eine leichtere Ptose beobachtet. Die Einteilung der Migränefälle in eine angiospastische und angioparalytische, wie sie auf Grund der hier angeführten Reiz- oder Lähmungserscheinungen vorgenommen wurde, ist aber schon aus dem Grunde ungerechtfertigt, weil im Einzelfall neben Reizsymptomen gleichzeitig Lähmungserscheinungen bestehen können. Auch findet man am häufigsten nur vereinzelte Symptome von seiten des Halssympathicus.

Hierher gehören als durch den Halssympathicus bedingte Zirkulationsstörungen, vorübergehende Schwellungen im Haut- und Schleimhautgebiet des Kopfes, die Ähnlichkeit mit dem QUINCKE-Ödem aufweisen. Diese Schwellungen in umschriebenen Bezirken der Kopfhaut, in den Augenlidern, Lippen treten gewöhnlich während des Anfalles, manchmal auch vor dem Kopfschmerz auf. Ein analoger Vorgang kann sich auch in der Rachenschleimhaut und in der Nasenschleimhaut abspielen, wobei der sog. vasomotorische Schnupfen oder Rachenkatarrh entsteht. Gewöhnlich ist die der schmerzenden Kopfhälfte entsprechende Nasenhälfte angeschwollen; ein wäßrig schleimiger Ausfluß aus diesem Nasenloch pflegt diesen vasomotorischen Schnupfen zu beenden, der zumeist nur wenige Stunden andauert. Manchmal besteht nur eine leichte Schwellung ohne Ausfluß. Als vasomotorische Störungen können die Blutungen aufgefaßt werden, die während des Anfalles am Gesicht, in der Nase, oder auf der Netzhaut beobachtet wurden; diese kommen aber nur selten vor. M. ULRICH sah unter ihren 500 Fällen fünfmal halbseitiges Schwitzen am Gesicht, nur zweimal auf der Seite des Kopfschmerzes.

2. Erscheinungen von seiten der übrigen Sympathicusabschnitte. Als solche sind vor allem die Herzbeschwerden aufzufassen, die sich in der Aura oder während des Anfalles einstellen. Ein sehr häufiges Begleitsymptom ist die Beschleunigung der Herzaktion mit dem subjektiven Gefühl des Herzklopfens; Neigung zu Tachykardie besteht bei diesen Kranken auch in der anfallsfreien Zeit (nach Aufregungen, Übermüdung). Andere klagen über quälende Schmerzsensationen in der Herzgegend (Stiche, Beklemmung, Angstgefühl). Seltener ist eine Bradykardie während des Anfalles. CURSCHMANN beschrieb unter dem Namen Angina pectoris vasomotoria ein aus heftigem Herzklopfen, Schmerz und Druck in der Herzgegend und Todesangst bestehendes Herzsyndrom als Begleiterscheinung des Migräneanfalles, welches manchmal auch als selbständige Migräneäquivalente auftreten kann. THOMAS stellt die von seiten der Brustorgane beobachteten Krankheitssymptome als „Brustmigräne" der Bauchmigräne zur Seite und nimmt innige Beziehungen auch zwischen paroxysmaler Tachykardie und Migräne an.

Von Darmstörungen kommen Diarrhöen häufiger als Stuhlverstopfung vor. Nach CURSCHMANN begleiten solche nur die schweren Anfälle; BERGER beschrieb wäßrige Stuhlentleerungen im Anfall. Häufig handelt es sich um das Zustandsbild einer Colitis mebranacea. Darmkoliken können bei Migränekranken als periodisch auftretende Äquivalente in Erscheinung treten. CURSCHMANN beobachtete einen 13jährigen Jungen, der seit dem 11. Lebensjahr zweiwöchentlich an Darmkolikanfällen litt, die gewöhnlich von einem Asthmaanfall begleitet waren; mitunter gesellten sich rechtsseitige Migräneanfälle hinzu. Nicht wenige Kranke klagen über einen lästigen Harndrang während des Anfalles, der sie häufig zur Miktion zwingt, wobei ein heller Urin in dünnem Strahl entleert wird (spastischer Urin). Seltener begegnet man der Erscheinung, daß die Kranken während des Anfalles überhaupt keinen Harn entleeren und ein ausgiebiges Urinieren das Ende des Anfalles ankündigt. Quälende, lang anhaltende Erektionen ohne Libido kommen während des Anfalles öfters vor.

Als Sympathicusreizerscheinungen an den Gliedmaßen beobachtet man öfters schmerzhafte Parästhesien, Kaltwerden der Hände und Füße, Schweißausbrüche, seltener eine Pulsverkleinerung an der kontrahierten Arteria radialis. Schon FÉRÉ beobachtete lokale Asphyxie und Akrocyanose an den Fingern oder Zehen.

CURSCHMANN sah bei einem 42jährigen Arzt während des Anfalles linsen- bis pfenniggroße Bläschen in der linken Hohlhand und im linken vierten Finger sowie auf der vierten Zehe des linken Fußes; vor dem Auftreten der Bläschen bestand heftiges Jucken an den genannten Stellen. Der Kranke zeigte in der anfallsfreien Zeit Ödeme und Urticaria. Alleinstehend ist auch eine andere Beobachtung von CURSCHMANN, die eine 28jährige Frau betrifft, bei welcher während ihrer selten auftretenden aber schweren Migräneanfälle (Übelkeit, Erbrechen, Fernsehen und rechtsseitiges Scotom) eine Anschwellung der Brustdrüse mit Sekretion von Colostrum beobachtet wurde.

Temperaturerhöhungen wurden während des Migräneanfalles von mehreren Autoren (FLATAU, GOWERS, CURSCHMANN) beobachtet, besonders bei Kindern und thermolabilen Menschen; DETERMAN beschrieb Anfälle mit regelmäßigen Temperaturen bis 40° C.

3. Reizsymptome von seiten der Hirnnerven. Auch solche gehören zu den häufigen Begleitsymptomen des gewöhnlichen Migräneanfalles. Der Reizzustand des Trigeminus und Vagus ist eine regelmäßige Begleiterscheinung des Anfalles, als deren Symptome der Schmerz im Stirn- und Augenast, die Lichtscheu, die Druckempfindlichkeit des Nervus supraorbitalis, sowie Brechreiz und Erbrechen schon früher erwähnt wurden. Seltener kommt es vor, daß der Kopfschmerz sich auch auf das Gebiet des zweiten und dritten Trigeminusastes erstreckt und flüchtige Parästhesien am Gesicht oder in einer Zungenhälfte auftreten. Auch die Überempfindlichkeit der Kopfhaut (Haarweh) wurde beobachtet. Als Vagusreizsymptom kann auch das Gähnen und Niesen aufgefaßt werden, die allerdings selten vorkommen (FLATAU). Ein relativ häufiges Begleitsymptom des gewöhnlichen Migräneanfalles bildet der Schwindel. Manchmal tritt er in Begleitung von Ohrensausen auf, öfters jedoch ohne dieses. Eine mit der Seite des Kopfschmerzes zusammenhängende Gesetzmäßigkeit in der

Richtung des Schwindels konnte nicht festgestellt werden. Es handelt sich nicht um einen Drehschwindel, sondern zumeist um ein subjektives Unsicherheitsgefühl, welches die Kranken zwingt, sich niederzulegen. Manchmal erscheint der Schwindel nur im Beginn des Anfalles, manchmal besteht er stundenlang (Weiteres hierüber bei der ophthalmoplegischen Migräne).

Als Reizsymptom des Nervus facialis wurden tickartige Bewegungen, Zuckungen und Spasmen in einzelnen Gesichtsmuskeln mehrfach (CORNU, FÉRÉ, FLATAU, MEIGE) beschrieben, am häufigsten Blepharospasmus. MEIGE erblickt in den Gesichtsspasmen solcher Leute die früher an Migräneanfällen litten, Äquivalente dieser Anfälle. Häufig geht mit dem Gesichtskrampf eine lebhafte Rötung des Gesichts einher. Die Gesichtskrämpfe können halb- oder beiderseitig auftreten. Die halbseitigen werden als Reizzustand des Gesichtsnervs aufgefaßt, die beiderseitigen führt SICARD auf einen Sympathicusreiz zurück. FLATAU nimmt für manche Fälle einen corticalen Ursprung an. Auch von seiten des Sehnerven wurden mehrfach Reizerscheinungen beschrieben, die sich aber von der Sehstörung des ophthalmischen Migräneanfalles zumeist dadurch unterscheiden, daß die Sehstörung eine sehr flüchtige ist und meistens nur ein Auge betrifft. Es treten dabei schwarze oder leuchtende Punkte im Gesichtsfeld auf, oder es tritt eine Verschleierung des Sehens, Verdunkelung des ganzen Gesichtsfeldes auf. Wiederholt wurde in solchen Fällen ein Spasmus der zentralen Netzhautarterie festgestellt. In einem Fall von Voss kam es zu einer dauernden Erblindung, verursacht durch eine Blutung aus dem zentralen Netzhautgefäß. Geruchs- und Geschmacksparästhesien (Metallgeschmack, Veilchenduft) beschrieben LIVEING, NICATI, ROBIOLIS u. a.

Allgemeine Überempfindlichkeit der Sinnesorgane kennzeichnet die meisten Migräneanfälle; stärkere Sinneseindrücke auf optischem, akustischem, olfaktorischem und gustatorischem Gebiet werden von den meisten Migränekranken im Anfall schlecht vertragen.

Das Ende des Anfalles fällt mit dem Aufhören des Kopfschmerzes zusammen; bei allmählicher Abnahme des Kopfschmerzes tritt zumeist ein tiefer Schlaf ein, aus welchem die Kranken in einem Zustand körperlichen Wohlbehagens erwachen. Seltener kommt es vor, daß Kranke nach schweren Anfällen noch am folgenden Tag über eine gewisse Benommenheit im Kopf klagen. Wahrscheinlich spielt bei diesen Zuständen die reichliche Einnahme von analgetischen Mitteln am Vortage auch eine Rolle.

3. Die Augenmigräne.
(Migraine ophthalmique).

CHRISTIANSEN erblickt im ophthalmischen Migräneanfall den kompletten, voll entwickelten Migräneanfall und faßt den gewöhnlichen Anfall nur als eine rudimentäre Offenbarung der Migräne auf. Er weist darauf hin, daß Leute, die Jahre hindurch an gewöhnlichen Migräneanfällen leiden, einmal oder einigemal typische, ophthalmische Anfälle bekommen und betont, daß alle Symptome der Augenmigräne vereinzelt auch beim einfachen Anfall vorkommen. Bei Anerkennung seiner Argumente möchte ich eine gewisse Sonderstellung der verschiedenen Anfallsarten schon deshalb aufrecht halten, weil sie in prognostischer Hinsicht doch nicht gleichmäßig beurteilt werden können. Die Augenmigräne ist im Verhältnis zur einfachen Migräne eine seltene Anfallsform und es käme die richtige Beurteilung der Krankheit zum Schaden, wenn man die gewöhnlichen Migräneanfälle, unter welchen es auch sehr schwere Formen gibt, als nicht zur Vollentwicklung gelangte Manifestationen betrachten würde. Die Statistiken über die Häufigkeit der Augenmigräne bringen recht breit variierende

Verhältniszahlen, so daß sie in dieser Hinsicht nicht leicht verwertbar sind. LIVEING fand unter 60 eigenen Migränefällen 37mal Sehstörungen, MOEBIUS unter 130 Fällen 14, FLATAU bei 500 Fällen 12%, meine eigene Statistik ergibt kaum 10%. Die Fälle, wo in der Aura des Anfalles leichte, einige Sekunden oder Minuten lang andauernde Sehstörungen und leuchtende Erscheinungen auftreten, die einmal da sind, das anderemal fehlen, können nicht zur Augenmigräne gerechnet werden, bei welcher die Sehstörung einen zeitlich und gegenständlich recht scharf begrenzten Zustand darstellt, der einen wesentlichen Bestandteil des Anfalles ausmacht. Das erste Auftreten der Augenmigräne wird am häufigsten zwischen dem 20. und 40. Lebensjahr beobachtet, doch sind Fälle verzeichnet, die auf ein früheres Einsetzen hindeuten (LECLERC beobachtete in 12 Fällen den Beginn zwischen 9 und 19 Jahren, FLATAU und ich sahen das erste Auftreten im 5. Lebensjahr). Bemerkenswert ist, daß im vorgerückten Alter die ophthalmische Migräne häufiger auftritt, als die gewöhnliche; GALEZOWSKI beobachtete in einem Fall das Auftreten des ersten Migräneanfalles im 80. Lebensjahr, MEIGE im 73. Lebensjahr. Bei einem von mir beobachteten 63jährigen Arzt, der früher an gewöhnlichen Migräneanfällen litt, trat nach einer 10jährigen Pause der erste Anfall von Augenmigräne auf; die offenkundige allgemeine Gefäßsklerose, die in diesem Falle vorlag, unterstützt den Verdacht, daß es sich hier schon um eine symptomatische Migräne handelte. Überhaupt lehrt die allgemeine Erfahrung, daß hinter den im vorgerückten Alter auftretenden oder sich häufenden ophthalmischen Migräneanfällen zumeist eine organische Gehirnschädigung im Hintergrunde steht.

Der Augenmigräneanfall setzt häufiger ohne Prodromalerscheinungen ein als der gewöhnliche, doch können auch hier die bei der gewöhnlichen Migräne bekannten Auraerscheinungen den Anfall einleiten. FÉRÉ verzeichnet unter diesen eigentümliche Träume visuellen Inhaltes (Brand, Vulkanausbrüche).

Die die Augenmigräne kennzeichnenden Sehstörungen sind von zweierlei Art: es gibt einfache Störungen des Sehvermögens und flimmernde, leuchtende Erscheinungen. Die ersteren können sich von einem leichten Nebel bis zur völligen Amaurose steigern, wobei die Sehstörung mehr-minder gleichmäßig auf das ganze Gesichtsfeld sich erstreckt; eine andere Form der einfachen Sehstörung stellen fleckförmige Ausfälle im Gesichtsfeld (Skotome) dar, die gewöhnlich im peripheren Gesichtsfeld beider Augen auftreten und sich allmählich vergrößernd die homonym hemianopische Form der Sehstörung annehmen. Das Skotom erreicht zumeist auch bei der vollentwickelten homonymen Hemianopsie nicht die Mittellinie, die Macula bleibt ausgespart; nach LAPERSONNE pflegt auch das Maculagebiet inbegriffen zu sein. Zentrales Skotom kommt nur äußerst selten vor (ANTONELLI), ist auch halbseitig (GRÜNSTEIN). CHARCOT beobachtete einmal eine binasale Hemianopsie (mit Taubheitsgefühl in beiden Händen). PANDELESCO-DUMITRESCO beschrieb einen Fall mit bitemporaler Hemianopsie; CASTERS und VAN BOGAERT einseitige nasale Hemianopsie und ringförmiges peripapilläres Skotom im temporalen Gesichtsfeld mit absoluter Pupillenstarre (Rückgang sämtlicher Erscheinungen in 4 Tagen). Beim Skotom wird gewöhnlich über ein Nichtsehen berichtet (negatives Skotom). Das Skotom ist nicht stabil, es vergrößert und verkleinert sich. Eine genaue Beschreibung der Skotombewegung gibt O. SITTIG (Eigenbeobachtung). Auch die Intensität des Skotoms wechselt (absolutes und relatives Skotom). Viel charakteristischer sind die Flimmererscheinungen, die zu den Skotomen hinzutreten. Diese Form der Sehstörung kommt weit häufiger vor. M. ULRICH fand sie in einem Drittel ihrer Migränefälle. Es sind hier vermerkt: Hin- und Herbewegen leichter Nebel und Schleier, vibrierender Luft, also eine Art oszillatorischer Sehstörung; Auftreten von brillanten Figuren, goldenem Regen, farbigen, sich wurmartig bewegenden Bändern, leuchtenden, weißen oder in den Spektralfarben variierenden, konzentrischen Ringen, oder von leuchtenden, an Fortifikationsmauer erinnernden Zickzacklinien, die das Skotom umgrenzen oder auch durchbrechen. Das sog. Flimmerskotom (Scotoma scintillans) vereinigt in sich flimmernde Erscheinungen mit dem Skotom. Über die zahlreichen Variationen des Flimmerskotoms sind wir aus zahlreichen fachmännischen Selbstbeobachtungen aus älterer und jüngerer Zeit (JOLLY, AIRY, SCHULTZE, PARALT, ROHRER, KRÄMER, BEYER, GRÜNSTEIN usw.) gut unterrichtet. Die häufigste Form ist die, wo an einer umschriebenen Stelle des Gesichtsfeldes, meistens in der Nähe der Mittellinie, ein leuchtender Punkt auftritt, der immer größer wird und sich zickzackförmig ausbreitend und fortwährend bewegend allmählich an der Peripherie verschwindet. Die Zickzackfigur begrenzt das Skotom. JOLLY beobachtete eine völlige Schließung des Skotoms durch die Flimmerfigur, nach CHARCOT ist der Ring nie geschlossen. Die Flimmererscheinungen treten zumeist halbseitig und in beiden Augen auf, doch gibt es einzelne Beobachtungen, wo nur das eine Auge betroffen ist (GALEZOWSKI, DETERMAN, FLATAU). Zentrale Flimmerskotome beschrieben FLATAU, HILPERT, BEYER.

Die Sehstörung weist bei ein und derselben Person eine gewisse Gleichmäßigkeit sowohl im Auftreten der Skotome wie auch der Flimmererscheinungen auf. Doch können die einzelnen Anfälle diesbezüglich manche Unterschiede aufweisen. BARALT z. B. beobachtete bei sich einmal einfache Skotome, das andere Mal leuchtende Skotome. Die Frage, ob Skotome oder flimmernde Erscheinungen zeitlich früher auftreten, kann nach den vorliegenden Beobachtungen nur so entschieden werden, daß beides vorkommen kann. Nach LIVEING soll häufiger das Skotom früher einsetzen als die Sehstörung. In einem von mir beobachteten Fall traten zuerst leuchtende weiße Ringe auf, dann kamen Zickzackfiguren und etwa 10 Minuten später begann allmählich das Sehvermögen zu verschwinden und es trat eine etwa $^1/_2$ Stunde lang andauernde vollkommene Amaurose auf. Bei dem echten Flimmerskotom scheinen jedoch Flimmern und Sehstörung auch zeitlich eng aneinander geknüpft zu sein. Die Dauer der Sehstörung erstreckt sich von einigen Minuten bis etwa eine halbe Stunde.

Die für die Augenmigräne charakteristischen Sehstörungen leiten den eigentlichen Kopfschmerzanfall ein. Es gibt aber einzelne Beobachtungen, welche darauf hinweisen, daß die Sehstörung auch allein, ohne von Kopfschmerz oder anderen Anfallssymptomen begleitet zu werden, auftreten kann. Solche Bruchteile des Migräneanfalles werden als Migräneäquivalente aufgefaßt. So sah ich bei einem Kollegen im 32. Lebensjahr eine etwa 10 Minuten lang andauernde rechtsseitige homonyme Hemianopsie, welcher erst ein halbes Jahr später ein echter ophthalmischer Migräneanfall folgte. Ähnliche formes frustes der Augenmigräne beobachteten GALEZOWSKI, MOEBIUS, AIRY, CHARCOT, FÉRÉ.

Der Kopfschmerz ist bei der ophthalmischen Migräne gewöhnlich sehr heftig. Seine Lokalisation entspricht der bei der gewöhnlichen Migräne beschriebenen. Neben der Augen- und Stirngegend möchte ich gegenüber CHRISTIANSEN besonders das häufige Betroffensein der Nacken- und Hinterhauptgegend betonen. Besteht eine hemianopische Sehstörung, so sitzt der Kopfschmerz auf der entgegengesetzten Seite. Dieser Beobachtung, die von den meisten Forschern bestätigt wurde, widersprechen die Selbstbeobachtung von JOLLY, sowie die Angabe von M. ULRICH, die unter 16 Fällen achtmal den Kopfschmerz auf der Seite des Skotomes verzeichnete. Bei einseitigem Skotom wird die Augengegend der betroffenen Seite als Sitz des Kopfschmerzes angegeben. Im allgemeinen setzt der Kopfschmerz nach Ablauf der Sehstörung ein, zumeist von Schwindel, Brechreiz oder Erbrechen begleitet. Ganz selten (FÉRÉ, GALEZOWSKI) kommt es vor, daß der Kopfschmerz früher auftritt als die Sehstörungen, oder daß letztere während des Kopfschmerzes in Erscheinung treten (FLATAU). Die Dauer und der weitere Verlauf des ophthalmischen Migräneanfalles zeigt gegenüber der gewöhnlichen Migräne keinen wesentlichen Unterschied.

Das abwechselnde Vorkommen von gewöhnlichen und ophthalmischen Migräneanfällen bei ein und derselben Person ist eine ziemlich häufige Erscheinung und bestätigt die innige Zusammengehörigkeit beider Anfallsformen; die ophthalmischen Anfälle zeichnen sich hier durch besondere Intensität des Kopfschmerzes und der übrigen Begleiterscheinungen aus.

CHARCOT und FÉRÉ bezeichneten als *dissoziierte Form der Augenmigräne* solche Anfälle, wo Teilsymptome des Anfalles (Sehstörung, Kopfschmerz, Schwindel) nicht zeitlich zusammenhängen, sondern durch freie Intervalle unterbrochen in Erscheinung treten.

Eine häufige Begleiterscheinung der Augenmigräne sind halbseitige, sensible Reiz- und Ausfallserscheinungen, welche schon von CHARCOT und FÉRÉ beschrieben und als kombinierte oder *assoziierte Form der Augenmigräne* bezeichnet wurden. Sie treten manchmal schon zu Beginn des Anfalles gleichzeitig mit der Sehstörung auf, in anderen Fällen erscheinen sie erst in der Periode des Kopfschmerzes. Betrifft die Gefühlsstörung die rechte Körperhälfte, dann ist sie häufig mit einer Sprachstörung verbunden; es gibt aber einige Beobachtungen, wo diese auch bei linksseitiger Hemiparästhesie auftrat. Unter den Gefühlsstörungen werden Kribbeln, Taubheitsgefühl, Herabsetzung der Tast- und Druckempfindlichkeit, Störung des Muskel- und Lagesinnes angegeben. Die von manchen Kranken geklagte „Lähmung" der Extremität wird durch die Ungeschicklichkeit der Bewegungen vorgetäuscht, deren Ursache in der Störung des Muskel- und Lagesinnes liegt. Die Gefühlsstörung erstreckt sich am häufigsten auf die eine Gesichtshälfte, Zungenhälfte und die obere Extremität. Äußerst selten ist die untere Extremität einbezogen. Die Seite der Gefühlsstörung ist regelmäßig der Seite des Kopfschmerzes entgegengesetzt und wenn es sich gleichzeitig um eine homonyme Hemianopsie handelt, mit der Seite dieser letzteren identisch. Eine ziemlich häufige Erscheinungsform der Gefühlsstörung ist nach CHRISTIANSEN die aufsteigende Parästhesie, die von den Fingern längs des Armes auf das Gesicht und die Zunge schleicht und als charakteristisch hebt er das langsame Tempo der Ausbreitung hervor. Oft dauert es 10 Minuten, bis die Parästhesie die Zunge erreicht.

In der Selbstbeobachtung von GRÜNSTEIN, wo die Parästhesie sich ganz allmählich von einem Finger auf den andern erstreckte, dauerte es 10—20 Minuten, bis die Parästhesie vom Kleinfinger aus den Daumen erreichte. Objektiv ließ sich taktile Anästhesie, Hyperalgesie und Herabsetzung der Temperaturempfindung im jeweiligen Auragebiet feststellen. In diesem Fall traten die Parästhesien noch vor den Skotomen auf.

Mitunter erstreckt sich die Gefühlsstörung auf beide Körperhälften und wird von einem diffusen, beiderseitigen Kopfschmerz begleitet.

Die Sprachstörung dauert gewöhnlich 10—15 Minuten. Sie tritt allmählich auf; zuerst fällt dem Kranken das Sprechen schwer, er bringt die Worte mühsam hervor, später bringt er unverständliche oder unrichtige Worte heraus und kann sich überhaupt nicht verständigen, zuletzt stammelt er nur die Worte „ja" und „nein" vor sich hin. Das Wortverständnis ist gut erhalten, das Nachsprechen oft gestört. Seltene Fälle von Worttaubheit beschrieben CHARCOT, PICK, SCHOB. Aphasie mit Agraphie und Paragraphie beschrieben PICK, FÉRÉ, DETERMAN u. a. Eine Kombination von Hemiparästhesie, Aphasie und homonymer Hemianopsie beschrieben SIEGRIST, MEIGE, H. ROGER (18 Fälle).

Motorische Reiz- und Ausfallserscheinungen kommen sowohl bei der Augenmigräne wie bei der gewöhnlichen Form nur äußerst selten vor. Was die Reizerscheinungen betrifft, muß mit Nachdruck betont werden, *daß die als motorische Rindenreizerscheinungen bekannten tonisch-klonischen Krämpfe bisher bei Migräneanfällen noch nie beobachtet wurden* [1]. FLATAU erwähnt in seiner Monographie einige Fälle, wo er im Anfall kurze, blitzartige Zuckungen im Gesicht oder in den Gliedern zumeist wahllos, manchmal auch halbseitig auftreten sah; auch berichtet er über myoklonische faszikuläre Zuckungen, die er regellos in verschiedenen Körpergebieten beobachtete. Ich sah solche niemals, dagegen wiederholt eine gewisse mimische Unruhe im Gesicht ohne rhythmischen Charakter. Es sind einige Fälle bekannt, wo im Verlauf einer Migräneattacke eine vorübergehende *Hemiplegie oder Hemiparese* auftrat. Interessant ist die Beobachtung von CLARK, in welcher mehrere Mitglieder einer Familie an Migräne mit Hemiplegie litten. Die regelmäßig wiederkehrenden Anfälle verliefen mit einseitigem Kopfschmerz, Erbrechen, Sehstörungen und Hemianopsie; Hemiplegie und motorische Aphasie traten als Auraerscheinungen vor dem Kopfschmerz auf. Das Bewußtsein war immer erhalten, Zuckungen, Spasmen, Sphincterlähmungen waren niemals vorhanden. Von den drei eigenen Beobachtungen über transitorische Hemiplegie bei Migräne soll hier folgender Fall kurz registriert werden.

43jähriger Fabriksbeamter, von mütterlicher Seite hereditär schwer belastet, leidet seit dem 12. Lebensjahr an periodisch auftretenden typischen Migräneanfällen mit wechselnder Seite. Seit 2 Jahren werden die Anfälle häufiger und intensiver. In der letzten Zeit nur linksseitige Anfälle, manchmal mit ophthalmischem Charakter. Nach Angabe seiner Frau erlitt er vor einigen Wochen bei einem solchen überaus heftigen Kopfschmerzanfall mit Sehstörung eine Lähmung der rechten Körperhälfte und verlor die Sprache. Das Bewußtsein blieb ungestört, Krämpfe wurden nicht beobachtet. Der Zustand hielt 10 Minuten lang an, worauf der Kranke seine rechten Glieder wieder anstandslos bewegen konnte und auch die Sprache zurückgewonnen hat. 3 Wochen später wiederholte sich dieser Zustand und dauerte etwa 1 Stunde lang. Die Sprachstörung war vom Charakter einer motorischen Aphasie; der Kranke verstand jedes Wort, konnte sich aber nicht ausdrücken und murmelte unverständliche Laute vor sich hin. Ich sah den Kranken unmittelbar nach Ablauf des Anfalles. Die Sprache war noch etwas verlangsamt, die rechtsseitigen Glieder schon gut beweglich, Triceps-, Knie- und Achillesreflex waren rechts lebhafter als links, keine Pyramidenzeichen, Sensibilität normal. Die allgemeine Untersuchung gab außer einer Anämie nichts Pathologisches.

Unter allen anderen Migräneformen ist es die Augenmigräne, die sich am häufigsten mit Epilepsie kombiniert.

Die Periodizität ist bei der Augenmigräne viel weniger ausgesprochen als bei der gewöhnlichen Migräne. Die Anfälle treten meist in größeren Intervallen, 6—12 Monaten, auf; es kommt vor, daß die Anfälle jahrelang ausbleiben und sich dann wieder häufen. Das bevorzugte Befallenwerden des weiblichen Geschlechtes ist bei der Augenmigräne weniger ausgesprochen als bei der gewöhnlichen Migräne.

Durch eine Reihe von Beobachtungen wird es bestätigt, daß nach Anfällen von Augenmigräne einzelne Funktionsausfälle nach dem Anfall weiter bestehen und kürzere oder längere Zeit hindurch nachgewiesen werden können. Dauerdefekte im Gesichtsfeld beschrieben PICHLER, RENTZ; ich sah in einem Fall eine quadrante Hemianopsie im linken oberen nasalen Gesichtsfeld, die erst nach drei Wochen verschwand. Permanente homonyme Hemianopsie beobachteten ORMOND, THOMAS, WIENER. FÉRÉ beobachtete die Stabilisierung der Aphasie nach einem Anfall. Es ist aber hier vor Augen zu halten, daß bei der Augenmigräne gar nicht selten organische Hirnveränderungen hauptsächlich vasculärer Natur das Krankheitsbild komplizieren.

---

[1] KRISCH beobachtete bei einigen Migränefällen choreatische Bewegungen in den Gliedern, die er auf einen Reizzustand des extrapyramidalen Systems zurückführt.

Wichtig ist in dieser Hinsicht der Fall von ALAJOUANINE, PETIT-DUTAILLIS und MONBRUN, wo bei einem 47jährigen Kranken seit dem 10. Lebensjahr Anfälle von ophthalmischer Migräne bestanden, zwischen dem 16. und 40. Lebensjahr ausblieben und dann wieder in der gleichen Art auftraten. Es bestand linksseitige Hemianopsie im unteren Quadranten, beiderseitige Stauungspapille, im Ventrikulogramm blieb das rechte Hinterhorn ungefüllt. Die Operation ergab ein Hämangiom des rechten Occipitallappens, nach dessen Entfernung die Krankheitssymptome verschwanden.

Dauerveränderungen im Auge wurden beschrieben von GALEZOWSKI, der in vier Fällen Thrombose und Embolie der Netzhautgefäße mit dem Augenspiegel feststellen konnte; WEGNER fand in zwei Fällen mit Erblindung Spasmus der Arteria centralis retinae, venöse Blutungen und Ödem des Augenhintergrundes. Ob diese Augenveränderungen mit der ophthalmischen Migräne selbst im Zusammenhang stehen, oder nur begleitende, akzidentelle Schädigungen darstellen, darüber soll bei der Besprechung der Pathogenese einiges gesagt werden.

4. Die ophthalmoplegische Migräne.

Die Streitfrage, ob diese Form der Migräne eine von den übrigen Migränearten abweichende selbständige Krankheit darstellt oder nicht, kann auch heute noch nicht als endgültig entschieden betrachtet werden. MOEBIUS verteidigte als erster die Sonderstellung dieser von ihm als ,,periodisch wiederkehrende Oculomotoriuslähmung" bezeichneten Fälle und seine Ansicht wurde von weiteren Forschern, so von MANZ und MAUTHNER, PALLET, MINGAZZINI unterstützt, wobei folgende Unterscheidungsmerkmale als Unterlagen zur Absonderung dieser Migräneform dienten: 1. Das seltenere Vorkommen der hereditären Belastung, 2. das Fehlen von Sehstörungen (Flimmerskotom im Anfall), 3. es kommt nicht zum Wechsel der Seite des Kopfschmerzes und der Lähmung, 4. die lange Dauer der Anfälle und unregelmäßige Perioden zwischen den Anfällen, 5. die Lähmung ist einseitig und total, 6. die Lähmung tritt erst nach Ablauf des Kopfschmerzes auf, sie kann im Intervall noch lange bestehen und oft zu dauernden Ausfallserscheinungen führen. CHARCOT verfocht als erster den gegenteiligen Standpunkt, nämlich daß die von ihm als ,,ophthalmoplegische Migräne" bezeichnete Form mit gleicher Berechtigung zur echten Migräne eingereiht werden kann, wie die ophthalmische oder assoziierte Migräne. CHARCOT stützte sich dabei als Hauptargument auf die allgemein bekannte Erfahrung, daß Kranke mit ophthalmoplegischer Migräne regelmäßig auch gewöhnliche Migräneanfälle aufweisen. MOEBIUS faßte diese zwischen den ophthalmoplegischen Anfällen auftretenden gewöhnlichen Migräneanfälle als unvollständige ophthalmoplegische Anfälle auf, in welchen es nicht zur Lähmung kam. CHARCOTS Standpunkt beherrschte die Stellungnahme der meisten Autoren in dieser Frage, auch FLATAU unterstützt in seiner Monographie diese Auffassung. Erst in den letzten Jahren mehren sich wieder die Stimmen, welche die unitarische Auffassung von CHARCOT bekämpfen und für die ophthalmoplegische Migräne eine Sonderstellung verlangen. Gerade der Kongreß der Französischen Neurologischen Gesellschaft, welcher im Jahre 1925 als Hundertjahrfeier dem Andenken CHARCOTS gewidmet war und als Thema die Migräne behandelte, zeigte sowohl die Referenten (CHRISTIANSEN, VALLERY-RADOT) als auch andere Teilnehmer auf der Seite der dualistischen Theorie. Maßgebend für diesen Umschwung waren zweifellos eine Anzahl von kasuistischen Beobachtungen der letzten Jahre, in welchen nach ophthalmoplegischer Migräne organische Veränderungen an der Hirnbasis oder an einzelnen Hirnnerven gefunden wurden. Es ist zuzugeben, daß unter den ophthalmoplegischen Migränefällen ein größerer Prozentsatz auf organisch bedingte sog. symptomatische Migränefälle fällt als bei den anderen Migräneformen, doch bilden auch diese Fälle nur einen geringen Bruchteil des gesamten klinischen Materials und ich möchte auf Grund eigener Erfahrungen bemerken, daß die ophthalmoplegische Migräne eine häufiger vorkommende Anfallsform darstellt, als man auf Grund der vorliegenden Literaturangaben anzunehmen geneigt ist. FLATAU zählt (bis 1911) 97 hierher gehörige Fälle. Ich besitze in meinem Krankenmaterial, welches ungefähr 2000 Fälle von Migräne umfaßt, 12 Beobachtungen von ophthalmoplegischer Migräne mit negativem organischen Befund, unter welchen natürlich nicht nur die Fälle von Oculumotoriuslähmung, sondern auch die mit Lähmung der übrigen Augenmuskelnerven einbezogen sind.

Der ophthalmoplegische Migräneanfall tritt gewöhnlich bei solchen Leuten auf, die schon früher an gewöhnlichen Migräneanfällen gelitten haben; nur selten ist die Verlaufsart verzeichnet, daß schon der erste Anfall ein ophthalmoplegischer war, welchem später gewöhnliche Migräneanfälle folgten (KARPLUS, KOLLARICH, SPILLER-POSEY). Auch im weiteren Verlauf treten zwischen den einzelnen ophthalmoplegischen Attacken vulgäre Migräneanfälle auf. Bezüglich des Alters, in welchem die ophthalmoplegische Migräne auftritt, kann der von MOEBIUS vertretene Satz, diese betreffe vornehmlich Kindheit und Jugend, angesichts der Literaturangaben nicht mehr aufrechterhalten werden; dieselben Schwankungen, die man bei der gewöhnlichen Migräne antrifft, lassen sich auch hier feststellen. Die zeitliche Distanz, die zwischen Beginn der gewöhnlichen Migräne und dem Auftreten der ersten ophthalmoplegischen Attacke besteht, zeigt auch große Schwankungen. Neben Fällen, in welchen beide Anfallsarten ungefähr gleichzeitig in Erscheinung traten, gibt es Beobachtungen, wie z. B. die von BOUCHARD, in welcher die Patientin mit 12 Jahren an gewöhnlicher Migräne erkrankte und ihren ersten ophthalmoplegischen Anfall im 60. Lebensjahr bekam. Ich beobachtete den ersten ophthalmoplegischen Anfall bei einer 62jährigen Frau, die seit 25 Jahren an gewöhnlicher Migräne litt.

Der ophthalmoplegische Anfall verläuft ebenso wie der gewöhnliche Migräneanfall, mit dem Unterschied, daß er von einer Augenmuskellähmung begleitet oder gefolgt wird. Der Kopfschmerz ist gewöhnlich einseitig und sehr heftig. In der überwiegenden Mehrzahl der Fälle wird er auch von heftigem Brechreiz und Erbrechen begleitet. Die Augenmuskellähmung tritt erst auf, wenn der Kopfschmerz 1—2 Tage lang angehalten hat; gewöhnlich flaut der Kopfschmerz bald nach dem Einsetzen der Lähmung ab. Nicht selten tritt die Lähmung überhaupt erst nach dem Verschwinden des Kopfschmerzes auf. Neben diesem Verlaufstypus gibt es einen anderen, wo die Augenmuskellähmung überhaupt nur während des Kopfschmerzes besteht. Ich sehe keinen Grund, diese Fälle von kurzdauernder Augenmuskellähmung aus dem Bereich der ophthalmoplegischen Migräne auszuschließen und die Zahl solcher Fälle dürfte gar nicht gering sein. Schon CHARCOT beschrieb einen Fall, wo mit dem Kopfschmerz immer eine Ptose eintrat und verschwand. M. ULRICH fand unter 500 Fällen 12 solche, die manchmal oder stets während ihrer Anfälle Doppeltsehen gehabt haben. Ähnliche Angaben bekam ich wiederholt bei meinem Migränekrankenmaterial. Es bedarf also die von MOEBIUS gemachte Feststellung, wonach die Augenmuskellähmung immer erst nach Ablauf des Kopfschmerzes auftritt, einer Revision. Die Beobachtungen von ROMANO, KARPLUS, SCHMIDT-RIMPLER, HUDOVERNIG, H. EHLERS zeigen, daß bei der ophthalmoplegischen Migräne Sehstörungen, wie sie für die ophthalmische Migräne charakteristisch sind, ebenfalls vorkommen können. Auch ich fand in zwei Fällen von ophthalmoplegischer Migräne Sehstörungen flimmernder Art. Der Kopfschmerz und die Augenmuskellähmung betreffen bei ein und demselben Individuum gewöhnlich nur eine und immer dieselbe Seite, doch auch da gibt es Ausnahmen. Neben früheren Beobachtungen von ZIEHEN, CHABBERT, CHARCOT, HUDOVERNIG erwähne ich den Bericht von AGNELLO, der unter 5 Fällen 2 solche fand, in welchen die Lähmung mit dem Kopfschmerz die Seite wechselte.

Ich beobachtete bei einer 52jährigen Frau, die seit ihrer Kindheit an abwechselnd halbseitigen Kopfschmerzen mit Erbrechen und Sehstörungen leidet, die nur während der Schwangerschaft ausblieben, innerhalb von 2 Jahren zwei Anfälle: einen linksseitigen Kopfschmerzanfall mit linksseitiger Oculomotoriuslähmung (Ophthalmoplegia externa) und 1 Jahr später einen rechtsseitigen Kopfschmerzanfall mit totaler (inkompletter) Oculomotoriuslähmung rechts. Eine 38jährige Frau, die seit Kindheit an Kopfschmerzen von wechselnder Seite leidet, hatte vor 9 Jahren ihren ersten Anfall mit Doppelsehen (Seite unbekannt), vor 2 Jahren hatte sie einen rechtsseitigen Kopfschmerz mit Doppelbildern beim Schauen nach rechts; ich beobachtete bei ihr einen linksseitigen Kopfschmerzanfall mit Doppelbildern beim Schauen nach links.

In den Fällen von ANDERSON, JACKSON, CHABBERT und E. MENDEL waren gleichzeitig beide Seiten betroffen.

Die Dauer des Kopfschmerzes ist im allgemeinen länger, als bei der gewöhnlichen Migräne. Nicht selten hält er einige Tage lang an, in manchen Fällen besteht er durch mehrere Wochen (4 Wochen, $2^1/_2$ Monate). Die Dauer der Lähmung zeigt noch größere Schwankungen. Abgesehen von den früher erwähnten abortiven Fällen, wo die Ptose oder das Doppeltsehen nur während des Kopfschmerzanfalles besteht oder gar nur einige Minuten lang anhält, pflegt sie sich in der Mehrzahl der Fälle nach einigen Tagen oder nach 1—2 Wochen zurückzubilden. Es ist aber gar nicht selten, daß die Lähmung sich auf mehrere Wochen oder Monate erstreckt. In dieser Hinsicht besteht eine große Variabilität auch bei ein und demselben Kranken: Im allgemeinen beobachtet man, daß die Lähmung sich nach den ersten Anfällen rascher zurückbildet und mit der Häufung der Anfälle die funktionelle Wiederherstellung immer längere Zeit in Anspruch nimmt. Es gibt Fälle, wo bei den späteren Anfällen keine völlige Restitution mehr zustande kommt. Manchmal bleiben schon nach der zweiten oder dritten Attacke leichte Residualerscheinungen zurück, die mit den folgenden Anfällen immer zunehmen. In anderen Fällen treten solche nach jahrzehntelangem Bestehen der ophthalmoplegischen Migräne erst im vorgerückten Alter auf. Die Störungen der äußeren Augenmuskeln scheinen rascher abzuklingen als die Bewegungs- und Reflexstörungen der Pupille.

Recht große Schwankungen zeigen die Intervalle, in welchen die ophthalmoplegischen Anfälle auftreten. Neben zahlreichen Fällen, wo eine für die gewöhnliche Migräne charakteristische Periodizität (z. B. alle 4 Wochen) besteht, gibt es eine beträchtliche Anzahl von Beobachtungen, in welchen das Intervall viel länger ist (mehrere Monate, ein- bis zweimal im Jahr), nicht selten trennen mehrere Jahre (6—10 Jahre) zwei ophthalmoplegische Attacken voneinander, wobei im Intervall gewöhnliche Migräneanfälle regelmäßig auftreten können. Es gibt Migränekranke, die nur ein- bis zweimal im Leben eine ophthalmoplegische Attacke hatten. Im allgemeinen kann man sagen, daß die Periodizität auch bei der ophthalmoplegischen Migräne nicht die Regelmäßigkeit aufweist, wie man sie bei der gewöhnlichen Migräne findet.

Die Augenmuskellähmung betrifft am häufigsten den Oculomotorius, seltener die übrigen Augenmuskelnerven. Isolierte Abducenslähmung wurde von BERNHEIMER, ORMEROD, MARINA, BORNSTEIN beschrieben.

Neuerdings teilte A. STERN den Anfall einer 28jährigen Frau mit, die seit 20 Jahren an periodisch auftretenden rechtsseitigen Kopfschmerzanfällen mit rechtsseitiger Abducenslähmung leidet. Unter meinen 12 Fällen von ophthalmoplegischer Migräne fand ich 3 Fälle mit isolierter Abducenslähmung und einen Fall von Abducenslähmung mit Hemiplegia alternans facialis. Die Abducenslähmung dürfte also keineswegs so selten vorkommen.

Isolierte Trochlearislähmung beschrieben LUTZENBERGER, BORNSTEIN und A. FUCHS. Die Kombination von III. und IV. beschrieb MARIN AMAT, die Kombination von III. und VI. beschrieben CHARCOT, SOUQUES, F. MENDEL; beiderseitige Lähmung von III. und VI. beschrieb DEL RIO.

Die Läsion des Oculomotorius ist in den meisten Fällen eine totale: weite, absolut starre Pupillen, gesenktes Oberlid, das Auge nach außen oder nach außen unten gedreht und nur in dieser Richtung beweglich. Seltener tritt die Lähmung in den ersten Attacken nur mit Teilerscheinungen auf und erst später entwickelt sie sich zu einer mehr-minder kompletten Lähmung. Die am frühesten und häufigsten beobachtete Lähmungserscheinung ist die Ptose, die oft Jahre hindurch als isolierte Ausfallserscheinung der Attacke bestehen kann.

Im Falle von E. SUSMANN trat die Ptose im 14. Lebensjahr bei der ersten Attacke auf, wiederholte sich durch 3 Jahre bei jedem Anfall und blieb im 17. Lebensjahr permanent; jetzt traten Strabismus divergens und erweiterte Pupille mit träger Reaktion hinzu.

Vielleicht dürften, wenigstens teilweise, jene Beobachtungen, die von WESTPHAL als paroxysmale Lähmungen selbständig gemacht wurden, in welchen eine anfallsweise, ohne Kopfschmerz auftretende Ptose das einzige Krankheitssymptom bildete, auch als Äquivalente der ophthalmoplegischen Migräne aufgefaßt werden. Ähnliche Beobachtungen bringen K. E. SCHMIDT und CURSCHMANN. Manchmal ist die Ptose mit Lähmung eines einzelnen Augenmuskels verbunden, wobei die übrigen, vom III. versehenen Augenmuskeln funktionstüchtig bleiben oder es können andere äußere Augenmuskeln isoliert gelähmt sein. Betrifft die Lähmung alle vom III. versorgten Muskeln, dann gibt es auch Unterschiede im Grade der Lähmung. Die Lähmung des III. bei ophthalmoplegischer Migräne kann also eine totale oder partielle und komplette oder inkomplette sein. Eine isolierte Lähmung des Musculus sphincter iridis mit Verschonung der äußeren Augenmuskeln beschrieben ROTTMANN, TRÖMNER. Ich beobachtete in 3 Fällen eine isolierte Lähmung sämtlicher vom III. versorgten äußeren Augenmuskeln bei Verschonung der Pupille; CHABBERT und WOHLWILL beobachteten auch solche Fälle; im Falle von VOGELSANG waren auch nur die äußeren Muskeln betroffen, mit Ausnahme des Levators.

Es ist charakteristisch für die Fälle von ophthalmoplegischer Migräne, daß bei diesen auch von seiten anderer Hirnnerven Ausfallserscheinungen viel häufiger auftreten als bei der gewöhnlichen oder ophthalmischen Migräne. Namentlich sind es der Trigeminus und Facialis, welche nicht selten mitbeteiligt sind. Zahlreich sind die Beobachtungen, in welchen auf der Seite der Augenmuskellähmung Parästhesien in der Stirnhälfte, in einer Nasenhöhle nebst Hypästhesie, Analgesie, Hyperästhesie, Hyperalgesie im Hautgebiet eines oder aller drei Trigeminusäste, Unempfindlichkeit der Hornhaut, Parästhesie und Hypalgesie der einen Zungenhälfte verzeichnet sind.

In einem von mir beobachteten Fall von rechtsseitiger Migräne, in welchem der Anfall von einer Ophthalmoplegia externa gefolgt war, trat schon während des Kopfschmerzes ein Kribbeln und dumpfe Berührungsempfindung im Hautgebiet des Unterlides, des Nasenrückens und Oberkiefers auf; ähnliches Gefühl empfindet die Kranke auch im Munde beim Kauen, im rechten oberen Caninus und in beiden oberen Prämolarzähnen. In einem anderen Fall begleiten überaus intensive Schmerzen im Gebiete des I. und II. Trigeminusastes die Augenmuskellähmung; objektiv ließ sich nur eine lebhafte Druckempfindlichkeit dieser Austrittspunkte feststellen.

In einem Fall von KNAPP war blutig-eitriger Ausfluß aus dem auf der Kopfschmerzseite liegenden Nasenloch zu beobachten. Blutungen in der Netzhaut und in den Augenlidern beschrieben BRASCH und LEWINSOHN; Blutungen in der Nase und Orbita TRÖMNER.

Die Lähmung des Nervus facialis als Begleiterscheinung der ophthalmoplegischen Migräne beschrieben CANTALAMESSA, MINGAZZINI, PADERSTEIN und HUDOVERNIG. MUSSO-FOURNIER beobachteten bei einer 47jährigen Frau mit chronischem Hypothyreoidismus in der Menopause 2 Migräneanfälle mit linksseitiger Facialis- und Abducenslähmung, die nach einigen Wochen verschwand. C. DE LANGE teilt den Fall einer 60jährigen Frau mit, die seit ihrem

28. Lebensjahr nach einem Erysipel 12 Anfälle mit Kopfschmerz und Ptosis von wechselnder Seite, oder beiderseitig und darunter 3 mal mit Facialislähmung hatte.

Zwei einschlägige eigene Beobachtungen möchte ich hier etwas ausführlicher mitteilen, weil in beiden vorkommende Symptomenkomplex einer Hemiplegia alternans facialis bei Migräne bisher noch nicht beschrieben wurde.

Frau F. K., 62 Jahre alt, keine hereditäre Belastung. Patientin leidet seit 25 Jahren an halbseitigen, immer rechtsseitigen typischen Migräneanfällen. Wa.R. im Blut und im Liquor wiederholt untersucht, immer negativ. Die Kranke meldete sich zuerst im Jahre 1922 mit der Klage, daß sie seit einer Woche wieder heftige Kopfschmerzen habe, vor den Augen farbige Kreise sieht, lichtscheu ist und seit 2 Tagen das rechte Oberlid nicht heben kann. Bei der Untersuchung fand ich rechts vollkommene Ptose, der Augapfel ist nach rechts gedreht und kann nur in dieser Richtung bewegt werden. Nach allen übrigen Richtungen sind die Bewegungen äußerst eingeschränkt. Kein Nystagmus. Pupillen mittelweit, gleichmäßig rund, prompt reagierend. Nach Angabe der Patientin hatte sie eine solche Lähmung noch nie gehabt, während farbige Kreise und Lichtscheu bei den früheren Anfällen schon öfters auftraten. Die Untersuchung der inneren Organe ergab außer einer mäßigen Arteriosklerose nichts Pathologisches. Harn normal. Der Zustand der Kranken blieb etwa 4 Wochen lang unverändert, während welcher Zeit auch die Kopfschmerzen mit zeitweiligen Unterbrechungen bestanden. Diese blieben erst im 2. Monat aus und gegen Ende des 3. Monats konnten wir die vollständige Restitution des rechten Auges feststellen. Ungefähr 1 Jahr später meldete sich die Kranke wieder und gab an, daß der Kopfschmerz, welcher seit der vorjährigen Erkrankung fast vollständig ausblieb, seit 3 Wochen von neuem mit großer Stärke eingesetzt hat und abweichend von den bisherigen Anfällen sich nicht nur auf die rechte Nacken-, Schläfen- und Stirngegend erstreckte, sondern auch die rechte Gesichtshälfte betraf. Allmählich bemerkte sie dann, daß die rechte Gesichtshälfte sich nicht so gut bewegte wie die linke. Dies fiel ihr besonders bei der Nahrungsaufnahme auf, seit 2 Tagen rinnt beim Trinken das Wasser aus dem rechten Mundwinkel, seit einigen Tagen beobachtete sie auch, daß sie beim Gehen das linke Bein nach sich zieht und die linke Hand bei feineren Bewegungen sie im Stich läßt. Auch klagt sie über krampfhafte Schmerzen im linken Bein, besonders nachts. Sehstörungen hatte sie diesmal nicht. Die Untersuchung ergab eine hochgradige Parese des rechten Facialis, an welcher auch der Stirnast beteiligt war. Intensive Schmerzen im Gebiet des rechten I. und II. Trigeminusastes ohne nachweisbare Sensibilitätsstörung. Pupillen prompt reagierend. Rechts Lagophthalmus, sonst Augenbewegungen frei. Die gestreckte Zunge weicht etwas nach rechts ab. Velum gut beweglich. Der linke Arm ist ungeschickt, die Muskelkraft laut Angabe der Kranken schwächer als früher. Beim Gehversuch bemerkt man, daß nach einigen richtig ausgeführten Schritten das linke Bein geschleift wird. Die linksseitigen Triceps-, Knie- und Achillesreflexe sind deutlich lebhafter als rechts. Im linken Fuß zeitweise positives BABINSKI- und OPPENHEIM-Zeichen vorhanden. Kein Fußklonus. Bauchdeckenreflexe auslösbar. Unter Einführung einer Papaverin-Luminalkur allmähliche Abnahme der Kopfschmerzen und der Lähmungserscheinungen, nach 2 Monaten völlige Restitution. Die Patientin hatte die Papaverin-Luminalkur etwa 1 Jahr lang fortgesetzt und es zeigte sich bis zur letzten Vorstellung, die im Herbst 1929 erfolgte, überhaupt kein Kopfschmerzanfall mehr.

Die 36jährige Musiklehrerin E. L., deren Mutter seit ihrer Jugend an halbseitigen Kopfschmerzen leidet, ist selber seit ihrer Kindheit kopfleidend. Ihre Anfälle kommen immer nach der Menstruation und nehmen in den letzten Jahren an Heftigkeit zu. Vor 5 Jahren hatte sie einmal während des Anfalles Doppeltsehen, sowie Kribbeln und Schwäche im rechten Arm gefühlt; diese Erscheinungen wiederholten sich bei einem Anfall vor 2 Jahren, in welchem sie 20 Minuten überhaupt nichts sah. Die Kranke meldete sich im November 1926 mit der Angabe, daß der übliche postmenstruelle Anfall mit nicht so heftigen Kopfschmerzen einherging, wie die vorausgehenden, dagegen trat in Begleitung von einem überaus heftigen Schwindelgefühl und Brechreiz, der schon seit einigen Tagen bestand, Doppeltsehen und Gesichtsverzerrung auf. Die Untersuchung ergab folgenden Befund: Korrespondierend mit dem linksseitigen Kopfschmerz linksseitige Abducenslähmung, linksseitige Facialisparese (auch Stirn- und Augenast inbegriffen), horizontaler Nystagmus beim Schauen nach rechts, ausgesprochene Parese des rechten Beines, welches beim Gehen geschleift wird, erhöhte Sehnenreflexe rechts, Fußklonus rechts, fehlende Bauchdeckenreflexe rechts, kein BABINSKI. Sensibilität erhalten, auch keine Parästhesien in den Gliedern. Sprache gut. Im rechten Arm ist keine Schwäche nachweisbar. Pupillen normal. Trigeminusdruckpunkte links druckempfindlich. Die Prüfung des Vestibularis ergab eine Herabsetzung der Erregbarkeit links. Beim Gehen und Stehen mit geschlossenen Augen leichtes Wanken ohne bestimmte Richtung. Gehör gut. Die vorgenommene Blut- und Liquoruntersuchung ergab normalen Befund. Nach Einführung einer Papaverinluminalkur allmählicher Rückgang der Erscheinungen, nach 6 Wochen vollkommene Restitution sämtlicher Erscheinungen, so auch der Vestibulariserregbarkeit. Die Kranke steht seit 4 Jahren unter meiner Kontrolle, sie hatte während dieser Zeit 3 postmenstruelle linksseitige Migräneanfälle, die nur mit leichteren Parästhesien im linken Trigeminusgebiet einhergingen.

Im ersten der hier mitgeteilten Fälle entwickelte sich also bei einer seit 25 Jahren an typischer Migräne leidenden Frau zuerst ein Anfall von ophthalmoplegischer Migräne mit rechtsseitiger III. Lähmung und 1 Jahr später ein Anfall, bei welchem eine rechtsseitige Facialislähmung (von nucleärem Typus) mit Hemiparese der linken Extremitäten kombiniert war. Auch bestanden in diesem Fall Reizsymptome von seiten des rechten Trigeminus. Im zweiten Fall traten bei einer seit Kindheit an hereditärer Migräne leidenden Frau im Anschluß an eine Kopfschmerzattacke linksseitige Abducenslähmung, linksseitige Facialislähmung (von nucleärem Typus), linksseitige Vestibularisläsion und eine spastische Schwäche des rechten Beines auf. Es kann keinem Zweifel unterliegen, daß in beiden Fällen eine Hemiplegia alternans facialis bestand, die nur durch einen in der Brücke sich abspielenden krankhaften Prozeß erklärt werden kann. Wir wollen noch auf die Bedeutung dieser Beobachtungen bei der Besprechung der Pathogenese zurückkommen.

Isolierte Facialislähmungen als Begleitsymptome gewöhnlicher Migräneanfälle beschrieben NEUMANN, ROSSOLIMO und BERNHARDT (die Fälle von MOEBIUS und EULENBURG mit rezidivierender Facialislähmung gehören nicht hierher, weil in diesen keine Migräne vorlag). In ROSSOLIMOS Fall bestand bei einer 28jährigen Frau mit hereditärer Belastung vom 16. Lebensjahr an eine menstruelle Migräne; sie hatte in den letzten 9 Jahren 4 solche Migräneanfälle, die von einer Facialislähmung begleitet waren, und zwar 2mal links und 2mal rechts, immer gleichzeitig mit dem Kopfschmerz. Auch ich sah 2 Fälle von isolierter Facialislähmung bei Migräne immer gleichzeitig mit dem Kopfschmerz auftreten. In einem Fall bildete sich die Lähmung binnen 14 Tagen zurück, in einem zweiten Fall war noch nach 5 Monaten eine Parese der linken Gesichtshälfte mit beginnender Kontraktur und herabgesetzter elektrischer Erregbarkeit feststellbar. BERNHARDT faßte diese Fälle als *Hemicrania facioplegica* zusammen.

Vereinzelte Beobachtungen führen als Begleiterscheinungen der ophthalmoplegischen Migräne Reiz- und Ausfallserscheinungen des Acusticus, Hypoglossus (SIL), vasomotorische und sekretorische Störungen im Gesicht (Conjunctivitis, Ödem der Lider, Tränen, Nasenlaufen) an. In einigen Fällen begleitete Fieber die Anfälle (CANTALAMESSA, WADSWORTH, JOACHIM, BALLET, und der jüngst mitgeteilte Fall von PANDELESCO-DUMITRESCO). Über die Kombination von ophthalmoplegischer Migräne mit epileptischen Zuständen berichten JOACHIM, ZIEHEN, SCHWEINITZ, GIEBLER. Hierher gehört ein Fall von PÁKOZDY, welcher auch ansonsten interessante Züge aufweist.

Eine 43jährige Frau, deren Vater seit seiner Jugend an Migräne leidet, hat seit 30 Jahren Kopfschmerzanfälle, die sich in 4 verschiedenen Anfallstypen zeigen: 1. Kurzdauernde linksseitige Kopfschmerzen mit Erweiterung der linken Pupille, Ptosis, auf der Höhe des Anfalles totale III. Lähmung links. Der Kopfschmerz zieht von der Stirn nach hinten und dauert 2—10 Minuten, die Lähmung nur einige Sekunden. 2. Kurzdauernde rechtsseitige Kopfschmerzen mit oder ohne Lähmung. (Leichte Ptosis und Erweiterung der Pupille.) 3. Kurzdauernde Augenmuskellähmung links ohne Kopfschmerz. 4. 2—3 Tage anhaltende gewöhnliche Migräneanfälle ohne Augenmuskellähmung. Die Patientin hat außer diesen Anfällen seltener kurzdauernde Zustände von Bewußtseinstrübung bzw. Bewußtlosigkeit ohne Krämpfe mit Amnesie und nachheriger leichter Benommenheit und Taubheitsgefühl in der linken Körperhälfte. Die Einreihung dieses Falles zur reinen ophthalmoplegischen Migräne wird dadurch erschwert, daß im neurologischen Befund Knie- und Achillessehnenreflexe fehlen. Wa.R. im Blut und Liquor negativ, im Liquor keine Zellvermehrung, Pándy ++, Nonne-Apelt +, Goldsol unspezifisch.

Über psychotische Zustände bei ophthalmoplegischer Migräne berichten GUBLER, ZIEHEN, PADERSTEIN.

Bevor wir zur eingangs erwähnten Frage, ob die ophthalmoplegische Migräne im Sinne von MOEBIUS als eine gesonderte Erkrankungsform angesehen werden muß oder nach Ansicht von CHARCOT nur eine durch ihre Symptomatologie spezifisch gezeichnete Form der echten Migräne darstellt, Stellung nehmen wollten, erscheint es geboten, über jene Fälle von ophthalmoplegischer Migräne zu berichten, in welchen offenkundige, durch die Sektion nachgewiesene anatomische Veränderungen des Gehirns und der Hirnhäute vorlagen. Wie schon früher erwähnt, ist die Zahl dieser zweifellos als symptomatische ophthalmoplegische Migräne anzusehenden Fälle im Vergleich zu den übrigen Migräneformen recht groß. Auch die Erkrankungen, welche der Sektionsbefund als Grundlage der ophthalmoplegischen Migräne erkennen ließ, sind mannigfach. So erwähnen GUBLER, MASSALONGO basale meningitische Prozesse, ZIEHEN Pachymeningitis haemorrhagica, WEISS tuberkulöse Granulationen und eine besondere Erwähnung verdienen drei gleichlautende Beobachtungen von THOMSEN-RICHTER, KARPLUS und SHIONOYA, in welchen eine Geschwulst des III. Stammes bei seinem Eintritt in den Duralsack als Ausgangspunkt der ophthalmoplegischen Migräne hingestellt werden konnte. Es soll hier gleich bemerkt werden, daß in letzteren drei Fällen das klinische Bild alle Unterschiede erkennen läßt, welche MOEBIUS zur Abgrenzung der ophthalmoplegischen Migräne gegenüber der vulgären hervorhebt. Natürlich wird man auch hier annehmen müssen, daß der Tumor an sich nicht die sich zeitweise wiederholenden und wieder zurückbildenden Anfälle verursacht, sondern daran denken müssen, daß Geschwülste am III. Stamm den Ausgangspunkt für ophthalmoplegische Migräneanfälle bilden können, wobei aber für die Auslösung des Anfalls derselbe pathophysiologische Mechanismus Geltung hat, wie bei den übrigen Formen.

Man wird den Standpunkt von SICARD als berechtigt anerkennen müssen, daß diejenigen Fälle, in welchen die Liquoruntersuchung eine Lymphocytose und Eiweißvermehrung aufweist, als symptomatische Migräneanfälle anzusehen sind. Rechnet man aber auch diese Fälle ab, so bleibt noch immer eine beträchtliche Zahl von ophthalmoplegischen Migräfällen zurück, deren Absonderung gegen die übrigen Migräneformen keineswegs begründet ist, weil für sie die von MOEBIUS hervorgehobenen Unterscheidungsmerkmale eine nur sehr beschränkte Gültigkeit aufweisen. Mit Ausnahme von ganz wenigen Beobachtungen ist das Krankheitsbild der ophthalmoplegischen Migräne mit gewöhnlichen Migräneanfällen vermischt, wobei es nebensächlich bleibt, ob letztere vor oder nach der ersten ophthalmoplegischen Attacke auftraten. Die Heredität, und zwar die gleichartige, beträgt auch bei der ophthalmoplegischen Migräne einen bedeutenden Prozentsatz; wenn er nicht so groß ist, wie bei der vulgären Migräne, so liegt der Grund darin, daß unter den Fällen von ophthalmoplegischer Migräne tatsächlich verhältnismäßig mehr symptomatische Fälle vorkommen. Eine im engsten Sinne genommene Heredität (also Übertragung der ophthalmoplegischen Migräne von Eltern auf Nachkommen) ist nie beobachtet worden; läge eine solche vor, so würde diese eher die Sonderstellung der ophthalmoplegischen Migräne unterstützen. Die Einseitigkeit der ophthalmoplegischen Migräne ist eine häufige, aber keine gesetzmäßige Erscheinung. Auch Sehstörungen kommen bei der ophthalmoplegischen Migräne vor. Die lange Dauer der Anfälle bildet ein charakteristisches Zeichen der ophthalmoplegischen Migräne; man muß aber hier in Erwägung ziehen, daß die anatomische Schädigung, welche zur Augenmuskellähmung führt, gerade durch das längere Anhalten jenes pathophysiologischen Zustandes hervorgerufen wird, der dem

Migräneanfall zugrunde liegt und daß die inzwischen auftretenden gewöhnlichen Migräneanfälle eben infolge ihrer kürzeren Dauer eine solche Ernährungsstörung nicht aufkommen lassen. Ich möchte mich also im Einklang mit FLATAU der Ansicht CHARCOTS anschließen, nach welcher die ophthalmoplegische Migräne nur eine besondere Erscheinungsform der echten Migräne darstellt und keine selbständige nosologische Einheit bildet; gleichzeitig aber betonen, daß innerhalb dieser Anfallsform die Fälle von symptomatischer ophthalmoplegischer Migräne, unter welchen die Geschwulstbildung am III. Stamm als organische Erkrankung eine besondere Rolle spielt, relativ häufiger vorkommen.

Eine Identifizierung der ophthalmoplegischen Migräne mit der „rezidivierenden III. Lähmung" ist schon aus dem Grunde unstatthaft, weil, wie die mitgeteilten Beobachtungen zeigen, auch die übrigen Augenmuskelnerven manchmal in Mitleidenschaft gezogen sind; wenn man noch in Betracht zieht, daß die Läsion des Trigeminus und Facialis auch zu den häufigen Begleiterscheinungen der ophthalmoplegischen Migräne gehört und daß in 2 Fällen von ophthalmoplegischer Migräne das Syndrom der Hemiplegia alternans facialis in Erscheinung trat, dann glaube ich, daß diese Anfallsgruppe eine einheitlichere Zusammenfassung erhält, wenn man, das Lokalisationsprinzip vor Augen haltend, diese Fälle als „ponto-mesencephale" Form der Migräne bezeichnet.

Anschließend mögen kurz als gesonderte Gruppe der Migräne diejenigen Fälle zusammengefaßt werden, in welchen

Schwindel und Gleichgewichtsstörungen

im Mittelpunkt des klinischen Anfallsbildes stehen. Subjektives Schwindelgefühl am Beginn oder im Verlauf des gewöhnlichen Migräneanfalles gehört zu den häufigen Begleiterscheinungen. Isolierte, ohne Kopfschmerz auftretende Schwindelanfälle bei Migränekranken wurden schon von ESCAT, PEZZI, DWIGHT und PARRY als Migräneäquivalente aufgefaßt. Zahlreiche Beobachtungen von OPPENHEIM, HEVEROCH, FLATAU bestätigen dies. Überzeugend ist auch folgende eigene Beobachtung:

32jähriger Mann, mit Migräne erblich belastet, leidet seit seinem 5. Lebensjahr bis zum Alter von 28 Jahren an selten auftretenden ophthalmischen Migräneanfällen: Beginn mit Sehstörung (Skotom, halbstündige Amaurose), dann folgt Erbrechen und Durchfall, Herzklopfen, Schwindel auf kurze Zeit und nachher ein heftiger, beiderseitiger Kopfschmerz einige Stunden lang. Zwischen dem 28. und 30. Lebensjahr waren keine Anfälle; seit 2 Jahren traten sie von neuem, aber in anderer Form auf: das Hauptsymptom ist ein überaus heftiger Schwindel, welcher ohne Sehstörung, Erbrechen und Kopfschmerz stundenlang besteht, beim Liegen unerträglich wird und nur sitzend abgewartet werden kann; manchmal tritt gleichzeitig Herzklopfen, Schweißausbrüche, Gesichtsröte auf. Vor einem solchen Anfall hatte er eine kurzdauernde Sehstörung.

CHRISTIANSEN bringt auch zwei Beobachtungen. Die eine betrifft eine 50jährige Frau mit hereditärer Belastung, die bis zu ihrem 34. Lebensjahr einfache typische Migräneanfälle hatte und nach einem Intervall von 14 Jahren 3—4 monatlich Schwindelanfälle ohne Kopfschmerzen: der Boden wankt unter ihren Füßen, sie muß sich an den Möbeln im Zimmer festhalten oder niederlegen. Der Schwindel dauert auch im Liegen fort, so daß sie die Augen schließen muß, weil die Möbel, Plafond, Wände sich vor ihren Augen bewegen. Brechreiz und Erbrechen machen dem Anfall ein Ende. Der Anfall dauert einen Tag. Für den Migränecharakter dieser Anfälle spricht die Tatsache, daß die Kranke zwischen diesen Anfällen hin und wieder einen typischen Migräneanfall bekommt. Der zweite Fall betrifft eine 34jährige Frau mit 2 migränekranken Schwestern, die 3—4monatlich an Schwindelanfällen in der Dauer von 6—8 Stunden leidet. Der Schwindel tritt ohne Prodrome auf, sie muß sich in eine bequeme Lage bringen, weil sie diese im Laufe des Anfalles nicht mehr ändern kann. Auf der Höhe des Anfalles heftiges Erbrechen.

HEVEROCH berichtet über 38 Fälle, in welchen Schwindel und Gleichgewichtsstörungen in der Dauer von einigen Minuten bis einigen Tagen das Hauptsymptom des Migräneanfalls bildeten. Er fand unter diesen: 1. Fälle, in welchen die Prüfung des Gehörs und des Vestibularisapparates normale Ergebnisse zeigte; er nimmt in diesen Fällen eine Drucksteigerung in den Bogengängen an; 2. Fälle, wo eine Steigerung oder Herabsetzung der Reizbarkeit des Vestibularisapparates nachgewiesen wurde. Er sondert diese Fälle von der Gruppe der MENIÈRE-Krankheit durch das vollkommne Fehlen einer Gehörsverschlimmerung ab; auch während der Anfälle ist dieses nicht gestört. In einer Reihe von Fällen trat die vestibulare Migräne als echtes Äquivalent zwischen gewöhnlichen und ophthalmoplegischen Migräneanfällen auf. FLATAU betrachtet den ohne Kopfschmerz auftretenden Schwindel als eine nicht seltene interparoxysmale Erscheinung der Migräne, bestätigt aber die Beobachtung, daß der Schwindelanfall als ein Äquivalent vikariierend für den Migräneanfall auftreten kann, namentlich in solchen Fällen, wo der Kopfschmerz im späteren Verlauf des Anfalles auftritt oder wenigstens angedeutet ist.

Eng schließt sich den hier erwähnten Beobachtungen jener Fall OPPENHEIMS an, den er als *Hemicrania cerebellaris* bezeichnete: im Anfall war das Stehen und Gehen überaus unsicher, der Kranke taumelte wie ein Betrunkener, hatte heftigen Schwindel und die Empfindung, sein Körper oder einzelne Teile seien verdoppelt. Die Gleichgewichtsstörung schwand mit dem Anfall. Andere, auf Kleinhirnschädigung hinweisende Symptome wurden nicht verzeichnet. Über ähnliche Beobachtungen mit ausgesprochenem Halbseitencharakter berichtet I. SCHUSTER. Einen hierhergehörigen Fall beschrieb PHILLIPS.

Ich beobachtete folgenden Fall: Der 41jährige Aufseher H. L., dessen Familienanamnese belanglos ist und bezüglich Migräne keine hereditäre Belastung aufweist, erkrankte im 20. Lebensjahr an einem manischen Erregungszustand und war damals 3 Monate in einer geschlossenen Heilanstalt; seither geistig gesund. Er hat vier gesunde Kinder. Im Alter von 29 Jahren traten zum erstenmal typische ophthalmische Migräneanfälle auf, die sich 2—3wöchentlich wiederholten und nach einem halben Jahr aufhörten. Erst im Sommer 1933 hatte er wieder 2 typische Anfälle mit Sehstörung und Erbrechen. Am 24. 10. 33 tritt in Begleitung von Augenflimmern heftiges Erbrechen und Schwindel auf und dieser Zustand hielt schon fast ununterbrochen seit 14 Tagen an, als er auf die Ohrenabteilung des Spitals gebracht wird. Er erbricht täglich öfters galligen Schleim, kann sich überhaupt nicht ernähren und liegt unbeweglich mit nach links gebeugtem Kopf im Bett. Versucht er den Kopf zu wenden, tritt immer heftiger Schwindel und Erbrechen auf. Nachdem die Ohrenuntersuchung einen vollkommen normalen Befund des akustischen Apparates feststellte, wurde der Kranke auf die Nervenabteilung überführt. Der neurologische Befund ergab folgendes: Von seiten der Hirnnerven nichts Pathologisches, kein Nystagmus. Deutliche Ataxie, Hypotonie und geschwächte Sehnenreflexe an den linksseitigen Gliedmaßen, Adiadochokinesis links. Bauchreflexe erhalten; keine Pyramidensymptome. Sensibilität erhalten. Augenhintergrund normal. Vollkommen normaler Liquorbefund. Blutwassermann negativ. Normales Blutbild. Fieberfrei. Intravenöse Dextroseinjektionen einer 40% Lösung werden täglich gemacht. Nach einigen Tagen unbeweglichen Liegens auf der linken Seite hört das Erbrechen allmählich auf, nach 1 Woche kann er schon eine gerade Liegestellung einnehmen. Wendung nach rechts oder der Versuch des Aufsitzens bringt Schwindel und Erbrechen wieder zum Vorschein. Zeitweise tritt auch jetzt noch ein linksseitiger Kopfschmerz durch einige Stunden auf. Die Schädelröntgenuntersuchung zeigte Dolichocephalie und eine Verbreiterung der Lambdanaht. Das Gesichtsfeld ist vollkommen erhalten. Neben Dextroseinjektionen wird Papaverin und Luminal verabreicht. Erst in der 4. Woche des Spitalsaufenthaltes kann der Kranke eine kurze Zeit am Bettrand sitzen, den Kopf noch immer nach links gerichtet. Jetzt ist die Ataxie des linken Armes und Beines kaum nachweisbar, auch die Hypotonie und Reflexschwäche kaum angedeutet. Bei den ersten Gehversuchen in der 5. Woche machte er mit weitgespannten Füßen kurze Schritte und neigt deutlich nach links. Bei längerem Stehen fällt er nach links. Vorbeizeigen nach links. In der 6. Woche ein neuerlicher linksseitiger Kopfschmerzanfall (in der Scheitel- und Schläfengegend) mit lebhaftem Augenflimmern und neuerlichem Erbrechen, kann durch eine intravenöse Papaverininjektion in 1 Stunde behoben werden. Die nachfolgende rasche Besserung sämtlicher Symtome ermöglicht es, daß der Kranke nach 8 Wochen vollkommen symptomfrei das Spital verläßt. Von einem leichten Migräneanfall abgesehen, der nach 3 Monaten auftrat und in einigen Tagen (ohne Schwindel) verlief, ist der Kranke auch seither beschwerdefrei.

Im Anschluß an einen linksseitigen ophthalmischen Migräneanfall trat hier ein linksseitiges Kleinhirnsyndrom auf.

OPPENHEIM beschrieb auch eine Form von Dauerschwindel, die er der Dauermigräne (Hemicrania permanens) gleichstellt; auch FLATAU sah solche Fälle bei älteren Leuten, die in ihrer Jugend an heftiger Migräne litten.

All diese Beobachtungen deuten darauf hin, daß auch Schwindel und Gleichgewichtsstörungen manchmal das beherrschende Symptom des Migräneanfalles bilden können. Der Ausgangspunkt der Funktionsstörung kann sehr verschieden sein: er erstreckt sich von den Bogengängen (HEVEROCH) über den Vestibularis und seinen Kern (Pons) bis zum Kleinhirn.

5. Die mit Epilepsie kombinierte Migräne.

Auch in der Frage, ob diese beiden Krankheitsbilder in einem innigeren Zusammenhang miteinander stehen, gehen die Ansichten der verschiedenen Autoren weit auseinander. Die statistischen Zusammenstellungen der verschiedenen Autoren lassen diesen schroffen Gegensatz deutlich erkennen. FLATAU fand unter 500 Migränekranken 36 Fälle, also 7,2% Epileptiker, M. ULRICH 17, also 3,4%, ich fand nur 12 Fälle, also 2,4%. CHRISTIANSEN und SCHULTZE betrachten aber diese Verhältniszahlen gegenüber den Erfahrungen der allgemeinen Praxis zu hoch und lehnen jede, über das zufällige Zusammentreffen dieser beiden ziemlich häufigen Erkrankungen hinausgehende Kombination ab. Zu einer ähnlichen Stellungnahme gelangt auf Grund seiner statistischen Erhebungen W. ALLAN, der unter 4000 Patienten ohne Auswahl 0,85% Epileptiker, unter 400 Migränekranken 0,75% Epileptiker fand. Trachtet man näher nach den Ursachen dieser großen statistischen Unterschiede, so muß man vor Augen halten, daß in der überwiegenden Mehrzahl der vorliegenden Beobachtungen die Kombination von Migräne und Epilepsie sich derart gestaltet, daß zuerst Migräneanfälle auftreten und erst im vorgerückten Alter epileptische Anfälle hinzutreten. Prüft man also bei Migränekranken einfach anamnestisch darnach, ob sie vorher epileptische Anfälle hatten, so bekommt man schwerlich ein richtiges Bild über die Kombination dieser beiden Anfallsarten. Wahrheitsgetreuere Verhältniszahlen erhält man, wenn man bei Epileptikern darnach prüft, ob sie früher Migräneanfälle hatten. A. BUCHANAN bringt eine solche Statistik, in welcher 29% seiner Epileptiker an Migräne gelitten haben. Als ein weiterer Beweis für den innigen Zusammenhang zwischen Migräne und Epilepsie werden die Ergebnisse der Heredität- und Familiaritätsprüfung angeführt. Es bestehen mannigfache substituierende hereditäre Beziehungen zwischen Migräne und Epilepsie. Man findet in Epileptikerfamilien relativ häufiger Migränekranke und vice versa. Interessant ist in dieser Beziehung die Statistik DEJERINES, die die Aszendenz von 350 Epileptikern berücksichtigt und in 51,6% der Fälle Alkoholismus, in 24,5% Migräne und in 21,2% Epilepsie nachweist. BOURNEVILLE konnte bei Verwandten von Epileptikern die Migräne in 24% der Fälle feststellen. FÉRÉ fand in der Aszendenz von 308 Epileptikern 88mal Migräne des Vaters und 116mal Migräne der Mutter. A. BUCHANAN zeigte, daß 75% seiner Epileptiker von migränekranken Eltern stammten. Von neueren Untersuchern sei auf die wertvollen Statistiken von ELY und COBB hingewiesen, welche die innigen hereditären Wechselbeziehungen zwischen Migräne und Epilepsie sinnfällig beleuchten.

Andere Forscher, wie MOREAU, REVINGTON, LIVEING und FLATAU wiesen auf das häufige Nebeneinander der beiden Krankheiten innerhalb einer Familie hin. Ähnliche Beobachtungen konnte auch ich wiederholt machen.

So sah ich die 16jährige Tochter einer an Migräne schwer leidenden Mutter, die seit 2 Jahren typische prämenstruelle Migräneanfälle zeigt und deren 5 Geschwister (2 Mädchen, 3 Knaben) nach Angabe der Mutter alle an typischen epileptischen Krämpfen leiden. Vater gesund, kein Trinker, für Lues besteht kein Anhaltspunkt. In einer anderen Familie beobachtete ich eine überaus schwere, vulgäre Migräne bei einem 30jährigen jungen Mann, dessen Mutter als Mädchen und junge Frau ebenfalls an Migräne litt, seit 20 Jahren die Migräne gänzlich verlor, dagegen halbjährlich einen typisch epileptischen Anfall bekommt; eine jüngere Schwester litt ebenfalls seit Kindheit an schwerer Migräne, hatte im letzten Jahr zwei epileptische Anfälle und endete 28jährig durch Selbstmord.

Solche Einzelbeobachtungen von Familien, in welchen alle oder fast alle Mitglieder der Familie von der einen oder anderen Anfallsform befallen sind, scheinen mir am meisten überzeugend zu sein dafür, daß die Kombination von Migräne und Epilepsie doch nicht auf einer rein zufälligen Koinzidenz der beiden Anfallsarten beruhen dürfte.

Die Kombination der beiden Anfallsarten zeigt eine recht große Abwechslung. Die zeitliche Priorität der Migräne ist in der überwiegenden Mehrzahl der Fälle nachweisbar. Die Migräneanfälle treten gewöhnlich in der Kindheit auf und erst im späteren, reifen Alter der erste epileptische Anfall. Manchmal treten als Übergangssymptome Petit-mal-Anfälle auf. FLATAU hebt hervor, daß unter den verschiedenen Migräneformen besonders die ophthalmische und assoziierte Migräne sich häufig mit Epilepsie kombiniert; dies wird auch von anderen bestätigt. Es ist auch eine allgemeine Erfahrung, daß mit dem Auftreten der epileptischen Anfälle die Migräneanfälle seltener kommen und milder auftreten, sehr oft auch gänzlich verschwinden. Dieses vikariierende Auftreten von Migräne und Epilepsie kann sich sogar öfters wiederholen.

So fand ich in der Krankengeschichte einer 22jährigen Frau, daß sie als kleines Kind an halbseitigen Kopfschmerzanfällen litt, die mit dem Eintritt der Menses aufhörten und an ihre Stelle typische epileptische Krampfanfälle traten in 5—6monatlichem Intervall; seit 3 Jahren blieben diese aus und seit dieser Zeit traten wieder schwere ophthalmische Migräneanfälle auf, die sich durch ihre lange Dauer (auch 10 Tage lang) auszeichnen. Die Mutter der Patientin litt als junge Frau an halbseitigen Kopfschmerzen. Die körperliche Untersuchung (auch Liquor) erwies sich als vollkommen negativ.

In einer Reihe von Fällen treten Migräne und Epilepsie ungefähr gleichzeitig auf, wobei aber der selbständige Charakter der beiden Anfallsarten bewahrt bleibt. Nur vereinzelte Beobachtungen gibt es, wo die epileptischen Anfälle früher auftreten als die Migräneanfälle (Fälle von FÉRÉ, KOVALEWSKY, FLATAU).

Auch ich beobachtete eine 33jährige Frau, die im Alter von 25 Jahren während der zweiten Gravidität einen mehrstündigen schweren Status epilepticus hatte. Nachher normale Geburt. 11 Monate nach dem ersten Anfalle kam ein neuerlicher Status epilepticus mit 15, nacheinander folgenden epileptischen Anfällen; seither leidet an typischen linksseitigen Migräneanfällen, die anfangs nur vor der Menstruation, später auch in der Zwischenzeit auftraten; selten betrifft der Anfall die rechte Seite. Über Heredität nichts bekannt, körperliche Untersuchung (auch Liquor) vollkommen negativ.

Der epileptische und der Migräneanfall pflegen sich manchmal auch zeitlich miteinander zu verbinden, so daß beiderlei Syndrome „wie angegliedert und miteinander verkettet" (FLATAU) erscheinen. Diese Fälle bezeichnet FLATAU als Migräneepilepsie. Am häufigsten kommt es vor, daß ein epileptischer Anfall während des Migräneanfalls, und zwar auf der Höhe desselben sich entwickelt, oder daß prodromale Migränesymptome einen epileptischen Anfall einleiten. Insbesondere wurden die einleitenden Erscheinungen der ophthalmischen Migräne (Flimmerskotom) häufig als Aura eines epileptischen Anfalls beobachtet. In anderen Fällen vermischen sich die Symptome der beiden Anfälle, so, daß es schwer fällt, sie voneinander zu trennen. Den Ausklang eines epileptischen Anfalls in einem Migräneanfall beschrieb KRAFFT-EBING.

Auch ich beobachtete ein 20jähriges Mädchen, dessen Mutter und zwei Schwestern an typischer Migräne leiden, bei welchem im 13. Lebensjahr 10 Tage nach der ersten Periode, nachts ein typischer epileptischer Anfall auftrat und am folgenden Morgen ein heftiger halbseitiger Kopfschmerz mit Erbrechen folgte. Die Anfälle zeigten sich seither regelmäßig nach jeder Periode und in derselben Reihenfolge.

Außer dieser innigen Verflechtung der Anfallssymptome kann man noch auf zahlreiche gemeinsame Züge der allgemeinen klinischen Offenbarung hinweisen, die sich bei beiden Anfallsarten kundgeben. Das erste Auftreten in der Jugend, der anfallsartige Verlauf, das häufige Einsetzen mit Auraerscheinungen, die Periodizität der Anfälle, das Auftreten von protrahierten Anfallszuständen bei beiden Erkrankungen (Status hemicranicus-status epilepticus) sind Kennzeichen, die auf eine innigere Zusammengehörigkeit der beiden Anfallsformen hindeuten. Eine weitere Ähnlichkeit besteht auch darin, daß nach dem epileptischen Anfall, ebenso wie nach dem Migräneanfall, postparoxysmale, durch Herdläsion bedingte Ausfallserscheinungen zurückbleiben und eine gewisse Zeitlang bestehen können, wenn auch zwischen diesen klinisch erhebliche Unterschiede bestehen. Ein nicht zu vernachlässigendes Argument für die Zusammengehörigkeit der beiden Krankheiten bietet endlich auch ihre gemeinsame therapeutische Beeinflußbarkeit (Brom, Luminal).

Werden also von einem Teil der Forscher die hier angeführten Tatsachen, also die innige hereditäre Verflechtung, das prozentuell nachgewiesene, häufigere Vorkommen beider Anfallsarten in einer Familie oder bei ein und demselben Individuum, der nicht selten beobachtete kontinuierliche Übergang zwischen beiden Anfallsarten und die angedeuteten vielfachen analogen Züge in der klinischen Erscheinungsweise beider Anfallsarten als Argumente für eine nahe, wesentliche Verwandtschaft zwischen Migräne und Epilepsie angeführt, so bildet für andere, namhafte Autoren den stärksten Einwand gegen diese Auffassung die Tatsache, daß das klinische Bild des epileptischen Anfalls von jenem des Migräneanfalls vollkommen abweicht. Tatsächlich bieten die kardinalen Züge des epileptischen Anfalls die Bewußtlosigkeit und Muskelkrämpfe von tonisch-klonischem Charakter solche Symptome, die dem Migräneanfall vollkommen fremd sind. Es wäre nicht richtig, wenn man die leichteren Bewußtseinstörungen der epileptischen Petit-mal-Anfälle und die bei schweren Migräneanfällen manchmal beobachteten Dämmerzustände als Übergang betrachten wollte, die diesen krassen Unterschied in der Symptomatologie beider Anfallsarten überbrücken könnten. Man muß hier in Betracht ziehen, daß unter den Migränekranken eine gewisse Anzahl von Psychopathen sich befindet, bei welchen geistige Alterationen eben auf dieser psychopathischen Grundlage entstehen können (CHRISTIANSEN). Anderseits aber kann man auch die Möglichkeit nicht von der Hand weisen, daß die Migräne, wie eben davon die Rede ist, sich nicht selten mit Epilepsie kombiniere, daher psychische Alterationen bei Migräne auch auf eine Kombination mit der epileptischen Komponente zurückgeführt werden können. Die motorischen Reizerscheinungen des epileptischen Anfalles, die tonisch-klonischen Krämpfe fehlen gänzlich aus dem Symptomenbild des Migräneanfalls. Auf diese Tatsache wurde schon früher die Feststellung gestützt, daß die im Migräneanfall auftretenden Hemiparesen unmöglich auf die Läsion der motorischen Rinde zurückgeführt werden können. Auch das Gebiet der inneren Kapsel müssen wir aus dem Läsionsbereich des Migräneanfalls ausscheiden und zu demjenigen des epileptischen Anfalls einreihen.

Als Beweise für diese Annahme dienen Beobachtungen, welche die Folgezustände des epileptischen Anfalles betreffen. Nach REDLICHS Zusammenstellungen sind bisher folgende Zustände beobachtet worden. a) Aphasische Störungen seltener motorischer, häufiger sensorischer oder amnestischer Art. b) Spastische Erscheinungen, die oft nur die eine Seite betreffen, wo die Krämpfe häufiger waren. c) SCHILDER beschreibt eigenartige Spannungszustände im postparoxysmalen Stadium, die er nach ihrer Erscheinungsweise (gleichmäßiges Befallen von Agonisten und Antagonisten ohne spastische Phänomene) auf eine Schädigung des Corpus striatum zurückgeführt. d) KNAPP fand Bilder, die teils an Pseudobulbärparalyse, teils an Paralysis agitans erinnern. Pseudobulbäre Erscheinungen beobachteten schon früher RAYMOND, ROSE, VOISIN, bei Kindern nach gehäuften Anfällen ZAPPERT.

Wir sehen also unter den Folgezuständen des epileptischen Anfalls neben Hemiparesen Nachbarschaftssymptome, die auf das Gebiet der inneren Kapsel und der Zentralganglien hinweisen. Diese Zustandsbilder wurden bei Migräne überhaupt nie beobachtet, dagegen festgestellt, daß hier die Hemiparesen sich häufig mit Augenmuskellähmungen verbinden und in meinen zwei früheren Beobachtungen von Hemiplegia alternans facialis wurde der strikte Beweis erbracht, daß die Hemiparese auf eine Brückenläsion zurückzuführen ist. Diese Erwägungen machen die Annahme wahrscheinlich, daß auch die motorischen Ausfallserscheinungen bei Epilepsie und Migräne Unterschiede erkennen lassen, die auf eine verschiedentliche Lokalisation der cerebralen Schädigung hindeuten; beim epileptischen Anfall ist die motorische Hirnrinde und das Gebiet der inneren Kapsel und der Zentralganglien als Sitz der Läsion anzunehmen, beim Migräneanfall jener Abschnitt der zentralen motorischen Bahn, welcher die tieferliegenden Hirnteile (Mittelhirn, Brücke) passiert.

Unterstützt wird diese Ansicht auch durch die Unterschiede, welche die Sprachstörung bei Migräne und Epilepsie aufweist. Bei Migräne handelt es sich fast immer um eine motorische Aphasie, seltener um dysarthrische Beschwerden; aphasische Störungen von corticaler Natur fehlen im Krankheitsbild der Migräne; dagegen ist es bekannt und wurde erst unlängst von F. SCHÖNE darauf hingewiesen, daß die im epileptischen Anfall oder postparoxysmal beobachteten Sprachstörungen in überwiegendem Maße rein corticale Ausfallserscheinungen darstellen.

Eine gewisse Annäherung im klinischen Bild weisen die Fälle von ophthalmischer, assoziierter Migräne auf, bei welcher der Anfall außer den Lichterscheinungen durch halb- oder beiderseitige Gefühlsstörungen, Parästhesien und Hypästhesien eingeleitet oder begleitet wird, CHARCOT bezeichnet diese Fälle als „Epilepsie sensitive". Die Ähnlichkeit dieser Anfallsform der Migräne mit den sog. sensiblen JACKSON-Anfällen der Epilepsie ist auch deshalb bemerkenswert, weil es vorkommt, daß bei beiden Formen der Anfall sich manchmal über diese einleitenden Symptome hinaus nicht weiter entwickelt. CHRISTIANSEN hebt als Unterscheidungszeichen hervor, daß die Parästhesien bei der assoziierten Migräne sich nur sehr langsam ausbreiten, während beim sensiblen JACKSON-Anfall diese Auraerscheinung rasch abläuft. Er hebt weiter hervor, daß bei der Migräne die Gefühlsstörung vornehmlich die Arme, die Zunge und das Gesicht betrifft, die unteren Glieder aber regelmäßig verschont, ihren Sitz auch während des Anfalls oft wechselt und häufig beide Körperseiten betrifft. Diese Eigentümlichkeiten fehlen beim sensiblen JACKSON-Anfall.

Die Analyse der klinischen Symptome muß also zu dem Ergebnis führen, daß die Läsion, welche dem Migräneanfall zugrunde liegt, ganz andere Territorien des Gehirns betrifft wie diejenige, die den epileptischen Anfall verursacht. Es ist aber fraglich, ob diese verschiedentliche Lokalisation, die sich in der abweichenden Symptomatologie kundgibt, allein ausreicht, um jene Wesensverwandtschaft zwischen beiden Neurosen völlig abzulehnen, die durch eine Reihe von anderen Argumenten unterstützt wird. Namhafte Forscher befinden sich in beiden Lagern. MARSHALL, HALL, LIVEING, CHARCOT, FÉRÉ, GOWERS, MOEBIUS, OPPENHEIM, MINGAZZINI, CURSCHMANN, FLATAU, M. ULRICH u. a. befürworten die Annahme eines gewissen Zusammenhangs zwischen Epilepsie und Migräne, den auch REDLICH (Erg.-Bd. zu LEWANDOWSKYS Handbuch 1923) sich zu eigen macht, indem er sagt: „Es reicht meines Erachtens nicht aus, den Zusammenhang zwischen Epilepsie und Migräne einfach damit erklären zu wollen, daß beide Erkrankungen durch hereditäre Belastung ausgelöst sind, zur sog. Famille neuropathique gehören. Vielmehr bestehen zweifellos nähere pathogenetische Beziehungen, die genauer zu präzisieren darum so große

Schwierigkeit hat, weil die Pathogenese beider Erkrankungen eigentlich noch so wenig bekannt ist". KOVALEWSKY, FÉRÉ, LIVEING, LASEGUE und CORNU nehmen sogar eine Substitution oder Umwandlung der einen Neurose in die andere an; SIEVEKING und SIKLE identifizieren beide Krankheiten. EPSTEIN betrachtet die Migräne als ein Äquivalent der Epilepsie, BOLTEN nimmt nur einen quantitativen Unterschied zwischen Migräne und Epilepsie an, die Migräne sei eine abgeschwächte Form der Epilepsie. LÖWENFELD und JACKSON identifizieren nur die Fälle von assoziierter Augenmigräne mit den epileptischen. Auch im Lager der Gegner dieser Auffassung gibt es verschiedene Schattierungen. Neben Forschern, die nur die Annahme eines innigeren Kontaktes bekämpfen (SCHAFFER, GRADLE, v. SARBÓ), steht die Mehrzahl auf einem absolut ablehnenden Standpunkt, indem sie die Kombination von Migräne und Epilepsie als zufällige Koinzidenz, wie sie bei zwei gar nicht seltenen Krankheiten vorkommen kann, betrachten (KRAFFT-EBING, KARPLUS, BERNHARDT, BORDONI, FORNI) und eine scharfe Trennung fordern. Eine Anzahl neuerer Forscher hat sich der letzteren Auffassung angeschlossen (CHRISTIANSEN, RADOT, PETZ, PHILLIPS u. a.). SCHULTZE fordert ebenfalls eine strikte Absonderung; die Analogien reichen nach ihm nicht aus, um eine Wesensverwandtschaft zu begründen: „Schmetterlinge sind noch keine Vögel, bloß weil sie Flügel haben"[1]. Er betont als wesentliche Unterschiede, daß die Migräne in höherem Alter ausheilt oder sich vermindert, daß sie keine Verblödung hinterläßt; auch im Nachweis des BABINSKI-Zeichen nach dem epileptischen Anfall erblickt er ein wichtiges Absonderungsmerkmal gegenüber der Migräne. KRAFFT-EBING will eine engere Beziehung nur zwischen den schweren ophthalmischen Migräneformen und Epilepsie zulassen und glaubt, daß es sich in diesen Fällen zumeist um symptomatische Zustände handelt, denen organische Gehirnschädigungen zugrunde liegen. Zu ähnlicher Ansicht gelang VALLERY-RADOT, der bemängelt, daß in den Beobachtungen, wo Migräne und Epilepsie in Kombination vorkommen (zumeist handelt es sich auch nach ihm um ophthalmische Migräneanfälle), die Untersuchung des Liquors fehlt. Er beruft sich auf zwei Beobachtungen von SICARD, wo positive Liquorveränderungen eine organische Gehirnerkrankung als Grundlage dieser Kombination ergaben. RADOT betrachtet die zahlreichen Ähnlichkeiten in der Pathogenese und Verlaufsart der beiden Krankheiten als einfache Analogien, aus welchen weitere Konsequenzen nicht gezogen werden dürfen. FLATAU formuliert seine Ansicht dahin, daß er einen innigeren Zusammenhang zwischen Migräne und Epilepsie nur für diejenigen Fälle annimmt, wo die beiden Neurosen bei ein und demselben Individuum auftreten. Hier könne es sich nach ihm nicht um eine bloße Koinzidenz und noch weniger um eine zufällige Kombination handeln. Auch ich möchte mich in dieser Frage im wesentlichen der FLATAUschen Ansicht anschließen und dabei betonen, daß dieser vermutete innigere Zusammenhang sich nicht so sehr auf die Krankheiten Migräne und Epilepsie, vielmehr auf die beiden Anfallssyndrome des migränösen und epileptischen Anfalls beziehe. Bei der Besprechung der Pathogenese werde ich es versuchen, auf die gemeinsamen Züge im Entstehungsmechanismus der beiden Anfallsarten hinzuweisen und darzulegen, daß der Unterschied, der sich in der Symptomatologie der beiden Anfallsarten zeigt, lediglich auf einer verschiedentlichen Lokalisation des pathologischen Vorgangs im Gehirn beruht. Die Ätiologie der Migräne ist heute noch ebensowenig klargelegt, wie die der Epilepsie; als gesichert müssen wir aber annehmen, daß sie nicht einheitlich ist. Diejenigen ursächlichen Faktoren, die in der Ätiologie der Migräne eine Rolle spielen, stehen auch bei der Epilepsie zur Diskussion.

---

[1] Ein nicht sehr glücklicher Vergleich, wenn man bedenkt, daß die beiden Anfallsformen gerade in ihrer äußeren Erscheinungsweise den größten Unterschied zeigen.

Die Annahme erscheint also nicht gewagt, daß es Fälle gibt, wo ein bestimmter ursächlicher Faktor beide Anfallsarten hervorbringen könne. Daß dieser ursächliche Faktor ein erbbedingter sein müsse, beweisen die früher angeführten Daten über substituierende Heredität zwischen Migräne und Epilepsie und noch deutlicher der familiäre Rahmen, in welchem die innige Verflechtung beider Anfallsformen beobachtet wird. Ich möchte also den innigen Zusammenhang zwischen Migräne und Epilepsie nicht als eine die beiden Krankheiten allgemein kennzeichnende Eigenschaft betrachten, sondern nur annehmen, daß innerhalb beider Erkrankungsformen je eine Gruppe existiert, bei welcher ein erbbedingter ursächlicher Faktor sich ambivalent auswirken kann, so daß er sich unter den Mitgliedern einer Familie bei einigen in Migräneanfällen, bei anderen in epileptischen Anfällen äußert, oder daß er bei ein und demselben Individuum beide Anfallsarten hervorzubringen vermag. Beachtenswert sind in dieser Hinsicht die erbanalytischen Ergebnisse, zu welchen SZONDI bei der Prüfung der Verwandtschaft von 70 Stotterern gelangte. Er fand, daß Stottern, Epilepsie und Migräne in einem engen, erbbiologischen Zusammenhang stehen, der einen besonderen Erbgang erkennen läßt. Näheres über diesen als gemeinsam aufgefaßten erbbedingten ursächlichen Faktor können wir vorderhand nicht aussagen, nur soviel, daß er durch seine ambivalente Wirkung spezifisch gekennzeichnet ist. Er bildet aber nur einen der zahlreichen ursächlichen Faktoren, die bei der Migräne und Epilepsie sonst noch wirksam sein dürften.

6. Psychische Störungen bei Migräne.

Die bei der Migräne beobachteten seelischen Alterationen weisen eine breite Skala auf, die sich von der einfachen Depression bis zu den schwersten Verwirrtheitszuständen erstreckt. Über die den Migräneanfall einleitende oder begleitende und nur selten nachfolgende Gemütsverstimmung wurde schon bei der Beschreibung des gewöhnlichen Migräneanfalls erwähnt, daß sie eine häufige Begleiterscheinung darstellt und als eine elementare psychische Reaktion anzusehen ist, die nicht notwendigerweise durch die übrigen peinlichen Migränesymptome verursacht wird, kündigt sie doch nicht selten als einziges Zeichen den kommenden Anfall an. Der autonome Charakter dieser Gemütsverstimmung, wie ihn neuerdings wieder CHRISTIANSEN betonte, wird von anderen Autoren (SCHULTZE) geleugnet.

Depressionszustände kommen bei Migränekranken häufig auch im interparoxysmalen Stadium zur Erscheinung. FLATAU fand sie in einem Viertel seiner Fälle, sie kommen anfangs nur sporadisch vor und dauern erst einige Stunden oder Tage, später treten sie häufiger auf und haben eine längere Dauer. In selteneren Fällen nehmen sie die Form einer dauernden Stimmungslage an, die Jahre und Jahrzehnte hindurch ununterbrochen anhalten kann. Neben der traurigen Gemütsstimmung ist die Arbeitsunlust dieser Kranken auffallend, so daß auch die Tagesarbeit nur mit der größten Anstrengung erledigt werden kann; vollständige Interesselosigkeit der Umwelt gegenüber beherrscht diese Zustände, welche manchmal noch durch Selbstanklage, Versündigungsgedanken, Gewissensbisse gefärbt sind. Angstzustände treten nur selten auf.

Die psychischen Störungen, die mit dem Anfall zeitlich zusammenhängen, können von verschiedener Art sein. FLATAU, der die bis 1912 in der Literatur niedergelegten Fälle gesammelt hat, gibt folgende Zusammenfassung: Die häufigsten Formen der migränösen psychischen Störung sind Dämmerzustände und Verwirrtheitszustände, die durch Angstgefühl, psychische, motorische Unruhe und schreckhafte Halluzinationen beherrscht werden. Ein psychisches Trauma spielt dabei nur selten eine Rolle. Die Psychose begleitet am häufigsten den Anfall selbst, entsteht oft schon zu Beginn des Anfalles oder auf der Höhe desselben. Der Kopfschmerz wird durch den psychotischen Zustand verdeckt. Es gibt aber Fälle (LÖWENFELD), wo die Psychose eine so kurze Dauer hat, daß noch nachher der Kopfschmerz folgen kann. Nur ganz wenige Fälle sind bekannt, wo die Psychose nach dem Anfall auftrat. Noch seltener ist es, daß die Psychose vor dem Anfall auftritt. Im sog. Dämmerzustand sind die Kranken benommen, erscheinen desorientiert, lassen häufig Gesichts- und Gehörshalluzinationen erkennen, die fast immer einen schreckhaften Charakter haben, wodurch die Kranken in einen Erregungszustand versetzt werden, in welchem es zu Suicidversuchen und gewalttätigen Handlungen an Personen der Umgebung kommen kann. Die Psychose entwickelt sich in kurzer Zeit, manchmal wenigen Stunden. Die Schwere der Verwirrtheit ist verschieden. In leichteren Fällen ist es nur eine ängstliche Unruhe, dabei gewisse Krankheitseinsicht, in schweren Fällen vollständige Desorientiertheit, halluzinatorisches Delir (MINGAZZINI). Die Dauer der Psychose ist im allgemeinen kurz; sie reicht von einigen Stunden bis einige Tage. In seltenen Fällen bleibt sie längere Zeit (Monate lang) bestehen. Die Erinnerung an die geistige Störung ist eine summarische und lückenhafte, oft besteht vollständige Amnesie. Die Psychosen treten gewöhnlich in großen Zeitintervallen auf.

Eine besondere Besprechung verdienen die sog. *psychischen Äquivalente der Migräne*.

Schon CORNU machte in einigen Fällen die Beobachtung, daß die Migräneanfälle zeitweise verschwinden und an ihrer Stelle Zustände von Melancholie mit Versündigungs- und Verfolgungsgedanken auftreten, die er als Äquivalente der Migräneanfälle auffaßt. FLATAU nimmt eine solche nur dort an, wo die periodische Abwechslung zwischen Migräne und psychischer Alteration eine Regelmäßigkeit erkennen läßt und den für die Migränepsychosen typischen Charakter zeigt; auch zählt er zu den Postulaten der Migräneäquivalente, daß sie von kurzer Dauer sei, keine Progressivität im psychischen Verhalten zeige, im Intervall normales psychisches Bild bestehe, ferner das Fehlen von Merkmalen einer epileptischen oder hysterischen Konstitution. JAHRREIS berichtet über periodisch sich wiederholende, anfallsweise auftretende Zustände von Bewußtseinstrübung bei einem 40jährigen Mann, der übrigens vollkommen gesund ist. Leichte Benommenheit, taumelnder Gang, aphasische und dyspraktische Störungen, die von Kopfschmerz begleitet und gefolgt werden und durch einen langen Schlaf beendet werden. Er nimmt für diese Migränedämmerzustände eine Sonderstellung an und findet Berührungspunkte mit der manisch-depressiven Erkrankung. F. MOERSCH, der unter seinen Migränefällen psychische Störung in 15—26% der Fälle vorfand, bestätigt ebenfalls die Existenzberechtigung der psychischen Äquivalente, unter welchen er nicht nur Zustände von Verstimmung, Erregung, Verwirrtheit, sondern auch Zwangshandlungen (Kleptomanie) beobachtete. J. M. NIELSEN berichtet über den Fall eines 37jährigen Arztes, ohne hereditäre Belastung, bei dem sich seit dem 18. Lebensjahr jährlich 1—2mal anfallsweise auftretende psychische Zustände zeigen, die 3—6 Stunden lang andauern und dann spurlos verschwinden. Die Störung ist durch Gemütsverstimmung und eine eigenartige Denkstörung gekennzeichnet indem bei vollkommen erhaltenem Bewußtsein und guter Perzeption die assoziative Funktion schwer gestört ist; das Bewußtsein ist immer nur auf einzelne Gesichtsfelder eingestellt, die er miteinander nicht in Beziehung zu bringen vermag. Unabhängig von diesen Attacken leidet er auch an Anfällen von Sehstörung in der Form einer homonymen Hemianopsie oder Quadrantenhemianopsie mit Spektralerscheinung (selten auch Fortifikationsfiguren). Nie waren die geschilderten Anfälle von Kopfschmerz, Erbrechen oder Brechreiz begleitet.

Eine einschlägige eigene Beobachtung soll hier kurz angeführt werden. 52jähriger Kaufmann, verheiratet, 2 Kinder, erblich nicht belastet, leidet seit 27 Jahren an Anfällen von seelischer Verstimmung mit Arbeitsunlust, Menschenscheu: der am Vortag noch fleißige, lebensfrohe Mann ist nicht aus dem Zimmer zu bringen, er will niemanden sprechen, kann seiner Frau in geschäftlichen Sachen keinen Rat geben, spricht überhaupt nur selten, verschließt sich vor seiner Familie. Der Anfall wird manchmal von 1—2tägigem beiderseitigem Kopfschmerz mit Brechreiz eingeleitet und immer mit einem ähnlichen Kopfschmerz beendet. Anfänglich kamen die Anfälle nur ganz selten, in 2—3 Jahren, und dauerten 3—4 Tage lang, allmählich wurden sie häufiger und länger. Im Jahre 1929 hatte er schon acht solche Anfälle in der Dauer von 10—30 Tagen. Einigemal kam die Depression nach stattgehabtem Coitus. Der Beginn und das Aufhören dieser Zustände erfolgt plötzlich; am ersten Tag, wo er wieder ins Geschäft geht, ist er der tüchtige, arbeitsfrohe Kaufmann von früher.

Einigemal kamen abortive Anfälle vor, die nur einen halben Tag dauerten. Der die Depression beendende Kopfschmerz erfolgt so regelmäßig, daß die Angehörigen dieses Symptom schon als günstiges Zeichen zu verwerten pflegen. Die körperliche Untersuchung ergab gar keine pathologische Veränderung. Ich möchte diesen sehr einleuchtenden Fall von anfallsweise auftretender Gemütsdepression um so eher für eine Migräneäquivalente auffassen, weil hier auch andere rudimentäre Symptome des Migräneanfalles verzeichnet sind.

Die hier angeführten Beobachtungen weisen darauf hin, daß psychische Krankheitszustände als substituierende Symptome den Migräneanfall vertreten können. Doch ist die Frage, ob diese psychischen Störungen zum engeren Krankheitsbild der Migräne gehören, nicht leicht zu beantworten. Die Schwierigkeit, der man hier begegnet, hängt damit zusammen, daß die Migräne sich nicht selten mit einer allgemeinen psychopathischen Anlage verbindet und daß auch eine epileptische Kombination nicht außer acht gelassen werden darf. CHRISTIANSEN z. B. führt die leichteren Formen der psychischen Störung (Depression) als psychogen bedingte Störung auf die psychopathische Anlage zurück. Für die schweren Formen nimmt er eine organische Grundlage an. KRAFFT-EBING kommt auf Grund seiner zahlreichen Kasuistik zur Ansicht, daß der größte Teil der die Migräne begleitenden psychischen Störungen einer larvierten Epilepsie zugeordnet werden muß; dies gilt besonders für die Augenmigräne und die mit sensiblen Erscheinungen einhergehenden Anfälle. Dieser Auffassung gegenüber betont MINGAZZINI auch in seiner letzten, über dieses Thema veröffentlichten Arbeit die Sonderstellung der Migränepsychosen, die er unter dem Namen Dysphrenia hemicranica selbständig macht. Als charakteristisch für diese Zustände hebt er hervor, daß hauptsächlich diejenigen Fälle von ophthalmischer Migräne mit Psychosen einhergehen, in welchen der Kopfschmerz den Sehstörungen zeitlich vorausgeht und nicht nachfolgt und daß ein strenger Parallelismus in der Intensität zwischen Kopfschmerz und Sehstörung einerseits und der Psychose andererseits besteht. Er erblickt in der die Psychose begleitenden Halluzination, welche die übrigen psychotischen Erscheinungen verursacht, die höchste Steigerung jener Gesichtserscheinungen, welche als einfache Phosphene den ophthalmischen Migräneanfall einleiten. MINGAZZINI unterscheidet eine kurzdauernde und vorübergehende Störung von einer Dysphrenia permanens, welche er der Hemicrania permanens gleichstellt (mit periodischen Schwankungen, wie sie auch der Kopfschmerz bei Dauermigräne zeigt).

Stützt also MINGAZZINI die Sonderstellung der psychischen Migräne auf einen sich in der Zeitdauer und Intensität kundgebenden Parallelismus zwischen Migräneanfall und Psychose (ein Standpunkt, der nur wenig Anerkennung fand), so beruht die ablehnende Haltung KRAFFT-EBINGs und der meisten Forscher hauptsächlich darauf, daß die bei Migräne beobachteten psychischen Störungen nach den Beobachtungen von KRÄPELIN, ASCHAFFENBURG, BINSWANGER u. a. auch bei Epileptikern sehr häufig angetroffen werden. Hält man sich noch vor Augen, daß es eine große Anzahl von Migränekranken gibt, die trotz des langen Bestandes ihrer Migräne gar keine psychische Alterationen aufweisen, unter denen sogar eine Reihe von geistig hervorragenden Männern sich befanden (CHARCOT, DUBOIS, REYMOND, HALLER, LINNÉ, MIRABEAU, NAPOLEON usw.), so wird man dem Gedanken, daß der Migräneanfall als solcher zu geistigen Störungen führe, widerstreben. Ich möchte mich auch hier zu der Ansicht bekennen, die ich bei der Kombination der Migräne mit Epilepsie betonte. Die Fälle mit psychischer Migräne repräsentieren eine eigene Gruppe unter den Migränekranken, mit welchen sie nur das Syndrom des Migräneanfalles gemeinsam haben. Wenn man auch zugeben muß, daß psychische Störungen einen integrierenden Bestandteil des Migräneanfalles bilden können, sogar als psychische Äquivalente den Migräneanfall vertreten können, muß man anderenteils daran festhalten, daß in *diesen Fällen die psychische Färbung der Anfälle nicht der Migränekrankheit als solcher, sondern ihrer anderweitigen konstitutionellen Anlage zuzuschreiben ist.* Zweifellos gibt es unter den Fällen von psychischer Migräne eine große Anzahl, in welcher die epileptische Anlage für diese Störungen verantwortlich gemacht werden kann; bei den übrigen Fällen wird man eine allgemeine psychopathische Konstitution hierfür beschuldigen müssen.

7. Hysterische Reaktionen bei Migräne.

Da sowohl Migräne wie Hysterie krankhafte Zustände darstellen, welche das weibliche Geschlecht bevorzugen, müßte man, wenn ein innigerer Zusammenhang zwischen Migräne und Hysterie bestehen würde, diese Kombination viel häufiger antreffen, als es in Wirklichkeit der Fall ist. Mit Recht betont FLATAU, daß die Berührungspunkte zwischen Migräne und Hysterie geringer sind, als zwischen Migräne und Epilepsie. Französische Autoren, wie CHARCOT, BABINSKI u. a. behaupten, daß die Migräne unter Umständen als hysterisches Symptom auftreten könne, BABINSKI vertritt sogar die Ansicht, daß die „hysterische Augenmigräne" auf demselben angiospastischen Prozeß beruhe, wie die echte ophthalmische Migräne. Die hysterische Veranlagung kann sich vielfach in das Migränesyndrom hineinspielen und diesem eine eigenartige Prägung geben. Hysterische, die gleichzeitig an Migräne leiden, können hysterische Zustandsbilder hervorbringen, die dem wahren Migräneanfall ähnlich sind. Auch können im Zusammenhang mit dem Migräneanfall andere hysterische Erscheinungen, Weinkrämpfe, spasmodische Zustände, Arc de cercle usw, auftreten. OPPENHEIM sah bei Hysterischen während ihrer Migräneanfälle Hemianästhesien auf Seite des Kopfschmerzes, die man sehr wahrscheinlich als hysterische Manifestation wird auffassen können. KRAFFT-EBING und FLATAU teilen Fälle mit, wo protrahierte hysterische Anfälle echte Migräneanfälle auslösten [1]. Es liegen auch zahlreiche Beobachtungen vor, in welchen nach Anfällen von Augenmigräne sich postparoxysmale hysterische Zustände entwickelten und ein oder mehrere Symptome der Augenmigräne eine hysterische Fixierung erhielten; so sah man, daß sich auf das Symptom der migränösen Sehstörung eine hysterische Amblyopie mit Dyschromatopsie und konzentrischer Gesichtsfeldeinschränkung (GALEZOWSKI) oder einseitige hysterische Muskelspasmen aufpfropften. MOEBIUS und BABINSKI beobachteten öfters die hysterische Fixierung der sensiblen Epilepsie bei Augenmigräne. Eine lehrreiche eigene Beobachtung gehört auch hierher.

Frl. I. P., Pädagogin, 34 Jahre alt, ohne nachweisbare hereditäre Belastung, leidet seit 4 Jahren an linksseitiger Migräne mit Brechreiz und kurzer Sehstörung. Die Anfälle zeigen sich in Intervallen von 3—4 Monaten und dauern gewöhnlich einige Tage. Im April 1930 ereilte sie der Anfall in einer Gesellschaft, und zwar so, daß zuerst eine von der rechten Seite des Gesichtsfeldes herantretende und wie ein Vorhang das Gesichtsfeld von rechts her absperrende Sehstörung eintrat, welche sich bis zu einem Nichtsehen durch einige Minuten steigerte; kurz nachher trat ein heftiges Kribbeln im rechten Arm und Bein, sowie im rechten Gesicht auf, welches ungefähr eine halbe Stunde lang dauerte und eine Ungeschicktheit der rechtsseitigen Glieder zurückließ. Nach Hause gebracht, beobachtete sie, daß ihre Sprache erschwert ist; sie bringt die Worte nach Silben gegliedert hervor. Jetzt konnte sie auch eine vollkommene Unempfindlichkeit der rechten Körperhälfte gegen Berührung und Schmerzempfindung feststellen. Der linksseitige Kopfschmerz trat erst 3 Stunden nach Beginn des Anfalles auf und dauerte auch diesmal mit besonderer Heftigkeit 4 Tage lang, während welcher Zeit sie im Bette lag, rechten Arm und Fuß ungeschickt bewegte, im Sprechen stark verhindert war und auch über eine Sehstörung klagte. Eine Woche nach dem Anfall fand ich bei der Patientin folgendes Bild: Pupillen mittelweit, gleichmäßig gut reagierend, Facialis beiderseits gleich gut innerviert. Rechtsseitige homonyme Hemianopsie mit Aussparung der Maculagegend. Anästhesie und Analgesie der ganzen rechten

---

[1] M. ULRICH fand unter ihren 500 Migränefällen 48 Fälle, wo Migräne und Hysterie unabhängig von einander bestanden, 13 Fälle, wo sich hysterische Reaktionen dem Migräneanfall überlagerten und 11 Fälle von „hysterischer Migräne".

Körperhälfte genau bis zur Mittellinie für alle Gefühlsqualitäten. Hochgradige hysterische Inkoordination der willkürlichen Bewegungen bei erhaltener motorischer Kraft im rechten Arm und Bein. Feinere Handbewegungen können überhaupt nicht ausgeführt werden, beim Gehen bleibt das rechte Knie gespannt, der Gang zeigt alle Merkmale einer hysterischen Dysbasie. Reflexe auf beiden Seiten gleich, nur die Bauchdeckenreflexe rechts abgeschwächt. Bei Prüfung auf Babinski- und Oppenheimzeichen rechts keine Bewegung der Zehen, links normale Plantarflexion. Sprache etwas verlangsamt, die Worte werden saccadiert, manchmal spastisch-explosiv hervorgebracht. Keine Andeutung einer motorischen Aphasie. Die Kranke wurde auf meiner Spitalsabteilung isoliert und faradisch behandelt. Allmählicher Rückgang sämtlicher Erscheinungen binnen 10 Tagen, zuletzt blieb eine angedeutete Quadrantenhemianopsie im linken nasalen Gesichtsfeld, welche nach 3 Wochen verschwand.

8. Interparoxysmale Erscheinungen bei Migräne.

Von diesen sollen hier nur diejenigen Symptome eine kurze Erwähnung finden, welche mit dem Migräneanfall irgendwie in einem pathogenetischen Zusammenhang stehen. FLATAU berücksichtigt vor allem die Krankheitserscheinungen, welche auf einen Sympathicusreiz zurückzuführen sind. Er erwähnt Gesichtsödeme mit Jucken, OPPENHEIM vasomotorischen Schnupfen, CURSCHMANN Hautödeme im Gesicht, an den Händen, am Rumpf; er beobachtete auch kleine Bläschen an den Fingerspitzen und am ganzen Körper. Eine ebenfalls als trophische Störung zu betrachtende Veränderung sah ich bei einer an linksseitiger Migräne leidenden Frau, die unabhängig von den Anfällen zeitweise ein mit Jucken auftretendes Geschwür bekam auf der linken Zungenspitze und in der linken unteren Mundschleimhautfalte; das Geschwür, am meisten einem Mal perforant ähnlich (ohne entzündliche Umrandung), verschwand in 4—5 Tagen spurlos. In zwei eigenen Fällen beobachtete ich Heuasthma. Sympathicusbedingte Schmerzanfälle bei Migränekranken wurden von OPPENHEIM, LAMACQ, FREUD und E. MENDEL an verschiedenen Körperstellen beschrieben. Sie dauern von einigen Minuten bis zu einigen Stunden, werden manchmal von Speichelabsonderung, Brechreiz oder Erbrechen gefolgt. Es wurde schon erwähnt, daß Schmerzanfälle im linken Hypochondrium, im Epigastrium, in der Nabelgegend von neueren Autoren als Migräneäquivalente aufgefaßt werden. Seitens des Herzens sind Tachykardie, Arythmie mit Oppressionsgefühl, sowie Anfälle von Angina pectoris vasomotorica (CURSCHMANN) beobachtet worden. Auch Asthmaanfälle sind als interparoxysmale Erscheinungen verzeichnet. FLATAU erwähnt auch Gähn- und Nieskrämpfe. Von cerebralen Ausfallserscheinungen erwähnen LIVEING und FLATAU interparoxysmale aphasische Störungen.

II. Pathogenese der Migräne.

Je mehr sich unsere Kenntnisse über die Pathogenese der Migräne erweitern, um so verwickelter erscheint dieses Problem und um so stärker drängt die Erkenntnis durch, daß die Entstehungsursachen und Bedingungen dieser Krankheit nicht einheitlich zusammengefaßt werden können. Der Überblick über diese komplexe Frage wird einigermaßen erleichtert, wenn man die Pathogenese der Migräne in zwei selbständig zu behandelnde Probleme sondert. Das erste Problem richtet sich auf den Pathomechanismus des Migräneanfalles selbst und gipfelt in der Frage, was für ein pathophysiologischer Vorgang im Organismus sich abspielt, wenn ein Migräneanfall sich einstellt. Das pathogenetische Problem des Migräneanfalles ist für alle Migräneformen gemeinsam, also nicht nur für die früher geschilderten verschiedenen Erscheinungsformen der echten Migräne, sondern auch für die symptomatische Migräne, da die wesentliche Übereinstimmung in der Symptomatologie und im Verlauf zwischen echter und symptomatischer Migräne zur Annahme zwingt, daß auch bei der letzteren dem Migräneanfall derselbe pathophysiologische Vorgang zugrundeliegen müsse, wie bei der echten Migräne. Die zweite Frage richtet sich auf die eigentliche Ätiologie der Migräne und sucht vor allem die Kennzeichen der spezifischen Beschaffenheit jener Individuen zu ermitteln, in welchen es zu migränösen Offenbarungen kommt, also die Merkmale jener Struktureigentümlichkeit, die wir mit dem Namen „Migräneanlage" zu bezeichnen pflegen; sie bezieht sich aber hauptsächlich auf unsere Kenntnisse über die anfallsauslösenden Ursachen, seien diese exogen oder endogen bedingt.

1. Pathomechanismus des Migräneanfalles.

Die ältesten Theorien über das Zustandekommen des Migräneanfalles suchten den Entstehungsort außerhalb des Schädelraumes. Nach den mehr spekulativen Ansichten von GALEN, FERNELL u. a. brachte TISSOT (1813) als erster die sog. „Reflextheorie" in die Diskussion; er faßte die Migräne als eine besondere Form der Trigeminusneuralgie auf, welche durch den Reiz des Magens, der sich auf die Kopfnerven reflektorisch ausbreitet, zur Entstehung gelangt. Später wurden andere Organe, wie die Gallenblase, die Gebärmutter als Entstehungsorte für die reflektorische Migräne in Erwägung gebracht. Auch Erkrankungen der Nase und der Nebenhöhlen, sowie Augenkrankheiten, Refraktionsanomalien spielten bei manchen Autoren eine wesentliche Rolle als reflektorisch wirksame Ursachen des Migräneanfalles. Die Unzulänglichkeit dieser Theorien wurde schon seit langem erkannt; es fehlten die experimentellen, anatomischen und physiologischen Grundlagen für die Annahme eines solchen Reflexvorganges.

Eine zweite Theorie, welche die Ursache und den Entstehungsort des Migräneanfalles außerhalb des Schädelinnenraumes suchte, ist die sog. *myalgische Theorie*. Sie fand schon seit langem und in den verschiedensten Ländern Vertreter (BALFOUR, ROSENBACH, EDINGER, PERITZ, NÖRSTROM, KINDBERG, neuerdings MÜLLER, HARTENBERG-DIDSBURY). ROSENBACH führt gewisse Formen der Migräne auf myalgische Zustände und Schwielenbildung an den Ansatzpunkten der Kopfmuskeln (Mm. frontalis, occipitalis, cucullaris, sternocleidomastoideus) zurück, die er von den nervösen Formen unterscheidet: Muskelmassage beeinflußt günstig diese Migräne. MÜLLER nimmt überhaupt nur einen muskulären Ursprung an, nach ihm bestehe ein Hypertonus der Kopfmuskulatur, welcher von den kleinen Knötchen an den Muskelansatzpunkten ausgeht und zu einer Behinderung des venösen und Lymphabflusses führt. HENSCHEN spricht von einer rheumatischen Form der Migräne, bei welcher eine Verdickung in der Umgebung des Trigeminus und N. occipitalis (Perineuritis) den Kopfschmerz verursacht, er nimmt aber auch eine andere Form an, bei welcher die entzündlichen Veränderungen in der Tiefe der Dura und Pia sich abspielen. ROSE führt die Hypertonie der schmerzhaften Muskeln auf eine latente Arthritis der oberen Halsgelenke zurück. HARTENBERG und DIDSBURY sprechen von einer subakuten oder chronischen Myositis; bei der chronischen Form findet man harte Schwielen in den Muskeln, manchmal Lymphdrüsenschwellungen in der Nachbarschaft sowie Infiltration und Verdickung der Haut. Die Muskelveränderungen verursachen in der Nachbarschaft der Nerven einen Reizzustand, der sich in der Druckempfindlichkeit an den Austrittsstellen kundgibt. HARTENBERG bemerkt aber, daß diese Muskelveränderungen den Migräneanfall nicht erklären können, es müsse auch ein Reizzustand des Halssympathicus angenommen werden, welcher von den erkrankten Muskeln ausgeht. LORENZ und STOCKMANN untersuchten mikroskopisch die Muskelinfiltrate und fanden in diesen eine Bindegewebswucherung mit Endoperiarteriitis. AUERBACH unterscheidet den Schwielenkopfschmerz von der Migräne. HARTMANN meint, daß unter den Migränekopfschmerzen zahlreiche Fälle von „gelöser Erkrankung" der Weichteildecke als solche unerkannt bleiben. Man wird die Ansichten von HARTMANN und AUERBACH anerkennen, diesen oft verkannten Schwielenkopfschmerz aber vom Migräneanfall streng absondern. Von den Gründen, die gegen die myalgische Theorie sprechen, soll hier nur angeführt werden, daß die genannten Muskelveränderungen gewöhnlich im vorgeschrittenen Alter aufzutreten pflegen, während die Migräne vorwiegend eine Krankheit der Jugend und des mittleren Alters bildet. Auch ist es nicht verständlich, daß eine chronische Muskelerkrankung die unmittelbare Ursache von periodisch auftretenden Anfällen sein sollte.

Die zahlreichen cerebralen Begleiterscheinungen des Migräneanfalles (Skotome, Aphasie) könnten auch schwerlich bei dieser Theorie eine Erklärung finden. Zum Schluß soll aber der wichtigste Einwand erhoben werden, daß in den meisten Fällen von Migräne die von den genannten Autoren beschriebenen Muskelveränderungen überhaupt nicht nachweisbar sind.

Die Erklärungsversuche, welche den Migräneanfall auf einen im intrakraniellen Raum sich abspielenden pathophysiologischen Vorgang zurückführen, sind überaus zahlreich und beziehen sich auf alle Gewebsschichten dieses Raumes. Von den Hirnhäuten hat man besonders die Dura in den Mittelpunkt gestellt, weil es bis vor kurzem angenommen wurde, daß sie allein unter den Hirnhäuten sensible Fasern besitze. *Die Hirnrinde* wurde zuerst von MOEBIUS als Sitz des Migränevorganges in Erwägung gezogen; er nahm an, daß die Auraerscheinungen in der Hirnrinde infolge Alteration der Zellen gewisser Rindenpartien entstehen und der nachfolgende Kopfschmerz durch ein Überspringen des Reizes von der Rinde auf die benachbarte Hirnhaut. Er stellte also die Aura als den wesentlichen Teil des Anfalles hin und in den Fällen, wo Auraerscheinungen fehlen, nahm er an, daß der Rindenreiz ein stummes Gebiet betraf. KRAFFT-EBING sprach von einer Neurose der Rindenfelder, ROMBERG von einer cerebralen Neuralgie, SCHULTZE nahm eine besondere Erregbarkeit der Hirnrinde an, SCHOTTIN eine erhöhte Empfindlichkeit der sensiblen und sensorischen Zentren, die er auf Phosphorarmut der Gehirnzellen zurückführt. *Jaquet* und *Jourdanet* sprechen von Überempfindlichkeitskrisen der Gehirnsubstanz, welche vom Magen ausgelöst werden, LIVEING von „nervösen Stürmen" usw. Eine Reihe von Theorien sucht den Sitz des Migräneanfalles in anderen Gehirnsegmenten. TEED und später KOVALEWSKI betrachten das Kerngebiet des vierten Ventrikels, THOMAS und CORNU das Kerngebiet des Trigeminus als Sitzort des Migränevorganges; nach CORNU erkläre der Reizzustand dieses Kernes die Kopfschmerzen, das Erbrechen, die vasomotorischen und sekretorischen Störungen, die anderen Migränesymptome dürften durch eine Ausstreuung des Reizzustandes in andere Hirnsegmente entstehen. Eine ähnliche Auffassung findet sich bei L. LEVI, der ein sog. „*Migränezentrum*" im sensiblen Kerngebiet des V. am Boden des 4. Ventrikels annimmt, von wo aus der krankhafte Reiz durch nervöse Wellenbewegung auf die benachbarten Kerne des IX., X., Deiters und des vasomotorischen Zentrums ausstrahlt. BONNIER wählte das Kerngebiet des VIII., speziell den Deiterskern, als Ausgangspunkt des Migräneanfalles. Er betrachtet als Syndrom des Deiterskernes den Schwindel mit Gleichgewichtsstörung und führt die übrigen Migränesymptome als reflektorische Übertragung des Reizes auf die Hirnnerven III., IV., VI., VIII., IX. und X. zurück, welche mit dem Deiterskern in Verbindung stehen. BRISSAUD, THOMAS, F. LEVI nehmen eine Neuralgie der intrakraniellen Trigeminuswurzelfasern an, EULENBURG der Durafasern des Trigeminus, BABONNEIX und H. DAVID sprechen von einer Radikulalgie des Trigeminus, wobei die Druckerhöhung des Liquors auf die Wurzelfasern einen schmerzhaften Reiz ausübt, der sich auf die meningealen Zweige ausbreitet.

Der große Mangel dieser Theorien liegt darin, daß sie nur das Lokalisationsprinzip berücksichtigen, über den pathophysiologischen Vorgang aber nichts aussagen. Stellt man sich bei diesem einen erhöhten Erregbarkeitszustand der genannten Zentren vor, dann müßte man auch bei anderen Erkrankungen der Hirnrinde oder der Oblongatazentren Migränezustände als ständige Begleiterscheinungen erwarten.

An diese sog. zentralen Theorien reiht sich die *Hypophysentheorie*. DEYL hat (1900) als erster eine Erklärung gegeben, nach welcher der Migräneanfall durch den ersten Ast des Trigeminus aufrechterhalten wird, welcher bei Migränekranken durch Anschwellung der Hypophyse in der Falte zwischen Carotis und der Drüse gedrückt und gezerrt wird. Die Schwellung der Hypophyse soll durch erhöhten Blutzufluß und verhinderten Abfluß des venösen Blutstroms im Gehirn verursacht werden. PLAVEC nimmt ebenfalls eine Schwellung der Hypophyse als Primum movens an, durch welche die benachbarten sympathischen Geflechte, der Plexus caroticus und cavernosus gedrückt werden; diese geben die Symptome der gewöhnlichen Migräne ab. Eine besondere anatomische Disposition muß vorliegen, wenn auch der Oculomotorius in das Druckgebiet gelangt (ophthalmoplegische Migräne). Die Halbseitigkeit der Anfälle sei durch eine Asymmetrie der Hypophyse bedingt. Die Theorie, daß der Migräneanfall durch eine vorübergehende Volumvergrößerung der Hypophyse bedingt ist, wird von mehreren Autoren (FISHER, CHARLES, HODGES, SEDILLOT, LORD DAVSON, PAULIAN, POUSSEPP, KAST) auch heute noch verfochten. PAULIAN nimmt eine spezielle Migräneform an, die durch anatomische Veränderungen an der Hirnbasis in der Hypophysengegend aufrechterhalten wird; Röntgenbilder solcher Fälle lassen eine Deformation der Sella, Schwund und Verdickung des Processus clinoideus, sowie Knochenneubildungen in dieser Gegend erkennen. THOMSON fand in 17 unter 25 Fällen von menstrueller Migräne am Röntgenbild eine abnorme Gestaltung der Sella durch Verknöcherung des Diaphragma sellae; die menstruelle Schwellung der Hypophyse führe in diesen Fällen, wo das Diaphragma nicht ausweicht, zu einer Drucksteigerung in der Hypophyse und dadurch zum Migräneanfall. Die angeführten und auch voneinander abweichenden Röntgenbefunde dienen eigentlich als einzige Beweise für die hypophysären Theorien. Dagegen möchte ich hier nur darauf hinweisen, daß vorübergehende Hypophysenschwellung klinisch bisher hauptsächlich in der Gravidität festgestellt wurde, in einer Periode also, wo erfahrungsgemäß die Migräneanfälle auszubleiben pflegen. Auch konnte ich mich von der Richtigkeit der Angabe einiger Autoren, nach welcher Krankheitszustände, die mit einer Hypophysenvergrößerung einhergehen, oft von Migräneanfällen begleitet werden, nicht recht überzeugen.

Störungen der Liquorzirkulation werden in den Theorien von SPITZER und QUINCKE als Ausgangspunkt des Migräneanfalles hingestellt. Nach SPITZER wird der Migräneanfall durch einen plötzlichen, vorübergehenden Verschluß des Foramen interventriculare MONROI hervorgerufen auf die Weise, daß der vom Plexus chorioideus in die Seitenventrikel sezernierte Liquor keinen Abfluß findet und auf die Gehirnhemisphären einen Druck ausübt, welcher das Gehirn gegen die Dura drückt und durch diesen Druck die Migränesymptome herbeiführt. Chronisch entzündliche Veränderungen am Foramen MONROI dürften die Ursache dieser absoluten oder relativen Verengung sein, in diesen liege das pathologisch-anatomische Substrat der Migränekonstitution. Die Auraerscheinungen sind auf Zerrung und Zerreißung der Piabalken an der Hirnrinde zurückzuführen. SPITZERS Erklärung fand viel Interesse, doch wenig Anklang. Bei der von ihm vermuteten grob mechanischen Entstehungsweise des Migräneanfalles müßte man die von ihm zur Grundlage dieser Theorie gemachten pathologisch-anatomischen Veränderungen in den Seitenventrikeln und auf der Rindenoberfläche irgendwie schon nachgewiesen haben.

Nach QUINCKE sei der Migräneanfall eine Form von angioneurotischem Hydrocephalus, wo neben der Innervationsstörung der Gefäße auch ein akuter Meningealerguß am Prozeß beteiligt wäre. Er führt den Kopfschmerz auf Krampf- und Lähmungszustände begrenzter Gefäßgebiete zurück, während die schweren Migränesymptome, Schwindel, Erbrechen, Unfähigkeit zum Denken, durch den Meningealerguß bedingt wären. Als Beweis führt er 3 Fälle an, von welchen bei zweien die während des Anfalles ausgeführte Lumbalpunktion eine Linderung der Kopfschmerzen herbeiführte. Der angioneurotische Komplex bestehe außer einer erhöhten Liquorproduktion in einer Hyperämie der Hirnhäute und einem umschriebenen Ödem der Dura. QUINCKES Auffassung wurde von vielen

Autoren zustimmend aufgenommen. STRÜMPELL faßte die Migräne in diesem Sinne als eine besondere Form der exsudativen Diathese auf. Auch L. R. MÜLLER, ASSMANN, LÖWENTHAL, FLATAU, KÄMMERER u. a. stellen die exsudativen Vorgänge im Gehirn oder an den Gehirnhäuten in den Mittelpunkt der Pathogenese. Eine wesentliche Förderung erhielt die exsudative Theorie durch die in neuester Zeit gewonnenen Kenntnisse über die sog. anaphylaktischen Migräne, weil der im Gehirn vermutete exsudative Prozeß als anaphylaktische Erscheinung eine gute Erklärung finden konnte. So spricht KÄMMERER von anaphylaktogenen Eiweißstoffen, welche teils vasokonstriktorisch (tyramin), teils vasodilatorisch und exsudativ (hystamin) wirken und setzt das Substrat des Migräneanfalles einer rasch abklingenden Urticaria der betroffenen Hirnteile gleich, wodurch die Flüchtigkeit der Erscheinungen eine Erklärung findet. F. KENNEDY erblickt ebenfalls in einem „lokalisierten intrakraniellen Ödem" das pathologische Substrat des Migräneanfalles, wobei eher die Hirnhäute als das Hirngewebe selbst Sitzort der Schwellung sein dürften. KOCHER bezieht sich auf Experimente CUSHINGs und führt den Anfall auf eine durch Liquorvermehrung verursachte Druckerhöhung im Schädelinnern zurück, welche von einem gewissen Grade an eine Kompression der Venen im Schädelinnern erzeugen und dadurch zur Stauung und weiteren Vermehrung des intrakraniellen Druckes führe. Der Kopfschmerz tritt nach CUSHING bereits im ersten Stadium des Hirndruckes auf durch Reiz der Durafasern des Trigeminus. FLATAU schließt sich zum Teil dieser Auffassung an, wobei er neben dem Gefäßkrampf eine Druckerhöhung des Liquors annimmt, die durch ihre verschiedentliche Auswirkung an verschiedenen Zentren des Gehirns die abwechslungsreiche Symptomatologie der Migräne hervorbringt. AUERBACH und SCHÜLLER sehen die Ursache der Migräne in einem dauernden Mißverhältnis zwischen Schädelkapazität und Schädelinhalt, in einer abnormen Größe des Gehirns zum Schädel. SCHÜLLER führt auf Röntgenbildern nachgewiesene Veränderungen, Druckusuren, Hyperostosen und destruktive Knochenprozesse als Beweise für diese Annahme an. Er erwähnt auch, daß Leute mit Turmschädel oft an Migräne leiden.

So einleuchtend auch die Annahme eines exsudativen Vorganges als Grundlage des Migräneanfalles, besonders bei den Fällen von anaphylaktischer Migräne, erscheint, fehlen bisher jegliche Beweise für eine solche. Man wird aber allen Theorien, welche den Migräneanfall mit einer Druckerhöhung im Schädelinnern in Zusammenhang bringen, mit größter Skepsis entgegentreten müssen, wenn man die von allen Seiten bestätigte Erfahrung vor Augen hält, daß die Liquorentnahme, also die Druckentlastung, entgegen den zitierten Beobachtungen von QUINCKE, keinen mildernden Einfluß auf den Migräneanfall ausübt. Zahlreiche eigene Beobachtungen bestätigen diese Erfahrung. Ich konnte im Gegenteil in einigen Fällen eine Zunahme der Anfallssymptome unmittelbar nach der Lumbalpunktion beobachten. Und wenn es auch vorkommt, daß Gehirnprozesse, die mit Drucksteigerung im Schädelinnern einhergehen, manchmal Migränesyndrome hervorrufen, so ist auch zweifellos, daß die bekannten Symptome der allgemeinen Hirndrucksteigerung etwas vom Migränesyndrom gänzlich Abweichendes darstellen.

Unter allen Theorien, die als Erklärung für das Zustandekommen des Migräneanfalles vorgebracht wurden, steht heute zweifellos die zuerst von DUBOIS-REYMOND inaugurierte *angiospastische Theorie* im Vordergrund. Nachdem schon vorher PARRY und MARSHALL HALL Störungen der Blutzirkulation beim Migräneanfall in Erwägung brachten, und zwar PARRY eine arterielle Hyperämie, einen Blutandrang zum Kopf, welcher auch die Ursache der Epilepsie, Hysterie und verschiedener paroxysmaler Psychosen bilden sollte, MARSHALL HALL dagegen eine venöse Hyperämie annahm, gelangte DUBOIS (1860) auf Grund von Eigenbeobachtungen zu der Erkenntnis, daß die Migräne auf einem Krampf (Tetanus) der vom Halssympathicus innervierten Hirn- und Kopfgefäße beruhe. Er gründete seine Ansicht auf erkennbare Begleiterscheinungen des Migräneanfalles, wie Blässe des Gesichts auf der Seite des Kopfschmerzes, niedrigere Temperatur im äußeren Gehörgang dieser Seite, Erweiterung der Pupille und Zusammenziehung der Schläfenschlagader. Diese Symptome sind seit den Untersuchungen von CLAUDE BERNARD als Reizsymptome des Halssympathicus bekannt. Der Kopfschmerz sei nach DUBOIS durch den Gefäßmuskelkrampf selbst bedingt, das Erbrechen durch Schwankungen des intrakraniellen Blutdruckes. DUBOIS machte diese Erklärung nur für eine Gruppe von Migräneanfällen geltend, die er als Hemicrania sympathicotonica von den übrigen Fällen absonderte. Für eine andere Gruppe gab MÖLLENDORF (1867) als Ursache des Anfalles eine paroxysmale Lähmung des Halssympathicusabschnittes an, der sich äußerlich in Gesichtsröte, erhöhter Temperatur im äußeren Gehörgang, Verengung der Pupille, Erweiterung der Schläfenarterie und der Retinalgefäße und Injektion der Bindehaut zu erkennen gibt, wesentlich aber auf einer Anenergie der die Carotis beherrschenden vasomotorischen Nerven beruht, wodurch die Arterien erschlaffen und ein Blutandrang zum Gehirn steigt.

Als Beweis führte er an, daß die Kompression der Carotis auf der schmerzenden Seite den Kopfschmerz augenblicklich aufhebt, mit Nachlaß des Druckes setzt dieser wieder ein; umgekehrt wird durch die Kompression der Carotis auf der entgegengesetzten Seite und der Subclavia auf derselben Seite der Kopfschmerz gesteigert, da durch Abschneiden dieser Zuflüsse eine größere Pulswelle in die schlaffe Carotis gelangt. Nach MÖLLENDORF werden die Migränesymptome teils durch den Blutandrang in das Gehirn, teils durch den Druck des vergrößerten Gehirns auf die Basis und Wände verursacht. Die Anenergie der Gefäßwand wird im Wege des Sympathicus durch Reize verschiedener Art herbeigeführt. Die Erblichkeit der Migräne beruhe daher auf schwacher Entwicklung der Gefäße und leichter Erschöpfung der vasomotorischen Nerven.

EULENBURG, BERGER, HOLST und HAMMOND glaubten beide Theorien in der Pathogenese der Migräne verwerten zu können, indem sie eine blasse (Hemicrania sympathicotonica) und eine rote (Hemicrania sympathicoparalytica) Migräne annahmen. LATHAM brachte Gefäßkrampf und Gefäßerweiterung miteinander in Verbindung, indem er die Auraerscheinungen des Anfalles als Effekt der Anämie, den Kopfschmerz als Folgezustand der Hyperämie deutete; ähnliche Erklärung brachten JACCOUD, PEMBERTON PEAKE.

VALLERY-RADOT, der die Angaben von MÖLLENDORF über die Wirkung der Kompression auf den Kopfschmerz nachprüfte, fand, daß nach Kompression der Carotis auf der Seite des Kopfschmerzes dieser sofort verschwand, aber nur auf die Dauer von 40—50 Sekunden. Setzt man aber den Druck fort, dann tritt er wieder auf, zuerst allmählich, gewinnt aber rasch an Intensität; die Kompression der Carotis der anderen Seite hat zumeist keinen Effekt oder bringt eine leichte Verringerung des Kopfschmerzes. Nach RADOT sei der Carotisdruck ein recht verwickelter Vorgang, bei welchem auch die Jugularis und das sympathische Geflecht gedrückt werden, so daß es schwer ist, zu beurteilen, auf welche Faktoren die erwähnte Wirkung zurückzuführen ist.

Die vasomotorische Theorie von DUBOIS wurde im Anfang heftig bekämpft. Es wurde vor allem in Zweifel gezogen, daß der Halssympathicus an der vasomotorischen Innervation der Gehirngefäße überhaupt beteiligt ist. Die Untersuchungen von WEBER, HÜRTHLE, WIECHOWSKY haben diese Frage endgültig geklärt, indem sie nachwiesen, daß sämtliche vasokonstriktorischen Nerven der Gehirngefäße aus dem Halssympathicus stammen, von wo sie im Verband des Plexus caroticus und Plexus vertebralis mit den gleichnamigen Arterien zum Gehirn hinaufsteigen. WEBER konnte aus weiteren Versuchen den Schluß ziehen, daß die sympathischen Fasern für die Hirngefäße nicht dem allgemeinen Vasomotorenzentrum in der Oblongata unterstehen, sondern einem besonderen, im Großhirn gelegenen. Die von HILL aufgestellte These, daß die Hirngefäße aktiv ihr Lumen nicht zu ändern vermögen, wurde durch zahlreiche Experimente, insbesondere durch den Adrenalininjektionsversuch von BIEDEL und

REINER, ferner von COBB u. a. widerlegt[1]. Die Annahme, daß der dem Migräneanfall zugrunde liegende Gefäßkrampf auf einer primären Alteration des Halssympathicus beruhe, erhält eine Unterstützung durch die häufig beobachteten mannigfachen Begleiterscheinungen des Anfalles, die als erkennbare Reizsymptome des Hals- und Kopfsympathicus im klinischen Teil angeführt wurden. Es soll aber hier gleich bemerkt werden, daß ihr Vorhandensein in einem gegebenen Fall keinesfalls als eine obligate Erscheinung angesehen werden darf, da es sehr gut möglich ist, daß ein Reizzustand der die Hirngefäße innervierenden sympathischen Bahnen auch ohne Beteiligung der die Gesichtsgefäße versorgenden Fasern bestehen kann. Auch muß man sich gegenüber der Beweisführung von MÖLLENDORF skeptisch verhalten, wenn er die Existenz einer angioparalytischen Migräne auf Symptome (Gesichtsröte, Miosis) stützt, die auf eine Verringerung des Sympathicotonus im Gesicht oder im Auge hindeuten. Man wird hier vor Augen halten müssen, daß die Innervation der Gefäße auf ein feines Reziprozitätsspiel eingestellt ist: spastische Zustände in einem bestimmten Gefäßbezirk vermögen auf dem Wege der vasovasalen Reflexe, vielleicht durch aktive Reizung der Dilatatoren zur Gefäßerweiterung in einem benachbarten Gefäßbezirk führen. Beachtenswerte Angaben macht diesbezüglich F. HARE. Die von DUBOIS betonten Sympathicuserscheinungen wurden seither von den meisten Autoren beobachtet und bestätigt. Die Erweiterung der Pupille ist als eine den Migräneanfall ziemlich häufig begleitende Erscheinung bekannt: ihr Einsetzen am Beginn des Anfalles und Verschwinden am Ende des Anfalles konnte ich wiederholt feststellen (s. auch S. 173). Die Gesichtsblässe während des Anfalles ist vielleicht eine noch häufigere Erscheinung, während die Gesichtsröte (MÖLLENDORF) nach RADOT zumeist nur am Beginn oder Ende des Anfalles auftritt. Für die Beteiligung des Sympathicus am Migräneanfall kann auch die von OPPENHEIM, BRUNNER, BERGER u. a. nachgewiesene Druckempfindlichkeit der sympathischen Halsganglien auf der Seite des Kopfschmerzes angeführt werden. Auch ich fand eine solche Druckempfindlichkeit, die sich aber bis in die untersten, dem Druck zugänglichen Partien des Halssympathicus erstreckte und besonders im medialsten Teil der Fossa supraclavicularis ausgesprochen war.

Sprechen also eine Reihe von Beobachtungen für eine aktive Rolle des Halssympathicus beim Zustandekommen des hemikranischen Anfalles, so wird man der Frage nähertreten müssen, ob es sich hier um einen Reiz- oder Lähmungszustand handelt, ob also ein Gefäßkrampf oder eine Gefäßerweiterung die unmittelbare Ursache des Anfalles bildet. Unwahrscheinlich sind ab ovo die Theorien, welche für eine Gruppe der Migräneanfälle einen Gefäßkrampf, für die andere eine Gefäßerweiterung in Erwägung ziehen, da man sich nicht gut vorstellen kann, daß ein typisch wiederkehrendes Anfallssyndrom durch zwei so entgegengesetzte Elementarvorgänge verursacht werden sollte. Für die Annahme eines Gefäßkrampfes sprechen zahlreiche Beobachtungen, in welchen analoge angiospastische Erscheinungen auf anderen Sympathicusgebieten vermerkt sind, die bei Migräne gleichzeitig vorkommen. GOLDBLADT und STERLING sahen intermittie-

---

[1] Die von HERING entdeckte Reflexwirkung des am Bulbus caroticus liegenden Nerven (sinus caroticus)-geflechtes auf den allgemeinen Kreislauf scheint durch Untersuchungen der letzten Jahre immer mehr an Bedeutung zu gewinnen. Experimentelle Arbeiten von HEYMANS und BOUCKAERT deuten darauf hin, daß die Sinusreflexe nicht nur herzhemmend und blutdrucksenkend wirken, sondern auch das Atem- und Vasomotorenzentrum des Gehirns direkt beeinflussen. Nach GOLLWITZER-MEIER und SCHULTZE wird die an sich schwache, eigene Vasomotorik des Gehirns vornehmlich vom Sinus-caroticus-reflex beeinflußt. MARINESCO-KREINDLER und DANIELOPOLOU fanden bei Epilepsie eine geschwächte Reflextätigkeit des Sinusgeflechtes und führen die Instabilität der Gehirnvasomotorik, in welcher sie die Ursache der Epilepsie erblicken, auf die herabgesetzte Funktion der Sinusreflexe zurück. Über verändertes Verhalten der Sinusreflexe bei Hypertonie, Arteriosklerose berichten REGNIERS, COBB u. a.

rendes Hinken bei Migräne; CURSCHMANN erblickt in der von ihm als häufige Begleiterscheinung beschriebenen Angina pectoris vasomotoria ein mit dem Migräneanfall pathogenetisch zusammenhängendes Symptom. Als experimenteller Beweis für die angiospastische Genese kann der Fall von CURSCHMANN gelten, wo bei einem 19jährigen Mädchen, welches beim Waschen in kaltem Wasser sowohl Absterben der Hände und Ohrmuscheln als auch einen linksseitigen Kopfschmerzanfall mit Flimmern und Erbrechen bekam, durch Einwirkenlassen von Kälte auf die Hände dieses Syndrom künstlich hervorgerufen werden konnte. VALLERY-RADOT und BLAMOUTIER konnten bei zwei Migränekranken durch Anlegen von Eis auf der Stirn Kopfschmerzen mit dem Charakter ihrer Migräneanfälle hervorrufen. Die Wahrscheinlichkeit, daß der Migräneanfall durch einen Gefäßkrampf, also durch einen gesteigerten Sympathicotonus verursacht wird, bestätigen zahlreiche Beobachtungen, nach welchen während des Anfalles der allgemeine Blutdruck erhöht ist. Zur Feststellung des gesteigerten Sympathicotonus empfiehlt KERPPOLA die intravenöse Einspritzung von 0,005 mg Adrenalin, welches bei Normalen den Blutdruck kaum beeinflußt, bei Migräne häufig Blutdruckanstiege um 20—30 mm Hg auszulösen pflegt. HADLICH, der sich mit dieser Frage beschäftigte, betont, daß es bei jugendlichen Personen auf migränöser Basis zu Hypertonien von langem Bestand kommen kann und hebt die Neigung dieser Kranken zur Angina pectoris und Nephrosklerose im späteren Alter hervor; in der Vorgeschichte der essentiellen Hypertonien spiele nach ihm die Migräne eine Hauptrolle. Auch THAYSEN macht auf die Kombination von Migräne mit essentieller Hypertonie aufmerksam. Dagegen fanden KERPPOLA und MOEHLIG normale Blutdruckwerte bei Migräne. Einen wichtigen und auch vom diagnostischen Standpunkt wertvollen Beweis für die vasokonstriktorische Erregbarkeit bei Migräne brachte O. MUCK (1924). Sein Sondenversuch besteht darin, daß man mit einem in 1°/$_{00}$ Adrenalinlösung getauchten, auf eine Sonde befestigten Wattebausch an der Schleimhaut der vorderen Partie der unteren Nasenmuschel einen Strich zeichnet. Bei Normalen tritt eine rötliche Strichzeichnung auf, bei Migränekranken ein auffallend weißer Strich. Bei einseitiger Migräne tritt die weiße Strichzeichnung nur auf der vom Anfall heimgesuchten Seite auf, während die andere die normale rötliche Färbung zeigt. Es soll hier noch bemerkt werden, daß MUCK diesen positiven Ausfall des Sondenversuches außer der Migräne auch bei Epilepsie konstant nachweisen konnte. Seine Angaben wurden von mehreren Seiten nachgeprüft und in jeder Hinsicht bestätigt; auch ich konnte sie in etwa 30 Fällen von Migräne bestätigen, bei halbseitigen Fällen auch das gesetzmäßige Befallenwerden der kranken Seite feststellen.

Eine bedeutsame Unterstützung erhielt die angiospastische Theorie des Migräneanfalles durch J. PALs Lehre von den *Gefäßkrisen*. PAL faßte unter diesem Begriff mannigfaltige, bisher ungeklärt gebliebene Krankheitszustände in einem gemeinsamen, pathologischen Rahmen zusammen, als welchen er anfallsartig auftretende Gefäßwandkrämpfe in bestimmten Gefäßbezirken bezeichnete. Der Sympathicotonus, welcher als der hauptsächliche Regulator des Vasomotorenspiels betrachtet werden kann, kann in einem umschriebenen Gefäßbezirk auf beschränkte Zeit eine krankhafte Erhöhung erfahren, die sich in einem Gefäßkrampf innerhalb dieses Gebietes äußert und klinisch in der Form von Reiz- und Ausfallserscheinungen des betreffenden Körpergebietes oder Organs zum Ausdruck kommt. Das pathologisch-anatomische Substrat dieser Symptome dürfte in der lokalen Ischämie des betreffenden Zirkulationsgebietes gegeben sein, welches infolge des Gefäßkrampfes eine ungenügende Blutzufuhr erleidet. Es wurde bekannt, daß namentlich zwei Gefäßbezirke eine besondere Disposition zu solchen Gefäßkrisen besitzen: der in das Innervationsgebiet des Splanchnicus gehörende Bauchgefäßtrakt und das Gefäßsystem des Gehirns. Die bisher so rätselhaften, ohne organische Veränderungen auftretenden, oft bedrohlich aussehenden Bauch- und Nierenkrisen erhielten auf diese Weise ihre pathogenetische Klärung; wir gewannen auch einen besseren Einblick in die Entstehungsart gewisser Formen von intermittierendem Hinken, bei welchen eine organische Gefäßwanderkrankung nicht nachgewiesen werden konnte. Die Untersuchungen von PAL, ROSENSTEIN u. a. machen es auch wahrscheinlich, daß die im Anschluß an Bleivergiftung vorkommenden Kopfschmerzen, Sehstörungen usw., die übrigens eine unverkennbare Ähnlichkeit mit den migräneartigen Symptomen haben, ebenfalls auf Gefäßkrämpfe im Gehirn zurückzuführen sind. Im Sinne der VOLHARDschen Theorie über die Pathogenese gewisser Nierenerkrankungen gewinnt heute die Auffassung immer mehr Boden, daß ein großer Teil der bei Urämie auftretenden Gehirnsymptomen durch einen Gefäßkrampf und nicht durch eine unmittelbare Gehirnintoxikation bedingt sind. Die große Bedeutung der Lehre von den Gefäßkrisen für die Pathogenese der Migräne liegt darin, daß sie eine gut fundierte pathologische Grundlage schuf für eine Reihe von Krankheitsbildern, unter welchen der hemikranische Anfall mit seinen Reiz- und Ausfallserscheinungen als Gefäßkrampf im Gehirn seinen richtigen Platz findet. Die Feststellung, daß ein periodisch sich wiederholender, auf einen bestimmten Gefäßbezirk beschränkter Gefäßkrampf im betreffenden Organ oder Körperteil gewisse, sich typisch wiederholende Symptome hervorrufen kann, gibt dem Migräneanfall als einem cerebralen Gefäßkrampf eine plausible Erklärung, während für angioparalytische Zustände eine solche klinisch-pathologische Grundlage gänzlich fehlt. Der wichtigste Einwand gegen die Gefäßkrampftheorie, welcher seinerzeit von MOEBIUS u. a. erhoben wurde, bezog sich darauf, daß das Hauptsymptom des Migräneanfalles, der Kopfschmerz, durch einen Gefäßkrampf nicht bedingt sein könne. Dieser Einwand wurde durch die Untersuchungen von PH. STÖHR beseitigt. Ihm ist der Nachweis gelungen, daß sämtliche Blutgefäße der Pia und des Plexus chorioideus mit Nerven versorgt sind, die teils aus dem Plexus caroticus und vertebralis, teils aus feinen Ästen verschiedener Hirnnerven stammen; die Gefäße führen neben den vasomotorischen Nerven auch sensible Bahnen, die aus dem pialen Nervengeflecht herrührend sich den Gefäßen anlegen. ODERMATH konnte feststellen, daß nur bei Reizung der Adventitia, nicht aber der inneren Wandschichte der Gefäße Schmerzen ausgelöst werden. Die experimentellen Untersuchungen von FRÖHLICH und MEYER deuten darauf hin, daß die Schmerzempfindlichkeit der verschiedenen Gefäßarten Unterschiede aufweist, indem die Zusammenziehung der Präcapillaren keine Schmerzen hervorruft, dagegen der Krampf der mittleren Arterien schmerzhaft ist; in Übereinstimmung mit dieser physiologischen Feststellung fanden STÖHR und MÜLLER, daß die kleinen Arterien des Gehirnparenchyms keine Nervenbahnen besitzen. Auf die Überempfindlichkeit der Kopfvenen bei Migräne hat DÖLLKEN hingewiesen. Die Klinik bietet andererseits zahlreiche Beispiele für die Schmerzhaftigkeit solcher Vorgänge, die auf einem Gefäßkrampf beruhen (Angina pectoris, intermittierendes Hinken, schmerzhafte Bauch- und Nierenkrisen). FOERSTER hält den Migränekopfschmerz für das markanteste Beispiel des Gehirngefäßschmerzes, besonders zu Beginn des Anfalles, wo er etwas absolut Eigenartiges an sich hat, das ihn vom gewöhnlichen Kopfschmerz deutlich unterscheidet und seine angiospastische Genese deutlich erkennen läßt. „In der Folge allerdings", sagt FOERSTER, „wenn die Migräne anhält, geht auch der Migräneschmerz in den gewöhnlichen tiefen und zuletzt auch oberflächlichen Kopfschmerz über, was bei der engen Verknüpfung aller afferenten Nerven des Schädelinnern und Schädeläußern in den Kernsäulen des V. im Nucleus solitarius und den Hinterhörnern der oberen Halssegmente nicht wundernehmen kann."

Es ist mit dem heutigen Stand unserer Kenntnisse am besten zu vereinbaren, wenn man im Migräneanfall einen paroxysmal auftretenden Gefäßkrampf im

Gehirn erblickt, welcher durch irgendeinen Reiz des Halssympathicus verursacht wird. Wie sich dieser Gefäßkrampf im Gehirngewebe abspielt, ob außer der Ischämie auch andere Störungen des Saftverkehrs und Stoffwechsels bei der Entstehung des Anfallsyndroms eine Rolle spielen, bleibt einstweilen eine offene Frage. Bemerkenswert finde ich aber den von SEPP angegebenen Unterschied, welcher zwischen den Gehirncapillaren und den Capillaren des übrigen Gefäßsystems besteht. Nach SEPP besitzen die Gehirncapillaren eine eigene elastische Membran und unterscheiden sich von den Capillaren der anderen Organe dadurch, daß sie sich nicht erweitern und eine Transsudation nicht ermöglichen; diese Rolle beim Saftaustausch im Gehirn übernehmen die präcapillaren Arteriolae und die postcapillaren Venulae. Die erwähnte Eigentümlichkeit im Gefäßbau dürfte sich in den Auswirkungen des Gefäßkrampfes im Gehirn darin kundgeben, daß die Erweiterung der Capillaren, welche bei Gefäßkrämpfen in anderen Körperabschnitten dem Arterienspasmus zu folgen pflegt, im Gehirn nicht stattfindet. Es wurde früher hervorgehoben, daß einige Autoren (KÄMMERER u. a.) das Wesen des Migräneanfalles neben dem Gefäßkrampf auch in einem exsudativen Gewebsvorgang erblicken, welcher als anaphylaktische Gewebsveränderung durch eine Transsudation aus den erweiterten Capillaren entsteht; die chemische Substanz, welcher diese Wirkung zugeschrieben wird, sei das capillarerweiternde Hystamin. Die von SEPP hervorgehobene Eigentümlichkeit im Aufbau der Hirncapillaren läßt es als unwahrscheinlich erscheinen, daß im Hirngewebe solche anaphylaktische Gefäßreaktionen zustande kommen wie im übrigen Körper. Gegen die Annahme eines exsudativen Vorganges in der Pathogenese des Migräneanfalles spricht auch, daß, wie wir sehen werden, nur ein Bruchteil der Migränefälle als anaphylaktische Migräne aufgefaßt werden kann, wo ein exsudativer Gehirnprozeß in Frage käme. Bei den übrigen Migräneformen liegen für eine solche Annahme keine Anhaltspunkte vor; würde also bei der anaphylaktischen Migräne ein exsudativer Vorgang auch eine Rolle spielen, dann müßte man zwischen den anaphylaktischen und den nichtanaphylaktischen Migräneanfällen deutliche Unterschiede erkennen.

Es sprechen also gewichtige Argumente für die Annahme, daß dem Migräneanfall ein durch einen örtlichen Sympathicusreiz bedingter Gefäßkrampf zugrundeliegt. Nun tauchen gleich folgende Fragen auf: 1. Erstreckt sich der den Anfall auslösende Gefäßkrampf auf das ganze Gehirn oder nur auf gewisse Abschnitte desselben ? 2. Welche Gehirnsegmente muß der Gefäßkrampf betreffen, um die für den Anfall charakteristischen Symptome in lokalisatorischer Hinsicht verständlich zu machen ? 3. Läßt der anatomische Aufbau der Hirngefäßinnervation eine solche Annahme zu, nach welcher ein durch zeitweilige Erhöhung des Sympathicotonus bedingter Gefäßkrampf nur diese Gehirnsegmente befällt, ohne sich auf die übrigen Teile des Großhirns auszubreiten ?

Bei Beantwortung der ersten Frage wird man die auffallende Tatsache berücksichtigen müssen, daß zwei der häufigsten und aus der Pathologie des Gehirns am meisten bekannten Reiz- und Ausfallserscheinungen beim Migräneanfall regelmäßig fehlen: es sind dies die Störung des Bewußtseins und die tonisch-klonischen Krämpfe. Das Fehlen der letzteren ist besonders in solchen Fällen auffällig, wo im Anschluß an einen Migräneanfall motorische Ausfallserscheinungen im Bilde einer Hemiparese auftreten. Über die Lokalisation des ischämischen Vorganges in solchen Fällen wurde schon früher hervorgehoben, daß dieser in der motorischen Rinde deshalb nicht gesucht werden kann, weil die kennzeichnenden Symptome des motorischen Rindenreizes, die tonisch-klonischen Krämpfe fehlen. Es wurden dort Beweise für die Annahme gebracht, daß die Läsion der Pyramidenbahn bei Migräneanfall den Abschnitt vom Hirnschenkel bis zur Oblongata zu betreffen pflegt. Die corticale Natur der

Bewußtseinsstörungen steht ebenfalls außer Zweifel, wobei die verschiedenen Rindengebiete des Gehirns erfahrungsgemäß nicht dieselbe Bedeutung besitzen. Man darf, ohne ein lokalisatorisches Prinzip dabei vertreten zu wollen, annehmen, daß das Erhaltenbleiben des Bewußtseins vor allem an die Funktionstüchtigkeit des Stirnhirns gebunden ist. Berücksichtigt man also das Fehlen der Bewußtlosigkeit und der tonisch-klonischen Krämpfe, so erscheint die Folgerung, daß beim Migräneanfall namhafte Abschnitte der Hirnrinde, namentlich das Stirnhirn und die motorische Rindenregion, vom pathologischen Vorgang des Migräneanfalles verschont bleiben, als zulässig.

Bei der Beantwortung der zweiten Frage, welche Gehirnabschnitte beim Migräneanfall vom Gefäßkrampf befallen werden, wird man vor allem die Symptomatologie der verschiedenen Migränefälle in Betracht ziehen müssen. Diese setzt sich aus subjektiven Beschwerden (Kopfschmerz, Erbrechen usw.) und aus objektiv feststellbaren Ausfallserscheinungen zusammen. Bei der Lokalisierung des Gefäßkrampfes im Gehirn dürften uns die letzteren einen besseren Dienst erweisen, als die subjektiven Beschwerden, welche, wie z. B. der Kopfschmerz, verschiedentlich gedeutet werden können. Versucht man nun die in der reichlichen Migränekasuistik enthaltenen Ausfallserscheinungen im Gehirn näher zu lokalisieren, so ergeben sich lediglich zwei größere Gehirnabschnitte als solche, in welchen die abwechslungsreiche Symtomatologie der Migränefälle lokalisatorisch untergebracht werden kann. Das eine Gebiet umfaßt das sog. Mittel- und Nachhirn vom Hirnschenkel bis zur Oblongata. Hier müssen wir den Sitz der anatomischen (ischämischen) Schädigung annehmen in den Fällen mit III-Lähmung (Hirnschenkelgebiet), mit IV-, V-, IV-, VII-Lähmung (Ponsgebiet), mit VIII—X-Lähmung (Oblongata) und endlich in den Fällen mit Kleinhirnstörung. Ob der Sitz der Schädigung im intracerebralen Kern- oder Wurzelgebiet der genannten Hirnnerven oder im extracerebralen intrakraniellen Abschnitt liegt, zu dieser auch heute noch unentschiedenen Streitfrage wäre folgendes zu bemerken: Ich brachte mehrere Beobachtungen von III.-Lähmung, in welchen nur die zu den äußeren Augenmuskeln gehenden Äste betroffen waren. Auch die von anderen Autoren gemachte Feststellung, daß bei der ophthalmoplegischen Migräne häufig nur ein einziger Augenmuskel betroffen wird, spricht dafür, daß die Zirkulationsstörung nicht den extrakraniellen Stamm des Nerven, sondern das Kerngebiet betrifft, wo die äußere Muskelkerngruppe ihre eigene, von der inneren gesonderte Gefäßversorgung besitzt. Unzweideutig ist der interkranielle Sitz der Schädigung bewiesen durch die mitgeteilten zwei Fälle von Hemiplegia alternans facialis, welche eine andere Lokalisation als im Kerngebiet der Brücke nicht zuläßt. Diese Beobachtungen führen mich in dem Streit, ob der Sitz der Schädigung bei der ophthalmoplegischen Migräne im intracerebralen Kerngebiet oder im extracerebralen Nervenstamm liegt, in das Lager jener Autoren (CHARCOT, MOEBIUS, ROTTMANN, TRÖMNER usw.), die den krankhaften Vorgang, der sich beim Migräneanfall abspielt, in die Kerne der betroffenen Hirnnerven verlegen. Diese Erklärung kann auch für diejenigen Anfälle eine Gültigkeit haben, wo gleichzeitig mehrere Hirnnerven einer Seite betroffen werden, wenn man annimmt, daß die diese Kerne versorgenden kleinen Arterien auf einmal in einen Gefäßkrampf geraten. Die Annahme einer nucleären intracerebralen Schädigung wird noch dadurch bekräftigt, daß es auch andere Migräneausfallserscheinungen gibt (Hemianästhesien, Aphasie), welche nur durch eine intracerebrale Schädigung verursacht werden können.

Der zweite Gehirnabschnitt, welcher bei der Lokalisation der Reiz- und Ausfallserscheinungen im Migräneanfall in Betracht kommt, betrifft *den Sitzort der Sehstörungen*. Bei der Länge der Sehbahn und ihren zahlreichen Umschaltstationen ist es nicht verwunderlich, daß die mannigfachen Sehstörungen des Migräneanfalles auf verschiedene Abschnitte der Sehbahn lokalisiert wurden. Neben der Iris wurde hauptsächlich die Retina als Ausgangsort der ophthalmischen Migräne beschuldigt, eine Theorie, die sich hauptsächlich auf den Augenspiegelbefund mancher Migränefälle, wo ein Krampf der Arteria centralis retinae beobachtet und auf anatomische Befunde stützte, in welchen eine Thrombose der Netzhautgefäße festgestellt wurde. Andere Autoren zogen den Nervus opticus, das Chiasma und den Tractus opticus mit den äußeren Kniehöckern (JOLLY) als Sitzort des Vorganges in Erwägung. FÉRÉ war der erste, der darauf hinwies, daß die Symptome der ophthalmischen Migräne, besonders die sensiblen Halbseitenerscheinungen und Aphasie, die als häufige Begleiterscheinungen dieser Anfälle bekannt sind, mit einer Annahme im extracerebralen Abschnitt der Sehbahn nicht gut vereinbart werden können. Er vermutete den Prozeß im Gebiet des Carrefour sensitive, wo die zentrale Sehbahn mit der sensiblen Bahn eng benachbart ist. Andere Autoren, ANTONELLI, FUCHS, SAHLI, SIEGRIST und die überwiegende Mehrzahl der späteren Autoren betrachten als Sitzort der Sehstörungen die Sehrinde im Hinterhauptslappen. Die flimmernden Erscheinungen werden als Rindenreizsymptome und die Sehstörungen als Ausfallserscheinungen infolge des Gefäßkrampfes der Arteria cerebri posterior aufgefaßt.

Zugunsten der corticalen Theorie wurde angeführt, daß das negative Skotom von DUFOUR (Nichtssehen), welches bei Migräne häufig beobachtet wird, auf die Läsion des corticalen Sehzentrums hindeutet, zum Unterschied vom positiven Skotom (Dunkelsehen), welches bei Störungen der Sehbahn beobachtet wird. Von einigen Autoren wird heute die Richtigkeit des DUFOURschen Satzes bezweifelt. Das wichtigste Argument dafür, daß die Sehstörungen nicht im Auge und nicht im Sehnerv ihren Sitz haben können, ist der am häufigsten beobachtete homonym hemianopische Typus der Sehstörung. Lehrreich ist in dieser Hinsicht eine Beobachtung von KELLER, der in einem Migräneanfall eine solche homonyme Hemianopsie beobachtete, bei welcher die hemianopische Pupillenreaktion erhalten blieb, ein Befund, der darauf hinweist, daß die Affektion in diesem Falle eine solche Stelle der zentralen Sehbahn betraf, die occipitalwärts von dem zum III.-Kern abzweigenden Reflexfasern liegt. Für den zentralen bzw. corticalen Ursprung der Sehstörungen spricht auch der Fall von RAULLET: Bei einer 28jährigen Frau, die an kompletter tabischer Opticusatrophie litt, traten bei den Migräneattacken leuchtende Erscheinungen auf. Die Anhänger der corticalen Theorie führen als weiteren Beweis an, daß bei der homonymen Hemianopsie das Maculagebiet ausgespart wird, ferner daß die Sehstörung nicht selten die Form einer Quadrantenhemianopsie aufweist. Unentschieden ist die Frage, ob die im Anfall auftretenden flimmernden Erscheinungen, wenn sie auf beiden Seiten auftreten, immer in den gleichen Gesichtsfeldhälften erscheinen. Nach FLATAU soll dabei das ganze Gesichtsfeld in Mitleidenschaft gezogen sein. Es gibt Beobachtungen, wo Skotome und Flimmererscheinungen nur eine Seite betrafen, dann solche, wo der Migräneanfall von einer bitemporalen Hemianopsie begleitet wurde, oder eine Amblyopie des einen Auges auftrat. Wir müssen aber diese Beobachtungen als Ausnahmefälle betrachten gegenüber der regelmäßigen Sehstörung, welche im Bilde der homonymen Hemianopsie sich abspielt. Vom Standpunkt der uns hier beschäftigenden Fragen ist es eigentlich irrelavant, ob wir die Sehrinde oder die in sie einstrahlende zentrale Sehbahn als Sitzort der Sehstörungen betrachten; bei der Annahme eines Gefäßkrampfes wird man überhaupt ein solches Auseinanderhalten als unmöglich ansehen, da doch Sehrinde und der letzte Abschnitt der zentralen Sehbahn von demselben Blutgefäß versorgt werden. Wichtig ist nur die Feststellung, daß nach dem heutigen Stand unserer Kenntnisse und nach Ansicht der meisten Autoren die Sehstörungen bei Migräne auf eine Schädigung der Sehrinde und der zentralen Sehbahn zurückzuführen sind. Klinische Erscheinungen, Augenspiegelbefunde und Sektionsbefunde, welche auf die peripheren Stellen der Sehbahn als Ursprungsorte der Sehstörung hinweisen, erhalten als angiospastische Begleitsymptome des Migräneanfalles dieselbe Bedeutung, wie die früher besprochenen Sympathicusreizerscheinungen am Gesicht. Bemerkenswert ist in dieser Hinsicht die Erfahrung des Augenarztes SEDAN, welcher bei Besprechung der mit Gefäßspasmen einhergehenden Sehstörungen betont, daß er in Fällen von retinalem Gefäßspasmus nie Kopfschmerzen sah.

Wir können also auf Grund der bisherigen Feststellungen zwei Gehirnabschnitte als solche bestimmen, in welchen die Ausfallserscheinungen des Migräneanfalles lokalisiert werden können. Es sind dies: das Mittel- und Nachhirn einerseits und der Hinterhauptslappen des Großhirns andererseits. Betrachten wir diese Hirnsegmente vom Standpunkt der von uns aufgestellten dritten Frage, so zeigt sich, daß die beiden erwähnten Gehirnsegmente aus einem vasomotorisch gemeinsam innervierten Gefäßsystem ihre Blutzufuhr erhalten.

Bekanntlich erfolgt die Blutversorgung des Gehirns aus zwei verschiedenen Hauptaderquellen. Der größte Teil der beiden Hemisphären, die Zentralganglien und der überwiegende Teil des Zwischenhirns erhalten ihre Blutgefäße aus den beiden Arteriae carotis internae, welche die Aae. cerebri anterior und media in die Hirnsubstanz senden; die in der hinteren Schädelgrube lagernden Hirnteile: Occipitallappen, Kleinhirn, Hirnschenkel, Pons und Oblongata erhalten ihre Gefäße aus dem Aderstamm, welcher sich aus den beiden Aae. vertebrales als Arteria basilaris zusammensetzt und in den beiden Aae. cerebri posteriores endet. Die Aae. vertebrales geben Gefäßäste ab an die Oblongata und zum Teil zum Kleinhirn; die Art. basilaris versieht Kleinhirn und Brücke. Der ausgebreitete Ernährungsbezirk der Art. cerebri posterior gestaltet sich nach der genauen Beschreibung von DURET folgendermaßen: a) Im Mittelhirn das ganze Hirnschenkelgebiet; aus dem Gefäßgeflecht der Substantia perforata posterior steigen dünne Äste (Arteriae radicinae) mit den einzelnen Bündeln des III. bis zum Kern hinauf; die Arterien der einzelnen III. Kerne stammen aus den Gefäßen der Lamina quadrigemina, welch letztere ebenfalls aus der Art. cerebri posterior abgehen. b) Im Zwischenhirn die Zirbeldrüse, der Hinterteil des Thalamus und der Plexus chorioidea des 3. Ventrikels. c) Von den Großhirnhemisphären eine variable Beteiligung an der Blutversorgung der dritten Schläfenwindung, des Gyrus hypocampi und fusiformis, während der Hauptast als Art. calcarina in der Fissura calcarina zum Hinterpol des Occipitallappens zieht und die ganze weiße und graue Substanz des Hinterhauptlappens versorgt.

Welche Bedeutung gewinnen nun die hier angeführten Daten bei einer Erklärung über das Zustandekommen des Migräneanfalles? Wenn wir den Migräneanfall im Sinne von PAL als eine cerebrale Gefäßkrise betrachten, also als einen anfallsartig auftretenden Gefäßwandkrampf, welcher durch eine isolierte, örtlich begrenzte Tonuserhöhung eines Sympathicusabschnittes verursacht wird, dann ergibt sich aus der Analyse der Migränesymptome, daß der Migräneanfall sich mit allen seinen Symptomen in jenem Hirngebiet abspielt, welches aus dem System der beiden Aae. vertebrales seine Gefäße erhält. Das Einheitliche dieses Blutgefäßsystems (welches doch durch den Circulus arteriosus Willisii mit dem Blutgefäßsystem der Carotis in innigster Verbindung steht und bei Zirkulationsstörungen im Gehirn eine rege wechselseitige Kompensation aufrecht hält), liegt also nicht in der Abgeschlossenheit ihres Ernährungsbezirkes, sondern in ihrer einheitlichen sympathischen Innervation, die vom Sympathicussystem der Carotiden unabhängig ist. Bekanntlich stammen die sympathischen Fasern der beiden Aae. vertebrales aus dem unteren Cervicalganglion des Grenzstranges und ziehen als Plexus vertebralis mit dem Gefäß zum Gehirn, wo sie sich auf die Arteriae basilaris und cerebri posterior sowie auf die einzelnen Gefäßäste derselben fortsetzen. Es besteht also anatomisch die Möglichkeit, daß ein sympathicotonisch bedingter Gefäßkrampf im Gehirn jene und nur jene Gebiete erfasse, die als Lesionsstellen des Migräneanfalles erkannt wurden und die übrigen Gehirnsegmente freiläßt. Die sympathische Innervation des Carotidensystems erfolgt aus dem obersten Cervicalganglion des Halsstranges, von wo aus der Plexus caroticus zum Gehirn hinaufsteigt. Wenn wir also mit PAL annehmen, daß bei den sog. Gefäßkrisen verschiedene Sympathicusabschnitte selbständig in einen erhöhten Reizzustand gelangen können, *dann wird man im Migräneanfall den Effekt eines Reizzustandes erblicken, welcher im unteren Halsganglion, oder in dem aus diesem entstammenden Plexus vertebralis sich abspielt und lediglich einen angiospastischen Zustand im Gefäßgebiet des Vertebralissystems darstellt, dessen Intensität und verschiedentliche lokale Akzentuiertheit die jeweiligen subjektiven Beschwerden und objektiven Ausfallserscheinungen bestimmt.*

Bei dieser Annahme erhalten die verschiedenen Anfallsformen eine plausible Erklärung. Bezüglich des Kopfschmerzes habe ich schon in meiner früheren Arbeit eine Deutung in Erwägung gebracht, welche mit der oben zitierten Ansicht FOERSTERs im wesentlichen übereinstimmt, indem ich annehme, daß dieser zum Teil als ein direkter Gefäßwandschmerz aufgefaßt werden muß. Ich habe dies besonders für den im Hinterhaupt- und Nackengebiet sitzenden Kopfschmerz in Erwägung gebracht, von welchem gesagt wurde, daß er ein überaus häufiges und für den Migräneanfall kennzeichnendes Symptom darstellt und oft den Anfall einleitet. Die sensiblen pialen Nervengeflechte, welche den Gefäßwandschmerz weiterleiten, entstammen aus dem Trigeminus und Vagus und führen die Schmerzimpulse zu den Oblongatakernen dieser Hirnnerven, wo eine Irradiation dieses Reizzustandes auf das ganze sensible Kerngebiet dieser Hirnnerven und auf die Hinterhörner der oberen Halssegmente erfolgt, wodurch sich der primäre Gefäßwandschmerz in einen allgemeinen tiefen oder oberflächlichen Kopfschmerz umwandelt. Die Schmerzzustände in der Stirn, Augenhöhle, Schläfe und Gesicht, die Lichtscheu sind Reizzustände des Trigeminuskernes. Der Brechreiz und das Erbrechen erhalten als Vagusreizsymptome ihre Erklärung, der Schwindel als Reizzustand des benachbarten Vestibulariskernes. Die Symptome des gewöhnlichen Migräneanfalles beruhen also auf einem Gefäßwandschmerz und aus den durch diesen bedingten Reizerscheinungen gewisser Hirnnerven, haben aber noch keine ischämische Ernährungsstörung zur Voraussetzung. Eine solche tritt erst auf, wenn der Gefäßkrampf eine besondere Intensität erhält, oder durch längere Zeit anhält, wie wir dies bei der ophthalmoplegischen und ophthalmischen Migräne annehmen können. Hier führt die durch den Gefäßkrampf bedingte Ischämie zu Ernährungsstörungen, die schon eine zeitweilige Aufhebung der Funktion mit sich bringen. Der größte Teil der im Anfall auftretenden Funktionsstörungen wird allmählich wieder behoben, nur in seltenen Fällen, wo die Intensität des Gefäßkrampfes oder die lange Dauer desselben aus der ischämischen Ernährungsstörung eine irreparable anatomische Schädigung hervortreten ließ, bleiben die Ausfallserscheinungen endgültig zurück. Die Mannigfaltigkeit der Migränesymptome, sowohl der subjektiven Beschwerden wie auch der objektiven Störungen, läßt vermuten, daß der angiospastische Zustand nicht in allen Gefäßästen des Vertebralissystems gleichmäßig stark auftritt, vielmehr dürften in dieser Hinsicht zwischen den einzelnen Fällen große Differenzen bestehen. Stellt sich z. B. im Laufe eines Migräneanfalles eine isolierte Abducenslähmung ein, da wird man sich diese so erklären können, daß der Gefäßkrampf in dem kleinen, zum Abducenskern führenden Gefäßast eine besondere Intensität erreichte und eine solche Ernährungsstörung hervorrief, daß der Nerv gelähmt wurde. Man kann also die verschiedenen Migränesymptome nach der wechselnden Intensität und Dauer des Gefäßkrampfes im Vertebralissystem in drei Gruppen einteilen. Die leichteste Form veranschaulichen die Fälle mit gewöhnlichem Migräneanfall, die nur durch subjektive Beschwerden (als Reizerscheinungen von seiten des Trigeminus und Vagus) gekennzeichnet sind, die mittlere Gruppe repräsentieren die Fälle, wo im Verlauf des Anfalles auch objektive Ausfallserscheinungen als Ausdruck einer ischämischen Ernährungsstörung im Bilde erscheinen, sich jedoch nach Ablauf des Gefäßkrampfes allmählich, in einigen Tagen oder Wochen zurückbilden. Die dritte Gruppe umfaßt die nur selten beobachteten Fälle mit dauernden Ausfallserscheinungen, welchen eine irreparable anatomische Schädigung (ischämische Erweichung) zugrunde liegt. Ein mikroskopisch genau untersuchter Fall von OSTERTAG (apoplektischer Insult bei einer 26jährigen Hypertonikerin) kann als Beweis dafür gelten, daß ein rein funktioneller Gefäßverschluß anämische Gewebsnekrosen und Erweichungsherde verursachen kann.

Bezüglich der Sehstörungen, welche als Aura der ophthalmischen Migräne auftreten, erscheint die Erklärung am nächsten liegend, daß hier der Gefäßkrampf nicht an den Blutgefäßen der Hirnbasis, sondern im Endgebiet der Art. cerebri posterior einsetzt und sich erst später auf die basalen Gefäße fortsetzt. Hierfür spricht, daß die Sehstörung regelmäßig vor dem Kopfschmerz auftritt; daß die angiospastischen Zustände der kleinen Gefäße des Hirnparenchyms mit keinen Schmerzen einhergehen, geht auch aus den früher zitierten Befunden von STÖHR und MÜLLER hervor. Die flimmernden Erscheinungen können am leichtesten als ischämische Reizerscheinungen der Sehrinde aufgefaßt werden, die homonyme Hemianopsie als ischämische Funktionsstörung der Sehrinde, oder als Leitungsunterbrechung der zentralen Sehstrahlung. Das verschiedene Verhalten der Maculagegend bei der Hemianopsie zwingt zu der Annahme, daß sowohl die Sehrinde als auch die zentrale Sehstrahlung selbständiger Sitzort der ischämischen Lesion sein kann. Für diejenigen Fälle, in welchen homonyme Hemianopsie mit Hemiparästhesie verbunden ist, kommt im Sinne von FÉRÉ das Fasergebiet des Carrefour sensitive als einheitlicher Focus dieser Schädigung in Betracht. Für die motorische Aphasie und Hemiparesen wurde schon früher auseinandergesetzt, daß hier eine Schädigung der Pyramidenbahn in der motorischen Rinde oder im Gebiet der inneren Kapsel unwahrscheinlich ist, dagegen der Abschnitt vom Pedunculus bis zur Oblongata auch deshalb gut in Betracht kommt, weil in einigen Beobachtungen nachgewiesene Nachbarschaftssymptome eine solche Lokalisation bestätigen. Inwieweit die sich an Migräneanfälle anschließenden psychischen Zustände mit dem Gefäßkrampf in ursächliche Beziehung gebracht werden können, ist schwer zu beurteilen. Die Möglichkeit, daß Zirkulationsstörungen im Gehirn bei Veranlagten psychische Störungen hervorrufen können, ist nicht von der Hand zu weisen. Ein Gefäßkrampf im Hinterhauptslappen, wie wir ihn bei ophthalmischer Migräne annehmen, könnte auch in den übrigen Großhirnsegmenten eine gewisse Stoffwechsel- oder Funktionsstörung hervorrufen, die bei entsprechend Labilen psychische Alterationen zur Folge haben kann. Daß der psychopathischen Anlage hier eine bedeutende Rolle zukommt, wurde schon früher betont.

Es ist vielleicht nicht ohne Interesse, vom Standpunkt der hier angeführten angiospastischen Pathogenese die Beziehungen zwischen Migräneanfall und epileptischem Anfall noch einmal zu prüfen. Es wurde schon früher auf die Tatsachen und Erfahrungen hingewiesen, welche eine innigere Verwandtschaft zwischen Migräne und Epilepsie beweisen. Auch bezüglich der Pathogenese lassen beide Erkrankungen zahlreiche gemeinsame Züge erkennen. Bei beiden stehen in der Frage der Pathogenese dieselben ursächlichen Faktoren im Mittelpunkt der Diskussion. Die beim Migräneanfall von DUBOIS angeführte angiospastische Theorie wurde zur Erklärung der Entstehung des epileptischen Anfalles von NOTHNAGEL aufgestellt und im Laufe der Zeit vielfach angefochten, konnte sie kaum durch eine bessere ersetzt werden, erhielt sogar in der letzten Zeit durch experimentelle Erfahrungen (FISCHERs Nebennierenreduktionsversuche) und besonders in der letzten Zeit durch die histopathologischen Befunde SPIELMEYERs und Stoffwechseluntersuchungen von WUTH eine kräftige Unterstützung. Wie ist es nun möglich, daß zwei Anfallsarten, die man gemeinsam auf einen Gefäßkrampf im Gehirn zurückführt, in ihrer Symptomatologie so große Unterschiede aufweisen, wie sie zwischen Migräneanfall und epileptischem Anfall bestehen? Die Analyse des epileptischen Anfalles zeigt als die zwei wesentlichsten Komponenten desselben die Aufhebung des Bewußtseins und die tonisch klonischen Krämpfe. In lokalisatorischer Hinsicht weisen beide Symptome auf die Hirnrinde als Lesionsstelle des Gehirns hin. Es ist vor allem das Stirnhirn, welchem an der Erhaltung des Bewußtseins eine Bedeutung zuerkannt werden muß. Die tonisch klonischen Krämpfe werden aber allgemein als Reizerscheinungen der motorischen Hirnrinde aufgefaßt. Die mydriatische Pupillenstarre, eine typische Begleiterscheinung des epileptischen Anfalles, wird man nach den Darlegungen von BUMKE ebenfalls als eine Rindenreizerscheinung auffassen können. Der typisch epileptische Anfall muß daher auf einen pathologischen Vorgang zurückgeführt werden, der sich wesentlich in der Hirnrinde, und zwar vornehmlich des Vorderhirns abspielt. Hält man sich an die uns hier zunächst beschäftigende Gefäßkrampftheorie und will den epileptischen Anfall auf einen ischämischen Reiz der Hirnrinde zurückführen, so muß man den Sitz des Gefäßkrampfes in das System der beiden Arteriae carotis internae verlegen. Diese versorgen nämlich mit Ausnahme des Occipitallappens, die ganze Hirnrinde sowie die Zentralganglien und den überwiegenden Teil des Zwischenhirns. Man wird im Sinne PALS auch hier einen selbständigen, nur auf das Carotissystem beschränkten Gefäßkrampf annehmen können, welcher durch die Tonuserhöhung des im Plexus caroticus verlaufenden sympathischen Faserabschnittes zustande kommt. Es ist bekannt, daß der Plexus caroticus aus dem obersten Ganglion des Halsstranges entstammt und, mit den Carotiden in die Schädelhöhle hinaufsteigend, sich in die Arteriae cerebri anterior und media verzweigt. Die wechselnde Intensität und lokale Akzentuiertheit offenbart sich im epileptischen Anfall ebenso wie wir es beim Migräneanfall sehen. Wird das Gefäßgebiet der motorischen Rinde verschont, so bildet die Bewußtseinsstörung das alleinige Symptom des Anfalles. Die wechselnde Intensität der Bewußtseinsstörung (von Petit mal bis zur schweren Bewußtlosigkeit) dürfte ein Gradmesser für die quantitativen Schwankungen des durch den Gefäßkrampf bedingten ischämischen Zustandes bilden. Die anfänglich allein bestehenden tonisch-klonischen Krämpfe der JACKSON-Anfälle lassen vermuten, daß der Gefäßkrampf zu Beginn nur im Gebiet der motorischen (bei sensiblen Reizerscheinungen der sensiblen) Hirnrinde bestand und sich erst allmählich auf das Gefäßgebiet des übrigen Rindenterritoriums erstreckte. Bei solchen JACKSON-Anfällen, die ohne Bewußtseinsstörungen verlaufen, bleibt der Gefäßkrampf bis zum Ende auf die motorische oder sensible Rindenpartie beschränkt. Verläuft der Anfall im Bilde einer reinen Bewußtseinsstörung (Absencen), dann wird man den Sitz des Gefäßkrampfes im Stirnhirn vermuten, welches durch die Arteria cerebri anterior mit Blut versorgt wird. Vielleicht entsprechen die in der epileptischen Aura so häufig wiederkehrenden Geruchsparästhesien einer Reizung des unter dem Stirnhirn liegenden Lobus olfactorius, welcher ebenfalls durch die Arteria cerebri anterior versorgt wird. Eine wichtige Stütze findet diese Annahme in den Beobachtungen, welche die Folgezustände des epileptischen Anfalles betreffen. Wir haben diese schon früher angeführt; es zeigten sich Ausfallserscheinungen, die lokalisatorisch auf die Hirnrinde, auf das Gebiet der inneren Kapsel und der Zentralganglien zurückgeführt werden können. Alle drei erwähnten Hirnabschnitte gehören ausschließlich zum Gefäßversorgungsgebiet der Arteria carotis interna.

Ich bin weit entfernt davon, den hypothetischen Charakter dieses Erklärungsversuches zu verkennen, insbesondere bei der Pathogenese des epileptischen Anfalles, wo wir im Sinne der Darlegungen von FOERSTER noch weitere anfallsauslösende Faktoren in Erwägung ziehen müssen. Daß aber der Gefäßkrampf des Gehirns beim Zustandekommen des epileptischen Anfalles eine bedeutende Rolle spielt, wird heute allgemein angenommen und in dieser Hinsicht dürfte der hier gegebene Erklärungsversuch einen heuristischen Gedanken enthalten, welcher einerseits die zweifellose Wesensverwandtschaft zwischen Migräne und Epilepsie, die sich in der Kombination beider Anfallsformen und zahlreichen Analogien kundgibt, anderseits den großen Unterschied in der Symptomatologie beider Anfallsformen unserem Verständnis näherbringt. Wir kommen dabei zu der Schlußfolgerung, daß der Migräneanfall ebenso wie der epileptische Anfall, zwei spezielle Formen der cerebralen Gefäßkrisen (im Sinne PALS) repräsentieren. Der Migräneanfall spielt sich im Gefäßgebiet des Vertebralissystems ab, welches seine sympathische Innervation vom unteren Cervicalganglion erhält. Der epileptische Anfall ist durch einen Gefäßkrampf im Gebiet des Carotissystems bedingt; die sympathische Innervation des letzteren stammt aus dem oberen Ganglion des Halsstranges. Die nosologische Selbständigkeit der beiden Krankheiten findet ihre Erklärung in der Definition PALS, wonach einzelne Abschnitte des sympathischen Nervensystems isoliert in einen erhöhten Erregungszustand gelangen können, welcher zu einem umschriebenen Gefäßkrampf des diesem Abschnitt untergeordneten Gefäßsystems führt. Migräne und Epilepsie hängen also in diesem Sinne miteinander nicht inniger zusammen als Migräne und Raynaudkrankheit oder intermittierendes Hinken, in welchen wir ebenfalls

Gefäßkrisen vermuten. Die den Migräneanfall oft begleitenden Sympathicusreizerscheinungen am Gesicht, die Erscheinungen der Bauchmigräne usw. deuten darauf hin, daß gleichzeitig mit dem im Vertebralissystem sich abspielenden Gefäßkrampf auch andere Sympathicusabschnitte in einen Reizzustand geraten können. Die Kombination der Migräne mit Epilepsie könnte daher so erklärt werden, daß der den Sympathicusreiz verursachende ätiologische Faktor einmal den Symphaticusabschnitt des Vertebralissystems, das anderemal den des Carotissystems oder wenn beide Anfälle sich eng miteinander verbinden, zuerst den einen und später den anderen Sympathicusabschnitt angreift.

Mein Erklärungsversuch über das Zustandekommen des Migräneanfalles weicht von den meisten heute anerkannten Erklärungen dadurch ab, daß ich nicht den ganzen Halssympathicus, sondern nur den untersten Abschnitt desselben mit dem Plexus vertebralis für den Migräneanfall verantwortlich mache. Die zum eigentlichen Syndrom des Migräneanfalles gehörenden Symptome entstehen als unmittelbare Folgeerscheinungen eines Gefäßkrampfes im Vertebralissystem. Die übrigen Sympathicusreizerscheinungen am Gesicht, im Auge usw. sind zwar häufige Begleiterscheinungen des Migräneanfalles, gehören aber nicht zum legitimen Anfallsbild, ebensowenig, wie die Sympathicusreizerscheinungen in anderen Körpergebieten. Dies gilt z. B. für die Blässe des Gesichts, Spasmus der Arteria centralis retinae oder der Arteria temporalis usw. Daß solche begleitenden Reizsymptome der höheren Halssympathicusabschnitte bei Migräne häufiger vorkommen als bei den übrigen Sympathicusbahnen, findet vielleicht in ihren näheren anatomischen Beziehungen eine Erklärung.

Zum Schluß sollen als Beweise des hier gegebenen Erklärungsversuches kurz zwei Krankengeschichten mitgeteilt werden, in welchen das Migränesyndrom akzidentell auftrat. Sie bringen auch neue Daten für die Entstehungsmöglichkeiten der sog. symptomatischen Migräne, die bisher nur bei Erkrankungen des Gehirns beobachtet wurde, da in beiden Fällen pathologische Veränderungen im untersten Abschnitt des Halssympathicus den Migränezustand aufrechthielten.

1. Die 32jährige Frau suchte im Juni 1925 unsere Spitalsambulanz mit der Beschwerde auf, daß sie seit etwa 5 Jahren an heftigen Kopfschmerzen leide, die schon von mehreren Fachärzten als Migräne bezeichnet wurden. Ausgesprochen rechtsseitige Kopfschmerzen hauptsächlich im Nacken und im Auge sowie in der Stirn. Optische Reizerscheinungen hat sie nie beobachtet, dagegen Lichtscheu, stechende Schmerzen in der Herzgegend, bei intensiven Anfällen Übelkeit und Schmerzen in der ganzen rechten Gesichtshälfte. Die Anfälle wiederholten sich anfangs 2—3mal monatlich, im letzten Jahr wöchentlich und seit 3 Monaten fast täglich. Auch die Intensität des Kopfschmerzes hat in der letzten Zeit wesentlich zugenommen und das schmerzende Gebiet sich vergrößert, indem nicht nur die rechte Kopfhälfte sondern auch die rechte Schulter und der rechte Arm von heftigen Schmerzen befallen werden; manchmal wird der Arm ganz blaß, sie empfindet ein lebhaftes Kribbeln und kann dann die Finger durch einige Stunden schlecht bewegen. Ihre Periode war immer regelmäßig. Ein zeitlicher Zusammenhang der letzteren mit den Anfällen war auch im Anfang, wo die Anfälle noch selten kamen, nicht zu bemerken. Sie gibt an, daß die ersten Anfälle während ihrer einzigen Gravidität aufgetreten sind. Zwei artifizielle Aborte vor der Geburt ihres 5jährigen Knaben. Eine hereditäre Veranlagung fehlt. Ich fand in der großen Familie der Patientin weder Migräne noch Epilepsie. Die körperliche Untersuchung ergab außer einer Druckempfindlichkeit des ersten und zweiten Trigeminusastes rechts eine lebhafte Schmerzempfindlichkeit im medialsten Gebiet der rechten Fossa supraclavicularis; auch in der Schulter und im rechten Arm gab sie eine stärkere Druckempfindlichkeit an. Die grobe motorische Kraft erschien hier etwas herabgesetzt, die Hautfarbe der rechten Hand etwas dunkler rot. Schon bei der ersten Untersuchung fiel es auf, daß die Stelle der rechten Articulatio sternoclavicularis von einer etwa nußgroßen glatten knochenharten Erhebung eingenommen wird, die von normaler Haut bedeckt und nicht klopfempfindlich war. Nach Angabe der Patientin habe sie diese Erhebung etwa nach der Geburt ihres Kindes bemerkt und ein Größerwerden seit dieser Zeit nicht beobachtet. Die Röntgenaufnahme ergab über diese Stelle folgenden Aufschluß: ,,Der distale Teil des rechten Schlüsselbeines ist stark verdickt, die sternale Epiphyse ist besonders verbreitet, die Gelenksfläche uneben, in der Epiphyse sind mehrere kleine, auf Knochenzerfall hinweisende rare und kondense Schattenflecke zu sehen. Die sternale Gelenksfläche ist glatt. Diagnose: Osteochondritis." Wa.R. im Blute negativ und im übrigen ein normaler Blutbefund. Im Harn nichts Pathologisches.

Das klinische Bild faßten wir als ein rechtseitiges Migränesyndrom auf, welches sich in der letzten Zeit mit Schmerzparoxysmen im rechten Arm komplizierte; auch hier zeigten sich Symptome, die auf angiospastische Zustände im rechten Arm hinwiesen. Die zeitliche Übereinstimmung im Auftreten der Migräneanfälle und der Knochengeschwulst legten uns schon vom Anfang an einen kausalen Zusammenhang zwischen beiden Erscheinungen nahe, der auf Grund unserer oben besprochenen pathogenetischen Erklärung als plausibel erschien. Die Lage der Knochengeschwulst entsprach einer solchen Stelle wo durch Druck der tiefer gelegenen Gewebe der Anfangsabschnitt des Plexus subclavius in Mitleidenschaft gezogen werden konnte. Die Annahme wurde noch mehr wahrscheinlich gemacht durch die Tatsache, daß die Kranke in der letzten Zeit auch im rechten Arm Symptome bot, die einem angiospastischen Zustand entsprachen.

Gegen die Annahme eines direkten Druckreizes auf den Halsstrang selbst sprach die größere Entfernung von der Geschwulst, sowie das Fehlen einer Pupillenerweiterung rechts. Die symptomatische Natur der Migränefälle wurde auch durch das Fehlen einer hereditären Belastung und die Unabhängigkeit der Anfälle von der Menstruation bekräftigt. Wir faßten also den Fall als eine symptomatische Migräne auf, die aus einem, durch die Knochengeschwulst bedingten mechanischen Reizzustand im rechtseitigen Plexus subclavius bzw. vertebralis zur Entstehung kam und legten der Patientin die operative Entfernung der Geschwulst nahe. Die Zunahme der Zahl und Intensität der Schmerzanfälle ließen darauf schließen, daß die Geschwulst sich gegen die Tiefe vergrößerte. Nach einigen ergebnislosen Heilversuchen mit verschiedenen Medikamenten wurde im November 1925 die vorgeschlagene Operation ausgeführt. Das sternale Ende des Schlüsselbeins wurde freigelegt und reseziert. Es war auf mehr als das Doppelte des Normalen verdickt und usurierte die darunterliegende 1. Rippe, deren knorpeliger Anteil verknöchert und auch auf das Doppelte verdickt war; auch von der Rippe wurde dieser verdickte Teil in einer Länge von 6 cm abgetrennt. Glatte Heilung der Wunde in 8 Tagen. Die histologische Untersuchung des entfernten Knochens ergab den Befund einer Ostitis hyperplastica.

Die Wirkung der Operation zeigte sich prompt und in absolut überzeugender Weise. Die Kopfschmerzanfälle zeigten sich seit der Operation überhaupt nicht mehr, ebenso blieben die Schmerzen und übrigen Beschwerden der rechten Hand vollständig aus. Die einzige Beschwerde der Kranken nach der Operation war, daß sie beim Liegen auf dem Rücken in der Nackengegend rechts einen dumpfen Schmerz verspürte, so daß sie anfangs nur auf der Seite liegen konnte. Nach 2 Monaten ist auch dieser Schmerz gewichen. Die Patientin ist seit 9 Jahren vollkommen beschwerdenfrei.

Bei der Beurteilung des Falles war ich bestrebt, alle Einwände, die gegen die Richtigkeit des von mir angenommenen kausalen Zusammenhanges zwischen Knochengeschwulst und Kopfschmerzen sprechen konnten, eingehend zu berücksichtigen. Ich fand bei der Patientin keinen Anhaltspunkt für eine hysterische Konstitution, welche ähnliche Symptome hervorbringen könnte, wobei auch die suggestive Heilwirkung der Operation verständlich wäre. Der Kopfschmerz war ein typischer Migränekopfschmerz und konnte auf psychogene Art nicht beeinflußt werden. Durch den vollen Erfolg der Operation, welcher bereits seit 9 Jahren unverändert besteht, ist es bewiesen, daß der rechtseitige angiospastische Zustand, welcher die Migräneanfälle und später die Armparoxysmen herbeiführte, durch den Druck der Knochengeschwulst auf den Plexus vertebralis bzw. Plexus subclavius verursacht wurde.

2. Ein 54jähriger Mann ohne hereditäre Belastung, Vater von 4 gesunden Kindern; nie geschlechtskrank gewesen, kein Trinker. In der Anamnese außer einem Schlüsselbeinbruch, der etwa 3 Monate vor seiner Erkrankung glatt abheilte, nichts von Belang. Plötzliche Erkrankung mit heftigen Kopfschmerzanfällen, die nur die rechte Kopfhälfte, hauptsächlich Stirn und Augenhöhle betrafen, oft von Brechreiz, manchmal von Herzklopfen begleitet und in den letzten Tagen auch Augenflimmern, wobei er leuchtende Ringe vor den Augen sah. Bei der körperlichen Untersuchung war der medialste Abschnitt der rechtsseitigen Supraclaviculargrube hinter dem Sternocleidomastoideus überaus druckempfindlich; ebenso der Austrittspunkt des rechten N. supraorbitalis. Als einziges Symptom fanden wir, daß die rechte Pupille stark erweitert, fast doppelt so weit war wie die linke, mit guter Reaktion, doch erfolgte nach anfänglicher Verengung bald wieder die Erweiterung. Blut-Wa.R. negativ, Harn normal. Dieses Krankheitsbild, also rechtsseitige Migräneanfälle und rechtsseitige Mydriasis, bestand etwa 4 Wochen lang unverändert. Wir faßten den Fall wieder als eine symptomatische Migräne auf, wobei die am Röntgenbild sichtbare schiefe Verwachsung des gebrochenen Schlüsselbeines als die Ursache eines auf den unteren Halssympathicus ausgeübten Reizes in Erwägung gezogen wurde. Die weitere Gestaltung des Krankheitsbildes ließ uns aber von dieser Annahme abkommen, es entstand nämlich 4 Wochen nach Beginn der Kopfschmerzen plötzlich eine Heiserkeit, bedingt durch eine rechtsseitige totale Recurrenslähmung. Nach weiteren 3 Wochen ändert sich das Krankheitsbild, indem die Migräneanfälle nachlassen und bald gänzlich aufhören, dagegen von neuem heftige Schmerzen in der rechten Schulter und

Schulterblattgegend auftreten mit Parästhesien im rechten Arm und eine deutliche Pulsdifferenz zwischen beiden Arteriae radiales, indem die rechte schwächer fühlbar ist als die linke. An Stelle der erweiterten Pupille rechts traten jetzt ausgesprochene Myosis mit deutlicher Ptose und Enophthalmus. Bei der operativen Freilegung wurde im medialsten Abschnitt der oberen Schlüsselbeingrube eine harte Geschwulst tastbar, die aus dem hinteren Mediastinalraum gegen den Hals hinaufdringt. Nachdem eine Entfernung der Geschwulst als unausführbar erschien, wurde die Operation beendet. Nach einer tiefen Bestrahlung, die der Operation folgte, beobachteten wir nicht nur keine Besserung, sondern eine raschere Zunahme der Geschwulst, die 6 Wochen später den medialsten Abschnitt der Schlüsselbeingrube deutlich emporwölbte. Die Schmerzen in der Schulter und im rechten Arm nahmen immer mehr zu und erforderten heroische Morphindosen. Im objektiven Befund bemerkten wir 4 Wochen nach der Operation, daß das Hornertrias bis auf eine leichte Ptose zurückging, der Radialispuls beiderseits gleich war, nur die Recurrenslähmung blieb unverändert. Der Migränekopfschmerz wiederholte sich nicht. Wir sahen den Kranken zuletzt vor seinem Transport in die Heimat in schwer kachektischem Zustand, welcher durch eine hinzutretende Schluckstörung (Kompression durch die Geschwulst) verschärft wurde. Die epikritische Betrachtung des Falles zeigt, daß eine aus dem hinteren Megiastinum gegen die rechte Halsseite hinaufwachsende Geschwulst als erste Symptome rechtsseitige Migräneanfälle und Mydriasis hervorrief. Die Pupillenerweiterung als Reizsymptom des Halssympathicus ist allgemein bekannt. Das gleichzeitige Auftreten der Migräneanfälle läßt diesen dieselbe Bedeutung zukommen und bekräftigt durch vorliegenden Fall meinen Erklärungsversuch über die Bedeutung des unteren Halsganglions bei der Pathogenese des Migräneanfalles. Die erwähnten zwei Symptome traten am frühesten auf, sie waren die ersten Reizsymptome, die durch den Druck der emporwachsenden Geschwulst auf das rechte untere Halsganglion ausgelöst wurden. Im späteren Verlauf verschwanden beide Symptome und an ihre Stelle tritt als Lähmungserscheinung von seiten des Sympathicus das Hornertrias. In der vorübergehenden Pulsdifferenz müssen wir eine Reizerscheinung des Plexus subclavius erblicken. Die Schulter- und Armschmerzen, die bis zuletzt anhielten und sich fortwährend steigerten, dürften eher mit einem Druck der Geschwulst auf die Nerven des Armgeflechts zusammenhängen. Die Recurrenslähmung gehört als Nachbarschaftssymptom zum Krankheitsbild.

Eine kurze Besprechung verdient das Verhalten der Augensymptome in beiden Fällen. Im ersten Fall lokalisierten wir die Stelle des Sympathicusreizes auf den Anfangsteil des Plexus subclavius oder direkt auf den Plexus vertebralis und lehnten die direkte Beteiligung des unteren Halsganglions deshalb ab, weil Pupillenerweiterung fehlte. Im zweiten Fall erschienen Migräne und Mydriasis gleichzeitig und ließen den Sitz der Erkrankung direkt im Halsstrang vermuten. Bekanntlich nehmen die aus dem untersten Zervikalmark austretenden sympathischen Fasern des Centrum ciliospinale ihren Weg durch das unterste Halsganglion des Grenzstranges und ziehen im Grenzstrang zum obersten Ganglion, wo der präganglionäre Abschnitt dieser Bahn sein Ende findet. Das zweite postganglionäre Neuron entstammt aus den Ganglienzellen des obersten Halsganglions und gelangt durch Plexus caroticus, Plexus ophthalmicus usw. zu den Endorganen des Auges. Aus dieser Tatsache geht hervor, daß ein Reiz, der den Grenzstrang des Halssympathicus betrifft, ob er nun auf das oberste oder das unterste Ganglion einwirkt, immer Pupillenerweiterung verursacht. Betrifft der Reiz das unterste Halsganglion, so gesellen sich zu den Augensymptomen als weitere Reizerscheinung Migräneanfälle hinzu, so wie wir es in unserem zweiten Fall beobachten konnten. Der Reizzustand des unteren Halsganglions ist also durch Migräneanfälle und Pupillenerweiterung gekennzeichnet. Aus dieser Betrachtung könnte man vielleicht auch bezüglich der Pathogenese der gewöhnlichen Migräneanfälle einige Schlüsse ziehen. Wir sahen früher, daß in gar nicht seltenen Fällen der Migräneanfall von einer gleichseitigen Pupillenerweiterung gefolgt wird, welche den Anfall regelmäßig begleitet. In anderen Fällen fehlt dieses Symptom. Man könnte daran denken, daß bei der ersten Gruppe der Reizzustand des Sympathicus, welcher den Anfall verursacht, aus dem unteren Halsganglion selbst seinen Ausgang nimmt. Bei den übrigen Fällen, die übrigens die Mehrzahl der Migränefälle bilden, dürfte der Reizzustand in der Gefäßbahn selbst, also im Plexus vertebralis sich abspielen. Die klinischen Beobachtungen weisen darauf hin, daß auch die Ausbreitung des Gefäßkrampfes beim Migräneanfall nicht immer in gleicher Weise erfolgt. Bei der ophthalmischen Migräne, wo zuerst die Sehstörungen und nachher der Kopfschmerz auftritt, dürfte der Gefäßkrampf in den kleinen Gefäßen der Sehrinde und Sehbahn einsetzen und sich erst später auf die Gefäßstämme der Hirnbasis fortsetzen. Bei der ophthalmoplegischen Migräne, wo gewöhnlich der Kopfschmerz früher einsetzt und bedeutend später die Augenmuskellähmung, ist anzunehmen, daß der Gefäßkrampf sich zuerst in den größeren Arterien der Hirnbasis abspielt und erst nachher auf die kleinen Gefäße der Hirnnervenkerne übergreift.

Mein hier erörterter Erklärungsversuch kann nur darauf Anspruch erheben, daß er die von Dubois inaugurierte, rein angiospastische Theorie des Migräneanfalles von neuem begründet. Bemerkt soll werden, daß schon DUBOIS den Reizzustand des Sympathicus in den Abschnitt des Centrum ciliospinale, also in jene Sympathicusbahn verlegte, welche mit dem unteren Halsganglion und den aus diesem austretenden Sympathicusbahnen korrespondiert. Er berief sich als Beweis auf die Druckempfindlichkeit der Dornfortsätze der unteren Hals- und oberen Brustwirbel, die er bei Migräne konstatierte. Überblickt man die von den neueren Autoren zur Geltung gebrachten Anschauungen über die Pathogenese des Migräneanfalles, so findet man, daß es auch heute noch 2 Richtungen gibt. Die rein angiospastische Auffassung wurde von V. RADOT auf dem Kongreß der französischen Neurologischen Gesellschaft 1925 vertreten. Auch CURSCHMANN und M. ULRICH hält sie für die am meisten plausible; andere Autoren, wie FLATAU, HARTMANN, KÄMMERER, die ebenfalls in den Zirkulationsstörungen des Gehirns die Grundlage des Migräneanfalles erblicken, wollen neben den angiospastischen, auch den vasodilatativen Vorgängen sowie transsudativen Veränderungen im Gebiet der Zirkulationsstörung eine Rolle zuschreiben.

2. Ätiologie der Migräne.

Wir haben im Migräneanfall ein Syndrom kennengelernt, welches durch den Angiospasmus eines bestimmten Abschnittes des Hirngefäßsystems entsteht und für diesen Gefäßkrampf einen zeitweilig erhöhten Reizzustand jenes Sympathicusabschnittes verantwortlich gemacht, welchem die vasomotorische Innervation dieses Gebietes unterstellt ist. Bei der Prüfung der Frage, wodurch diese erhöhte Gefäßkrampfbereitschaft bedingt ist, wollen wir zuerst jene *wesentlichen inneren Ursachen* berücksichtigen, die im Begriff der *Anlage zur Migräne* zusammengefaßt werden und dann jene ursächlichen Faktoren behandeln, die als periodisch auftretende *auslösende Ursachen* in Betracht kommen.

Die *Anlage zur Migräne* ist in der überwiegenden Mehrzahl der Fälle vererbt. Die große Bedeutung des hereditären Momentes ist schon den ältesten Forschern bekannt gewesen. SYMMONDS, LIVEING und GOWERS fanden in etwa der Hälfte ihrer Fälle die Migräne vererbt: E. MENDEL berichtet über 80%, HEYERDAHL über 85%, MOEBIUS über 90% hereditäre Fälle. W. ALLAN fand, daß von 318 Kindern, deren Eltern (56 Paare) beide an Migräne litten, 240 (83,3%) Migräne hatten. Unter 750 Kindern, wo einer der Eltern (141 Paare) an Migräne litt, waren 342 (61%) von Migräne befallen; unter 485 Kindern migränefreier Eltern (98 Paare) waren 18 (3,7%) mit Migräne behaftet. BUCHANAN fand in 100 Familien, wo einer der Eltern migränekrank war, 143 kranke und 481 nichtkranke Kinder, also nur 22,6% Migränekranke; in 3 Familien, wo beide Eltern an Migräne litten, beobachtete er bei sämtlichen 15 Kindern Migräne. WILDBRANDT-SÄNGER beobachteten ophthalmische Migräne in 4 Generationen; ähnliche Beobachtungen machten LASEGUE und OPPENHEIM. In der überwiegenden Mehrzahl der Fälle ist der *Vererbungsmodus ein dominanter*. JENS CHR. SMITH behauptet, daß die Migräne sich im Sinne des MENDELschen Gesetzes vererbt; auch BUCHANAN vertritt diese Ansicht. Es wird allgemein anerkannt, daß das weibliche Geschlecht beim Übertragen der hereditären Anlage eine viel größere Rolle spielt als das männliche. FLATAU fand bei migränekranken Männern, daß in 79% die Mütter und 21% die Väter die Migräne übertrugen; bei migränekranken Frauen fand er in 63% die Mütter, in 30% die Väter und in 7% beide Eltern an der Übertragung beteiligt. Für die überwiegende Mehrzahl der **Migränefälle ist die *homologe, gleichsinnige* Vererbung bezeichnend.** Bei einer heterologen Vererbung kann heute eine reale Bedeutung nur der Epilepsie zuerkannt werden, wie es die früher angeführten Statistiken beweisen. Frühere Autoren, wie BOUCHARD, TROUSSEAU, CHARCOT, DÉJERINE u. a. nahmen eine sehr weitgefaßte heterologe Vererbbarkeit an, indem sie die Migräne in eine Krankheitsgruppe einreihten, in welcher Psychoneurosen, Ekzem, Asthma, Rheumatismus, Gicht, Diabetes, Tuberkulose, Carcinom und noch zahlreiche andere Krankheiten Platz fanden. CHARCOT faßte diese Gruppe als Famille neuroarthritique zusammen, BOUCHARD bezeichnete sie als Krankheiten mit verlangsamtem Stoffwechsel. Bei beiden Gruppen stand die Gicht und die gichtische Anlage im Mittelpunkt der Krankheitsgruppe. Es gibt auch heute noch Autoren, welche einen innigeren Zusammenhang zwischen Gicht und Migräne annehmen (FLATAU, HAIG, CROFTAN, CAPPARONI), von der überwiegenden Mehrzahl der Autoren wird aber ein solcher entschieden abgelehnt. Der viel zitierte englische Major von TROUSSEAU wird von CHRISTIANSEN mit Recht als „rara avis" bezeichnet, dem er auch nur einen einzigen Fall aus seiner Erfahrung gleichzustellen vermochte. In den Ländern, wo die Gicht eine seltene Krankheit ist, findet man überhaupt nicht weniger Migränefälle und der von englischen und französischen Autoren behauptete Zusammenhang wurde hier immer mit Skepsis aufgenommen. Ich fand in einem Krankenmaterial von 2000 Migränekranken keinen einzigen Fall, wo sich Migräne mit einer gichtischen Anlage paarte. Berücksichtigt man also einerseits, daß der Hauptrepräsentant dieser Krankheitsgruppe, die Gicht, eine äußerst seltene und nur als Zufall aufzufassende Erkrankung im Reiche der Migräne darstellt und findet man andererseits, daß eine Reihe von Erkrankungen, wie Urticaria, Asthma, Ekzem, welche früher zur neuroarthritischen Krankheitsgruppe gezählt wurden, heute die gut gekennzeichnete Gruppe der allergischen Erkrankungen bilden, in welcher auch der Migräne ein Platz gebührt, dann erkennt man erst die Haltlosigkeit jener früheren Gruppierung und auch die Unzulässigkeit dessen, daß eine heterologe Vererbung der Migräne auf die sog. neuroarthritischen Erkrankungen ausgedehnt werde.

Die gleichsinnige dominante Vererbung, die sich bei der Migräne in einem so hohen Prozentsatz nachweisen läßt, wie bei keiner anderen Nervenkrankheit (MOEBIUS), macht die Annahme wahrscheinlich, daß die wesentliche innere Ursache, die Anlage zur Migräne an die Erbmasse gebunden ist. Diese konnatale Bedingtheit der Migränebereitschaft wird man auch für die wenigen Migränefälle nicht ganz ausschließen können, wo eine direkte Heredität nicht nachweisbar ist. Wenn man noch vor Augen hält, daß die sog. symptomatische Migräne auch eine gewisse Auswahl erkennen läßt, indem dieselbe organische Hirnerkrankung bei einem Kranken Migräneanfälle auslöst, bei einem anderen nicht, dann müssen wir die Grenzen der Migränebereitschaft noch weiter fassen, als es durch die nachweisbare Heredität bestimmt ist.

Eine weitere Frage, die sich hier aufstellt, in welchem Organ diese vererbte Anlage verankert ist, läßt uns vorderhand über Vermutungen nicht hinauskommen. Früher wurde die angeborene Schwäche der Gefäße (arterielle Heredität von HUCHARD, neurovasculäre Diathese von OPPENHEIM, zuletzt Gefäßdyspraxie von HAHN und STEIN) als die sich vererbende Anlage aufgefaßt, heute erscheint es geläufiger, in der Schwäche und Reizbarkeit des vegetativen Nervensystems die inhärente Eigenschaft der Erbmasse zu erblicken. So spricht M. ULRICH von einer angeborenen, spezifisch verminderten Widerstandsfähigkeit des Sympathicussystems, in welcher sie das Wesen der „hemikranischen Diathese" erkennt. Auch V. RADOT spricht von einer erhöhten Reizbarkeit des Sympathicus, die auf einer Labilität des neurovegetativen Gleichgewichts beruht. Hier wäre aber zu bemerken, daß es heute kaum mehr angängig ist, einen solchen Schwächezustand nur für den Sympathicus anzunehmen und den Parasympathicus dabei unberücksichtigt zu lassen; zeigten uns doch sowohl klinische als experimentelle Untersuchungen, daß die von EPPINGER und HESS aufgestellten sympathicotonischen und vagotonischen Konstitutionstypen in Wirklichkeit nicht existieren, sondern daß sich eine Menschengruppe dadurch von den Normalen unterscheidet, daß ihr ganzes vegetative Nervensystem eine erhöhte Reizbarkeit aufweist, wobei aber sympathicotonische und vagotonische Erscheinungen gleichzeitig und nebeneinander auftreten können. In welcher Richtung der vegetative Tonus in einem bestimmten Organ sich verschiebt, das hängt vor allem vom Zustand des Erfolgsorgans ab; befindet sich dieses in einer sympathicotonischen Bereitschaft, so erfolgt hier bei jeder Störung des vegetativen Gleichgewichtes, sei es, daß die Tonusschwankung in sympathicotonischer oder vagotonischer Richtung erfolgt, immer der sympathicotonische Effekt. Diese Erkenntnis, zu der man bei der Prüfung der übrigen neurovegetativen Störungen gelangte, müssen wir auch bei der Migräne zur Geltung bringen, wenn wir eine Reihe von Beobachtungen nicht ungeklärt lassen wollten. Es bliebe nämlich ein Rätsel, wieso der Migräneanfall, in dem wir einen sympathicotonisch bedingten Gefäßkrampf erblicken, manchmal von solchen Symptomen begleitet wird, die auf einen geschwächten Sympathicotonus und erhöhten Vagotonus zurückgeführt werden müssen (Gesichtsröte, Myosis); auch die Kombination des Migräneanfalles mit dem Asthmaanfall, also einem rein vagotonischen Symptomenkomplex, wäre unerklärt. Man müßte auch Bedenken haben, wenn man im Migräneanfall einen allergischen Vorgang erblicken sollte analog der Urticarie und dem Asthma, wo doch bei allergischen Zuständen gewöhnlich eine Erhöhung des Parasympathicustonus angenommen wird. Hält man noch vor Augen, daß unter den Migränekranken gar nicht selten Leute mit ausgesprochenen vagotonischen Zeichen vorkommen, dann zeigt sich wohl recht die Unhaltbarkeit jeder Theorie, die die Migräne einseitig auf eine erhöhte Reizbarkeit des Sympathicus zurückführen möchte. Diese Gegensätze verschwinden aber sogleich, wenn man, wie bei den anderen vegetativen Neurosen, auch bei der Migräne eine allgemeine erhöhte Reizbarkeit des vegetativen Nervensystems als den grundsätzlichen krankhaften Zustand betrachtet, wobei aber eine lokale, sympathicotonische Organbereitschaft des Vertebralisgefäßsystems das Wesentliche der Migräneanlage bildet. So wird es erklärlich, daß neben dem sympathicotonischen Gefäßkrampf, welcher den Migräneanfall verursacht, in anderen Organen vagotonische Syndrome auftreten, oder daß auch bei sog. Vagotonikern sich Migräneanfälle einstellen können. Die erbbedingte Migräneanlage würde also in diesem Sinne eine erhöhte Erregbarkeit des ganzen vegetativen Nervensystems bedeuten, die sich in einer Neigung zu Tonusschwankungen, in einer Gleichgewichtslabilität kundgibt, wobei aber gleichzeitig eine spezielle, sympathicotonische Organbereitschaft des Vertebralisgefäßabschnittes besteht.

Neuere Beobachtungen von BEECHER, SCIMONE u. a. deuten aber darauf hin, daß nicht immer die oben gekennzeichnete „Migräneanlage" den sich vererbenden Faktor darstellt. Sie wiesen nämlich darauf hin, daß die familiäre Anamnese von solchen Migränekranken, die an einer allergischen Migräne leiden, eine auffallend hohe, erbliche, allergische Belastung aufweist, indem sich zahlreiche Mitglieder dieser Familien durch Neigung zu anderen allergischen Krankheiten auszeichnen.

BALL fand bei einer in dieser Richtung geführten Untersuchung, daß in den Familien von 261 Migränekranken Asthma in 60 Fällen (22,9%), Heufieber in 35 Fällen (13,4%), Urticaria in 73 Fällen (27,9%), Ekzem in 25 Fällen (9,5%) vorkam und nur in 70 Fällen (26,8%) war neben der Migräne keine andere allergische Erkrankung in der Familie nachweisbar. MOLONEY fand, daß in den Familien der von ihm untersuchten Migränefälle allergische Manifestationen in 47% der Fälle nachweisbar waren, dreimal häufiger als in den übrigen untersuchten

Fällen. BALYEAT und RINKEL fanden sogar in 82% ihrer Fälle (202 an der Zahl) allergische Erkrankungen bei den Vorfahren der Migränekranken. GOVIN berichtet über eine familiäre Allergieanamnese in 85% seiner Fälle (60 Fälle von Migräne). ROVE (130 Fälle) fand allergische Heredität in 69,2% seiner Fälle. BALYEAT und RICHARDS machten auf Grund ihrer durch Fragebogen erhaltenen Daten (55 Familien mit je 2—3 Generationen) schon einige Angaben über die Gesetzmäßigkeiten der allergischen Heredität: Nach ihnen handle es sich um eine unregelmäßige, inkomplette, dominante Vererbung, wobei die einzelnen Formen von Allergien in bunter Variabilität auftreten; Spezialgene, welche den Charakter der Allergie bestimmen, werden abgelehnt. Ein eineiiges Zwillingspaar zeigte dieselben 3 Formen von Allergie.

Der Enthusiasmus, mit welchem die amerikanischen Autoren die allergische Natur der Migräne verfechten, mahnt jedenfalls zu einer gewissen Vorsicht. Wir haben schon einen solchen „ersten Ansturm" wiederholt in der Medizin erlebt; es hat den Anschein, als wolle man die allergische Migräne einfach in die früher allesbeherrschende Stellung der „neuroarthritischen" Migräne einsetzen.

Als nicht sehr gangbar erwiesen sich bis heute die Bestrebungen, die sich um die Feststellung eines für die Migräne charakteristischen *Konstitutionstypus* bemühten. HAHN und STEIN glauben einen solchen gefunden zu haben im Habitus asthenicus (STILLER) mit kleinem Herzen und schmalem Gefäßtrakt, bei welchem Typus die hereditäre Lues eine gewisse Rolle spiele. LAUDENHEIMER stellt die Partialkonstitution des vasomotorischen und endokrinen Systems in den Vordergrund, wobei er im asthenischen Habitus mit Vasolabilität, vornehmlich vagotonischen Symptomen und Zeichen von Hypothyreoidismus die kennzeichnenden Merkmale der Migränekonstitution erblickt. CURSCHMANN lenkt die Aufmerksamkeit auf die hypoparathyreoide Konstitution, die sich in der nicht seltenen Paarung von Tetanie und Migräne, besonders bei Kindern kundgibt. In ähnlichem Sinne spricht KRAMSZTYK von einer calcipriven Konstitution, die durch den asthenischen Habitus, kombiniert mit dem CHOVSTEK- und ERBschen Phänomen, stigmatisiert ist. Diesen Beobachtungen gegenüber weist KÄMMERER mit vollem Recht darauf hin, daß man bei Migräne neben den hier geschilderten auch andere Typen, wie Pykniker, Hyperthyreotiker usw. finden kann. Wer Gelegenheit hat, eine größere Anzahl von Migränekranken zu untersuchen, muß zu der Überzeugung kommen, daß die geschilderten Konstitutionstypen bei Migräne wohl vorkommen, aber keinesfalls in einer solchen Häufigkeit, daß sie für die Gesetzmäßigkeit des einen oder des anderen Konstitutionstypus die notwendige Grundlage bieten könnten. Dieser Vorbehalt ist auch am Platze, wenn man die Beziehungen der neuro- und psychopathischen Anlage zur Migräne prüft. Zweifellos gibt es unter den Migränekranken eine gewisse Anzahl von Kranken, die neben ihrer Migräne neuro- und psychopathische Reaktionen aufweisen oder Kennzeichen einer solchen vererbten Anlage erkennen lassen. Wie hoch diese Gruppe unter den Migränekranken vertreten ist, darüber fehlen zuverlässige Daten; jedenfalls dürften Psychopathen und Epileptiker zusammen auch nur einen geringen Bruchteil der Migränekranken ausmachen. Die Migränekonstitution — wenn von einer solchen gesprochen wird — kann mit der neuro- oder psychopathischen Konstitution keineswegs indentifiziert werden.

Wenig aussichtsreich blieben bis heute auch diejenigen Untersuchungen, welche durch Prüfung der *Stoffwechselvorgänge* dem Wesen der Migräneanlage näherzukommen trachteten. Im Vordergrund stand früher das Verhalten der Harnsäure. STECKEL, HAIG, HOLMES berichteten über Harnsäureretention und Harnsäureüberschuß; CROFTAN fand, daß die endogene Harnsäure vermindert,

die exogene in der Ausscheidung verschleppt ist. LICHTY, sowie V. RADOT und
LAUDAT fanden dagegen normale Harnsäurewerte. RÉMOND und ROUZAUD
fanden bei Migränekranken die Vermehrung des Cholesterins, der Gallenfarb-
stoffe, des Harnstoffes, des Reststickstoffes und der Harnsäure im Blut und eine
geringe Vermehrung des Blutzuckers; bei Untersuchung des Zirkulationsapparates
fanden sie eine Erhöhung der Blutviskosität und eine geringere Differenz zwischen
systolischem und diastolischem Blutdruck. Sie nehmen einen toxischen Zustand an, bei welchem die Störungen des Stickstoff-Stoffwechsels die Hauptrolle
spielen. V. RADOT und LAUDAT haben diese Angaben nachgeprüft und fanden
mit Ausnahme des Blutcholesterins, welches auch in ihren Fällen eine Erhöhung
zeigte, ansonsten normale Werte. LOEPER konstatierte Oxalämie in drei Migränefällen. THOMAS und POST haben die Vermutung ausgesprochen, daß bei der
Migräne die Störung des Stoffwechsels darin bestehe, daß die Gewebe das
Oxygen nicht gut aufbrauchen, so daß sich saure Stoffwechselprodukte im Körper
anhäufen. R. und S. WEISSMANN-NETTER untersuchten das Verhalten der
Alkalireserve und die Verschiebung des Basen-Säuregleichgewichts und fanden
in einigen Fällen eine erhöhte Alkalose vor dem Anfall. MARGOLIS macht auf
die Beziehungen aufmerksam, die zwischen Migräne und chronischer Pentosurie
bestehen; letztere geht häufig mit vagotonischen Symptomen einher und verhält sich in mancher Beziehung wie die allergischen Erkrankungen. RATSHFORD
beobachtete Vermehrung des Paraxanthins im Urin; PFAFF und PUTNAM haben
diesen Befund nicht bestätigt. Auch die Angaben über die Bedeutung des Blutcalciumspiegels bei Migräne sind heute noch vielfach einander widersprechend
und kaum zu verwerten (BERENCSY, GAISBOCK, BILLIGHEIMER, ROTHLIN, DA-
VANZO, POPOVICIU und POPESCU, PERITZ, STERLING). V. RADOT und seine Mitarbeiter betrachten als die wesentlichste Stoffwechselveränderung, welche dem
Migräneanfall vorausgeht, die sog. ,,hämoklasische Krise", welche bei Asthma
und Urticaria von WIDAL beschrieben wurde (Leukocytensturz und Inversion
des Blutbildes, Senkung des refraktometrischen Index und des Blutdruckes).
Diese brüsk einsetzende physikalisch-chemische Veränderung soll durch Störung
des neurovegetativen Gleichgewichts den Migräneausfall herbeiführen. Nach
RADOT spiele das humorale Syndrom der hämoklasischen Krise nicht nur bei
der anaphylaktischen Migräne eine Rolle, sondern auch bei der Mehrzahl der
übrigen Migräneformen; nach ihm gebe es nur wenige Fälle, wo ein direkter
Sympathicusreiz den Migräneanfall auslöst.

Aussichtsreicher sind die Bestrebungen, welche durch die Erforschung der
auslösenden Ursachen des Migräneanfalles in die Ätiologie der Migräne einen
Einblick zu gewinnen versuchen. Diese Kenntnisse unterscheiden sich von den
früheren, mehr hypothetischen Annahmen dadurch, daß sie zumeist auf klinische Beobachtungen, biologische Reaktionen und therapeutische Erfolge aufgebaut
sind. Es soll gleich bemerkt werden, daß wir heute erst am Beginn dieser neuen
Ära stehen und weit davon entfernt sind, jeden Migräneanfall durch Eruierung
seiner auslösenden Ursachen in eine bestimmte Gruppe einzureihen; sicher
ist aber, daß dies bei vielen Migränefällen heute schon möglich ist und daß wir
hiedurch wertvolle Aufschlüsse für eine kausale Behandlung erhalten. Es wurde
früher darauf hingewiesen, daß eine Absonderung der Migränefälle auf Grund
des klinischen Anfallsbildes keine Berechtigung besitzt. Auch sahen wir,
daß die erbbedingte Anlage zur Migräne, in der wir die wesentliche innere
Ursache dieser Erkrankung erblicken, eine für sämtliche Migränefälle gemeinsame Eigenschaft repräsentiert. Anders steht es, wenn wir auf Grund der auslösenden Ursachen eine Gruppierung innerhalb der Migräne vorzunehmen versuchen. Es können nämlich auf diese Weise schon heute einige gut umschriebene
Gruppen voneinander abgesondert werden, die nicht nur von pathogenetischem

Standpunkt erhebliche Unterschiede aufweisen, sondern auch unserem therapeutischen Vorgehen ein Individualisieren vorschreiben. Im Vordergrund steht die Lehre von der *anaphylaktischen* oder richtiger *allergischen Migräne*. Bahnbrechend waren auf diesem Gebiet die Untersuchungen von RADOT, PAGNIEZ und NAST (1919). Sie fanden, daß der Migräneanfall in gewissen Fällen nichts anderes als eine anaphylaktische Krise darstellt und dem Asthmaanfall oder der Urticaria gleichzusetzen ist, deren allergische Natur schon von früher her bekannt war. RADOT und seine Mitarbeiter führten zur Stütze ihrer Ansicht klinische, biologische und therapeutische Erfahrungen heran. Sie beriefen sich in erster Linie auf die bekannte Tatsache, daß bei Migränekranken nicht selten Asthma, Urticaria, flüchtige Ödeme beobachtet werden, und zwar entweder unabhängig von den Migräneanfällen oder im Verlauf des Anfalles. Das häufige Zusammentreffen von Asthma und Migräne wurde auch von STRÜMPELL, CURSCHMANN, GAENSSLEN und F. COKE bestätigt. Noch mehr überzeugend für die allergische Theorie waren die Beobachtungen, daß bei gewissen Migränekranken die Einnahme eines bestimmten Nahrungsmittels, Medikamente oder die Einatmung eines bestimmten Duftes regelmäßig einen Migräneanfall auslöst. In diesen Fällen ist die allergische Natur des Anfalles auf die Überempfindlichkeit des betreffenden Organismus gegen eine bestimmte chemische Substanz zurückzuführen. Seit den ersten diesbezüglichen Beobachtungen von PAGNIEZ und NAST, die sich auf Schokolade bezog (LASEGUE beschrieb — schon früher — einen solchen Fall), haben sich die diesbezüglichen Mitteilungen wesentlich vermehrt, in der neueren Literatur werden diese Fälle schon summarisch behandelt. Es zeigte sich, daß eine ganze Reihe von Substanzen eine anaphylaktogene Wirkung besitzt, die sich in einem Migräneanfall kundgibt. Auch hier stehen, wie bei den übrigen allergischen Reaktionen, Milch, Eier, manche Fleisch- und Fischsorten, Weizenmehl, sowie einige aromatische Stoffe im Vordergrund. In einem Fall von LUBBERS trat der Migräneanfall nach Genuß von Hülsenfrüchten (Bohnen, Erbsen) auf. Ich beobachtete einen Fall von anaphylaktischer Migräne nach Genuß von mit Rahm bereiteten Speisen und einen anderen nach Genuß von Sardellen. Lehrreich ist der Fall von BERGH.

Ein junger Maschinenführer, der bei der Teerung einer Straße verwendet wurde, erkrankte das erstemal am 8. Tag und das zweitemal, als er wieder die Arbeit aufnahm, am ersten Tag seiner Beschäftigung an einem Schnupfen mit Atemnot und linksseitigem Kopfschmerz mit Übelkeit und Erbrechen, Augentränen, Flimmern und Schwindel. Beim Versuch mit Einatmung von Steinkohlenteer gelang es regelmäßig, diesen allergischen Zustand, welcher aus asthmaähnlicher Atemnot und linksseitiger Migräne bestand, zu provozieren. Am sechsten Versuchstag konnte die Zunahme der eosinophilen Zellen von 1% bis auf 12% festgestellt werden. Vorherige Injektion von Aphenil milderte den Anfall. Bei Kontrollpersonen trat nur eine geringe Bindehautreizung auf.

Die allergische Natur mancher Migräneanfälle konnte auch durch biologische Vorgänge bekräftigt werden. PAGNIEZ und NAST fanden in ihrem Fall nach Einnahme von 60 g Schokolade auf nüchternen Magen das Auftreten einer hämoklasischen Krise (Leukocytensturz, Inversion des Blutbildes) und nachher trat der Migräneanfall auf. Auch LUBBERS konstatierte in seinem Fall Leukocytensturz vor dem Migräneanfall. RADOT macht darauf aufmerksam, daß der Nachweis dieser Blutveränderungen nur dann im Sinne einer allergischen Reaktion verwertet werden kann, wenn diese dem Anfall vorausgehen und nicht während des Anfalles beobachtet werden.

Der Wert der hämoklasischen Krise als Indikator einer allergischen Reaktion wird verschiedentlich beurteilt. ERDMANN u. a. halten sie nicht für spezifisch. Auch bewiesen eine Reihe von Untersuchungen, daß die Verschiebung der Blutveränderungen in einer entgegengesetzten Richtung, als es WIDAL angab, bei anaphylaktischen Vorgängen ebenso häufig vorkommt und als positives Zeichen aufgefaßt werden muß (BRACK). Von anderer Seite (MIBELLI, TÖRÖK-RAJKA-LEHNER) wird die Ansicht von WIDAL und RADOT, nach welcher die humoralen Veränderungen die primären sind und erst durch diese die anaphylaktische Reaktion hervorgerufen wird, bekämpft, in dem sie sie als koordinierte, humorale Veränderungen den anaphylaktischen Zellvorgängen gleichstellen.

Als ein weiterer Beweis für die anaphylaktische Natur des Migräneanfalles wird die von mehreren Autoren gefundene Erhöhung der eosinophilen Zellen im Blutbilde angesehen, die auch bei anderen allergischen Erkrankungen als positives Zeichen gedeutet wird. Die erste diesbezügliche Mitteilung stammt von NEUSSER, der in einem Fall von schwerer Migräne während des Anfalles Eosinophilie beobachtete. GAENSSLEN prüfte das Blutbild in 42 Migränefällen und fand bei 31 eine Vermehrung der Eosinophilen von 5—16%, in 11 Fällen, wo die Migräne mit anderen Krankheiten kombiniert vorkam, erhielt er normale Werte. GAENSSLENs Befund wurde seither von mehreren Autoren (MILLER-RAULSTON, WEITZ) bestätigt. RADOT und BLAMOUTIER fanden dagegen unter 18 Fällen nur dreimal eine erhöhte Zahl (über 5%) und bezweifeln die Verwertbarkeit dieses Befundes. RADOT beruft sich noch auf Versuche von VAN LEEUWEN und ZEYDNER, die im Blut von Migränekranken eine Substanz fanden, welche in der glatten Muskulatur des Katzendarms ähnliche Kontraktionen hervorrief, wie man sie durch Pilocarpin beobachtete; sie fanden diese Substanz auch bei Urticaria, Asthma und Epilepsie und vermuten in ihr die eigentliche Ursache des allergischen Zustandes. Weitere Angaben über die allergische Migräne enthalten die Arbeiten von MILLER und RAULSTON, CURTIS-BROWN, KENNEDY, DATTNER, BOLTEN, VAUGHAN, CURSCHMANN u. a.

Eine zweite, schon lange bekannte Gruppe innerhalb der Migräne bilden die Fälle, wo die auslösende Ursache der Migräneanfälle in einer *Funktionsstörung des Verdauungstraktes* vermutet wird. Dabei können Unregelmäßigkeiten in der Nahrungsaufnahme, schlechte Zusammenstellung der Nahrung ebenso eine Rolle spielen wie die eigentlichen Funktionsstörungen im Verdauungstrakt. Es gibt Erfahrungen, nach welchen reichliche Mahlzeiten einen Migräneanfall auslösen können. LORD DAWSON of PENN macht diesbezüglich auf die Sonntagsmigräne aufmerksam, bei deren Zustandekommen neben der kopiösen Mahlzeit auch die darauf folgende sportliche Überlastung des Körpers eine Rolle spiele. Auch das rasche Essen (Tachyphagie) wird von einigen Autoren beschuldigt. In beiden Fällen nimmt RADOT an, daß durch die ungenügende Einwirkung der Verdauungsfermente auf die Nahrung der weitere Abbau durch die Leber gestört wird, wodurch toxische Produkte des intermediären Stoffwechsels in den Blutstrom gelangen und dort eine, den Anfall provozierende kolloidoklasische Krise herbeiführen. Die schädliche Zusammensetzung der Nahrung steht schon seit langem in der Reihe der den Migräneanfall auslösenden Ursachen. KELLOG machte schon in 1895 auf die mangelhafte Verdauung von Fleisch und Amylazeen aufmerksam. Von den meisten Autoren wird die reichliche Kohlenhydratzufuhr und animalische Eiweißnahrung beschuldigt (BROWN, BOND, MINOT u. v. a.), während die fettige Nahrung im allgemeinen als unschädlich, von einigen Autoren sogar als vorteilhaft angesehen wird; eine Störung des Purinstoffwechsels, die früher in der Ära der gichtischen Migräne viel diskutiert wurde, wird heute kaum mehr in Erwägung gezogen. RADOT bezweifelt, daß eine gesteigerte Kohlenhydratzufuhr bei der Auslösung des Migräneanfalles eine Rolle spiele, dagegen sah er mehrere Fälle, wo tierisches Eiweiß anfallsauslösend wirkte. Er setzt diese Fälle zur allergischen Migräne in nahe Beziehung; auch BALYEAT äußert diese Ansicht, indem er annimmt, daß hier eine Überempfindlichkeit dem tierischen Eiweiß gegenüber bestehe, die sich deshalb nicht immer prompt und so regelmäßig wie bei der allergischen Migräne bemerkbar macht, weil die Anfallsbereitschaft bei den Migränekranken eine wechselnde ist, die Kranken sich nicht immer „im Bereich der Migräne"

(PAGNIEZ) befinden. Die Bedeutung der Obstipation als anfallsauslösender Ursache wird auch heute öfters betont (MINOT, LAING, BASTEDO, RUPPERT, WILSON und ROGER-CREMIEUX); durch diese sollen besondere Gärungsprozesse im Darm entstehen und Darmtoxine die unmittelbare Ursache des Migräneanfalles bilden. HARTSOCK beschuldigt die Stauung im Duodenaltrakt als eine Funktionsstörung, welche häufig zu Migräneanfällen Anlaß gibt; bei Kranken, wo der Anfall mit einem galligen Erbrechen endet, dürfte nach ihm durch die Beseitigung der Stase im Duodenum die toxische Wirkung aufgehoben sein. Auch Enteroptose und Darmadhäsionen können nach HARTSOCK durch Aufrechterhalten eines Stauungszustandes im Duodenum Migräne verursachen; LEWEN beschuldigt die Magenptose. ROGER und CREMIEUX berichten über einen Fall von assoziierter Augenmigräne, in welchem Störungen des Digestivtraktes, verursacht durch eine Senkung und Verzogensein des Colon transversum, bestanden und die Beseitigung der letzteren auch die Migräne zur Heilung brachte. Auch chronische Appendicitis könne einen Migränezustand aufrechterhalten.

Immer zahlreicher werden die Beobachtungen, welche auf die innigen Beziehungen zwischen Migräne und Leberfunktionsstörung hinweisen. Es ist mehr eine allgemein ärztliche, als statistisch erwiesene Erfahrung, daß cholecystopathische Zustände öfters mit Migräneanfällen verknüpft sind. In diesem Sinne sprechen die von mehreren Autoren nachgewiesene Erhöhung des Blutcholesterins und die von HETÉNYI und FODOR gefundene Hyperbilirubinämie bei Migräne, die auch von DIAMOND bestätigt wurde. CHIRAY und TRIBOULET fanden in zahlreichen Migränefällen eine Gallenstauung (stase vesiculaire) infolge Blasenatonie, die sich am Röntgenbild in der Erweiterung der Gallenblase, sowie in der dunklen, dickflüssigen Beschaffenheit der Galle kundgibt. Sie betrachten diese Gallenstauung als die auslösende Ursache der Migräneanfälle und brachten die Duodenalsondierung als Heilmethode für diese Fälle in Vorschlag. McCLURE und HUNTZINGER betonen das häufige Zusammentreffen und den innigen Zusammenhang zwischen Migräne und Cholecystopathien, wobei sie darauf hinweisen, daß unter ihren 72 untersuchten Fällen nur in einem Bruchteil eine Cholecystitis oder Gallensteinbildung sich zeigte; oft erwies sich auch die operative Behandlung als erfolglos, sie konnten fast in allen Fällen eine Dysfunktion der Leber feststellen. FRIEDLÄNDER und PETTOW halten den Migräneanfall für den Effekt einer Shockwirkung, die durch cholangiopathische Zustände im intermediären Stoffwechsel ausgelöst wird, wobei sie im unzerstört in den Blutstrom gelangten Histamin den unmittelbaren anfallsauslösenden Faktor erblicken.

Neuere Untersuchungen von FODOR machen es wahrscheinlich, daß ein Teil der cholecystopathischen Zustandsbilder selbst nichts anderes, als eine allergische Reaktion darstellen, ebenso, wie der Migräneanfall oder der Asthmaanfall. Schon KELLING betrachtete manche typische Gallenkrampfanfälle als Migräneäquivalente. FODOR fand bei einem Material, welches 264 Fälle von Gallenerkrankungen in sich faßt, daß cholecystopathische Zustände sich häufig mit den bekannten allergischen Zuständen (Asthma, Urticaria, Ekzem, Migräne, Prurigo, Colitis) assoziieren. Nach ihm stelle der allergische Gallenkrampfanfall im Sinne von BERGH und WESTPHAL einen dyskinetischen Zustand der Gallenwege dar, an dessen Zustandekommen vor allem Innervationsstörungen im betreffenden Sympathicus- und Parasympathicusabschnitt verantwortlich sind.

Eine dritte Gruppe der anfallsauslösenden Ursachen bilden *die Funktionsstörungen des endokrinen Apparates*. Der zeitliche Zusammenhang des Anfalles mit der periodischen Funktion der weiblichen Genitalorgane ließ einen solchen Zusammenhang schon seit langem als sehr wahrscheinlich erscheinen. Eine theoretische Unterstützung erhielt diese Lehre durch die Erkenntnis, daß dem Migräneanfall eine Gleichgewichtsstörung im vegetativen Nervensystem zugrunde liege, da letzteres bekanntlich mit den endokrinen Drüsen in engster funktioneller Verbindung steht.

Bei der *ovariellen Migräne* unterscheidet RADOT dreierlei Beziehungen: 1. Die eigentliche menstruelle Migräne, die mit der Pubertät einsetzt, nur bei Menstruation (vor oder während der Menses) auftritt, während der Gravidität und oft auch während der Laktation ausbleibt und mit der Menopause aufhört. Hier spiele nach ihm eine Hyperfunktion der Ovarien eine Rolle. L. LEVI und STEVENS glauben, daß in diesen Fällen auch eine Funktionsstörung der Schilddrüse (Hypothyreoidismus) mitspiele. Bei Besprechung der Entstehungsarten des ovariellen Migräneanfalles erörtert RADOT die Möglichkeit einer Shockwirkung, welche durch die plötzlich in den Blutstrom gelangenden Produkte des Corpus luteum ausgelöst wird; hierfür sprechen das manchmal auftretende Fieber oder Urticaria; auch eine brüske Gleichgewichtsstörung im vegetativen Nervensystem oder im kolloido-plasmatischen Gleichgewicht durch die Sekrete des Eierstockes wird in Erwägung gezogen, wodurch bei veranlagten Individuen der Migräneanfall ausgelöst wird; hier dürfte also die Menstruation nicht als direkt auslösender, sondern nur als prädisponierender Faktor wirken. 2. Die indirekt wirkende, nur prädisponierende Beteiligung der Menstruation am Migräneanfall ist offenkundig in solchen Migränefällen, wo nicht nur die Menstruation, sondern auch andere ursächliche Momente den Anfall auslösen können. In diesen Fällen tritt die Migräne gewöhnlich schon vor dem Einsetzen der Regel auf und besteht oft während der Gravidität und auch in der Menopause. 3. Die dritte Gruppe umfaßt die Fälle von ausgesprochener Funktionsstörung der Ovarien (Anovarie, Hypovarie, Dysfunktion der Ovarien). Der unmittelbare Zusammenhang zwischen Migräne und Funktionsstörung der Ovarien ist in diesen Fällen, deren Zahl übrigens nicht groß ist, zweifellos, besonders dort, wo die Anfälle erst in einem späteren Alter, gleichzeitig mit dem Eintreten der Funktionsstörung (Unregelmäßigkeiten der Menses, Kastration usw.) auftraten. Eine Besserung des Genitalzustandes führt gewöhnlich zur Besserung der Migräne.

Die Bedeutung der Ovarien beim Zustandekommen der Migräne wird von einigen Autoren entschieden überschätzt. LÜHRS glaubt aus der Erfahrung, daß die Migräne während der Gravidität ausbleibt, die Theorie aufstellen zu können, daß die menstruationshemmenden Substanzen des Corpus luteum graviditatis und der Placenta die anfallsauslösende Wirkung des Ovariums paralisieren; er bringt auch eine Behandlung der Migräne mit diesen Substanzen in Vorschlag. CHARLES glaubt, daß bei der ovariellen Migräne auch die zugleich einsetzende Schwellung des vorderen Hypophysenlappens bei der Auslösung des Migräneanfalles mitwirkt.

RILEY, BRICKNER und KURZROK machten fortlaufende Harnuntersuchungen bei 11 weiblichen und 2 männlichen Migränekranken und fanden, daß das Follikelhormon (Femal sex hormon) bei den weiblichen Kranken im Urin fehlt oder nur in geringer Menge vorhanden war, dagegen konnte das Prolan (Hypophysenvorderlappenhormon) bei 20 von den beobachteten 29 Migräneattacken 1—2 Tage vor dem Anfall im Urin nachgewiesen werden. Auch bei einem männlichen Patienten fanden sie das Prolan vor dem Migräneanfall. Injektion von Follikelhormon löste bei 7 von 9 Frauen einen typischen Migräneanfall aus. Die Autoren nehmen an, daß eine hypophysäre Hyper- und eine ovarielle Hypofunktion bei der Entstehung des Migräneanfalles eine bedeutende Rolle spielen dürfte.

Die Beziehungen *der Schilddrüse* zur Migräne werden auch heute noch lebhaft diskutiert. HERTOGHE hat als erster die Ansicht verfochten, daß die Migräne ein Symptom des hypothyreoiden Zustandes sein könne. Diese Ansicht wurde dann durch LEVI und ROTSCHILD durch mehrere Beobachtungen unterstützt, in welchen die Migräne sich nach Behandlung mit Schilddrüsensubstanz besserte. APERT und CONSIGLIO zeigten, daß in solchen behandelten Fällen die Migräne wieder zum Vorschein kommt, wenn man die Thyreoidinbehandlung aussetzt. Weitere bestätigende Beobachtungen brachten MUSSO-FOURNIER, CHARRIN, RIBBIÉRE, BOUVEYRON, GORDON, FRANZ, PARHON, LEY u. a. In LAUDENHEYMERs Fall traten die Migräneanfälle nach Thyreoidektomie auf und wurden durch Schilddrüsenbehandlung beseitigt; auch er nimmt bei einer Gruppe der Migränefälle die Schilddrüseninsuffizienz als wesentliche Ursache der Migräne an. Der eifrigste Verfechter dieser Theorie ist auch heute noch L. LEVI, der auf Grund seiner therapeutischen Erfolge annimmt, daß die Kindermigräne fast immer und die Männermigräne in der Mehrzahl der Fälle mit einem Hypothyreoidismus zusammenhängen. Die ophthalmische Migräne reagiere nach ihm besonders günstig auf Schilddrüsenbehandlung. LEVI glaubt, daß die Dysfunktion der Schilddrüse auch bei der menstruellen Migräne und in gewissen Fällen von allergischer Migräne eine Rolle spielt. CURSCHMANN lehnt diese Ansichten ab, wobei er sich darauf beruft, daß die Migräne in ausgesprochenen Fällen von Schilddrüseninsuffizienz (Myxödem) und Hyperthyreoidismus (Basedow) nur selten vorkommt. Auch sah er nie Erfolge von der Thyreoidinbehandlung bei Migräne. Man wird mit RADOT recht tun, wenn man in dieser Frage eine Mittelstellung annimmt und einerseits die Möglichkeit, daß eine Dysfunktion der Schilddrüse einen Migränezustand aufrechterhalten kann, nicht ausschließt, andererseits aber die von LEVI angenommene überwiegende Bedeutung der Schilddrüse als zu weitgehend betrachtet.

Die *Hypofunktion der Nebenschilddrüse* als gelegentlicher ursächlicher Faktor der Migräne erscheint durch die Beobachtungen von CURSCHMANN, KRAMSZTYK, STERLING, PARHON u. a. als bewiesen; sie spielt besonders bei der Kindermigräne eine Rolle. Das gleichzeitige Vorkommen von Migräne und Tetanie, sowie andere Zeichen des latenten kalziprivien Zustandes und die günstige Beeinflussung der Migräne durch Kalkpräparate (CURSCHMANN) machen es wahrscheinlich, daß auch die Hypofunktion der Nebenschilddrüse als anfallsauslösende Ursache in Betracht komme.

Die Bedeutung der *Hypophyse* in der Pathogenese der Migräne wird heute von zahlreichen Forschern lebhaft verfochten. Die Theorien, in welchen eine vorübergehende Schwellung der Drüse als die den Anfallsmechanismus auslösende unmittelbare Veränderung hingestellt wird, sind schon früher erwähnt worden. Auch die Dysfunktion der Hypophyse, und zwar sowohl die Hyperals auch die Hypofunktion wird von mehreren Autoren als anfallsauslösende Ursache aufgefaßt (HARTUNG, HAHN und STEIN, RILEY, BOUVEYRON u. a.). TIMME und PARDEE berichten über akromegale Skeletveränderungen bei Migränekranken.

Die *reflektorische Migräne*, die in den Darstellungen der älteren Autoren so häufig erörtert wurde, hat viel von ihrer Bedeutung eingebüßt. Die Mehrzahl der früher hierher eingereihten Fälle wird man heute in den früher besprochenen Gruppen unterbringen können. Es bleiben aber doch Fälle zurück, in welchen gewisse Organerkrankungen mit der gleichzeitig bestehenden Migräne ursächlich zusammenhängen dürften, wobei die „reflektorische" Wirkung etwa so aufgefaßt werden kann, daß eine chronische Krankheit bei veranlagten Individuen zeitweilige Sympathicusreizzustände entfachen könne. Manche chronischen Erkrankungen des Magendarmkanals, des Genitalapparates, Augenerkrankungen (besonders das Glaukom), Refraktionsfehler der Augen, Erkrankungen der Nebenhöhlen sind als prädisponierende Zustände in diesem Sinne bekannt.

Daß die Einwirkung von *Kältereiz* auf den Körper einen Migräneanfall auslösen kann, ist nicht nur aus den Selbstbeobachtungen vieler Migränekranken bekannt, sondern durch die früher erwähnten Beobachtungen von CURSCHMANN und RADOT auch experimentell bewiesen. Der rasche Eintritt des Migräneanfalles nach der Kälteeinwirkung in diesen Experimenten deutet darauf hin, daß die Kälte als direkter Gefäßreiz wirkt. Die Möglichkeit einer allergischen Reaktion ist aber auch nicht ganz auszuschließen, wenn man die Versuche von SOUQUES und MOREAU, sowie von LEHNER und RAJKA berücksichtigt, die den exakten Beweis lieferten, daß es auch eine echte Kälteanaphylaxie gibt. Der Wärmereiz spielt als auslösender Faktor eine viel geringere Rolle; in den wenigen Fällen, wo eine solche vermutet wird, dürfte die Erweiterung der Hautgefäße durch reziproke Innervation den Gefäßkrampf im Gehirn hervorrufen.

Als *gelegentliche auslösende Ursachen* des Migräneanfalles sind noch bekannt: körperliche Übermüdung, starke geistige Arbeit, unregelmäßiger Schlaf, manchmal langer Schlaf am Tag, sexuelle Exzesse, manchmal auch normaler Coitus (bei Männern). Die anfallsauslösende Wirkung des Alkohols ist allgemein bekannt; auch nach meinen Erfahrungen gibt es diesbezüglich unter den Migränekranken nur selten eine Ausnahme (SCHULTZES Eigenbeobachtung). Bezüglich des Nicotins sind die Erfahrungen keineswegs so gleichlautend. Nach FRANKL-HOCHWART ist es nur im höheren Alter als anfallsauslösende Schädlichkeit wirksam. Nach Selbstbeobachtungen von HAHN kann das Einatmen von Tabakrauch einen Anfall auslösen. Manche Migränekranke reagieren lebhaft auf Wetterwechsel und Schwankungen des Luftdruckes. Allgemein bekannt ist die Bedeutung des Klimas, welche sich in der oft bewährten, ärztlich empfohlenen Luftveränderung kundgibt. Welche Momente hier eine Rolle spielen, ist unbekannt; die Höhenlage eines Ortes dürfte hier kaum bestimmend sein, denn man findet diesbezüglich die größten individuellen Unterschiede. RADOT und Mm. WEISSMANN vermuten auch hier allergische Vorgänge.

Eine eigene Beobachtung scheint dies zu bestätigen: eine 32jährige Frau, die immer auf dem Lande (unweit von Budapest) lebte, bekommt seit etwa 10 Jahren jedesmal, wenn sie in die Großstadt fährt, schon im Eisenbahnzug, wenn dieser die äußeren Fabriksviertel der Stadt passierte, ein mit heftigen Jucken einhergehendes Ödem der Augenlider oder Lippen, welches erst dann gänzlich verschwindet, wenn sie sich aus dem Bereich der Hauptstadt wieder entfernte; einigemal hatte sie während eines solchen Aufenthaltes typische halbseitige Kopfschmerzanfälle mit Brechreiz und Herzklopfen. Bei einem einzigen Besuch in einer anderen Großstadt (Wien) hat sich dieser Zustand wiederholt.

Auch heftige seelische Erregungen können gelegentlich einen Migräneanfall verursachen. M. ULRICH fand, daß unter 500 Migränefällen in sieben Fällen eine seelische Erschütterung den ersten Migräneanfall auslöste und in acht Fällen eine wesentliche Verschlimmerung des Migränezustandes herbeiführte. Nach F. HURST handelt es sich hier um eine allgemeine Sympathicuserregung, die durch eine gesteigerte Adrenalinproduktion noch verstärkt wird. Natürlich hat ein solcher, durch psychische Shockwirkung ausgelöster Migräneanfall mit der psychogenen Pseudomigräne (Salonmigräne) mancher Hysterischen nichts gemeinsam. Erwähnt soll noch werden, daß SCHULTZE bei sich, durch Blendung mit grellem Licht, einen typischen ophthalmischen Migräneanfall experimentell erzeugen konnte. Bei Bewertung der auslösenden Ursachen, auf welche die Patienten ihren ersten Migräneanfall zurückführen, mahnt CURSCHMANN mit recht zu einiger Vorsicht, die angesichts des bekannten Kausalitätsbedürfnisses der Kranken als begründet erscheint. Hervorzuheben wäre hier die Bedeutung der verschiedenen akuten Infektionskrankheiten, welche nicht mit Unrecht als den ersten Anfall provozierendes Ereignis öfters erwähnt werden. In diesem

Sinne spricht die ärztliche Erfahrung, nach welcher eine bis dahin leichte Migräne nach einer Infektionskrankheit sich deutlich verschlimmert; ich hatte wiederholt Gelegenheit in solchen Fällen einen schweren Status hemicranicus zu beobachten. Ob den in der Anamnese von Migränekranken so oft erwähnten Kopftraumen dieselbe Bedeutung zukommt, ist zweifelhaft. M. ULRICH fand unter 500 Fällen 56, die ein Kopftrauma erlitten, allerdings waren davon 29 mit Migräne erblich belastet. Sie spricht auch dem Geburtstrauma eine gewisse Bedeutung zu, indem sie dieses als einen vollständig neuen Erwerb der Migränekonstitution betrachtet. Auch CHRISTIANSEN rechnet das Kopftrauma zu den auslösenden Ursachen der Migräne, er rechnet aber diese Fälle nicht zur echten Migräne.

Nach Aufzählung der bis heute bekannten Auslösungsursachen erscheint es notwendig, zu ihrer richtigen Bewertung einige Bemerkungen hinzuzufügen. Es soll zuerst darauf hingewiesen werden, daß eine scharfe Trennung der Migränefälle auf Grund der hier abgesonderten Gruppen oft nicht möglich ist. Viele Beobachtungen bestätigen, daß in ein und demselben Migränefall zwei oder noch mehr der angeführten auslösenden Ursachen wirksam sein können. Ich beobachtete einen Fall von typisch menstrueller Migräne, in welchem zwei heftige Migräneanfälle durch Genuß von Sardellen ausgelöst wurden; hier bestand also eine Ambivalenz für allergische und endokrine Beeinflussung. In einem andern Fall lag die Sache noch komplizierter: Die Kranke leidet seit Kindheit an postmenstrueller Migräne; für ihre allergische Veranlagung spricht, daß sie heufieberkrank ist und es besteht bei ihr erhöhte Anfallsempfindlichkeit gegenüber dem geringsten Kältereiz, der den Kopf trifft.

Die Wirksamkeit der anfallsauslösenden Faktoren ist nicht immer die gleiche. Das erkennt man am besten bei den Gelegenheitsursachen, die sich das eine Mal geltend machen, das andere Mal nicht. RADOT vermutet hier eine durch den Anfall erworbene Immunität, welche allmählich abnimmt und auf diese Weise die Periodizität der Anfälle aufrecht hält; dieser Schutzzustand sei aber nach ihm nicht eine anaphylaktische Immunität, wie man sie im Tierversuche beobachtet (eine solche gibt es bei der menschlichen Anaphylaxie nicht). Auch CHURCH und PETERSON sprechen von einer „Klärung der Atmosphäre" durch den Anfall in diesem Sinne. Die wichtigste Einschränkung erhalten aber die hier angeführten Erfahrungen dadurch, daß es eine beträchtliche Anzahl von Migränefällen gibt, in welchen keine der hier angeführten ursächlichen Faktoren als Ursache der Migräne nachgewiesen werden kann. Es ist mit Sicherheit anzunehmen, daß die künftige Forschung auf diesem Gebiet weitere positive Erkenntnisse bringen wird und durch Verbesserung unserer Untersuchungsmethoden die Zahl dieser Migränefälle immer geringer wird. Man muß aber auch damit rechnen, daß es solche im engsten Sinne des Begriffes „genuine" Fälle gibt, bei welchen die Entstehung eines Anfalles nicht an einen den Körper irgendwie schädigenden Einfluß gebunden ist, sondern auch durch die gesetzmäßigen Schwankungen der normalen Lebensvorgänge bedingt sein kann.

Es ergeben sich aus obigen Ausführungen über die Pathogenese der Migräne einige Schlußfolgerungen, die vielleicht geeignet sind, das Verhältnis der hereditär bedingten Anlage zu den verschiedenen anfallsauslösenden Ursachen besser zu beleuchten. Sie könnten etwa folgendermaßen zusammengefaßt werden: Der Migräneanfall ist kein Symptom einer bestimmten Krankheit, sondern ein Syndrom, in welchem wir eine spezifische, im Organismus gewissermaßen vorgebildete Reaktionsform des menschlichen Körpers erblicken. Der Anfall selbst besteht in einem Gefäßkrampf des Gehirns und wird durch einen zeitweiligen Reizzustand eines bestimmten Sympathicusabschnittes verursacht, er stellt im Sinne von PAL eine Gefäßkrise des Gehirns dar. Ob neben dem Gefäßkrampf auch noch andere Zirkulationsstörungen (Gefäßerweiterung, Transsudation) am Anfallsprozeß beteiligt sind, ist noch umstritten; daß das Hauptgewicht jedoch auf dem Gefäßkrampf liegt, wird heute allgemein angenommen. Die Migräne als Krankheit ist durch eine in der überwiegenden Mehrzahl der Fälle erblich stigmatisierte Bereitschaft zum Migräneanfall gekennzeichnet, die wir mit dem Begriff der Migräneanlage identifizieren. Die Migräneanlage ist nach unseren heutigen Kenntnissen durch eine gesteigerte Erregbarkeit des vegetativen Nervensystems und Gleichgewichtslabilität desselben gekennzeichnet, wobei eine sympathicotonische Organbereitschaft in demjenigen Hirngefäßabschnitt vorliegt, in welchem der den Anfall auslösende Gefäßkrampf sich abspielt. Neben dieser Anlage sind noch eine Reihe krankhafter Vorgänge oder schädigender Einwirkungen als anfallsauslösende Faktoren am Zustandekommen des Migräneanfalles beteiligt. Das Wechselverhältnis zwischen Anlage und auslösenden Faktoren ist sehr verschieden. Ist die erblich erworbene Anfallsbereitschaft groß, dann tritt die Bedeutung der auslösenden Faktoren in den Hintergrund, so sehr, daß letztere in vielen Fällen gar nicht festzustellen sind. Die Anlage zur Migräne muß auch in solchen Fällen eine starke sein, wo mehrere auslösende Ursachen gleichzeitig wirksam sind. Eine geringere Anfallsbereitschaft müssen wir in den Fällen vermuten, in welchen nur ein bestimmter und intensiv einwirkender Auslösungsfaktor eine Rolle spielt.

Anhang.
Symptomatische Migräne.

Mit diesem Namen werden Krankheitsfälle bezeichnet, in welchen bei von Migräne bis dahin verschont gebliebenen Menschen im Laufe einer organischen Erkrankung (vornehmlich des Gehirns) Migräneanfälle auftreten. Alle bekannten Anfallsformen der Migräne, also sowohl der gewöhnliche als auch der ophthalmische und ophthalmoplegische Anfall können dabei in Erscheinung treten. Auch der mit dem epileptischen kombinierte Migräneanfall ist wiederholt als symptomatische Migräne beschrieben worden. Am häufigsten werden aber der ophthalmoplegische und ophthalmische Anfall beobachtet. Symptome und Verlauf der Anfälle zeigen eine bis in die Einzelheiten gehende Ähnlichkeit mit den echten Migräneanfällen, wenn nicht schon andere Symptome der organischen Grundkrankheit das Bild komplizieren. Im allgemeinen tritt aber die symptomatische Migräne als früheste, oft durch längere Zeit als die einzige Krankheitserscheinung auf, so daß ihre Unterscheidung von der echten Migräne recht schwierig sein kann. Bei der Pathogenese der symptomatischen Migräne muß vor allem betont werden, daß es keine einzige solche organische Erkrankung gibt, die gesetzmäßig mit einer symptomatischen Migräne einhergeht. Auch der Sitz und die Schwere der Erkrankung sind dabei nicht bestimmend. Man muß also eine latente Migränebereitschaft annehmen auch dann, wenn sie hereditär nicht nachweisbar ist. Der Anfallsmechanismus ist derselbe wie bei der echten Migräne, es kann sich auch hier nur um einen Gefäßkrampf im Gehirn handeln, von welchem wir aber zum Unterschied von der echten Migräne anzunehmen haben, daß er nicht durch einen primären Reizzustand des Halssympathicus verursacht wird, sondern den Effekt eines direkten Gefäßreizes darstellt, welcher von der organischen Schädigung auf die periadventitielle Sympathicusbahn eines im Bereiche des Krankheitsherdes liegenden Gefäßes ausgeübt wird. Eine solche Möglichkeit nämlich, daß der krampferzeugende Reiz nicht immer aus dem Sympathicusganglion ausgehen müsse, sondern durch Reizung der vasomotorischen Bahn an irgendeiner Stelle auch autonom einsetzen könne, haben wir auch bei der echten Migräne in Erwägung gebracht.

Die Sympathicusbahnen begleiten die Gefäße bis ins Gehirn. Es ist also leicht vorstellbar, daß eine organische Erkrankung des Gehirns durch eine unmittelbar auf ein Gefäß ausgeübte Reizwirkung den ganzen Pathomechanismus des Migräneanfalles ins Werk setzen kann. Entsprechend dem von mir gegebenen Erklärungsversuch über den Sitz des migränösen Gefäßkrampfes wäre anzunehmen, daß nur solche organische Schädigungen eine symptomatische Migräne hervorzubringen imstande sind, die ihren Sitz innerhalb des vom Vertebralissystem versorgten Gehirnterritoriums haben. Von den Sektionsbefunden, die über symptomatische Migräne vorliegen, können diesbezüglich diejenigen, die diffuse meningitische Veränderung an der Hirnbasis zeigten, nicht verwertet werden. Als Beweise dienen aber die früher zitierten Fälle, in welchen eine Geschwulst am Oculomotoriusstamm gefunden wurde, wo es nicht bezweifelt werden kann, daß die Geschwulst durch einen direkten Gefäßreiz die Anfälle auslöste. Auch in den Fällen von symptomatischer ophthalmischer Migräne weisen die späteren Dauerveränderungen auf eine Erkrankung des Occipitallappens hin. In diesem Sinne kann auch die von CURSCHMANN gemachte Beobachtung verwertet werden, daß unter den Gehirngeschwülsten besonders diejenigen der hinteren Schädelgrube migräneartige Kopfschmerzanfälle auszulösen pflegen. Es liegen aber auch Beobachtungen über eine andere Lokalisation vor; nach FRANKL-HOCHWART sollen die Geschwülste der Hypophyse nicht selten mit ophthalmischen Migräneanfällen einhergehen. Der Annahme, daß bei Gehirngeschwulsten der Migräneanfall durch den allgemeinen Hirndruck ausgelöst wird, widerspricht die Erfahrung, daß die Migräne häufig das frühzeitigste Symptom der Erkrankung darstellt, der Stauungspapille oft lange vorauseilt und im späteren Verlauf der Erkrankung verschwindet. CURSCHMANN und URECHIA beobachteten bei Hydrocephalus und bei Zuständen von Hirnschwellung typische Migräneanfälle; auch bei Hirnabscessen wurden Migräneanfälle beschrieben.

Die Bedeutung der Gefäßwanderkrankung beim Zustandekommen der symptomatischen Migräne erhellt daraus, daß sie am häufigsten bei solchen Allgemeinerkrankungen auftritt, die mit Affektion der Gefäßwand einhergehen. CURSCHMANN lenkt die Aufmerksamkeit auf die primäre, sekundäre und arteriosklerotische Schrumpfniere, die sich nicht selten Jahre voraus durch Migräneanfälle ankündigen, welche später in den urämischen Kopfschmerz übergehen. Die symptomatische Migräne ist eine häufige Begleiterscheinung der Cerebrosklerose. Sie kommt auch bei den verschiedenen chronischen Meningitiden vor, besonders dort, wo der entzündliche Prozeß sich im Bereich der basalen Gefäße abspielt (Meningitis basilaris tuberculosa, luetica usw.). Die Lues kann sich in allen Stadien und bei allen nervösen Affektionen mit einer symptomatischen Migräne verbinden. HALBAN und NONNE machen in diesem Zusammenhang auf die hereditäre Lues aufmerksam. A. LERI sah Migräneanfälle bei Luetikern, die nur eine Lymphocytose und positive Wa.R. im Liquor zeigten; energische antiluische Behandlung brachte die Anfälle zum Verschwinden. Die verschiedenen Formen der Hirnlues, die Endarteriitis luetica, Meningitis basilaris luetica, Encephalomeningitis luetica zeigen oft als Begleitsymptom Migräneanfälle. Häufig bilden ophthalmische Migräneanfälle das einleitende Symptom der Paralyse schon zu einer Zeit, wo von der organischen Erkrankung noch nichts zu bemerken ist. Als Begleitsymptom der Tabes tritt sie seltener auf; MOEBIUS, NONNE und FLATAU bezweifeln den Zusammenhang zwischen Tabes und Migräne. Ich sah einige Fälle ohne hereditäre Belastung, wo die Migräne im vorgerückten Alter gleichzeitig mit der Tabes auftrat. Bei multipler Sklerose beschrieben CURSCHMANN u. a. Migräneanfälle. Von den Infektionskrankheiten wurde früher (TISSOT, WHYTT) die Malaria als eine mit symptomatischer Migräne einhergehende Krankheit bezeichnet; nach THOMAS können Migräneanfälle eine larvierte Malaria anzeigen. Die Kopfschmerzanfälle bei chronischer Bleivergiftung zeigen eine große Ähnlichkeit mit Migräneanfällen; in der Pathogenese der durch Bleivergiftung verursachten Hirnschädigungen spielen bekanntlich (PAL, ROSENSTEIN) Gefäßkrämpfe eine große Rolle. Symptomatische Migräne wurde noch beobachtet von ESCAT bei gewissen Fällen von Otosklerose; von TROUSSEAU beim Glaukom. Meine früher mitgeteilten zwei Fälle zeigen, daß auch organische Erkrankungen in der Nachbarschaft des Halsstranges symptomatische Migränezustände auslösen können.

III. Zur Differentialdiagnose.

Die Unterscheidung des Migränekopfschmerzes von andersartigen Kopfschmerzen begegnet in der überwiegenden Mehrzahl der Fälle keinen besonderen Schwierigkeiten, wenn man die zahlreichen klinischen Eigentümlichkeiten vor Augen hält, die den Migränekopfschmerz kennzeichnen. Als solche sind bekannt das anfallsmäßige Auftreten, die erbliche Veranlagung, die mehrweniger ausgesprochene Periodizität, die Halbseitigkeit und endlich als das wichtigste Erkennungszeichen die mit dem Kopfschmerz einhergehenden Begleiterscheinungen (Magenerscheinungen, vasomotorische Störungen, psychische Alterationen usw.). Ganz selten sind nur die Fälle, in welchen der Migränecharakter des Kopfschmerzes bei Berücksichtigung dieser Momente verdeckt bleibt. Vom differentialdiagnostischen Standpunkt aus kann manchmal die Trigeminusneuralgie zu Verwechslungen Anlaß geben, weil es sich auch hier nicht selten um zeitlich begrenzte Schmerzanfälle handelt, die gewöhnlich halbseitig verlaufen und hauptsächlich deshalb, weil der Migränekopfschmerz sich gar nicht selten im Stirn und Augenastgebiet des Trigeminus festsetzt, also eine ähnliche Ausbreitung zeigt wie der Kopfschmerz bei der Supraorbitalisneuralgie. Die Kopfschmerzen pflegen bei Migräne manchmal auch in den zweiten und dritten Trigeminusast auszustrahlen. Gewöhnlich werden die beiden Zustände so verwechselt, daß die Migräne für eine Trigeminusneuralgie gehalten wird. Ich beobachtete zwei Fälle von typischer Migräne, in welchen Alkoholinjektionen und operative Ausreißung des ersten Trigeminusastes erfolglos vorgenommen wurden. Zur Unterscheidung der beiden Anfallsarten sei außer den oben für die Migräne angegebenen Kennzeichen besonders die Lokalisation des Migränekopfschmerzes im Hinterhaupt hervorgehoben, die, wie früher betont wurde, fast immer nachweisbar ist und bei der Trigeminusneuralgie fehlt. Auch sind die Intervalle bei der letzteren gewöhnlich viel kürzer als bei der Migräne und die Schmerzanfälle haben auch eine kürzere Dauer. Der Schmerz ist bei der Gesichtsneuralgie schärfer, stechender als im Migräneanfall.

Von dem *myalgischen* Kopfschmerz, der seinen Sitz in den Nackenmuskeln hat, ist der echte Migränekopfschmerz in den meisten Fällen leicht zu unterscheiden.

Die größte Schwierigkeit kann sich aber ergeben, wenn man in einem gegebenen Fall zu entscheiden hat, ob es sich um eine echte oder um eine symptomatische Migräne handelt. Es wurde schon erwähnt, daß symptomatische Migräneanfälle sehr oft als das einleitende und einzige Symptom einer organischen Erkrankung auftreten. Die Fälle, wo die ersten Anfälle schon in höherem Alter (jenseits des 40. Lebensjahres) auftreten, sind in dieser Hinsicht mit größter Vorsicht zu beurteilen und unter dauernder Kontrolle zu halten. Als nützlicher Wegweiser bewährt sich hier die von SICARD empfohlene diagnostische Lumbalpunktion; findet man im Liquor Eiweißvermehrung und Erhöhung der Zellzahl, dann muß man den Anfall als eine symptomatische Migräne behandeln.

IV. Prognose.

Die echte Migräne wird im allgemeinen als eine gutartige Krankheit angesehen, deren günstige Prognose auf die Erfahrungstatsache gestützt ist, daß bei der überwiegenden Mehrzahl der Migränekranken die Anfälle mit zunehmendem Alter seltener werden und milder verlaufen und nach dem 50. Lebensjahr gewöhnlich verschwinden, ohne irgendwelche Schädigung der körperlichen oder psychischen Verfassung hinterlassen zu haben. Eine solche günstige Voraussage erlauben vor allem diejenigen Migränefälle, in welchen gewöhnliche Anfälle vorkommen. Bei der häufigsten Form der menstruellen Migräne der Frauen fällt der Zeitpunkt, in welchem die Anfälle aufhören, zumeist mit dem Wechsel zusammen. Doch gibt es Fälle, wie die Beobachtungen von MATHIEU und ROUX sowie RIVIÈRE zeigen, wo die menstruelle Migräne im Präklimax oder Klimax an Intensität zunimmt. Die Anfälle können dabei mit dem Abklingen der übrigen klimakterischen Beschwerden wieder verschwinden, in anderen Fällen begleiten sie aber die Kranken bis in das späte Alter hinein, wo es bei den gewöhnlich schon nachweisbaren hypertonischen und arteriosklerotischen Veränderungen oft schwer zu unterscheiden ist, ob diese Migräneanfälle des späten Alters noch die Fortsetzung der früheren echten Migräne bilden, oder aber schon symptomatische Migräneanfälle darstellen, die durch die organische Erkrankung der Hirngefäße bedingt sind. Mit dieser Möglichkeit muß man besonders in denjenigen Fällen rechnen, wo die echten Migräneanfälle sich im späteren Alter in ophthalmische, ophthalmoplegische oder epileptische Migräne umwandeln. Eine ernstere Prognosenstellung ist bei der ophthalmischen, ophthalmoplegischen, epileptischen und psychischen Migräne angezeigt, nicht nur deshalb, weil unter diesen Fällen sich verhältnismäßig häufiger symptomatische Migränefälle mit schweren organischen Veränderungen verbergen, sondern auch aus dem Grunde, weil, wie die Erfahrung zeigt, hier nervöse und psychische Dauerschädigungen auftreten können, die man mit der Migränekrankheit in Verbindung setzen muß. Auf welche Weise diese Dauerschädigungen zustande kommen, darüber kann man heute mangels verwertbarer Befunde nichts Sicheres aussagen. Es ist aber naheliegend, daran zu denken, daß die sich oft wiederholenden schweren Zirkulationsstörungen, die diesen Migräneanfällen zugrunde liegen, im Laufe der Jahre allmählich eine immer tiefergreifende Dauerveränderung des Hirnparenchyms herbeiführen. Wenn dies in den Migränefällen mit vulgären Anfällen viel seltener vorkommt, so liegt die Ursache darin, daß beim gewöhnlichen Migräneanfall der Gefäßkrampf viel leichter ist und die ischämische Ernährungsstörung nicht so tiefgreifend ist, daß es zu Ausfallserscheinungen kommt, wie es bei der ophthalmischen und ophthalmoplegischen Migräne der Fall ist. Ich möchte also die Behauptung mancher Autoren, daß der Migränezustand als solcher keine Dauerveränderungen herbeizuführen imstande ist, nicht als allgemeingültig betrachten, vielmehr bei diesen schweren Formen die Möglichkeit einer anatomischen Schädigung als Folgezustand der gehäuften, tiefgreifenden Zirkulationsstörungen ins Auge fassen. Man wird die Möglichkeit, daß es solche, durch angiospastische, nutritive Schädigungen bedingte organische Parenchymläsionen gibt, nicht von der Hand weisen können, wenn man den früher zitierten Fall von OSTERTAG und die von SPIELMEYER beschriebenen laminären Rindenveränderungen in Epileptikergehirnen berücksichtigt, die der Autor nur als vasculär (ischämisch) bedingt erklären konnte.

Naheliegend ist eine solche Annahme für die Migräne in dem früher erwähnten Fall von C. DE LANGE, wo bei einer ophthalmoplegischen Migräne Gefäßwucherung und Hypoplasie im Kerngebiet des Oculomotorius gefunden wurde. Die Autorin nimmt an, daß die Kernhypoplasie einen angeborenen Defekt darstellt, es kann sich aber auch um einen sekundären Kernschwund handeln, der durch die sich wiederholenden Gefäßkrämpfe allmählich verursacht wurde. Die Feststellung, daß der Kernschwund auch dort nachweisbar war, wo keine Gefäßsklerose bestand, kann nach meiner Ansicht nicht als Argument gegen diese zweite Entstehungsmöglichkeit angeführt werden. Die Sklerose der Gefäßwand kann man ohne weiteres mit den Gefäßkrämpfen in Verbindung bringen, weil es naheliegend ist, daß die häufigen und langdauernden Gefäßkontraktionen auch zu Ernährungsstörungen in der Gefäßwand führen, als deren Folge die sklerotische Umwandlung der Gefäße anzusehen ist (OSTERTAG). Die ungünstige Prognose der schweren Migränefälle liegt eben darin, daß sie sich häufig mit Hypertonie und Gefäßwanderkrankungen kombinieren.

Eine ernstere Beachtung vom prognostischen Standpunkt verdienen die Zustände vom Status hemicranicus, die manchmal unter beängstigenden Symptomen verlaufen; es sind auch Todesfälle beschrieben, in welchen als letzte Todesursache eine Herzschwäche auftrat.

V. Therapie der Migräne.

Eine kausale Therapie der Migräne hat es bis vor kurzem überhaupt nicht gegeben; die meisten Ärzte trachteten danach, ihre Migränekranken mit „allgemein roborierenden" Methoden und Vorschriften zu erledigen. Bei einer in 80% der Fälle erblich bedingten Krankheit, wie es die Migräne ist, kann dieser therapeutische Nihilismus, der sich aus der Überzeugung von der absoluten Unbeeinflußbarkeit des Leidens ergab, gar nicht wundernehmen. Viele Ärzte denken auch heute noch so, wie seinerzeit MONTAIGNE sich mit seiner Migräne abfand, indem er meinte, «qu'il faut souffrir doucement les lois de notre condition». Schuld an diesem Mangel eines ernsten therapeutischen Vorgehens ist auch der allgemein ärztlich verbreitete Glaube, die Migräne sei keine gefährliche Krankheit; so werden auch die Klagen dieser Kranken sehr oft nicht entsprechend gewürdigt. Die im Intervall beim Arzt vorsprechenden Patienten, bei denen natürlich nichts Krankhaftes gefunden wird, erhalten die üblichen Weisungen über Roborantien, Klimawechsel, Diätregelung, für den Anfall ein Kopfschmerzpulver, womöglich aus der Schar der sich immer vermehrenden, vielversprechende Namen tragenden Spezialitäten. Wird der Arzt zu einem Anfall gerufen, so erledigt er ihn rasch mit der Morphiumspritze. Die Zahl der Migränekranken, deren Leiden wegen der Seltenheit und geringeren Intensität ihrer Anfälle ein ernstes therapeutisches Eingreifen nicht notwendig macht, ist sicherlich eine sehr große; diese kommen aber meistens auch nicht zum Arzt. Es gibt aber Fälle, und auch ihre Zahl ist nicht gering, deren Schmerzen und Qualen und die die Anfälle begleitenden Lähmungserscheinungen einen höchst beunruhigenden Zustand darstellen und eine ernste zielbewußte Beschäftigung mit dem Leiden notwendig machen. Die zweifelhafte Prognose mancher dieser Fälle macht es ebenfalls zur Forderung, daß alles geschehe, um die Anfälle zu beseitigen oder wenigstens einer Besserung zuzuführen. Die neu gewonnenen Erkenntnisse über das Wesen des Migräneanfalls und über die Pathogenese der Migräne brachten eine Reihe von therapeutischen Ideen und Vorschlägen hervor, die sich in einer großen Anzahl der Migränefälle schon nutzbringend erwiesen haben. Jedenfalls stehen wir heute diesem Leiden gegenüber nicht mehr so machtlos da, als es noch vor wenigen Jahrzehnten der Fall war.

Bei der recht verzweigten Pathogenese der Migräne ist es angezeigt, bei der Aufstellung eines Behandlungsplanes systematisch vorzugehen. Es muß vor allem entschieden werden, ob es sich um eine echte oder symptomatische Migräne handelt. In letzterem Fall ist das organische Grundleiden zu behandeln. Dort, wo die symptomatische Migräne durch luische Affektion des Gehirns, der Hirnhäute oder der Gefäße bedingt ist, erzielt man durch die antiluische Behandlung in den meisten Fällen ein rasches Zurückgehen und gänzliches Verschwinden der Migräneanfälle.

Handelt es sich um eine echte Migräne, dann ist unsere nächste Aufgabe, festzustellen, ob und in welche der nach den bekannten Auslösungsursachen gesonderten Migränegruppen der Fall eingereiht werden kann. Wie schon erwähnt, erhalten wir diesbezüglich nicht selten von den Kranken selbst verwertbare Angaben. Einige wissen genau die Nahrungsmittel, Gerüche usw. anzugeben, die bei ihnen Anfälle auslösen; bei anderen erfährt man über allergische Begleiterscheinungen der Anfälle oder über selbständig auftretende allergische Zustände (Asthma, Urticaria, Ödem), die die Einreihung des Falles zur Gruppe der allergischen Migräne ermöglichen. Unterstützen kann uns bei der Feststellung einer allergischen Migräne der Nachweis von Eosinophilie im Blute oder, wenn es ausführbar ist, der Nachweis des humoralen Syndroms, der hämoklasischen Krise im präparoxysmalen Stadium. Eingehende Untersuchung erfordert im weiteren die Funktion des Verdauungsapparates. Auch hier bringen nicht selten die Patienten über die Menge und Zusammensetzung ihrer Nahrung, Störungen der Stuhlordnung oder andere Verdauungsbeschwerden verwertbare Aufschlüsse. In verdächtigen Fällen möge eine systematische Untersuchung des Verdauungstraktes nicht unterlassen werden. Bei der Funktionsprüfung des endokrinen Apparates sind Ovarien und Schilddrüse an erster Stelle zu berücksichtigen, aber auch die übrigen innersekretorischen Drüsen können eine Bedeutung erhalten. Eine allgemeine körperliche Untersuchung zwecks Ausschließung anderweitiger Organerkrankungen bildet natürlich die Voraussetzung einer jeden Spezialbehandlung.

Bei der Behandlung der allergischen Migräne ist als wichtigster Grundsatz das prophylaktische Fernhalten der schädlichen Substanz zu betrachten, wenn eine solche bekannt ist oder ermittelt wird. Als anaphylaktogene Substanzen (für die Migräne) sind bekannt: Schokolade, Vanille, Eier, Weizenmehl, Roggenmehl, Oliven, Milch, Rahm, manche Fleisch- und Fischarten (Tunfisch, Sardellen), Gerüche mancher Blumen (Veilchen, Rosen, Lilien), manche Parfüms, Essenzen (Terpentin), Naphthalin, Steinkohlenteer. BERGH, CORNIL und VAUGHAN konnten mit Exaktheit des Experiments durch Zufuhr der schädlichen Substanzen die Anfälle von neuem zum Erscheinen bringen. In den meisten Fällen ist aber die schädliche Substanz nicht zu ermitteln und hier läßt auch die Hautreaktion mit den verschiedenen allergischen Proteintesten nicht selten im Stich. So erhielten negative oder unverwertbare Resultate von der Testprüfung BROWN, LUBBERS und RADOT; auch ich versuchte die Kutireaktion in 2 Fällen mit einem negativen und einem unverwertbaren positiven Befund. Dagegen berichtet RAMIREZ über 3 Migränefälle, in welchen er mittels der Hautreaktion eine Überempfindlichkeit gegen Schokolade, Sellerie und Eiweiß feststellen konnte; Entfernung dieser Substanzen aus der Nahrung des betreffenden Kranken brachte in allen 3 Fällen die Migräneanfälle zum Verschwinden. VAUGHAN fand unter 35 Migränefällen bei 10 positive Hautreaktion und konnte durch Beseitigung der schädlichen Substanzen gute therapeutische Wirkung erzielen. Über therapeutisch gut verwertbare Testproben berichten GOVIN, ROVE, MCCLURE und HUNTSINGER, sowie BALYEAT und RINKEL durch Entfernung der allergisch wirkenden Nahrungsmittel aus der Diät der Kranken. Interessant ist ein von RINKEL beschriebener Fall, in welchem periodische Kopfschmerzanfälle durch periodisch auftretende Sensibilisierung gegen gewisse Nahrungsmittel (Äpfel, Getreide) auftraten. Über die Wirksamkeit einer spezifisch-sensibilisierenden Vaccinebehandlung, die sich auf die allergische Hautreaktion stützt, sind bei Migräne noch keine Erfahrungen bekannt. Um so zahlreicher sind die günstigen Berichte, die über die Heilwirkung einer *allgemeinen Desensibilisierung* bei Migräne vorliegen. NAST, RADOT und PAGNIEZ waren die ersten, die eine präventive Behandlung der Migräne auf diese Art versuchten, indem sie den Kranken eine Stunde vor jeder der drei Mahlzeiten 0,5 g Pepton verabreichen ließen und mit dieser Behandlung in einer beträchtlichen Anzahl ihrer Fälle gute Resultate erhielten. Die Autoren erklären die Wirkung des Peptons so, daß es die hämoklasische Krise, welche durch die in den Stoffwechsel gelangten schädlichen Substanzen verursacht wird, verhindere. Die fortgesetzte Behandlung unterdrücke aber nicht nur die jeweilig fällige Krise, sondern führe zu einer dauernden Desensibilisierung. Die günstige Wirkung der Peptonbehandlung wurde seither von zahlreichen Autoren (VIDAL, ABRAMI, JOLLTRAIN, WEISSMANN, LUBBERS, SCHLESINGER, COKE, ALDA, KERPPOLA) bestätigt. RADOT empfiehlt auch subcutane Injektionen aus einer 5%igen Peptonlösung in längeren Serien täglich oder jeden 2. Tag. Dagegen hält er die intervenöse Peptonbehandlung für nicht ganz gefahrlos. MILLER und RAULSTON behandelten 25 Fälle mittels intravenöser Injektionen aus einer 7%igen Lösung von Armours Peptonum siccum und erzielten in 9 Fällen Anfallsfreiheit, in 12 Fällen Besserung des Zustandes, nur 4 Fälle blieben unbeeinflußt. Unangenehme Begleiterscheinungen haben weder diese Autoren, noch F. BALL beobachtet, der die intravenöse Behandlung aus einer 5%igen Peptonlösung (mit steigenden Dosen von 0,25 cm³ bis 1,25 cm³) bei 20 Migränekranken ausführte und dabei 3 geheilte und 7 erheblich gebesserte Fälle erhielt. Auch VEGAS berichtet über gute Wirkung bei einem mit dieser Methode behandelten Fall.

Als weitere allgemeine Desensibilisierungsmethoden wurden empfohlen: die Behandlung mit Alttuberkulin (VAN LEEUWEN, KERPPOLA), die Eigenblutbehandlung (KÄMMERER, LIPPMANN, GUTTMAN, RADOT), die Behandlung mit Eigenserum (FLANDIN), Milchinjektionen (MARIN AMAT, SICARD, PARAF und HAGUENAU), Typhusvaccine (DATTNER). BOUCHÉ und HUSTIN erblicken im Migräneanfall einen „choc vasotrophique", der aus einer angiospastischen Phase und aus einem durch Parasympathicusreiz bedingten Syndrom bestehe, halten ihn aber ebenfalls für einen anaphylaktischen Vorgang, welcher durch systematisch provozierte kleine anaphylaktische Reaktionen hintangehalten werden kann. Sie machen wöchentlich einmal subcutane Injektionen von 1 cm³ Pferdeserum oder 0,2 mg Crotolin; bei lange (auch über 1 Jahr) fortgesetzter Behandlung erhielten sie gute Resultate. In günstigem Sinne äußert sich über diese Methode SPUZIC. SICARD empfahl intervenöse Injektionen von Natrium bicarbonicum, mit welchem er als Präventivmaßregel gegen Salvarsanschädigungen und Serumkrankheit Erfolge hatte, auch zur Verhütung der allergischen Migräne.

Auch bei der durch *Verdauungsstörungen* bedingten Migräneform wurden die allgemein-desensibilisierenden Methoden vielfach angewandt. FRIEDLÄNDER und PETOW führen die Wirksamkeit des Peptons auf seinen Histamingehalt zurück und verabreichen dem Prinzip „Similia similibus" folgend: Histamin per os in den Mengen von 0,001—0,01 mg jeden 2. Tag; sie berichten über ausgezeichnete Erfolge bei solchen Migränefällen, die gleichzeitig Symptome einer Gallen- oder Leberdysfunktion zeigten. F. COKE erhielt gute Resultate mit Pepton und einer aus Darmtoxinen hergestellten Vaccine. LEISCHNER sah gute Erfolge von längerer Behandlung mit Decholin (2 Fälle), O. MÜLLER ebenfalls in einem schweren Fall.

Großes Gewicht wird von den meisten Autoren auch heute auf die richtige Auswahl der Nahrung und Regelung des Stuhlgangs gelegt. FLATAU, der in seiner Monographie noch an der gichtischen Natur der Migräne festhält, stellt in seiner Diätvorschrift die purinfreie Nahrung als die wichtigste Präventivmaßregel hin. Sie müsse monate-, sogar jahrelang beibehalten werden. Er schreibt eine ovolakto-vegetabilische Kost vor bei strenger Vermeidung von

Fleisch und Fischen, Hülsenfrüchten und Pilzen. Von den neueren Autoren wird die purinfreie Nahrung nur mehr selten (REMOND und ROUZAUD) in Vorschlag gebracht. Im allgemeinen wird die kohlehydratreiche und viel tierisches Eiweiß enthaltende Kost verboten. Eine vorwiegend vegetabilische Diät hat auch viele Befürworter. HARTSOCK empfiehlt bei Ausschaltung von Weißbrot, Kartoffeln, Milch und Eier, häufige Fettmahlzeiten. Eine ketogene Diät, die oft allein zur Besserung der Krankheit führen soll, wird auch von anderen Autoren (BARBORKA, POLLOCK und BARBORKA, F. HARE, MINOT, BOYDEN) empfohlen. BROWN empfiehlt zuerst eine kohlehydratfreie, später eine pflanzliche Kost. GERSON rühmt die Erfolge seiner mineralogenen Diät besonders bei Migräne; nach seiner Ansicht fällt der Zustand der Anfallsbereitschaft mit der Kochsalzretention im Körper zusammen, nach Ablauf des Anfalls erfolge eine Ausschwemmung der Chloride.

Auch die Stuhlregelung wird von vielen Autoren als wichtiger präventiver Behelf angesehen. Sie soll möglichst durch entsprechende Diät, schlackenreiche Kost erreicht werden. Wo dies nicht gelingt, sollen Einläufe gemacht werden. Abführmittel werden von einigen Autoren perhorresziert. HARTSOCK empfiehlt systematische Leibesübungen, Klysmen und monatlich ein- bis mehreremal Kalomel und ein salinisches Abführmittel.

Besondere Erwähnung verdient die *Behandlung mit der Duodenalsonde,* die von CHIRAY und TRIBOULET eingeführt wurde. Sie bezweckt eine Behebung der Gallenstauung, die nach den genannten Autoren eine der wichtigsten auslösenden Ursachen der Migräne bildet. Nach Einführung der Duodenalsonde werden 10—30 cm³ einer $33^1/_3$%igen Magnesiumsulfatlösung eingespritzt. Die günstigen Erfolge von CHIRAY und TRIBOULET wurden auch von anderer Seite bestätigt. MCCLURE und HUNTZINGER behandelten 29 Patienten, die an Migräne und Leberfunktionsstörungen litten und konstatierten einen Parallelismus in der Besserung der Migräne und der Leberfunktion. RADOT und BLAMOUTIER behandelten 22 Migränefälle ohne Auswahl bezüglich der auslösenden Ursache und erhielten nach 2jähriger Beobachtung 7 vorzüglich gebesserte, 8 deutlich gebesserte Fälle und 7 Versager; unter den letzteren nur solche Fälle, deren Anfälle weder von Brechreiz noch von Erbrechen begleitet waren, während bei den gebesserten Fällen diese Begleitsymptome vorhanden waren. Die Autoren stützen daher die Indikation dieser Behandlungsmethode auf das Vorhandensein von Magensymptomen. Die Duodenalsondierung soll anfangs jeden 2. Tag durch mehrere Wochen, später wöchentlich einmal durch viele Monate durchgeführt werden. In einem besonders schweren Fall, wo die Anfälle seit 37 Jahren jeden 5. Tag auftraten, brachte sie eine 2 Monate lang geführte Behandlung mit der Duodenalsonde zum Verschwinden, die Behandlung mußte aber auch weiterhin fortgesetzt werden (97 Duodenalsondierungen), weil der Versuch, sie auszusetzen, zu Rückfällen führte. Auch G. LYON empfiehlt diese Behandlung. Ich habe diese Methode bei einigen schweren Fällen, wo die Migräne mit cholecystopathischen Zuständen kombiniert vorkam, versucht und erhielt fast in allen eine merkliche Besserung des Zustandes; zu einer völligen Beseitigung der Anfälle kam es aber in keinem Fall.

Über die kausale Behandlung der durch endokrine Störungen verursachten Migränefälle gehen die Ansichten recht weit auseinander. Einige Autoren (zuletzt CHRISTIANSEN, SCHULTZE) lehnen eine solche als absolut unwirksam ab. Andere sind begeisterte Befürworter einer solchen. Sicher ist, daß selbst in solchen Fällen, wo die endokrine Genese der Migräneanfälle sehr warscheinlich ist, die therapeutische Wirkung der Hormonbehandlung oft ausbleibt. Der ursächliche Zusammenhang zwischen endokriner Störung und Migräneanfällen scheint ein viel verwickelter zu sein, als daß man von einer Substitutionsbehandlung die gesetzmäßig erfolgende Beseitigung der Anfälle erwarten könnte. Eine strenge Kritik bei der Auswahl der zur Behandlung geeigneten Fälle ist notwendig, wenn man sich größere Täuschungen ersparen will. Als allgemeine Regel sollte gelten, daß nur in solchen Fällen eine aktive Substitutionstherapie zur Anwendung gelange, wo sichere Kennzeichen einer herabgesetzten Funktion der betreffenden innersekretorischen Drüse vorliegen. Dies ist vor allem bei der Behandlung der menstruellen Migräne vor Augen zu halten. RADOT hat diese Fälle in drei Gruppen eingeteilt; die ersten zwei Gruppen umfassen die Fälle, wo die Anfälle zwar periodisch mit der Menstruation zusammenfallen, wo aber gar keine Anzeichen einer herabgesetzten Ovariumfunktion vorliegen, in manchen eher eine Hyperfunktion angenommen werden kann. Es ist also auch theoretisch unbegründet, in solchen Fällen ein Ovariumpräparat anzuwenden. Dagegen scheint dies angezeigt bei der dritten Gruppe, wo auch andere Zeichen eines Hypovarismus bestehen oder wo die Migräne bei einer vorher gesunden Frau gleichzeitig mit den Symptomen einer herabgesetzten Eierstockstätigkeit in Erscheinung trat. LEVI und STEVENS empfehlen bei der ovariellen Migräne immer eine kombinierte Behandlung von Eierstockpräparaten und Schilddrüsensubstanz. LÜHRS versuchte auf Grund seiner früher erwähnten Annahme eine Behandlung mit Corpus luteum- und Placentaextrakt (MERCK) und erzielte bei 7 von 8 Patienten nach einer 3monatigen Behandlung Aufhebung der Anfälle. Über günstige Erfolge mit Eierstockpräparaten berichten SAJITZ (Progynon), THOMSON (Theelin), STUKOVSKY (Thelygan).

Die Schilddrüsentherapie ist in solchen Fällen angezeigt, wo auch andere Anzeichen eines Hypothyreoidismus nachweisbar sind. Die Fälle von LAUDENHEIMER, APERT und CONSIGLIO bestätigen die therapeutische Wirksamkeit der Schilddrüsenbehandlung in solchen Fällen. Ein so breites Anwendungsgebiet, wie L. LEVI für die Schilddrüsentherapie bei der Migräne annimmt, dürfte kaum vorhanden sein. Hier wäre eine strengere Auswahl der zu behandelnden Fälle auch deshalb zu empfehlen, weil die Schilddrüsenbehandlung bekanntermaßen schädliche Folgezustände mit sich bringen kann. In Fällen von Hyperthyreoidismus ist die Röntgenbehandlung der Schilddrüse nach FRÄNKEL zu versuchen.

CURSCHMANN sah bei hypoparathyreoiden, kalzipriven Migränefällen, vornehmlich bei Kindern, gute Erfolge von einer lange fortgesetzten Kalkbehandlung. TIMME und PARDEE, KLAUSNER und CRONHEIM, HARTUNG, SCHOTTMÜLLER sowie BOUVEYRON berichten über günstige Wirkung nach Behandlung mit Hypophysenpräparaten. KUPFERBERG sah von Röntgenbehandlung der Hypophyse gute Erfolge.

Die bisher angeführten Behandlungsmethoden, in welchen wir eine kausale Therapie der Migräne auf Grund der auslösenden Ursachen erstreben, können heute wohl nur bei einer Minderzahl der Migränefälle Anwendung finden. In der Mehrzahl der Fälle ist die auslösende Ursache entweder unbekannt oder aber es sind mehrere auslösende Ursachen gleichzeitig wirksam, so daß eine strikte Indikation im obigen Sinne nicht aufgestellt werden kann. Wir stehen aber auch diesen Fällen gegenüber nicht mehr ratlos da. Die Erfahrungen lehren, daß auch die erbbedingte migränöse Anfallsbereitschaft bekämpft werden kann. Wir erkannten im Migräneanfall einen örtlich begrenzten Gefäßkrampf, der durch einen Sympathicusreiz bedingt ist; es ist also naheliegend, die migränöse Gefäßkrampfbereitschaft mit solchen Mitteln zu bekämpfen, die aus der Pharmakodynamik als spezifisch gefäßkrampflösende Arzneien bekannt sind. Eine solche Wirkungsweise kann man bei der schon von den älteren Autoren eingeführten *Brombehandlung* annehmen. CHARCOT ließ seine Migränekranke 6—12 Monate lang täglich 3—6 g Brom nehmen. GILLES DE LA

TOURETTE empfahl sogar, mit der Bromdosis so lange zu steigen, bis Vergiftungserscheinungen auftreten. GOWERS verordnete 1—1,5 g Brom zweimal täglich mit kleinen Dosen von Phenozon oder Cannabis indica. Auch MOEBIUS tritt für die chronische Brombehandlung in steigenden und fallenden Dosen ein. Die Bromtherapie hat sich im Laufe der Zeit immer mehr Anhänger erworben und gehört auch heute als gut bewährtes Mittel zum Arzneischatz der Migränetherapie. Ihre Anwendung wurde in der letzten Zeit nur dadurch eingeschränkt, daß uns im Luminal (Gardenal) ein gefäßkrampflösendes Mittel zur Verfügung gestellt wurde, welches an Wirksamkeit das Brom weit übertrifft. Zahlreiche Veröffentlichungen bestätigen seine ausgezeichnete Wirkung bei Migräne. STRASBURGER nimmt hier eine spezifische Wirkung des Mittels an, welche sich nicht nur in der Abnahme der Zahl und Intensität der Anfälle kundgibt, sondern die Kranken auch im Intervall frischer und leistungsfähiger macht. Unangenehme Nebenwirkungen hat er, von einer anfänglichen Schläfrigkeit abgesehen, nicht beobachtet, auch keine Angewöhnung. Er empfiehlt 0,10 g abends oder in zwei Teilen zu 0,05 g tagsüber einzunehmen. Die Behandlung soll 2 Jahre lang dauern. Ähnliche günstige Wirkungen beobachteten STIEFLER, LINDENMEYER (bei ophthalmischer Migräne), REICHE (bei Kindern Tagesdosen von 0,03—0,1; nach 3 Tagen 2 Tage Pause), STROOMANN, VAN SCHELVEN, HARRIS (mehrmals täglich kleine Dosen, zuerst auf-, dann absteigend), KÄMMERER. Die Tagesdosis von 0,10 g wird von den meisten Autoren nicht überschritten.

Eine weitere wichtige Bereicherung unseres Arzneimittelbestandes an gefäßkrampflösenden Medikamenten bedeutet die Einführung des Papaverins, welches bei Migräne von mehreren Autoren (FREUND, HAHN und STEIN, RICHTER) empfohlen wurde. Ich habe das Papaverin in Verbindung mit Brom und Luminal seit mehr als 8 Jahren bei einigen hundert Fällen von Migräne angewendet und konnte mich von der ausgezeichneten Wirkung dieser Behandlungsart, wenn sie systematisch durchgeführt wird, in den meisten Fällen überzeugen. Die Wirkung des Papaverins kommt aber nur in entsprechend hohen Dosen zur Geltung. Es herrscht diesbezüglich eine gewisse Ängstlichkeit in weiten ärztlichen Kreisen. Ich verordne in schweren Fällen (bei erwachsenen Leuten mit normalem Körpergewicht) das salzsaure Papaverin (MERCK) dreimal täglich zu Einzeldosen von 0,10 g mit je 0,5 g Bromnatrium und lasse abends vor dem Schlafengehen 0,10 g Luminal nehmen. In leichteren Fällen, sowie bei Jugendlichen und Unterentwickelten verordne ich 0,05 g Papaverin dreimal täglich und abends 0,05—0,10 g Luminal. Schädliche Nebenwirkungen habe ich bei dieser Dosierung nie gesehen. Eine Schläfrigkeit oder Mattigkeit, die sich in den ersten Tagen einzustellen pflegt, beunruhigt die Kranken nicht, wenn sie darauf vorbereitet werden; nach 8—10 Tagen verschwindet sie gewöhnlich; manchmal genügt die Herabsetzung der Luminaldosis auf die Hälfte, um diese zu beheben. Die pünktliche Einnahme der vorgeschriebenen Medikamente möglichst zur selben Tagesstunde wird den Kranken eindringlich zur Pflicht gemacht. Die Wirksamkeit der Kur zeigt sich gewöhnlich erst etwa nach 4 Wochen, bis dahin sind die Medikamente auch während der Anfälle pünktlich zu nehmen, ausgenommen die Fälle mit Erbrechen. Wenn der 2. Monat anfallsfrei blieb, dann vermindere ich die Dosis nach folgender Vorschrift: Für die nächsten 2 Monate zweimal 0,10 g Papaverin mit 0,5 g Brom (früh und mittags), und abends 0,10 Luminal, für die folgenden 2 Monate (5. und 6. Monat der Behandlung) 0,10 Papaverin morgens und 0,10 Luminal abends; die letzten 2 Monate (7. und 8. Monat der Behandlung) nur 0,10 g Luminal abends. Die Behandlung nimmt also in einem günstigen Fall 8 Monate in Anspruch. Zeigt sich aber in den ersten 2 Monaten nur eine geringe Besserung, dann verlängere ich die erste Dosierung auf 3 oder auch 4 Monate und behalte diese längeren Termine auch beim späteren Abbau. Auf Grund meiner Erfahrungen möchte ich die hier angegebene Behandlungsart in jedem Migränefall zum Versuch empfehlen, wo die auslösende Ursache der Migräne nicht bekannt ist, oder nicht beseitigt werden kann, oder wenn die früher besprochenen spezifischen Methoden keinen Erfolg brachten. Es ist aber zu erwägen, bevor man eine mehrmonatige systematische Kur einleitet, ob die durch die Migräne verursachten Beschwerden so beträchtlich sind, daß der Kranke die Last dieser mit gewissen Mühseligkeiten immer doch verbundenen Kur auf sich zu nehmen bereit ist. Einen Mangel an Ausdauer, der die Wirksamkeit dieser Kur in erster Linie in Frage stellt, habe ich besonders bei psychopathisch Veranlagten gesehen. Auch sah ich einige Male bei solchen ,,anbehandelten" Fällen eine gewisse Verschlimmerung des Migränezustandes.

Als gefäßkrampflösende Mittel fanden auch die verschiedenen Nitrokörper Anwendung bei der Migräne. Schon GOWERS empfahl das Natrium nitrosum und das Nitroglycerin, ROSENTHAL (bei Augenmigräne) das Amylnitrit. E. MENDELS Vorschrift lautet: Nitroglycerin 0,1, Spiritus vini, Acidi phosphor āā 10,0 zweimal täglich zwei Tropfen. Von neueren, auf die Gefäßwirkung eingestellten Mitteln sollen erwähnt werden: Benzylbenzoat (DELORME, CASTERS-VAN BOGAERT), Ergotamintartrat (nach TZANCK bis zur täglichen Dosis von 6 mg per os oder zweimal 0,5 mg subcutan, bei Basedow kontraindiziert), Gynergen (als sympathicushemmendes Mittel von E. TRAUTMANN empfohlen). Das von DÖLLKEN eingeführte *Moloid* (Sächsische Serumwerke) enthält eine Nitrokörpermischung; vorgeschrieben sind zwei halbe Tabletten zu je 0,5 mg, nach dem Frühstück und Mittagessen, mehrere Monate lang. VIELLI empfiehlt eine Kombination von Papaverin und Atropin (Spasmalgin). DEJEAN sah gute Erfolge bei ophthalmischer Migräne von intramuskulären Injektionen des Acetylcholins (0,1 mg).

Roborierende Kuren bildeten vor einigen Jahrzehnten die wichtigste Behandlungsmethode der Migräne. OPPENHEIM rühmte die lange fortgesetzte Arsenbehandlung, fallweise mit einer Eisenbehandlung kombiniert (Serien von 30 Arseninjektionen jährlich 2—3mal wiederholt), auch Strychnin wurde häufig verordnet. BING empfahl Pillen nach folgender Vorschrift: Chinin. sulf. 1,0, Acid. arsen. 0,10, Extr. cannabis ind. 0,45. Extr. et pulv. rad. Valer. ad Pill. 30, abends eine Pille. CURSCHMANN sah manchmal von einer Behandlung mit reinem Chinin (3 × 0,25) Nutzen.

Operative Behandlungsmethoden wurden bei der Migräne erst mit dem Auftauchen der Gefäßkrampftheorie in Vorschlag gebracht, die erste von JONNESCU (1910): er resezierte bei einem 10jährigen Mädchen, welches seit 3 Jahren an Migräneanfällen litt, den sympathischen Halsstrang und das obere dorsale Ganglion; nach der Operation hatte die Kranke während der folgenden 2 Jahre nur einen einzigen Anfall und im Jahre 1923 bestätigt JONNESCU die weitere Anfallsfreiheit. DEBRÈZ berichtet (1922) über eine 42jährige Frau, die seit 20 Jahren an häufigen, intensiven Migräneanfällen mit wechselnder Seite litt, bei der er die Exstirpation des rechten oberen Halsganglions und eine periarterielle Sympathektomie an der Carotis interna vornahm; die Kranke hatte während der folgenden 9 Monate nur einen leichten Anfall. HELLWIG (1924) empfahl auf Grund tierexperimenteller Beobachtungen, die ihn zu der Ansicht führten, daß der Schmerz beim Gefäßkrampf sekundär durch Zerrung und Zug auf die periarteriellen Nervenelemente entstehe, die periarterielle Sympathektomie an der Carotis communis und interna. WITZEL sah das Verschwinden der Anfälle in einem Migränefall, wo er die Carotis communis in einer Länge von 3—4 cm und die Carotis externa bis zur Arteria lingualis und die Carotis interna so hoch wie nur erreichbar sympathektomiert hat. SICARD und LERMOYEZ machten periarterielle Sympathektomie an der oberflächlich liegenden Arteria temporalis (in $1^{1}/_{2}$ cm Länge) und haben das Gefäß nachher abgebunden. Die Anfälle blieben 6 Monate aus, dann kamen sie wieder. BRÄUCKER berichtet über erfolglose Operationen am Sympathicus bei einem Fall von ophthalmoplegischer Migräne. DANDY hat in 2 Fällen von Migräne das untere cervicale und erste thorakale Sympathicusganglion auf der Seite des Kopfschmerzes entfernt, und erzielte in beiden Fällen Schmerzfreiheit, die in einem Fall seit 7, im anderen seit 4 Monaten anhielt. In einem der Fälle exstirpierte er zunächst das obere Cervicalganglion und erst nachdem dieser Eingriff erfolglos blieb, entfernte er das untere. DICKERSON hat in 7 Fällen nach einer subtemporalen Trepanation und Freilegung der Dura die Arteria meningea media mit 2 Klammern gefaßt und das Zwischenstück excidiert; er berichtet über gute Erfolge in allen Fällen.

Es ist sehr schwer, auf Grund dieser spärlichen und ihrer Zielsetzung nach recht verschiedenen Eingriffe sich ein Urteil über den Wert der operativen Behandlungsmethode bei der Migräne zu verschaffen. Der große Enthusiasmus, mit welchem die periarterielle Sympathektomie bei anderen angiospastischen krankhaften Zuständen aufgenommen und eine Zeitlang als die Methode der Wahl betrachtet wurde, ist heute schon sichtlich abgeflaut. Besonders seitdem es bekannt wurde, daß ihre gefäßkrampflösende Wirkung nur auf proximale Gefäßabschnitte beschränkt ist, weil die Sympathicusbahn der distalen Gefäßabschnitte längs ihres Verlaufs aus den benachbarten cerebrospinalen Nerven frische Fasern zugeführt erhält, ihre Leitungsfähigkeit also durch die Sympathektomie an einem vom Krampfgebiet entfernteren Abschnitt der Gefäßbahn nicht sehr beeinträchtigt wird. Prinzipielle Bedenken gegen die Wirksamkeit operativer Eingriffe am Sympathicus müssen auch entstehen, wenn man sich des klassischen Versuchs von LEWANDOWSKY erinnert. Wenn man bei der Katze das obere sympathische Halsganglion elektrisch reizt, erweitert sich die Pupille an dieser Seite. LEWANDOWSKY zeigte nun, daß, wenn man das obere Halsganglion exstirpiert und die Katze in einen psychischen Erregungszustand versetzt, die Pupille sich auch auf der operierten Seite erweitert (sogar noch mehr als auf der nicht operierten Seite), dagegen bleibt die Pupillenerweiterung auf psychische Erregung aus, wenn man vorher die beiden Nebennieren der Katze entfernt hat. Dieser Versuch, der von anderen Autoren und auch an anderen Organen bestätigt wurde, kann nur so gedeutet werden, daß die Pupillenerweiterung auf psychische Erregung durch erhöhte Adrenalinproduktion und eine reichlichere Ausschwemmung desselben in die Blutbahn zustande kommt; diese hormonale Reizwirkung kann sich aber im vegetativen Endorgan auch dann geltend machen, wenn die leitende Sympathicusbahn ausgeschaltet ist. In Analogie zu diesem Versuch muß man daran denken, daß der den Migräneanfall verursachende Gefäßkrampf im Vertebralissystem auch dann zustande kommen kann, wenn seine Sympathicusbahn unterbrochen oder sein sympathisches Zentrum ausgeschaltet ist; die hormonalen oder humoralen anfallsauslösenden Reize können ihre Wirkung unmittelbar an den Sympathicusendigungen der Gefäßwand ausüben. Besteht aber eine solche Möglichkeit, dann kann man weder von den Operationen am Sympathicushalsstrang, noch von einer periarteriellen Sympathektomie am Plexus subclavius und Plexus vertebralis eine therapeutische Beeinflussung der Migräne erwarten.

Operative Eingriffe zur Beseitigung der Migräne wurden auch aus anderen Indikationen ausgeführt. Es gab eine Zeit, wo die krankhaften Veränderungen im Nasen- und Rachenraum und in ihren Nebenhöhlen zu allererst als Ursache der Migräne einer radikalen Behandlung unterzogen wurden. OPPENHEIM, HARTMANN berichten über günstige Wirkung von Tonsillotomien. Auch bei den mit Verdauungsstörungen einhergehenden Migränefällen wurden operative Eingriffe mit Erfolg versucht. HIGGINS beobachtete, daß von 17 Kranken, die er wegen Erweiterung des Duodenums operierte (eine Duodenojejunostomie ausführte), bei 13 Kranken die gleichzeitig bestehenden Migräneanfälle verschwanden. LEWEN sah gute Erfolge von der operativen Beseitigung der Magenptose. DUVAL und ROUX erreichten die Heilung der Migräne in 3 Fällen durch operative Beseitigung der gleichzeitig vorliegenden Duodenalstenose. STROHMEYER sah in einem Fall nach Herausmeißelung eines schräg gewachsenen Zahnes das Verschwinden der Migräneanfälle.

Die Behandlung des Migränekranken im Anfall selbst ist natürlich eine rein symptomatische. Die meisten Kranken bringen sich selbst zur Ruhe, legen sich in einem stillen dunklen Zimmer nieder, vermeiden körperliche Bewegungen und auch geistige Arbeit. In leichten Fällen kann eine nicht anstrengende geistige Betätigung lindernd wirken. In der Frage, ob der Kopfschmerz zu Beginn des Anfalles mit Medikamenten kupiert werden solle oder nicht, nimmt FLATAU den Standpunkt ein, daß die Unterdrückung des Anfalles zu vermeiden ist, Migränemittel nur im Notfall bei sehr starken Kopfschmerzen angewendet werden sollen. Er meint, daß die Anfälle, wenn sie mit Mitteln kupiert werden, immer heftiger werden und auch daß die Intervalle sich günstiger gestalten, wenn der Anfall sich ausgetobt hat. Mit CURSCHMANN und anderen Autoren möchte auch ich der entgegengesetzten Ansicht beipflichten, nämlich daß jeder Anfall sobald als möglich behandelt werden solle. Man hört überaus häufig von Migränekranken, daß bei rechtzeitiger Einnahme eines Kopfschmerzpulvers der Anfall sich nicht bis zu seiner gewohnten Intensität entwickelt, manchmal wesentlich verkürzt oder rasch unterdrückt wird. Auch ist es allgemein bekannt, daß der vollentwickelte Anfall, wenn überhaupt, so nur mit den drastischesten Mitteln einigermaßen gelindert werden kann. Übrigens macht hier FLATAU die Rechnung ohne den Wirt, weil die meisten Kranken zu Beginn ihres Anfalles eines der ihnen momentan am bewährtesten, schmerzlindernden Mittel einzunehmen pflegen. Unter diesen Mitteln stehen auch heute Antipyrin, Aspirin, Pyramidon, Phenacetin, Migränin sowie die Kombination dieser Mittel mit Coffein an erster Stelle. Die Wirksamkeit dieser Kopfschmerzmittel ist zeitlich beschränkt und deshalb ist von Zeit zu Zeit ein Wechsel vorzunehmen. Die viel gelobten Spezialitäten besitzen kein Anrecht zu einer besonderen Bevorzugung. Manche Kranke empfinden eine Erleichterung nach dem Genuß von schwarzem Kaffee. Auch die Massage der Hals- und Nackenmuskulatur bringt zuweilen eine Milderung des Kopfschmerzes. HARTMANN empfiehlt in einem jeden Fall einen Versuch mit der von ihm propagierten anatomischen Massage am Kopf, Hals, Schulter und Armen, bei Übelkeit und Erbrechen auch eine Massage im Magendermatom. Kalte und warme, nasse Kompressen auf den Kopf werden vielfach angewendet. OPPENHEIM sah von heißen Fußbädern Gutes, BONNAL von einer heißen Luftbehandlung mit Föhn. GOWERS empfahl eine einmalige Dosis von $2^1/_2$ g Brom zu Beginn des Anfalles, was sich ihm besonders bei ophthalmischer und epileptischer Migräne bewährte. Auch Einatmung von Amylnitrit kann eine Linderung bringen (2—5 Tropfen auf ein Tuch geträufelt zu Beginn des Anfalles), KOLLE sah gute Erfolge von Paracodin (KNOLL), die Einnahme von 2—4 Tabletten bei beginnendem Anfall kann diesen wesentlich vermindern. KOLLEs Erfahrungen, die er bei ophthalmischer Migräne machte, bestätigte bei der gewöhnlichen Migräne FAHRENKAMP. BONN empfiehlt intervenöse Papaverininjektionen während des Anfalles; auch ich sah von solchen

(0,04—0,05 Papaverin) einigemal eine deutliche Besserung der Anfallsbeschwerden. STROOMANN bringt intravenöse Luminalinjektionen in Vorschlag. Es ist jedenfalls angezeigt, einen Versuch mit Papaverin oder Luminal zu machen, bevor man zum Morphium greift, dessen Anwendung nur für die schwersten Fälle vorbehalten bleiben und bei Anfällen mit Erbrechen möglichst vermieden werden sollte. CURSCHMANN sah im Status hemicranicus einigemal Nutzen von der Lumbalinjektion. Ich konnte mich von der therapeutischen Wirksamkeit dieses Eingriffes, den ich früher öfters vornahm, nie recht überzeugen.

Die der Prophylaxe dienenden allgemeinen Verhaltungsmaßregeln für Migränekranke bezwecken eine in jeder Hinsicht geregelte, ruhige Lebensführung. Geregelte Nahrungsaufnahme (nicht übermäßige Mahlzeiten), geregelte Speisestunde; wiederholt sah ich bei Migränekranken, die schon seit langem anfallsfrei waren, den Ausbruch eines Anfalles an einem Fasttag oder unmittelbar darauf folgend. Die Regelung des Stuhlganges ist ebenso wichtig. Auch der Zeitpunkt des Schlafengehens soll möglichst nicht sehr gewechselt werden. Neben einer genügenden Dauer des Nachtschlafes soll der Nachmittagsschlaf möglichst nicht lang sein. Geistige Überarbeitung ist zu vermeiden (dieser Umstand ist auch bei der Berufswahl zu berücksichtigen), besonders geistige Arbeit in den Nachtstunden. Ungünstig wirkt langer Aufenthalt in schlecht gelüfteten Räumen; Bewegung im Freien und leichte sportliche Betätigung ist in jedem Fall angezeigt. Die günstige Wirkung des Orts- und Klimawechsels hält nicht selten noch mehrere Monate nach der Rückkehr an. Eine der wichtigsten diätetischen Maßregeln ist das absolute Alkoholverbot. Die weitaus überwiegende Mehrzahl der Migränekranken vermeidet den Alkohol aus eigener Erfahrung, so daß der Arzt nur selten dazu kommt, den Alkoholgenuß zu verbieten. Die Schädlichkeit des Rauchens ist nach meinen Erfahrungen nicht so allgemein geltend. Auch hier gibt es Fälle von ausgesprochener Nikotinempfindlichkeit, wie der Fall von ROSENFELD, der nach Aufgabe des Rauchens seine Migräne verlor und nach 2 Rauchrezidiven sie immer wieder zurückbekam. Im allgemeinen wäre aber ein mäßiges Rauchen nicht zu verbieten. Über die Schädlichkeit des Genusses von schwarzem Kaffee oder Tee konnte ich mich nicht überzeugen; eine Übertreibung ist auch hier zu vermeiden.

Literatur.

ADIE: Lancet **1930 II**. — AGNELLO, F.: Riv. otol. ecc. **1929**. — AIRY: Philos. trans. roy. Soc. Lond. **1870**, 160. — ALDA: Brit. med. J. **1920**. — ALLAN, W.: J. nerv. Dis. **1927**. — Arch. of Neur. 18 (1927). — Arch. int. Med. 42 (1930) — Arch. of Neur. 27 (1932). — ANDERSON-JACK: Glasgow med. J. **1894**. — ANTONELLI: Arch. de Neur. 24 (1892). — APERT: Soc. méd. Hôp. Paris, 12. Mai 1906. — ASSMANN: Krkh.forsch. 4 (1927). — AUERBACH: Fortschr. Med. 31 (1913).

BABINSKI: Arch. de Neur. 20 (1890). — BABONNEIX et DAVID: J. Méd. et Chir. pract. **1918**. — BALL, F. E.: Amer. med. Sci. 173 (1927). — BALLET: Méd. moderne **1896**. — BALYEAT and RICHARDS: Genetics 18 (1933). — BALYEAT and RINKEL: Ann. int. Med. 5 (1931).— Amer. J. Dis. Childr. 42 (1931). — BARALT: Thèse de Paris 1880. — BARBORKA: J. amer. med. Assoc. 95 (1930). — BASTEDO: J. amer. med. Assoc. 77 (1921). — BEECHER: Illinois med. J. 55 (1929). — BEHMAK: Z. Neur. 114 (1928). — BERENCSOY: Klin. Wschr. **1929, 1930**. — BERG, H. J. VAN DEN: Endocrinology 5 (1921). — BERG, W.: Klin. Wschr. **1928 I.** — BERGER: Berl. klin. Wschr. 1871. — Virchows Arch. 59 (1874). — BERNHARDT: Berl. klin. Wschr. **1889 II**. — BERNHEIMER: GRAEFE-SAEMISCHs Handbuch der gesamten Augenheilkunde, 2. Aufl., 39. Lief., 1902. — BEYER: Neur. Zbl. 1 (1895). — BIEDL u. REINER: Pflügers Arch. 79 (1900). — BILLIGHEIMER: Klin. Wschr. **1929**. — BING, R.: Lehrbuch der Nervenkrankheiten, 3. Aufl. Wien u. Berlin: Urban & Schwarzenberg 1924. — BLIZSTEIN u. BRAMS: J. amer. med. Assoc. 86 (1926). — BOLTEN: Über Genese und Behandlung der exsudativen Paroxysmen. Abh. Neur. **1925**, H. 31. — BOND: Trans. Assoc. amer. Physicians 37 (1922). — BONN: Med. Klin. **1926 I**. — BONNIER: Presse méd. **1903**. — BORNSTEIN: Mschr. Psychiatr. 25 (1907). — BOUCHAUD: Presse méd. **1897**. — BOUCHÉ et HUSTIN: Bull. Acad. Méd. Belg. 30 (1920). — BOUVEYRON: Rev. Hyg. et Med. infant. **1911**. — BRÄUCKER:

Ref. 18. Verslg Ges, dtsch. Nervenärzte Hamburg. **1928**. — BRASCH u. LEVINSOHN: Berl. klin. Wschr. **1898 II**. — BROWN, T. R.: Trans. Assoc. amer. Physicians **44** (1929). — BUCHANAN: New York med. J. **113** (1921). — Boston med. J. **192** (1925). — CAESAR: Med. Klin. **9** (1913). — CANTALAMESSA (Zit. nach WILDBRAND-SAENGER.): Boll. Sci. med. **1891**. — CAPPARONI: Policlinico **33** (1926). — CASTERS et VAN BOGAERT: J. de Neur. **26** (1926). — CHABBERT: Progrès méd. **15** (1895). — CHARCOT: Leçons du mardi à la Salpêtiere, 2. Ausg. Paris 1892. — Revue neur. **8** (1897). — CHARLES: Practitioner **91**, No 3. — CHIRAY-TRIBOULET: Presse méd. **33** (1925). — CHRISTIANSEN: Rapport sur la migraine (Etude clinique). Revue neur. **32** (1925). — CHURCH and PETERSON: Nervous and mental diseases. Philadelphia: Saunders, ed. 1914. — CLARK: Brit. med. J. **1910**. — COBB: Arch. int. Med. **7** (1933). — COBBS: Arch. of Neur. **27** (1932). — COKE, F.: Asthma, by Wright. Bristol 1923) — COMBY: Arch. Méd. Enf. **24** (1921). — CORNIL: Revue neur. **1925**. CONSIGLIO: Semaine méd. **1904**. — Gazz. Osp. **1904**. — CORNU: Thèse de Lyon 1902. — CROFTAN: Internat. med. J. **1912**. — CURSCHMANN: Dtsch. Z. Nervenheilk. **38** (1910). — Kopfschmerz, Migräne und Schwindel. Handbuch der inneren Medizin von BERGMANN-STAEHELIN. Berlin: Julius Springer 1926. — Nervenarzt **4** (1931). — CURTIS-BROWN: Brit. med. J. **1** (1925).
DANDY: Bull. Hopkins Hosp. **48** (1931). — DATTNER: Wien, klin. Wschr. **1930 II**. — DAVSON OF PENN, LORD: Brit. med. J. **1927**. — DAVANZO: Riv. ital. Ginec. **8** (1929). — DEBRÉ, R.: J. des Prat. **1925**. — DEBREZ: J. Chir. et Ann. Soc. belge Chir. **29** (1922). — DELORME: Arch. d'Ophthalm. **40** (1924). — DEJEANE: Presse méd. **1932 II**. — DEJERINE: L'heredité dans les maladies du systéme nerveux. Paris 1886. — DETERMANN: Dtsch. med. Wschr. **1896 I**. — DEYL: 13. Congr. internat. Paris 1900, Sect. neur. — DIAMOND: Amer. J. med. Sci. **174** (1927). — DICKERSON: J. nerv. Dis. **77** (1933). — DIDSBURY: Le Concours med., Sept.-Okt. 1924. — DÖLLKEN: Münch. med. Wschr. **1928**. — DUANE: Arch. of Ophthalm. **52** (1923). — DUBOIS-REYMOND: Arch. Anat. u. Physiol. **4** (1860). — DUFOUR: Rev. Suisse **8** (1889). — DUVAL et ROUX: Soc. Gastroenterol. Paris, 10. Dez. 1923.
EDINGER: Von den Kopfschmerzen und der Migräne. Deutsche Klinik am Eingang des XX. Jahrhunderts, 1901. — EHLERS: Acta psychiatr. (Københ.) **3** (1928). — EPSTEIN: Neur. Zbl. **1904, 1905**. — ESCAT: Revue Neur. **1904**. — EULENBURG: Berl. klin. Wschr. **1873**. — Wien. med. Press. **28** (1887). — ELY: Arch. of Neur. **24** (1930).
FABRE: Revue neur. **1905**. — FÉRÉ: Rev. Méd. **1881**; **12** (1882); **23** (1903). — Belg. méd. **13** (1906). — FECHT: Med. Welt **4** (1930). — FISHER: Brit. J. Ophthalm. **1919**. — FLATAU: Die Migräne. Berlin: Julius Springer 1912. — FODOR-KUNOS: Arch. Verdgskrkh. **51** (1932). — FOERSTER: Die Leitungsbahnen des Schmerzgefühls und die chirurgische Behandlung der Schmerzzustände. Wien u. Berlin: Urban & Schwarzenberg 1927. — FORNI: Revue neur. **1907**. — FRAENKEL: Zbl. Gynäk. **48** (1924). — FRANZ: Amer. J. Physiol. **19** (1909). — FRIEDLÄNDER-PETOV: Med. Klin. **1927 I**. — FUCHS: Wien. klin. Wschr. **1930 I**.
GÄNSSLEN: Med. Klin. **17** (1921). — GAISBÖCK: Arch. f. exper. Path. **141** (1929). — GALEZOWSKY: Arch. gén. Méd. **1** (1878). — Rec. d'Ophtalm. **1** (1883). — GERSON: Verh. dtsch. Ges. inn. Med. **42** (1930). — GIEBLER: Über rezidivierende Oculomotoriuslähmung. Diss. Dresden 1897. — GOLLWITZER-MEYER u. SCHULTZE: Naunyn-Schmiedebergs Arch. **165** (1932). — GORDON: Internat. Clin. **1** (1924) — GOWERS: Brit. med. J. **1906**. — Diseases of the nervous system, 2. Aufl. London 1883. — GRADLE: Med. News **1904**. — GRASSET-RAUZIER: Traité pratique des maladies du systeme nerv., 1886. — GRIMES: Med. J. a. Rec. **134** (1931). — GRÜNSTEIN: Sovrem. Psichonevr. (russ.) **1** (1925). — Zbl. Neur. **44** (1926). — GUBLER: Gazette des hôpit. 1860.
HADLICH: Dtsch. Z, Nervenheilk. **75** (1922). — HAHN: Med. Klin. **1930 I**. — **1932 II**; HAHN u. STEIN: Dtsch. Z. Nervenheilk. **77** (1923). — HAIG: Harnsäure als ein Faktor bei der Entstehung von Krankheiten (übersetzt von BIRCHER-BENNER.) Berlin 1902. — HALBAN, V.: Jb. Psychiatr. **1901**. — HAMBURGER: Münch. med. Wschr. **1923**. — HAMMOND: N. Y. med. J. **38** (1883). — HARE: Med. Press a. Circ. **130** (1905). — HARRIS: Brit. med. J. **1922**, Nr 3226. — HARTENBERG: Presse méd. **1906, 1912**. — HARTMANN: Der Kopfschmerz. Neue Deutsche Klinik, 1932. — HARTSOCK: J. amer. med. Assoc, **89** (1927). — HARTUNG: N. Y. State J. Med. **27** (1927). — Med. J. a. Rec. **132** (1927). — HELLWIG: Arch. klin. Chir. **128** (1924). — HENSCHEN: Jubilarband für BIANCHI-Catania 1913. — HERTOCHE: Nouv. iconogr. alpêtriere 1899. — HETÉNYI: Arch. Verdgskrkh. **31** (1923). — HEVEROCH: Revue neur. **1925**. — HEYERDAHL: Ref. Jber. Neur. **11**, 853. — HEYMANOWITSCH: Nervenarzt **4** (1931). — HEYMANS-BOUCKAERT: Monogr. Rev. Belg. Sci. Méd. **1929**. — HILBERT: Zbl. Augenheilk. **22** (1898). — HILL: The Physiology and Pathology of the cerebral circulation. London 1896. — HODGE: Virginia med. monthly **48** (1921). — HUDOVERNIG: Orv. Hetil. (ung.) **1894**. — HURST: Brit. med. J. **1917**.
JACCOUD: Traité de pathologie interne, 1876. — JACKSON: Lancet **1875**. — JACQUET et JOURDANET: Rev. Méd. **1909**. — JAHRREISS: Verh. dtsch. Ver. Psychiatr.. Ref. Zbl. Neur. **48** (1928). — JOACHIM: Dtsch. Arch. klin. Med. **44** (1889). — JOLLY: Berl. klin. Wschr. **1902**. — JONNESCO: Le sympathique cervicothoracique. Paris: Masson et Cie. 1923.

KÄMMERER: Münch. med. Wschr, **1925**. — KARPLUS: Jb. Psychiatr. **22** (1902). — Wien. klin. Wschr. **1903**. — KAST: Bull. N. Y. Acad. Med. **2** (1925). — KELLER: Neur. Zbl. **1920**. — KELLING: Arch. Verdgskrkh. **30** (1922). — KENNEDY: Internat. Clin. III. s. **41** (1931). — KELLOGG: Semaine méd. **178** (1895). — KERPPOLA: Mschr. Psychiatr. **51** (1926). — KLAUSNER-CRONHEIM: Dtsch. med. Wschr. **1931**. — KNAPP: Boston med. J. **1894**. — KOCHER: Hirnerschütterung, Hirndruck und chirurgischer Eingriff bei Hirnkrankheiten. NOTHNAGELS Spezielle Pathologie und Therapie, 1901. — KOLLARITS: Dtsch. Z. Nervenheilk. **26** (1904). — KOLLE: Münch. med. Wschr. **77** (1930). — KOVALEWSKY: La migraine et son traitement. Paris 1902. — Revue neur. **1904**. — KRAFFT-EBING: Arb. Psychiatrie u. Neuropath. **1** (1897. — KRÄMER: Wien. med. Wschr. **1924**. — KRAMSZTYK: Polska Gaz. lek. **3** (1924). — KRISCH: Z. Neur. **98** (1925).

LABARRAQUE: Essai sur la cephalalgie et la migraine. Thèse de Paris 1837. — LAING: Med. Clin. N. Amer. **11** (1927). — LAMACQ: Presse méd. **1896**. — LANGE, C. DE: Dtsch. Z. Nervenheilk. **96** (1927). — LAPERSONNE: Revue neur. **1925**. — LASEGUE: Etudes medicales, Tome 2. Paris 1884. — LATHAM: On nervous or sick head-ache. Cambridge 1873. — LAUDENHEIMER: Ther. Gegenw. **24** (1922). — LÉVI, L.: Revue neur. **13** (1905). — Soc. de Biol. **1912**. — Soc. de Therapie 1913, 1914. — Bull. Soc. méd. Hôp. Paris **1923**. — Bull. Soc. Med. Paris **1928**. — LEHNER-RAJKA: Krkh.forsch. 8. H. 2. — LEHNER-RAJKA-TÖRÖK: Arch. f. Dermat. **153** (1927). — LEISCHNER: Med. Klin. **1930** I. — LECLERC: Lyon méd. **1909**. — LEVI, A.: Revue neur. **1925**. — LÉVI, L. et H. DE ROTSCHILD: Bull. Soc. méd. Hôp. Paris **1906**. — Rev. Hyg. et Med. infant. **1911**. — LEWANDOWSKY: Funktionen des Nervensystems. Jena 1907. — Bericht der Berliner Akademie, 1900. Nr 52. — LEY: J. de Neur. **31** (1931). — LINDENMEYER: Klin. Mbl. Augenheilk. **79** (1927). — LippMANN: Soc. Méd. Paris **1923**. — LIVEING: On megrim, sick-headache and some allied disorders. London: Churchill 1873. — LOEPER: 13. Congr. franç. Méd. Paris 1912. — LÖWENFELD: Neur. Zbl. **1882**. — Arch. f. Psychiatr. **1890**. — LUBBERS: Nederl. Tijdschr. Geneesk. **62** (1921). — LÜHRS: Dtsch. med. Wschr. **1923** II. — LUZENBERGER: Il Manicomio **1897**.

McCLURE and HUNTSINGER: New England J. Med. **199** (1928). — Arch. int. Med. **43** (1929). MACKAY: Amer. J. Ophthalm. **12** (1929). — MANGELSDORF: Berl. klin. Wschr. **1903**. — MANZ: Berl. klin. Wschr. **1885**. — MARBURG: Der Kopfschmerz und seine Behandlung. Wien: Moritz Perles 1926. — Margolis: Amer. J. med. Sci. **177** (1929). — MARIN AMAT: Arch. Ophtalm. hisp.-amer. **22** (1922). — Siglo méd. **69** (1926). — MARINA: Über multiple Augenmuskellähmungen, 1896. Zit. nach SCHMIDT-RIMPLER. — MARINESCO-KREINDLER-BRUCH: Z. exper. Med. **79** (1931). — MASSALONGO: Riforma med. **1891**. — MATHIEU et ROUX: Gaz. Hôp. **1903**. — MAUTHNER: Die Lehre von den Augenmuskellähmungen. Wiesbaden 1889. — MEIGE, H.: Revue neur. **1925**. — MENDEL, E.: Dtsch. med. Wschr. **1906**. — MENDEL, K.: Neur. Zbl. **1910**. — MILLER-RAULSTON: J. amer. med. Assoc. 80 (1923). — MINGAZZINI: Z. Neur. **101** (1926). — Mschr. Psychiatr. **1** (1897). — MINOR: Ref. Zbl. Neur. **55** (1930). — MINOT: Med. Clin. N. Amer. **7** (1923). — MOEBIUS: Die Migräne. Wien: Alfred Hölder 1894. — Über periodisch wiederkehrende III. Lähmung. Neurologische Beiträge von MÖBIUS, H. 4. Leipzig 1895. — Die Migräne. NOTHNAGELS Spezielle Pathologie und Therapie, Bd 12. 1899. — MOEHLIG: Endocrinology **15** (1931). — MÖLLENDORF: Virchows Arch. **41** (1867). — MOERSCH: Amer. J. Psychiatr. **3** (1924). — MOLONEY: Arch. Neur. **19** (1928). — MORENAS et DECHAUME: J. Méd. Lyon **10** (1929). — MUCK: Münch. med. Wschr. **1924**. — MUSSO-FOURNIER: Revue neur. **1925**. — MÜLLER, A.: Dtsch. Z. Nervenheilk. **40** u. **44**. — MÜLLER, L. R.: Die Lebensnerven, Berlin: Julius Springer 1924. — MÜLLER, O.: Med. Klin. **1931**.

NEUMANN: Arch. de Neur. **1887**. — NICATI et ROBIOLIS: C. r. Soc. Biol. Paris **1884**. — NIELSEN: Amer. J. Psychiatr. **9** (1930). — NÖRSTROM: Der chronische Kopfschmerz und seine Behandlung durch Massage. Leipzig: Georg Thieme 1910. — NONNE: Syphilis und Nervensystem, 5. Aufl. Berlin: S. Karger 1924.

ODERMATH: Bruns' Beitr. **1922**. — OPPENHEIM: Mschr. Psychiatr. **29** (1911). — Berl. klin. Wschr. **1884**. — Lehrbuch der Nervenkrankheiten, 1912. — OSTERTAG: Verslg dtsch. Naturforsch. Hamburg 1928.

PADERSTEIN: Dtsch. Z. Nervenheilk. **15** (1899). — PÄSSLER: Münch. med. Wschr. **1902**. — PAGNIEZ: Presse méd. **1921**. — PAGNIEZ-NAST: Presse méd. **28** (1920). — PÁKOZDY: Klin. Wschr. **1929**. — PAL, J.: Die Gefäßkrisen. Leipzig 1905. — PANDELESCO et DUMITRESCO: Bull. Soc. méd. Hôp. Bucarest 9 (1927). — PARHON et HORTOLOMEI: Bull. Soc. Neur. Jassy **1919**. — PAULIAN: Spital (rum.) 44 (1924). Ref. Zbl. Neur. **41** (1925). — Spital. (rum.) **45** (1925). — Ref. Zbl. Neur. **41** (1925). — PELZ: Z. Neur, **12** (1912). — PEMBERTON, PEAKE: Lancet **1890**. — PERITZ: Med. Klin. **1906**; **23** (1927). — PEZZI: Revue neur. **1907**. PHILLIPS: J. amer. med. Assoc. **78** (1922). — PHILLIPS, W.: Lancet **1932** II. — PICHLER: Z. Augenheilk. **51** (1919). — PICK: Berl. klin. Wschr. **1894**. — PIORRY: Zit. nach TISSOT. — Plavec: Dtsch. Z. Nervenheilk. **32** (1907). — POLLAK, E.: Der Kopfschmerz und seine Behandlung. Leipzig: Franz Deuticke 1929. — POLLOCK and BARBORKA: Med. Klin. N. Amer. **11** (1928). — POPOVICIU-POPESCU: Z. exper. Med. **69** (1929/30). — PUTNAM: Trans. Assoc. amer. Physicians **15** (1896).

Quincke: Dtsch. Z. Nervenheilk. **9** (1897); **40** (1910).
Rachford: Amer. J. med. Sci. **115**. — v. Rad: Münch. med. Wschr. **73** (1926). —
Ramirez: s. bei P. Vallery-Radot et Blamoutier: Presse méd. **24** (1925). — Raullet:
Etude sur la migraine ophthalmique. Thèse de Paris **1883**. — Redlich: Wien. klin. Wschr.
39 (1926). — Reese: Pensilvania med. J. **33** (1929). — Regniers: Rev. Belg. Sci. Méd. **2**
(1930). — Reichardt: Handbuch der normalen und pathologischen Physiologie, Bd. 10.
1927. — Reiche: Dtsch. med, Wschr. **1927**. — Rentz: Berl. klin. Wschr. **1914**. —
Remond et Rouzaud: Rev. Mél. **38** (1921). — Richter, A.: Arch. f. Psychiatr. **18**
(1887). — Richter, H.: Z. Neur. **97** (1925); **113** (1928). — Riley: Bull. neur. Inst.
N.-Y. **2** (1932). — Riley, Brickner and Kurzrok: Bull. neur. Inst. N.-Y. **3** (1933). —
Rinkel: J. Allergy **4** (1933). — Rio, Del: Giorn. Clin. med. **2** (1921). — Rivière: De la
migraine tardivement aggravée. Thèse de Bordeaux **1911**. — Roger: Rev. d'Otol. etc.
6 (1928). — Roger-Cremieux-Robert: Progrés méd. **1929**II. — Rohrer: Med. Klin.
1915. — Romberg: Münch. med. Wschr. **77** (1930). — Rose: Semaine méd. **1911**. —
Rosenbach: Dtsch. med. Wschr. **1886**. — Rossolimo: Neur. Zbl. **20** (1901). — Rothlin:
Z. exper. Med. **70** (1930). — Rothmann: Neur. Zbl. **1903**. — Rove: California Med. **33**
(1930). — Rupert-Wilson: Amer. J. Med. Assoc. **152** (1919).

Sajitz: Med. Welt **4** (1930). — Saundby: Lancet **1882**. — Schelven, van: Nederl.
Tijdschr. Geneesk. **65** (1921). — Schlesinger: Schweiz. med. Wschr. **1923**. — Schmidt-
Rimpler: Rezidivierende Oculomotoriuslähmung. Nothnagels Spezielle Pathologie und
Therapie, Bd. 21. 1898. — Schob: Z. Neur. **35** (1916). — Schöne, F.: Arch. f. Psychiatr.
71. — Schottin: Münch. med. Wschr. **1911**. — Schottmüller: Münch. med. Wschr.
1931. — Schüller: Wien. klin. Wschr. **1909**. — Schultze: Die Migräne. Erg. inn.
Med. **21** (1922). — Schuster, J.: (Aussprache zum Referat Stiefler: Ges. dtsch. Nerven-
ärzte.) Dtsch. Z. Nervenheilk. **81** (1924). — Schwartz: Schweiz. med. Wschr. **1930**. —
Schweinitz: Amer. ophthalm. Soc. Trans. **1895**. — Scimone: Minerva med. **10** (1930). —
Sedan: Aussprache zum Vortrag von Beauvieux, Pichaud et Rudeau, Straßburg 1929.
Ref. Zbl. Neur. **55** (1930). — Sedillot: Presse méd. **37** (1929). — Monde méd. **39** (1929). —
Sepp, E.: Die Dynamik der Blutzirkulation im Gehirn. Berlin: Julius Springer 1928. —
Shionoya: Dtsch. Z. Nervenheilk. **42** (1911). — Sicard, Paraf et Forestier: Bull. Soc.
méd. Hôp. Paris **1921**. — Sicard-Paraf-Hageneau: Revue neur. **1925**. — Siegrist: Mit-
teilungen aus Kliniken und medizinischen Instituten der Schweiz, 1. Reihe. 1894. — Sil:
Arch. bohem. Med. clin. **8**. — Simon: Mschr. Psychiatr. **68** (1928). — Sittig: Med. Klin.
1923 I. — Smith, Jens Chr.: Bibl. Laeg. (dän.) Aug. **1922**. — Souques: Bull. Soc. méd.
Hôp. Paris **38** (1922). — Souques-Moreau: Academie de Méd. **1920**. — Spiller: Amer.
J. med. Sci. **119** (1900). — Spiller-Posey: Amer. J. med. Sci. **1905**. — Spitzer, A.: Über
Migräne. Jena 1901. — Spuzic: Serb. Arch. Med. **28**, Nr 4. — Sterling: Polska Gaz. lek.
8 (1929). Ref. Zbl. Neur. **56** (1930). — Stevens: New England. J. Med. **201** (1929). —
Stiefler: Dtsch. Z. Nervenheilk. **81** (1924). — Storm van Leeuwen and Zeydner: Brit.
J. exper. Path. **3** (1922). — Stöhr: Die Nervenversorgung der zarten Hirnhaut, der Rücken-
markshaut und der Gefäßgeflechte des Gehirns. L. R. Müllers Die Lebensnerven. Berlin:
Julius Springer1924. — Strasburger: Klin. Wschr. **1923** I. — Strohmayer: Neur. Zbl.
1902. — Stroomann: Fortschr. Ther. **2**, H. 10. — Strümpell: Dtsch med. Wschr. **1921** II. —
Lehrbuch der speziellen Pathologie und Therapie der inneren Krankheiten, 25. Ausg.
Leipzig: F. C. W. Vogel 1926. — Stukovsky: Münch. med. Wschr. **1925**. — Susmann:
Med. J. Austral. **1929** II. — Szondi: Konstitutionsanalyse psychisch abnormer Kinder.
Halle a. S.: Carl Marhold 1933.

Terrien: Progrès méd. **1930** I. — Thaysen: Ugeskr. Laeg. (dän.) **83** (1923). — Thomas:
La migraine. Paris: Delahaye et Lecrosnier 1887. — Thomas, W. A. and W. E. Post:
J. amer. med. Assoc. **84** (1925). — Thomsen: Neur. Zbl. **1884**. — Thomson: Lancet **1932** II. —
Timme: Brit. med. J. **1926**. — Tissot: De la migraine. Oevres complétes. Nouv. Edit.
Paris 1813. — Trautmann: Münch. med. Wschr. **1928** I. — Trömner: Neur. Zbl. **1899**. —
Trousseau: Clinique medical de l'Hôtel-Dieu, 1865. — Tzanck: Bull. Soc. méd. Hôp.
Paris **53** (1929).

Ulrich: Mschr. Psychiatr. **31**, Erg.-H. (1912). — Urechia et Apostol: Arch. internat.
Neur. **47** (1928).

Vallery-Radot, P.: Rapport sur la pathogenie des migraines. Revue neur. **32** (1925). —
Vallery-Radot et Blamoutier: Bull. Soc. méd. Hôp. Paris **49** (1925). — Presse méd. **33**
(1926). — Vaughan: J. amer. med. Assoc. **88** (1927). — Vietti: Folia med. (Napoli) **8**
(1922). — Vogelsang: Z. Augenheilk. **77** (1932).

Weber, E.: Der Einfluß psychischer Vorgänge auf den Körper, Kap. VII. Berlin 1910. —
Wegner: Klin. Mbl. Augenheilk. **76** (1926). — Weiss: Wien. klin. Wschr. **1895** II. —
Weissmann-Netter: C. r. Soc. Biol. Paris **92** (1925). — Westphal: Neur. Zbl. **1913**. —
Widal-Abrami: Presse méd. **32** (1924). — Wiechowsky: Arch. f. exper. Pathol. **48** (1902). —
Wiener: Med. Rec. **100** (1921). — Wildbrand-Sänger: Die Neurologie des Auges, 1900. —
Witzel: Zbl. Chir. **1924**.

Vasomotorisch-trophische Erkrankungen.

Von R. CASSIRER † und R. HIRSCHFELD-Berlin[1].

Mit 16 Abbildungen.

I. Die RAYNAUDsche Krankheit.

Im Jahre 1862 erschien die Monographie von RAYNAUD «De l'asphyxie locale symétrique des extrémités». In dieser wies RAYNAUD nach, daß es eine Varietät der trockenen Gangrän gibt, die an den Extremitäten sitzt und nicht durch eine Verstopfung der Gefäße zu erklären ist, eine Varietät, die charakterisiert ist ganz besonders durch eine bemerkenswerte Tendenz zur Symmetrie derart, daß sie immer gleichgelegene Teile affiziert, die beiden oberen oder unteren Extremitäten oder alle vier auf einmal, in manchen Fällen die Nase und die Ohren; ihre Ursache bezieht er auf eine fehlerhafte Innervation der Capillargefäße; als Ursache der Synkope und Asphyxie locale sieht er einen infolge dieser fehlerhaften Innervation auftretenden Capillarkrampf an, während er die Gangrän auf die dadurch entstehende Abwesenheit des Blutes oder die Anwesenheit eines zur Ernährung unzweckmäßigen Blutes zurückführt. Vor RAYNAUD hatte schon eine Reihe von Autoren ähnliche Fälle publiziert; aber diese Beobachtungen hatten nur den Wert interessanter Kuriosa, deren Bedeutung eine höchst zweifelhafte war, bis RAYNAUD, zum Teil auf diese Beobachtungen gestützt, mehr aber noch auf Grund eigener Erfahrung, das Krankheitsbild der symmetrischen Gangrän kennen lehrte. Historisch bedeutsam sind ferner die Arbeiten von WEISS (1882), HOCHENEGG (1885), CASSIRER (1900), wo alle detaillierten Literaturangaben über das ganze Gebiet zu finden sind; im gleichen Jahre hat MONRO die RAYNAUDsche Krankheit behandelt. Die letzte eingehende Beschreibung der RAYNAUDschen Krankheit stammt aus der Feder des Dermatologen V. MUCHA.

Die kritische Durchsicht der Einzelbeobachtungen lehrt, daß viele Fälle dem ursprünglichen Typus der Krankheit recht fern stehen und zu Unrecht hierher gerechnet werden. Wir beginnen in der Schilderung mit der Beschreibung der klassischen Fälle; auf die zahlreichen, in wichtigen Punkten abweichenden Beobachtungen werden wir später zurückzukommen haben.

Die Nomenklatur hat schon RAYNAUD selbst Schwierigkeiten gemacht. Er hat mehrfach in seiner Namengebung gewechselt und hat schließlich den Namen «Asphyxie et gangrène locale symétrique des extrémités» beibehalten. Später hat man sich zumeist mit der Bezeichnung „RAYNAUDsche Krankheit" begnügt, nachdem andere Namen, z. B. „Jugendliche Gangrän", mit Recht als verfehlt zurückgewiesen worden sind. STRAUS hat den Namen „Angiospastische Gangrän" vorgeschlagen, der auch sonst schon benutzt worden war. Wir lehnen diesen Namen ab, weil er zuviel präjudiziert. Bei der Schwierigkeit, für diese Krankheit einen kurzen, prägnanten Namen zu finden, ziehen wir es vor, den Namen RAYNAUDsche Krankheit zu verwenden.

Ätiologie.

Die RAYNAUDsche Krankheit ist wohl eine seltene Erkrankung, stellt aber auch in ihren typischen und ganz ausgebildeten Fällen keineswegs eine Rarität dar.

Es werden häufiger Frauen als Männer betroffen; unter 150 Fällen fanden ALLEN und BROWN die Krankheit nur in 11% bei Männern. Das Leiden

---

[1] Neubearbeitung des Beitrages von R. CASSIRER im Handbuch der Neurologie, herausgegeben von M. LEWANDOWSKY, V. Band, erschienen 1914.

betrifft die ersten Lebensjahrzehnte bis zum 50. Lebensjahr ungefähr gleichmäßig; eine Bevorzugung des Kindesalters, wie früher vermutet wurde, scheint nicht vorhanden zu sein. Nach dem 50. Lebensjahre tritt die Erkrankung recht selten auf. Die frühesten Fälle sind bei wenigen Wochen und Monaten alten Säuglingen beobachtet worden (REISS, BECK-KOLISCH, FRIEDEL, BJERING, JOHNSON, DEFRANCE, DUPÉRIÉ).

CASTANA berichtet über einen Säugling, der bei der Geburt eine starke Cyanose zeigte, danach setzte eine Woche lang Blutverlust aus dem Nabel ein; nach diesem Zeitpunkt wurde die Hautfarbe normal. Am Ende des ersten Monats stellte sich stundenweise Cyanose der Finger und Zehen ein. Die Anfälle nahmen allmählich an Intensität und Dauer zu; es trat Gangrän auf, von der äußersten Peripherie der Nägel an der linken oberen Extremität an den Vorderarm aufsteigend. Allmählich bildete sich eine starke Verstümmelung der Hand heraus. Im geringeren Grade bestanden auch Störungen am linken Bein. BEJARANO schildert das Krankheitsbild bei einem 3jährigen Mädchen; es fanden sich Verfärbung der Zehen beiderseits, rechts stärker als links, Ulcerationen, Schmerzen; ob es sich um einen echten *Raynaud* gehandelt hat, ist zweifelhaft angesichts der Tatsache, daß das Kind an Lues congenita litt[1].

DUPÉRIÉ schildert zusammenfassend das Auftreten der RAYNAUDschen Krankheit beim Säugling. Aus seiner Schilderung ist zu entnehmen, daß die Erkrankung schon am 6. Lebenstage beginnen kann, hereditär und familiär auftritt. Kälteschäden, Infektionen und Intoxikationen haben sich oft ätiologisch nachweisen lassen. Die Prognose ist bei dem Säugling infaust, wofern nicht Syphilis im Spiele ist. Daß auch bei Greisen die RAYNAUDsche Krankheit beobachtet wird, beweist ein Fall von HENRY. Er betrifft eine 77jährige Frau.

Als wichtiger ätiologischer Faktor macht sich eine *hereditäre Disposition* geltend, zunächst in Form einer allgemeinen neuropathischen Belastung. So war in einem unserer Fälle eine Schwester geisteskrank, eine taubstumm, eine Schwester litt an Migräne. Auch der Fall von RÜLF zeigte starke neuropathische Belastung. Noch bemerkenswerter sind die Fälle direkter Vererbung, die vielfach (RAYNAUD, MONRO, eigene Beobachtung, ULLRICH) konstatiert werden konnte. Sehr interessant ist folgende Kombination: die Schwester einer unserer Kranken litt an Sklerodaktylie, eine andere Schwester an Basedow, der Bruder war an Basedow gestorben. GROTE hat die RAYNAUDsche Krankheit bei 4 Personen in 2 Generationen beobachtet (zit. nach SIEMENS). Nach BLOMFIELD und WEBER (zit. nach MUCHA) wird die Erkrankung bei russischen und polnischen Juden auffallend häufig beobachtet. GEWIN beobachtete sie bei einem 43jährigen Farbigen; sie trat zunächst an den Zehen auf, die amputiert werden mußten, später auch an den Fingern, die gangränös wurden. MUCHA spricht von der Möglichkeit einer vererbten Überempfindlichkeit gegen Kälte (familiäres Auftreten von Pernionen).

Stand und *Beschäftigung* haben nur insofern irgend einen Einfluß, als die Betätigung in der Kälte oder mit kalten und nassen Gegenständen provozierend wirkt. Mehrfach ist chronische Bleiintoxikation beobachtet worden (RAYNAUD, SAINTON, MADER, DECLAUX, GERBIS, eigene Beobachtungen). SIMON führte in einem Falle das Auftreten der RAYNAUDschen Krankheit auf eine toxische Wirkung von unter der Haut befindlichen kleinen Kupfersplitterchen zurück. KRAETZER sah die Erkrankung bei einer Frau sich einstellen, die 14 Jahre hindurch mit arsenhaltigen Insektenmitteln gearbeitet hatte.

Merkwürdig und nicht eindeutig ist der von TOENNIES beobachtete Fall: Wenige Stunden nach einer störungslos verlaufenen Pantopon-Äthernarkose trat bei einem Kranken eine

---

[1] ULLRICH berichtet über einen 2 Monate alten Knaben mit langsam fortschreitender ulceröser Zerstörung der Nasenspitze, bei dem nach einem weiteren Monat Asphyxie und Schwellung an den Händen und am linken Ohr, symmetrische Gangrän der Acren auftrat. Nach vorübergehender Heilungstendenz im Anschluß an eine Infektion Wiederaufflackern des Prozesses mit Gangrän am Penis und Kopf. Eine ältere Schwester habe die gleiche Erkrankung durchgemacht.

mit heftigsten Schmerzen verbundene starke Cyanose beider Hände auf, die am nächsten Tage rechts zurückging. Links stellte sich Nekrose der zweiten Fingerkuppe und der halben Endglieder des 4. und 5. Fingers ein. Histologisch fanden sich Thromben in allen Stadien der Organisation. Verf. entscheidet sich bei diesem Falle für die Annahme eines Angiospasmus im Sinne einer RAYNAUDschen Gangrän.

Chlorose, Anämie, Blutverluste z. B. durch Magengeschwür, erhebliche körperliche Anstrengung mögen gelegentlich wohl auslösend wirken. Hin und wieder werden *Traumen* als Ursache der Krankheit angegeben. Ein Kranker von BRASCH hatte sich im Laufe von vielen Jahren eine große Anzahl leichter Verletzungen der Finger durch seine Beschäftigung bei einer Säge zugezogen; auch SCHÄFFER sah einen Fall traumatischer Genese, HÜBNER hat bei einem 4jährigen Kinde symmetrische Gangrän beider Beine nach Fall von einem Baume auftreten sehen.

Auch *psychische Erregungen* und Erschütterungen können den Anstoß zum Auftreten der Krankheit geben. Auffallend häufig wurde ein jäher Schreck angeschuldigt (DEFRANCE, GARRIGUES, HOESSLIN, DEHIO, CLAUDE und TINEL). Eine unserer Kranken bekam ihren ersten Anfall gelegentlich des Brandes ihres Hauses und des damit verbundenen Ausbruches einer Psychose bei ihrem Bruder. Bei einer unserer Patientinnen sahen wir in demselben Moment eine absolute Synkope aller Finger beider Hände eintreten, in dem sie der Blutentnahme einer anderen zusah.

Als auslösendes Moment sind ferner *Kälte* und *Nässe* zu beschuldigen. Bei LÄHRS kam der erste Anfall zustande, als der Kranke in einer kalten Winternacht, vom Tanzen erhitzt, ins Freie kam. Besonders ungünstig scheint feuchte Kälte oder Waschen mit kaltem Wasser, kaltes Baden usw. zu wirken (KUNTZ, HNATEK, HOLST, URBANTSCHITSCH, BECK, DUERDOTH).

Gelegentlich kann auch *Wärme* ungünstig wirken, wenn auch viel seltener. Aber schon RAYNAUD berichtet von der häufigeren Entstehung der Krankheit in den Hundstagen. Sehr oft wird über Fälle berichtet, in denen sich die RAYNAUDschen Symptome im Anschluß an *Infektionskrankheiten* entwickelten. SLAUGHTER hat die aus der Literatur bekannten Beobachtungen zusammengestellt. Solche sind beschrieben worden nach Flecktyphus (ESTLÄNDER, FISCHER), Typhus abdominalis (BRÜNNICHE, BORETIUS, HASTREITER, SCHULZ u. a.), Cholera (REICHE, GAILLARD), Diphtherie (POWELL), Pneumonie (SEIDELMANN, DUFOUR, WANDEL), Influenza (VERDELLI, BATMAN, DARDIGNAC, LAURENTI, RENDU, ISAAC-GEORGES), Erysipel (ANGELESCO, HOLM, RAYNAUD u. a.), Pocken (DEFRANCE, RAYNAUD), Scharlach (DIXON, MONRO, HOYEN), Masern M'CALL, ANDERSON, GASPARDI u. a.), Rubeola (NOBECOURT), Keuchhusten (PHOCAS, HENNECAUT), Eiterungen. Eine Reihe von diesen Fällen ist durchaus typisch. In anderen handelt es sich aber nicht um das echte Bild der RAYNAUDschen Krankheit, sondern um durch marantische Thrombosen bedingte Gangrän, die ganz zu Unrecht als RAYNAUDsche Gangrän beschrieben wurde. Wieder andere Fälle sind schwierig zu klassifizieren, vor allem diejenigen, bei denen symmetrische Gangrän oder symmetrische Asphyxie im Laufe einer Infektionskrankheit zu einer Zeit auftrat, wo keinerlei sonstige Zeichen auf eine allgemeine Schwäche der Zirkulation hinwiesen, also namentlich im Beginn der betreffenden Krankheit.

Wichtig sind die Beziehungen zwischen *Malaria* und RAYNAUDscher Krankheit. RAYNAUD selbst hat bereits 3 solcher Fälle beschrieben; andere Beschreibungen stammen aus der Feder von MARCHAND, FISCHER, MOURSON, CALMETTE, PETIT und VERNEUIL, SLAUGHTER. Auch in der Monographie MONROs findet sich darüber eine ausführliche Erörterung. Die vasomotorischen Erscheinungen können mit den Fieberattacken zusammenfallen oder sie können unabhängig von der Zeit des Fieberanfalles auftreten, ihm folgen, ihn ersetzen oder mit ihm abwechseln (MITCHELL und ALLEN).

Ebenso wie im Verlauf akuter kommt der RAYNAUDsche Symptomenkomplex auch im Verlauf *chronischer* Infektionskrankheiten vor. Namentlich ist von vielen, besonders französischen Autoren auf die wichtige Rolle aufmerksam gemacht worden, die die Tuberkulose in der Ätiologie der RAYNAUDschen Krankheit spielen soll. In unseren Fällen haben wir schwere tuberkulöse Erscheinungen fast nie gesehen, und wir können auf Grund der eigenen Erfahrungen nicht zugeben, daß die Intoxikation mit dem Gift des KOCHschen Bacillus die RAYNAUDsche Krankheit häufig hervorruft. In der Tat sind die Stimmen, die dieser Ätiologie das Wort reden, seltener geworden; zuletzt haben sich BERNARD und PELLISSIER für diese Ätiologie eingesetzt und weisen dabei auf die Häufigkeit hin, mit welcher die Tuberkulose das sympathische System schädigt.

Die im Anschluß an *Lues* sich einstellenden RAYNAUDschen Erscheinungen werden zusammen mit den Fällen behandelt, in denen irgendwelche anderen Gefäßveränderungen vorliegen, da die Lues jedenfalls in vielen Fällen durch Vermittlung der Gefäßerkrankung ihre Wirksamkeit entfaltet. Diese Kombination, wie die Kombination von RAYNAUDschen Symptomen mit Erscheinungen von Seiten der Niere (Albuminurie, Mellituire, Hämoglobinurie) sollen erst später geschildert werden, ebenso wie die Beziehungen zur Gicht, zum chronischen Alkoholismus und Nikotinismus.

Als Rarität mag noch der folgende Fall von BENNETT und POULTON erwähnt werden: Ein 60jähriger Mann erkrankte mit symmetrischer Gangrän an den Händen, mit Schmerzen und Cyanose der Finger. Die Exstirpation des Ganglion cervicale inferius war erfolglos; während der periarteriellen Sympathektomie starb der Kranke. Anatomische Diagnose: Carcinoma ventriculi. Im Ganglion cervicale inferius fanden sich Carcinomzellen.

Symptomatologie.

Es erscheint zweckmäßig, an den Beginn dieses Abschnittes die aus der ersten RAYNAUDschen Abhandlung entnommene Beschreibung eines Falles zu setzen, der uns von der Gesamtheit der Symptome und dem Verlaufe der Krankheit ein anschauliches Bild gibt.

27jährige Frau, Hände im Sommer meist rot, oft Trockenheit der Finger. Neigung zu Frostbeulen. 3 Monate nach der 2. Entbindung Paraesthesien in den Fingern. Bald traten Schmerzen in diesen auf, die sich in wenigen Tagen zu einer ungemeinen Heftigkeit steigerten und der Kranken trotz Opium die Nachtruhe nahmen. Zugleich wurden einzelne Finger taub und sahen totenblaß aus, später nahmen die Endphalangen eine so intensiv schwarze Färbung an, als wären sie in Tinte getaucht worden. Als die Kranke auf RAYNAUDs Rat die Hände für kurze Zeit in ein Senfbad steckte, wurden diese und die Unterarme sofort tiefschwarz. Auch die Nasenspitze wurde, ohne selbst der Sitz schmerzhafter Empfindungen geworden zu sein, während der heftigen Schmerzen an den Fingern schwarz. Einen Monat später fand sich dasselbe an den Füßen, die Zehen wurden schmerzhaft, die Endphalangen schwarz. Nach weiteren 4 Wochen traten an den Nagelphalangen der Finger, und zwar an der Pulpa, oberflächliche, stecknadelkopfgroße Brandschorfe auf, während an der Dorsalseite der 4 letzten Zehen die Epidermis in Form von sanguinolentes Serum enthaltenden Brandblasen emporgehoben wurde, die nach und nach zu schwarzen Schorfen vertrockneten. Später bot sich dasselbe Bild auch an beiden großen Zehen. Auch an einer Hinterbacke zeigten sich kleine Schorfe. An den Fingern blieb die Gangrän auf die oberflächlichen Cutisschichten beschränkt; an den Zehen dagegen schritt die Gangrän der Fläche und Tiefe nach weiter vor; allmählich waren die Nagelphalangen aller 4 Zehen beider Füße gangränös; es hatte sich eine Demarkation gebildet, so daß sie „wie angeheftete Kohlenstückchen" von den gesundgebliebenen Phalangen herabhingen. Die nekrotischen Phalangen wurden entfernt, worauf die Vernarbung in kurzer Zeit erfolgte. Die Veränderungen waren überall vollkommen symmetrisch. Der Puls war stets normal, solange die symmetrische Gangrän vorhanden war, während vor und nach dieser Periode gelegentlich Unregelmäßigkeiten des Pulses beobachtet wurden. Am Herzen war nie etwas abnormes festzustellen. Urin frei von pathologischen Bestandteilen. Temperatur stets normal. Keine Ergotinvergiftung. Die Frau blieb in der Zukunft gesund.

Der vorstehende Fall ist typisch; er zeigt uns Symptomatologie und Verlauf der Affektion in klassischer Weise.

Das Krankheitsbild setzt sich aus folgenden Symptomen zusammen:

1. vasomotorische Symptome in Form der Syncope locale, Asphyxie locale und lokalen Hyperämie;
2. trophische Störungen in Form der umschriebenen Gangrän oder diffuser oder umschriebener dystrophischer Prozesse, die in Verhärtung, Verdichtung, Schwellung der Haut und der tiefer liegenden Teile, zum Teil in sklerodermatischer Veränderung der betreffenden Gebiete bestehen;

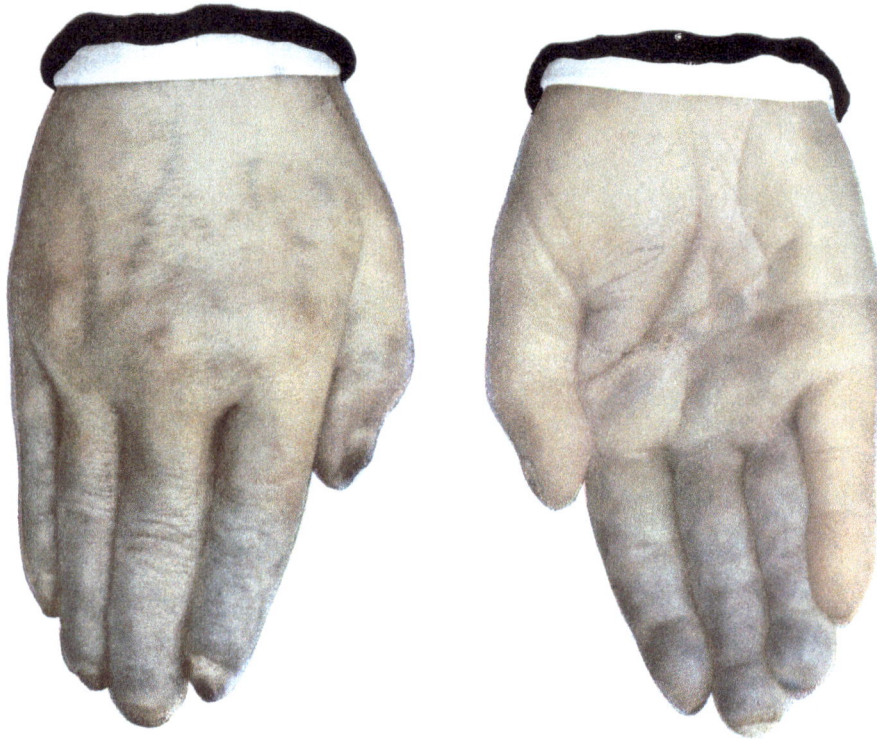

Abb. 1a und b. RAYNAUDsche Krankheit. (Moulage der Universitäts-Hautklinik Breslau).

3. sensible Symptome in Form von Parästhesien, namentlich Thermoparästhesien, Schmerzen, seltener in Form von Hypalgesien oder Hyperalgesien;
4. sekretorische Störungen: Anhydrosis oder Hyperhydrosis. Dazu kommen gelegentlich motorische Störungen, ferner die Erscheinungen, die wir auf eine allgemeine Störung des Nervensystems, insbesondere des autonomen Systems, zu beziehen haben: vasomotorische Instabilität, vasomotorische Ataxie COHENs oder, wie er es später nennt, ,,autonomic-endocrin imbalance".

Das Bild der *lokalen vasomotorischen* Störungen wird in den typischen Fällen eingeleitet durch die Syncope locale (Anémie locale [HARDY], lokale Ischämie [WEISS], lokale Asphyxie [JOHANSON]): die befallenen Teile, ein oder mehrere Finger, seltener Zehen, gelegentlich die Ränder der Ohren oder der Nasenspitze werden plötzlich auffallend weiß und kalt. Die Farbenveränderung kann verschiedene Nuancen aufweisen; bald besteht eine wirkliche Totenblässe, ein

Weiß mit einem grünlichen Ton, ein andermal modifiziert eine leichte Beimischung von blau oder einem hellen Rot den Farbenton; man hat die Finger wachsbleich oder totenbleich genannt, die Nasenspitze erschien kreideweiß. Mit der Farbenveränderung geht regelmäßig eine erhebliche Temperaturerniedrigung einher, wodurch der Eindruck des ,,doigt mort", des Totenfingers, noch verstärkt wird. Die Temperaturerniedrigung soll bis 20° betragen können. GARRIGUES fand im Stadium der Synkope am Rücken des dritten rechten Fingers 15°, HNATEK über den Fingern rechts 21°, links 27°. Wir fanden in einem unserer Fälle am 5. rechten Finger 33,9°, am linken 33,1°, am Daumen beiderseitig 23°, am 3. rechten Finger 17°. Sorgfältige Temperaturmessungen hat in letzter Zeit FULTON angestellt, die auch aus dem Grunde Interesse verdienen, weil sie vor und nach der Ramisektion ausgeführt sind. Die Temperatur kann selbst unter die der umgebenden Luft sinken, offenbar durch starke Verdunstung. Die Dauer dieser Erscheinungen ist wechselnd, von Minuten bis zu Stunden. Sie treten also anfallsweise auf, die Anfälle können sich mehrere Male am Tage bis zu 20- oder 30mal wiederholen. Die Rückkehr zur Norm vollzieht sich in verschiedener Weise, bisweilen plötzlich, manchmal über das Durchgangsstadium einer reaktiven Röte hin. Aus der Syncope locale entwickelt sich die Asphyxie locale (regionäre Cyanose [WEISS]), die aber auch primär auftreten und so das erste Symptom bilden kann. Dann erscheint die Haut bald weiß-blau, bald violett-grau und ist von eigentümlich durchsichtiger Beschaffenheit; die blaue Farbe kann sich mehr nach dem Schwarz hin vertiefen oder eine etwas stärkere Beimischung von Rot bekommen; erst kürzlich habe ich einen Kranken beobachtet, bei dem im Anfall sämtliche Finger aussahen, als ob sie in blasse Tinte getaucht worden waren. Bei Druck bleibt ein weißer Fleck längere Zeit bestehen. In den an die betroffenen Teile anstoßenden Partien findet sich oft eine bläuliche Marmorierung, die sich ausnahmsweise weiter ausdehnen und über den ganzen Körper ausbreiten kann. Zu der Farbenveränderung gesellt sich regelmäßig, mit der Dauer der Cyanose zunehmend, eine Temperaturerniedrigung in den befallenen Teilen, die allerdings nicht so erheblich zu sein pflegt, wie im Stadium der Syncope locale.

Oft tritt auch gleichzeitig mit der Asphyxie locale ein gewisser Grad von Schwellung auf; die Umfangszunahme ist meist nur eine mäßige, sie beträgt Bruchteile eines Zentimeters. Bei Nadelstichen in das Gebiet der lokalen Asphyxie erhielt BERNHARDT aus der asphyktischen rechten Hand ein dunkelblaurotes Blut, aus der linken normalen kam hellrotes Blut heraus. Die Cyanose verschwindet durch mechanischen Druck momentan und kehrt langsam wieder. Hochhalten der Hände, Eintauchen in Wasser kann verschiedene, zum Teil paradoxe Reaktionen hervorrufen.

Neben der typischen Asphyxie kommt auch spontan eine Reihe von Modifikationen der vasomotorischen Erscheinungen vor. Die Haut bekommt eine himbeer- bis fuchsinrote Färbung, wie WEISS, RAYNAUD, HOLM, FISCHER und wir selbst beobachtet haben; häufig findet man die Zeichen einer aktiven *Hyperämie*, nicht immer nur als Reaktionsstadium. Da wo diese stärker ausgebildet ist und länger anhält, erinnert das Bild an die Symptomatologie der Erythromelalgie, wie z. B. in einer Beobachtung ROLLESTONs.

Synkope und Asphyxie locale sind einander sehr verwandte Zustände, die, wie schon erwähnt, engste Beziehungen zueinander haben und nebeneinander und durcheinander bei demselben Individuum beobachtet werden. In helles Licht gerückt wird diese Verwandtschaft durch die capillarmikroskopischen Beobachtungen OTFRIED MÜLLERs, von denen später noch die Rede sein soll. Die Dauer der Zustände von Asphyxie ist sehr verschieden und äußerst wechselnd: wenige Minuten, aber auch in vereinzelten Beobachtungen Stunden und Tage.

Die Anfälle kommen ein- oder mehrmals am Tage wieder, können aber auch in mehrtägigen und noch längeren Zwischenräumen auftreten. Die Asphyxie hält meist länger an als die Synkope.

In seltenen Fällen kann man gelegentlich im Gebiet der Asphyxie eine Verengerung größerer Venen sehen. So notiert WEISS, daß wiederholt einzelne Venen des Fußrückens allmählich ihr Lumen veränderten und schließlich ganz verschwanden, während die Zehenrücken in dieser Zeit allmählich cyanotisch wurden.

Im Anschluß an die eben geschilderten vasomotorischen Symptome entsteht als *trophische* Störung in den typischen Fällen die *Gangrän*, und zwar auf verschiedene Weise; es kann zur Bildung kleiner Bläschen kommen, die mit serös blutigem, bisweilen schwärzlichem Inhalt gefüllt sind; diese öffnen sich und lassen kleine Excoriationen und Geschwüre zurück, die allmählich unter Bildung fester, oft dunkel pigmentierter Narben heilen. Ein andermal platzen die Bläschen nicht, sondern trocknen ein, die Oberhaut löst sich fetzenweise los. Auch ohne Bläschenbildung kann sich eine Verdichtung und Verdickung der Haut und eine Ablösung in festen braunen Schuppen ausbilden; es bleiben dann kleine, stecknadelkopf- bis linsengroße, verhärtete, meist etwas dunkler gefärbte Fleckchen und Borken zurück; geht der Prozeß weiter in die Tiefe, so entstehen größere Blasen und entsprechend größere Geschwüre, die nur sehr langsam heilen. Oder es kommt ohne Geschwürsbildung direkt zu einer meist trockenen Gangrän von verschiedenem Umfang; doch geht sie selten über eine ganze Phalange hinaus. Die Demarkation braucht für gewöhnlich lange Zeit, bei Ergriffensein einer ganzen Phalange dauert der Prozeß bis zur Vernarbung viele Monate. Die Gangrän betrifft meist *symmetrische* Stellen der Akra, Finger, Zehen, Ohren, Nase und ist seltener asymmetrisch. Die Verteilung der Gangrän ist im ganzen äußerst wechselnd und zeigt die mannigfaltigsten Kombinationen, ebenso übrigens auch die Verteilung der vasomotorischen Störungen. Es können alle Finger und Zehen betroffen sein, dazu auch Nase und Ohren; oder nur die Zehen oder Finger, Zehen und Nase; es gibt auch Fälle, in denen nur die Nasenspitze und Ohren oder auch nur die Nasenspitze oder nur die Ohren, besonders die Helices, befallen sind. MARCHAND und USSE beobachteten in monatlichem Zwischenraum bei einem Kranken zwei Krisen: in der ersten Krise waren Zehen, Nase, Ellenbogen betroffen; der zweite Anfall war viel milder und betraf die Lider. In seltenen Fällen kann die Gangrän eine erhebliche Ausdehnung bekommen; es ist klar, daß sich hier besonders leicht diagnostische Bedenken erheben, aber es unterliegt keinem Zweifel, daß auch solche Fälle vorkommen (BARLOW, AFFLECK, BEGG, ARNING).

Bei der zur Zeit der Untersuchung 31jährigen Patientin von ARNING stellten sich 10 Jahre vorher die ersten Spuren symmetrischer Gangrän an den Fingerspitzen ein; später traten geschwürige Prozesse an der Nasenspitze und den Ohrmuscheln auf, dann auch an den Füßen, stets begleitet von sehr heftigen Schmerzen. Bei der Untersuchung fanden sich von beiden Händen nur noch Stümpfe, an der kleinen verschrumpften Mittelhand saßen noch kurze, unförmliche Reste der Finger; nur die Daumen waren noch etwas besser erhalten.

Sehr instruktiv ist der folgende Fall, den GERMES und ISAAC-GEORGES beobachtet haben: 44jährig. Im Anschluß an eine Infektionskrankheit Auftreten der RAYNAUDschen Krankheit mit Gangrän: an beiden Händen traten in streng symmetrischer Anordnung gangränöse Stellen auf; am stärksten am Zeige- und kleinen Finger, schwächer am Mittelfinger, in ganz geringem Grade am Ringfinger; die Daumen blieben verschont. Patientin war Schleiferin in einer Metallfabrik; bei der Arbeit hielt sie Daumen und Ringfinger volarwärts gebeugt, während die übrigen Finger der ständigen Einwirkung des Wassers ausgesetzt waren; diese letzteren Finger wurden später gangränös.

Fälle von einseitiger, mehr oder minder ausgedehnter Gangrän sind in nicht allzu geringer Zahl beschrieben worden. So von COLSON, DOMINGUEZ, EICHHORST, MINOR u. a. In einem diagnostisch sehr schwierig zu beurteilenden Fall von BENDERS, den der Autor als halbseitige angiospastische Gangrän bezeichnet, fand sich eine bis zur Mitte des rechten Unterschenkels erstreckende Gangrän, während an den Fingern der rechten Hand sich eine mehr umschriebene Gangränbildung einstellte.

Über den Modus des Zustandekommens der Gangrän ist häufig diskutiert worden, ohne daß Klarheit geschaffen worden ist; einzelne Autoren führen sie auf die Wirkung des Angiospasmus zurück (RAYNAUD, MONROE, NIEKAU), eine Annahme, die uns mit Rücksicht auf die Fälle unbewiesen erscheint, in denen der Gangrän vasomotorische Erscheinungen nicht vorausgehen. KREIBICH (zit. nach MUCHA) hält die Gangrän für die Folge eines auf dem Nervenwege übermittelten Gefäßshocks, währenddessen das Gefäß dem von außen wirkenden Gewebs- oder Exsudatdruck durch einige Zeit nicht entgegenarbeiten könne und der vasomotorischen Anämie verfalle.

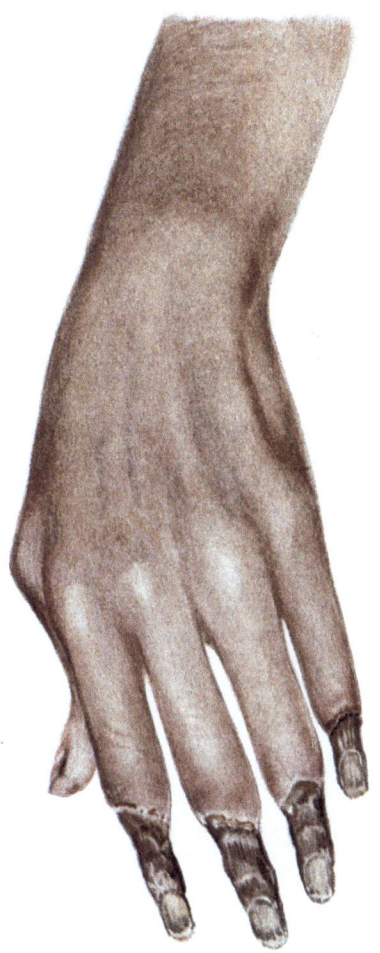

Abb. 2. Gangrän der Endphalangen bei RAYNAUDscher Krankheit. (Nach CASSIRER).

Die Gangrän ebenso wie die Asphyxie locale können sich ausnahmsweise an jeder beliebigen Stelle des Körpers lokalisieren. An der Zunge wurden mehrfach derartige Erscheinungen konstatiert. Einer unserer Patienten bekam häufig mit Synkope der Hände und Füße zusammen eine solche der Zunge. Bei einer Kranken, die HOESSLIN beobachtete, wurde im Anfall die ganze vordere Hälfte der Zunge weiß, ihr Volumen schien vermindert. An den Mamillae beobachtete RAYNAUD eine Asphyxie locale, FOX eine Synkope. Ähnliches wurde gesehen an den Lippen, an den Wangen, an den Nates, der Kreuzbeingegend, den Augenlidern. Eine Gangrän des Penis haben wir einmal beobachtet bei einem Manne, der früher an Malaria gelitten hatte, seit Jahren typische Migräneanfälle hatte, an Colitis membranacea litt, bei dem plötzlich unter furchtbaren Schmerzen eine Gangrän der Spitze des Penis eintrat, die mehrere Monate dauerte. Später hatte er Asphyxie an den Zehen, an den Händen eine leichte Neigung zur Cyanose. Die Schleimhaut der großen Labien ist befallen gewesen in dem Fall von WEISS, die der großen und kleinen Labien und der Vagina in dem Fall von LUSTIG. Vereinzelte oder multiple gangränöse Stellen sind zum Teil in ausgesprochen symmetrischer Verteilung auch an den Proximalteilen der Extremitäten und auch am Rumpf beobachtet worden. Einen hierhergehörenden Fall beschreibt MUMFORD: Im Anschluß an eine fieberhafte Erkrankung traten gangränöse Stellen an den Ohren, den kleinen Zehen, den Knien und an der Vorderseite des linken Oberschenkels auf; typische RAYNAUD-Erscheinungen gingen voraus. In einer Reihe derartiger Fälle (wir nennen die von KÖSTER,

SMITH, HUTCHINSON, RENHAW und DIDIER) fehlten alle vorausgehenden vasomotorischen Symptome. Sie bilden den Übergang zur multiplen neurotischen Hautgangrän bzw. gehören sie dieser an.

In sehr zahlreichen Fällen fanden sich neben den typischen Erscheinungen der Gangrän, zum Teil aber auch ohne solche, *sklerodermatische* Veränderungen an den gipfelnden Teilen, insbesondere an den Fingern, also eine Sklerodaktylie. In vielen dieser Fälle weicht das Bild sonst von der typischen RAYNAUDschen Krankheit in keiner Beziehung ab, in anderen nähert es sich, namentlich durch den von vornherein chronischen Verlauf, mehr den gewöhnlichen Bildern der Sklerodaktylie. Über die besonders engen Beziehungen, die zwischen diesen Erkrankungsformen herrschen und jede schärfere Abgrenzung unmöglich machen, ist an anderer Stelle noch zu sprechen (s. S. 327).

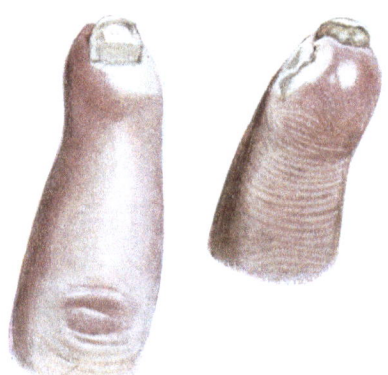

Abb. 3. RAYNAUDsche Krankheit. 65jähr. Frau. Nagelveränderungen. (Nach HELLER.)

Neben den gangränösen und sklerodermatischen Veränderungen treten anderweitige trophische Störungen zurück, fehlen aber doch nicht ganz. Es handelt sich dann häufig um eine dauernde Vermehrung des Bindegewebes, die in eine Verhärtung der befallenen Partien ausgeht, in anderen Fällen mehr um einen entgegengesetzten Zustand, der in einer übermäßigen Auflockerung des Gewebes besteht und zu einer abnormen Weichheit, zu einer Art Pseudoödem führt. Auf diese Weise werden in manchen Fällen die Hände und Füße größer. Starke Grade dieser Vergrößerung kommen selten zur Beobachtung. Gewöhnlich betrifft die Vergrößerung nur die Hände oder die Füße, über eine Vergrößerung der Nase berichten AKA und LAFON. Der Ernährungszustand der Nägel leidet vielfach. Sie werden abnorm brüchig, verdickt, längs gerieft, sie sind von vorn nach hinten gebogen, haben die Tendenz ins Fleisch einzuwachsen, werden geradezu klauenartig. Es finden sich subunguale Hyperkeratosen und Pachyonychien (MONTGOMERY, KLAPPENBACH), Leukonychien (BECKMANN). HELLER hat sich ausführlich mit diesen Fragen beschäftigt. Er stellt fest, daß die Nagelveränderungen in zwei Formen auftreten können, einerseits durch Gangrän in der Umgebung des Nagelorgans mit Übergreifen der Ernährungsstörung auf dieses; andererseits ist der Vorgang mehr direkt von den neurotrophischen Störungen abhängig. Er weist darauf hin, daß diese Tatsache auch aus der röntgenologisch leicht nachweisbaren trophischen Störung der Nagelphalanx hervorgeht, die eintritt lange bevor von dem klinischen Bild einer Gangrän die Rede ist.

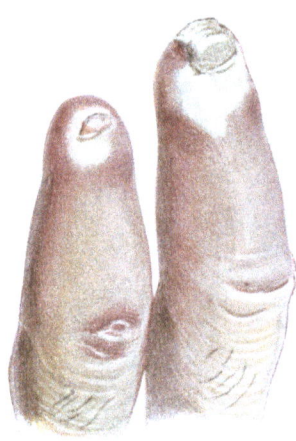

Abb. 4. RAYNAUDsche Krankheit. 65jährige Frau. Chronische rezidivierende Form ohne Nekrosebildung. (Nach HELLER.)

Zu erwähnen ist ferner noch das im Laufe der RAYNAUDschen Krankheit häufiger beobachtete Auftreten von Panaritien. Wir haben eine ganze Reihe derartiger Fälle gesehen. Es handelte sich zumeist um wenig umfangreiche Panaritien mit geringer Eiterproduktion, manchmal mit Knotenbildung in den

Fingerspitzen, die auch Kalkkonkremente enthalten (ORMSBY und EBERT, DAVIS), die zum Teil äußerst schmerzhaft waren und nur sehr langsam mit Hinterlassung kleiner, fester, strahliger Narben heilten. Die Schmerzhaftigkeit unterscheidet diese Panaritien von denen bei Syringomyelie.

Die Untersuchung mit *Röntgenstrahlen* hat uns weitgehende Aufklärung über das Verhalten der tieferen Teile, insbesondere der Knochen gebracht (OPPENHEIM, CASSIRER, LIPPMANN, BECK, LUSTIG, ALBERS-SCHÖNBERG, FOX, PHLEPS u. a.).

Diese Veränderungen können sehr frühzeitig auftreten, wahrscheinlich zugleich mit dem Auftreten der übrigen trophischen Störungen. Sie beschränken sich keineswegs nur auf die distalen Abschnitte der betreffenden Partien, also etwa nur auf die Endphalangen, sondern sind in viel größerer Ausdehnung nachweisbar, selbst bis zum Handgelenk hin; sie bestehen im wesentlichen in atrophischen Prozessen, die zu einer Verdünnung der Corticalis, zur Erweiterung der Zwischenräume und zu einer schärferen Zeichnung der Spongiosa führen. Bei stärkerer Ausbildung kommt es zum Verschwinden ganzer Knochenpartien; Teile von Phalangen, ja selbst ganze Phalangen gehen zum Teil offenbar durch wirkliche Resorption, nicht auf dem Wege der Nekrose und der Eliminierung nach außen verloren. Neben den atrophischen Prozessen kommen, wenn auch in viel geringerer Ausdehnung, auch hypertrophische Prozesse vor. Diese Veränderungen sind der Rückbildung fähig (PHLEPS). BORAK fand bei 12 Fällen in 40% pathologische Befunde, ohne daß etwa gleichzeitig eine Gangrän nachweisbar war. Die Veränderungen sind in der Hauptsache an den Spitzen der Endglieder lokalisiert, seltener an der Basis derselben oder an den anderen Phalangen. Es handelt sich um Substanzverluste, die durch Resorption nekrotisch gewordener Knochenteile zustandekommen müssen. In der Nachbarschaft dieser Resorptionsherde sieht man eine diffuse Kalkverarmung.

Betrachten wir nunmehr die bei der RAYNAUDschen Krankheit auftretenden *sensiblen* Erscheinungen. In der Mehrzahl der typischen Fälle sind *Schmerzen*, und zwar von beträchtlicher Intensität, vorhanden. Sie können von vornherein sehr hochgradig sein, sind nicht gerade selten überhaupt das erste Zeichen der Affektion. Sie können erst allmählich zu voller Höhe aufsteigen und dann ganz der Kurve der vasomotorisch-trophischen Anfälle folgen. Aber oft genug sind sie wenigstens während des größten Teiles der Krankheit nicht so sehr intensiv. Sie sind stets mehr oder weniger diffus, schlecht begrenzt, nehmen bald ein größeres, bald ein kleineres Gebiet ein, sind aber niemals in die Bahn eines Nerven gebannt. Sie sitzen oft anscheinend tief in den Knochen. Arm an Schmerzen oder ganz frei von solchen sind am ehesten diejenigen Fälle, in denen sich mehr allmählich eine Asphyxie entwickelte. Oft genug klagen die Kranken zuerst über Ameisenlaufen und Kältegefühl, die periodisch auftreten, besonders bei Eintritt der Kälte, während diese Erscheinungen in der warmen Jahreszeit nachlassen.

Auch die *objektiven Sensibilitätsstörungen* sind wechselnd und mannigfaltig; sie halten sich nicht an die Grenzen eines bestimmten peripheren Nerven oder radikulärer oder spinaler Segmente, sondern betreffen die gipfelnden Teile in verschiedener Ausdehnung. Meist handelt es sich um eine Abstumpfung der Berührungsempfindung, seltener sind auch die übrigen Qualitäten stärker betroffen. In der Mehrzahl unserer Fälle fanden wir aber überhaupt keine Sensibilitätsstörung. Wo sie vorkommt, ist sie nicht immer dauernd vorhanden, schwankt im Laufe der Beobachtung. In einigen unserer Fälle fanden wir eine ausgesprochene Druckschmerzhaftigkeit des Ganglion cervicale supremum.

Von *sekretorischen* Störungen spielen Anomalien der Schweißsekretion eine große Rolle. Es kommt Hyperidrosis und Anidrosis vor. Häufiger wird das

Vorliegen einer Hyperidrosis verzeichnet (RAYNAUD, RHAM, VULPIAN, MONRO). Im Fall von PHLEPS bestand ein so erhebliches Schwitzen der Hohlhand, daß der Schweiß in Tropfen ablief.

Über primäre *motorische* Störungen ist nicht viel zu berichten. Lähmungen bestimmter Muskeln und Muskelgruppen gehören nicht zum Bilde der Krankheit. Nur WEISS sah einmal eine atrophisch degenerative Parese der Musculi interossei und der Muskeln am kleinen Finger- und Daumenballen in seinem auch sonst außerordentlich merkwürdigen Fall, in dem vorübergehend Anfälle von syringomyelitischer Sensibilitätsstörung, von Aphasie, von Nekrosen an verschiedenen Stellen des Körpers, von oculopupillären Symptomen eintraten. Sonst sind gelegentlich leichtere Atrophien im Gebiete der vasomotorischen Störungen beobachtet worden (RIVA, SCHEIBER, OPPENHEIM, PHLEPS, BENDER, eigene Beobachtung). Die Atrophie pflegt in diesen Fällen meist stärker zu sein als die Funktionsstörung. Degenerative Veränderungen der elektrischen Erregbarkeit finden sich nicht, wohl aber quantitative Störungen derselben, die ebenso wie die Funktionsstörung von der größeren oder geringeren Intensität der vasomotorischen Störungen sich abhängig erweist. In einigen unserer Fälle wurde über leichte motorische Reizerscheinungen, über ein krampfhaftes Verziehen der Finger und Zehen geklagt.

Sehr interessant ist das Vorkommen passagerer Kontraktionszustände in den größeren Arterien, das zuerst von RAYNAUD beschrieben worden ist, der in einem seiner Fälle eine Kontraktion der Arteria centralis retinae und ihrer Verzweigungen beobachten konnte. Damit parallel ging eine Trübung des Sehvermögens. Diese Anfälle wechselten mit den Anfällen von Asphyxie an den Extremitäten ab. Ähnliche Beobachtungen sind von MORGAN, BLAND, WARREN, ROQUES, FRIEDEMANN, GARRIGUES, MANTLE, ROGER-SEDAN-AYMÈS gemacht worden. CALHOUN berichtet über einen Fall, bei dem neben den RAYNAUDschen Symptomen auch eine Erythromelalgie bestand. Es fand sich ferner eine Cyanose der Retina: der Fundus war dunkler als gewöhnlich, die nasale Papillenseite verschwommen und leicht ödematös, die retinalen Gefäße wiesen eine Vermehrung auf. APPELBAUM und LERNER sahen einen Patienten, der als erstes Symptom Migräneanfälle und Sehstörungen darbot. Es fand sich später im Raynaudanfall beiderseits Stauungspapille, Hämorrhagien und Exsudatbildung in der Netzhaut. Die Augensymptome bildeten sich zurück. Übrigens konnten auch außerhalb des Gebietes der RAYNAUDschen Krankheit gelegentlich von WAGENMANN, WEISS, BENSON solche passageren Kontraktionen der Netzhaut konstatiert werden. BLAAUW hat diese Fälle einer scharfen Kritik unterzogen, die uns aber über das Ziel hinauszuschießen scheint. BORGHESAN sah anfallsweise Labyrinthstörungen als vasomotorische Erscheinung auftreten. Auch an der Arteria radialis sind mehrfach ähnliche Beobachtungen angestellt worden (BERNHARDT, FUCHS, HOLST, PASTEUR, CARP, CUSHING u. a.).

Sehr bemerkenswert ist ein Fall von WESTPHAL: Bei einer an Epilepsie und Demenz leidenden Kranken kam es im Anschluß an Erregungen zum Auftreten von schmerzhaften, tonischen Krampfanfällen an den unteren Extremitäten und zugleich zu Anfällen von Asphyxie und Syncope locale. Während der Anfälle verschwanden die Fußpulse, die in den anfallsfreien Zeiten deutlich fühlbar waren. Das ist also eine Analogie zur Kontraktion der Retinalarterien während der vasomotorischen Anfälle.

Der *Blutdruck* in den anfallsfreien Zeiten ist meist normal. Untersuchungen während der Schmerzattacken geben aus naheliegenden Gründen keine einwandfreien Resultate. MONTGOMERY und CULVER fanden an der befallenen Extremität einen Blutdruck von 170 mm gegen 180 mm auf der gesunden Seite; erst allmählich wurde der Blutdruck auf beiden Seiten gleichmäßig, und zwar in dem Maße, in dem die Schmerzen und Beschwerden abnahmen. RUD stellte niedrigen Blutdruck (100/60), subnormale Temperaturen (36,8 rectal), langsamen Puls, niedrige Blutzuckerwerte (0,065 und 0,078) fest und bezog diese Symptome auf eine Nebenniereninsuffizienz. Messungen des peripheren Blutdruckes an den Fingern vermittels des GÄRTNERschen Tonometers zeigten uns häufig das Resultat, daß die durch Umschnürung hervorgerufene künstliche Syncope locale den mechanischen Reiz, bzw. die mechanische Blutabschnürung oft für lange Zeit überdauerte, so daß nach Abnehmen des Ringes eine vollkommene Blutleere bestand und der Blutdruck in den Fingerarterien so für eine Weile noch Null blieb. Die mit dem GÄRTNERschen Apparat angestellten Untersuchungen ergaben fernerhin zahlenmäßige Belege für die Größendifferenzen der in den peripherstern Partien der Finger herrschenden Blutdruckverhältnisse, indem bei nebeneinanderliegenden Fingern Zahlen zwischen 0 und 100 vorkamen.

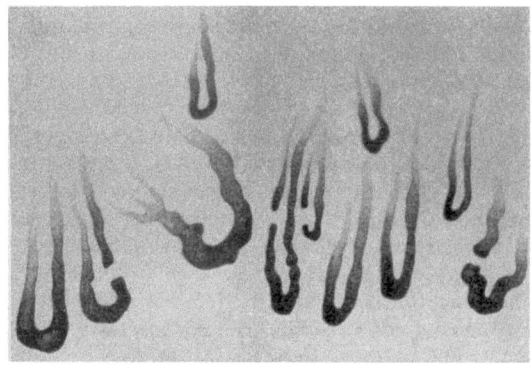

Abb. 5. Verlängerte, stark erweiterte und deformierte Capillaren bei RAYNAUDscher Krankheit. Vergr. 70 fach. Nagelrand. (Aus O. MÜLLER: Capillaren. 1922.)

Plethysmographische Untersuchungen sind von VEDRELLI, CASTELLINO und CARDI, CURSCHMANN, STEPHENS, LANDIS und besonders von PHLEPS und SIMONS vorgenommen worden. SIMONS fand auch im Latenzstadium, d. h. also außerhalb der Anfälle, eine funktionelle Schwäche der vasomotorischen Zentren, die sich im Schwanken der Reflexe, dem versteckten Hinken der Zentren, in einer anderen Verarbeitung der Reize, einer rascheren Ermüdung, einer paradoxen Reaktion verriet. Ein völliges Fehlen der Gefäßreflexe, das CURSCHMANN gefunden haben wollte, besteht nicht; das hat auch STURSBERG betont.

Ein besonderes Interesse beanspruchen die capillar-mikroskopischen Beobachtungen, welche in den letzten Jahren Gegenstand der Forschung gewesen sind (HOLLAND und MEYER, WEISS, PARRISIUS, HALPERT u. a.). Die Untersuchungen wurden vor, während und nach den Anfällen ausgeführt. HALPERT fand neben erheblich erweiterten Riesenschlingen im gleichen Gesichtsfeld fadenförmig dünne Capillaren. Die Strömung im Intervall war träge, körnig, zeitweise trat Stase ein. Im Anfall zeigten bis auf einige wenige Schlingen mit langsamer, körniger Strömung alle Schlingen Stase und bläulich-violette Färbung. Außerdem beobachtete die Verfasserin während des Anfalls Auswüchse und Vorbuckelungen der Capillaren, die mehrere Minuten bestehen blieben; daneben waren ganz leere Gefäßabschnitte zu sehen. Anscheinend war dieses Bild durch eine äußerst langsam verlaufene Peristaltik oder durch einen lang anhaltenden lokalen Spasmus der Capillaren bedingt. Die Reaktion auf lokale Wärme- und Kälteeinwirkung trat langsamer als in normalen Fällen auf. Nach einem heißen Bad erfolgte keine Erweiterung der Capillaren, zeitweise vielmehr eine Verengerung. Dagegen kam bei längerer Wärmeeinwirkung in allen Schlingen, auch in den gestauten Riesenschlingen, eine manchmal recht erhebliche Beschleunigung der Strömung in Gang. Auch WEISS fand schwere zirkulatorische Störungen: Stase in den Capillaren mit enorm erweiterten, gestauten, manchmal schon nach Auftropfen von Öl makroskopisch sichtbaren Capillarschenkeln, vollkommene Unterbrechung der Blutsäule. Auch LERICHE und POLICARD berichten über die Veränderungen der Capillarzirkulation bei der RAYNAUDschen Krankheit: im Augenblick des Anfalls werden die Capillaren fast unsichtbar. Die seitlichen Teile der Gefäßbucht werden fadenförmig und sind fast kaum mehr wahrzunehmen. Der Scheitel der Bucht verändert sich nicht, sondern bleibt gut durchblutet. Nach einiger Zeit beginnen sich die seitlichen Teile wieder mit Blut zu füllen. Nach dem Abklingen des Anfalles sind sowohl die seitlichen Teile als auch der Scheitel der Gefäßbucht stärker mit Blut angefüllt.

CLAUDE und TINEL machten die Beobachtung, daß der Spasmus in den peripheren Capillaren beginnt und sich langsam proximalwärts ausbreitet; dabei erfolgte eine erhebliche Verminderung der Amplitude des Radialpulses. GRENET und ISAAC-GEORGES haben, wie die vorher genannten Autoren, versucht, auf dem Wege der oscillatorischen Methode das Vorhandensein arterieller Schädigungen nachzuweisen. In 5 Fällen haben sie Messungen angestellt. Sie stellten fest, daß im Verlauf der ischämischen Krise die vasokonstriktorischen Spasmen nicht nur die terminalen Arterien ergriffen, sondern auch die großen Arterien des Vorderarmes. Alle 5 Kranken zeigten eine gewisse Asymmetrie in der Verteilung der vasomotorischen Störungen. Bei wiederholten Prüfungen zwischen Anfällen wurde stets eine oscillometrische Asymmetrie festgestellt nebst einer mangelhaften Zirkulation auf der Seite, auf die die Erscheinungen des Raynaud übergingen. In allen Fällen zeigte sich zwischen den Anfällen eine Zirkulationsstörung an den Gefäßen dort, wo sich im Verlauf die spasmodischen Phänomene offenbarten. Sie stellen fest, daß für dieses Phänomen die einzige Erklärung in dem Bestehen arterieller Schädigungen zu suchen ist [1].

RUD sah deutliche Unterschiede während und außerhalb des Anfalles; während des Überganges von der Synkope zur Asphyxie sah er stark erweiterte Capillaren; wurde dieselbe Gegend 5 Minuten lang in Wasser gewärmt, so waren nur noch wenige Capillaren erweitert. BROWN sah in der anfallsfreien Zeit erweiterte Schlingen und Riesenschlingen. Während des Anfalls verschwanden einige Schlingen oder waren nur teilweise mit stagnierendem Blute gefüllt. Darauf erfolgte Erweiterung und starke Anfüllung der Capillaren mit cyanotischem, stagnierendem Blute. Im letzten Stadium beobachtete man starke Durchblutung. Ähnliche Bilder sahen LERICHE und POLICARD, NIEKAU, MALCHERS. Besonders wichtig erscheint der klinisch und anatomisch einwandfrei durchuntersuchte Fall von RIEDER. Über die anatomischen Ergebnisse wird an der entsprechenden Stelle berichtet werden.

Es handelte sich um eine 36jährige Kranke, bei der als erstes Symptom während der Schwangerschaft Kribbeln in den Fingerspitzen auftrat; nach einem Jahr bot sie das Bild einer ausgesprochenen RAYNAUDschen Krankheit. Das capillarmikroskopische Bild war vor der Operation ungefähr mit dem identisch, das die anderen Autoren beschrieben haben (PARRISIUS, O. MÜLLER). Nach der operativen Entfernung des Ganglion stellatum zeigte sich eine wesentliche Erweiterung der Capillaren an der operierten Seite. Die Strömung in den Capillaren wurde langsamer, die Stasenbildung hörte auf. Auf der linken Seite blieb das capillarmikroskopische Bild auch nach der Operation unverändert.

Alle diese Beobachtungen bestätigen die von O. MÜLLER bereits 1922 geäußerte Ansicht, daß häufig im Capillarsystem spastische und atonische Schlingen zusammenliegen, daß sich also Reizung und Lähmung je nach den momentan vorliegenden inneren und äußeren Einflüssen kombinieren, wenn auch zuzugeben sei, daß im allgemeinen während der Synkope die Spasmen der Arterien, Capillaren und Venen vorherrschen, während bei der Asphyxie arterielle Atonien und venöse Spasmen auftreten. Eindeutige Schlüsse seien aus den vorhandenen Befunden nicht zu ziehen. Eine ähnliche Auffassung vertritt auch PARRISIUS in seiner mit zahlreichen instruktiven Abbildungen versehenen Arbeit.

---

[1] Zit. nach dem Referat von STIEFLER: Zbl. Neur. 44, 617.

Die Beobachtungen über die abnorme Kleinheit und Enge der Arterien sind bei Ausführung der Sympathektomie von vielen Beobachtern, auch von uns selbst und zuletzt von KÜMMELL gemacht worden. Zweifellos handelt es sich dabei mindestens zum Teil um eine angeborene Kleinheit (Hypoangie), wie sie in ganz identischer Form schon früher beim intermittierenden Hinken nachgewiesen ist. Das *Herz* ist in den unkomplizierten Fällen normal. Der Puls ist außerhalb der Anfälle stets deutlich fühlbar, oft beschleunigt, gelegentlich kommt es zu Attacken von paroxysmaler Tachykardie.

Es gibt aber eine große Reihe von Fällen, in denen *neben* den Symptomen der RAYNAUDschen Krankheit solche einer organischen Erkrankung des *Herzens* und der *Gefäße* vorlagen. MONRO fand sie unter 180 Fällen 22 Mal.

In allen diesen Fällen macht die Rubrizierung des Leidens erhöhte Schwierigkeiten, da auch eine andersartige endarteriitische, arteriosklerotische oder embolische Gangrän Erscheinungen hervorrufen kann, die in sehr vielen Beziehungen den RAYNAUDschen ähneln. Zweifellos ist eine Reihe von Fällen dieser Art als RAYNAUDsche Krankheit beschrieben worden, die nicht als eine solche aufgefaßt werden darf.

So erwähnt z. B. BARMWATER die Beobachtung bei einem neugeborenen Mädchen, das hochgradig cyanotisch war. Nach Eintreten einer Extremitätengangrän erfolgte Exitus nach 9 Tagen. Die Sektion ergab Hypertrophie des Herzens und Mißbildung desselben: Defekt im Septum atriorum, offenen Ductus Botalli, Isthmusstenose der Aorta.

Auf der anderen Seite gibt es aber doch Fälle, in denen neben den typischen RAYNAUDschen Symptomen und unabhängig von ihnen ein organisches Herzleiden vorliegt (CHALIER, CUNNINGHAM). Auch die Kombination einer diffusen *Arteriosklerose* mit Erscheinungen der RAYNAUDschen Krankheit, wo diese in typisch intermittierender Weise beobachtet wurden, kommt ganz bestimmt vor. Und was die *Lues* angeht, so gibt es Fälle akquirierter (MORGAN, RIVA, PHLEPS, eigene Beobachtungen, GHELFI, LISSER und zahlreiche andere) oder hereditärer (HUTCHINSON, KRISOWSKI, RIETSCHEL, SPIELER, STÖLTZNER, BOSANYI u. a.) Lues, auf deren Boden wahrscheinlich durch Vermittlung einer spezifischen Gefäßerkrankung typische Erscheinungen RAYNAUDscher Krankheit sich entwickeln können. In manchen dieser Fälle wird der enge Zusammenhang durch den günstigen Einfluß einer spezifischen Therapie deutlich demonstriert. In der Mehrzahl der mitgeteilten Beobachtungen ist aber entweder die Diagnose nicht einwandfrei oder die ätiologische Bedeutung der Lues nicht sichergestellt.

Aus den letzten Jahren stammen einschlägige Beobachtungen von MARCUS: Mutter Tabes, Pat. leidet an Lues congenita mit luischer Meningitis im unteren Cervicalsegment, Raynaudsymptome an der linken Hand, Miosis. Auf Jodkali Besserung. ALURRALDE und SPOTA: Raynaud an der rechten Hand, später auch an der linken, Hypaesthesia dolorosa der Hände ohne objektive Gefühlsstörung.

Ähnliche Schwierigkeiten macht das Vorkommen RAYNAUDscher Symptome zusammen mit den Erscheinungen einer *Schrumpfniere* (eigene Beobachtung, KRONER, GIBERT, ATKIN, ROQUES, COLSON, BLAND). Daß die Syncope locale häufig eine Erscheinung der Nephritis ist, ist bekannt. In diesen Fällen hat sie einen direkt toxischen Ursprung. Bei der Schrumpfniere finden sich ja auch ganz ähnliche Sehstörungen wie beim Raynaud, die zum Teil vielleicht auch auf einer Kontraktion der Arteria centralis retinae beruhen, besonders als Vorläufer bzw. Teilerscheinung urämischer Komplexe. Unter diesen Verhältnissen haben die RAYNAUDschen Symptome natürlich nur einen akzidentellen Wert. PARRISIUS weist darauf hin, daß die Mikrocapillarbilder bei Nephritiskranken oft ganz ähnliche Befunde zeigen wie bei der RAYNAUDschen Krankheit. In manchen Fällen handelt es sich auf der anderen Seite doch wieder um die Kombination zweier voneinander unabhängiger Symptomenbilder. Gelegentlich ist auch eine intermittierende Albuminurie beobachtet worden, wo bei den

Schwankungen der RAYNAUDschen Krankheit auch der Eiweißgehalt des Urins schwankte. Auch Melliturie bzw. Diabetes mellitus ist festgestellt worden. Ebenso wird auch ein Diabetes insipidus erwähnt. Vereinzelt wurden RAYNAUDsche Symptome bei Arthritis urica beobachtet; auch wir haben diese Kombination gesehen und sind geneigt, gewisse Beziehungen zwischen einer individuellen oder familiären Disposition zur Gicht und dem Auftreten von gewissen paroxysmalen vasomotorischen Erscheinungen vom Typus Raynaud oder vom anderen Typus (angioneurotische Ödeme) anzunehmen. Eine ähnliche Ansicht vertritt noch ASSMANN, dessen Kranker gleichzeitig QUINKEs Ödem und periphere Gefäßstörungen darbot.

Besonders interessante Beziehungen bestehen zwischen der paroxysmalen *Hämoglobinurie* und der RAYNAUDschen Krankheit; derartige Beobachtungen sind vielfach beschrieben worden (SOUTHEY, DRUITT, HUTCHINSON, OSLER, PRESTORA u. a.). Das Verhältnis dieser beiden Erscheinungsreihen ist ein wechselndes. In der einen Gruppe stechen durchaus die RAYNAUDschen Symptome hervor und die der Hämoglobinurie kommen nur gelegentlich zum Vorschein. In anderen Fällen ist es umgekehrt. Auch das zeitliche Verhältnis ist mannigfachen Variationen unterworfen. Es gibt Fälle, in denen die Hämoglobinurie der Asphyxie locale vorausgeht, während später dann beide Affektionen zusammen vorkommen; Fälle, wo erst die Anfälle von Asphyxie locale erscheinen und dann sich zu ihnen die von Hämoglobinurie gesellen, wo dann beide Symptomenkomplexe weiter regelmäßig zusammen auftreten, und schließlich solche, wo Hämoglobinurie und Asphyxie locale stets alternieren. Über einen sehr charakteristischen Fall, in dem paroxysmale Hämoglobinurie jahrelang vorausgegangen war und später noch das sehr typische Bild der RAYNAUDschen Krankheit bestand, haben wir berichtet. Es gibt eine Reihe von Erklärungsmöglichkeiten für die Tatsache des häufigen Zusammenvorkommens von Raynaud und Hämoglobinurie. In einer Anzahl der mitgeteilten Fälle gewinnt man durchaus den Eindruck, daß die Hämoglobinurie nur eine Teilerscheinung eines allgemeineren Leidens ist, als das man die RAYNAUDsche Krankheit anzusehen hätte *(Abercrombie)*. Die Hämoglobinurie könnte dabei auf doppelte Weise entstehen. Den einen Erklärungsmodus können wir von Versuchen ableiten, die schon früher von EHRLICH und BOAS angestellt wurden. BOAS fand nämlich bei gewissen Personen, daß, wenn sie den vermittels einer elastischen Ligatur abgebundenen Finger einer Hand eine Viertelstunde lang in Eiswasser steckten, in jeder dem Finger entnommenen Blutprobe die charakteristischen Kennzeichen der Hämoglobinurie vorhanden waren, während die Untersuchung des übrigen Körperblutes ein fast ganz negatives Resultat ergab. So könnte man annehmen, daß sekundär in gewissen Fällen von Asphyxie locale von den asphyktischen Extremitätenenden aus eine Hämoglobinämie und dadurch eine Hämoglobinurie erzeugt wird. MONRO ist geneigt, diese Erklärung ganz allgemein zu akzeptieren. Eine zweite Möglichkeit wäre die, daß es durch einen Vorgang analog dem, der sich in den Arterien der Gliedmaßen abspielt und hier zur äußerlich sofort sichtbaren Asphyxie locale und zu bisweilen nachweisbaren Blutveränderungen führt, in den Nierenarterien oder anderen Arterien innerer Organe direkt zur Hämoglobinämie käme; diese Erklärung würde besonders für die Fälle sich eignen, in denen die Hämoglobinurie der Asphyxie locale vorausgeht (HENRY, eigene Beobachtung) oder wo beide Zustände miteinander alternieren. MONRO widerspricht freilich einem solchen Erklärungsversuch; er meint, es müßte in einem solchen Falle nicht Hämoglobinurie, sondern Hämaturie die Folge sein; die geringen Beimischungen körperlicher Blutbestandteile, die sich im Urin in mehreren Fällen fanden, bezieht er auf die durch das ausgeschiedene Hämoglobin bedingte sekundäre

Hyperämie der Nieren. HAIG sucht sowohl die Anfälle von Asphyxie locale als auch die von Hämoglobinurie auf eine Anhäufung von Harnsäure im Blut zurückzuführen, wodurch einerseits ein die peripheren Arterien zur Kontraktion bringender Reiz, andererseits ein Zerfall der roten Blutkörperchen mit ihren Folgen herbeigeführt würde; hiernach wären RAYNAUDsche Erscheinungen und Hämoglobinurie Folgen derselben Ursache, also koordiniert, und ständen nicht im Verhältnis von Ursache und Wirkung. Doch hat diese Erklärung sicher nur ganz beschränkte Geltung.

In vielen Fällen wird man annehmen müssen, daß die Grundkrankheit die RAYNAUDsche Krankheit ist, und daß die befallenen Individuen durch eine auffallende Resistenzunfähigkeit ihrer roten Blutkörperchen ausgezeichnet sind; dadurch kommt es von den Nieren oder von den peripheren Teilen her zur Hämoglobinämie oder Hämoglobinurie. Wodurch diese abnorm geringe Vitalität der roten Blutkörperchen bedingt ist, ist hier, wie aber auch sonst in den Fällen von paroxysmaler Hämoglobinurie, zweifelhaft. Man hat an den schädigenden Einfluß früherer Lues und Intermittens (BYWATER, TOLESA u. a.) gedacht und mit der betreffenden spezifischen Therapie auch Erfolge erzielt. Auch in einzelnen Fällen von RAYNAUDscher Krankheit plus Hämoglobinurie findet man diese Krankheiten in der Anamnese. Wir möchten im übrigen nicht behaupten, daß diese Erklärung von der Rolle der sekundären Hämoglobinurie überall ausreicht, Das Bestehen einer primären Intoxikation des Blutes, die zur Hämoglobinämie führt, und die dann ihrerseits erst wieder die lokale Asphyxie bedingen könnte, muß ebenfalls in Erwägung gezogen werden. Sichere Hinweise für eine solche Annahme im einzelnen Falle besitzen wir nicht, wenn wir nicht das zeitliche und Intensitätsverhältnis der beiden Erscheinungsreihen dafür gelten lassen wollen. BOGAERT und DELBECKE, auch CHVOSTEK fanden Hypocholesterinämie und Störung der Urinmengenausscheidung. IWAI, SEISHIRO und NINHEI-SAI fanden in einem einzigen Fall im Serum ein Autoagglutinin, das in der Kälte die Erythrocyten zum Verkleben brachte; der Vorgang war in der Wärme reversibel. Sie bauten auf diesen Befund die Theorie auf, daß eine durch agglutinierte rote Blutkörperchen hervorgerufene Versteifung der Capillaren in ihrem Falle die Symptome der RAYNAUDschen Krankheit hervorgebracht habe.

In einer Reihe von Fällen, in denen über RAYNAUDsche Krankheit berichtet wird, finden sich zugleich noch Symptome, die auf Erkrankung des zentralen oder peripheren Nervensystems hinweisen. Unter den Erscheinungen eines organischen Hirnleidens waren es am häufigsten Symptome der Hemiplegie, die sich mit solchen Erscheinungen verbanden (HOCHENEGG, RAYNAUD, BEADER, OSLER, SIMPSON, DUKEMAN u. a.), aber auch eine Pseudobulbärparalyse (BRISSAUD und SALIN), eine Dementia paralytica (ISOVESCO, NAUDASCHEW, ALLESSANDRI und MINGAZZINI), Hydrocephalus (BARLOW, BRENGUES), Paralysis agitans (STOLKIND) wurden beobachtet. Gliosis fanden HOCHENEGG, GOWERS, POSPELOFF, TEDESCO, CHIAVUTTINI, Tabes HOCHENEGG, KORNFELD, PERRIN, multiple Sklerose STRAUSS, Poliomyelitis anterior chronica McBRIDE und BARKER LEWELLYS, Tetanie MARGOLIN. CALMAN sah einmal die Erscheinungen eines Tumor medullae spinalis, in einem zweiten Fall solche eines Tumor der Cauda equina. Die Kombination mit Pachymeningitis cervicalis hypertrophica erwähnt BUSY; MARCUS sah gleichzeitig Horner links und Raynaud linke Hand; dann traten Paresen und Atrophien an der linken Hand und am Arm auf; er nimmt eine luische Meningitis im unteren Cervicalsegment an. Die Kombination mit einer Radiculitis chronica sahen GILBERT und VILLARET, Dermatomyositis GRUSZECKA. Viermal haben wir die Kombination von RAYNAUDscher Krankheit mit Dystrophia musculorum progressiva beobachtet. Zweimal handelte es sich dabei um voll ausgebildete Krankheitsbilder, die ziemlich gleichmäßig progredient waren. Es ist nicht wahrscheinlich, daß das nur eine zufällige Kombination ist.

Rülf fand bei einem neuropathisch stark belasteten Individuum, das in der Kindheit an Tics gelitten hatte, neben Raynaudschen Symptomen Migräne, eine intermittierende Gangstörung, Stenokardie und Erythromelie der Nasenspitze. Das Entstehen oder Verschwinden der Raynaudschen Symptome wurde durch psychische Momente beeinflußt. Heuk hat ausgerechnet, daß $4^1/_2\%$ aller Fälle von Raynaud eine Verbindung mit geistigen Störungen zeigen. Bland und Macpherson sahen Raynaudsymptome bei akuter Manie, Shaw und Targowla bei Melancholie, Ritti bei zirkulärer Psychose, Dide und Ducocher bei Katatonie, Marchand und Usse bei seniler Demenz. Im Falle Macphersons bestand ein auffallender Parallelismus zwischen vasomotorischen Erscheinungen und psychischem Verhalten. Die Kranke Heuks zeigte allgemein nervöse Symptome, periodische Melancholie, hysterische Krampfanfälle und Störungen der inneren Sekretion; die vasomotorischen Erscheinungen setzten meist ungefähr zu gleicher Zeit wie die Depression ein. Keineswegs in allen diesen Fällen ist die Bezeichnung „Raynaudsche Krankheit" für die gefundenen vasomotorisch-trophischen Symptome berechtigt. Am interessantesten ist die Kombination von Syringomyelie und Raynaudsymptomen wegen des Streiflichtes, das von hier aus auf die Pathogenese des Leidens fällt.

In der Literatur ist auch vielfach die Rede von einem Zusammenvorkommen von peripherer Neuritis und Raynaudscher Krankheit. Wenn man schärfer zusieht und sich auch die Kriegserfahrungen vergegenwärtigt, so ergibt sich das Resultat, daß Symptome, die den Raynaudschen ähnlich sind, gelegentlich auch durch eine Neuritis hervorgebracht werden können, wodurch aber keineswegs bewiesen ist, daß die Raynaudsche Krankheit selbst von einer Neuritis abhängt. In dieses Gebiet gehören auch die Fälle, bei denen der Raynaudsche Symptomenkomplex im Anschluß an eine Halsrippe aufgetreten ist.

Schon in dem Kapitel „Ätiologie" ist betont worden, daß die Symptome der Raynaudschen Krankheit sich häufig bei Personen finden, die mehr oder minder deutliche Zeichen einer allgemeinen oder speziellen funktionellen Erkrankung des Nervensystems darbieten. Dieser Punkt bedarf noch einer besonderen Berücksichtigung. Ängstliche, nervöse, aufgeregte Menschen sind die Mehrzahl der Kranken, die die Symptome der Raynaudschen Krankheit darbieten, aber doch nicht alle.

In einer Gruppe dieser Fälle treten neben den lokalen Erscheinungen der Raynaudschen Krankheit die Symptome *vasomotorischer* und *kardialer* Labilität sehr in den Vordergrund. Viele dieser Kranken bieten Erscheinungen dar, die von Herz und Solis-Cohen unter dem Namen der vasomotorischen Ataxie zusammengefaßt sind. Es handelt sich bei diesen Kranken um einen Zustand von Instabilität des Mechanismus der Blutzirkulation, der durch die Leichtigkeit der Störung und die langsame Restitution des Gleichgewichts in den Funktionen des Herzgefäßapparates charakterisiert ist. Die Erscheinungen sind am auffälligsten am Herzen und den peripheren Gefäßen, aber, wie man annehmen darf, kommen auch analoge Zustände in den Gefäßen der Drüsen und Eingeweide, besonders an den Nieren, am Magendarmapparat, am Gehirn vor. Die Phänomene sind entweder spastischen oder paretischen Charakters, oft finden sich beide Arten der Störung bei dem gleichen Patienten. Sie sind stets in gewissem Grade paroxysmal und treten in den mannigfaltigsten klinischen Erscheinungen zutage. Es sind asthmatische Attacken dahin gerechnet worden, Heufieberanfälle, gastrische und enterale Schmerzanfälle und Sekretionsstörungen, Polyurie, Menorrhagien, die verschiedene Formen der kardiovasculären Störungen, die paroxysmale Tachykardie, Angina pectoris vasomotoria (Schott), allerhand anderweitige Ungleichmäßigkeiten in der Verteilung des Blutes in der Haut. Neuere Forschungen haben sich bemüht, für die Genese dieser Erscheinungen, die bis dahin einfach als Ausdruck einer vasomotorischen Ataxie oder einer vasomotorischen Instabilität galten, speziellere Bedingungen ausfindig zu machen und sind in Anlehnung an die differenten pharmakologischen Eigenschaften der verschiedenen Unterabteilungen des großen vegetativen Systems dazu übergegangen, diese Einzelsymptome schärfer zu definieren und abzugrenzen; es ist der Begriff der Vagotonie und Sympathicotonie geschaffen worden, es ist eine Gegensätzlichkeit zwischen vagotonischen und sympathicotonischen Erscheinungsreihen angenommen worden. Es hat sich aber alsbald herausgestellt, daß die supponierte Gegensätzlichkeit in Wirklichkeit nicht existiert, daß es also nicht angeht, auf diesem Boden neue Krankheitsbilder zu schaffen. Dagegen unterliegt es keinem Zweifel, daß diese neuen Forschungen zu einer Vertiefung unserer Kenntnisse von der Entstehung und Bedingtheit der einzelnen Symptome beigetragen haben.

Im allgemeinen wird man annehmen dürfen, daß in der Pathologie der RAYNAUDschen Krankheit *sympathicotonische* Symptome überwiegen, und zwar, wie wir bisher schon gesehen haben, *Reizerscheinungen* im Bereich des sympathischen Systems im engeren Sinne. Dafür sprechen die zahlreichen konstriktorischen und dilatatorischen Gefäßphänomene, die im Mittelpunkt der Krankheit stehen, dafür aber auch eine Reihe von Nebensymptomen.

Ausführlichere Untersuchungen über die Toleranz Raynaudkranker gegenüber den verschiedenen pharmakologischen Agentien, dem Adrenalin, dem Atropin, dem Pilocarpin, liegen bisher nur in geringer Zahl vor. Wir selbst haben nur vereinzelte Untersuchungen angestellt, die kein einwandfreies Resultat ergeben haben, bzw. auch hier erkennen ließen, daß teils sympathicotrope, teils vagotrope Dispositionen vorhanden sind. PARRISIUS hat eine Reihe Untersuchungen nach dieser Richtung hin angestellt. Bei 25 Patienten hat er Adrenalininjektionen von 1 cmm subcutan vorgenommen. Blutdruck und Puls wurden alle 3 Minuten beobachtet. Die meisten haben sehr schwach darauf reagiert. Bei einigen fehlte sogar Steigerung von Blutdruck und Pulsfrequenz. Nur in zwei schwereren Fällen mit anfallsweiser Asphyxie und Synkope der Finger (einer hatte auch symmetrische Gangrän) erzielte er stärkere Reaktionen. Bei dieser wurde die Farbe der vorher scharlachroten Brust cyanotisch. Mikroskopisch beobachtete er enge arterielle Schenkel der Capillaren bei weiten venösen und weiten Gefäßen des subpapillären Plexus und Stagnieren des Blutstromes, der vorher gut von statten gegangen war; die andere bekam einen Anfall von schwarzblauer Verfärbung der Finger, dem PARRISIUS jedoch geringe Bedeutung beimißt, da bei ihr schon geringe psychische Einflüsse das gleiche bewirkten. Auf *Atropin* bei einmaliger Injektion von 1 mg subcutan sah er bei 15 Patienten keinen nachweisbaren Erfolg, weder im Allgemeinzustand, noch an den Capillaren, hat aber beobachtet, daß längerer Atropingebrauch die Beschwerden dieser Patienten wesentlich linderte. Besonders stark war die Wirkung auf Pilocarpin bei den an schwereren vasomotorischen Störungen leidenden Patienten; enormer Schweißausbruch und Speichelfluß, die vorher asphyktischen blauen Finger ziegelrot, Erbrechen oder jedenfalls Würgen. HÖSSLIN beobachtete Zurückgehen der Anfälle von lokaler Synkope auf Pilocarpin. HEUK injizierte einer Raynaudkranken (ohne Gangrän) $^3/_4$ mg Adrenalin subcutan ohne Effekt, fand aber auf 0,0075 Pilocarpin eine das normale Maß zweifellos übersteigende Wirkung. PARRISIUS spricht von einer Disharmonie im Antagonismus zwischen Sympathicus und Vagus; je nachdem gerade dieser oder jener überwiegt, wird man eine stärkere Wirkung auf Adrenalin oder Pilocarpin haben. RUD fand bei der pharmakodynamischen Prüfung im Adrenalin- und Atropinversuch Hyperfunktion des N. vagus. Pilocarpinwirkung trat zwar erst nach 10—15 Minuten auf, war aber sonst normal. STRADIN untersuchte das Blut, Plasma und Serum während der Durchströmung des isolierten Kaninchenohres auf vasokonstriktorische Substanzen, fand aber nur regellose Werte zwischen Erweiterung und Verengerung, so daß er zu keinem Resultat kommt.

Bemerkenswert ist die Kombination mit *Basedow*, die von uns und anderen Beobachtern gesehen wurde (PIAZZA, MÖBIUS). Viel häufiger als die Kombination der ausgebildeten Typen ist das Vorkommen von Basedowsymptomen im Laufe der RAYNAUDschen Krankheit. Mehrfach hatte sich eine weiche, bisweilen pulsierende Struma entwickelt; es wurde von Exophthalmus berichtet, von Hitzegefühl, Herzklopfen, Tremor der Hände, dabei aber keine Struma. Die Kombination von Migräne, Raynaudsymptomen und Dysthyreoidismus ist von LEOPOLD LÉVY und DE ROTHSCHILD beschrieben worden. Migräne und RAYNAUDsche Krankheit sind auch sonst mehrfach, auch von uns selbst beobachtet worden; in einem dieser Fälle kam es im Laufe der Zeit zu passagerer Amaurose. Sehr bemerkenswert ist die Kombination von RAYNAUDscher Krankheit mit Anschwellung der *Speicheldrüsen* und der *Tränendrüsen*, also die Kombination von RAYNAUDscher und MIKULICZscher Krankheit in einem Falle eigener Beobachtung. Die Anschwellung der Speichel- und Tränendrüsen war in diesem Falle keine kontinuierliche, sondern eine intermittierende, ohne daß ein Parallelismus zwischen den RAYNAUDschen und den Speicheldrüsensymptomen bestand. Über eine ähnliche Beobachtung berichten DAUNIC und LAURENTIER, welche die Ansicht aussprechen, daß die Parotisläsion die Ursache des Syndroms darstelle. Sie vermuten, daß die Parotis und die Speicheldrüsen eine in diesem Sinne sich betätigende hormonale Wirkung entfalten. Es bleibt späterer Forschung überlassen zu erkunden, inwieweit diese Kombination auf gemeinsame Ursachen zurückzuführen ist. Daß eine solche vorliegt, bezweifeln wir nicht im Hinblick auf die Erfahrungen, die wir auch bei anderen Erkrankungen unseres Gebietes in bezug auf die Beteiligung des Speicheldrüsensystems gemacht haben.

Flüchtige Ödeme und Urticaria zusammen mit RAYNAUDscher Krankheit sind wiederholt beobachtet und beschrieben worden. Recht oft sahen wir diese Kombination. Über die Beziehungen zwischen RAYNAUDscher Krankheit und Akroasphyxia chronica sowie der Erythromelalgie wird an anderer Stelle die Rede sein.

LEHRNBECHER sah als sekundäre Folge der RAYNAUDschen Krankheit eine Calcinosis interstitialis bei einer Frau in den Gewebsteilen auftreten, die wegen RAYNAUDscher Krankheit doppelseitig sympathektomiert waren.

Einmal wird das Auftreten von Achylia gastrica im Verlauf der RAYNAUDschen Krankheit erwähnt. Die Achylie trat an den asphyktischen Tagen auf (FRIEDMANN). FRIEDENWALD und LOVE sahen einen Fall, der mit Magengeschwür kompliziert war. Sie halten es für denkbar, daß diese Zirkulationsstörungen in Gefäßspasmen derselben Art bestehen, wie sie an den Extremitäten zum RAYNAUD führen.

Endlich verdienen die Beobachtungen von GOUGEROT und BURNIER Erwähnung, die bei einem Raynaudkranken an Armen und im prästernalen Dreieck zahlreiche rote Teleangiektasien und Lipomatose der oberen Gliedmaßen sahen.

Verlauf.

Das Charakteristikum des Verlaufs der RAYNAUDschen Krankheit ist ihr Auftreten in *Anfällen*. Zunächst stellen sich meist allmählich zunehmende Erscheinungen von lokaler Synkope mit lokaler Asphyxie ein. Daß es sich da nicht um getrennte Stadien handelt, ist bereits erwähnt worden. Die Dauer der einzelnen Paroxysmen ist sehr verschieden; sie braucht sich nur auf wenige Minuten zu erstrecken, aber es gibt Anfälle von stundenlanger Dauer der Asphyxie, während Synkope meist kürzer ist. Unter immer größerer Intensität der Lokalerscheinungen der Asphyxie locale und unter Zunahme der Schmerzen kommt es dann meist an den Spitzen der Finger oder Zehen zu einer oberflächlichen Gangrän. Während nun hier die Elimination des toten Gewebes beginnt, kann im Verlauf erneuter heftiger Asphyxieanfälle an anderer Stelle sich die Gangrän von neuem etablieren. Der gesamte Anfall hat nach RAYNAUD meist eine Dauer von 3—4 Monaten; er kann sich aber noch viel länger hinziehen. Eine sehr wenig umfangreiche gangränöse Stelle bei einem unserer Kranken heilte erst nach 5 Monaten.

Die Krankheit kann sich in einem einzigen Anfall erschöpfen; das soll nach WEISS auch die Regel sein; er fand dieses Verhältnis in 71% der Beobachtungen. In, wie uns scheint, zahlreicheren Fällen traten zwar schwerere trophische Störungen nur in einer Attacke auf, aber leichtere oder schwerere vasomotorische Störungen wiederholten sich doch nach Abklingen des einen Anfalles sehr häufig. Aber es gibt auch Fälle mit jahrelang auseinanderliegenden Anfällen von typischer Gangrän. Wir sahen einen solchen, bei dem die zweite typische Nekrose der ersten am entsprechenden Finger der anderen Hand nach einem Dezennium folgte. Anfälle von Asphyxie locale können sehr lange, oft viele Jahre lang immer wieder kommen, bis es einmal zu einem Anfall kommt, in dem die Gangrän eintritt. Es werden Kranke mit einer 40jährigen Beobachtungszeit beschrieben. Das Gegenstück dazu geben die Fälle ab, in denen die Affektion sich in ganz kurzem Zeitraum, im Verlauf weniger Tage, entwickelte und ablief. Der paroxysmale Verlauf gehört zu den bedeutsamsten Zeichen der Krankheit, wenigstens in seinen ersten Entwicklungsperioden; später ändert sich das oft in dem Sinne, daß geringe Störungen, namentlich eine geringe Asphyxie, dauernd vorhanden sind, aber Exacerbationen sind noch immer die Regel. Es gibt aber auch Fälle, in denen sich die Asphyxie (für die Synkope ist das nicht bekannt) von vornherein rein progressiv entwickelt, in denen weiterhin das Bild dann doch in den typischen Raynaud ausmündet. Das sind die Fälle, die die Übergänge zu der Akroasphyxia chronica progressiva darstellen und im nächsten Abschnitt beschrieben werden sollen.

In vielen Fällen kann die Syncope locale ganz fehlen. Nur sehr viel seltener fehlt zwischen Syncope locale und Gangrän das Mittelglied der lokalen Asphyxie. Sehr häufig kommt es überhaupt nie zur Gangrän, es treten nur Anfälle von Synkope und Asphyxie oder auch nur von letzterer auf. Eine Andeutung gangränöser Prozesse ist dann häufig noch insofern nachweisbar, als sich an den Fingerspitzen kleinste Substanzverluste bemerkbar machen.

Die Krankheit als solche bedroht das Leben nicht. In keinem Falle von echter RAYNAUDscher Krankheit war diese direkt als Todesursache zu bezeichnen. Auch die Prognose quoad sanationem ist insofern günstig, als es oft bei einem oder einigen wenigen Anfällen bleibt. Wenn einmal Gangrän eingetreten war, so ist es natürlich immer eine Heilung mit Defekt, doch sind die Narben bei der oberflächlichen Art der Gangrän meist unscheinbar und wenig störend. An ihnen findet noch oft jahrelang eine Krustenbildung statt. Nach Ablauf der Gangrän bleibt häufig ein chronischer Zustand von Asphyxie locale mit gelegentlicher passagerer Steigerung der vasomotorischen und sensiblen Erscheinungen zurück. Das scheint der häufigste Typ zu sein. Wo Gangrän sich nicht einstellt, können Anfälle von Asphyxie locale sich jahre- und jahrzehntelang wiederholen, oft ohne die betreffenden Kranken gar zu sehr zu belästigen. Die Anfälle können aber auch nach mehrjährigem Verlauf dauernd verschwinden.

Pathologische Anatomie und Pathologie.

Pathologisch-anatomische Untersuchungen bei Raynaudkranken sind zwar in einer nicht geringen Anzahl von Fällen ausgeführt worden, die verwertbare Ausbeute ist jedoch ziemlich dürftig. Das hat folgende Gründe: einerseits ist eine ganze Reihe von Fällen zu Unrecht der RAYNAUDschen Krankheit zugezählt worden; die anatomischen Befunde dieser Fälle sind in die Literatur übergegangen und haben dort Verwirrung in der Frage nach der Pathologie der RAYNAUDschen Krankheit angestiftet. CASSIRER hat zuerst in seiner Monographie diese Fälle kritisch gesichtet. In den Einzelfällen krankt die Untersuchung an einem Mangel an Genauigkeit; nur in wenigen, unlängst publizierten Fällen finden sich z. B. die anatomischen Befunde, die an den Gefäßnerven und Gefäßzentren erhoben sind. In einer großen Anzahl klinisch typischer Fälle war der Sektionsbefund völlig negativ, wobei allerdings beachtet werden muß, daß die anatomische Untersuchung meist keine vollständige gewesen ist.

Die erhobenen positiven Befunde sind sehr mannigfaltig; es fanden sich Veränderungen des *Nervensystems* und des *Gefäßsystems*, bzw. beider gleichzeitig. In der Regel waren jedoch weder Veränderungen des Herzens, noch der größeren Gefäße, noch grobe Veränderungen des Zentralnervensystems nachweisbar und dort, wo sie gefunden wurden, konnten sie als pathogenetisch bedeutsam nicht angesehen werden. An den kleineren Gefäßen und den Verzweigungen der Nerven wurden bei einer Reihe von Sektionen Veränderungen gefunden. Aber auch dieses Vorkommnis ist durchaus kein konstantes. Sie können ganz fehlen; die Gefäße können allein, die Nerven können allein und beide können zusammen ergriffen werden, ohne daß klinisch ein sicherer Unterschied zwischen den einzelnen Fällen in die Augen springt. Solche Ungleichheiten in den Einzelbefunden mahnen naturgemäß infolge der Regellosigkeit ihres Auftretens zu besonderer Vorsicht bei der Verwertung der positiven pathologisch-anatomischen Ergebnisse.

Es fanden sich Veränderungen des *Zentralnervensystems* in den Fällen von HOCHENEGG (Syringomyelie), STRAUSS (multiple Sklerose), CALMANN (Tumor in den Wurzeln der Cauda equina). Veränderungen im Sinne einer *Neuritis* waren nachweisbar in den Fällen von AFFLEEK, DE GRAZIA, MOUNSTEIN, KORNFELD, PITRES und VAILLARD, WWEDENSKY, WIGGLESWORTH. GAGEL und WATTS fanden bei einem an Carcinoma pylori gestorbenen 48jährigen Manne, der an RAYNAUDscher Krankheit litt, zwar keinen pathologischen Befund an den Ganglien des Grenzstranges, aber im Rückenmark an den Zellen der Seitenhorngruppe Veränderungen im Sinne der von NISSL beschriebenen sog. primären Reizung. Sie erblicken in diesen Veränderungen einen wichtigen ätiologischen Faktor für die Entstehung der symmetrischen Gangrän.

Alterationen der peripheren Gefäße fanden sich in den Fällen von CASTELLINO und CARDI, LYLE und GREIWE, BECK und KOLISCH. In letzterem Falle war eine hochgradige hyperplastische Intimaverdickung an den Gefäßen der erkrankten Partien, aber auch an den Gehirnarterien nachweisbar. PFISTER (zit. nach MUCHA) fand Endarteriitis der Fingerarterien, SACHS Endarteriitis obliterans, DOVE abnorme Gefäßverdünnung und interstitielle Bindegewebsvermehrung (zit. nach MUCHA). GRENET und ISAAC-GEORGES fanden in drei Fällen ausgesprochene Veränderungen der cutanen Arteriolen im Sinne einer Verdickung des Endothels. Die Zellen hatten kubische Gestalt und lagen übereinandergeschichtet; in einem Falle hatten sie vollkommenen Gefäßverschluß herbeigeführt. An den größeren Arterien war eine Infiltration der Tunica media sichtbar.

Veränderungen in den Endverzweigungen sowohl der Gefäße als der Nerven wurden von BERVOETS, GIOVANNI, DEHIO, COLLIER, zuletzt von ALLAN und

BROWN, CUNNINGHAM, GRENET und ISAAC-GEORGES beschrieben. In keinem der Fälle ist übrigens eine genügende Untersuchung der hauptsächlich in Frage kommenden Gewebe vorgenommen worden. Insbesondere fehlt überall die Untersuchung der Gefäßnerven. In einem Falle fanden wir als bemerkenswertes Resultat eine Hypoplasie der Aorta und der gesamten Gefäßgebiete, worauf auch sonst schon aufmerksam gemacht worden ist; es ist besonders bemerkenswert, daß auch beim intermittierenden Hinken vielfache Erfahrungen auf eine solche allgemeine Hypoplasie des Gefäßsystems hinweisen.

In den letzten Jahren hat sich die Aufmerksamkeit besonders den Untersuchungen der sympathischen Ganglien zugewendet. LAIGNEL-LAVASTINE fand in zwei Fällen ausgesprochene Sklerose der Bauchganglien; BENNETT und POULTON stellten bei einem 60jährigen Mann mit symmetrischer Gangrän an den Händen im erfolglos exstirpierten Ganglion cervicale inferius Carcinomzellen fest.

STAEMMLER fand bei RAYNAUDscher Gangrän Degeneration der Ganglienzellen, die mit lymphocytären Infiltraten, Kapselzellwucherungen und Bindegewebsvermehrung vergesellschaftet waren. Aus seinen Befunden schließt STAEMMLER, daß bei den vasomotorischen Neurosen der chronisch-entzündlich-degenerative Prozeß in den Ganglien die Ursache der peripheren Gefäßspasmen ist. Mit Recht machen ERNST RUHEMANN und PARISOT und CORNIL darauf aufmerksam, daß STAEMMLER die gleichen Ganglienveränderungen bei einer Reihe infektiöser Prozesse findet und daß dadurch die Befunde stark an Beweiskraft einbüßen. Zu ähnlichen Resultaten kommt TERPLAN, der in 70 Fällen bei den verschiedensten Krankheiten das Ganglion cervicale superius, Ganglion stellatum und das Ganglion coeliacum untersuchte. Er berichtet, daß er, je länger er untersuchte, desto weniger Befunde feststellen konnte, die man mit Sicherheit als spezifisch für bestimmte Krankheiten bezeichnen konnte. Ähnliches erwähnten CRAIG und KERNAHAN. PALLASSE-DECHAUME-ARNAUD fanden in einem Falle von RAYNAUDscher Krankheit mit allmählich eingetretener symmetrischer Gangrän an Zehen und Fingern entzündliche Veränderungen an den Ganglien des Grenzstranges: lymphocytäre Infiltration und als Ersatz für zugrunde gegangene Ganglienzellen, Wucherung von Trabantzellen nach Art einer Neurogliawucherung. Sie erblicken in diesen Veränderungen die Grundlage für die RAYNAUDsche Krankheit und sind der Ansicht, daß die Gefäßläsionen sekundär bedingt sind.

Pathologisch-anatomisch bedeutungsvoll erscheint der von ASSMANN und E. RUHEMANN beschriebene Fall von angioneurotischer exsudativer Diathese:
Der 26jährige Patient bot multiple vegetative Störungen, nämlich Hydrops articulorum intermittens, QUINCKEsches Ödem, Migräne, multiple angiospastische Zustände mit RAYNAUDscher Gangrän, epileptiforme Anfälle, außerdem Urinblutungen, Hodenschwellungen. Eine beachtenswerte Veränderung des Blutbildes trat immer nur für die Zeit der Anfälle auf. Während derselben polynucleäre Leukocytose mit Zurücktreten der Eosinophilen; außerhalb der Anfälle normale Leukocyten, Vermehrung der Lymphocyten, Eosinophilie von 8—12%. Bei der Sektion fanden sich infarktartige anämische und hämorrhagische Nekrosen in den verschiedensten Organen, ferner Blutungen unter anderem im linken Großhirnschenkel. Die größeren Arterien waren intakt; an einzelnen mittelgroßen Arterien war eine mäßige elastisch-muskuläre Hypertrophie und eine Verkalkung der Elastica interna nachweisbar. Dagegen waren in zahlreichen Venen frische, sowie ältere organisierte und rekanalisierte Blutpfröpfe vorhanden. Im Gehirn hyaline Wandquellung einiger kleiner Arterien im verlängerten Mark, ferner mäßiges Ödem, in 2 Spinalganglien degenerative Atrophie der Ganglienzellen; auch an den Grenzstrangganglien zeigten sich zahlreiche Ganglienzellen atrophisch, einige auch gebläht; es bestand eine gleichmäßige bindegewebige Induration, hyaline Quellung der Wand zahlreicher Venen, im Plexus coeliacus spärliche Rundzellinfiltrate. Auffallend war das Fehlen der VATER-PACCINIschen Körperchen an den Gefäßen. Die Nebenniere zeigte Hyperplasie von Mark und Rinde; außerdem fand sich eine accessorische, aus Mark und Rindensubstanz bestehende Nebenniere im Plexus coeliacus [1].

---

[1] Zit. nach Ref. WOHLWILL: Zbl. Neur. **51**.

Recht zahlreich sind die bioptischen Untersuchungen des Materiales, das durch Operation gewonnen wurde. Über einen besonders bemerkenswerten Fall hat jüngst RIEDER berichtet, der nach allen Richtungen hin eingehend bioptisch und später anatomisch untersucht wurde.

Es handelt sich um eine Patientin mit echter RAYNAUDscher Erkrankung, bei der das Ganglion stellatum auf der rechten Seite entfernt wurde. Die Patientin starb nach ungefähr 1 Jahr an einer interkurrenten Grippepneumonie. Es fanden sich bei der mikroskopischen Untersuchung in einem Teil der Ganglienzellen feinkörniger Zerfall, Fehlen oder Randständigkeit des Kerns, selten stark geblähte Nervenzellen, ferner ausgedehnte lymphocytäre, plasmacelluläre Ganglieninfiltrate, die meist um die kleinsten Gefäße herumlagen. An Gehirn und verlängertem Mark konnte kein krankhafter Befund festgestellt werden. In der Nebenniere bestanden vereinzelte Infiltrate, wie man sie normalerweise öfters zu sehen gewohnt ist.

RIEDER kommt zu dem Resultat, daß die beschriebenen Ganglienzellveränderungen und lymphocytären Herde nicht ausreichen, um die Ursache der RAYNAUDschen Krankheit zu erklären, obwohl man sich vorstellen könnte, daß so ausgedehnte pericapilläre Infiltrate einen funktionellen Reizzustand sympathischer Fasern und damit charakteristische vasomotorische Reizerscheinungen hervorrufen könnten.

Nach dem Gesagten unterliegt es jedenfalls keinem Zweifel, daß in den bisher beschriebenen pathologisch-anatomischen Befunden eine ausreichende Erklärung für das gesamte Krankheitsbild der RAYNAUDschen Krankheit *nicht* zu finden ist. Wir haben oben versucht die Pathogenese der einzelnen Symptome, die das Krankheitsbild zusammensetzen, so weit als möglich aufzuklären. Wir wiederholen aus dem dort Gesagten nur, daß sowohl die lokale Synkope als auch die lokale Asphyxie auf Reizungen irgendeines Abschnittes des vasomotorischen Systems zurückzuführen sind, daß die Gangrän mit ihnen wie mit den sensiblen Symptomen in einen engen Zusammenhang zu bringen ist, ohne daß es jedoch erlaubt ist, sie einfach als Folge der vasomotorischen Störungen aufzufassen, daß die sensiblen Reizsymptome an sich auf Beziehungen zum Vasomotorenzentrum hinweisen, offenbar Reizzustände vasosensibler Fasern sind, und daß auch die übrigen Symptome, die gelegentlich auftretenden Muskelatrophien, die sekretorischen Symptome, die allgemeinen Krankheitserscheinungen auf *Alterationen* des *vegetativen Systems* zu beziehen sein dürften.

Alles weist also auf dieses System hin. Offenbar sind es in erster Linie die der *Vasokonstriktion* dienenden Bahnen und Zentren, diejenigen also, die aus dem sympathischen System im engeren Sinne stammen, die den Locus morbi darstellen. Sie sind in einem Zustand erhöhter Ansprechbarkeit versetzt; dieser kann bedingt sein durch eine kongenitale abnorme Anlage, die auch sonst in nervöser Heredität oft ihren Ausdruck findet. Sie kann aber auch erworben sein durch langanhaltende und wiederholt einwirkende schädigende Einflüsse, wie häufige Kältereize, rheumatische Erkrankungen, somatische und psychische Traumen. Erhöhte Reizbarkeit kann ferner ohne vorhandene Anlage und besonders bei solcher direkt hervorgerufen werden durch Intoxikationen und Infektionen und reflektorisch durch Erkrankungen peripherer Organe, meist der Gefäße und seltener der Nerven. Einen ähnlichen Standpunkt hinsichtlich der Pathogenese vertritt auch MUCHA.

Daß experimentelle Untersuchungen geeignet sind, uns die Beantwortung einiger hierhergehöriger Fragen näher zu bringen, beweisen die interessanten Untersuchungen von H. MARCUS. Dieser hat bei 42 Kaninchen zur Erzielung eines angiospastischen Zustandes subcutane Adrenalininjektionen während einer längeren Zeit 2mal täglich in das eine Ohr gemacht. In die Randvene des anderen Ohres oder in eine Beinvene wurden Streptokokkenkulturen injiziert. In fast allen Fällen entstand eine Gangrän des adrenalisierten Ohres. Adrenalininjektionen oder Streptokokkeninjektionen *allein* vermochten keine Gangrän hervorzurufen. Es wurde also offenbar auf diesem Wege eine „Opportunität zur Nekrose" geschaffen, die man auch vordem schon postuliert hatte. MARCUS glaubt, daß die eigentliche

RAYNAUDsche Krankheit durch eine pathologische Einwirkung auf den Sympathicus entstehe, und daß die Gangrän von einer zu dieser Störung hinzutretenden allgemeinen Infektion verursacht werde. Zu diesen Versuchen wurde er durch die Beobachtung veranlaßt, daß das letzte schwere Stadium, die symmetrische Gangrän, bei der RAYNAUDschen Krankheit erst auftrat, als eine schwere septische Infektion die Kranken befiel. Diese Versuche sind von einem Mitarbeiter ASSMANNs, SCHMIDT-WEYLAND, wiederholt und ergaben ebenfalls das Auftreten von Gewebsschädigungen, freilich von etwas geringerem Ausmaß, im Bereiche des adrenalisierten Bezirks. ASSMANN weist jedoch darauf hin, daß der entzündungsfreie Charakter der trockenen Mumifikation nicht ohne weiteres eine Analogie mit den Tierversuchen zuläßt. Derselben Meinung ist auch MUCHA. Ähnliche Gedankengänge wie bei MARCUS finden sich auch schon vorher bei BRESLAUER.

ZIERL spricht von Reizzuständen von Gefäßnervenbahnen und Zentren, die auf Grund einer besonderen Disposition zustande kommen, welche im vasomotorischen System selbst, im Stoffwechsel oder in einem besonderen Chemismus der Haut begründet liegt. Die große Rolle, welche die begleitenden, manchmal äußerst heftigen Gemeingefühle (allerdings nicht in allen Fällen) im klinischen Bilde spielen, deuten auf eine wesentliche Beteiligung des vasosensiblen Systems hin. Auch RIEDER faßt den Raynaud als konstitutionelle Allgemeinerkrankung auf, die schwächliche, konstitutionell minderwertige Individuen mit herabgesetzten Capillarreaktionen der Haut befällt. Das Auftreten der Symptome an den distalen Körperteilen erklärt er in der Weise, daß die Blutzirkulation hier schwieriger sich abwickelt als an anderen Körperstellen und daß der Blutstrom eine Umschaltung erfährt. Er faßt den Zustand als einen krankhaften Reizzustand im vegetativen System auf, der in den autonomen Zentren oder in der Wand der Präcapillaren und Capillaren sich lokalisieren kann. Der Reiz kann aber auch über das cortico-spinale System auf dem Wege der Vasokonstriktoren zu den capillären Netzen geschickt werden oder auch auf dem Blutwege rein cellulär zustande kommen. Die innige Verknüpfung des endokrinen mit dem vegetativen System durch das Gefäßsystem bringt es mit sich, daß beim Krankheitsbereiten eine korrelative Dysfunktion eintritt. Ähnliche Anschauungen vertreten GRENET und ISAAC-GEORGES, die der anatomischen Veränderung der Endarteriolen eine besondere Bedeutung zusprechen. BOROVSKY spricht sich auf Grund von vier Beobachtungen, die eine einheitliche Genese erkennen lassen, dahin aus, daß eine Schädigung der höheren vegetativen Zentren im Gebiet der subcorticalen Ganglien mit primärer oder sekundärer Störung des Kalkumsatzes in seinen Fällen angenommen werden mußte. POLLAK vertritt die Auffassung, daß die RAYNAUDsche Krankheit einer Störung der Zentren des vegetativen Systems am Boden des dritten Ventrikels ihre Entstehung verdanke.

Bei allen diesen Störungen muß man auch daran denken, daß Störungen in der sensiblen Versorgung der Haut mit zu den beobachteten Veränderungen führen können. Neuere Untersuchungen, vor allem von THOMAS LEWIS[1], weisen nämlich darauf hin, daß für den normalen Tonus der Hautgefäße nicht nur das vegetative System sondern vor allem die Unversehrtheit der sensiblen Nerven maßgebend ist. Er konnte z. B. zeigen, daß die bekannte Erweiterung der Hautgefäße, die bereits auf geringe Kältegrade auftritt, durch einen Axonreflex in den sensiblen Fasern hervorgerufen wird und ausbleibt, wenn die sensiblen Fasern degeneriert sind. Dabei nimmt gleichzeitig die Hauttemperatur um mehrere Grade zu. Der erweiternde Axonreflex in den sensiblen Fasern hat nach THOMAS LEWIS vor allem an den Acren eine große Bedeutung. Wie stark physiologische Veränderungen in der Gefäßweite von den sensiblen Nerven abhängen, geht auch aus folgenden Beobachtungen im Tierexperiment hervor. Reibt man ein Kaninchenohr, so tritt nach kurzer Zeit eine Erweiterung der Gefäße ein; sind die sympathischen Fasern zu den Ohrnerven degeneriert, so tritt die Erweiterung bereits viel schneller ein [2]; sind dagegen auch die sensiblen Fasern degeneriert, so gelingt es nicht, durch noch so starkes Reiben eine Erweiterung zu beobachten. Der Unterschied zeigt sich auch, wenn man das Ohr anschneidet. Während das normale Ohr dann stark blutet, erhält man vom denervierten Ohr kaum

---
[1] THOMAS LEWIS: Heart **16**, 177 (1930). Brit. med. J. **1932**, Nr 3733, 136—138.
[2] FELDBERG: J. of Physiol. **61**, 518 (1926).

einen Blutstropfen [1]. Diese schlechtere Durchblutung ist durch das Fehlen der sensiblen Nervenversorgung verursacht. Über den genauen Mechanismus, wie die gefäßerweiternden Fasern die Gefäßerweiterung bedingen, herrscht noch keine Klarheit. THOMAS LEWIS nimmt an, daß alle Schädigungen, z. B. auch geringe Temperaturerniedrigungen, einen histaminähnlichen Stoff (H-Substanz) in der Haut frei machen, welcher die sensiblen Nervenendigungen erregt. Die sensiblen Fasern sollen dann die Gefäße direkt erweitern, während nach KROGH auch an den Gefäßendigungen der sensiblen Fasern wieder gefäßerweiternde Stoffe frei werden, welche erst die Erweiterung bedingen. Es herrscht auch keine Übereinstimmung darüber, ob die sensiblen Fasern des Axonreflexes mit den bei der antidromen Gefäßerweiterung erregten Fasern identisch sind. Diese sind nach KURÉ wahrscheinlich parasympatischer Natur [2].

Die anatomisch nachgewiesenen Erkrankungen des Zentralnervensystems und der peripheren Nerven sind gewiß nicht als gleichgültig für die Entstehung der RAYNAUDschen Krankheit anzusehen, aber sie sind nur Hilfsursachen, sie sind keine notwendige Voraussetzung für die Entstehung der Krankheit. Von hierher gehörigen modernen Arbeiten soll diejenige von BORAK Erwähnung finden, welcher der Ansicht ist, daß die RAYNAUDsche Gangrän auf eine zentral nervöse Erkrankung des Rückenmarks zurückzuführen ist. Zu dieser Auffassung gelangt er durch die Beobachtung therapeutischer Erfolge bei Röntgenbestrahlung der Wirbelsäule in der Höhe der Rückenmarkssegmente, die den erkrankten Gefäßgebieten entsprechen. Diese Beobachtungen bedürfen einer Nachprüfung.

Was von den Nervenerkrankungen soeben gesagt ist, gilt auch für die Erkrankung der peripheren Gefäße; naturgemäß ist die anatomische Erkrankung der Gefäße für den weiteren Verlauf der Krankheit von größter Bedeutung, indem sie die Opportunität zur Nekrose steigert, aber auch den Gefäßerkrankungen kann nur die Rolle einer Hilfsursache für die Entstehung der RAYNAUDschen Gangrän zukommen.

Ähnliche Gedankengänge hat schon vor Jahren KRAUS geäußert, denen wir jedoch nicht folgen können, um so weniger als bei der Beobachtung von KRAUS die Untersuchung des Gehirns und des autonomen Systems fehlt.

Es ist sehr wahrscheinlich, daß bei der RAYNAUDschen Krankheit auch *endokrine* Störungen eine Rolle spielen. MÖBIUS hat diesen Standpunkt schon früher vertreten. SOLIS-COHEN hat unter Hinweis auf die Beziehungen zum Morbus Basedowii im speziellen eine Störung der Funktion der Schilddrüse angenommen. Ganz ähnlich haben auch LEOPOLD LÉVI und DE ROTHSCHILD eine Parafunktion der Schilddrüse behauptet. (Siehe auch BÜCHLER, WEDROV.) Wir werden auf diese Frage gelegentlich der Besprechung der Pathologie der Sklerodermie noch näher einzugehen haben. PRIBRAM sah einen Kranken mit RAYNAUDscher Krankheit, bei dem sich eine ganz bedeutende Vergrößerung der Hypophyse im Röntgenbild nachweisen ließ. Er sowohl wie SANNICANDRO und BLOCH sprechen von einem hypophysären Raynaud. Auch KOPF sah im Röntgenbilde erhebliche Vertiefung und Verbreiterung der Sella und Abflachung der Processus clinoidei post. BÜCHLER sah die Kombination von Basedow- und Addisonsymptomen bei einer 36jährigen Frau, die auch das Bild der Erythromelalgie und Sklerodermie bot. Auch hier zeigte sich im Röntgenbilde eine abnorm tiefe Sella. BOGAERT und DELBEKE sahen ein akromegales Symptombild ohne Veränderung des Türkensattels, verbunden mit schmerzhaften symmetrischen Anfällen von Syncope locale an den Fingern. Sehr merkwürdig ist die Beobachtung von HOLSCHAW und BOOTH, die in diesem Zusammenhang Erwähnung verdient: ein einjähriges Kind wurde wegen schwerer Ernährungsstörung mit Pituitrininjektionen behandelt, die irrtümlicherweise in zu großen

---

[1] STERNBERG: Z. exper. Med.
[2] Literatur bei FELDBERG u. SCHILF: Histamin. Berlin: Julius Springer. — Siehe auch die ähnliche Gesichtspunkte vertretende Arbeit von MIVERGHI.

Dosen dargereicht wurden; es entwickelte sich eine symmetrische Gangrän an Händen und Füßen; der Sektionsbefund war negativ. WEDROW beobachtete eine 27jährige Kranke mit auffallend dunkler Haut, Pigmentverschiebungen, Haarausfall, Sklerodaktylie und Raynaudsymptomen. Die Erscheinungen gingen auf Schilddrüsendarreichung erheblich zurück. CATTANEO sah eine Verbindung mit Katarakt. FORNERO und DAL MASO beobachteten Dysmenorrhöe, RUD Impotenz und Hodenschmerzen, Pigmentverschiebungen, Bronzehaut an Hals und Gesicht, Vitiligo. PAULINY-TÓTH sah nach einer Entbindung unter Dysmenorrhöe und Amenorrhöe einen Raynaud auftreten.

Nach unserer Überzeugung schweben, sobald es sich um detailliertere Angaben handelt, alle diese Dinge noch völlig in der Luft. Von dem Nachweis einer einheitlichen Störung irgendeiner endokrinen Drüse kann noch nicht die Rede sein. Auch uns ist es nicht zweifelhaft, daß eine Reihe von endogenen oder exogenen toxischen Stoffen eine besondere Affinität zu den vegetativen nervösen Zentren hat und unter Mitwirkung einer angeborenen oder erworbenen Instabilität dieser Zentren für die Entstehung der Krankheit von Bedeutung sein kann. Man hat ferner zu berücksichtigen, daß in neuerer Zeit darauf hingewiesen wurde, daß in den Organen selbst, also in der Peripherie, unabhängig von irgendwelcher Regulation Nervenstoffe entstehen, die in regulativem Sinne die Gefäßweite oder das Organ selbst beeinflussen (tissue products LEWIS-LANDIS, Gewebshormone FELDBERG-SCHILF). Solche chemischen Körper können, wenn sie unter pathologischen Bedingungen frei werden, die Alteration im Sinne eines Raynaud verursachen. Gerade das *anfallsweise* Auftreten der Erscheinungen läßt sich dahin interpretieren, daß die Summation der Einwirkung chemischer Produkte auf das bereits geschädigte vegetative System für die Periodizität der klinischen Erscheinungen mit verantwortlich zu machen ist. Denn es ist sonst nicht einzusehen, warum ein chronischer Prozeß im Nervengewebe immer gerade anfallsweise Zustandänderungen im Sinne eines Raynaud bedingt. Wieweit diese eine Rolle spielen können, beweist der Fall von RIEDER, nach dem Raynaudanfälle auch dann noch aufgetreten sind, nachdem sämtliche Nervenverbindungen zu dem betreffenden Gewebe durchtrennt waren. Es ist ferner darauf hinzuweisen (TH. LEWIS), daß pathologisch veränderte Gefäße gegen Reize der Außenwelt (Kälte) überempfindlich werden und im Sinne eines Raynaud reagieren. Eine ähnliche Ansicht äußern MORTON und SCOTT. Alle Einzelheiten, auf die eine solche Annahme sich zu stützen hätte, fehlen noch. Immer ist dabei mit der Möglichkeit zu rechnen, daß, selbst wenn solche endokrinen bzw. gewebshormonalen Störungen nachgewiesen werden, sie ihrerseits auf eine Störung der nervösen Zentren dieser Drüsen zurückzuführen sind, zumal wir jetzt sicher wissen, daß das vegetative System auch die Sekretion zumindest einiger endokriner Drüsen beherrscht. Bei den gegenseitigen engen Beziehungen, die nach den neueren Anschauungen zwischen den einzelnen endokrinen Apparaten herrschen, ergeben sich die verschiedensten Möglichkeiten und Wechselwirkungen, die uns vorläufig unentwirrbar zu sein scheinen, wobei wir nochmals darauf hinweisen müssen, daß in einzelnen Fällen ein Nachweis von Störungen im endokrinen System überhaupt nicht gelingt, auch wenn alle neueren zur Verfügung stehenden Methoden angewendet werden.

So war es z. B. in einem Falle, den wir im KRAUS-BRUGSCHschen Handbuch mitgeteilt haben.

Der Vollständigkeit halber seien noch die Anschauungen von IWAI SAISHIRO und NIN MEISAL und TOKARSKI erwähnt. Erstere bestreiten, daß die RAYNAUDsche Krankheit eine vasomotorische Neurose ist; sie sehen sie vielmehr an als Folge einer Agglutination des Eigenblutes. Sie haben bei einem Patienten, der wegen Schrumpfniere aufgenommen wurde, ein wirksames Autoagglutinin nachgewiesen und wollen durch Kälteversuche festgestellt haben, daß er an Raynaud leide. Die Erythrocyten werden agglutiniert und die Blutcapillaren mechanisch verstopft. Derartige Beobachtungen sind sonst von keinem Autor erwähnt.

TOKARSKI glaubt aus einer Beobachtung schließen zu dürfen, daß auf dem Boden einer Leberinsuffizienz durch akute Einwirkung eines Giftes eine hämoklasische Krise sich einstellte mit sympathisch-spinaler Vasokonstriktion. Diese symmetrisch gelagerte Gefäßverengerung verursachte das akute RAYNAUDsche Syndrom.

In der Mehrzahl von Fällen der RAYNAUDschen Krankheit schreiben wir dieser die Bedeutung einer *selbständigen Affektion* zu. Es ist aber nicht zu leugnen, daß die RAYNAUDschen Symptome gelegentlich nur einen Teil der Symptomatologie eines andersartigen umfassenderen Krankheitsbildes darstellen. Es handelt sich da meist um Erkrankungen des Nervensystems zentraler oder peripherer Genese. Wir fanden solche Symptome bei einigen Fällen von Rückenmarkstumor, bei der Syringomyelie, vielleicht auch bei einzelnen Neuritiden. Besonders häufig kommen RAYNAUDsche Symptome bei einer Anzahl von Neurosen und Psychosen vor. Hier treten sie oft so weit zurück, daß wir ihnen nur noch symptomatischen Wert zubilligen können. Auf der anderen Seite sind die Übergänge zu anderen vasomotorisch-trophisch-sensiblen Symptomenkomplexen von intermittierendem Charakter fließende, indem die spezifischen und besonders charakteristischen Symptome der RAYNAUDschen Krankheit, in erster Linie die Gangrän, verblassen, die Allgemeinerscheinungen der nervösen Reizbarkeit und Erschöpfung in den Vordergrund rücken, wobei die auf dem Gebiete der Vasomotilität bzw. der vegetativen Funktion überhaupt sich abspielenden Krankheitszeichen besonders ausgeprägt zu sein pflegen. Es gibt also einerseits nahe Beziehungen der RAYNAUDschen Krankheit zu den allgemeinen Neurosen, andererseits sind die engsten Verbindungen zu den anderen vasomotorisch-trophischen Erkrankungen vorhanden. MARTINET bestreitet überhaupt das Vorkommen einer einheitlichen RAYNAUDschen Krankheit, indem er auf die Verschiedenheit der Ursachen dieses Symptomenkomplexes hinweist, auch JELIFFE nähert sich dieser Auffassung.

Diagnose.

Bei allen diagnostischen Erwägungen wird man sich, wie auch MUCHA betont, darüber klar sein müssen, daß das Einzelsymptom bei der RAYNAUDschen Krankheit manchmal völlig fehlen kann und daß man daher stets genötigt ist, den gesamten sich darbietenden Symptomenkomplex zu berücksichtigen.

Die Hauptschwierigkeiten ergeben sich bei der Abgrenzung der RAYNAUDschen Krankheit im engeren Sinne von gewissen vasomotorisch-trophischen Symptomen, die sich im Verlauf organischer Erkrankungen des Nervensystems, des Herzgefäßapparates und von Nierenerkrankungen (VOLHARD) entwickeln.

Unter den ersteren kommt die *Syringomyelie* in erster Reihe in Betracht. Bei der Syringomyelie (und besonders ist da der sog. MORVANsche Typus dieser Krankheit zu berücksichtigen) entwickeln sich die vasomotorisch-trophischen Störungen meist ganz allmählich. Die Ausdehnung der überhaupt nicht häufigen umschriebenen Gangrän ist eine größere; die charakteristischen intermittierenden vasomotorischen Symptome fehlen, ebenso fehlen meistens Schmerzen. Hingegen tritt die Anästhesie viel deutlicher hervor und ebenso die degenerativ atrophische Muskellähmung. Die bei der Syringomyelie sehr häufigen Panaritien kommen bei der RAYNAUDschen Krankheit, wie wir sahen, auch vor, besonders in den mit Sklerodaktylie kombinierten Fällen, aber sie sind meist außerordentlich schmerzhaft, während das bei der MORVANschen Krankheit doch selten der Fall ist.

Von BRAMANN, BRUNS, OEHLECKER, NEKAM, STEWART, PRICE, GOEBELL und RUNGE sind Fälle beobachtet worden, bei denen ein familiäres Auftreten schwerer trophischer ulcerativer und gangränöser Prozesse sich kombinierte mit vasomotorischen und sensiblen Störungen an den unteren und oberen Extremitäten. Die Krankheit ist eine familiäre. Von der RAYNAUDschen Krankheit weichen diese Fälle durch das Fehlen vasomotorischer Reizerscheinungen ab, während sie an die RAYNAUDsche Krankheit mehr als die gewöhnlichen Fälle von Syringomyelie durch die Betonung tropischer Störungen erinnern. Es scheint sich um progressive organische Veränderungen im untersten Rückenmarksabschnitt zu handeln. Eine völlige Aufklärung ist erst von einem Sektionsbefund zu erwarten.

Daß die vasomotorischen Störungen, welche als *Folgeerscheinung von Nervenverletzungen* auftreten, Raynaud-ähnliche Symptome hervorrufen können, beweisen die Beobachtungen einer Reihe von Autoren, besonders O. FÖRSTERs. Dieser erwähnt Nekrosen, cyanotische Verfärbung, Weißfärbung, Bilder, die an die ,,Doigts morts" erinnern; er hat sie besonders bei Medianuslähmung und bei gleichzeitiger Medianus- und Ulnaruslähmung, sowie bei Ischiadicusunterbrechung beobachtet. Ähnliche Befunde stammen von GRUGENT, BLUM, ZHA und von LORTAT JACOB und SÉZARY, die ein typisches Raynaudsyndrom mit Gangrän der Finger und Zehen bei Nervenverletzungen beobachteten, die mit Obliteration der großen Gefäße gepaart waren (zit. nach O. FÖRSTER). Der Nachweis der Nervenverletzung wird sich in solchen Fällen ohne Schwierigkeit erbringen lassen.

Wiederholt sind ferner Raynaudsymptome, wie bereits oben erwähnt, als Folgeerscheinung einer *Halsrippe* beobachtet worden. In diesen Fällen wird in der Regel die Röntgenaufnahme Klärung bringen. Zuletzt haben LOESSL, BENEDECK, BOMBI, TELFORD und STOPFORD über derartige instruktive Fälle berichtet. Die letztgenannten Autoren vertreten die Auffassung, daß die Druckwirkung der Halsrippe einen Reizzustand in den Vasokonstriktoren hervorruft im Sinne eines Dauerspasmus, der nach operativer Entfernung der Rippe schwindet.

Die Vertrautheit mit dem Krankheitsbilde gewisser gewerblicher Angioneurosen wird vor Verwechslungen mit der RAYNAUDschen Krankheit schützen; es handelt sich dabei um Gesundheitsschädigungen durch Anklopfmaschinen, wie sie in der Schuhindustrie haptsächlich verwendet werden. Publikationen stammen von GERBIS, GROS, MEYER, BRODNITZ, ROBINSON, sowie von KOELSCH. Es handelt sich hier meist um Gefäßkrämpfe, die durch die fortgesetzten starken Erschütterungen der den Schuh haltenden, in krampfhafter Stellung befindlichen Hände hervorgerufen werden. Man beobachtet Gefäßstörungen an den Händen mit Weißwerden, Pelzigsein, Gefühllosigkeit, Kältegefühl. Kalte Temperatur und Alkoholgenuß wirken auf die Entstehung des Leidens begünstigend.

Bei manchen Fällen von *Polyneuritis*, namentlich bei der Beriberi treten vasomotorische Reiz- und Lähmungserscheinungen und auch trophische Störungen mehr in den Vordergrund als sonst in den anderen Formen der Neuritis. Es sind Fälle von symmetrischer Gangrän bei Beriberi beschrieben worden. Aber die fundamentalen Symptome der Neuritis fehlen bei der typischen RAYNAUDschen Krankheit durchaus. Auch die *Lepra* (E. WOLFF u. a.) kann ähnliche Erscheinungen machen; doch wird wohl auch hier die Diagnose ohne jede Schwierigkeit gelingen.

Die Abgrenzung von der *postinfektiösen* und *kachektischen* Gangrän kann gelegentlich Schwierigkeiten machen. Das beweist z. B. ein Fall von SEIDELMANN, wo die Gangrän im Anschluß an eine Infektionskrankheit auftrat, in einem Zuge ohne eigentliche Attacke verlief, aber eine außerordentliche exakte Symmetrie und vasomotorische Störungen doch die Ähnlichkeit mit der RAYNAUDschen Gangrän hervortreten ließen. Auch der Patient von IMPERIALE gehört in diese Gruppe.

Wir haben bereits erwähnt, daß recht häufig RAYNAUDsche Erscheinungen sich im Anschluß an LUES einstellen; in diesen Fällen wird man meist die für Lues charakteristischen Gefäßveränderungen nachweisen können. In Zweifelsfällen wird die Blut- und Liquoruntersuchung der Diagnose näher bringen; gelegentlich hat auch die Einleitung einer spezifischen Kur, welche eine überraschende Besserung brachte, den Verdacht auf das Vorliegen einer Lues bestätigt.

Die Bilder, die durch die *Endarteritis obliterans* hervorgebracht werden, können der RAYNAUDschen Gangrän einigermaßen ähnlich sehen. Das sicherste Unterscheidungsmerkmal bieten zweifellos die vasomotorischen Phänomene. Wenn solche bei der endarteriitischen Gangrän auch keineswegs zu fehlen brauchen, so ist doch das eigentümliche Spiel lokaler Synkope und Asphyxie nur der RAYNAUDschen Krankheit eigen. Bei der endarteriitischen Gangrän ist Ischämie bei Hochlagerung und Rötung bei herabhängenden Beinen so gut wie regelmäßig zu erzeugen. Die Symmetrie der Gangrän ist bei der endarteriitischen Gangrän nur ganz ausnahmsweise so ausgesprochen wie bei der RAYNAUDschen Krankheit. Die Pulslosigkeit spricht zugunsten der endarteriitischen Gangrän, namentlich wenn sie eine dauernde ist, während ein passageres Verschwinden des Pulses ja auch bei der RAYNAUDschen Krankheit vorkommt; und wenn die Pulslosigkeit sich weit bis in die großen Gefäße hinein erstreckt, ist RAYNAUDsche Krankheit sicher auszuschließen. Die Gangrän bei Raynaud pflegt meist viel weniger umfangreich zu sein, wie die Endarteritis. Es unterliegt keinem Zweifel, daß in einer Reihe von Fällen, die als RAYNAUDsche Gangrän bezeichnet worden sind, eine Verwechselung mit der endarteriitischen Gangrän vorgekommen ist. Eine Abhandlung von BROWN schildert die differentialdiagnostischen Erwägungen, die zwischen vasomotorischen Störungen und organischen Gefäßerkrankungen Platz greifen müssen. Eine für die Abgrenzung der RAYNAUDschen Krankheit gegenüber der Thrombangitis obliterans bedeutungsvolle Abhandlung liefern ALLAN und BROWN: in ungefähr 5% der Fälle von Thrombangitis obliterans, welche die Verfasser an der Mayoklinik beobachteten, konnten sie an der Arteria dorsalis pedis und tibialis postica eine abnorme Pulsation nicht feststellen; der Gefäßverschluß hatte vielmehr die digitalen und interossealen Arterien ergriffen und dehnte sich aus auf die plantaren, metatarsalen und tarsalen Arterien, so daß die Zeichen des Gefäßverschlusses auf die distalen Abschnitte von Fuß und Zehen beschränkt waren. An der Hand von 4 Fällen weisen die Verfasser nach, daß die Gefahr besteht, in solchen Fällen fälschlich RAYNAUDsche Krankheit zu diagnostizieren und empfehlen dringend, stets alle zugänglichen Arterien am Körper zu palpieren. In einer vor kurzem erschienenen Arbeit über periphere Gefäßstörungen im jugendlichen und mittleren Lebensalter geht ASSMANN auf die Unterscheidungsmerkmale zwischen RAYNAUDscher Gangrän und der jugendlichen Spontangangrän ein und betont beim Raynaud klinisch das anfallsweise und symmetrische Auftreten sowie die trockene Beschaffenheit der Gangrän gegenüber der jugendlichen Spontangangrän, während im anatomischen Bilde beim Raynaud im Gegensatz zur anderen Gangrän die Arterien sich histologisch normal verhalten. Er erklärt jedoch, daß es andererseits nicht ausgeschlossen ist, daß die verschiedenen Krankheitsursachen sich auch in verschiedenartiger Weise miteinander verknüpfen können, die manchmal eine sichere Einreihung in eine der genannten Gruppen schwierig, ja manchmal auch gar nicht gerechtfertigt erscheinen lassen. Ähnliche Gedankengänge enthält auch die sehr kritische Arbeit von G. GRUBER, der auf Grund seiner pathologisch-histologischen Untersuchungen zu folgenden Resultaten kommt: „Die Endarteriitis obliterans ist immer nur ein formender Ausdruck von Folgen anderer, vorausgegangener Gefäßwand- und Gefäßlichtungsstörungen; diese Störungen können aber verschieden sein, rein zirkulatorischer Art, also abhängig von einer neurovaskulären örtlichen bzw. reflektorischen Leistungsunregelmäßigkeit, sie können auch Folge infektiös toxischer Beeinflussung sein, sie können den Ausdruck eines organisierenden Umbaues nach Wandthrombose darstellen." In der Überzeugung, daß in Fällen sog. juveniler Gangrän dem verschließenden Wandprozeß im befallenen Gefäßgebiet zirkulatorische Leistungsstörungen nach dieser oder jener exogenen Schädigung bei besonders empfindlicher Reaktionsbereitschaft des neurovaskulären Apparates vorausgingen, erklärt er, daß der Gegensatz zwischen dem Heer der Trophovasoneurosen und den Fällen der juvenilen Spontangangrän (mit dem Befund der Endarteriitis obliterans) nicht mehr unüberbrückbar erscheinen wird, daß es sich vielmehr letzten Endes doch um *ein* großes Gebiet handeln wird. In diesem Sinne sprechen auch Fälle, wie sie TOLOSA beschrieben.

Mit der RAYNAUDschen Krankheit hat das *intermittierende Hinken*, namentlich in seiner von OPPENHEIM geschilderten benignen Form, große Ähnlichkeit. Das intermittierende Hinken steht in seiner typischen Ausbildung und in seiner gewöhnlichen Form geradezu in der Mitte zwischen der endarteriitischen Gangrän und der RAYNAUDschen Krankheit. Es entlehnt beiden Krankheiten Züge, die Lebhaftigkeit der vasomotorischen Reizerscheinungen nähert es der RAYNAUDschen Krankheit, die Veränderungen, die klinisch in dem dauernden Fehlen des Pulses in Erscheinung treten, der endarteriitischen Gangrän. Unsere Auffassung, daß für die Entstehung des Symptomenbildes des intermittierenden Hinkens zwei Komponenten von Wichtigkeit sind, die organische Veränderung der Gefäße und die funktionelle Komponente einer vasomotorischen Übererregbarkeit, läßt diese Mittelstellung sehr gut verstehen, und wenn der benignen Form von OPPENHEIM das angiosklerotische Moment fehlt, so ist auf diese Weise noch mehr eine Annäherung an die RAYNAUDsche Krankheit geschaffen; das einzige Unterscheidungsmerkmal ist und bleibt dann der zwischen der Ausübung der Funktion des Gehens und dem Auftreten der pathologischen Erscheinungen bei dem intermittierenden Hinken bestehende enge Zusammenhang. Wir möchten der Vermutung Ausdruck geben, daß diese Differenz nur eine solche der Lokalisation sein dürfte.

Es gibt noch eine Gangränform, die große Ähnlichkeit mit der RAYNAUDschen Gangrän hat, nämlich die durch *Ergotismus* bedingte Gangrän. Zuletzt hat sich KAUNITZ mit dieser Frage beschäftigt. Hier werden die Extremitäten kühl, blaß, cyanotisch, schließlich kommt es an den verschiedenen Stellen der Haut zu Ernährungsstörungen, Blasenbildung, Auftreten von trockener Gangrän, die meist Finger und Zehen befällt. Es liegt nahe, bei der großen Ähnlichkeit des klinischen Bildes beider Affektionen an eine ähnliche pathologische Grundlage zu denken und zu versuchen, aus der Pathologie der Ergotinintoxikation Anregungen für die Auffassung der RAYNAUDschen Krankheit zu entnehmen. Leider lassen uns aber auch unsere Kenntnisse bezüglich der Einzelheiten der Pathogenese des Ergotismus im Stich.

Ein weiteres bei der Diagnosenstellung zu berücksichtigendes Moment, das den RAYNAUDschen Erscheinungen ähnliche Symptome hervorzurufen vermag, sind Kälteschäden. Hier wird außer der anamnestischen Feststellung intensiver Kälteeinwirkung das Fehlen charakteristischer vasomotorischer Symptome, oft auch die große Ausdehnung der Gangrän die Diagnose ermöglichen, wobei man auf die von BOADMANN erwähnte Tatsache zu achten hat, daß Kälteapplikation die durch die Kälte hervorgerufenen Beschwerden stets bessert.

Von der RAYNAUDschen Krankheit zu trennen sind die von WIETING im Türkischen Heere beobachtete Massenerkrankung in Form von fast stets symmetrisch auftretender Gangrän der Zehen bzw. der Füße. Die Kranken waren unterernährt, starken Kälteeinflüssen ausgesetzt und hatten meist an Dysenterie gelitten. Es handelte sich um Gefäßlähmung durch schwere Schädigung der Gefäßinnervation mit schließlicher Stase und Thrombose. In diese Gruppe sind auch die von SCHALABUTOFF publizierten Fälle zu rechnen. TOLOSA erörtert diese Fragen an Hand eines einschlägigen Falles, bei dem die Entscheidung, ob es sich um ein Frosterythem oder um einen Raynaud handelt, offen bleiben mußte. Über die diagnostischen Erwägungen, die man bei der Abgrenzung der RAYNAUDschen Krankheit gegenüber den anderen vasomotorischen Erkrankungen anzustellen hat, verweisen wir auf die betreffenden Abschnitte.

Therapie.

Die Behandlung der RAYNAUDschen Krankheit hat die verschiedensten Gesichtspunkte zu berücksichtigen. Man wird zunächst darauf bedacht sein, eine Hebung und Kräftigung des Allgemeinzustandes herbeizuführen, unter besonderer Berücksichtigung der durch die allgemeine neuropathische Diathese bedingten Erfordernisse. Auf diesen Teil der Behandlung brauchen wir hier nicht näher einzugehen; sie ist wie die der allgemeinen Neurosen.

Diätetische Ratschläge gibt MORRIS (zit. nach MUCHA), der Fleischnahrung und Trinken von heißem Wasser zur Verhinderung der Darmgärung empfiehlt, während SHOEMAKER vegetabilische Kost anwendet. MUCHA rät, den Kranken Alkohol und Tabak zu verbieten.

Die *physikalische* Behandlung ist in den verschiedensten Formen angewandt worden. Unter den gegen die Krankheit selbst gerichteten Behandlungsmethoden ist die *elektrische* Behandlung ehemals mit den größten Hoffnungen aufgenommen worden; sie hat aber leider diese bei weitem nicht erfüllt, obwohl an einem wohltätigen Einfluß der lokalen Anwendung der Elektrizität nicht zu zweifeln ist. Wir empfehlen galvanische Hand- und Fußbäder in lauwarmem Wasser in einer Dauer von 10 Minuten. Auch faradische Handbäder haben wir, namentlich in leichteren Fällen mit gutem Erfolg angewandt. TOBY COHN empfiehlt ebenfalls warme galvanische Handbäder, ist jedoch der Ansicht, daß periphere Faradisation nicht ratsam sei. KAHANE und SILLEY haben von der Anwendung der Diathermie Erfolge gesehen. BROOKE hingegen hält letztere in schweren Fällen für kontraindiziert. Manchmal erzielt man, wie LAQUEUR mitteilt, eine Besserung, wenn man Hochfrequenzfunken örtlich appliziert.

Von weiteren physikalischen Prozeduren ist neben lokalen lauwarmen und allgemeinen Bädern am ehesten Erfolg von der Heißluftbehandlung zu erwarten. Wir haben einige Fälle unter Heißluftbehandlung besser werden sehen; auch SCHREIBER empfiehlt dieselbe, verbunden mit Massage jeden 2. Tag je 5 Minuten. Natürlich ist sehr große Vorsicht in der Applikation wegen der geringen Widerstandsfähigkeit der betreffenden Teile am Platze; auch bei der Massage ist größte Vorsicht notwendig. GRAHAM sah bei der Massage Besserung der Zirkulationsstörung und Linderung der Schmerzen. Er massiert in der Richtung nach abwärts, um dem Blutstrom den Weg in die Arterie zu erleichtern; auch empfiehlt er abwechselnde Flexion und Extension von Hand und Fuß anzuwenden; HAMMER hält Schleudern der Hände für zweckmäßig. TOBY COHN wendet die Effleurage und das Tapotement an und macht darauf aufmerksam, daß die Kranken dieselben instinktiv und spontan selber im Anfalle ausführen. Aus theoretischen Erwägungen heraus wendet KERR eine Art Übungstherapie der Gefäße an: die betroffenen Gliedmaßen werden regelmäßig mit Bädern allmählich zunehmender Kälte behandelt, die die normale Hyperämie hervorrufen und so die Stase verhindern sollen (in der ersten Woche 3mal 10 Minuten lang täglich Bad von 10^0, in der zweiten von 8^0, in der dritten von 6^0, in der vierten von 5^0 und in der fünften von 4^0).

PICK will in der Annahme, daß die RAYNAUDsche Krankheit zum Teil auf einer konstitutionellen Minderwertigkeit des Herzens und der Gefäße beruht, eine Beschleunigung und Vermehrung des gesamten Blutumlaufes in die Wege leiten, um auch der Peripherie genügend Blut zuzuführen. Er wendet Herz- und Gefäßgymnastik an und das Luftdruckdifferenzverfahren. Durch dasselbe zwingt er die Lungen durch Unterdruck, der in Gestalt einer Einatmungserschwerung angewendet wird, unmittelbar zu einer größeren Energieleistung und will dadurch eine energischere Stromgeschwindigkeit des Blutes erreichen. CUSHING empfahl als erster die Stauung durch Anwendung des Tourniquet. Wir haben das Verfahren viel und wie es schien, meist mit zufriedenstellendem Erfolge angewendet. Wir ließen eine Cambricbinde so fest um den Oberarm wickeln, bis eine deutliche venöse Stauung eintrat, der arterielle Puls aber fühlbar blieb. Gelegentlich kam es dabei allerdings zu starker Erhöhung der Schmerzen und einer Anschwellung der ganzen Hand, meist aber war der Erfolg ein guter. Auch CRICHLOW u. a. empfehlen Saugglockenunterdruckbehandlung. BRAEUCKER empfiehlt zur konservativen Behandlung folgendes Verfahren: die Extremität wird bis zum Ellenbogen bzw. bis zum Knie luftdicht in ein Hohlgefäß, eine Art Saugglocke eingeschlossen, woraus dann die Luft abgesaugt wird. Der Unterdruck saugt das Blut in die eingeschlossene Extremität hinein, sie schwillt an und füllt sich strotzend mit Blut. Die passive Gefäßerweiterung wird zuerst $1/2$ Stunde, später 1—2 Stunden aufrecht erhalten. Die Gefäße werden stark erweitert, Spasmen und abnorme Gefäßreflexe werden durch die Blutfülle überwunden, und der Einfluß krankhafter Innervationsvorgänge wird durch eine passive und lange anhaltende Dehnung der Gefäßwände beseitigt. Solches Training der Gefäßwände vermag nach seiner Ansicht allmählich die abnormen nervösen Vorgänge im perivasculären Nervennetz zu überwinden und bei anhaltender Übung über längere Zeit hinaus schließlich zum Schwinden zu bringen. Mit diesem Verfahren hat BRAEUCKER 19 Fälle mit meist günstigem Erfolge behandelt.

Ähnliche Erwägungen liegen dem von NÖSSKE empfohlenen Verfahren zugrunde: bei einem Fall von schwerer RAYNAUDscher Krankheit wurden die stark cyanotischen Finger in Lokalanästhesie inzidiert und darauf in der Saugglocke einem negativen Druck von 10 ccm Hg ausgesetzt. Unmittelbar nach der Incision entleerten sich einige Tropfen dunklen Blutes. Der Erfolg war auffallend gut. Eine weitere Fortsetzung dieser Behandlung ergab dieselben günstigen Resultate. In einem von CASSIRER beobachteten Falle wurde mit dieser Methode ein allerdings nur vorübergehender Erfolg erzielt. SCHREIBER hat in einem Falle nach anfänglicher Besserung eine Verschlimmerung des Leidens mit dieser Behandlungsmethode gesehen.

LAPINSKY, der die Symptome der RAYNAUDschen Krankheit auf Entzündungen bzw. Zirkulationsstörungen in den Bauchorganen zurückführt, empfiehlt lange Zeit fortgesetzte heiße Applikationen auf den Bauch.

Eine Reihe von Autoren empfehlen *Strahlenbehandlung:* Blaulichtbestrahlung (LAQUEUR), ultraviolette Strahlen (PARISOT und CORNIL). BORAK hat bei 18 Kranken in der Annahme, daß es sich bei der RAYNAUDschen Krankheit um eine Affektion spinalen Ursprungs handelt, eine Röntgenbestrahlung der die erkrankten Extremitäten versorgenden Rückenmarksabschnitte vorgenommen und mit diesem Verfahren gute Erfolge erzielt. Es kamen immer nur sehr schwache Bestrahlungen zur Anwendung. In 3 Sitzungen in 4—9 tägigen Intervallen wurde ein Drittel der Hauteinheitsdosis (4 H-180 primäre R) bei 0,5 mm Zinkfilter und 170 kV aus 30 cm Abstand auf den erkrankten Rückenmarksabschnitt bei einer Feldgröße von etwa 8—10 cm Breite und 15 cm Länge appliziert. Mittelpunkt des Feldes bei Erkrankung der oberen Extremitäten der 7. Halswirbel, bei Erkrankung der unteren der 1. Lendenwirbel. Nach etwa 4 Wochen wurde die Bestrahlungsserie wiederholt, womit die Behandlung in einem Teil der Fälle beendet war. Mehr als 3 Serien in 4—6wöchentlichen Intervallen kamen nicht zur Anwendung. Er rühmt dieser Methode nach, daß sie die krampfartigen Schmerzen sehr günstig beeinflußt und daß die trophischen Störungen zum Verschwinden gebracht werden. Über ähnliche Erfolge berichten SCHÖNHOF, KRISER und LENK (Literatur bei BORAK). GOUIN und BIENVENUE sahen bei peripherer gefilterter Bestrahlung Hypoleukocytose auftreten, bei zentraler ungefilterter Bestrahlung Hyperleukocytose, MARBURG und SGALITZER haben bei fortgeschrittenen Fällen leichte Besserung gesehen; leichtere Geschwürsbildung wurde gut beeinflußt, am besten die Fälle, bei denen noch keine Geschwürsbildung eingetreten war. MONIER, VINARD, DELHERM und BEAU berichten ebenfalls über Erfolge nach Röntgenbestrahlung, und zwar wenden sie folgendes Verfahren an: Bestrahlung der Hals-Brustwirbelsäule bis D 2 bei Erkrankung des Gesichts und der oberen Extremitäten, wobei die Halsanschwellung und gleichzeitig das Ganglion cervicale inferius getroffen werden. Bei Erkrankung der Zehen wird die untere Brust- und Lendenwirbelsäule bestrahlt, um die Lendenanschwellung und die paravertebralen Ganglien längs der Wirbelsäule zu erreichen. Methodik: Ein Feld auf jeder Seite. EE = 25 cm Distanz. Antikathode = 25 cm. Al = 5 mm. 400 R für die Sitzung, 3 Sitzungen in der Woche, 1200—1600 R für jede Bestrahlungsserie mit einer Ruhepause von mindestens 3 Monaten zwischen jeder Serie. In den Pausen empfehlen die Autoren Diathermiebehandlung.

Chemische gefäßerweiternde Mittel sind vielfach versucht worden, das Amylnitrit (auch als 10%ige Salbe angewandt), das Nitroglycerin, das Trinitrin und in jüngster Zeit das Acethylcholin (10 Injektionen zu 0,1) (GOUGEROT und BURNIER), nach GAUCH, SOHIER und DE COURRÈGES) in einer Dosis von 0,05 subcutan, und verwandte Mittel. RANDAK empfiehlt die intravenöse Darreichung von Akineton. Mit dem Vasotonin haben wir ziemlich umfangreiche Versuche angestellt, aber nur in einzelnen Fällen Erfolge gesehen. MONTGOMERY und CULVER wollen mit einer Darreichung von Calcium lacticum 50 : 300 3mal täglich einen Teelöffel gute Erfolge erzielt haben. Andere Autoren haben Afenilinjektionen empfohlen. HÖSSLIN beobachtete ein Zurückgehen der Anfälle von lokaler Synkope auf Pilocarpin; doch war nach dem Aussetzen des Mittels alles wieder beim alten. Von allen inneren Mitteln empfehlen wir am meisten das Arsen, entweder in Injektion oder in Form der FOWLERschen Lösung. Chinin empfiehlt HERZ. Das theoretisch kontraindizierte Ergotin wird von BROCK gerühmt. Die bisweilen enorm intensiven Schmerzen erfordern häufig ein Eingreifen. Die Antineuralgika, unter denen namentlich das Pyramidon zu erwähnen ist, haben sich uns mehrfach als ganz ausgezeichnete Mittel bewährt. Manchmal sind Narkotika nicht zu entbehren, die enormen Schmerzen trotzen oft selbst hohen Morphiumdosen.

Wo Malaria oder Lues in Frage kommt, zeigen die entsprechenden spezifischen Mittel oft vorzügliche Resultate. In den Fällen, in denen als ätiologische Momente Arteriosklerose oder Nierenkrankheiten eine Rolle spielen, wird man zweckmäßig die Grundkrankheiten behandeln.

Den supponierten Beziehungen zwischen der RAYNAUDschen Krankheit und Störungen der endokrinen Drüsen ist therapeutisch oft Rechnung getragen worden. SOLIS-COHEN verwendet den Nebennierenextrakt; auch das Thyreoidin, bzw. das Jodothyrin wurde einige Male mit Erfolg angewandt (HIRSCH, WEDROV, JELLIFFE and OSBORNE). PRIBRAM hat bei seinem oben erwähnten Fall einen überraschenden Erfolg mit Hypophysininjektionen erzielt. Über ähnliche Erfolge berichten KOPF, BLOCH, SANNICANDRO, RUD, ferner wandten CLAUDE und TINEL Hypophysen- und Ovarialpräparate an. SILBERSTEIN (zit. nach MUCHA) macht darauf aufmerksam, daß bei Schwangeren eine drohende Gangrän durch Schwangerschaftsunterbrechung inhibiert wird, und führt diese Tatsache auf eine endokrine Umstimmung zurück. In den letzten Jahren ist von FREY die Aufmerksamkeit auf die Wirkung des *Kallikreins* (Padutin), eines Kreislaufhormons des Pankreas, gelenkt worden. Kallikrein führt zu Blutdrucksenkung und Erweiterung der Arteriolen, Präcapillaren und Capillaren. Durch Verabreichung von 2—4 Einheiten täglich intragluteal gelingt es nicht nur, den Prozeß oft zum Stillstand zu bringen, sondern auch eine auffallend schnelle Abheilung der trophischen Geschwüre zu erzielen. Die Behandlung muß längere Zeit durchgeführt werden. MESSING wandte bei einem Kranken, bei welchem die periarterielle Sympathektomie erfolglos geblieben war, Insulin an (100 Injektionseinheiten p. o. subcutan) mit sehr günstigem und anhaltendem Erfolge; GIROUX-KISTHINIOS berichten von der Anwendung insulinfreien Pankreasextrakten (Angioxyl).

Ist die Gangrän einmal eingetreten, so ist nach den allgemein gültigen Gesetzen der Chirurgie zu verfahren. Vor einer frühzeitigen Abtragung der nekrotischen Teile ist zu warnen, da die Nekrose im weiteren Verlauf sich meist sehr beschränkt und die Gefahr einer Sepsis nach Art und Ausdehnung der Gangrän nicht vorliegt.

In den letzten Jahren ist die *chirurgische* Behandlung der RAYNAUDschen Krankheit in den Brennpunkt des Interesses gerückt, seitdem LERICHE durch eine *periarterielle Sympathektomie* Erfolge erzielt hat. Auf die theoretischen Erwägungen, die zu der Anwendung dieser Operation geführt haben, wird an anderer Stelle eingegangen werden. Die Operation versagte allerdings gerade bei schweren Fällen, und zwar aus dem Grunde, weil die periarterielle Sympathektomie nur die vasomotorischen Hilfsbahnen unterbricht, die Hauptbahn aber verschont (BRAEUCKER). LERICHE empfahl später sämtliche der Läsion entsprechenden Rami communicantes zu durchschneiden. In der Erwägung, daß die sympathischen Dermatome an den Extremitäten ebenso geordnet sind wie die sensiblen, durchtrennt BRAEUCKER nur noch die Rami communicantes derjenigen Dermatome, in denen Krankheitsäußerungen vorhanden sind: beim Raynaud an der Hand die Rami communicantes von D 1, C 8 und C 7, bei größerer Ausbreitung der Erkrankung auch C 6. Er betont, daß der Ramus communicans von D 1 unbedingt durchschnitten werden müsse, da er den ulnaren Rand der Hand versorge. BRAEUCKER erklärt, daß bei exakter Durchschneidung dieser Wurzeln geradezu schlagartig alle Erscheinungen der Krankheit verschwinden; um das perivasculäre Nervengeflecht auszuschalten, fügt er noch ihre Unterbrechung hinzu, weil erst dadurch die Ausschaltung der vasomotorischen Leitungsbahnen eine vollständige ist. Aber auch in diesem Falle braucht der Erfolg kein absoluter zu sein; so berichtet er über eine Patientin mit schwerem Raynaud der linken Hand, bei der die Krankheitserscheinungen nach Unterbrechung der zugehörigen Rami communicantes und des perivasculären Nervengeflechts vollständig schwanden. Ungefähr ein Jahr später entwickelten sich zur Zeit des Einsetzens klimakterischer Beschwerden an der rechten nicht operierten Hand Zeichen lokaler Asphyxie, ebenso an den Zehen beider Füße; und nun traten auch in der operierten linken Hand Kältegefühl und ziehende Schmerzen im Arm ein ohne sichtbare Zirkulationsstörungen. BRAEUCKER kommt in seinen Untersuchungen zu dem Resultat, daß die Unterbrechung der sympathischen Leitungsbahn zu den Extremitäten in allen Fällen, in denen eine Erkrankung in den vegetativen Zentren oder in den zentralen Abschnitten der Leitungsbahn lokalisiert ist, zu einem vollen Erfolge führen muß. Hat aber die Erkrankung ihren Sitz auch noch in der Peripherie der Leitungsbahn, so kann die Leitungsunterbrechung infolge des Persistierens der sympathischen Endgeflechte ihre Auswirkungen nicht völlig zum Verschwinden bringen. Die Literatur über dieses Thema ist in den letzten Jahren sehr stark angewachsen. Besonders von amerikanischer Seite sucht man sich die physiologischen Erfahrungen zunutze zu machen (LEWIS, ADSON, BROWN und SIMPSON, FAY, TAKATS, DU BOSE) und modifiziert die Operation nach den verschiedensten Richtungen, die an dieser Stelle nicht im einzelnen angeführt werden brauchen. Wir erwähnen die Arbeiten von BRÜNING, BECK, FEILING, KÜMMEL jr., LAWSON, MAYO und ADSON, ALLAN, ROYLE, FULTON, MESCHEDE, W. LEHMANN, DURANTE; der letzte Autor betont, auf Grund von Erfahrungen in 3 Fällen, daß die periarterielle Sympathektomie der kleinen Extremitätenarterien ebenso wirksam sei wie die der großen. LERICHE selbst hat in den letzten Jahren wiederholt in der Frage der Anwendung der periarteriellen Sympathektomie das Wort genommen. Er berichtet über eine ganze Reihe von Dauerheilungen bei der RAYNAUDschen Krankheit, ist aber sehr vorsichtig in seinen Ausführungen hinsichtlich der Indikationsstellung für die periarterielle Sympathektomie. Wenn man die Literatur der letzten Zeit durchmustert, fällt einem auf, daß die kritische Einstellung gegenüber den Dauererfolgen der LERICHschen Operation recht ausgesprochen ist; diese Auffassung kommt besonders in einer Arbeit von DEMEL aus der EISELSBERGSCHEN Klinik zum Ausdruck. Der Autor hat weder Erfolg bei der RAYNAUDschen Krankheit mit der periarteriellen Sympathektomie gesehen, noch mit der von DOPPLER empfohlenen Sympathicodiaphtherese. Wichtig und interessant ist der bereits mehrfach erwähnte Fall RIEDERs, weil er auch einen wertvollen Beitrag zur Lehre von der Capillarfunktion und der Autonomie der peripheren Gefäßnetze liefert. Bei der Kranken mit echter RAYNAUDscher Krankheit wurden alle die rechte Hand versorgenden faßbaren Sympathicusäste entfernt (Ganglion stellatum und thoracale) im Zusammenhang mit einem Teil des Halsgrenzstranges rechts, alle periarteriellen Sympathicusästchen mitsamt dem periarteriellen Gewebe der Arteria subclavia. Der ausgezeichnete Erfolg hielt 4 Monate an; danach trat Akrocyanose am Zeige- und Ringfinger der rechten Hand, nach weiteren 3 Monaten Ulcerationen auf. Die Sektion der an einer intercurrenten Krankheit gestorbenen Kranken bewies, daß die beabsichtigte Ausschaltung des Sympathicus in vollem Umfange gelungen war. BRÜNING berichtet über Erfolge nach Exstirpation des Ganglion stellatum, desgleichen KOLODAN und BOGGON, die raten, auch das zweite Thorakalganglion mit zu entfernen.

Wir selbst haben in einer Reihe von Beobachtungen die Erfahrung gemacht, daß die Erfolge durchaus nicht immer befriedigende sind. Wir haben vollkommene Mißerfolge gesehen, in anderen Fällen nur eine vorübergehend Minderung der Beschwerden und Erscheinungen erzielen können. In einem Falle ist die Exstirpation der Halsganglien erfolgreich gewesen, wenn auch selbst dabei noch immer das Bedenken bestehen bleibt, daß nach der Abstoßung der nekrotischen Partien auch spontan oft genug eine Besserung eingetreten ist.

DE BOVIS sah in 2 Fällen RAYNAUDscher Gangrän einen guten Erfolg von der Nervendehnung. Über die von TRINCAS vorgeschlagene Arterio-venöse Anastomose bestehen noch keine ausreichenden Erfahrungen.

OPPEL berichtet über Erfolge bei 7 Kranken, bei welchen er die Epinephrektomie ausgeführt hat. Von anderer Seite wird diese Operation als theoretisch unbegründet abgelehnt (DEMEL).

II. Die Akroasphyxia chronica (Akrocyanose).

Es gibt eine Anzahl von Beobachtungen, in denen das hauptsächlichste Symptom eine meist von Kindheit an allmählich sich entwickelnde Asphyxie der Extremitätenenden ist. Diese Asphyxie entspricht in ihrem äußeren Habitus und ihrer Lokalisation dem Bilde der lokalen Asphyxie, wie wir sie bei der RAYNAUDschen Krankheit kennen gelernt haben, so daß sie an dieser Stelle nicht nochmals eingehend beschrieben zu werden braucht. Es besteht aber in der Entwicklung dieses Symptoms in den Fällen dieser Art insofern ein Unterschied, als sie sich hier allmählich ohne ausgesprochene Anfälle herausbildet. Neben der *Asphyxie* zeigen die Extremitätenenden meist noch andere Symptome, sei es auf dem Gebiete der *Trophik*, sei es auf dem der *Sensibilität*.

Diesen Symptomenkomplex hat 1896 CROCQ unter dem Namen „Akrocyanosis" als ein selbständiges Krankheitsbild beschrieben und trotz wichtiger gemeinsamer Berührungspunkte von der RAYNAUDschen Krankheit und anderen vasomotorisch-trophischen Erkrankungen abgetrennt. Im Jahre 1900 und in der Folgezeit erweiterte und vertiefte R. CASSIRER unter Beibringung neuer Kasuistik das Krankheitsbild, dem er nach den es hauptsächlich charakterisierenden Symptomen den Namen „Akroasphyxia chronica" beilegte. In den folgenden Jahrzehnten hat diese Erkrankung wiederholt das Interesse der Forscher, besonders in Frankreich auf sich gezogen. 1929 hat LAYANI eine monographische Darstellung herausgegeben, die ein ansehnliches Literaturverzeichnis enthält, die Kasuistik um eine Reihe nach den modernsten Methoden untersuchter Fälle bereichert, das Krankheitsbild jedoch sehr weit faßt.

In der Regel sind die Hände und das untere Drittel der Unterarme Sitz der asphyktischen Verfärbung, öfters auch die Füße und das untere Drittel des Unterschenkels. In seltenen Fällen ist auch die Nase befallen (LAYANI). LAIGNEL-LAVASTINE und PARRISIUS machen darauf aufmerksam, daß ein nach Fingerdruck innerhalb des asphyktischen Bezirkes entstehender anämischer Fleck auffallend lange Zeit braucht um sich auszugleichen. Als Begleiterscheinung findet sich besonders an den Vorderarmen und Unterschenkeln, aber auch am übrigen Körper, eine Cutis marmorata. Die befallenen Teile sind im Gegensatz zu den Fällen von Erythromelalgie kalt, nach LAYANI, der Temperaturmessungen vorgenommen hat, 2—3⁰ kälter als die gesunden Körperteile. Die Kranken sind besonders empfindlich gegen Kälte; die Hände sind stets auffallend feucht.

Die begleitenden *trophischen* Symptome bestehen meist in einer mehr oder minder hochgradigen Hypertrophie der Weichteile der betroffenen Gebiete, während die Knochen unverändert bleiben *(Akroasphyxia hypertrophica)*. In einer kleinen Anzahl von Fällen findet sich an Stelle dieser Hypertrophie eine Neigung zur Verkleinerung, zur Verschmälerung der Extremitätenenden *(Akroasphyxia atrophica)*. Meist sind die Erscheinungen symmetrisch an beiden Händen und Füßen entwickelt, erhebliche Asymmetrien fanden sich z. B. in den Fällen von ROTHFELD.

Die begleitenden *sensiblen* Symptome tragen insofern ein besonders Gepräge, als die die RAYNAUDsche Krankheit sehr häufig charakterisierenden Schmerzen meist fehlen. Dafür findet sich in einigen dieser Fälle eine sehr eigentümliche *Sensibilitätsstörung*, die in bezug auf ihre Ausbreitung und Intensität von den Sensibilitätsstörungen, die gelegentlich bei der RAYNAUDschen Krankheit vorkommen, abweicht. Es läßt sich in diesen Fällen an Händen und Füßen, im wesentlichen im Gebiet der vasomotorischen Störungen, eine erhebliche Herabsetzung der Sensibilität für alle Qualitäten, am stärksten ausgesprochen für Kälte und Schmerz, nachweisen. Die Kranken selbst leiden unter Stechen und Kribbeln in den befallenen Extremitäten und unter einer Erschwerung der Ausführung feinerer Bewegungen. Wir haben diese Sensibilitätsstörung sowohl bei der Akroasphyxia hypertrophica, als auch bei der Akroasphyxia atrophica gefunden und haben sie auch einmal in einem Falle gesehen, der in vieler Beziehung an die Sklerodermie erinnerte. Ganz ähnliche Sensibilitätsstörungen fanden ROTHFELD und KARTJE in ihren Fällen. Die Erklärung derselben macht erhebliche Schwierigkeiten. Diesen Beobachtungen stehen andere von LAYANI und MARAÑON gegenüber, die sie, wenn überhaupt, nur angedeutet feststellen konnten. In einem Falle von COHN traten auf der Dorsalseite der Finger und Hände mit wäßrigem Inhalt gefüllte Blasen auf, wie auch in einem von uns beobachteten Falle.

Fälle von *Akroasphyxia chronica hypertrophica* sind außer von CASSIRER von NOTHNAGEL, PÉHU, ROTHFELD, URECHIA und OBREGIA, LAYANI, BARKER und SLADEN, von KARTJE, STERNBERG, HOFFMANN, CROCQ, GASNE und SOUQUES beschrieben worden. PÉHU hat eine zusammenfassende Studie darüber unter Anführung eines eigenen Falles mitgeteilt.

In der Symptomatologie sind mancherlei Abstufungen erkennbar: Die Hypertrophie braucht nicht stark entwickelt zu sein, sondern im wesentlichen in einer Auflockerung, stärkeren Durchtränkung der gipfelnden Teile zu bestehen. Die Sensibilitätsstörung ist keineswegs eine regelmäßige Erscheinung, sondern nur in einer Anzahl von Fällen, dann aber immer in der hier geschilderten eigentümlichen Ausprägung vorhanden. Auf diese Weise reduziert sich das Krankheitsbild öfters auf eine chronische, einfache Asphyxie, die den Patienten wenig Beschwerden zu machen braucht, mit der sie, namentlich wenn sie schon sehr lange besteht, rechnen und die demgemäß auch häufig in den leichteren Fällen gar nicht zur Kenntnis des Arztes kommt. Es sind das die Fälle, in denen die Patienten dann nur gelegentlich darüber Auskunft geben, daß sie immer blaue oder rote, häufig etwas schwitzende Hände haben.

Wie schon erwähnt, gibt es nun noch einzelne Beobachtungen, in denen neben dauernden vasomotorischen Symptomen namentlich neben permanenter Asphyxie der Haut, Ernährungsstörungen sich finden, die nicht einem hypertrophischen, sondern einem *atrophischen* Typus entsprechen. Derartige Fälle haben wir wiederholt beobachtet. Von SCHÜTZ u. a. ist etwas Ähnliches mitgeteilt worden; es handelt sich jedoch hier zweifellos um recht seltene Beobachtungen, die am meisten Beziehung zur Sklerodermie bzw. Sklerodaktylie haben.

Bevor wir uns den differentialdiagnostischen Betrachtungen zuwenden, ist es zweckmäßig, an dieser Stelle die Resultate der Untersuchungen von LAYANI zu referieren, der unter dem Titel ,,Les Acrocyanoses" den von uns geschilderten Symptomenkomplex weiter faßt und das pathophysiologische Bild der Akrocyanose auf Grund seiner Untersuchungen in 3 Gruppen einteilt: 1. Störungen von seiten des Sympathicus (Insuffizienz oder Hypotonie). 2. Störungen von seiten des endokrinen Systems mit allgemeiner Untererregbarkeit des neurovegetativen Systems (meist Verminderung des Grundumsatzes). 3. Störungen von seiten des kardiovasculären Systems (Tropfenherz, Hypotonie und venöse Hypertension). Diese verschiedenen Äußerungen wachsen auf dem Boden hereditärer vasomotorischer Instabilität. Manchmal spielt auch die Tuberkulose eine Rolle. Die klinischen Formen teilt er ein in symptomatische und assoziierte Formen. Zu den symptomatischen Formen rechnet er die anästhetischen bzw. hypästhetischen, die hypertrophischen und amyotrophischen Krankheitsbilder, zu den assoziierten die Formen, die Verknüpfungen mit den von ihm genannten Ektosympatosen zeigen, d. h. mit der RAYNAUDschen Krankheit, der Erythromelalgie, den Akroparästhesien, der Sklerodermie usw., andererseits mit dem visceralen vasomotorischen Symptomenkomplex, d. h. der Augenmigräne, der paroxymalen Tachykardie, der Enterocolitis mucomembranacea und anderen gewissen Störungen von seiten des Verdauungstractus.

Als organisch bedingte Akrocyanosen, die durch eine Läsion der zentralen sympathischen Bahnen hervorgerufen sind, bezeichnet LAYANI diejenigen Fälle, die infolge von mesencephalen Störungen und bei der Katatonie festgestellt worden sind. CLAUDE und BARUK bezeichnen sie als orthostatische Akrocyanose; sie erscheint plötzlich in vertikaler Stellung und verschwindet in horizontaler Lage. Dieses Phänomen soll nur bei Katatonikern vorkommen, während es bei Dementia simplex und Hebephrenie fehlt. Auf solche Fälle haben ferner bereits CROCQ, OBREGIA und URECHIA, endlich DE JONG aufmerksam gemacht.

Ätiologisch ist zu bemerken, daß die Erkrankung bei Frauen häufiger vorzukommen scheint, als bei Männern. Die hypertrophische Form fand LAYANI 6mal bei Frauen, 4mal bei Männern. TOOMY sah die Erkrankung bei 2 Säuglingen im Alter von 7 und 9 Monaten, THOMAS fand sie bei Schulkindern am häufigsten am Alter von 12 Jahren. Das Syndrom der Akrocyanose wurde besonders häufig bei in der Pubertät stehenden Individuen, aber auch relativ oft in der Menopause beobachtet (zuletzt von KREINDLER-ELIAS berichtet).

Nach SIEMENS ist die Akroasphyxie in ihrer gewöhnlichen Form oft erbbedingt. Er hat sie bei eineiigen Zwillingen übereinstimmend gefunden; er betont jedoch, daß es auch Formen gibt, die weitgehend unabhängig von den Erbanlagen sind.

FRENKEL-TISSOT fand die Erkrankung bei 2 Schwestern, die auch noch andere Symptome einer Störung des vegetativen Systems darboten. Schon LEGROS hat die familiäre Disposition erkannt. Wiederholt ist die abnorme Disposition zu Kälteschäden in den Familien der Akroasphyktiker beobachtet worden. SIEMENS, MARTINET u. a. weisen in diesem Zusammenhange auf das familiäre Auftreten der Frostschäden in diesen Familien hin, sowie darauf, daß die Akroasphyxie den idiodispositionellen Boden für Erfrierungen und Tuberkulide abgibt. So spielt offenbar die Einwirkung von Kälteschäden bei der Ätiologie der Erkrankung eine nicht unerhebliche Rolle (CASSIRER, ROTHFELD, NOBÉCOURT, HERTOGHE, ETIENNE, WEISSENBACH, MAY, LAYANI). Sehr instruktiv ist eine Mitteilung von MAY und DREYFUSS-SÉE: Bei dem von der Erkrankung befallenen Patienten traten die Erscheinungen zu der Zeit auf, in der er einen neuen Beruf ergriff, in welchem er täglich am Schmiedefeuer stand und seine Hände von Zeit zu Zeit in kaltes Wasser tauchen mußte. Bei den von THOMAS beobachteten Fällen traten die Symptome hauptsächlich in der kalten Jahreszeit oder zur Zeit des Wechsels der Saison auf. Ähnliches erwähnt auch KARTJE. Die ungünstigen Einwirkungen von Temperaturschäden werden von BEJLIN bestritten.

Auch dem emotionellen und anaphylaktischen Shock weist LAYANI eine ätiologisch bedeutsame Rolle zu.

Wiederholt ist die Erkrankung im Verlaufe von Infektionskrankheiten aufgetreten. CASSIRER sah sie nach einer schweren Osteomyelitis, MAY im Verlaufe der Encephalitis lethargica bei einem jungen Mädchen, LAYANI im Anschluß an den Typhus unter schweren psychischen Erscheinungen sich einstellen. Die Lues congenita wird gelegentlich als ätiologisches Moment angeführt, wesentlich häufiger findet jedoch die Tuberkulose Erwähnung. LAYANI konnte bei 6 seiner Kranken eine sichere Tuberkulose nachweisen, macht aber darauf aufmerksam, daß bei seinen Kranken die Akrocyanose bereits lange manifest war, bevor die Tuberkulose nachgewiesen werden konnte, so daß er der Tuberkulose jedenfalls keine unmittelbare ätiologische Bedeutung zuschreibt.

Eine Reihe von Autoren hat auf die bedeutsame Rolle hingewiesen, die die Dysfunktion des endokrinen Systems bei der Erkrankung spielt. Störungen der *Schilddrüsentätigkeit* beobachteten LÉVY und DE ROTHSCHILD, HERTOGHE, VINCENT, LAYANI. Letzterer fand bei einer Kranken bei vermindertem Grundumsatz eine deutliche Insuffizienz der Thyreoidea, ebenso BEJLIN, MATHEZ und THOMAS, die in zahlreichen Fällen Kropfbildung konstatierten. CASTELLINO und PENDE beobachteten Hypothyreose. Eine Insuffizienz der *Hypophyse* scheint nach den Angaben von LAYANI nicht selten zu sein; er selbst hat 3 Fälle beobachtet. In dem einen Fall hat sich hypophysäre Fettsucht, Infantilismus, bilaterale Hemianopsie, Erweiterung des Türkensattels gefunden. In einem weiteren Falle findet er sehr große Hände und Füße, auffallendes Wachstum, Prognathie, große Nase und Zunge ohne Türkensattelveränderungen, sowie Verminderung des Grundumsatzes. LEREBOULLET hat ähnliche Beobachtungen gemacht. BEJLIN und GALENKO haben *Nebenniereninsuffizienz* festgestellt. Am bedeutungsvollsten jedoch erscheinen die seitens des *Ovariums* festgestellten Störungen, über die eine Reihe von Autoren übereinstimmend berichtet. In erster Linie sind hier die Arbeiten von MARANON zu nennen, der seine Fälle unter der Bezeichnung *Hypogenitale Hand* publiziert. Er weist auf die mangelhafte ovarielle Funktion der Betroffenen hin, auf die Häufigkeit des Auftretens in der Periode unmittelbar nach der Pubertät und im Klimakterium. Auch BEJLIN beobachtet Hypofunktion der Geschlechtsdrüsen, schwach entwickelte sekundäre Geschlechtsmerkmale, verminderte oder fehlende Libido. Ähnliches berichten VILLARET und ST. GIRONS und HAY. LAYANI beobachtet Dysmennorrhoe, Amennorrhoe, verzögertes Eintreten der Menses. Er stellt auf Grund seiner Untersuchungen fest, daß es sich bei den Kranken in der Regel um eine pluriglanduläre Insuffizienz handelt, und zwar besteht am häufigsten eine thyrreoovarielle Störung. Ähnliche Befunde erhebt auch BEJLIN. Den Grundumsatz findet LAYANI in der Regel um 10—34% vermindert. Interferometrische Studien (MAY-LAGARDE-LAYANI) sprachen jedoch eher für eine Beteiligung des Hypophysen-Nebennierensystems als des thyreo-ovariellen Systems.

Bei *diagnostischen* Erwägungen wird man sich vergegenwärtigen müssen, daß die Akroasphyxie enge Beziehungen zu anderen vasomotorisch-trophischen Erkrankungen unterhält. Die Abgrenzung gegenüber der RAYNAUDschen Krankheit kann natürlich keine ganz scharfe sein. Wir haben ja gesehen, daß es auch bei der RAYNAUDschen Krankheit Fälle gibt, in denen wenigstens im späteren Verlaufe die Anfälle sich immer mehr verwischen und mehr ein gleichmäßiger Zustand sich bildet. Wo aber von vornherein die Progression eine ganz allmähliche ist, haben wir doch unseres Erachtens die Pflicht, eine Abgrenzung von der RAYNAUDschen Krankheit vorzunehmen. CROCQ trennt die Erkrankung scharf von der RAYNAUDschen Krankheit, indem er darauf hinweist, daß im Gegensatz zu letzterer niemals Gangrän auftritt. Die gleiche Auffassung vertritt LAYANI. Wir können dieser Auffassung nicht ohne weiteres beipflichten.

Die Differentialdiagnose gegenüber den Arteriitiden wird leicht zu stellen sein, wenn man sich das bereits bei Besprechung der Diagnose der RAYNAUDschen Krankheit gesagte vergegenwärtigt.

Wichtiger sind die Beziehungen zu der sog. *submalleolaren Erythrocyanose* und dem *Erythema indurativum* (BAZIN). Die tuberkulöse Ätiologie der zuletzt genannten Erkrankung kann als gesichert gelten (TACHAU). In Zweifelsfällen kann der positive Ausfall der Tuberkulinreaktion für die Diagnose ausschlaggebend sein. Die Erythrocyanosis crurum puellarum ist meist eine Erkrankung der jungen Mädchen. Es findet sich eine symmetrische blaurote cyanotische Verdickung der Unterschenkel meist an der Außenseite zwischen Fußknöchel und Wade. Die Haut läßt sich nicht in Falten abheben, ist teigig geschwollen und fühlt sich feucht und kalt an. Im cyanotischen Gebiet sind infolge größerer oder kleinerer Blutungen um die Follikel zinnoberrote Partien zu bemerken (zitiert nach STRANDBERG).

Von sonstigen differentialdiagnostischen Erwägungen kommen noch die folgenden in Frage: Die vasomotorisch-trophischen Störungen bei der *Syringomyelie* können zweifellos ein ähnliches Bild hervorbringen. Die Veränderungen erinnern oft an die ,,main succulente", die wir bei der Syringomyelie so häufig finden. Das Vorhandensein der Sensibilitätsstörung erhöht die Ähnlichkeit mit dieser Erkrankung. Doch ist die Lokalisation bei der Sensibilitätsstörung ja meist eine durchaus andere. Dazu kommt das Fehlen aller motorischen Störungen, sowohl der degenerativ atrophischen, als auch der spastischen Symptome. Doch mögen in einzelnen Fällen nicht alle Zweifel zu lösen sein, wie z. B. in einem Falle, den JOURDENS beschrieben hat.

Einige Fälle dieser Art ergeben der *Akromegalie* ähnliche Bilder. Der 1917 von OECONOMAKIS als Akroasphyxia chronica hypertrophica beschriebene Fall ist wohl mit Sicherheit als echte Gigantoakromegalie aufzufassen, bei der die Erscheinungen der Akroasphyxia chronica hypertrophica nur symptomatischen Wert haben. Über ähnliche Fälle berichtet auch LAYANI. BOETTIGER hat einen Fall als Akromegalie beschrieben, kompliziert durch Erscheinungen der RAYNAUDschen Krankheit; aber es fehlen alle die Akromegalie beweisenden Symptome in seiner Beobachtung: Der Kopfschmerz, die Vergrößerung des Unterkiefers, die Kyphose, die Sehstörung, überhaupt die Allgemeinerscheinungen der Akromegalie. An der Hypertrophie sind die Knochen nicht wesentlich beteiligt, wie auch das Röntgenbild in unseren Fällen erkennen läßt. Übrigens sprach auch der günstige Verlauf, die Rückbildung der Symptome nach einiger Zeit durchaus gegen die Diagnose ,,Akromegalie". Ein Fall von HOFFMANN, von dem Autor auch als Akromegalie aufgefaßt, zeigt ein ähnliches Bild.

Daß die *Polyneuritis*, namentlich gewisse Formen infektiöser Polyneuritis, wie die Beriberi, vasomotorisch-trophische Erscheinungen an den Extremitätenenden von ähnlichem Charakter wie bei der chronischen Asphyxie hervorrufen kann, ist nicht zu bezweifeln. Die Abgrenzung gegenüber diesen Formen wird gegeben durch das Fehlen aller neuritischen Symptome im engeren Sinne, das Fehlen der Druckschmerzhaftigkeit der Nerven, stärkerer Schmerzen, einer sich an die peripheren Nerven anschließenden Sensibilitätsstörung und aller atrophisch-degenerativen Lähmungserscheinungen. Dort, wo atrophische Veränderungen die Asphyxie begleiten, kann ein Bild sich herausbilden, daß der *Akrodermatitis chronica atrophicans* (HERXHEIMER und HARTMANN) ähnlich sieht. Die Symptome bestehen bei dieser Affektion in einer blauroten Verfärbung, einer Fältelung und Zerknitterung der Haut. Die Haut läßt sich leichter in Falten abheben, die sich langsam wieder ausgleichen. Die befallenen Teile sind arm an Haaren und schwitzen weniger. Die Extremitäten sind mit Vorliebe befallen, aber doch nicht die Extremitätenenden, sondern mehr Handrücken und Fingerrücken als die Fingerspitzen. Die Streckseite ist bevorzugt, der Prozeß schreitet mehr zentralwärts fort, häufig streifenförmig. Stets finden sich neben den atrophischen auch infiltrierte Stellen, die die früheren Stadien der Erkrankung darstellen und ihren entzündlichen Grundcharakter. Sensibilitätsstörungen und Schmerzen fehlen. Diese kurzen Angaben (bei HERXHEIMER und HARTMANN findet man eine ausführliche Schilderung der Symptome, der Histologie und auch die Literatur) genügen, um die Unterscheidung dieser Fälle sowohl von der chronischen Asphyxie als auch von der RAYNAUDschen Krankheit zu ermöglichen.

Die in diesem Abschnitte behandelten, vielfach differenten Fälle haben trotz aller Verschiedenheiten sehr intime gegenseitige Beziehungen. Die im Mittelpunkt stehenden Symptome sind solche von seiten der Vasomotilität, und zwar liegt stets eine chronische und meist progrediente Cyanose der Extremitätenenden vor. Sie lehnen sich klinisch mehr oder weniger eng an die RAYNAUDsche Krankheit, zum Teil auch an die Erythromelalgie an (CASSIRER, LAYANI, NOBECOURT), haben auch Beziehungen zur Akroparesthesie und zu den angioneurotischen Ödemen. Fast stets sind auch, wie aus den Krankengeschichten hervorgeht, *neuropathische Individuen* befallen. Man muß in diesen Fällen wohl zu der Annahme neigen, daß materielle, wenn auch recht feine Veränderungen, und zwar am ehesten diffuse, leichte Gliavermehrung in den zentralen Teilen des Vasomotorenapparates als Grundlage der dauernden Veränderungen der Vasomotilität und der Trophik anzusehen sind, und daß mit Ausbreitung dieser Störungen gelegentlich auch die geschilderten sensiblen Störungen zustande kommen. Auch LAYANI nimmt an, daß es sich bei den von ihm als organische Form der Akrocyanose bezeichneten Fällen um eine Schädigung des zentralen Neurons, der mesencephalen Zentren oder des peripheren Neurons handelt und setzt die Störung in Parallele mit der Akrocyanose, die beim thalamischen Syndrom des Parkinsonismus beobachtet ist. Es gibt Fälle chronischer lokaler Asphyxie, bei denen mit größter Sicherheit das Vorhandensein ausgesprochener anatomischer Veränderungen des Nervensystems angenommen werden muß. Solche Fälle sind beschrieben von JOHANNSEN unter dem Titel „lokale Asphyxie, kombiniert mit Funktionsstörungen von seiten des Gehirns", ebenso von BOECK, von SCHEIBER unter dem Titel „ein Fall von symmetrischer Asphyxie", endlich von ANDRÉ-THOMAS, der bei einem Falle von Hemiakrocyanose mit gleichzeitiger muskulärer Überdehnbarkeit und Muskelatrophie die Verknüpfung eines organischen Zustandes mit hysterischen Erscheinungen annimmt. Es leuchtet ein, daß auf der Grundlage organischer Veränderungen der Vasomotorenzentren, sei es nun des in der Medulla oblongata oder der an anderen Stellen gelegenen, dauernde Veränderungen in dem Blutgehalt der Körperteile sich einstellen können, so daß diese sich mit mannigfachen anderen organisch bedingten Veränderungen des Nervensystems kombinieren können. Wir wissen nur leider bisher außerordentlich wenig über solche Erkrankungen und können die hier zuletzt zitierten Fälle nur als Material für später zu erwerbende Kenntnisse betrachten.

In bezug auf die Therapie ist nur wenig zu sagen. In den Fällen, in denen pluriglanduläre Erscheinungen ausgeprägt sind, wird man es mit organo-therapeutischen Maßnahmen versuchen, im übrigen gegen die Gefäßstörungen die Mittel in Anwendung bringen, die bereits bei Besprechung der Therapie der RAYNAUDschen Krankheit Erwähnung gefunden haben.

III. Die Erythromelalgie.

Historisches. Im Jahre 1872 hat WEIR-MITCHELL eine Abhandlung verfaßt, die er "on a rare vasomotor neurosis of the extremities" betitelte und in der er das Krankheitsbild der Erythromelalgie zum ersten Male aufstellte und klinisch umgrenzte. Seine Hauptpublikation stammt aus dem Jahre 1878 und enthält die Krankengeschichten von 6 Fällen eigener Beobachtung, sowie eine Übersicht über die in der Literatur von anderer Seite mitgeteilten Fälle, welche nach seiner Ansicht zu dem von ihm beschriebenen Symptomenkomplex gehörten. Es sind dies Publikationen von GRAVES (1843), PAGET (1871), GRENIER (1873), VULPIAN (1875).

1880 hat dann MAURICE LANNOIS an der Hand einer kasuistischen Mitteilung die Aufmerksamkeit erneut auf das Krankheitsbild gelenkt und für dieses den Namen «Paralysie vasomotrice des extrémités» vorgeschlagen. 1894 haben zwei deutsche Forscher (LEWIN und BENDA) sich eingehend mit dieser Krankheit beschäftigt und sind auf Grund von kritischen Erwägungen zu der Auffassung gelangt, daß die Erythromelalgie als selbständiges Krankheitsbild nicht anzusehen sei. In der Folgezeit war die Erythromelalgie häufiger Gegenstand der Darstellung; einerseits hat WEIR-MITCHELL selbst seine Publikationen fortgesetzt, andererseits wurde die Kenntnis des Krankheitsbildes durch die Mitteilungen pathologisch-anatomischer Befunde erweitert (DEHIO, AUERBACH, WEIR-MITCHELL, SPILLER).

Abgesehen von den Zusammenfassungen, die in anderen Handbüchern zu finden sind, ist besonders zu erwähnen die umfassende Darstellung der Erythromelalgie von R. CASSIRER in seiner Monographie „die vasomotorisch-trophischen Neurosen" (2. Aufl. 1912).

Ätiologie.

Die Erkrankung ist in jedem Lebensalter beobachtet worden, am seltensten bei Kindern (HENOCH, KOPPIUS, STAEDTLER, SERIO, AVEZZU, NOBÉCOURT, ISHIDA), wiederholt im hohen Greisenalter (GRAVES, LÉVY). Es scheint, als ob das männliche Geschlecht häufiger an Erythromelalgie erkrankt als das weibliche. Nach einer Statistik der Mayoklinik kommt auf 200 Kranke mit peripherer vasculärer Erkrankung nur 1 Fall von primärer Erythromelalgie (BROWN).

Mannigfaltige Schädigungen werden für das Auftreten der Erkrankung verantwortlich gemacht. Oft hat sie sich im Anschluß an *berufliche Überanstrengungen* entwickelt; je ein Kranker von WEIR-MITCHELL und von MORGAN hatte seine Hand, die später von Erythromelalgie betroffen wurde, durch Klopfen mit einem kleinen Hammer längere Zeit hindurch angestrengt. Im Anschluß an anstrengende Märsche und intensives Maschinennähen ist die Erkrankung aufgetreten; SACHS & WIENER sowie SCHIRMACHER wollen festgestellt haben, daß der Schneiderberuf zu dieser Erkrankung disponiere. *Thermische Schädlichkeiten*, Kälte, Nässe und Hitze werden von LANNOIS, WEIR-MITCHELL, GERRARD, DEHIO, KELLY, SCHENK, u. a. angegeben. Der Kranke von BIKELES und RADONIČIČ war als Schiffsheizer raschen, exzessiven Temperaturunterschieden ausgesetzt. Im Falle von AVEZZU trat die Erkrankung im Anschluß an eine durch Erkältung bedingte Neuritis der beiden Medianusnerven auf. SPIELMEYER hat die Erythromelalgie in 4 Fällen von Medianusläsion beobachtet. Bei einem von uns beobachteten Falle trat das Leiden im Anschluß an eine Infanteriegeschoßverletzung am linken Unterschenkel auf. In einigen Fällen war ein lokales Trauma vorausgegangen. Eine interessante Beobachtung wird von BING-RAPOPORT publiziert: 2 Jahre nach einem Unfall mit Luxationsfraktur des 6. Halswirbels, wobei eine Kompression und Zerrung im Gebiete der letzten Cervical- und obersten Dorsalwurzeln erfolgt war, trat zunächst eine Neuralgie im betroffenen Nervenanteil auf, dem später eine Erythromelalgie in der Hand und der vom rechtsseitigen Halssympathicus versorgten Teile des Gesichts folgte (Erythroprosopalgie-BING).

Intoxikationen und Infektionen scheinen keine wesentliche Rolle zu spielen; NIELSEN sah nach einer Synergenvergiftung (15 Tabletten zu je 1 mg) ein erythromelalgieähnliches Krankheitsbild auftreten. Die Kranken von CAVAZZINI, BRACCHI und BIKELES waren maßlose Raucher. In einigen Fällen wurde Lues in der Vorgeschichte festgestellt (PERSONALI, LUZZATO, CASSIRER, KUNSTMANN, MAY, HILLEMAND, TSUJI). CEDERBERG sah sie familiär nach Bothriocephalusinfektion, HOSHINA bei Ascariden auftreten. In anderen Fällen waren Frauen im Klimakterium von der Erkrankung betroffen. LANDGRAF sah sie nach Myxödem, EICKEN nach Basedow auftreten. Einige französische Autoren beschrieben Fälle, in denen eine Nebennierenerkrankung als ätiologischer Faktor wirkte. Bei einer Patientin von HORIUCHI traten die Erscheinungen einige Tage nach der Entbindung auf, ein zweiter Anfall erfolgte einige Tage nach der zweiten Entbindung. Zwei Patienten von LAIGNEL-LAVASTINE waren ovarioektomiert.

Symptomatologie.

Wie schon der Name Erythromelalgie besagt, bestehen die hauptsächlichsten Merkmale der Erkrankung in Schmerzhaftigkeit und Röte an den Gliedern. Der *Schmerz* ist das beherrschende Symptom und steht im Beginn durchaus im Vordergrund des Krankheitsbildes. Er wird von den Kranken übereinstimmend als stechender, brennender Schmerz gekennzeichnet, der mit einer enormen Intensität auftritt. Manchmal setzen diese Schmerzen sofort mit voller Heftigkeit ein oder aber es kommt im Anfang zunächst nur zu unangenehmen Sensationen, Taubheitsgefühl, Kribbeln; zu diesen gesellt sich dann der immer stärker werdende Schmerz, der für die Kranken eine unerträgliche Marter bedeutet und sie infolge von Schlaflosigkeit in ihrem Allgemeinzustand erheblich herunterbringt. Im Beginn der Erkrankung hat der Schmerz oft intermittierenden Charakter, später ist er jedoch häufig dauernd vorhanden. Herabhängenlassen des schmerzenden Gliedes, Wärme und Anstrengung lösen die Schmerzattacken aus oder steigern die schon vorhandenen. Aber es wird auch über Fälle berichtet, welche Kälte schlecht vertrugen (BERNHARDT, EULENBURG, FINGER, PRENTIS, HAMILTON, WEBER) und bei denen trotz aller Versuche durch die eben erwähnten Kunstgriffe die Auslösung der Anfälle mißlang (GSTREIN und SINGER). Bei dem oben erwähnten Kriegsverletzten, den CASSIRER beobachtete, wurden die Schmerzen, je länger der Fuß herabhing, um so intensiver; jede Benutzung des Fußes zum Gehen war völlig unmöglich; der Kranke konnte eben mit der Fußspitze leicht auftreten. SAINTON und VÉRAN sahen in ihrem Falle bei Einsetzen der Schmerzkrisen, die bis zur Ellenbeuge ausstrahlten, vorübergehende Fingerkontrakturen.

Nachdem der Schmerz einige Zeit bestanden hat, gesellen sich als weitere Symptome die *Röte* und *Schwellung* hinzu. Oft beträgt das zeitliche Intervall zwischen dem Auftreten von Schmerz und Rötung 6—8 Wochen; es sind jedoch auch Fälle beschrieben worden, bei denen Schmerz und Rötung gleichzeitig in Erscheinung getreten sind (EULENBURG, PEZZOLI). Im Beginn der Erkrankung ist die Farbe der betroffenen Teile hellrot bis purpurfarben; es zeigt sich eben das Bild der aktiven Hyperämie, der Kongestionsröte. Die Haut ist turgescent, die Arterien klopfen und pulsieren, die Venen scheinen oft erweitert. Allmählich geht das Bild der aktiven Hyperämie in eine passive über; der Farbenton wird bläulichrot und später violett. Auf Druck schwindet die Verfärbung, um jedoch alsbald wiederzukehren. Bisweilen wird die dunkelrote Färbung der Haut von helleren Flecken unterbrochen. Die Rötung beschränkt sich im allgemeinen auf die schmerzempfindlichen Teile, also meist auf die Extremitätenenden. PARRISIUS hat mit dem Capillarmikroskop derartige Stellen bei Kranken untersucht; er fand in den hellroten Partien, daß immer gute Strömung vorhanden war, nicht das „va et vient" (ein Hin- und Herpendeln der Blutsäule), wie EBBECKE es beschreibt. Die arteriellen Schenkel der Capillaren waren zwar auch enger als die weiten und gänzlich schlaffen Gefäße des subpapillären Plexus, aber doch weiter als bei dem mit völliger Stase einhergehenden Zustand. Der Hauptunterschied war der, daß in den cyanotischen Partien Stase, in den ziegelroten gute Strömung herrschte. MINDLIN beschreibt Riesencapillaren mit reichlichen Anastomosen, neben Atonie und Erweiterung auch Spasmen. In dem später eingehender zu besprechenden Fall von GSTREIN und

SINGER, der mit Polyglobulie kompliziert war, zeigte die Capillaruntersuchung, daß die Capillaren der rechten gesunden Hand wohl leicht geschlängelt waren, was bei dem hohen Blutdruck nicht zu verwundern war; die Capillaren der erkrankten ulnaren Seite der linken Hand waren geradezu in Achtertouren gewunden und im Vergleich zur anderen Seite mächtig erweitert. Ähnliches beschreibt NIEKAU.

Meist kann man in den befallenen Partien eine Erhöhung der Hauttemperatur feststellen (G. BROWN). In einem Falle von STURGE betrug die Temperatur am Fuße außerhalb der Anfälle 24° C und stieg in den Anfällen auf 34,4° C. Auch LANNOIS fand stets eine ausgesprochene Temperaturdifferenz gegenüber dem gesunden Fuße. An diesem war meist die Temperatur 2—3° niedriger. Tritt im Laufe der Zeit livide Verfärbung und Cyanose ein, so läßt sich eine *Herabsetzung* der Temperatur an den erkrankten Gebieten beobachten.

Meist beobachtet man ein anfallsweises Auftreten der Erscheinungen; sehr oft sind sie durch Lageveränderungen der Gliedmaßen hervorzurufen. In einem Falle, den CASSIRER beobachtete, färbten sich in frappierender Weise noch in derselben Sekunde, in der die Kranke ihr Bein aus der horizontalen Lage in die senkrechte brachte, zuerst die Zehen tief dunkelrot und allmählich breitete sich diese Verfärbung in abnehmender Stärke bis zur Mitte der Wade aus. Gleichzeitig stellten sich Schmerzen und Temperatursteigerung ein; alle diese Erscheinungen kehrten augenblicklich zur Norm zurück, sobald das Bein wieder in die horizontale Lage versetzt wurde.

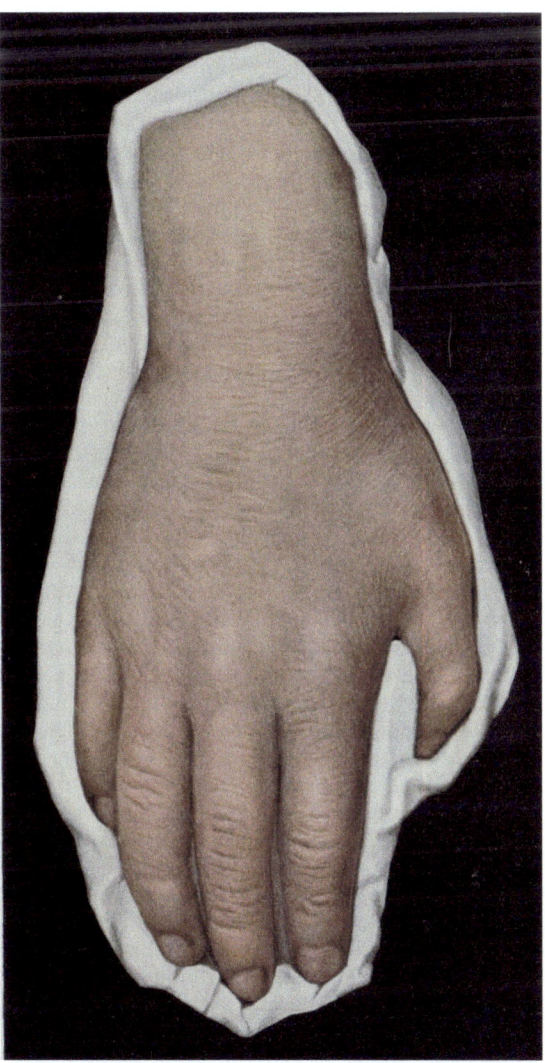

Abb. 6. Erythromelalgie. (Nach J. HOSHINA: Iconographia dermatologica, syphilidologica et urologica, 1932).

Der Lieblingssitz der Erythromelalgie sind die *Füße*. Doch werden die Erscheinungen auch an den Händen oder an allen 4 Extremitäten beobachtet. Ein hemiplegischer Typ war 3mal vertreten. Bei dem 45jährigen Kranken SCHIRMACHERs begann die Erkrankung mit starkem Schwitzen, Jucken und Kribbeln im linken Zeigefinger. Das Leiden ergriff später die übrigen Finger, den Oberarm, Rumpf, linken Fuß und beide großen Zehen. Bei einem Kranken von Lévi waren die Symptome an einem Ohrläppchen zu sehen, bei einer Beobachtung von Padilla waren außer den Händen und Füßen auch die Ohren, Nasenspitze und Wangen befallen. Schon früher haben Cavazzini und Bracchi an der Nasenspitze die Symptome der Erythromelalgie festgestellt.

Außer diesen Fällen werden noch solche beobachtet, in denen die Erscheinungen im wesentlichen an den Innervationsbereich eines oder mehrerer peripherer Nerven gebunden sind. In dem auch noch in anderer Hinsicht interessanten, schon erwähnten Falle von Gstrein und Singer fand sich eine hart an die Grenze des Innervationsbereichs des peripheren Teiles des Nervus ulnaris der linken Hand gebundene Hyperästhesie, Hyperalgesie und Thermhypästhesie mit Schweißsekretion im gleichen Gebiete; die Haut des Kleinfingers war dünn, glänzend und gespannt, die ulnaren Fingerkuppen heiß und lebhaft rot. Treten die Schmerzen überhaupt an mehr als einer Extremität auf, so beobachtet man fast immer, daß ein Glied nach dem andern befallen wird. Es können Jahre vergehen, bis der Schmerz seine örtlich größte Ausdehnung erreicht hat. Daß andere Teile als die Akra der Sitz des Schmerzes und der Rötung sind, ist selten. In einem Falle von Goette z. B. blieben diese aber ganz frei. H. Curschmann erwähnt einen Fall, bei welchem die Unterschenkel oberhalb der Knöchel allein betroffen waren.

Fast regelmäßig klagen die Kranken auch noch über eine gesteigerte Empfindlichkeit der befallenen Teile, insbesondere für Berührung. Sie können den Druck der Bettdecke nicht ertragen, das Tragen von Strümpfen und Stiefeln ist ihnen lästig, und besonders schmerzhaft ist das Gehen.

Bei einer ganz erheblichen Zahl von Kranken finden sich Störungen der *Schweißsekretion,* und zwar regelmäßig in Form der Hyperhidrosis (Collier, Weir-Mitchell, Eulenburg, Schirmacher). Oft trat sie in dem Augenblicke auf, in welchem der Schmerzparoxysmus seinen Höhepunkt erreichte.

Als weiteres lokales Symptom erwähnen wir die *trophischen Störungen.* Während die ersten Autoren auf das Fehlen trophischer Veränderungen aufmerksam machten (Lannois, Graves, Weir-Mitchell, Paget), lehrten spätere Beobachtungen, daß trophische Veränderungen verschiedenster Art vorkommen. In der Literatur sind erwähnt: diffuse oder knötchenartige Verdickungen der Haut, der Unterhaut, Auftreibung der Endphalangen der Finger und der Zehen, Verdickung und Verbiegung der Nägel (Grenier, Senator, Gerhardt, Lewin-Benda u. a.). Cassirer hat das Zusammenvorkommen von Erythromelalgie und Angiokeratomen, namentlich an den Fußsohlen, beobachtet. Wir halten diese Kombination deshalb für bemerkenswert, weil es sich bei den Angiokeratomen um eine Affektion des Hautgefäßapparats zu handeln scheint, die unter dem Einfluß thermischer Schädlichkeiten eintritt. Die Koinzidenz der beiden Erscheinungsreihen ist daher nicht als eine zufällige anzusehen, sondern deutet auf eine Insuffizienz bestimmter Apparate auf gemeinsamer Grundlage.

Wiederholt wurden ausgesprochene atrophische Veränderungen der Haut beobachtet. Diese sieht dann ganz ähnlich aus, wie die nach peripheren Verletzungen auftretende Glanzhaut (Weir-Mitchell, Dehio). Beobachtungen von Lassar und Schütz, die eine Kombination von Erythromelalgie mit Akrodermatitis atrophicans beschreiben, weichen so sehr vom Typus der Erythromelalgie ab, daß die Zugehörigkeit dieser beiden Fälle zur Erythromelalgie fraglich erscheinen muß. Auch Übergänge von Hauthypertrophie in Hautatrophie sind festgestellt worden, ferner glatte, spröde, rissige Haut (Eulenburg), glattes, glänzendes Aussehen der Finger (Lévi), pergamentartig veränderte Haut (Schwarz); auch die Nägel, Drüsen und Haare zeigen oft zahlreiche dystrophische Veränderungen.

Häufig werden auch die Knochen betroffen. Im Falle von WEIR-MITCHELL und SPILLER waren die Knochen der großen Zehe größer als die eines normalen Skelets. Bei einem Kranken, den wir beobachteten, war die Erkrankung im Anschluß an ein Trauma aufgetreten; der Prozeß hatte in der Hauptsache die linke große Zehe befallen, die geschwollen war. Im Liegen war sie blaß und die Geschwulst trat etwas zurück, während im Stehen Rötung und Hitze eintrat. Hier ergab das Röntgenbild, daß die beiden Phalangen und das Metacarpale I links gegenüber rechts erheblich verdickt war. In anderen Fällen fanden wir diffuse Knochenatrophie. In dem Falle von GSTREIN und SINGER fand sich im Röntgenbild konzentrische Atrophie der Handwurzelknochen und Entwicklungshemmung im Bereiche der Mittelhandknochen und der Fingerknochen. Die Karpalknochen waren konzentrisch verkleinert, und zwar betrug die Verkleinerung in allen Dimensionen und allen Durchmessern etwa 20% gegenüber der gesunden Seite. Sonst war eine Veränderung in der Struktur oder Form der Knochen nicht festzustellen. Die Länge der Mittelhand- und Fingerknochen entsprach der gesunden Seite, nur war der Durchmesser der Knochen um etwa 4% kleiner. KÖNIGSTEIN fand eine Haut-, Muskel- und Knochenatrophie einer Extremität bei gleichzeitiger Erythromelalgie und Hyperglobulie.

Während früherer Beobachter das Vorkommen von *Gangrän* bei Erythromelalgie ablehnten, haben spätere Erfahrungen gezeigt, daß es Fälle gibt, in denen zu einer typischen Erythromelalgie im späteren Verlauf plötzlich eine Gangrän sich einstellt, die ihrer Art und Ausdehnung nach durchaus der RAYNAUDschen Gangrän glich. So berichtet RADONIČIČ über einen Patienten, der vor mehr als einem Jahr an nächtlichen Schmerzen in den unteren Extremitäten erkrankte, die von den Zehen bis an den Oberschenkel zogen und durch Kälte gebessert wurden. Nach vorübergehender Besserung traten unter dem Einfluß der psychischen Erregungen und körperlichen Strapazen des Feldzuges die Erscheinungen wieder auf. Die Haut, namentlich des linken Fußes, war gerötet, hyperästhetisch und geschwellt. An den ersten drei Zehen entwickelten sich Geschwüre, an den distalsten Partien trat Analgesie und Hypästhesie auf. Auch andere Autoren haben Fälle beobachtet, in denen zu den typischen vasomotorischen Veränderungen der Erythromelalgie sich allmählich immer deutlicher werdende Symptome vom Raynaudtyp zugesellten, entweder in Form von Synkope und Asphyxie locale oder als Gangrän. In anderen Fällen waren nur die vasomotorischen Symptome der RAYNAUDschen Krankheit zu beobachten, während eine Nekrose sich nicht einstellte. Erst kürzlich habe ich einen Fall beobachtet, der neben den typischen Symptomen der Erythromelalgie eine typische RAYNAUDsche Geschwürsbildung zeigte. Der Prozeß war im wesentlichen im linken Fuß lokalisiert. Eine sehr eigenartige Beobachtung hat CALHOUN in einem Fall von Erythromelalgie mit Ausgang in RAYNAUDsche Krankheit gemacht. Er fand eine Cyanose der Retina; bei normalem Visus war der Fundus im ganzen dunkler rot als gewöhnlich; die temporale Hälfte der Papille scharf gezeichnet, die nasale dagegen verschwommen und leicht ödematös. Die retinalen Gefäße wiesen eine auffallende Zunahme an Zahl, Größe und Schlängelung auf. Die Arterien waren dunkler als normal; die Venen erweckten nach Umfang und Gestalt den Eindruck einer Masse von Würmern. Bei Übergang aus der aufrechten in die sitzende Stellung sah man deutlich Zunahme der Venenerweiterung. Verf. erklärt dieses Phänomen aus einem Mangel an vasomotorischem Tonus.

CASSIRER und auch andere Autoren (MILLS, MOREL-LAVALLÉE, POTAIN, SCHWARZ, ELSNER, ROST, MOLL, RADONIČIČ) sehen in allen diesen Fällen einen Beweis dafür, daß enge verwandtschaftliche Beziehungen zwischen der RAYNAUDschen Krankheit und der Erythromelalgie bestehen müssen.

Cassirer hat den Standpunkt vertreten, daß gerade in denjenigen Fällen häufig große symptomatische Ähnlichkeiten mit der RAYNAUDschen Krankheit sich ergeben, in denen die Erythromelalgie sich ganz und gar unter dem Bilde der Neurose darstellt, in denen also alle Zeichen einer Erkrankung organischer Art von seiten des zentralen oder peripheren Nervensystems oder des Gefäßapparates fehlen, so daß man wohl versucht sein könnte, die Erythromelalgie in diesem Sinne ganz als eine Varietät der RAYNAUDschen Krankheit anzusehen.

Auch zu anderen vasomotorisch-trophischen Erkrankungen bestehen mannigfaltige Beziehungen, über die in den entsprechenden Kapiteln berichtet werden wird. Enge Beziehungen zur *Sklerodermie* weisen die Fälle von STILLÉ und SAVILL auf; beide Fälle, die die Autoren zur Erythromelalgie rechnen, will CASSIRER dem Gebiete der Sklerodermie zuweisen.

Recht selten scheint die Kombination von Erythromelalgie und QUINCKEschem Ödem zu sein (H. SCHLESINGER u. a.). MAY berichtet über eine Kranke, die seit ihrer Kindheit an rezidivierendem QUINCKEschem Ödem litt. Später traten schmerzhafte Rötung und ödematöse Schwellung beider Beine auf. Außerdem bestanden Symptome von Tetanie und eine Arthritis deformans der Hände. Ein recht kompliziertes Krankheitsbild hat CASSIRER im Jahre 1905 beobachtet; es handelte sich um eine 46jährige Frau, die Symptome teils von RAYNAUDscher Krankheit, teils von Erythromelalgie, teils des angioneurotischen Ödems darbot.

Frühzeitig schon ist die Aufmerksamkeit der Forscher auf die Veränderung des *Blutbildes* bei Erythromelalgie gelenkt worden. Zahlreiche Veränderungen sind beschrieben worden, deren Wiedergabe sich jedoch im Hinblick auf ihre Mannigfaltigkeit erübrigt. Jedoch bedarf besonderer Erwähnung die Verbindung der Erythromelalgie mit der *Polycythämie*, welche in den letzten Jahren wiederholt Gegenstand der Forschung gewesen ist (PARKES WEBER, R. SCHMIDT, ROSENGART, SCHMELINSKI, GSTREIN und SINGER, KRAEGER, ZADEK, AVEZZU, HVAL, TSUJI; letzterer stellte in seinem Fall das Vorhandensein des BENCE-JONES-Eiweißkörpers im Urin fest). In dem Falle von GSTREIN und SINGER handelt es sich um eine 47jährige Frau; die Hauptsymptome ihrer Erkrankung waren einerseits Dystrophie der ulnaren Hälfte des linken Vorderarms, mäßige Atrophie des linken Hypothenar, Hyperästhesie im ulnaren Gebiet der linken Hand, Thermhypästhesie, starke Schmerzhaftigkeit, circumscripte Röte, erhöhte Temperatur und gesteigerte Schweißsekretion in den betroffenen Teilen; andererseits bestanden düsterrote Verfärbung der Gesichts-, Hals- und Brusthaut, der Schleimhaut des Mundes, Rachens, Kehlkopfes, Herzhypertrophie, starke gefüllte Halsvenen, stark erweiterte, geschlängelte Arterien, stark erhöhter Blutdruck und Zahnfleischblutungen, außerdem ein derber Milz- und Lebertumor. Die Zahl der roten Blutkörperchen betrug 10 000 000, die der weißen Blutkörperchen 19 000, Hämoglobin SAHLI 110%. Im Ausstrich hämoglobinarme anisocytotische Formen roter Blutkörperchen, 2 Normoblasten. Die weißen Blutkörperchen zeigten geringe Polynucleose. Am gesunden rechten Arm war der Blutdruck 200, am kranken linken Arm 160 mm Hg. Diese Differenz des Blutdrucks zwischen rechts und links erklären sich der Verfasser in der Weise, daß im erythromelalgischen Anfall eine beträchtliche Erweiterung der Blutgefäße eintritt, wobei die Verbreiterung des Stromgebiets eine Verringerung des inneren Widerstandes zur Folge hat und auf solche Weise die Blutsenkung bedingt. Für diese Erweiterung der Gefäße an der linken oberen Extremität sprach ferner die lebhafte aktive Hyperämie, die in einer flammenden Röte der ulnaren Hälfte der linken Hand ihren Ausdruck fand. Mit der Verschlechterung des Blutbildes ging auch eine Verschlechterung der erythromelalgischen Erscheinungen Hand in Hand und umgekehrt. Im Falle von AVEZZU fand sich eine Vermehrung der roten Blutkörperchen, beträchtliche Leukocytose unter Vermehrung der polynukleären Neutrophilen und Schleimhauthämorrhagien. HORIUCHI hat in seinen 3 Fällen starke Eosinophilie und Hyperglobulie festgestellt; ähnliche Befunde erhob KÖNIGSTEIN. HVAL beobachtete in einem ähnlichen Falle das Auftreten von Gangrän.

Im Falle von ZADEK traten die erythromelalgischen Symptome am rechten Bein erst auf, nachdem die Polycythämie 4 Jahre bestanden hatte. Es fand sich außerdem eine motorische Schwäche im rechten Arm und Bein. Das BABINSKIsche Zeichen war rechts positiv, die Reflexe der rechten unteren Extremität gesteigert. Dieses Zeichen einer organischen zentralnervösen Erscheinung veranlaßt ZADEK, die Hypothese auszusprechen, daß vorübergehende Gefäßstörungen im Zentralnervensystem auf Grund oder auf dem Boden der Polycythämie auch für die Erythromelalgie in Betracht kommen. Dieser Fall bildet den Übergang zu denjenigen Fällen, in denen neben der Erythromelalgie die Symptome einer *organischen Affektion* des *Zentralnervensystems* in Erscheinung treten, während bisher nur von solchen Fällen die Rede war, bei denen neben den im engeren Sinne als Erythromelalgie bezeichneten Symptomen nur noch Zeichen einer mehr oder weniger großen Labilität des gesamten Nervensystems und besonders des vegetativen Systems vorhanden waren. In diese zweite Gruppe gehören die Beobachtungen, bei denen eine Kombination von Erythromelalgie mit Hemiplegie (HENOCH, GRAVES, SMITH), Neuritis (VEDEL, PUACH und CHARDONNEAU), mit progressiver Paralyse (MACHOL, CASSIRER, LEWIN-BENDA), mit Tabes dorsalis (PERSONALI, AUERBACH, WOODNUT und COLLIER, CASSIRER, DUMAS und CHEVALIER), mit multipler Sklerose (COLLIER), mit Myelitis (COLLIER), nachweisbar war. SCHLESINGER beobachtete die Erythromelalgie einige Wochen hindurch bei einem extramedullären Tumor, POSPELOV bei Gliosis spinalis; TAUBERT und FERRANINI fanden sie bei Syringomyelie. In dem Falle von ROSS und BURY zeigte sich eine Kombination von Polyneuritis und den Symptomen der Erythromelalgie. HIROSE und SHINAZONO beschrieben erythromelylgieähnliche Symptome im Verlauf von Beri-Beri.

In einer Reihe von Fällen beschränken sich die Symptome der Erythromelalgie auf das Gebiet eines oder mehrerer bestimmter Nerven, ohne daß jedoch Symptome von Neuritis festzustellen waren; das gesamte Krankheitsbild zeigte sich in Rötung, Schmerzen, Schwellung der umschriebenen Nervengebiete (MORGAN, WEIR-MITCHELL, BOWEN, DÜNGER, HEIMANN, LEWIN, GSTREIN und SINGER). Einige dieser Fälle wiesen auch eine Druckschmerzhaftigkeit der entsprechenden Nerven auf, so daß das Krankheitsbild nur dadurch von der echten Neuralgie zu unterscheiden war, daß die vasosensiblen Fasern besonders stark in Mitleidenschaft gezogen waren.

Wie bei den anderen vasomotorisch-trophischen Erkrankungen, so finden sich auch bei den an Erythromelalgie leidenden Kranken die Anzeichen einer allgemeinen *neuropathischen Diathese:* Kopfschmerz, Migräne, Schwindel, Schlafstörungen, pathologische Stimmungsschwankungen, abnorme Erregbarkeit. Bei einer Reihe von Fällen wurden ausgesprochene Psychosen beobachtet (NIEDEN, CHRISTIANI, HORNOWSKI und RUDZKI). Auch der Zusammenhang dieser Erkrankung mit Hysterie ist zuweilen in der Literatur erwähnt. So berichtet H. CURSCHMANN über Erythromelalgie bei einer cyclischen Depression und bei schwerer Hysterie. Im Falle von MUMFORD standen hysterische Erscheinungen im Vordergrund; die Schwester litt an RAYNAUDscher Krankheit.

Kombinationen der Erythromelalgie mit endokrinen Störungen sind wiederholt beschrieben worden; beim Kranken von PRINCI bestand geringe Libido, das Fett an Brust, Gesäß, Armen und Hüften war vermehrt. PRINCI spricht von einer Keimdrüseninsuffizienz und will eine Besserung nach Darreichung von Testikelpräparaten und Adrenalin erzielt haben. PADILLA beobachtete bei seinen Kranken eine abnorme Reizbarkeit des vegetativen Systems, Hyperthyreoidismus, Hypopituitarismus, Hyposuprarenalismus und Hypogenitalismus. MAY sah eine Kombination mit Tetanie.

Endlich gibt es eine Reihe von Fällen mit Erkrankungen des *Herzens* und der *Gefäße*, bei denen Symptome von Erythromelalgie auftraten (DEHIO, WEIR-MITCHELL und SPILLER, SACHS und WIENER, ELSNER, HAMILTON, KELLY, LANNOIS und POROT, PARKES WEBER). SAINTON und VÉRAU sahen die Kombination von Erythromelalgie-Symptomen mit Aortitis, Mitralstenose und Basedow. Die Erythromelalgie setzte 6 Monate nach dem Auftreten der BASEDOWschen Krankheit ein. Diese Beobachtungen verdienen deswegen besonders registriert zu werden, weil sie beweisen, daß die erythromelalgischen Symptome als Begleiterscheinung einer organisch bedingten Erkrankung peripherer Gefäße, vor allem der Endarteriitis obliterans auftreten können. Häufig genug begleiten, wie CASSIRER wiederholt beobachtet hat, vasomotorische Reizerscheinungen die organische Erkrankung des Gefäßsystems, meist sind diese jedoch vasoconstrictorischen Charakters, führen zu Syncope locale und Asphyxie locale. Es kommen jedoch auch vasodilatatorische Reizphänomene als Begleiterscheinungen vor. In dieser Hinsicht bedeutungsvoll sind die oben erwähnten Capillaruntersuchungsbefunde. In solchen Fällen hat aber die Erythromelalgie nur symptomatische Bedeutung; demnach ist auch der Schluß, der verschiedentlich aus solchen Beobachtungen gezogen wurde, daß die Erythromelalgie immer oder häufig in einer organischen Erkrankung des Gefäßsystems ihre Ursache hat, zurückzuweisen. Ohne daß diese Beobachtungen einen Aufschluß über die Pathologie der eigentlichen Erythromelalgie geben, sind sie jedoch wohl geeignet, durch Hinzukommen von Erscheinungen, die den Symptomen der Erythromelalgie nahestehen, die Symptomatologie des intermittierenden Hinkens und der Endarteriitis obliterans zu bereichern.

Pathologische Anatomie und Pathogenese.

Nicht allzu zahlreich sind die pathologisch-anatomischen Untersuchungen, die bei der Erythromelalgie ausgeführt worden sind. Mitteilungen über Sektionsbefunde stammen von AUERBACH, ELSNER, LANNOIS und POROT, HAMILTON, SHAW, HORNOWSKI und RUDSKI. Bei einer größeren Anzahl von Fällen wurden Nervenstücke excidiert und untersucht, so von WEIR-MITCHELL, DEHIO, SPILLER, SACHS und WIENER, KUNSTMANN. In der kritischen Beurteilung dieser Fälle weist CASSIRER darauf hin, daß nicht alle sichere Erythromelalgie darstellen, sondern zum Teil dem Gebiete der Endarteriitis obliterans angehören. Es fanden sich folgende Veränderungen: Zellatrophie im Tractus intermediolateralis im Rückenmark (LANNOIS-POROT); Degeneration zahlreicher Wurzelbündel in der Cauda equina mit entsprechender aufsteigender Degeneration im Rückenmark (AUERBACH); Veränderungen in den peripheren Nerven (WEIR MITCHELL und SPILLER, SACHS und WIENER, HAMILTON). In diesen Fällen fanden sich auch schwere Gefäßveränderungen (Verlegung des Lumens unter schweren Erscheinungen an der Media, Intima und Elastica). Andererseits konnte man an anderen sehr ausgesprochenen Fällen keine Veränderungen in den peripheren Nerven nachweisen (2 Fälle von WEIR MITCHELL, DEHIO, ELSNER, SPILLER und KUNSTMANN, GRUBER), während Gefäßveränderungen in den Fällen von DEHIO, WEIR MITCHELL und SPILLER, SACHS und WIENER, GRUBER vorhanden waren. LANNOIS, POROT und HAMILTON berichten in ihren Fällen über eine allgemeine Arteriosklerose und Herzveränderungen. Im Falle von HORNOWSKI und RUDZKI bestanden die Veränderungen in einer Atrophie und

Zerreißung der radialen elastischen Fasern in den Gefäßwänden. Auch in der Epidermis waren die elastischen Fasern atrophisch. An den endokrinen Organen fanden sich sehr zahlreiche chromaffine Zellen in den sympathischen Ganglien und in der Marksubstanz der Nebenniere. Die Nebennieren waren sehr groß und schwer und ihre Marksubstanz sehr breit (HORNOWSKI und RUDZKI).

Die Darstellung der Pathogenese der Erythromelalgie läßt sich nicht auf den engen Rahmen dieses Krankheitsbildes beschränken; sie muß vielmehr im Zusammenhang mit den anderen vasomotorisch-trophischen Erkrankungen abgehandelt werden. Wir haben schon vorher darauf hingewiesen, daß zwischen den einzelnen vasomotorisch-trophischen Erkrankungen enge Beziehungen bestehen, daß ihre Grenzen ineinander übergehen, und daß sogar bei denselben Kranken verschiedenartige vasomotorisch-trophische Symptomenkomplexe zu beobachten sind. Andererseits muß betont werden, daß die soeben erwähnten pathologisch-anatomischen Befunde nicht einheitlich sind, daß im Gegenteil durchaus verschiedenartige anatomische Befunde dort erhoben werden, wo man nach dem klinischen Bilde gleiche Veränderungen erwarten müßte. Infolgedessen kann keine der aufgestellten Theorien einer strengen Kritik standhalten.

Einige Forscher sehen in der Erythromelalgie eine Angioneurose ohne gröbere anatomische Veränderungen. CAVAZZANI, ARACCI legen das Hauptgewicht auf die primäre Beteiligung der Vasodilatatoren. Eine spinale Grundlage für das Entstehen der Erythromelalgie nimmt unter anderen EULENBURG an und verlegt den Sitz der Erkrankung in die seitliche graue Substanz des Rückenmarks, in den Tractus intermedio-lateralis. Auch LANNOIS und POROT vertreten ähnliche Anschauungen. Von einigen Autoren wird das Leiden auf eine Erkrankung der peripheren Nerven bezogen (WEIR MITCHELL). SAINTON und VÉRAU sprechen von einer besonderen Anteilnahme der vasodilatatorischen Fasern des Sympathicus und sehen in der Rötung an Händen und Füßen eine Folge eines echten vasodilatatorischen Reflexes. Einige Autoren vertreten die Anschauung, daß die Erythromelalgie auf Erkrankung der peripheren Arterien zurückzuführen ist (SACHS und WIENER, SHAW, HAMILTON).

Wichtig und viel erörtert ist die Frage, ob die Erythromelalgie überhaupt eine Krankheit sui generis darstellt oder nicht. LEWIN und BENDA und zuletzt THOMAS LEWIS fassen sie als einen einfachen Symptomenkomplex auf, während EULENBURG, DEHIO u. a. ihr eine gewisse Selbständigkeit einräumen. Diesen Fragen hat CASSIRER in seiner Monographie besondere Aufmerksamkeit geschenkt. Er weist darauf hin, daß in einer nicht geringen Anzahl von Fällen zwar die erythromelalgischen Symptome nur beigeordnete Symptome irgendeines anderen Nerven- oder Gefäßleidens sind; andererseits findet sich in einer weiteren Reihe von Fällen außer einer anfangs wenigstens stets anfallsweise auftretenden schmerzhaften Röte und Schwellung an den gipfelnden Teilen mit trophischen Veränderungen und Hyperhydrosis keine andere wesentliche Störung. Die kritische Durchsicht dieser Fälle hat ihm gezeigt, daß sie sich insofern in 2 Gruppen teilen, als in der einen die lokalen Symptome der Bahn bestimmter Nerven folgen, in der anderen diffus auf alle oder die Mehrzahl der Endglieder verbreitet sind. In diesen Fällen faßt er die Erythromelalgie als Krankheit sui generis auf. Für die 1. Gruppe nimmt er als Grundlage der Erkrankung Reizzustände in den peripheren Nerven mit besonderer Bevorzugung vasomotorischer und speziell vasodilatatorischer und sekretorischer Fasern an. Auch die sensiblen Anteile der Nerven sind stets mit betroffen. Für die 2. Gruppe der selbständigen Erythromelalgie scheint ihm die Annahme einer zentralen nervösen Genese die am besten begründete zu sein. Es sind dieselben Teile befallen, wie bei der 1. Gruppe, also vasomotorische, sekretorische und sensible Elemente. Häufig gesellen sich trophische Störungen dazu. CASSIRER verlegt den Sitz der Störung in das sympathische System im engeren Sinne, läßt aber die Frage offen, welche Teile des Systems, ob die Ganglien des Sympathicus oder seine zentralen Ursprungsgebiete in Frage kommen. Die Disposition zur Erkrankung ist anscheinend oft angeboren. Nach ZIERL handelt es sich bei der Erythromelalgie ebenso wie bei den anderen Trophoneurosen im wesentlichen um Reizzustände an Gefäßnervenbahnen und -Zentren; diese kommen nur auf Grund einer besonderen Kombination zustande, die im vasomotorischen System selbst, im Stoffwechsel oder in einem besonderen Chemismus der Haut begründet liegt. Die große Rolle, welche die begleitenden, manchmal äußerst heftigen Gemeingefühle im klinischen Bilde spielen, deuten auf eine wesentliche Beteiligung des vasosensiblen Systems hin. THOMAS LEWIS nimmt als Ursache für den brennenden Schmerz an, daß eine Substanz aus den geschädigten Zellen frei wird, die die Enden der sensiblen Nerven angreift.

Diagnose.

Bei diagnostischen Erwägungen werden wir uns stets zu vergegenwärtigen haben, welche Hauptsymptome zur Erythromelalgie gehören. Wenn wir unser Augenmerk richten auf die Kombination von aktiver Hyperämie, Rötung, Schwellung mit heftigen Schmerzen und gelegentlich mit sekretorischen und trophischen Störungen, das paroxysmale Auftreten der Symptome, ihre Lokalisation, die meist die Extremitätenenden und oft genug diese ausschließlich betrifft, so wird die Diagnose nicht schwierig sein. CASSIRER legt besonderen Wert darauf, daß in der Tat auch wirkliche Schmerzen vorhanden sind; dadurch unterscheidet sich das Symptomenbild von einer Reihe anderer dermatologischer Affektionen. Die Erythromelie, die mit der Akrodermatitis chronica atrophicans identisch zu sein scheint (HERXHEIMER, HARTMANN, DIECK), befällt in der Regel Personen in den mittleren Lebensjahren und ist charakterisiert durch die Kombination von Erythrocyanose mit Hautatrophie. Sie beginnt meist an Hand- und Fußrücken und breitet sich nach der Basis des Gliedes aus. Zunächst zeigen sich Hypertrophie und Induration, später Hautatrophie und Versiegen der Schweißsekretion. Die Haut erhält eine zigarettenpapierartige Beschaffenheit. Die Erkrankung charakterisiert sich demnach als schmerzlose, vasodilatatorische Neurose an den Streckseiten der Gliedmaßen. Die Erythrodermie stellt eine lokal entzündliche Affektion dar, die viel gleichmäßiger verteilt ist, und zwar mehr auf den Stamm als auf die Extremitäten lokalisiert; die Rötung ist eine hellere; meist sind die Erythrodermien mit Lymphdrüsenschwellung verbunden (M. OPPENHEIM).

Die Differentialdiagnose gegenüber anderen mit heftigen Schmerzen verbundenen, besonders die Füße betreffenden Affektionen ist im Beginn des Leidens oft recht schwierig. Wir nennen die *Arthritis* der kleinen Gelenke, besonders die Gicht, die Gonorrhöe, die *Tarsalgien*, den entzündlichen *Plattfuß*, die *Metatarsalgien*. Man wird bei diesen Erkrankungen in der Regel die aktive Röte vermissen. Die Abgrenzung vom *Erysipel*, von der *Phlegmone*, vom entzündlichen *Ödem*, Krankheiten, die wiederum die der Erythromelalgie zukommende charakteristische Röte zeigen, kann nur im Beginn des Leidens ernsthafte Schwierigkeiten bereiten, da sich im Laufe der nächsten Wochen stets die für die genannten Krankheiten charakteristischen anderen Symptome entwickeln. Das gleiche gilt von der *Cyanose* der *Herzkranken*. H. CURSCHMANN weist darauf hin, daß der typische *Frost* der Füße manche Züge mit der Erythromelalgie völlig gemein hat, z. B. die Exacerbation bei Erwärmung und besonders beim Hängenlassen der Glieder. Das Erythem bei *Erythema exsudativum multiforme* zeigt fast stets eine symmetrische Anordnung der Efflorescenzen an den Prädilektionsstellen und meistens Allgemeinerscheinungen, welche auf das Bestehen eines inneren Leidens hinweisen.

Gewisse Formen von *Akromegalie* zeigen manchmal eine Ähnlichkeit mit der Erythromelalgie in den Fällen, in denen die Erythromelalgie eine erhebliche Vergrößerung der Hände und Füße herbeigeführt hat.

Recht schwierig kann die Unterscheidung von dem Krankheitsbilde des *intermittierenden Hinkens* sein. Man wird in diesen Fällen auf Veränderungen in den peripheren Arterien zu fahnden haben und daran denken müssen, wie häufig beim intermittierenden Hinken ein Fehlen der Fußpulse nachgewiesen worden ist, während die der Erythromelalgie zukommenden, in die Augen fallenden vasomotorischen Störungen recht selten beobachtet werden. Immerhin gibt es auch Fälle, in denen eine Kombination von intermittierendem Hinken mit Erythromelalgie nachgewiesen wurde (H. CURSCHMANN). Über die Beziehungen der *Thromangitis obliterans* zur Erythromelalgie und zur RAYNAUDschen Krankheit hat BÜRGER gearbeitet. Charakteristisch ist der langsame Verlauf dieser Erkrankung, die zunächst mit heftigen Schmerzen beginnt; nach Monaten oder Jahren stellen sich dann trophische Störungen ein, die in der Mehrzahl der Fälle zur Amputation wenigstens einer Extremität führen. PARKES WEBER betont, daß intermittierendes Hinken häufig von Erythromelalgie begleitet ist und weist darauf hin, daß eine nichtluische Endarteriitis der mittelgroßen Arterien sowohl die ischämischen Muskelkontrakturen bedingen kann, wie schmerzhafte Cyanose. Auch CASSIRER hat auf die bisweilen auftretenden symptomatologischen Ähnlichkeiten wiederholt hingewiesen.

Eine recht seltene Affektion, die gelegentlich bei größeren Epidemien beobachtet wurde, und die der Erythromelalgie äußerlich recht ähnlich sieht, ist die *Akrodynie* (synonymisches Erythrödem, PINK-Disease, FEERsche Krankheit „Encephalitis vegetativa"), die häufiger bei Kindern, als bei Erwachsenen vorkommt. SELTER und FEER haben dieser Erkrankung besondere Aufmerksamkeit geschenkt (zusammenfassend Fortschr. Med. 46, 537). Kürzlich ist die Erkrankung von ROCAZ monographisch bearbeitet worden. Unter unklaren Allgemeinsymptomen, Schweißausbruch, mit Miliaria rubra und Maceration der Epidermis entwickelt sich eine Cyanose der Hände und Füße unter heftigem Juckreiz und Kribbeln; sie werden feucht, gedunsen und kalt. Als Motilitätsstörungen stellt er fest: Schlaffheit der Beine, Tremor, Hypotonie. Bei Prüfung der Sensibilität findet er gelegentlich Hyperästhesie und Anästhesie, meist in den gipfelnden Teilen lokalisiert. Seitens des Zirkulationsapparates finden sich Pulsbeschleunigung, Steigerung des Blutdrucks, hohe Hämoglobinwerte, Vermehrung der Erythrocyten. An trophischen Störungen sind beobachtet: Zahnausfall, Speichelfluß, Entzündung der Finger mit Geschwürsbildung, der Zunge und Wangenschleimhaut. Weiterhin werden spastische Konstipation, gastrische Störung, Störungen der Harnentleerung, Hyperglykämie festgestellt. Hier werden die Allgemeinerscheinungen, welche auf das Bestehen einer Infektion hinweisen, den Ausschlag geben. Die Erkrankung hat im allgemeinen eine gute Prognose; die Erscheinungen gehen meist nach wenigen Wochen zurück. Wenn man sich die erwähnten Symptome vergegenwärtigt und bedenkt, wie selten die Erythromelalgie im Kindesalter vorkommt, wird die Diagnose gegenüber der Akrodynie keine Schwierigkeiten machen.

Auf die Tatsache, daß die Erythromelalgie oft symptomatisch bei Erkrankungen des Zentralnervensystems auftritt, ohne daß es sich um das klinisch abgeschlossene Bild der Erythromelalgie handelt, ist schon hingewiesen worden.

Die Unterscheidung von der Akroasphyxia chronica wird, wenn man sich die Symptome der beiden Erkrankungen vor Augen hält, in den ausgeprägten Fällen keine Schwierigkeiten machen; immerhin gibt es auch hier Übergangsformen, auf die jüngst LAYANI aufmerksam gemacht hat; dieser Autor beobachtet, daß im Gegensatz zu der Erythromelalgie die carmingefärbten Zonen bei der Akroasphyxie stets kühl bleiben.

Verlauf und Prognose.

Von einer typischen Verlaufsform des Leidens kann man nicht sprechen. Einige Autoren berichten, daß das Leiden akut eingesetzt und exacerbiert hat, um nach längerer oder kürzerer Dauer auf der Höhe zu bleiben; in manchen Fällen läßt sich dann eine allmähliche Besserung nachweisen. Bei anderen Kranken bleibt das Leiden durch Jahrzehnte stationär, um dann schließlich als Folge irgendeiner Gelegenheitsursache sich akut zu verschlechtern. In der Regel ist der Verlauf der Krankheit ein *chronischer* und *langsam progressiver*. Im Falle von MORGAN dauerte das Leiden 23 Jahre lang. Eine Reihe von Autoren berichtet über erhebliche Besserungen der Erythromelalgie im Laufe der Jahre; es gibt auch eine Reihe von Fällen, in denen von einer Heilung gesprochen werden kann. Indessen ist die *Prognose quoad sanationem* eine ziemlich zweifelhafte. Eine unkomplizierte Erythromelalgie birgt keine Lebensgefahr in sich; dagegen müssen die Aussichten der symptomatischen Erythromelalgie nach der Schwere des Grundleidens bewertet werden.

Therapie.

Wie so häufig in der Medizin steht die große Zahl der zur Beseitigung der Erythromelalgie empfohlenen Mittel im umgekehrten Verhältnis zu ihrer Brauchbarkeit. Angewandt worden sind fast sämtliche Prozeduren der physikalischen Therapie, die Organtherapie, Antineuralgica. Auch operative Eingriffe wurden versucht. Es ist stets mehr als zweifelhaft, ob die publizierten Heilerfolge wirklich auf die angewandten Heilmittel zurückzuführen sind.

Man wird sich bei der Behandlung des Kranken die klinische Erfahrung zunutze machen und ihm zunächst eine Ruhigstellung der befallenen Extremitäten und eine horizontale Lage empfehlen, sowie vor allem kühlende Prozeduren im Hinblick auf die schon erwähnte Tatsache, daß die Kranken in der kalten Jahreszeit eine Linderung ihrer Beschwerden erfahren. In 2 Fällen, die wir beobachtet haben, brachte der fortgesetzte Gebrauch von Aspirin, bzw. Pyramidon, die Anwendung des faradischen Stromes und der Kälte eine Linderung der Beschwerden. Schließlich kam es in beiden Fällen zu einer dauernden Besserung, ohne daß das Medikament weiter genommen werden mußte. Bei der Heftigkeit der Schmerzanfälle wird man um die Anwendung von Narkotica oft nicht herumkommen. SCHIRMACHER wandte Hydro- und elektrotherapeutische Maßnahmen an, und dauernd Salbenverbände: $1/2$ pro mille Adrenalin, 5%iges Cycloform āā. BENOIST injizierte Ergotin mit günstigem Erfolg, der aber dadurch zunichte gemacht wurde, daß dauernd mit der wirksamen Dosis in die Höhe gegangen werden mußte. Vorübergehende Erfolge wurden mit epiduralen Stovaininjektionen erzielt. STALKER hat mit Erfolg subcutane Injektionen von Collosol-Calcium angewendet (erste Injektion 0,25, dann aber weitere zu 0,5 in wöchentlichen Intervallen). H. CURSCHMANN verordnete mit Erfolg Kalk und Thyreoidin. STEINER will in einem Fall durch Insulin einen Erfolg erzielt haben, KAKU mit Eigenblutinjektionen.

Einige Male wurde ein operatives Heilverfahren eingeleitet. DEHIO resezierte ein Stück des Ulnaris ohne dauernden Erfolg. In einem Falle von WEIR-MITCHELL brachte die Operation (Resektion, bzw. Dehnung des Musculocutaneus und Saphenus major) Besserung. In einem 2. Fall trat Gangrän und Exitus ein. In sehr schweren Fällen könnte man Alkoholinjektionen versuchen. Die von SACHS und WIENER vorgenommene Amputation des erkrankten Beines am Oberschenkel betraf keinen reinen Fall; das gleiche gilt von dem Fall von KUNSTMANN. LAEWEN hat bei 2 Kranken die hohe Vereisung mit Erfolg angewendet. MAYESIMA hat bei einem Fall von Erythromelalgie mit Erfolg die FÖRSTERsche Operation ausgeführt. In einem Falle CASSIRERs wurde die periarterielle Sympathektomie angewendet, und zwar ohne entscheidenden Erfolg. Überhaupt ist auch wie bei den anderen vasomotorischen Erkrankungen die LERICHEsche Operation öfters versucht worden (LERICHE, BRÜNING und FORSTER, BRANDENBURG [Fall von KIRSCHNER]). Die Resultate waren wechselnd. Zu der Indikationsstellung der periarteriellen Sympathektomie bei Erythromelalgie nehmen BRÜNING und STAHL in ihrer Monographie „Die Chirurgie des vegetativen Nervensystems" eingehend Stellung. Mit Rücksicht auf die Tatsache, daß bei der Erythromelalgie der Angiospasmus keine Rolle spielt, sondern daß im Gegenteil bei ihr eine ausgesprochene Vasodilatation im Vordergrund steht und es sich somit nie um ein Zuviel, sondern eher um ein Zuwenig im Tonus im vegetativen System handelt, gehört nach ihrer Auffassung die Erythromelalgie nicht in das Indikationsgebiet der periarteriellen Sympathektomie. Demgegenüber wollen DAVIS, LOYAL und KANAVEL in einem Falle durch die lumbale Sympathektomie eine ganz wesentliche Besserung erzielt haben.

Dasselbe berichtet SAITO und teilt mit, daß die einseitige, sacrale Sympathektomie nicht nur auf der operierten Seite wirke, sondern auch auf der nicht operierten Seite. Die kontralaterale Wirkung dauere jedoch nicht lange Zeit, so daß also bei doppelseitiger Erythromelalgie auch eine lumbosacrale Sympathektomie indiziert sei.

CASSIRER hat bei einer Patientin, bei welcher das Leiden neben einer schweren Hysterie bestand, Psychotherapie vergebens angewandt, während MUMFORD in seinem Fall einen Erfolg zu verzeichnen hatte.

IV. Die Akroparästhesien.

Wenn wir die Erythromegalie in ihrer klassischen Form als Varietät der RAYNAUDschen Krankheit darstellen konnten, so vermögen wir auch das jetzt zu behandelnde Krankheitsbild der Akroparästhesien ohne weiteres aus der RAYNAUDschen Krankheit abzuleiten, wenn wir deren Symptomatologie ein wenig abändern bzw. vereinfachen. Die trophischen Störungen fehlen diesem Typus ganz, es bleiben nur die vasomotorisch-sensiblen übrig und von den vasomotorischen tritt mehr als bei der RAYNAUDschen Krankheit die Synkope gegenüber der Asphyxie in den Vordergrund. Aber auch die Synkope kann mehr und mehr verschwinden, wir haben es im wesentlichen dann nur mit Akroparästhesien zu tun. Der Name stammt von SCHULTZE; die erste ausführliche Beschreibung rührt aber von NOTHNAGEL her; vor NOTHNAGEL hat den Angaben BERNHARDTs zufolge verwandte Dinge MARTIN beschrieben. NOTHNAGEL erwähnt und beschreibt die beiden Erscheinungsreihen, das Gefühl der Vertaubung und Vertotung, meist zusammen mit einer Abnahme der Empfindungsschärfe, außerdem die Veränderung der Farbe der Finger, die blaß bis kreideweiß sind. Vor SCHULTZE haben auch JONES, PUTNAM, ORMEROD, SINKLER, SAUNDBY, BERNHARDT das Leiden beschrieben. Aus der späteren Zeit erwähnen wir die Publikationen von LAQUEUR, FRIEDMANN, FRANKL-HOCHWART, ferner von COLLINS, BALLET, HASCOVEC, SCHMIDT, CURSCHMANN, EGGER, DÉJÉRINE, PICK, BOLTEN. Unsere Erfahrungen bezogen sich bis 1914 auf 200 Fälle, haben sich aber seither erheblich vermehrt.

Ätiologie.

In überwiegendem Maße sind Frauen betroffen. COLLINS berechnet den Anteil der Frauen auf 70%. Wir fanden unter 155 Fällen, die wir daraufhin prüften, immerhin 24 Männer. H. CURSCHMANN fand unter 50 Fällen 7 Männer. Allerdings sind die Fälle bei ihnen häufig atypisch. Von 372 Fällen stammen aus dem Alter von 30—60 Jahren nicht weniger als 297, das Durchschnittsalter betrug in unseren Fällen bei Männern 43,5, bei Frauen 41,5 Jahre. Unsere jüngste Patientin war ein 7jähriges Mädchen. Die älteste Patientin, die von CURSCHMANN beschrieben ist, war 73 Jahre alt. H. CURSCHMANN glaubt, daß das Leiden im ersten Jahrzehnt nach der Geschlechtsreife relativ am häufigsten ist und zur Zeit der Klimax wieder eine starke Elevation erfährt. Ferner kann kein Zweifel sein, daß ein gewisser Zusammenhang zwischen dem Auftreten der Parästhesien und den Störungen der sexuellen Funktionen bzw. gewissen normalen Vorgängen des weiblichen Geschlechtslebens besteht. Die Affektion bevorzugt entschieden das *Klimakterium* und besonders interessant sind die Fälle, in denen sie in der Klimax praecox auftrat. Vor einiger Zeit beobachtete ich eine 44jährige Frau, die vor 3 Jahren eine Eierstockoperation durchgemacht hat, bei der im Anschluß an eine Degrasinkur ein Degrasinexanthem auftrat. Mit dem Auftreten des Exanthems stellte sich das Symptomenbild der Akroparästhesie im Sinne NOTHNAGELs ein. *Berufliche* Schädlichkeiten kommen soweit in Frage, als die Beschäftigung mit Wasser, namentlich die Beschäftigung mit kaltem Wasser, anscheinend disponierend wirkt (Waschfrauen).

Sonst sind die Akroparästhesien auch bei erschöpfenden Krankheiten zu beachten. Bei Männern wurde der Alkoholismus mehrfach beschuldigt. SCHMIDT hat eine Reihe von Beobachtungen veröffentlicht, in denen die Lungentuberkulose ätiologisch von Wichtigkeit war. Doch schied er selbst seine Fälle von der mehr selbständigen Form der Akroparästhesien. Vereinzelt wird ein Trauma als Ursache angegeben. In einem unserer Fälle war eine doppelseitige Halsrippe vorhanden.

Symptomatologie.

Im Vordergrund stehen die Angaben und Klagen über *unangenehme Empfindungen in den Händen, seltener in den Füßen*: Kribbeln, Jucken, Eingeschlafensein, Ameisenlaufen, das Gefühl des Geschwollenseins und Klammheit der Hand und der Finger, das Gefühl der Taubheit, als ob eine Haut über den erkrankten Teilen liegt. Diese Empfindungen strahlen oft nach Angabe der Kranken in die Unterarme aus. Von diesen unangenehmen Empfindungen finden sich ganz allmählich die Übergänge zu ausgesprochener Schmerzhaftigkeit, die so erheblich sein kann, daß sie die Kranken aus dem Schlafe weckt, daß diese vor Schmerzen laut schreien, und zum Gebrauch von Morphium gedrängt werden. Diese Empfindungen sind meist nicht kontinuierlich, sondern treten anfallsweise auf, am stärksten pflegen sie des Nachts und des Morgens beim Erwachen zu sein. Dann pflegt sich in den betroffenen Teilen auch eine gewisse Steifheit und Ungeschicklichkeit der Bewegungen einzustellen. Durch Reiben, Drücken, Schlagen werden die unangenehmen Empfindungen und die Steifigkeit gemildert. Meist sind beide Hände betroffen, oft eine mehr als die andere. Zuweilen beschränken sich die Parästhesien nur auf eine Hand, seltener nur auf einzelne Finger. Eine scharfe Begrenzung der Parästhesien auf das Gebiet eines peripheren Nerven wird nicht beobachtet. H. CURSCHMANN erwähnt, daß in seltenen Fällen auch Nase, Ohrmuschel und Wangen betroffen werden.

Der objektive Befund ist meist ein sehr dürftiger. Wir fanden unter 36 Fällen 22mal keine nachweisbaren Störungen. Wo solche vorhanden waren, handelte es sich meist um Hypästhesien, seltener um Hypalgesien von geringer Intensität und Ausbreitung, und zwar meist an den Fingern und Händen, ohne daß sie einen bestimmten Verbreitungstyp aufwiesen. Unseren Erfahrungen stehen die einiger neuerer Beobachter gegenüber, die die objektiven und subjektiven Sensibilitätsstörungen bei den Akroparästhesien in ganz bestimmten, scharf umschriebenen, der radiculären Innervation entsprechenden Gebieten fanden (DÉJÉRINE und EGGER, PICK, TROMBERT). Wir können bei Nachprüfung unseres Materials diese Angaben nicht bestätigen, sie stellen jedenfalls nicht die Regel dar, und wir haben den Verdacht, daß es sich zum mindesten in einem Teil der hierher gerechneten Fälle nicht um einfache Akroparästhesien gehandelt hat. Eine Druckempfindlichkeit der Nervenstämme pflegt zu fehlen.

Die Motilität weist niemals erhebliche Störungen auf. Die Sehnenphänomene zeigen ein normales Verhalten. In einer Reihe von Fällen beschränkt sich das Symptomenbild also rein auf die Parästhesien und Schmerzen. Es verbindet sich in der Minderzahl dieser Fälle mit leichten Störungen der Sensibilität, dazu kommen in einer zweiten Gruppe die schon erwähnten vasomotorischen Störungen. Wir schätzen die Zahl der mit vasomotorischen Störungen einhergehenden Parästhesien etwa auf $1/4$ der Gesamtzahl, und zwar handelt es sich da im allgemeinen um die in Attacken auftretenden Anfälle von Syncope locale. Blässe und Kälte der Haut wird meist abgelöst von reaktiver Röte und Brennen, mehrfach waren die Hände von vornherein mehr rot und brennend als weiß und kalt. Diese Fälle bilden, wie schon erwähnt, den Übergang zu den milden Formen der RAYNAUDschen Krankheit; eine scharfe Grenze zu ziehen ist hier unmöglich.

URECHIA-RETEZEANU fanden während der Anfälle 7,2—7,5 mg-% Calcium im Blut, im Intervall 8,5 mg-% und Vagotonie.

In der überwiegenden Zahl der Fälle entwickelt sich das Leiden ganz allmählich und aus geringen Anfängen heraus und entfaltet sich erst nach und nach zu voller Stärke. Es gibt aber auch akut einsetzende Fälle. OPPENHEIM sah einmal die Krankheit plötzlich entstehen, als ein Kranker im Sommer die schwitzenden Hände mit Eis in Berührung brachte. In diesen akuten Fällen können sich die Symptome auch rasch wieder zurückbilden. H. CURSCHMANN beobachtete, daß bei dem Abklingen des Anfalles eine reaktive Röte, Schwellung, subjektive und objektive Hitze, oft auch Hyperhidrosis der betroffenen Teile einsetzten. Sonst dauern die Beschwerden oft monate- und jahrelang fort; immer wieder kommen die Kranken, um in ermüdender Eintönigkeit dieselben Klagen zu wiederholen. Bei einer 60jährigen Frau bestanden die Beschwerden seit 10 Jahren dauernd, bei einer 48jährigen seit 5 Jahren mit Intermissionen. Eine 37jährige Frau hatte schon einmal vor 10 Jahren dieselben Beschwerden usw. Meist tritt das Leiden in einzelnen Anfällen auf; deren Lieblingszeit sind die Morgenstunden. Die Anfälle werden ferner ausgelöst durch Manipulationen im Wasser, durch Anstrengungen, durch Tragen von Lasten, Herabhängenlassen der Finger usw.

Pathologie.

Wie bei der RAYNAUDschen Krankheit läßt sich auch bei den Akroparästhesien feststellen, daß sie meist auf dem Boden einer allgemeineren Erkrankung oder vielmehr Disposition zur Erkrankung des Nervensystems stehen. In etwa $2/3$ unserer Fälle konnten wir Symptome einer allgemeinen *Neuropathie* bei den darauf untersuchten Patienten feststellen. In einem Drittel ließen sich solche Beziehungen nicht erkennen. Nicht selten waren es auch wieder Erscheinungen einer gesteigerten vasomotorischen oder vegetativen Irritabilität, die das allgemeine Krankheitsbild beherrschten. Einige Male wurde auch eine direkte *Heredität* oder *Familiarität* festgestellt. H. Curschmann hat sowohl ,,vasokonstriktorische", als auch allgemein vasoneurotisch veranlagte Familien gesehen. Auf diesem vorbereiteten Boden entstehen die spezielleren Erscheinungen der Akroparästhesien, deren Pathogenese wir nach dem schon früher gesagten hier nicht weiter zu erörtern brauchen. Auch hier handelt es sich um intermittierende Reizzustände in vasosensiblen, vasokonstriktorischen und seltener vasodilatatorischen Fasern bzw. Systemen. Auch hier bleibt der spezielle Sitz der Erkrankung zweifelhaft, auf die zentrale Genese weist auch hier die enge Verbindung mit allgemeinen neuropathischen Symptomen und im speziellen mit solchen eines gestörten Gleichgewichts im Vasomotoren- bzw. vegetativen System. Wir sahen da Kranke, bei denen fliegende Hitze, Rötung des Gesichts, Herzklopfen, Angina pectoris vasomotoria, Anfälle von Polydipsie und Polyurie, dyspeptische Beschwerden in Form von Sodbrennen, Brechreiz und Erbrechen (Heissen), gesteigerte vasomotorische Hauterregbarkeit vorkamen. Häufig vermischten sich die Akroparästhesien mit klimakterischen Erscheinungen zu einem unteilbaren Ganzen bzw. traten nur als mehr oder minder bedeutsame Symptome der klimakterischen Neurose auf, wie das vor längerer Zeit Windscheid beschrieben hat. Wir beobachteten Neigung zu Ohnmachten, sahen wiederholt die Kombination mit einer Struma. Savill teilt einen Fall mit, in dem der Morbus Basedowii mit Akroparästhesien einherging, und betont, daß er das häufiger gesehen hat. Auffällig oft sahen wir die Kombination mit Migräne oder fanden anamnestisch das frühere Auftreten von Migräne verzeichnet. Mehrfach waren leichte Störungen im Bereich des Halssympathicus zu konstatieren, Pupillen- und Lidspaltendifferenz, auch eine Druckschmerzhaftigkeit im Gebiet des Ganglion cervicale supremum. Einmal sahen wir einen an die Menièreschen Erscheinungen erinnernden Symptomenkomplex. Eine Kranke gab an, daß ihre Hände jetzt immer blaurot aussähen, objektiv ließ sich eine nur eine geringe Abweichung von der Norm erkennen. Diese Fälle bilden dann die Übergänge zu Kombinationen mit anderen vasomotorischen Neurosen. Hier verlieren die Akroparästhesien den Wert einer selbständigen Erkrankung und werden zu einfachen Symptomen. Wir sahen sie mehrfach sich mit angioneurotischem Ödem verbinden, Heissen mit Urticaria. Solis-Cohen erwähnt sie als ein Symptom seiner vasomotorischen Ataxie. Herz spricht von ihnen in seinen Erörterungen über Störungen der peripheren Kreislauforgane. Curschmann hat auf ihr Vorkommen bei der Angina pectoris vasomotoria aufmerksam gemacht, die ihrerseits im wesentlichen wiederum nur ein Ausschnitt aus dem größeren Gebiet der Neurasthenie mit vorwiegend vasomotorischen Symptomen darstellt. Heissen hat beobachtet, daß als Äquivalent Migräne und dyspeptische Beschwerden auftreten, wenn es gelungen war, die Akroparästhesien durch therapeutische Maßnahmen zu unterdrücken. Er beschreibt diese Anfälle, welche meist bei Frauen und Mädchen vorkommen, in der Weise, daß plötzlich oft nachts und morgens, nach Kälteeinwirkung, psychischen oder sexuellen Traumen, die Kranken von Kälte und Absterben der Hände und Füße befallen werden, die auch als Asphyxie und Synkope sichtbar ist; dabei tritt ein schmerzhaftes, mit Todesangst verbundenes Gefühl in der Herzgegend, oft mit Herzklopfen auf; der Puls ist gespannter als normal und etwas beschleunigt. Gegenüber diesen komplizierteren Fällen darf aber nicht vergessen werden, daß es Fälle gibt, in denen das Symptom der Akroparästhesien mit oder ohne vasomotorische Symptome ganz allein das Bild beherrscht.

Die Annahme, daß es sich um vasokonstriktorische Vorgänge handelt, gegen die Bolten sich ausgesprochen hat, ist durch O. Müllers direkte Beobachtungen bei der Capillaruntersuchung weiter befestigt worden. Die Parästhesien, die ja auch klinisch einen bestimmten Charakter tragen und am ehesten den durch starke Kälteeinwirkung hervorgerufenen Empfindungen gleichen, dürften auf Reizung vasosensibler Fasern zurückzuführen sein. Der supponierte Reizzustand des Vasomotorenapparates ist der Ausdruck einer hereditären Diathese (neuropathische Konstitution), die sich klinisch vielfach in allgemeineren oder spezielleren Erscheinungen bemerkbar macht, die durch eine Reihe von Momenten in manifeste Krankheitssymptome umgesetzt sind (thermische, toxische, endokrine Schädlichkeiten). Damit verliert das Syndrom in mancher Beziehung gewiß viel von seiner Selbständigkeit und wird zur Teilerscheinung eines größeren Ganzen; auf seine Abgrenzung ganz zu verzichten geht aber hier ebensowenig an wie bei anderen klinischen Erscheinungsformen, etwa bei der vielfache Ähnlichkeiten aufweisenden Migräne. PUTNAM versucht, wie schon andere Forscher vordem (L. R. MÜLLER), in dem die Nacht bevorzugenden Auftreten der Akroparästhesien eine Eigentümlichkeit der Erkrankungen des sympathischen Systems zu sehen. Während des Schlafes sei der Gefäßtonus erschlafft; derselbe steige beim Erwachen schnell an und gerade dann traten die Akroparästhesien am meisten auf.

Was das Verhältnis der sensiblen und vasomotorischen Reizerscheinungen angeht, so ist es nach unserer Ansicht nicht möglich, als primäres Moment stets den Vasomotorenkrampf anzusehen und den sensiblen Symptomen nur eine sekundäre Rolle zuzuschreiben, schon deswegen nicht, weil gar nicht selten Erscheinungen der lokalen Synkope ganz zurücktreten. Auch die von SIMONS festgestellte Tatsache, daß die Gefäßreflexe nie dauernd fehlen, spricht gegen eine solche Auffassung. Akrosynkope und Akroparästhesien müssen vielmehr als Manifestationen derselben Ursache angesehen werden, wobei es uns am wahrscheinlichsten ist, daß die sensiblen Reizerscheinungen durch eine Reizung der vasosensiblen Fasern, die vasomotorischen naturgemäß durch eine Reizung von vasokonstriktorischen produziert werden. O. MÜLLER und MÖBIUS haben sich im Gegensatz zu unserer Auffassung niemals von dem Vorkommen einer rein sensiblen Form überzeugen können und sind der Ansicht, daß die rein sensible Form von der NOTHNAGELschen vasokonstriktorischen Form nicht getrennt werden kann. Sie sahen bei ihren Patienten bei der Capillaruntersuchung stets Spasmen in einzelnen, manchmal in vielen arteriellen Capillarschenkeln. Die Cyanose rührte dann deutlich sichtbar von der partiellen Erweiterung der venösen Schenkel bzw. des subpapillären Plexus her. Ähnliche Beobachtungen machte HAHN. Auch BOLTEN und H. CURSCHMANN haben sich gegen die Trennung in 2 Gruppen ausgesprochen.

Man hat den Sitz der Erkrankung an verschiedenen Stellen gesucht. So hat z. B. SINKLER Störungen der Blutversorgung des Halsmarks angenommen. Wir glauben mit der Mehrzahl der übrigen Autoren nicht, daß an eine solche ganz bestimmte Lokalisation gedacht werden kann. Auf Grund der Lokalisation der Parästhesien und Hypästhesien in radikulären Gebieten kommen DÉJÉRINE und EGGER, ROASENDA, TROMBERT, zur Annahme einer irritativen Läsion der hinteren Wurzeln als Grundlage der Parästhesien. Die vasokonstriktorischen Phänomene betrachten sie als reflektorisch durch Übergang der Reizung von den hinteren auf die vorderen Wurzeln bedingt. Wäre diese Ausbreitung der Parästhesien sichergestellt, so wäre damit ja zweifellos ein fester Anhaltspunkt für die Lokalisation gegeben; wir haben aber bereits betont, daß unsere Erfahrungen uns bisher nicht erlauben, diese Ausbreitung als eine gesetzmäßige und gewöhnliche anzusehen. Die lokale Beschränkung der Symptome legt immer wieder den Gedanken nahe, daß periphere Abschnitte der Sitz der Erkrankung sein müssen, eine Ansicht, der wir uns auch selbst früher zugeneigt haben. Wir möchten jetzt jedoch das periphere Moment nicht allzusehr betont wissen, sondern meinen, daß durch eine ab origine vorhandene oder irgendwie erworbene Schwäche gewisser zentraler Abschnitte des Nervensystems in diesen eine Widerstandsunfähigkeit, eine Labilität erzeugt wird oder von vornherein vorhanden ist, die schon geringen Schädlichkeiten gegenüber einen krankmachenden Einfluß ausübt. Unter diesen Schädlichkeiten sind diejenigen zu verstehen, die ätiologisch und klinisch nach unserer Erfahrung überhaupt imstande sind, die Erscheinungen der Akroparästhesien hervorzurufen: Die Kälte, Überanstrengung, leichte Traumen, exogene Gifte usw. Damit rückt die Pathogenese der Akroparästhesien in diejenige nahe Nachbarschaft zur Pathogenese der RAYNAUDschen Krankheit, in die sie nach unserer Ansicht auf Grund der Ähnlichkeit des klinischen Bildes gehört. KARPLUS ist der Auffassung, daß meist durch periphere Schädlichkeiten reflektorisch über die vasomotorischen Zentren die Symptome ausgelöst werden, wobei in einzelnen Fällen eine neuropathische Konstitution mitspielen muß.

Auf die Beziehungen zu den Störungen der Funktion der endokrinen Drüsen weist die Tatsache, daß die Vorgänge der Pubertät, der Gravidität und namentlich des Klimakterium oft von Einfluß auf das Auftreten der Akroparästhesien sind. BALLERINI ist auf diese Frage näher eingegangen. Er erblickt in der Tatsache, daß die Erkrankung oft bei Frauen, und zwar vorwiegend in der Gravidität und im Puerperium, sowie in der physiologischen und künstlichen Menopause auftritt, den Beweis dafür, daß der Ausfall der Ovarialfunktion indirekt im endokrinen Apparat und im Gleichgewichtszustand des Nervensystems, speziell des vegetativen, entsprechende Veränderungen bei solchen Individuen hervorruft, die im Sinne einer Neurose dafür disponiert sind [1]. BORAK, der die Akroparästhesien bei klimakterischen Zuständen fand, setzt sie in Parallele zu den bei Akromelgalie vorkommenden (Zunahme der azidophilen Hypophysenzellen, die bei Bestrahlung verschwinden). Demgegenüber machen MARBURG und SGALITZER geltend, daß sich die Akroparästhesien doch häufig unter dem Einfluß lokaler Schädigungen und auch bei Jugendlichen finden.

Diagnose.

Schwierigkeiten macht bisweilen die Unterscheidung gegenüber den *professionellen Neurosen*, z. B. den in letzter Zeit häufig erwähnten sog. Anklopferkrankheit (GERBIS). Der durchgreifende Unterschied ist der, daß die professionellen Neurosen regelmäßig erst im Anschluß an eine bestimmte Arbeit entstehen, während bei den Akroparästhesien leichte Arbeit oft im Gegenteil von Nutzen ist, und nur die Einwirkung gewisser, mit der Arbeit verbundener Schädlichkeiten sie auslöst. Das Fehlen der typischen morgendlichen Anfälle bei den Beschäftigungsneurosen ist noch hervorzuheben. Immerhin gibt es Übergangsfälle, in denen eine exakte Unterscheidung nicht möglich ist. Gegenüber der *Neuritis* sind die Unterscheidungsmerkmale gegeben. Auch bei der reinen sensiblen Neuritis entstehen keine Schwierigkeiten, wenn man die Ausdehnung der Sensibilitätsstörung, die Druckschmerzhaftigkeit der Nervenstämme, das Zurücktreten vasomotorischer Erscheinungen berücksichtigt.

Schon vor längerer Zeit hat BERGER über eine eigentümliche Form von Parästhesien berichtet, die neben manchem Gemeinsamen doch auch viele Unterschiede von unseren Akroparästhesien aufweisen. Es handelt sich da meist um jugendliche Individuen, bei denen anfallsweise außerordentlich intensive Parästhesien auftraten, nach längerem Stehen oder auch nach wenigen Schritten. Sie ziehen von der Hüfte nach den Zehen, entweder gleich doppelseitig oder erst noch auf einer Seite. Regelmäßig besteht ein hochgradiges Schwächegefühl.

---

[1] Zit. nach Referat F. H. LEWY, Z. Neurol. **26**, 249.

Die Anfälle dauern einige Minuten, kommen oft, die unangenehmen Empfindungen breiten sich bis in die Hypochondrien aus. Vasomotorische Störungen fehlen. Die Affektion scheint nicht häufig zu sein, doch konnten wir einen Fall beobachten, auf den BERGERs Schilderung durchaus paßte. Die Unterschiede gegenüber den Akroparästhesien liegen auf der Hand.

Zur Unterscheidung von *Tetanie* und tetanoiden Zuständen gegenüber den Akroparästhesien macht FRANKL-HOCHWART folgende Angaben: Bei den ausgesprochenen Fällen besteht natürlich keine Schwierigkeit, man vergesse aber nicht, daß es auch Fälle gibt, bei denen die Leute nur über Parästhesien klagen, und weder Krämpfe noch TROUSSEAUsches Phänomen haben. Der Nachweis des CHVOSTEKschen Phänomens und die elektrische Übererregbarkeit sind Beweise für Tetanie. Meist handelt es sich um Schuster und Schneider. Der Ort, wo sie erkrankten, besonders Wien, wo die Tetanie endemisch ist, die Zeit März, April bringen auf die richtige Fährte. E. STRAUS und E. GUTTMANN haben dieser Frage besondere Aufmerksamkeit geschenkt und sind der Überzeugung, daß die eine vasokonstriktorische Form der Akroparästhesien eigentlich in das Gebiet der Vasoneurose gehört, während die andere rein sensible Form pathogenetisch der Tetanie nahesteht. Sie begründen ihre Auffassung unter anderem damit, daß die der Tetanie nahestehende Form meist eine elektrische und mechanische Übererregbarkeit analog dem Befunde bei der Tetanie zeige, während H. CURSCHMANN betont, daß solche Fälle die Diagnose nicht verdienen, sondern eben latente Tetanie sind. Auch CORNIL hat diese Fragen behandelt.

Wir machten früher darauf aufmerksam, daß Akroparästhesien häufig im Beginn der *Akromegalie* vorhanden sind. Von den *organischen* Krankheiten des Zentralnervensystems kommt sonst am ehesten die *Tabes* in Betracht, die gelegentlich mit Parästhesien in den oberen Extremitäten anfängt. Ähnliches wurde auch schon bei der Syringomyelie, ferner auch bei multipler Sklerose beobachtet. PERITZ bespricht die Differentialdiagnose der multiplen Sklerose gegenüber den Akroparästhesien. Auch an die kombinierten Systemerkrankungen ist zu denken. Gerade bei der perniziösen Anämie sind Akroparästhesien, und zwar solche der Zunge als Anfangssymptom nicht selten. In denjenigen Fällen, wo die Parästhesien in hemiplegischer Form auftreten, wäre an eine Verwechslung mit anatomisch bedingten Hirnleiden zu erinnern, soweit diese mit Schädigungen der sensiblen Bahnen in dem hinteren Teil der inneren Kapsel oder mit solchen der Schleife verbunden sind. Von Intoxikationen kommt der Ergotismus und der Alkoholismus in Frage.

Therapie.

Die Therapie besteht zunächst in der Ausschaltung der Schädlichkeiten und Vermeidung von Überanstrengungen, von Beschäftigungen mit Wasser usw. Sonst hat sich uns am besten die *Elektrizität* bewährt, besonders in der Form des elektrischen Pinsels, oder noch besser in der Form des elektrischen Handbades. Doch soll nicht verschwiegen werden, daß auch Mißerfolge zu verzeichnen sind. Ferner zeitigt zum Teil die *Heilgymnastik* und die *Massagebehandlung* gute Erfolge. Bei recht hartnäckigen Fällen hatten lokale lauwarme 1%ige Salzwasserbäder, die jeden Morgen 1—20 Min. lang genommen wurden, Erfolg. Bei anderen ließen wir während der Nacht einen PRIESSNITZ-Umschlag um den Arm machen, am besten in der Form, daß über einen dünnen, in Wasser getauchten Strumpf ein dicker, trockener Strumpf gezogen wurde. Auch Heißluftbehandlung hat sich uns und anderen bewährt. BORAK empfiehlt die Bestrahlung der Hypophyse, während MARBURG und SGALITZER nur die klimakterisch bedingten Akroparästhesien von der Hypophyse aus bestrahlen. In einem Falle haben sie auch durch periphere Erstarrung ein gutes Resultat erzielt.

In mehreren Fällen habe auch ich durch Bestrahlung der Hypophyse zufriedenstellende Resultate gesehen; doch waren diese nur temporär. Die medikamentöse Therapie ist dort in Anwendung zu bringen, wo die Akroparästhesien sich auf dem Boden einer Kachexie entwickeln. Hier sind die Tonika, in erster Linie Arsen, brauchbar. CURSCHMANN und HERZ rühmen besonders das Chinin (0,2 dreimal täglich), auch Adrenalinpräparate sind empfohlen worden (SOLIS-COHEN).

BOLTEN wendet eine kombinierte Organotherapie mit gutem Erfolge an: wie er angibt, schwanden bei solchen Fällen nach dem Gebrauch von relativ geringen Mengen von Ovarium-, Thyreoid- und Nebennierenpräparaten die Parästhesien vollständig nach wenigen Wochen. Setzte die Kranke die Medikamente jedoch 3—4 Wochen aus, traten die Beschwerden wieder auf, um nach Einnehmen der Präparate alsbald wieder zu verschwinden. BRÜNING berichtet, daß er auch bei Akroparästhesien die Sympathektomie mit Erfolg ausgeführt hat. Ähnliche Befunde haben W. LEHMANN und andere aufzuweisen.

V. Die multiple neurotische Hautgangrän.

Es sind in der Literatur einige Beobachtungen niedergelegt worden, in denen als hauptsächliches Krankheitszeichen eine multiple Gangränbildung eintrat, die sich weder aus dem Zustande des Gefäßsystems, noch dem der allgemeinen Ernährung, noch aus einer bakteriellen Invasion genügend erklärte. Eine Reihe von diesen Fällen hat enge Beziehungen zur RAYNAUDschen Krankheit. Wir haben schon gesehen, daß im Laufe der RAYNAUDschen Krankheit die Gangrän bisweilen über die Akra hinaus sich an verschiedenen Stellen des Körpers etablieren kann. Dort, wo die Bevorzugung der Akra ganz verschwindet, die Multiplizität der Nekrosen zunimmt, wo schließlich vasomotorische Störungen als Vorläufer der Gangrän ganz in den Hintergrund treten, dort resultiert das Krankheitsbild, dem man den Namen *multiple neurotische Gangrän* (multiple Hautgangrän [STUBENRAUCH, HINTNER], akute multiple Hautgangrän [DOUTRELEPONT], Herpes zoster gangraenosus hystericus [KAPOSI], Zoster cerebralis [WEISS], hysterische Hautgangrän [BAYET, GAUCHER, RIEHL]) gegeben hat, das an die RAYNAUDsche Gangrän, insbesondere noch immer durch die exakte Symmetrie der Nekrosen erinnern kann. Derartige Fälle sind beobachtet worden von LELOIR, SCHULZ, SINKLER, BRONSON, DIDIER, ZENGERLE, RENSHAW, CHAJES, SKLARZ, SAMADA, TOUTON, OPPENHEIM. Die Mehrzahl der genannten Fälle unterscheidet sich durch ein gemeinsames Kennzeichen von den typischen Fällen von RAYNAUD; sie verlaufen nämlich in einem einzigen Schube und tragen dadurch mehr den Charakter einer akuten Erkrankung. Sie stehen auf diese Weise der *Purpura rheumatica* nahe, die in Ausnahmefällen auch mit Nekrosen einhergehen kann, und würden auch zu gewissen Formen der Urticaria (RENAUT) in Beziehung zu setzen sein, bei der gelegentlich auch Nekrotisierungen vorkommen können.

Es gibt nun auch Fälle multipler neurotischer Gangrän, bei denen sich so enge Beziehungen zur RAYNAUDschen Krankheit nicht finden lassen. Man hat gegen die Mehrzahl dieser Fälle den Einwand erhoben, daß es sich überhaupt nicht um echte Krankheitszustände handele, sondern daß die Gangrän auf einem *Artefakt* beruhe, zumal die von ihr befallenen Kranken recht häufig hysterische Symptome aufwiesen. Es kann auch gar keinem Zweifel unterliegen, daß in einer großen Reihe von Fällen, in denen bei Hysterischen an einer oder mehreren Stellen sich eine Gangrän entwickelte, diese in der Tat artefiziell erzeugt war. Dieser Nachweis ist sehr häufig gelungen (CAVAGNES, THIBIERGE, GROSS, ZIELER, LITTLE, GUTFREUND, BETTMANN, SIEBEN, K. ALBRECHT u. v. a.). Es muß daher in der Tat die Forderung aufgestellt werden, daß überall, wo von multipler neurotischer Gangrän die Rede ist, zunächst eine Sicherung gegenüber dem Artefakt zu erfolgen hat. Diese Forderung ist gar nicht so einfach durchzuführen; es gehört dazu die allergenaueste Beobachtung, da der verschlagene und erfinderische Geist dieser Kranken immer wieder zu Täuschungsversuchen geneigt ist. Eine solche Beobachtung ist natürlich nur in der Klinik durchzuführen, dabei ist die Anlegung eines festen, dauernd kontrollierten Verbandes durchaus notwendig. Ein sicheres Kennzeichen für die nichtartefizielle Natur der Gangrän ist die Beobachtung, daß bei einer aus Bläschen entstehenden Gangrän durch die intakte Epidermis die nekrotischen tieferen Teile der Haut hindurchschimmern (KAPOSI); ZIELER hat sich nicht mit dem vielleicht doch nicht absolut zuverlässigen makroskopischen Nachweis dieser Integrität begnügt, sondern sie sogar an excidierten Nekrosen histologisch festgestellt; das ist der sicherste Weg, die Echtheit der Nekrosen nachzuweisen; es ist jedenfalls der dringende Wunsch auszusprechen, daß in Zukunft, wo die Frage neurotische oder artefizielle Gangrän zur Diskussion steht, die histologische Untersuchung excidierter Stücke erfolgen möge. Natürlich ist nicht zu übersehen, daß auch eine echte Gangrän zur frühzeitigen Nekrose der obersten Schichten führen kann. Ein weiteres sicheres Kennzeichen wäre das Auftreten von Nekrose an den Stellen, die der künstlichen Einwirkung der Kranken nicht zugänglich sind. Solche Fälle sind von DOUTRELEPONT und HINTNER beschrieben worden. Dazu gehört aber nicht das Auftreten von Nekrosen in der Vagina, die z. B. bei einer Patientin von GROSS künstlich hervorgerufen wurden. Ganz unzugänglich dürfte schließlich wohl überhaupt keine Stelle der äußeren Haut und der entsprechenden Schleimhäute für eine geschickte und erfinderische Kranke sein. In vielen Fällen drängt sich der Eindruck des Artefaktes ohne weiteres auf. Die Vielgestaltigkeit der Nekrosen, die Unregelmäßigkeit der Umgrenzung, die Tatsache, daß nur die linke Seite bei Rechtshändern von Nekrose befallen wird, das Aufhören der Nekrosenbildung bei Krankenhausbeobachtung und anderes mehr sprechen in diesem Sinne.

Aber wenn man die in der Literatur niedergelegten Fälle von multipler Gangrän auch noch so vorsichtig in Rücksicht auf die Frage des Artefaktes sichtet, so bleibt doch eine Reihe von solchen übrig, in denen ein Artefakt nicht vorgelegen zu haben scheint.

Diese Fälle haben viel Gemeinsames, zunächst in bezug auf die Ätiologie. Sehr häufig geht dem Eintritte der Gangrän ein Trauma mehr oder minder lange Zeit voraus. Nicht weniger als 17mal wurde unter 28 Fällen ein solches konstatiert. In 7 Fällen war es eine Verbrennung 2. Grades (HINTNER, KOPP, DINKLER, MÜLLER, VALOBRA, DEHIO, MOORMEISTER, PICK, BULLE und HASE). Eine Schwefelsäureverbrennung lag in den Fällen von JOSEPH und BAYET vor. In anderen Fällen handelte es sich um Einstoßen von Nägeln, Haken, Glassplittern usw. (DOUTRELEPONT, KREIBICH, BOLTEN.) FREY berichtet über eine 19jährige Kranke, die früher Neigung zu Pyodermie hatte. Im Anschluß an eine PIRQUETsche Tuberkulinreaktion trat die Erkrankung auf. Es bildeten sich allmählich große nekrotische Herde bis zu den Schultern hinauf. Ein Artefakt war nicht nachweisbar. Der Rachenreflex war aufgehoben, der Cornealreflex herabgesetzt. Das Gemeinsame dieser Verletzungen liegt darin, daß sie alle wohl geeignet waren, auf die Nerven der betreffenden Gebiete einen lang dauernden Reiz auszuüben und diese damit in einen Zustand einer gewissen Übererregbarkeit zu versetzen. Die Zeitdauer, in der die Gangrän dem Trauma folgt, ist sehr verschieden, sie schwankt von wenigen Tagen bis zu Jahren, wobei allerdings der Zusammenhang mehrfach durch immer erneutes Aufbrechen der Narben hergestellt wurde. Es ist ferner sicher, daß die multiple Hautgangrän meist nervöse Personen betroffen hat. Für eine Anzahl von ihnen erscheint auch die Diagnose „Hysterie" sichergestellt. Das vorliegende Material genügt aber keineswegs, um die multiple Gangrän zu einer echt hysterischen Affektion zu stempeln. Die Gangrän ist keine Teilerscheinung der Hysterie, sondern diese stellt nur die für die Entstehung der Gangrän förderliche Disposition dar (DINKLER).

Der Gesamtverlauf der Krankheit ist der folgende: Meist in der Nähe der von dem Trauma herrührenden Narbe bildet sich der erste gangränöse Fleck, dem in wechselnden Zwischenräumen neue, gewöhnlich zunächst in der Nachbarschaft der Verwundungsstelle folgen. Nachdem dann verschieden lange Zeit hindurch nur die verletzte Extremität Sitz des Krankheitsprozesses gewesen ist, breitet dieser sich weiter aus und geht auf die übrigen Teile der affizierten Körperhälfte über. Es können viele Monate vergehen, ehe es so weit kommt, es können aber auch schon nach einigen Tagen weit entfernte Stellen derselben Körperhälfte befallen werden. Der Prozeß kann sich dauernd auf die einmal befallene Seite beschränken, aber nach mehr oder minder langem Verlauf, oft erst nach vielen Monaten, kommt meist auch die andere Körperhälfte an die Reihe. Die Symmetrie der Nekrosen ist in den an den Raynaud erinnernden Fällen, wie oben erwähnt wurde, besonders ausgesprochen. Es kann in den schwersten Fällen allmählich der ganze Körper, eingeschlossen das Gesicht, Sitz der Nekrosen werden. Solche sind auch im äußeren Gehörgang und im Trommelfell gefunden

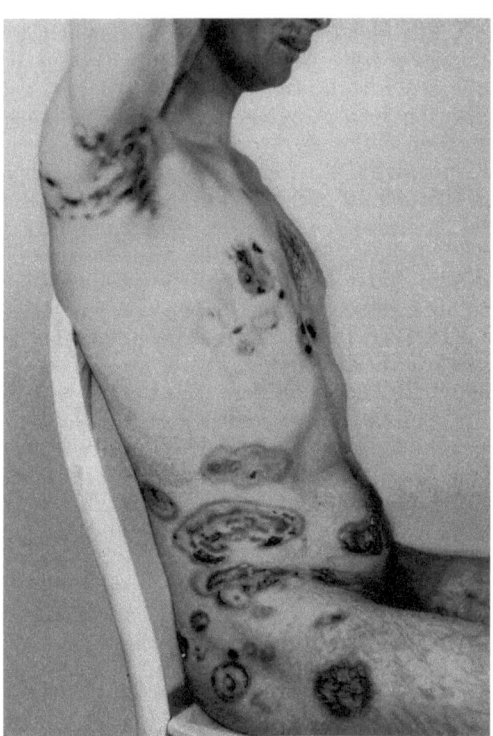

Abb. 7. Multiple neurotische Hautgangrän.
(Nach BODE.)

worden (HINTNER, TRUFFI), ferner an den Schleimhäuten, so in dem Falle von DOUTRELEPONT im Rachen, am harten und weichen Gaumen, an der Conjunctiva, auch an der Schleimhaut der äußeren Genitalien. Ähnliches berichten DINKLER, KREIBICH, TRUFFI. LÖBLOWITZ beschreibt als eine besondere Form eine neurotische Schleimhautgangrän und rechnet außer einer eigenen familiären Beobachtungsreihe hierher Fälle von JACOBI, SIBLEY, KICK, COURT.

Der zeitige Ablauf des Prozesses zeigt in den einzelnen Fällen die größten Divergenzen. Die Nekrosen können in sehr rascher Aufeinanderfolge entstehen. LELOIR berichtet, daß seine Kranke in der ersten Beobachtungszeit nicht 14 Tage, später nicht einmal 8 Tage hintereinander vom Auftreten neuer Schorfe verschont blieb und nach 3 Jahren war noch keine Besserung dieses Zustandes eingetreten. Kann sich so der Prozeß über Jahre hinziehen (so ist der Fall von TRUFFI 17 Jahre lang beobachtet worden, die Kranke hatte zuletzt 221 Narben), so ist in anderen Fällen der Verlauf ein kürzerer, erstreckt sich über einige

Monate, und wir haben schon erwähnt, daß es Fälle gibt, die in einem einmaligen Anfall sich erschöpfen. Im allgemeinen haben wir es also mit einer rezidivierenden, wenn auch in einzelnen, sehr unregelmäßigen Etappen ablaufenden Affektion zu tun.

Dem Auftreten der Nekrosen geht oft ein umschriebenes Brennen voraus, das die verschiedenen Patienten mehrfach in ganz gleicher Art schilderten; mit ihm zugleich sind häufig neuralgiforme diffuse Schmerzen beobachtet worden, meist nicht im Gebiet bestimmter Nerven, ebensowenig wie die Gangrän sich auf solche zu beschränken pflegt. Im Falle CHAJES' z. B. gingen leichte ziehende Schmerzen im Bein den Hautnekrosen an derselben Stelle voraus. Gelegentlich sind auch objektive sensible Ausfallserscheinungen festgestellt worden. Die nekrotischen Stellen sind anästhetisch, wie natürlich, aber die Anästhesie geht auch über das nekrotische Gebiet hinaus und sie kann einen großen Teil der befallenen Extremität in Anspruch nehmen. Die Narben sind zunächst meist überempfindlich, werden später erst normal empfindlich. Eine bestimmte Anordnung der Sensibilitätsstörung ist nirgends zu erkennen.

Die Gangrän entwickelt sich in verschiedener Form, entweder aus kleinen Bläschen, die weiter regressive Metamorphosen eingehen, oder durch direkte Nekrotisierung. Im Falle von CHAJES entwickelte sich zunächst ein bläschenförmiger Hautausschlag auf Brust und Rücken, der ausheilte. Wenige Monate später zeigten sich zahlreiche Geschwürs- und Schorfbildungen am rechten Unterschenkel, die immer wieder neu auftraten und durch Behandlung nicht merklich beeinflußt wurden. Trotz fester unverletzter Okklusivverbände traten wiederholt Bläschenbildungen mit oberflächlichen Hautnekrosen am rechten Bein auf. Im Falle von SKLARZ begann die Hautgangrän regelmäßig mit lokaler heller Rötung, dann kam es unter Exsudation zu Absterben der Epidermis und Nekrosenbildung. BODE sah die Erkrankung in periodisch einsetzenden Schüben verlaufen, und zwar bildeten sich verschiedene Primärefflorescenzen, die nacheinander in den einzelnen Krankheitsstadien auftraten: einerseits inmitten gesunder Haut discoide gerötete Flecke, in der Umgebung älterer Herde konzentrisch sich bildende bandförmige Erytheme, die nach eventuell eintretendem Substanzverlust abheilten, anderseits scheibenförmige Erytheme mit sekundärer zentraler Anämie, anämische Herde ohne vorangehende Entzündung, umschriebene Erytheme mit zentraler Anämie, die sämtlich zu tiefgreifender Gangrän führten. Auf weitere Einzelheiten gehen wir hier nicht ein, ebenso wie wir auf die Darstellung der genaueren histologischen Untersuchungen, wie sie von KREIBICH, CHAJES u. a. angestellt wurden, verzichten. Das Ende aller dieser in ihren Einzelheiten abweichenden Vorgänge ist jedenfalls die *Verschorfung*, deren Größe in ein und demselben Fall und sogar bei gleichzeitig oder rasch hintereinander auftretenden Nekrosen sehr wechselt. DINKLER beobachtete zehnpfennig- bis talerstück große Schorfe. KOPP sah in einem Falle Nekrosen von nicht mehr als Linsengröße und solche von 4 cm Länge und 1 cm Breite. Die Schorfe sind hart, pergamentartig, so fest, daß man sie nur mühsam mit einer Nadel durchstechen kann. Der Nekrosenbildung gehen Veränderungen des Blutgehaltes der betreffenden Teile nur selten voraus. Nicht selten kommen *Störungen* allgemeiner Art im Gebiete des *Vasomotorensystems* vor. Wiederholt wurde eine besonders starke Dermographie beobachtet. In einzelnen Fällen fanden sich auffallend große Differenzen der Temperatur zwischen beiden Körperhälften (RÖTHLER). Gelegentlich traten die Erscheinungen des flüchtigen Ödems auf. Einzelne Patienten waren besonders empfindlich gegen Pilocarpininjektionen (RÖTHLER, TRUFFI). Versuche, die vasomotorische Reaktion der Haut auf physikalische und chemische Reize hin zu prüfen und Abweichungen vom normalen Verhalten festzustellen, sind mehrfach gemacht worden. In einzelnen Fällen (HINTNER, DINKLER, KREIBICH, BETTMANN-LEWONTIN) sind auch positive Resultate erzielt worden. Die Nekrosen heilten oft unter Keloidbildung; doch ließ sich diese durch sorgfältige lokale Behandlung oft verhindern, sie ist also jedenfalls kein ausschlaggebendes Kriterium. Im Falle von SKLARZ erfolgte die Heilung teils ohne Narbenbildung, teils mit solcher unter Keloidbildung. Gelegentlich kommen auch in ganz typischen Fällen Störungen vor, die sehr an die Asphyxie locale erinnern und auf diese Weise nun doch auch wieder den Zusammenhang auch dieser Fälle mit der RAYNAUDschen Krankheit erkennen lassen.

Allgemeinsymptome fehlen oft völlig, doch konnten gelegentlich Temperaturanstiege, Übelbefinden, Appetitlosigkeit, Erbrechen beobachtet werden (BODE).

Eine Kranke DOUTRELEPONTS starb an Lungentuberkulose; die Untersuchung des Nervensystems hatte einen völlig negativen Befund. Sonst ist die Prognose quoad vitam absolut günstig.

Neben diesen *selbständigen Fällen* multipler neurotischer Hautgangrän gibt es solche, bei denen diese Erscheinungen im Zusammenhang mit *organischen Erkrankungen* des *Nervensystems* beobachtet wurden. Auf dem Boden der *Gliosis spinalis* wurde sie von POSPELOW, NEUBERGER, LESNÉ, wahrscheinlich auch von MÜLLER gesehen. In einem Falle von KREIBICH, bei dem die multiplen Nekrosen am linken Vorderarm saßen, in den sich die Kranke 2 Monate vorher einen rostigen Nagel eingestoßen hatte, bestanden die Symptome einer *Tabes*. Sie scheint ferner auch bei peripheren *Neuritiden*, bzw. *Nervenverletzungen* vorzukommen. Im Falle LÖHE-ROSENFELD fand sich eine ausgebildete Periarteriitis nodosa. Schließlich wollen wir hier noch wenigstens erwähnen, daß es auch Fälle des klassischen *Herpes zoster* gibt, in denen einige wenige oder seltener die Mehrzahl der Bläschen im weiteren Verlauf durch Verschorfung der Bläschendecke zu Ulcerationen werden (Herpes zoster gangraenosus). So ist die multiple neurotische Gangrän keine Krankheit sui generis, sondern ein unter verschiedenen Bedingungen sich findender Symptomenkomplex. Neben solchen Fällen, die wir eben erwähnten, wo sie als Symptom einer organischen Nervenkrankheit vorkommen, gibt es solche, in denen neben ihren Symptomen solche einer schweren *Urticaria* deutlich in den Vordergrund treten, so daß wir von Urticaria gangraenosa sprechen dürfen. Es gibt Fälle, in denen sie wie eine selbständige Infektion oder Intoxikation von der Art der gewöhnlichen Urticaria oder der von uns später näher zu charakterisierenden toxisch-infektiösen Form des angioneurotischen Ödems auftritt; endlich gibt es Fälle, die die Hauptgruppe darstellen und die Bezeichnung ,,neurotische Gangrän" deswegen ganz mit Recht tragen, weil sie offenbar auf dem Boden einer allgemeinen neuropathischen Diathese erwachsen.

In sehr vielen Fällen zeigt das Grundleiden deutlich die Züge der *Hysterie*. Es handelt sich oft um ausgesprochene und schwere Fälle von konvulsiver Hysterie. In anderen, weniger zahlreichen Fällen liegt keine ausgesprochene Hysterie, sondern nur eine allgemeine nervöse Labilität vor. Die außerordentlich große Seltenheit des Vorkommens der Gangrän bei Hysterie, ebenso wie der Mangel eines Nachweises dafür, daß selbst in den Fällen, wo Hysterie vorliegt, die multiple Gangrän ein hysterisches Symptom ist, läßt es geraten erscheinen, keine engeren Beziehungen zwischen der Neurose und dem nekrotisierenden Prozeß anzunehmen, die beiden Gruppen von multipler neurotischer Gangrän nicht zu trennen und in dem Vorhandensein der neuropathischen Diathese nur eine sehr häufige Voraussetzung für die Entstehung der Nekrosen zu sehen. Außer der *Disposition* ist in fast allen Fällen in der Vorgeschichte der Affektion ein Trauma vorhanden, dem man eine gewisse Bedeutung zusprechen muß. Es ist stets derart gewesen, daß es auf die peripheren Nervenenden für lange Zeit einen Reiz auszuüben imstande war. Es ist daher die Annahme statthaft, daß es auf reflektorischem Wege eine erhöhte Reizbarkeit entfernterer Nervengebiete produziert hat, die ihrerseits schon durch die kongenitale Disposition vorbereitet waren. Es bedarf keiner weiteren Begründung, daß wir für die Erklärung der speziellen Symptome der Nekrose auf eine besondere Beteiligung gewisser Abschnitte des *vegetativen Systems* unser Augenmerk richten müssen. Wir haben oft eine allgemeine Widerstandsunfähigkeit dieses Systems feststellen, aber auch noch einige spezielle Erscheinungen finden können; dahin sind die einige Male experimentell nachgewiesenen, einige Male klinisch deutlich gewordenen Zeichen der Labilität des Hautgefäßnervensystems, ferner die Empfindlichkeit gegen Pilocarpin zu rechnen. In diese Gruppe gehören die charakteristischen Fälle von SKLARZ und BOLTEN. Zur Unterstützung dieser Anschauungen dient es, daß enge Beziehungen der neurotischen Hautgangrän zur RAYNAUDschen Krankheit, übrigens auch zu anderen vasomotorisch-trophischen Neurosen, zur Erythromelalgie und zum flüchtigen Ödem vorhanden sind.

MUCHA vertritt den Standpunkt, daß hämatogen-toxische (wie z. B. im Falle FINKELSTEIN) und nervöse Momente vielfach nebeneinander ihre Wirksamkeit entfalten und erst dadurch das Krankheitsbild hervorrufen. Er hält jedoch die nervöse Komponente insofern für die wesentlichere, da sie in keinem Falle ohne weiteres abgelehnt wird, dagegen auf die Hineinziehung einer toxischen in manchen Fällen verzichtet werden konnte. Er schließt sich dem von uns und von CHVOSTEK vertretenen Standpunkt an, daß die multiple neurotische Hautgangrän keine Krankheit sui generis darstellt, daß aber andererseits nach Ausscheidung der auf anatomische Erkrankung des Nervensystems beruhenden Fälle Krankheitsbilder übrig bleiben, denen ein sichtlich verwandter, wenn nicht gemeinsamer Entstehungsmechanismus zugrunde liegt und deren Zusammenfassung in eine Gruppe nahegelegt wird. BODE neigt zu der Annahme einer einstweilen nicht erfaßbaren (haematogen-infectiös-) toxischen an den Gefäßen unmittelbar angreifenden Noxe.

Die *Diagnose* wird sich zunächst immer mit der Abwehr des Verdachts eines Artefaktes beschäftigen müssen. Daß dies in vielen Fällen große Schwierigkeiten macht, haben wir schon betont. Des weiteren wird das Augenmerk darauf zu richten sein, ob irgendwelche Erscheinungen eines organischen Nervenleidens (Gliosis spinalis, Tabes dorsalis, periphere Nervenverletzungen) vorliegen. Es gibt ferner eine Art von multipler Gangrän, die in ihrer Entstehung nichts mit dem Nervensystem zu tun hat, sondern auf dem Boden der Kachexie erwächst; es scheint sich da meist um infektiöse Ursachen zu handeln; von anderen wird diese Gangrän auf Thrombenbildung zurückgeführt. Neben der Kachexie bietet auch sonst der Allgemeinzustand charakteristische Merkmale; das Fieber ist intensiver, die Gangrän von sehr wechselnder Ausdehnung, oft ausgedehnter, als sie bei der neurotischen Gangrän zu beobachten ist. Die sensiblen Erscheinungen treten mehr zurück. Drüsenanschwellungen kommen vor (ROTHMANN u. a.).

Bezüglich der *Behandlung* ist nicht viel zu sagen. Bemerkenswert sind die Erfolge, die RÖTHLER mit BIERscher Stauung, TRUFFI mit lokaler Hyperämie (Sinapismen, Anwendung von heißem Wasser, Injektionen von Pilocarpin) erzielten. Schlechte Erfahrungen hat BRONSON mit Röntgenbehandlung gemacht. SKLARZ hat in der Annahme, daß infolge einer Hyperfunktion der Schilddrüse und des dadurch bedingten Kreisens von Toxinen im Blut die Gefäßwände alteriert werden und daß aus der gleichfalls erfolgenden Labilisierung des Sympathicus eine erhöhte Reflexbereitschaft der Vasomotoren resultiert, eine Antithyreoidinbehandlung angewandt, durch die der Krankheitsprozeß nach seiner Mitteilung rasch zum Stillstand gebracht wurde.

VI. Die Sklerodermie.

Die erste genauere Beschreibung dieser Krankheit stammt aus dem Jahre 1845 von THIRIAL. Aus den historischen Notizen, die EHRMANN und BRÜNAUER geben, geht hervor, daß bereits 1634 ZACUTUS LUSITANUS das Krankheitsbild richtig erkannt und dargestellt hat. 1872 hat BALL zuerst ausführlich die Sklerodaktylie, d. h. die im wesentlichen auf die Finger beschränkte Sklerodermie beschrieben. 1895 veröffentlichten LEWIN-HELLER die erste deutsche Monographie über die Krankheit; eine sehr ausführliche Zusammenstellung und Verwertung der Literatur, soweit Pathogenese und pathologische Anatomie in Frage kommen, ist von v. NOTHHAFFT geliefert worden. Es soll noch erwähnt werden die Darstellung von LUITHLEN im Handbuch für Hautkrankheiten, von R. CASSIRER in seiner Monographie 1912, endlich aus jüngster Zeit die ausgezeichnete und umfassende Darstellung der Sklerodermie und der ihr verwandten Prozesse von EHRMANN und BRÜNAUER.

Ätiologie.

Die Sklerodermie ist eine Erkrankung, die sich mit Vorliebe zur Zeit der höchsten körperlichen Reife entwickelt, aber sowohl das Kindesalter, als auch das Greisenalter (KREEGER und KAPOSI, NAEGELI u. a.) nicht verschont. Es werden Fälle berichtet, in denen echte Sklerodermie sich bei nur wenigen Wochen alten Kindern entwickelte; COCKAYNE berichtet über einen Fall von kongenitaler Sklerodermie und Sklerodaktylie bei einem Kinde mit Hydrocephalus. Die Diagnose wurde von PARKES WEBER bestätigt. HAUSHALTER und SPILLMANN, sowie EGGER beobachteten ähnliche Fälle. In einer Reihe von Fällen, die als Sklerodermie im Säuglingsalter beschrieben worden sind, handelt es sich jedoch um Sklerem und Sklerödem.

Das *weibliche* Geschlecht wird entschieden häufiger von der Krankheit befallen. LEWIN-HELLER fanden 67% Frauen. Nach EHRMANN-BRÜNAUER ist das weibliche Geschlecht 3—4mal häufiger beteiligt, wenn man die Sklerodermia diffusa und circumscripta zusammenrechnet. Auch KREN bemerkt die ungleich größere Häufigkeit des Vorkommens der Sklerodaktylie bei Frauen. ANSELMINO sah die Erkrankung in der Schwangerschaft auftreten und im Wochenbett wieder verschwinden. Die Krankheit ist im ganzen nicht selten. Statistische Berechnungen der Frequenz schwanken zwischen $1/2$% und 1,5% von Hautkrankheiten. Stand und Beruf sind im allgemeinen ohne Einfluß auf die Entstehung; AYRES berichtet indessen über 3 Fälle von allgemeiner Sklerodermie, bei denen chronische Arsenintoxikation eine Rolle spielte. BRAMWELL fand die Erkrankung häufiger unter Steinhauern verbreitet. Sie begann stets in der rechten Hand; er glaubt, daß dabei das ständige Halten des kalten Meißels in dieser Hand von Bedeutung gewesen ist.

In der Ascendenz oder Descendenz sowie familiär ist Sklerodermie wiederholt beobachtet worden (BAILEY). BAUER sah bei Vater und Tochter Sklerodaktylie, in Kombination mit Nekrose der Fingerspitzen bei Vater und ältestem Sohn, während die beiden jüngeren Söhne an Angiokeratoma Mibelli litten (zitiert nach H. W. SIEMENS). MONIER-VINARD-BARBOT sahen zwei Schwestern mit symmetrischer segmentaler Sklerodermie an den unteren Extremitäten mit Katarakt. KREBS-HARTMANN-THIÉBAUT beobachteten in zwei aufeinanderfolgenden Generationen der gleichen Familie bei mehreren Mitgliedern Sklerodermie und Canities praecox, infantile genitale Mißbildungen bei Erhaltensein der sexuellen Funktion, außerdem Katarakt, Basedowsymptome, Arthritis deformans, Erythrämie. LOUSTE-JUSTER-MICHELET sahen bei Mutter und Sohn Sklerodermie en bandes und en plaques, jedoch nicht an den gleichen Stellen.

Dabei bestanden Akroparästhesien und Akroasphyxie. Bei der Mutter war das Raynaudsyndrom rechts, die circumscripte Sklerodermie links. LEREBOULLET-LELONG sahen bei Mutter und Tochter multiple Kalkeinlagerungen in der Haut mit örtlicher Sklerdermie. TOEN (zit. nach EHRMANN-BRÜNAUER) berichtet über sklerodermatische Veränderungen bei zwei Brüdern und bei deren Mutter. Schwere *neuropathische* Belastung ist ziemlich häufig festzustellen und auch von uns mehrfach gesehen worden. So war die Mutter einer unserer Kranken tuberkulös, eine Schwester war geisteskrank, eine taubstumm, eine litt an Migräne. Der Bruder des Vaters war an Dementia paralytica erkrankt.

Vielfach sind vorausgegangene Krankheiten in ursächliche Beziehungen zur Entstehung der Sklerodermie gebracht worden. Es handelt sich da um *Infektions*-krankheiten verschiedenster Art, akute wie chronische; namentlich ist der Tuberkulose eine Rolle zugeschrieben worden. EHRMANN-BRÜNAUER haben diesem ätiologischen Faktor ihre besondere Aufmerksamkeit zugewandt und zitieren eine große Anzahl von Fällen, in denen teils die Pirquetreaktion positiv war, teils auch Tuberkulose an den inneren Organen festgestellt wurde. Sie selbst berichten über einen Fall, bei welchem Lupus vulgaris, Tuberkulose und Lichen scrofulosorum gleichzeitig vorhanden waren; die Patientin zeigte einen nicht einmal langsamen Übergang in typische diffuse Sklerodermie mit Erscheinungen von Akroasphyxie, sowie sklerodermatischen Veränderungen der Extremitäten, des Gesichtes und des Halses. EHRMANN-BRÜNAUER fassen ihre Ansicht in folgende Worte zusammen: ,,Wenn wir der Tuberkulose eine ätiologische Rolle bei der diffusen Sklerodermie einräumen möchten, so meinen wir damit nicht, daß Sklerodermie Tuberkulose ist, sondern daß durch die Tuberkulose als häufige Ursache eine Schädigung der innersekretorischen Organe und des mit diesen in engstem Zusammenhange stehenden autonomen Nervensystems bewirkt wird." Im Falle von POUSSEPP litt die Mutter an Tuberkulose, die Tochter an Drüsentuberkulose. Im Alter von 8 Jahren trat Sklerodaktylie und Sklerodermie en bandes auf.

In den letzten Jahrzehnten ist wiederholt die Frage des Zusammenhanges zwischen *Syphilis* und Sklerodermie diskutiert worden. Man stützte sich bei diesen Erwägungen auf das Zusammenvorkommen der Sklerodermie mit Lues congenita (ISOLA, BRUNSCHWEILER-FOREL, PETGES, JORDAN, WALDORP-BASOMBRIO u. a.). BERTIN hat sich mit diesen Fragen eingehend beschäftigt und ist der Ansicht, daß die ätiologische Bedeutung der Syphilis zwar selten, aber sicherlich bei gewissen Sklerodermien feststeht. Er weist im Einvernehmen mit anderen Autoren auf die Bedeutung der Liquoruntersuchung bei der Sklerodermie hin, sowie auf die anderen serologischen und klinischen Befunde, endlich auf die gelegentlich beschriebenen Fälle, in denen die spezifische Kur eine auffallend günstige Wirkung gehabt hat. Ähnliches berichten LORTAT-JACOB-LEGRAIN, LÉRI, BARTHÉLEMY-LINOSSIER u. a. LIEBNER fand histologisch bestätigte sklerodermische Herde bei einem Luiker, die teilweise eine gemeinsame Lokalisation mit Syphiliden hatten. Letztere wurden durch die antiluische Kur beseitigt, nicht aber die Sklerodermie. NAEGELI hat unter 20 Fällen von Sklerodermie niemals Lues in der Anamnese gefunden und betont die Wichtigkeit dieser Beobachtung, weil sie in der Schweiz gemacht sei, wo die Lues nicht sehr häufig sei. Angesichts der Tatsache, daß in einem syphilisreichen Lande das Zusammenvorkommen der Sklerodermie und Syphilis durchaus in den Bereich der Wahrscheinlichkeit gehört, muß diese Beobachtung besonders unterstrichen werden. ARTOM-FORNARA und JORDAN weisen auf den Zusammenhang der Sklerodermie mit Lues und mit endokrinen Störungen hin.

Erkältungen wurden oftmals beschuldigt, eine feuchte Wohnung, Arbeiten in der Nässe, ein Fall ins Wasser, ein kaltes Bad usw. In diesem Zusammenhang sei erwähnt, daß einzelne später an Sklerodermie erkrankte Individuen schon früher eine große Empfindlichkeit gegen Kälte zeigten. Diese dokumentierte sich manchmal in dem Auftreten von Frostbeulen.

Auch das *Trauma* ist als prädisponierendes Moment erwähnt worden. Wir selbst haben einen Fall gesehen, wo angeblich im Anschluß an einen schweren Unfall Sklerodermie entstanden sein soll. Aber hier wie in zahlreichen anderen Fällen, in denen die traumatische Entstehung in Erwägung gezogen wurde, ist der Zusammenhang nicht sicher. TESKE hat die Fälle angeblich traumatischer Genese zusammengestellt; er fand keinen mit einer die traumatische Genese zwingend erweisenden Vorgeschichte. Über Fälle angeblich traumatischer Genese berichten ferner KRAUS, GOLŠMID, ARONSTAM, ferner BARTHÉLEMY, GAUCH-SOHIER-DE COURRÈGES, WIGLEY, LHERMITTE-LÉVY. Interessant ist der Fall, den GRÖDEL-HUBERT beschrieben haben. Bei einem völlig gesunden 42jährigen Fabrikdirektor entwickelte sich im Anschluß an einen schweren Autounfall mit Frakturen und starken Blutergüssen in beiden Armen und Händen eine allmählich zunehmende Sklerodermie, die sich diffus ausbreitete, gleichzeitig mit Myosklerose und Gelenkerscheinungen. Beachtenswert sind die Fälle, in denen die sklerodermatischen Partien an den Stellen auftraten, die einem dauernden Druck von gewissen Kleidungsstücken ausgesetzt waren (CASSIRER, SPIEGLER, HUTCHINSON, ULLMANN, COVISA). Es gibt auch vereinzelte Erfahrungen, die lehren, daß bei schon entwickelter Sklerodermie aus irgendeinem anderen Grunde entstandene Narben sklerodermatisch entarten können.

Die Beobachtungen, in denen die von Sklerodermie befallenen Individuen lange vorher an einer allgemeinen funktionellen *Neurose* litten, sind häufig. Es wurde schon erwähnt, daß mehrfach neuropathische Belastung nachweisbar war. HERZOG glaubte in seinem Fall eine Anzahl von Degenerationszeichen feststellen zu können. Neben der allgemeinen Neuropathie fand sich wiederholt die Sklerodermie bei Epilepsie (FRÉMY), Chorea (ROGER, WHITE und BURNS, LOUSTE, CAILLIAU und LECLERC), Paralysis agitans (PANEGROSSI), Basedowscher Krankheit (siehe darüber Näheres unter Pathogenese). JOSEFOWITSCH sah ein 9jähriges Mädchen mit Anfällen rechtsseitiger JACKSONscher Epilepsie, die mit Zuckungen im Gesicht und konjugierter Deviation von Kopf und Augen nach rechts einsetzten; $1^1/_2$ Monate nach Beginn der Erkrankung trat eine rechtsseitige Gonitis auf und bald darauf ein sklerodermischer Herd an der rechten unteren Extremität. Später entwickelten sich sklerodermische Hautveränderungen an der rechten Seite des Körpers und der rechten oberen Extremität und fast gleichzeitig an der rechten Hälfte des behaarten Teiles des Kopfes und im Bereiche des linken Schulterblattes. Noch später stellte sich eine Hemiatrophia dextra linguae ein. Auch ausgesprochene geistige Störungen sind in der Anamnese derartiger Kranker notiert. Zwei unserer Patienten stotterten seit der Jugend, einer litt an schweren Infraorbitalneuralgien, einer hatte ausgesprochene Zwangsvorstellungen, die Mehrzahl der übrigen klagte über mehr oder minder stark hervortretende nervöse Erscheinungen. COURTOIS-ANDRÉ sahen sie bei Dementia praecox auftreten. LONGCOPE berichtet über das Auftreten von deliranten Zuständen mit Hypoglykämie. Es gibt aber auch Fälle, in denen die Symptome einer Störung des Nervensystems fehlen.

Relativ selten entwickelte sich die Sklerodermie bei Individuen, die an organischen Nervenkrankheiten litten. THIBIERGE-SPILLMANN-WEISSENBACH beobachteten ihr Auftreten bei Polyneuritis diphtherica. SCHULTZE sah sie bei Myelitis in den gelähmten Teilen entstehen, SENATOR, GUILLAIN und CELICE, LÉRI, BARTHÉLEMY und LINOSSIER beobachteten sie bei Tabes, CASSIRER bei progressiver Bulbärparalyse, KOPCZYNSKI sah sie mit bulbären Symptomen verknüpft, FRÉMY bei Tumor cerebri. Bei dem von TOMMASI beobachteten 32jährigen

Kranken entwickelte sich einige Monate nach Auftreten einer Encephalitis lethargica gleichzeitig mit den Erscheinungen des Parkinsonismus akut eine allmählich fortschreitende diffuse Sklerodermie mit ausgesprochener Vagotonie und Zeichen einer Insuffizienz der Schilddrüse. Im Falle STOLKIND entwickelte sich das Bild des Parkinsonismus ungefähr 20 Jahre nach dem Auftreten eines Raynaud mit Sklerodermie. CROSTI sah in dem sklerodermischen Gebiet einen Herpes zoster auftreten, ebenso VEROTTI. MANKOVSKIJ sah bei einem Kinde das an Poliomyelitis erkrankt war, in der gelähmten Körperregion typische sklerodermische Hautveränderungen sich entwickeln; ferner beobachtete er bei einem Kranken mit doppelseitiger Facialislähmung unter Beteiligung des Trigeminus nach 3 Wochen eine sklerodermische Hautveränderung an Stirn, Lidern, Wangen, Nase, Kinn und Lippen. Er ist der Ansicht, daß der sklerodermische Prozeß als Folge der primär erkrankten Nerven anzusehen sei. V. DECASTELLO beschreibt einen merkwürdigen Fall von perniziöser Anämie mit tabiformer Rückenmarksveränderung und diffuser Sklerodermie. Von seiten des endokrinen Systems fielen die auffallend kleinen atrophischen Hoden auf; die Schilddrüse war eher kleiner, der Türkensattel erschien radiologisch entschieden schmäler als normal. Wichtig und interessant sind die Angaben von MONTESANO, VERHOGEN, FEDOROW, SCHLESINGER, MORSELLI und POSPELOFF, die Sklerodermie bei Syringomyelie auftreten sahen. Freilich erscheint die Diagnose Gliosis nicht in allen diesen Fällen sicher. LHERMITTE und LÉVY sahen eine Sklerodaktylie mutilans an der linken Hand eines Kranken auftreten, der 30 Jahre vorher ein schweres Trauma dieser Hand erlitten hatte. Es bestanden außerdem Amyotrophie, vasomotorisch-trophische und sensible Störungen bis zu C 4 hinaufreichend. Die Autoren schließen die Diagnose Syringomyelie und Lepra aus und führen die Störungen auf eine im Anschluß an eine Sepsis aufgetretene ascendierende zentral nervöse Schädigung zurück. PER sah einen Fall von Sklerodermie en plaques in Verbindung mit atrophisch-neuritischen Erscheinungen. BRUNSCHWEILER und FOREL beobachteten einen sehr komplizierten Fall, in dem eine teratologische Strukturanomalie des Zentralnervensystems verbunden mit Sklerodermie, epileptischen Anfällen, endokrinen Störungen und psychischer Schwäche vorlag, wahrscheinlich auf dem Boden einer Lues congenita entstanden.

Einzelne Symptome organischer Läsion wurden von WESTPHAL, PAWLOWSKI, HERZOG, NAUNYN, RAYMOND, PETELIN u. a. beobachtet. Bemerkenswert ist ein Fall von BALLET und DELHELM, der eine Kombination von Dystrophia musculorum progressiva, Imbezillität und Sklerodermie darstellt. Auch ROGER berichtet über die Kombination mit Dystrophia musculorum progressiva. PATRZEK beschreibt einen Fall von Sklerodermie, der mit einer atypischen Form der Myasthenia gravis pseudoparalytica vergesellschaftet war. Sowohl die Myasthenie als auch die Sklerodermie waren im Gesicht lokalisiert. Ähnliches erwähnen MILIAN und RIMÉ, PARKES WEBER-BODE. Der Wert dieser Beobachtungen ist ein ungleichartiger; einige wenige können daran denken lassen, daß die Sklerodermie hier direkt als Folge der organischen Nervenkrankheit sich entwickelt habe. Man muß sich jedoch der Tatsache bewußt bleiben, wie unerhört selten bei den genannten doch häufiger zur Beobachtung kommenden organischen Nervenkrankheiten sklerodermische Prozesse zu beobachten sind. Andere Fälle weisen, falls man nicht an eine rein zufällige Koinzidenz denken will, nur auf eine gesteigerte allgemeine Vulnerabilität des Nervensystems hin. Auch schwere psychische Erregungen scheinen in der Anamnese eine gewisse Rolle zu spielen. Wir sahen eine Patientin, bei der sich in ziemlich nahem Zusammenhange mit dem Tode ihres Mannes eine Sklerodaktylie rasch entwickelte. Weitere Beobachtungen stammen von BALL, MAROTTE, COLLINS, LEWIN, RAYMOND, PER u. a.

Symptomatologie.

Als Sklerodermie im allerweitesten Sinne bezeichnen EHRMANN und BRÜNAUER in ihrer Darstellung „jene Prozesse, welche ohne Zellneubildung, ohne wesentliche Zellinfiltration durch Schwellung des Bindegewebes auf der Höhe ihrer Entwicklung die Haut so verändern, daß diese ihre Geschmeidigkeit, Haltbarkeit und Eindruckbarkeit einbüßt, sich derb, lederartig anfühlt, dabei ein weißliches, graugelbes oder pigmentiertes Aussehen bei sonst trockener, nicht nässender Oberhaut bekommt, um schließlich in Atrophie überzugehen".

Es ist vielfach auf Grund der Symptome der Sklerodermie versucht worden, diese Krankheit in eine Anzahl Unterabteilungen mit differenter Symptomatologie zu zerlegen (Sklerema neonatorum, Morphoea usw.). Die zuerst im Jahre 1871 von BALL beschriebene Sklerodaktylie wird allgemein als Form der Sklerodermie betrachtet. Diese Auffassung wird in letzter Zeit von SELLEI bestritten, der die Sklerodermie und die Sklerodaktylie (oder nach seiner Bezeichnung die Akrosklerose) als zwei voneinander verschiedene Krankheiten ansieht. Doch ist es zweifellos, daß sehr häufig beide Prozesse an einem und demselben Individuum beobachtet worden sind. LUITHLEN fand von 141 Fällen nur 35 isolierte Sklerodaktylie, 106 zeigen die Kombination mit Sklerodermie.

Man wird den bisher beschriebenen Differenzen demnach keine allzu große Bedeutung beilegen dürfen, und wir schließen uns denjenigen Autoren an, die einer einheitlichen Auffassung den Vorzug geben, wenn wir auch der Einteilung in weitere Unterabteilungen, wie sie auch EHRMANN und BRÜNAUER vorgenommen haben, durchaus nicht jeden Wert absprechen wollen. Im allgemeinen unterscheidet man je nach Ausdehnung und Begrenzung eine Reihe von Unterabteilungen, die untereinander fließende Übergänge zeigen: die Sklerodermia diffusa, die Sklerodermia circumscripta (en plaques und en bandes) und die Sklerodaktylie. Ihre Kombination, ihr Auftreten und in gewissen Fällen ihre Prognose wechselt in mannigfacher Weise. Es erscheint am meisten angemessen, mit der Analyse der Einzelsymptome zu beginnen.

Im Vordergrunde stehen die trophischen Störungen der Haut. Das erste Stadium der Hautveränderungen bildet das *Stadium oedematosum*. Es handelt sich hier um ein derbes Ödem; die Haut erhält eine fest-teigige Beschaffenheit, so daß der Fingerdruck nicht bestehen bleibt; dabei sieht sie über der ödematös infiltrierten Stelle glatt, glänzend und gedunsen aus. Dauer und Ausdehnung des Ödems wechseln sehr. OPPENHEIM berichtet in seinem Lehrbuch von einem Fall, in dem die Schwellung das vorherrschende Symptom war und eine fast universelle Verbreitung hatte. Dabei erhielt das Gesicht durch grobe Faltenbildung einen grotesken und derart gealterten Ausdruck, daß er das 17jährige Mädchen zunächst für die Mutter der sie begleitenden Mutter hielt. Über ähnliche Fälle eigener Beobachtung, die leicht zu diagnostischen Irrtümern führen, vermögen auch wir zu berichten. Daß das Ödem auch ganz fehlen kann, beweisen die Fälle, wo die Entwicklung immer neuer sklerotischer Flecke unter den Augen des Beobachters vor sich geht und trotzdem das Stadium ödematosum nicht beobachtet wurde. Es kann sich auf kleine Stellen beschränken, zudem rasch wechseln, abends stark entwickelt sein, um nachts oder morgens nicht mehr nachweisbar zu sein; es kann aber auch recht stabil werden. HEUSNER sah es $2^1/_2$ Jahre bestehen, ehe Zeichen von Induration bemerkbar wurden. H. CURSCHMANN betont, daß das Stadium des harten Ödems ganz inkonstant auftritt; er hat es nur vereinzelt gesehen und gibt an, daß es in der Vorgeschichte seiner Fälle nur selten zu eruieren war. Meist beginnt es an den Extremitäten symmetrisch, bleibt längere Zeit auf diese beschränkt und befällt dann Augenlider, Gesicht, Abdomen (EHRMANN-BRÜNAUER). Es gibt indessen auch noch andere Verbreitungsmöglichkeiten.

Eine größere Wichtigkeit beansprucht das *Stadium indurativum* und das diesem sich anschließende *Stadium atrophicum*. Im Stadium indurativum wird die Haut hart, fest gespannt, ist gar nicht oder nur schwer in Falten abhebbar, oft von einem spiegelnden Glanz, glasartig, durchsichtig, wie lackiert. Den Kranken macht sich diese Veränderung meist durch ein Spannungsgefühl bemerkbar. Die Konsistenz der Haut wird oft als knorpelhart, steinhart geschildert. Sie wird mit Leder, Holz, Alabaster, oft und treffend mit Pergament verglichen. Häufig hat man den Eindruck, als ob sie für die in ihr steckenden Teile zu kurz wäre, wie ein zu enger Handschuh. In Fällen ausgebreiteter, hochgradiger Sklerodermie hat die ganze Gestalt etwas mumienhaftes. Die kleinen Falten und Spaltlinien der Haut verschwinden, das Gesicht erhält durch die Unverschieblichkeit der Haut einen maskenartigen Ausdruck (sklerodermatische Maske). Der Anblick eines solchen Kranken mit den unbeweglichen, aber doch leidenden Gesichtszügen, der schmalen, spitzen, weit aus dem Gesicht hervortretenden Nase, dem zusammengezogenen Mund, den oft weit vorstehenden und nur mühsam zu schließenden Augen, dem leuchtenden Glanz der Haut, besonders an der Stirn, ist ungemein charakteristisch und bezeichnend. Im Stadium der *Atrophie* sinkt die Haut dann noch weiter zusammen, wird dünner als im normalen Zustand. Gewöhnlich hat man beide Stadien bei demselben Individuum vor sich. Diese Veränderungen der Haut können akut einsetzen, im Laufe weniger Tage und Wochen zu großer Intensität und Extensität anwachsen; sie können in jahrelangem, allmählichem Wachstum sich immer mehr ausbreiten. Die Ausbreitung kann von vornherein eine diffuse sein oder in

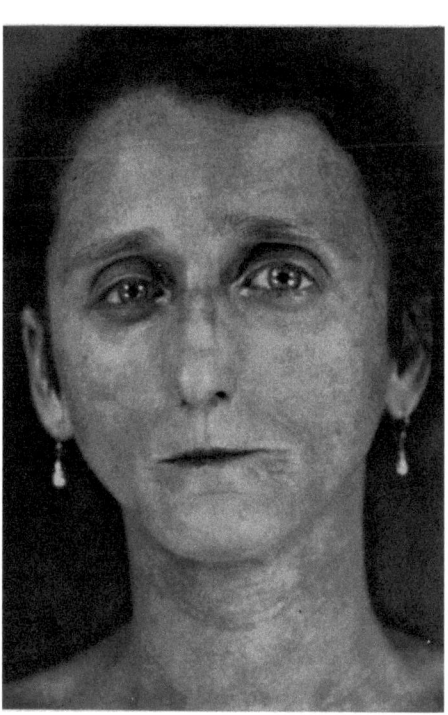

Abb. 8. Sklerodermie mit Pigmentverschiebungen. Maskengesicht.

großen Plaques vor sich gehen oder mit ganz kleinen Flecken beginnen. Bisweilen kommt es bei sehr starker Exudation zur Blasenbildung. In seltenen Fällen finden sich als klinisches Symptom der Sklerodermie *Tuberositäten*, die ganz verschiedener Art sein können. Zunächst sieht man gelegentlich, daß einzelne Herde von circumscripter Sklerodermie das Niveau der umgebenden Haut etwas überragen und dabei eine unebene, höckerige Oberfläche aufweisen können. Von den knotigen Vorwölbungen, die an ihrer Oberfläche anscheinend normale Haut zeigen, besteht ein Teil aus Ablagerungen von Kalksalzen (kohlensaurer und phosphorsaurer Kalk), welche im Röntgen- und mikroskopischen Bild leicht als solche erkennbar sind. Der andere stellt umschriebene Anschwellungen neben den typisch sklerosierten Hautpartien dar, die an verschiedenen Stellen des Stammes und der Extremitäten lokalisiert sein können. Diese Knoten sind mäßig hart anzufühlen, empfindungslos, mit der Haut verwachsen, über der Unterlage meist verschieblich, im einzelnen linsengroß oder größer. Die

Oberfläche ist glatt und nicht besonders verhärtet. Die Farbe ist verschieden, normal, bräunlich oder bläulich. Mikroskopisch zeigen sich in den tieferen Schichten der Haut charakteristische Veränderungen wie Verdichtung des kollagenen Gewebes, evtl. Gefäßveränderungen. Es handelt sich wahrscheinlich um Vorstadien eines späteren Übergreifens des sklerodermischen Prozesses vom subcutanen Gewebe auf die Haut (BRUHNS). Gelegentlich beobachtet man eine Ulceration dieser Knoten.

Mit den trophischen Veränderungen sind noch Störungen der *Schweißsekretion*, der *Vasomotilität* und der *Pigmentation* sehr häufig innig vergesellschaftet. Das Verhalten der Sekretion des Schweißes ist wechselnd. Die Schweißsekretion kann während des ganzen Verlaufes der Krankheit ungestört bleiben; einige Male wurde eine ganz allgemeine Hyperhydrosis beobachtet. Häufiger schwitzen die befallenen Hautpartien allein übermäßig stark (GRÖDEL-HUBERT u. a.). Am häufigsten aber war die Schweißsekretion an den befallenen Stellen herabgesetzt oder ganz unterdrückt, so weit, daß selbst Pilocarpin keine Schweißsekretion mehr hervorbrachte (HANDFORD, EULENBURG, HERXHEIMER, OSLER, VIDAL, ORLOF, ARADY, VUL, MANKOVSKIJ). DEVOTO fand erst Hyper-, später Anhydrosis; die Schweißdrüsen waren später atrophisch. SALKAN stellte in einem von ihm beobachteten Falle folgendes fest: Pilocarpin und Wärme riefen starkes Schwitzen bei der an diffuser Sklerodermie leidenden Kranken hervor, während die Aspirinprobe keine Schweißabsonderung bewirkte. Er schließt an diese Beobachtung die Erwägung, daß eine Störung des Zentralnervensystems im Tuber cinereum vorläge und begründet diese Theorie damit, daß das Pilocarpin auf die peripheren Schweißapparate wirke und das Aspirin die höheren Schweißzentren im Hypothalamus beeinflusse; MANKOVSKIJ dagegen konnte bei seinem Kranken, bei welchem zuerst eine doppelseitige Facialislähmung mit Beteiligung des Trigeminus, nach Wochen erst eine Sklerodermie des Gesichtes sich einstellte, ein Fehlen der Schweißsekretion im Gesicht feststellen; diese war auch nicht nach Pilocarpin zu erzielen. Ähnliche Erfahrungen hat schon KAPOSI gemacht. Im Einzelfall wird man darauf zu achten haben, inwieweit gerade der sklerodermische Prozeß an der Stelle, an der die Sklerosisanomalie festgestellt wurde, fortgeschritten ist. Wenig ist über die Änderung der Talgsekretion bekannt. Einige Male fiel die Trockenheit der Haut auf (NIELSEN, MORROW, DEVOTO u. a.), andere Autoren heben gerade das fettige Aussehen hervor.

Wichtiger als die Störungen der Sekretion sind die der *Vasomotilität*. Sie sind sehr früh vorhanden, oft sehr zahlreich und in die Augen springend; gelegentlich werden sie jedoch erst beobachtet, wenn der sklerodermische Prozeß voll ausgebildet ist (BROWN-O'LEARY-ADSON, SCOLARI). Hier treffen wir auf Symptome, die uns aus den früheren Schilderungen der RAYNAUDschen Krankheit und der Erythromelalgie schon geläufig sind. Oft gehen jahrelang Symptome von lokaler Synkope oder Asphyxie oder Hyperämie bestimmter Teile voraus. Besonders zeichnet sich die Sklerodaktylie dadurch aus, daß vasomotorische Symptome frühzeitig als Prodromalerscheinung auftreten und lange Zeit oder für immer dem Krankheitsbild treu bleiben (s. S. 327). Auch erythromelalgieähnliche Symptomenkomplexe kommen auf diese Weise zustande. Von sonstigen vasomotorischen Symptomen wurde von einigen Autoren Urticaria angegeben. Gelegentlich wurde eine auffällig starke Urticaria factitia gesehen. Übermäßige Hautvenenentwicklung wurde beobachtet, ebenso Teleangiektasien. Auf diese Erscheinung haben zuerst LEWIN und HELLER die Aufmerksamkeit gelenkt, später ist sie von zahlreichen Autoren beschrieben worden. Wir nennen unter anderem DUFOUR und DEBRAY, EHRMANN, PERNET, GOUGEROT-BURNIER, LORTAT-JACOB-BOUTELIER, DEVOTO, GOUGEROT-MEYER, SÉZARY. Sie sahen entweder erythematöse Fleckchen, oder angiomatöse Stellen. Im Falle GOUGEROT-BURNIER bestand eine Kombination mit Raynaudsymptomen und Telangiektasien, außerdem Lipomatose. GOUGEROT-MEYER sahen die Kombination von Sklerodaktylie, Raynaudsymptomen, Myxödem und multiplen Telangiektasien. KOGOJ glaubt, daß die Telangiektasien einerseits auf einen von außen wirkenden Druck des veränderten Bindegewebes, andererseits auf eine zirkulierende Noxe zu beziehen seien.

Im engen Zusammenhang mit den Veränderungen der Blutfüllung stehen auch die der *Temperatur* der befallenen Teile. Oft sind subjektiv Kälteempfindungen vorherrschend; es kommt bei Hyperämie natürlich auch das Gegenteil vor. In den späteren Stadien, in denen die Atrophie das Krankheitsbild beherrscht, ist meist Temperaturherabsetzung festzustellen; sie ist vielfach auch zahlenmäßig nachgewiesen worden (STEWART, BROWN-O'LEARY-ADSON, KOSMADIS). KOSMADIS hat 18 Messungen an drei Patienten vorgenommen und hat eine Herabsetzung der Temperatur bis zu $1,5^0$ an den von Sklerodermie betroffenen Hautpartien feststellen können. BROWN-O'LEARY-ADSON fanden beim normalen Menschen die durchschnittliche Oberflächentemperatur der Finger in einem Raume von $24—26^0$ gemessen zwischen 32 und 35^0 bei ihren Sklerodaktyliekranken zwischen 19,6 und $29,8^0$, im Durchschnitt $25,3^0$. Die Temperaturschwankungen der Akren sind offenbar durch den Hypertonus der Arteriolen bedingt.

Untersuchungen über die Wärmeabgabe hatten das Ergebnis, daß der Wärmeverlust durchschnittlich normalerweise 100 kleine Calorien, bei Sklerodermie 34 kleine Calorien beträgt.

Capillaroskopische Untersuchungen wurden in den letzten Jahren recht häufig angestellt. WEISS und FEDOROFF (zitiert nach KROLL) fanden abnorm stark gewundene Schlingen mit sehr engem arteriellen neben sehr weitem venösen Schenkel. Dazwischen liegen wieder zarte und weniger stark verunstaltete Schlingen. DEVOTO findet nur wenige Gefäße und in den Enden der Gefäßschlingen keinen sichtbaren Blutstrom (ähnlich TOLOSA). FENYES sieht schwerste Veränderungen, und zwar hypoplastische und archaisch-intermediäre Formen. BROWN-O'LEARY untersuchten die Hautcapillaren in 5 Fällen von Sklerodermie und in 5, in einer späteren Publikation in 16 Fällen von Raynaud mit Sklerodermie und fanden folgendes: bei diffuser Sklerodermie beträchtliche Verminderung der Capillarschlingen auf etwa ein Drittel, die um so erheblicher war, je größer sich die trophische Störung manifestierte. In der zweiten Gruppe fand er Dilatation, Krümmung, Stase und Permeabilitätsstörungen. MÉSZAROS beobachtete bei 8 Kranken starke Abnahme der Capillarzahl am Nagelfalz mit Auftreten von Capillaren, deren Schenkel auffallend weit voneinander standen und gleiche Weite hatten. Am Handrücken fiel ein starkes Hervortreten der plumpen Papillen auf, deren Spitze erweitert war. An der Brusthaut fehlten die Hautrinnen, der subpapilläre Plexus war gewaltig erweitert. PAUTRIER-ULLMO fanden eine Vergrößerung der interpapillaren Leisten und Verringerung der Capillarschlingen; an ihrer Stelle sind braune Flecke sichtbar, dagegen weder die Mündung eines Haares, noch einer Schweißdrüse zu sehen. Im allgemeinen sind es eben die gleichen Bilder, die sich auch sonst bei Vasoneurosen finden, ohne daß darum Haut- oder andere Weichteilverdickungen aufzutreten brauchen (O. MÜLLER).

Sehr häufig sind ferner Veränderungen der *Pigmentierung* der äußeren Decke, die nach L. R. MÜLLER in etwa 50% der Fälle auftreten. Es finden sich Verfärbungen, die einen braunen, einen gelben, einen grauen Farbton aufweisen. Die Stärke der Pigmentation steht zur Stärke der sonstigen Krankheitserscheinungen in keinem Verhältnis. Die Pigmentierung ist teils streifenförmig, teils fleckig, teils diffus. Sie findet sich auch an nicht sklerodermischen Stellen und kann dort auch als Vorläufer einer später sich entwickelnden Sklerodermie auftreten. Wir sahen eine Patientin, bei der im Verlauf einer über viele Jahre hinaus sich erstreckenden Beobachtung wiederholt das Auftreten einer unregelmäßig fleckweisen, ausgesprochen schmutzig-braunen Pigmentierung an vielen Stellen zur Beobachtung kam, ohne daß später immer gerade diese Partien sklerodermisch wurden. Die Pigmentierung kann sehr hochgradig sein, den größten Teil der Körperoberfläche einnehmen, wenn auch seltener und nicht sehr ausgedehnt, die Schleimhäute befallen. Fälle von hochgradiger allgemeiner Pigmentierung, in denen das Krankheitsbild dann der ADDISONschen Krankheit ähnlich ist, sind mehrfach beschrieben worden; wir kommen auf sie im Abschnitt ,,Diagnose" noch zurück. Im Gegensatz zur Pigmenthypertrophie kommt auch eine Pigmentatrophie vor (KREN). Bemerkenswert ist die Kombination mit vitiligoähnlichen Erscheinungen, über die in neuerer Zeit eine ganze Reihe von Autoren berichten (ROEDERER, JORDAN, JEANSELME - BURNIER, GOUGEROT, PERRIN-FILIOL, VOHWINKEL, HUFSCHMIDT). Im Falle GOUGEROT-PERRIN-FILIOL und von PAUTRIER-LEPINAY fanden sich auf dem Vitiligogebiet breite sklerodermatische Plaques und dunkelbraun pigmentierte Fleckchen teils auf den Plaques, teils am Rande derselben. BROWN sowie ROXBURGH, welche die Beziehungen der Vitiligo und der Alopecia areata zur Sklerodermie erörtern, äußern sich über diese Kombination sehr vorsichtig. EHRMANN-BRÜNAUER sprechen nur von einer Ähnlichkeit dieser Depigmentationsbezirke mit Vitiligo, glauben aber mit anderen Autoren, daß sie sich durch ihre Konsistenz von einer solchen unterscheiden lassen.

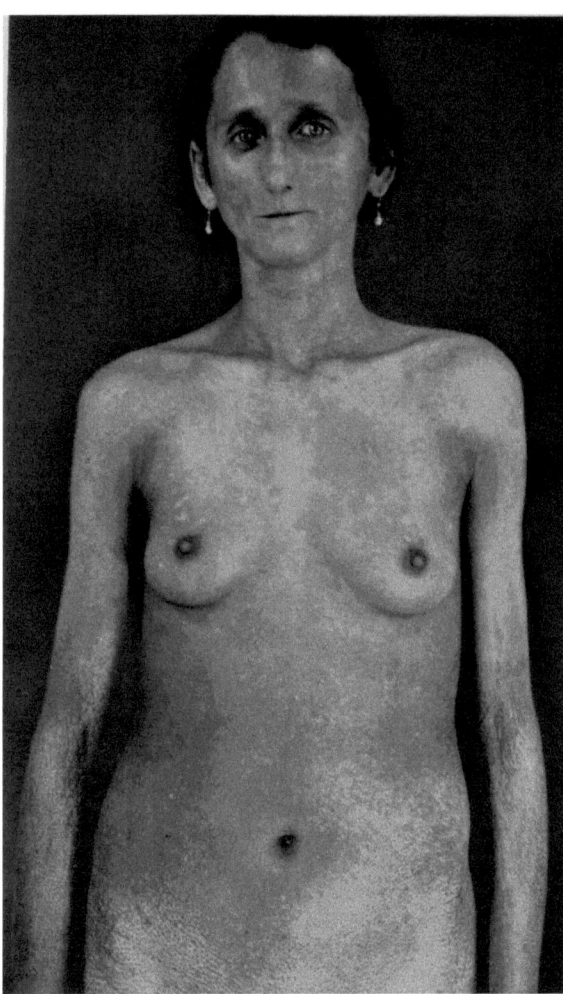

Abb. 9. Diffuse Sklerodermie mit Pigmentverschiebungen.

Die Reihe der trophischen Störungen ist mit den geschilderten sklerodermieartigen Veränderungen der Haut nicht abgeschlossen. Neben diesen kommt es häufig zu *Geschwürsbildungen*. Schon LEWIN und HELLER machten auf ihre

Häufigkeit aufmerksam und betonten, daß ihre Prädilektionsstelle die Knochenvorsprünge sind, in denen auch die Haut normal am leichtesten verletzbar ist. In den Fällen, wo sie erst spät auftreten, darf nicht daran gezweifelt werden, daß ihre Ursache in traumatisch-infektiösen Schädigungen zu suchen ist. Es kommen aber auch Panaritien und Ulcera an der Haut nicht veränderter Teile vor bzw. in der vasomotorischen Periode. Die Geschwürsbildung ist fast stets, was wichtig ist, mit Schmerzen verbunden; die Geschwüre sitzen oft symmetrisch und entwickeln sich gelegentlich zu schweren gangränösen und verstümmelnden Prozessen. Bisweilen zeichnen sie sich durch sehr geringe Heilungstendenz aus, während die Heilung ein anderes Mal rasch und anstandslos wie im gesunden Gewebe fortschreitet. KREN erwähnt, daß in einigen seltenen Fällen auch Geschwüre der Schleimhaut zur Beobachtung kamen.

Ernährungsstörungen der Anhangsgebilde der Haut kommen sehr häufig vor. LEWIN-HELLER fanden Störungen des *Haarwachstums*. Das Haar wird an den sklerodermischen Partien trocken, brüchig, dünner. Mehrere Male war ein totaler Haarverlust am ganzen Körper gleichzeitig mit der Sklerodermie aufgetreten (GRÜNFELD, HERRINGHAM, RILLE, NEUMANN). In anderen Fällen war der Behaarungstypus auffällig, eine Erscheinung, die von einigen Autoren als endokrine Komponente verwertet wurde (ARADY, JEANSELME und BURNIER u. a.). Es fand sich auch einmal halbseitige Alopecie (STERNTHAL), sowie die Kombination mit Alopecia areata (EDDOWES, GIBNEY, FORDYCE u. a.). Einige Male wurde partieller oder totaler Pigmentverlust der Haare beobachtet. Häufiger sind die Veränderungen der *Nägel*. Die Nägel werden längs oder quergestreift, brüchig, dabei auch dicker als normal, deformiert, bucklig oder hakenförmig gekrümmt. Ihr Oberhäutchen verdickt sich und verwächst so fest, daß es nicht zurückgeschoben werden kann. Am häufigsten sind atrophische Zustände, die Nägel schrumpfen zu kleinen Hornblättchen, sind nur linsengroß oder können auch vollständig verschwinden. Hochgradige Atrophie des Zahnfleisches und damit verbunden spontaner Ausfall der Zähne ist mehrfach beobachtet worden (HERRINGHAM, CROCHER, BOUTTIER).

Die subjektiven Störungen der *Sensibilität* treten bei der Sklerodermie sehr zurück. Es gibt viele Fälle, die ohne alle Schmerzen verlaufen und auch ohne alle Parästhesien. In anderen Fällen findet man häufig recht frühzeitig derartige Parästhesien, Brennen, Jucken, taubes Gefühl, Gefühl von Eingeschlafensein. Einige Male traten sie durchaus in der Form der Akroparästhesien auf. Die Schmerzen sind meist reißend, stechend, sitzen häufig in den von der Sklerodermie befallenen Gebieten und sind fast stets diffus, nicht auf ein Nervengebiet beschränkt. Nicht selten besteht eine gewisse Überempfindlichkeit gegenüber bestimmten Reizen, namentlich gegen Kälte. Demgegenüber sind sowohl objektive Hyperästhesien (neuerdings ORLOF), als auch Anästhesien ein recht seltener Befund. Die Empfindung kann selbst bei hochgradigster Veränderung der Haut noch immer völlig intakt sein, so daß z. B. DINKLERS Kranke mit ihren völlig sklerodermischen Fingern noch ohne jede Schwierigkeit Geld zählen konnte. Sonst findet sich wohl eine leichte Unterempfindlichkeit. Fälle mit stärkerer objektiver Sensibilitätsstörung sind im ganzen selten beschrieben worden. Wir haben einen solchen Fall gesehen, in dem es sich um eine diffuse Sklerodermie an Händen und Füßen handelte, bei dem gelegentlich Anfälle von Syncope locale, im weiteren Verlauf auch Ulcerationen und gangräneszierende Prozesse auftauchten, die mit intensiven Schmerzen einhergingen. Dazu gesellte sich eine schwere Sensibilitätsstörung in Form einer für alle Qualitäten ausgesprochenen Herabsetzung der Empfindung, die Hände und Füße gleichmäßig betraf und in der Mitte der Unterarme bzw. ungefähr am Knie, zirkulär abschloß. Wir erinnern daran, daß wir auch bei der Akroasphyxia chronica eine solche eigentümliche Sensibilitätsstörung, deren Erklärung sehr schwierig ist, beobachtet haben.

Die *Motilitätsstörungen* sind zum Teil rein sekundär durch die hochgradige Spannung und Verhärtung der Haut und eine daraus resultierende Behinderung der Bewegung in den Gelenken. Es können dadurch die größten Schwierigkeiten der Fortbewegung hervorgerufen werden, aber auch große Gefahren damit verknüpft sein, wenn z. B. der ganze Thorax in einen starren Panzer(GILMOOR) verwandelt ist. Als ein weiteres, die Beweglichkeit behinderndes Moment kommt in vielen Fällen die *sklerotische Veränderung der Muskeln* in Betracht. THIBIÈRGE hat zuerst eingehender die Ursache der Beteiligung der Muskulatur bei der Sklerodermie studiert. Es ist kein Zweifel, daß der sklerotische Prozeß von der Haut auf die Muskeln übergreifen kann; es ist aber ganz gewiß, daß die Muskeln auch primär unter unveränderter Haut erkranken können. Solche Beobachtungen sind von SCHULTZ, WESTPHAL, GOLDSCHMIDT, STERNTHAL, GUTH und ROSENFELD, PELIZÄEUS und von CASSIRER vielfach angestellt worden. Wir haben Fälle beobachtet, in denen z. B. die Veränderungen in den Muskeln des Unterarmes und der Hand gegenüber den Hautveränderungen sich ganz in den Vordergrund schoben. Wir haben solche Myosklerosen bei allen Formen der Sklerodermie gesehen. In dem Falle von GILMOOR wurde die erkrankte Brustmuskulatur die Todesursache. KREN macht darauf aufmerksam, daß auch Veränderungen der Zungenmuskeln vorkommen, die dann Kau-, Schluck- und Schlingbeschwerden hervorrufen; auch das können wir bestätigen. Einige Male ist die Zungenmuskulatur auch nur einseitig ergriffen worden (WESTPHAL, EBSTEIN, NATOUSEK u. a.). Beteiligung der Kaumuskulatur wurde von uns beobachtet, und auch der Muskulatur des oberen Augenlides, so daß eine Art Ptosis resultierte. Über Sklerodermie der Augenlider berichten auch MÜHSAM und ADAM. Störungen der Augenmuskeln stellten noch fest LOSETSCHNIKOW (Unbeweglichkeit des Bulbus), MORAWIECKA (Insuffizienz des Musculus rectus internus). Das Befallensein der Kehlkopfmuskeln notieren ARADY und KREN (mangelhafter Verschluß der Stimmbänder bei der Phonation). EHRMANN-BRÜNAUER machen darauf aufmerksam, daß nicht nur die Halsmuskeln oft auffallend verdünnt erscheinen und sich bei ihrer Kontraktion weniger vorwölben als beim Normalen, sondern daß auch die den Kehlkopf und die Luftröhre umgebende Muskulatur oft verdünnt, dabei aber starr und hart erscheint. HEIMANN-HATRY führen das Bestehen einer hochgradigen Schwerhörigkeit auf das Übergreifen des sklerodermischen Prozesses auf beide Trommelfelle zurück. Meist wurden bei Sklerodermie nur Störungen der quantitativen elektrischen Erregbarkeit der Muskulatur festgestellt; FENYES sowie TEDESCHI haben indes in ihren Fällen träge galvanische Zuckung bei guter faradischer Erregbarkeit gefunden. Über die Beziehungen der Myosklerose zur Dermatomyositis wird im Abschnitte „Diagnose" die Rede sein. NEUMARK hat die Muskelveränderungen, die bei Sklerodermie vorkommen, zusammengestellt. Er unterscheidet zwischen Myosklerose, Myatrophie und Myositis; auch Mischformen kommen vor. Er selbst beobachtete in einem Falle Myokymie in dem betroffenen Gebiete.

Über die Mitbeteiligung der Fascien, Sehnen und Sehnenscheiden äußern sich EHRMANN-BRÜNAUER dahin, daß man sie schon in einem relativ frühen Stadium beobachten kann, daß von der Tiefe aus sich eine mehr oder weniger starre Verbindung zwischen Haut und Sehnen sowie Fascien entwickelt. Die Autoren konnten an Präparaten feststellen, daß die Verbindung von innen nach außen hergestellt wird, also von den Sehnenscheiden gegen die Haut zu. Das gleiche gilt von der Verbindung zwischen Gelenkbändern und Haut. Die Kombination mit der DUPUYTRENschen Kontraktur sahen TOMMASI und LECHELLE,

BARUK und DOUADY; der Fall, den die letztgenannten Autoren beschreiben, zeigt eine DUPUYTRENsche Kontraktur beiderseits sowie Sklerodaktylie an Händen und Füßen. Die DUPUYTRENsche Kontraktur besteht auch bei dem Vater und Bruder.

Die Sklerodermie erstreckt sich aber nicht nur auf die Haut und die Muskeln, sondern auch auf andere Gewebe und Organe, man kann wohl sagen auf alle anderen Organe des Körpers. Die Erkenntnis von der Generalisierung des sklerotischen Prozesses ist im ganzen neueren Datums, wenn auch hierhergehörige Einzelbeobachtungen schon bei älteren Autoren sich finden. Am frühesten wendete sich die Aufmerksamkeit den *Knochenaffektionen* zu, die namentlich bei der Sklerodaktylie häufig sind. Es sind das meist atrophische Prozesse mit einer Verkürzung und Verdünnung der Knochen (Verschmälerung der Zwischenwirbelscheiben, Osteophytenbildung usw. GUARINI). Es kann ohne Geschwürsbildung zu einer ganz allmählichen und totalen Resorption einer Phalange kommen, oder wenn der Prozeß nicht so weit geht, werden die einzelnen Phalangen verkürzt und verschmälert. Darüber geben die Röntgenbilder gute Auskunft. Es resultiert auf diese Weise eine Art von Akromikrie, die mehrfach beschrieben wurde. In seltenen Fällen ist das Knochengerüst einer Seite im Wachstum zurückgeblieben, bei GRASSET sogar das ganze Knochensystem des Körpers zugleich mit allen übrigen Körpergeweben. Sehr merkwürdige Veränderungen an den verschiedensten Stellen des Knochengerüstes haben wir bei einer Patientin beobachtet, die viele Jahre lang in unserer Behandlung stand. Es ist eine typische Sklerodermie mit fleckweiser Verteilung der Veränderungen, mit starken Pigmentverschiebungen, bei der die Mutter im 14. Jahre ein Zurückbleiben des Wachstums der ganzen linken Schulter bemerkte; später sank eine Stelle der rechten Schläfen-Scheitelgegend ein, so daß hier eine Art Mulde entstand. Atrophische Veränderungen an den Knochen fanden sich im weiteren Verlauf der Beobachtung dann noch an den Händen und besonders an beiden Füßen, so daß man in diesem Falle wohl von einer Osteosclerosis disseminata (Ostéosclérose en plaques) sprechen kann. Es handelt sich überall in diesen Fällen um eine besonders die Spongiosa betreffende Rarefikation, wodurch die Struktur der Knochen eine abnorme Weitmaschigkeit erhält, die sich auf den Röntgenbildern durch eine übermäßig scharfe Zeichnung der Knochenbälkchen ausprägt. Neben atrophischen finden sich auch hypertrophische Veränderungen an den Knochen, Verdickungen, callöse Auftreibungen, Rauhigkeit. FLETCHER fand destruktive Veränderungen der Phalangealknochen am Rande der Gelenke. In einem Falle von ULLMANN scheint es zu einer Knochenneubildung in der Cutis gekommen zu sein. Über Ablagerungen von Kalkkonkrementen in den Geweben, die im Röntgenbilde sichtbar werden, berichten MEYER und HÜRLIMANN, ZADEK, DELHERM und MOREL, KAHN und COUPUT, AKOBDSZANJANZ u. a. EDEIKEN beschreibt eine Knochenabsorption an den Enden einiger distaler Phalangen bei vermehrtem Calciumgehalt in den proximalen Teilen der Phalangen und kalkhaltige Absonderungen in den Fingerspitzen. Das gleichzeitige Vorhandensein von Kalkdepots in den Weichteilen der Finger mit einer Knochenabsorption der Phalangealenden bezeichnet er als für Sklerodaktylie typisch. Recht instruktiv ist der von MILIAN, PÉRIN und HOROWITZ beobachtete Fall von Sklerodermie, Sklerodaktylie und Raynaudsyndrom durch die Lokalisation der knochenharten, nicht faltbaren sklerotischen Stellen an der Außenseite des Bauches, an den Hüften, bis ins obere Drittel des Oberschenkels hinabreichend; bei der Palpation waren kleine Knötchen bis zu Erbsengröße fühlbar. Die Verfasser machen darauf aufmerksam, daß diese an einer schweren Störung des Calciumstoffwechsels leidende Kranke die Kalkveränderungen am stärksten in den Regionen zeigt, die der Einwirkung ständiger Reibung ausgesetzt sind.

Die Röntgenaufnahme deckte hier interessante Veränderungen der Weichteile und des Skeletes auf: An den Weichteilen sieht man zahlreiche Calcifikationen (Gesäß, Oberschenkel, rechter Quadriceps); am Skelet findet man knöcherne Erosionen und Destruktionen (an den Fingern), Decalcifikationen (Hände, linker Fuß) und Hyperostosen (Calcaneus, Os cuneiforme).

Beteiligung der *Gelenke* an dem sklerosierenden Prozeß ist ebenfalls nichts seltenes. Es ist wahrscheinlich, daß die prodromalen Schmerzen, über die in einem Teil der Fälle geklagt wird, häufig der Ausdruck einer Gelenkaffektion sind. Durch die Mitbeteiligung der Gelenke kann die Ähnlichkeit zwischen den chronischen und subakuten Gelenkerkrankungen und der Sklerodermie in einzelnen Fällen recht erheblich werden, so daß eine sichere Diagnose nicht immer möglich erscheint (CASSIRER). ADRIAN und RÖDERER haben sich mit diesen Fragen eingehender beschäftigt. Sie unterscheiden auf Grund der Ergebnisse einer Literaturzusammenstellung 3 Gruppen: 1. Am häufigsten Fälle von einfachen und selbständigen Gelenkaffektionen, die mehr oder weniger lange der Sklerodermie voraufgehen. 2. Seltenere Fälle mit gleichzeitig auftretenden Gelenk- und Hautaffektionen. 3. Fälle, bei denen die Gelenkaffektion im Verlauf der Sklerodermie hinzukommt. Nach ihnen ist die Gelenkerkrankung ein relativ seltenes Ereignis. Alle Gelenke können betroffen werden. Den Erscheinungen können jahrelang Muskel-, Knochen- und Gelenkschmerzen voraufgehen. Die Erkrankungen der Gelenke nehmen meistens einen chronisch progredienten Verlauf ohne Remissionen. Komplikationen sind Muskelatrophien, Sehnenverkürzungen, seltener Schleimbeutelerkrankungen. Manchmal treten gleichzeitig Herzerkrankungen auf. Autoptische Befunde, sowie Röntgenaufnahmen zeigen Veränderungen der Knorpel und Knochen, Rarefikationen der Knochenlamellen bis zur Atrophie wie bei anderen destruktiven Gelenkprozessen, aber keine für die gleichzeitige Hauterkrankung charakteristischen Erscheinungen; der typische Befund der Arthritis deformans fehlt. In vorgeschrittenen Fällen stehen ankylosierende Prozesse im Vordergrund. Wahrscheinlich geht der Gelenkprozeß von der Synovia aus. DELHERM, MOREL, KAHN und COUPUT finden die Veränderungen hauptsächlich in den kleinen Gelenken lokalisiert, desgleichen REINER. Eine Reihe von Autoren diskutieren die Frage der pathogenetischen Beziehungen zwischen der Arthritis deformans und dem sklerodermischen Prozeß; eine Einigkeit in den Auffassungen besteht bisher nicht. Die Kombination mit STILLscher Krankheit beschreiben STEINITZ und CASPER-FÜRSTENHEIM.

Es wurden ferner einige Fälle von Sklerodermie beobachtet, bei denen eine Kyphoskoliose vorhanden war (SCHUBIGER, STEMBO, RAYMOND, MACHTOU u. a.). H. CURSCHMANN berichtet über eine Kombination mit Wirbelsteifigkeit.

Daß die Pigmentanomalien die *Schleimhäute* mitbetreffen, wurde bereits erwähnt; aber auch eine anderweitige Beteiligung der Schleimhäute ist kein ungewöhnliches Vorkommnis und verläuft hinsichtlich der Aufeinanderfolge der einzelnen Stadien ebenso wie wir es bei der Haut kennen gelernt haben. Nachdem früher nur einzelne Beobachtungen veröffentlicht waren, hat KREN diesem Vorkommnis seine besondere Aufmerksamkeit geschenkt. Er hat festgestellt, daß das Vorkommen der Schleimhauterkrankung viel häufiger ist, als man früher annahm. In den späteren Stadien der diffusen Sklerodermie sind die *Mundgebilde* sehr häufig ergriffen. Selten sind die ersten sklerodermischen Veränderungen an der Zunge zu treffen. Die Veränderungen sind diffus oder fleckförmig scharf umschrieben oder selten einseitig und zeigen oft Gefäßektasien (KREN, FUSS u. a.). Außer der Zunge sind noch andere Gebilde der Mundhöhle befallen; es kommt häufig zu einer Verkürzung des Frenulum, Schrumpfung der Uvula oder zu einer hochgradigen Veränderung des Mundbogens. Die Gaumenbogen werden ergriffen. Das Zahnfleisch und die Lippenschleimhaut werden befallen und verursachen gelegentlich Zahnausfall (STUDNICKA). HOPPE-SEYLER beobachtete eine Verengerung des Kehlkopfeinganges durch Verkürzung der aryepiglottischen Falten. Vielfach war die Schleimhaut des Kehlkopfes hochgradig blaß, die Stimmritze schloß sich nicht in normaler Weise. Artikulationsstörungen und Veränderungen der Stimmlage werden wiederholt beschrieben (ARADY). KREN fand Veränderungen der Kehlkopfschleimhaut, die sich durch Störung der Funktion nicht kenntlich gemacht hatten. Auch Veränderungen an der Schleimhaut des Oesophagus (EHRMANN-BRÜNAUER) mit Dysphagie (A. SCHMIDT, RAKE, FESSLER und POHL), der Bindehaut (KREN), der Vagina (HEKTOEN, HELLER, KRÖMER) sind beobachtet worden.

Besondere Aufmerksamkeit hat man dem Leitungswiderstand der Haut gegen elektrischen Strom gewidmet; die von EULENBURG, HERZOG, STERNTHAL, FRIEDHEIM, GRÜNFELD, KALISCHER, THIBIERGE angestellten Untersuchungen haben aber nicht zu einem einheitlichen Resultat geführt, so daß den Einzelbefunden keine Bedeutung zukommt.

Inwieweit auch die *inneren Organe* dem Einfluß der Krankheit unterliegen, darüber sind wir noch nicht genau unterrichtet. Immerhin besteht aber nach einigen pathologischen Befunden kein Zweifel, daß auch in den inneren Organen ein sklerosierender und atrophisierender, der Hautaffektion ähnlicher Prozeß zur Ausbildung kommen kann. Klinisch wird es nicht immer leicht und bisweilen auch ganz unmöglich sein, diese Symptome von denen zu unterscheiden, die sekundär durch die Krankheit bedingt sind. Das gilt insbesondere auch von der Kachexie, die in späteren Stadien recht häufig ist. Die Sklerodermie dokumentiert sich damit als eine *Allgemeinkrankheit*, deren am stärksten zutage tretenden Symptome die sklerodermatischen Veränderungen sind. Sie ist im größten Teil ihres Verlaufes sicher eine fieberlose Affektion. Einige Beobachtungen aber scheinen darauf hinzudeuten, daß namentlich da, wo die Krankheit akut oder subakut einsetzt, anfangs leichte Fiebersteigerungen eintreten können. Soweit Blutuntersuchungen vorliegen, haben sie bisher noch kein charakteristisches Verhalten des Blutes ergeben. Einige Blutbefunde seien hier angeführt: PEYRI und CARDENAL fanden rote Blutkörperchen 4 800 000, weiße 12 500, Lymphocyten 20%, Monocyten 28%, polynucleäre 51%, Metamyelocyten 1%. KREBS und HARTMANN, THIÉBAUT fanden 4 040 000 rote, 7 600 weiße, 54% Neutrophile, 3% Eosinophile, 39% Mononucleäre, 4% Übergangsformen. PARHON-CARAMAN, sowie HILLMANN fanden Lymphocytose. ORLOF und KANNO fanden Eosinophilie, die der letzte Autor bei circumscripter Sklerodermie vermißte. ČERKES fand das Blutbild normal. LORTAT und JAKOB messen dem Befund der Lymphocytose im Liquor eine gewisse Bedeutung zu und empfehlen bei einem solchen Befunde eine spezifische Kur zu versuchen. Über die Befunde, die bei Stoffwechseluntersuchungen erhoben worden sind, wird im Zusammenhang bei der Besprechung der Pathogenese berichtet werden. Das gleiche gilt von den pharmako-dynamischen Prüfungen.

Störungen im Bereiche des Digestionsapparates sind häufig, meist leichterer Natur, wiederholt im Sinne einer Achylie (BUSCHKE, EHRMANN und BRÜNAUER) beobachtet worden. RAKE fand Erweiterung des Oesophagus und des Colon; auch Störungen des Respirationsapparates sind nicht selten; sie beruhen zum Teil, wie schon erwähnt, auf mechanischer Behinderung der Atmung. Die Kombination mit tuberkulösen Prozessen der Lunge, der Bronchialdrüsen und der Pleura sind häufig erwähnt. Auch am Herzen sind eine Reihe von Veränderungen nachgewiesen worden, die jedoch weder konstant, noch besonders charakteristisch sind. Von ihnen wird noch im Abschnitt „pathologische Anatomie" die Rede sein.

Albuminurie wurde mehrfach beobachtet (FINLAY, STERNBERG u. a.); Glykosurie von DICKINSON und KELLER, ebenso von UHLENHUTH, der das Vorliegen einer nervösen Glykosurie diskutiert. EHRMANN stellte in 4 von 5 untersuchten Fällen alimentäre Glykosurie fest. AYRES hat im ganzen 6 Fälle von Sklerodermie gesammelt, in welchen im Urin Arsen nachgewiesen werden konnte. In einem Teil der Fälle konnte nicht festgestellt werden, daß der Kranke jemals mit Arsen in Berührung gekommen war. Ein derartiger Befund ist später nicht wieder erhoben worden.

Über Mitbeteiligung der einzelnen Organe berichten die Autoren noch manche Einzelheiten, worüber wir hier als prinzipiell nicht wichtige Befunde hinweggehen können. Nur eines Organes müssen wir noch gedenken, der *Schilddrüse*, wegen der Beziehungen, in die man die Sklerodermie zur Affektion dieser Drüse gebracht hat. Es wurde wiederholt bei der Sklerodermie Struma beobachtet. Hierbei sehen wir noch von den Fällen ab, wo die Struma zum Morbus Basedowii gehörte. Es wurde auch eine Atrophie der Schilddrüse gesehen, so von SCHÄFFER, RAYMOND, STERNTHAL, UHLENHUTH, GRASSET, JAMES u. a. Auf die Beziehungen der Schilddrüse sowie der anderen endokrinen Drüsen zur Sklerodermie gehen wir erst ein, wenn wir das Kapitel ,,Pathogenese" abhandeln.

An dieser Stelle soll jedoch noch eine kleine Anzahl von Publikationen Erwähnung finden, in denen das Vorliegen von Katarakt meist mit endokrinen Störungen verknüpft ist. ARADY fand doppelseitige Linsentrübungen bei einem 41jährigen Mann und erwähnt, daß die Starbildung bei Sklerodermie stets doppelseitig sei. MONIER, VINARD und BARBOT berichten von zwei Schwestern im Alter von 43 und 46 Jahren mit symmetrischer segmental angeordneter Sklerodermie an den unteren Extremitäten und Kataraktbildung. KREBS, HARTMANN und THIÉBAUT sahen in einer Familie Katarakt mit und ohne Sklerodermie, Basedowsche Krankheit, Infantilismus mit Spätpubertät, Arthritis deformans, Canities präcox und Erythrämie auftreten. Auch SÉZARY-FAVORY, MAMOU sahen eine Katarakt und endokrine Störungen bei Sklerodermie. Weitere Beobachtungen stammen von GUILLAIN, ALAJOUANINE und MARQUÉZY, SAINTON und MAMMOU, WERNER, VOSSIUS, ROTHMUND, EGUCHI.

Eine Sklerodermie des ganzen Körpers ist ziemlich selten, bisweilen wird aber nicht nur die ganze Oberfläche der Haut von dem Prozeß eingenommen, sondern auch Knochen, Gelenke, Muskeln werden davon ergriffen. Das Resultat ist der ,,*homme momie*", ein zwerghaftes, vertrocknetes Wesen, wie es GRASSET in Wort und Bild anschaulich geschildert hat. Ähnliche Fälle teilen auch BOMBARDA und MARINESCO mit. Von besonderen Lokalisationen der diffusen Sklerodermie ist die wichtig, in welcher nur eine Körperhälfte von dem Prozeß betroffen ist. Auch solche Beobachtungen sind nicht häufig; BERGSON, ANITSCHKOFF, PELIZAEUS, STEVEN, KOLB, DANILEWSKAJA und MARKOW, JOSEFOWICZ teilen solche Fälle mit. Ziemlich oft findet sich ein symmetrisches Auftreten der sklerodermatischen Prozesse, am häufigsten bei der Sklerodaktylie, bei der eine mehr oder minder ausgesprochene Symmetrie die Regel ist. Aber auch bei der Sklerodermie en plaques kommt sie vor.

Die *Sklerodaktylie* stellt eine ziemlich häufige Erscheinungsform der Sklerodermie dar. Sie ist außer durch die Lokalisation charakterisiert durch das häufige Ergriffenwerden der tiefer liegenden Gewebsteile, der Sehnen, Fascien, Muskeln, Gelenke und Knochen, durch die sehr häufig begleitenden erheblichen vasomotorischen sensiblen und trophischen Störungen mit einem vom gewöhnlichen Bilde abweichenden Typus, so daß SELLEI sie überhaupt von der Sklerodermie abzutrennen geneigt ist, wogegen MICHAELIS Stellung nimmt. Namentlich die schweren vasomotorischen Störungen erwecken hier unser Interesse.

Man findet sowohl lokale Cyanose, wie lokale Anämie oder Hyperämie. Diese Störungen treten anfallsweise auf, in stetem Wechsel und steter Aufeinanderfolge, ohne daß mit Sicherheit zu sagen wäre, daß ein Symptom zeitlich oder in bezug auf Intensität oder Extensität dominiert. Am stärksten ist meist freilich die Cyanose vertreten. Durch das Vorwiegen der vasomotorischen und zum Teil auch der sensiblen Störungen gewinnen diese Krankheitsbilder eine sehr große Ähnlichkeit mit der RAYNAUDschen Krankheit.

Die Beziehungen beider Krankheiten zueinander sind schon seit langem der Gegenstand eifriger Forschungen gewesen. Wir haben bereits im Kapitel

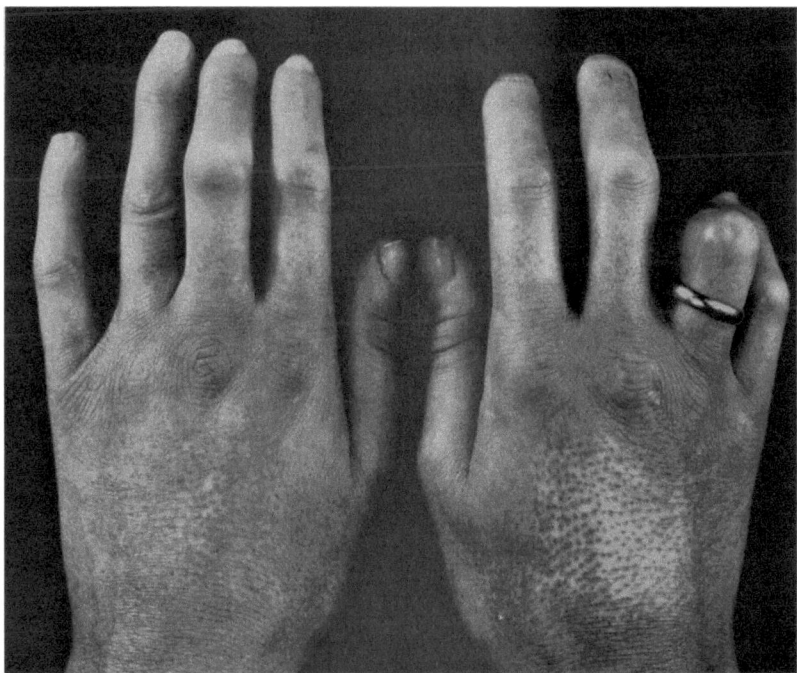

Abb. 10. Sklerodaktylie.

„RAYNAUDsche Krankheit" und bei Besprechung der Störungen der Vasomotilität in diesem Kapitel gesehen, daß im Verlauf dieser Affektion gelegentlich, zumal an den distalen Körperteilen, neben den typischen trophischen Störungen der Gangrän sich mehr chronisch dystrophische Prozesse abspielen, die im weiteren Verlauf zu einer Verhärtung und Verdickung der Haut und der tieferen Teile führen. In einer weiteren Reihe von Krankheitsfällen eröffnen die vasomotorischen Symptome der Asphyxie locale und der Syncope locale die Szene, herrschen lange allein vor, ganz in der typischen Weise wie bei der RAYNAUDschen Krankheit paroxysmal auftretend und miteinander abwechselnd. An die Stelle der die RAYNAUDsche Krankheit auszeichnenden nekrotischen Störungen treten nun chronische Veränderungen, oft unter Abschwächung der vasomotorischen Symptome, namentlich unter Verwischung der Anfälle und unter Rückgang der sensiblen Reizerscheinungen bildet sich eine typische Sklerodermie aus, die hier wie auch sonst sich nicht auf die distalen Körperteile zu beschränken braucht, sondern neben den Händen auch das Gesicht, selten auch noch andere Körperteile, Brust und Arme beteiligt. Es gibt Fälle, in denen die vasomotorischen Symptome sehr lange vorausgehen, selbst Jahrzehnte. Besonders aber ist die Gruppe von Fällen vertreten, in denen die vasomotorischen Symptome ganz allmählich und gleichzeitig mit den trophischen Symptomen sich entwickeln. BROWN, O'LEARY und ADSON sahen unter 15 Fällen 9 mal die vasomotorischen Störungen primär, in 4 Fällen Gefäßspasmen und Sklerodaktylie gleichzeitig, in 3 Fällen die Sklerodaktylie primär auftreten. Ähnliches beschreibt SCOLARI. Nicht immer ist es ferner möglich, einen sicheren Unterschied zwischen den nekrotischen und den sklerodermatischen Veränderungen zu statuieren. Auch andere dystrophische Prozesse kommen vor. Schon an der Haut finden sich trophische Störungen, die nicht immer sicher zu klassifizieren sind. Es entstehen kleine Geschwüre, die hartnäckig sind, langsam heilen und in eine derbe sklerotische Narbe ausgehen. Noch schwieriger wird die Beurteilung der trophischen Störungen sein, die die tieferen Teile betreffen. Es wurden bereits Fälle von Sklerodermie erwähnt, in denen es zum einfachen Schwund ganzer Phalangen gekommen ist. Ein ganz ähnliches Vorkommen ist auch bei der RAYNAUDschen Krankheit, wie wir gesehen haben, beschrieben worden. FRICK beobachtete z. B. eine 39jährige Frau, bei der sich seit etwa 15 Jahren nach Arbeiten in Kälte und Feuchtigkeit nacheinander Akroparästhesien, symmetrische Gangrän, Sklerodaktylie und diffuse Sklerodermie mit Maskengesicht entwickelten. GOUGEROT und BURNIER sahen bei einer 40jährigen Frau den RAYNAUDschen Symptomenkomplex, Sklerodermie des Gesichts, Lipomatose der Glieder und multiple Telangiektasien; ähnliches berichten LORTAT-JACOB und BOUTELIER.

So rollt sich vor uns in vielen Fällen ein Krankheitsbild auf, daß seine Symptome teils von der Sklerodermie, teils von der RAYNAUDschen Krankheit entnimmt. Es ist in diesen Fällen ein vergebliches Bemühen, eine scharfe Grenze zu ziehen; denn diese Mischformen gehen nun ihrerseits ganz allmählich und unter allen möglichen Abstufungen auf der einen Seite in die typischen Fälle der Sklerodermie, auf der anderen Seite in die ebenso typischen Fälle der RAYNAUDschen Krankheit über. Der erste, der die Beziehungen von RAYNAUDscher Krankheit und Sklerodermie näher ins Auge faßte, war GRASSET im Jahre 1878, nachdem schon vor ihm BALL, COLLIER, DUFOUR, HARDY solche Beobachtungen publiziert hatten, ohne jedoch ihre Bedeutung zu würdigen. Später berichteten VIDAL und POTAIN über ähnliche Fälle, ferner auch FAVIER, AIELLO. Weiterhin ist dann die Reihe derjenigen Autoren, die derartige Fälle beschrieben haben, sehr groß geworden. So beobachtete PARKES WEBER zwei in dieses Gebiet gehörende Fälle und wies darauf hin, daß die im Kriege beobachteten Schützengrabenerfrierungen und Schützengrabenfüße eine auffällige Ähnlichkeit mit der Sklerodaktylie der Füße zeigten, besonders in den Fällen, in denen die Neigung zu oberflächlicher Gangrän bestand, in denen aber das atrophische Stadium noch nicht zur Ausbildung gelangt war. Auf Grund eigener Beobachtungen müssen wir sagen, daß die Zahl dieser in der Mitte zwischen Sklerodermie und RAYNAUD stehenden Fälle recht bedeutend ist. Von Autoren, die sich in neuerer Zeit mit dieser Frage beschäftigt haben, erwähnen wir GOUGEROT und MEYER; SÉZARY, BORY, MICHAELIS; PETGES, LECOULANT und DELAS; LÉRI-BARTHÉLÉMY und LINOSSIER, GRIVEAUD, SCOLARI.

In vereinzelten Fällen sind auch erythromelalgische Prozesse beobachtet worden. So beobachtete SAVILL einen Fall, in dem neben Anfällen von Asphyxie locale und einer teils fleckförmigen, teils diffusen Sklerodermie an Händen und Füßen sowohl eine Gangrän einer Zehe unter sehr heftigen Schmerzen entstand, als auch anfallsweise von Schmerzen begleitete Kongestionen an den Händen zu beobachten waren. SAVILL berichtet auch über das Auftreten eines Falles typischer Sklerodermie in einer Familie, wo flüchtige Ödeme häufig waren und die Patientin selbst an solchen Anfällen litt. Eine Kombination mit Akrocyanose sahen GLASSER und LANZENBERG, ebenso DAHMEN, bei dessen Patienten sich die Sklerodermie mit Akroasphyxia chronica kombinierte. Der von TOMMASI beobachtete Kranke zeigte von frühester Kindheit an eine allgemeine symmetrische Atrophie der Haut am stärksten an den Händen, am Halse und im Gesicht bestand Sklerodermie. Ein örtlicher Reiz genügte, um an einer Stelle, die Hautatrophie zeigte, Sklerodermie hervorzurufen. Außerdem fiel eine erhebliche Neigung zu Keloidbildung auf. Die Kombination mit Hyperkeratosen beobachtete GRUTZ.

Die *Sklerodermie en plaques* (morphoea) beginnt mit einem kongestiven Fleck, der sich allmählich verbreitert, während das Zentrum sich entfärbt und verhärtet. RAYMOND schildert als besonders charakteristisch den Lilacring, der die einzelnen Flecke umgibt. Das allererste Stadium dieser Affektion schildern EHRMANN und BRÜNAUER derart, daß unter Jucken und Brennen Herde auftreten, welche ursprünglich vereinzelten gleichmäßig rosenroten, bläulich oder violett geröteten Flecken entsprechen. Sie legen besonderen Wert auf diese Tatsache und betonen, daß die ursprünglichen Erscheinungen das Bild eines Erythems darbieten. In der Regel gehen sie unmittelbar in das weißliche sklerodermatische Stadium über (EHRMANN und BRÜNAUER). Umschriebene Herde sind fast an jeder Stelle des Körpers beobachtet worden; die oberen Extremitäten werden am häufigsten ergriffen (LEWIN und HELLER). Es erübrigt sich, die Einzelheiten wiederzugeben; sie haben überwiegend dermatologisches Interesse und haben eine sehr eingehende Darstellung durch EHRMANN und BRÜNAUER gefunden.

Die *Sklerodermie en bandes* erweckt dadurch Interesse, daß ihre Streifen öfter dem Zuge von Nerven oder Gefäßen zu folgen scheinen. Schon LEWIN und HELLER haben 21 derartige Fälle zusammengestellt, in denen die Streifen dem Verlauf bestimmter peripherer Nerven (BLASCHKO, HALLOPEAU, PINKUS, SPILLMANN u. a.) folgten. Am häufigsten findet man sie im Ausbreitungsgebiet eines Trigeminus. Auch andere Autoren haben derartige Fälle beschrieben. BRISSAUD hob nachdrücklich hervor, daß sich die Ausbreitungsbezirke der Sklerodermie bisweilen nicht mit dem Ausbreitungsgebiet eines peripheren Nerven decken, sondern daß auch das Gebiet eines Wurzelterritoriums befallen sein könne, was WEST zuerst beschrieben hat. Derartige Fälle sind ferner unter anderen auch von BRUNS, HUTCHINSON, WAGNER gesehen worden. In den letzten Jahren ist ein hierher gehöriger instruktiver Fall von segmentaler Anordnung der Sklerodermien von VOHWINKEL beschrieben worden. In anderen Fällen waren die Herde entsprechend den HEADschen Zonen lokalisiert, ferner halbseitig oder symmetrisch. BRISSAUD geht aber noch weiter und behauptet, daß es in manchen Fällen die Ausbreitungsbezirke der spinalen medullären Metameren sind, mit denen sich die sklerodermatischen Bezirke decken. Die ganze Lehre dieser spinalen, von der radiculären abweichenden Metamerie ist aber allzu unsicher.

Es ist übrigens zuzugeben, daß die Anordnung der Streifen oft eine ganz regellose und willkürliche ist, die offenbar weder im Zusammenhang mit bestimmten Nerven, noch mit solchen größerer Gefäßterritorien steht (KAPOSI, HOFFA, EHRMANN, BLOCH u. a.). Interessante Beziehungen glaubte BETTMANN zwischen der bandförmigen Sklerodermie und der Naevuszeichnung aufgedeckt zu haben; ebenso sind in jüngster Zeit Zusammenhänge zwischen der umschriebenen Sklerodermie und den LANGERschen Spaltlinien wiederholt diskutiert worden und wahrscheinlich gemacht (EHRMANN-BRÜNAUER).

Hemiatrophia faciei progressiva.

Eine besondere Unterform der *Sklerodermie en bandes* stellt nach der Auffassung von CASSIRER die *Hemiatrophia faciei progressiva* dar, die er als eine im Trigeminusausbreitungsgebiet sich lokalisierende Sklerodermie auffaßt. Daß ihr einige Besonderheiten anhaften, gibt er zu; doch erscheinen sie ihm keineswegs so bedeutsam, daß sie eine völlige Abtrennung dieses Krankheitsbildes von den sonstigen Sklerodermien rechtfertigen würden. Diese Auffassung wird jedoch nicht überall geteilt, wie später auseinandergesetzt werden wird.

1846 hat ROMBERG in seinen Trophoneurosen die ersten Fälle von Hemiatrophie zusammengestellt. STILLING, BERGSON und besonders SAMUEL haben sich intensiv mit der Krankheit und ihrer Pathogenese beschäftigt. Weitere Beiträge rühren her von VIRCHOW und MENDEL, LOEBL und WIESEL, die über pathologisch-anatomische Untersuchungen berichten, ferner von MOEBIUS, der ihr eine monographische Darstellung widmete, welcher MARBURG eine zweite folgen ließ. Von anderen Autoren, die sich mit dem Gegenstand beschäftigt haben, nennen wir BOUVEYRON, JENDRASSIK, OPPENHEIM und namentlich BITOT und LANDE wegen der Besonderheit ihrer Auffassung der Krankheit, der sie auch einen eigenen Namen „Aplasie lamineuse progressive" gegeben haben.

Die Hemiatrophia faciei ist wohl im ganzen kein gar so seltenes Leiden, uns wenigstens ist sie auch in ausgeprägter Form oft vorgekommen. KORN hat 1910 in der Literatur 189 Fälle gefunden, von denen aber eine Anzahl nicht echt zu sein scheint. Das Leiden tritt vorwiegend in jugendlichem Alter auf. Nach KLINGMANN befanden sich unter 83 davon befallenen Kranken 29 im Alter von unter 10 Jahren, 37 zwischen 10 und 20 Jahren und 17 zwischen 20 und 30 Jahren. Nach BOST schwankt das Alter, in welchem die Erkrankung auftritt, zwischen 4 Monaten und 39 Jahren. Auch angeborene Fälle sind LÉVY und VALENSI, ELLENBROEK u. a. bekannt geworden. OPPENHEIM beobachtete eine angeborene Hemiatrophia faciei, bei der die linke Wangengegend tief eingesunken war, dünne Haut und spärliches Haarwachstum zeigte, sowie dünnere Knochen und Muskeln. Er faßte den Prozeß als örtliche Schädigung im Mutterleibe auf, hervorgerufen durch Druck des anderen Zwillings. Die Annahme, daß alle nach dem 30. Jahr aufgetretenen Fälle fälschlich der Hemiatrophie zugerechnet werden (MOEBIUS), hat sich als unrichtig erwiesen. Durchaus nicht selten ist auch ein späteres Auftreten beobachtet worden (MENDEL, HOFFMANN, ROTHMANN, WEINBERG und HIRSCH, HÄNEL, STIEF und TANKA, VAN BOGAERT und HELSMOORTEL). FRANKL-HOCHWART teilt einen Fall mit, der erst im 37. Lebensjahr begann, STIEFLER einen solchen im Alter von 56 Jahren. Das Leiden befällt, nach den neuesten Untersuchungen von ARCHAMBAULT und FROMM, Frauen kaum häufiger als Männer (nach einer Statistik MARBURGS 40% Männer gegen 60% Frauen, nach BORST unter 36 Fällen 16 Männer und 20 Frauen). Ebensowenig scheint, wie früher angenommen wurde, die linke Seite der häufigere Sitz der Hemiatrophie zu sein (61mal unter 83 nach der Statistik von KLINGMANN, 21mal unter 36 Fällen von BOST, während MARBURG ein viel geringeres Überwiegen der linken Seite annimmt, womit auch LADALLE, ARCHAMBAULT und FROMM übereinstimmen [400 Fälle]). Mit dieser Feststellung erübrigt sich ein Eingehen auf die Deutung von STIER, der alle hypoplastischen Bildungen bei Rechtshändern auf der linken Seite viel häufiger findet, zu denen nach seiner Auffassung auch die Hemiatrophie gehört, die er z. B. bei einem 11jährigen linkshändigen Kinde rechts, also auch hier auf der inferioren Seite fand. Eine gleiche Beobachtung machten STIEF und TANKA. Andererseits stellt STIER fest, daß die hypertrophischen Bildungen die superiore, bei Rechtshändern also die rechte Seite bevorzugen. So wurden die mehrfachen Mamillen in 39 von 43 Fällen rechts gefunden und ebenso saßen die Hemihypertrophien meist rechts. In Rücksicht auf die von ihm angenommene größere Frequenz der rechtsseitigen Hemiatrophie und auch auf das Vorkommen der doppelseitigen Hemiatrophie bezweifelt MARBURG diese Deutung von STIER, ebenso auch STIEFLER, HÜBNER, BÖNHEIM u. a.

Das *Trauma*, welches das Gesicht oder den Schädel betroffen hat, spielt in der Ätiologie der Hemiatrophie eine auffällig große Rolle. Es ist in etwa 30% der Fälle nachgewiesen worden (MARBURG, CASSIRER, BOST). Wenn der Zusammenhang zwischen Unfall und Krankheit zeitlich und örtlich ein enger ist, so wird man es nicht mit Stillschweigen übergehen können. Solche Fälle sind wiederholt publiziert worden (HOFFMANN, STILLING, FROMHOLD-TREU, KRACHT, später WAGNER, NEUSTAEDTER, STIEFLER, TRABAND, TRÖMNER). Wiederholt ist auch eine Zahnextraktion (ZIEGENWEIDT, E. BÖNHEIM) als auslösende Ursache der Erkrankung erwähnt; doch macht H. CURSCHMANN darauf aufmerksam, daß die Kranken wahrscheinlich meist bereits wegen trigeminusneuralgischer Zahnschmerzen den Zahnarzt aufgesucht haben, so daß anzunehmen ist, daß das Prodromalstadium der Erkrankung bereits vorlag. Oft ist auch das Vorausgehen lokaler infektiöser Prozesse oder einer *Infektionskrankheit* notiert, was bei einem so häufig im Kindesalter auftretenden Leiden nicht zu verwundern ist. Eine Beziehung zwischen der Infektionskrankheit und dem Leiden war aber niemals deutlich. Außer Masern, Scharlach, Diphtherie, Pneumonie, Erysipel, sind wiederholt der Typhus und besonders die Lungentuberkulose als ätiologische Faktoren angeschuldigt. Im Falle von POPOVA, der einen 18jährigen jungen Mann betraf, fand erst ein Kopftrauma statt, nach 2 Monaten erkrankte er an Typhus; im Anschluß an diesen trat eine Abmagerung der rechten Gesichtshälfte und dann der rechten Körperhälfte auf. STERLING sah die Erkrankung im Anschluß an Poliomyelitis und Encephalitis lethargica einsetzen. Sichere Hinweise auf eine Erkrankung der *endokrinen* Drüsen finden sich in der Ätiologie unserer Kranken nicht. Es ist gelegentlich von Schilddrüsenveränderungen die Rede, von kleinen Schwellungen derselben, von einem Zusammenhang mit der Pubertät oder Gravidität (zuletzt von POLLAK behauptet, der bei einer endokrin und spasmophil belasteten Frau das Auftreten des Leidens im Anschluß an eine Gravidität beobachtete). Aber alles das sind vielleicht doch nur Zufälligkeiten.

In 2 Fällen von OPPENHEIM war eine schwere *neuropathische Belastung* vorhanden. In einem dritten waren die Eltern blutsverwandt und eine Schwester litt an kongenitaler Hüftgelenksluxation. BEER schätzt die Häufigkeit neuropathischer Belastung auf 27% (zit. nach H. CURSCHMANN). Zwei unserer Patientinnen waren geistig zurückgeblieben, eine auch sonst wiederholt konstatierte Tatsache. Eine stotterte in erheblichem Maße seit der Jugend. Ein familiäres Auftreten, wobei nicht alle Fälle ausgebildete Typen darstellen, scheint vorzukommen (RAYMOND und SICARD, KLINGMANN, BOENHEIM, REISS, GEIST). Komplikationen mit anderen Erkrankungen des Nervensystems sind bei diesem Leiden nicht selten, es wurde zusammen mit Epilepsie vom idiopathischen sowie vom Jacksontyp (NEUSTAEDTER, BACKMANN, WARTENBERG, LAUBER, BOST, H. G. WOLFF, ARCHAMBAULT und FROMM), Psychosen, mit Chorea und Spasmen der Gesichts-, Kiefer- und Zungenmuskeln (B. SACHS, zuletzt von KRÜGER, NEMLICHER und RAPPOPORT, KIRSCHENBERG) mit Zwangsvorstellungen und psychasthenischen Krämpfen (HÜBNER, OPPENHEIM u. a.), mit angeborener Augenmuskellähmung und Facialislähmung, mit angeborenem Torticollis (SORSBY-SHAW) gesehen. In einem Falle von LÉRI und WEILL fand sich bei Mutter und Sohn das MARCUS-GUNNsche Phänomen (abnorme funktionelle Synergie zwischen den vertikalen und lateralen Bewegungen des

Unterkiefers und dem Heben des oberen Augenlides). Der Sohn litt an Hemiatrophia faciei. Wiederholt wird die Kombination mit Migräne angeführt (SALUS, REISS, SOUQUES und BOURGIGNON). Auf das Vorkommen von Hemiatrophie bei organischen Nervenerkrankungen soll später noch eingegangen werden.

Das wesentlichste Charakteristikum der Erkrankung ist die *Hautatrophie*. Sie beginnt meist unmerklich, es tritt eine kleine, rundliche oder streifenförmige Stelle auf, die sich verändert, blaß oder stärker pigmentiert gelblich bis bräunlich sich färbt, und sich ganz allmählich über die Gesichtshälfte ausbreitet, so daß zwischen gesunden Stellen atrophische Inseln entstehen (H. CURSCHMANN). Es kommt zu einer Verdünnung der Haut, die meist nicht derb und fest wie bei der Sklerodermie (das ist ein gewisser Unterschied), sondern dünner, verschieblicher, zerreißlicher, zum Teil fein gefältelt erscheint. Stellenweise, aber im ganzen selten, kommt es auch zu einer Infiltration der Haut, die aber z. B. von LÖBL und WIESEL auch bei der Obduktion vollkommen vermißt wurde. Sehr wichtig ist der Schwund des Unterhautbinde- und Fettgewebes, der manchmal den Veränderungen der Haut vorausgeht. Der Schwund dieses Gewebes schafft die charakteristischen Gruben an den Wangen und am Kinn, die rinnenförmigen Einsenkungen. Und weiterhin ist es für die Hemiatrophie charakteristisch, daß der Prozeß regelmäßig nicht an den Weichteilen Halt macht, sondern Knorpel und Knochen mitbetrifft. So ist z. B. der Nasenknorpel sehr häufig und früh befallen; die kranke Seite der Nase erscheint schmäler, der Eingang enger, auch Ohr-, Kehlkopf- und Lidknorpel können betroffen sein. Die Atrophie des Knochens betrifft zumeist und am ausgiebigsten das Jochbein und den Oberkiefer, doch werden auch alle anderen Gesichtsknochen von der Atrophie nicht verschont. Daß, je jünger das Individuum ist, desto größer die Knochenatrophie werden kann, ist schon von VIRCHOW betont worden und ohne weiteres verständlich. Die Knochenatrophie ist bald mehr gleichmäßig, bald mehr unregelmäßig und führt damit zur Rinnen- und Dellenbildung, zu mehr oder weniger tiefen Einsenkungen, wie wir sie z. B. in größerem Umfang an den Seitenteilen der Stirn fanden. Bisweilen verwächst die Haut fester mit den tiefer liegenden Gebilden, insbesondere mit den Knochen. Durch die verdünnte Haut schimmern die Gefäße stärker als in der Norm hindurch. In einer Anzahl von Fällen sind, wie auch bei der Sklerodermie, die Muskeln befallen (Gesichts-, Kau- und Zungenmuskeln). Darüber berichten ZIEGENWEIDT, KRACHT, MARBURG, HEINEMANN, BEER, HÜBNER, CALMETTE und PAGÈS u. a. Bei Prüfung der elektrischen Erregbarkeit der Muskulatur konnte niemals eine Entartungsreaktion festgestellt werden. Eine Beteiligung des Stimmbandes wird von SCHLESINGER und KÖRNER erwähnt. HÖFLMEYER, WILLIAMSON, HEINEMANN, sahen eine Atrophie des harten Gaumens, wobei die Atrophie linear in der Mitte abschnitt, während WARTENBERG darauf aufmerksam macht, daß das Abschneiden der Atrophie in der Medianlinie des Gesichts viel seltener ist, als in der Paramedianlinie. Er führt diese Erfahrung auf die Tatsache zurück, daß die mediane Partie bilateral innerviert wird. Einen halbseitigen Entwicklungsdefekt an Schlund und Nasenrachenraum, der mit einer Hemiatrophia faciei kombiniert war, beschreibt BOROWSKIJ. Sehr interessant ist der von LAUBER beschriebene Fall von linksseitiger Gesichtsatrophie, bei der die Weichteile und der Knochen besonders schwer ergriffen waren; es fand sich auf der kranken Seite eine Atrophie des weit hinten in der Orbita liegenden Augapfels mit Linsentrübung, die sich synchron mit der Erkrankung entwickelt hatte.

Die eben geschilderten Veränderungen verleihen dem Gesicht des Kranken ein charakteristisches Aussehen: Verkleinerung der Gesichtshälfte, Asymmetrie der Kiefer, Jochbeine, Nasenknorpel, Eingesunkensein des Auges, Furchen und Rinnen in der Wange mit abnormen Pigmentierungen (OPPENHEIM).

Die Anhangsgebilde der Haut zeigen häufig bemerkenswerte Veränderungen. Die Haare verlieren oft ihre Farbe; es besteht ausgesprochene Canities an den befallenen Stellen, Augenbrauen, Wimpern und Bart und Teile der Kopfhaare fallen aus. Wiederholt ist Alopecie beobachtet worden, die der Erkrankung vorausging. Veränderungen der Schweiß- und Talgdrüsensekretion werden oft notiert, anfangs im Sinne einer Vermehrung, später einer Verminderung und eines Versiegens (L. R. MÜLLER). Im Fall von JANSEN und EIBRINK war der Zahnwechsel auf der betroffenen Seite erheblich verzögert. Zuweilen besteht auch dauernde oder anfallsweise auftretende Gefäßerweiterung oder Gefäßverengerung (L. R. MÜLLER). BRÜNING fand in einem Fall die Pulsation der Arteria temporalis auf der erkrankten Seite sehr schwach, POLLAK bei capillarmikroskopischen Untersuchungen das Bild einer spastisch-atonischen Vasoneurose, und zwar trotz der Einseitigkeit des Prozesses an beiden Körperhälften lokalisiert. Einige Male wurde

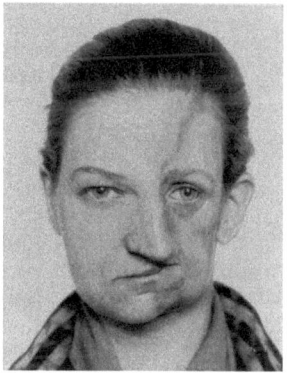

Abb. 11. Hemiatrophia Faciei progressiva. (Nach THIEL.)

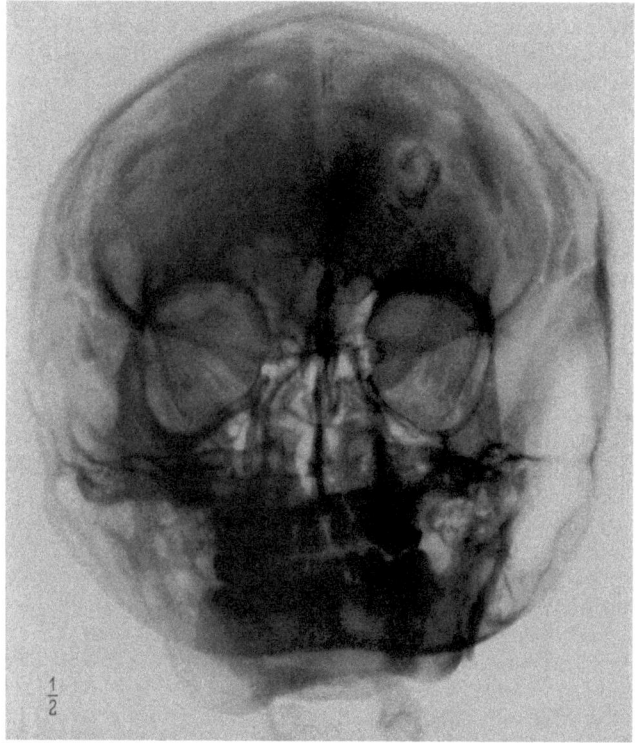

Abb. 12. P.-a.-Aufnahme. Asymmetrie des Gesichtsschädels. Orbitaeingang und Kieferhöhle links kleiner als rechts. Linker Jochbeinbogen fehlt. Kalklagerung im linken Stirnbein. (Nach THIEL.)

festgestellt, daß die Haut der atrophischen Seite nicht am Erröten teilnahm (zit. nach OPPENHEIM). In einigen Fällen fand sich ein Herpes (HÖFLMEYER).

Von besonderer Bedeutung für die Auffassung von der Entstehung des Leidens sind die Symptome, die einerseits auf eine Affektion des *Trigeminus*, andererseits des *Sympathicus* hinweisen. GOWERS glaubt, daß derartige Veränderungen in seinen Fällen sekundär dadurch entstanden seien, daß durch die Knochenatrophie die entsprechenden Kanäle und Foramina verkleinert seien und auf diese Weise ein Druck auf die sie durchziehenden Nerven ausgeübt würde, eine Theorie, die uns nicht einleuchtend erscheint. Schmerzen sind ziemlich häufig; sie können initial, oder aber auch dauernd bestehen, erreichen aber nur selten die Intensität echter Neuralgien. Sie können Monate oder Jahre lang dem Erscheinen der Hemiatrophie vorausgehen (HOFFMANN, SURAT). Häufiger ist von einer Hyperästhesie im Gebiet der atrophischen Hautpartie die Rede. BEER, der unter 148 Fällen 35mal Trigeminusaffektion fand, hat bei 54,5% Sensibilitätsstörungen verzeichnet, von denen etwa 40% Hyperästhesien waren. OPPENHEIM hat 2mal eine Anästhesie nachgewiesen, die die erkrankte Gesichtshälfte betraf, ohne sich streng an das Trigeminusgebiet zu halten. KRÜGER berichtet über einen Kranken, der eine Anästhesie und Analgesie im ersten bis dritten Ast des Trigeminus zeigte. Außerdem bestanden noch tonische und klonische Kaumuskelkrämpfe, die auf die erkrankte linke Seite beschränkt waren und sich reflektorisch nach Reizung der Haut dieser Gesichtshälfte einstellten. In dem interessanten Falle von STIEFLER traten unmittelbar nach dem Trauma anfallsweise heftige Schmerzen im gesamten peripheren Ausbreitungsgebiete des Quintus auf, später mit Anfällen von mehr oder minder lästigen Parästhesien verknüpft; es bestand umschriebene Druckempfindlichkeit der Austrittsstellen des oberen und mittleren Astes im Gesicht, Herabsetzung der Sensibilität im Gesicht für sämtliche Qualitäten im rechten Trigeminusbereiche. ARCHAMBAULT und FROMM stellen als vermutlich auf den Trigeminus zu beziehende Störungen aus der Literatur zusammen: rezidivierenden Herpes, rezidivierende Iridocyclitis, Keratitis neuroparalytica, Atrophie der Cornea und Bindehäute, partielle Katarakt.

Bemerkenswert sind andererseits die *Sympathicussymptome*. In mehreren Fällen eigener Beobachtung waren ausgesprochene oculopupilläre Symptome vorhanden. Ähnliche Sympathicussymptome wurden beschrieben von SEELIGMÜLLER, JENDRASSIK, LESKOWSKI, ZIEGENWEIDT, SÖDERBERGER, WILLIAMSON, SCHLESINGER, PAPARCONE, ANDREWS, BOUVEYRON. Auch in der neuesten Literatur begegnen wir häufig dem Hinweis auf dieses Symptom, ebenso auch auf eine Verfärbung der gleichseitigen Iris (L. R. MÜLLER, BUDINA). Auch wurde fast völlige Lichtstarre der Pupille beobachtet (OPPENHEIM, NOÏCA und VICOL, NEMLICHER und RAPPOPORT, SURAT). Die pharmakodynamischen Untersuchungen, die von verschiedenen Seiten ausgeführt sind (z. B. von STIEFLER, LÉRI, ČERNI, POPOVA) haben keine eindeutigen Resultate ergeben, teils verliefen sie völlig negativ. Daß das Ganglion cervicale supremum schmerzhaft ist, erwähnt OPPENHEIM. In einem seiner Fälle fand er außer einer erheblichen Druckempfindlichkeit der Sympathicusganglien eine geschwollene Drüse in der Gegend des Ganglion cervicale supremum; bei deren Exstirpation fand sich keine Verwachsung mit den Nerven; aber es trat zunächst eine Besserung ein, die nur 4—5 Wochen dauerte, um dann nicht weiter fortzuschreiten. Das erinnert an die Fälle, in denen sich direkt Veränderungen am Halssympathicus fanden und neben Reizerscheinungen und Ausfallserscheinungen dieses Nerven Andeutungen von Hemiatrophia faciei. Hierher gehören Fälle von BARREL, SOUQUES, BUDINA u. a. WEINBERG und HIRSCH haben 6 Fälle beschrieben, bei denen die Krankheit bei tuberkulöser Lungenspitzenaffektion auftrat. Das Leiden setzte während der chronischen Lungenaffektion ein. Sie halten einen Zusammenhang zwischen dem Lungenschrumpfungsprozeß und der Hemiatrophia faciei für sehr wahrscheinlich (s. auch LÖWY-HATTENDORFF, BUDINA). Andeutungen von Hemiatrophia faciei, die eine symptomatische Bedeutung zu haben scheinen, haben wir wohl in jedem Fall von Verletzung des Halssympathicus bei besonders darauf gerichteter Aufmerksamkeit gefunden, wobei das Maß der Ausprägung sehr wechselnd ist. Hierhin gehören auch die Fälle von SIEBERT (Schädigung der Halsdrüsen durch tuberkulöse Lymphdrüsen), JAQUET (Verwachsung des Ganglion cervicale supremum mit der schwielig verdickten Pleura), MANTHEY (Hemiatrophia faciei dextra et linguae nach zweimaliger Schilddrüsenoperation wegen Morbus Basedowii, ein halbes Jahr nach der Schilddrüsenoperation aufgetreten), HEILIGENTHAL, KURT MENDEL Kompression des Halssympathicus durch die vergrößerte Schilddrüse, ASCHER durch Halsrippe. Wir werden auf diese Fälle später noch zu sprechen kommen. Einige Autoren berichten auch über Fälle, in denen Trigeminus- und Sympathicuserscheinungen kombiniert vorgekommen sind (MARBURG, LÖWY-HATTENDORF u. a.).

Der Prozeß beschränkt sich nicht immer streng auf eine Gesichtshälfte. Einige Male dehnte er sich auch auf die andere Seite aus, welche jedoch meist nur in geringerem Grade betroffen war. (J. WOLFF, HILLER, OPPENHEIM, WASSERVOGEL, FRIEDMANN, SCHLESINGER, RAYMOND und SICARD, GERSUNY [zit. bei MARBURG], STIEFLER). Das Fortschreiten des Prozesses über das Gesicht hinaus bzw. über das Gebiet des Trigeminus wurde auch wiederholt beobachtet. So kann das vordere Halsdreieck schon im Beginn befallen werden (OPPENHEIM und O. FISCHER). Darüber hinaus wurden vereinzelte Veränderungen auch am Arm der gleichen Seite gefunden (COLLINS, BOUVEYRON). RAYMOND und SICARD unterscheiden 4 Typen: den Typus Hemiatrophia faciei, als eigentliche Hemiatrophie, den Typus hemifacioscapulohumerothoracicus, bei dem also ein Übergreifen auf den Arm und die Schultern beobachtet wurde (DEBRAY), weiter den alternierenden Typus, der im wesentlichen durch eine Beobachtung von LUNTZ dargestellt ist, der über eine Hemiatrophia cruciata berichtet. VOLHARD hat eine hierhergehörige Beobachtung publiziert, bei der auf der einen Seite die Hemiatrophia faciei, auf der anderen gekreuzte Pigmentanomalien in weitem Umfange bestanden. Eine gewisse Ähnlichkeit mit dem Falle von LUNTZ zeigt die Beobachtung von RATNER; unseres Erachtens läßt der Fall sich jedoch nicht mit Sicherheit von der Syringomyelie abgrenzen. BERNSTEIN beschreibt einen Fall von Hemiatrophia alternans faciei progressiva mit halbseitiger Alopecie, Pigmentverschiebung und Hautatrophie. Wahrscheinlich handelt es sich hier um eine zentrale Schädigung in der Gegend der Brücke, zumal die Kranke spastische Erscheinungen darbot. Eine ähnliche Lokalisation findet sich im Falle von MARINESCO, KREINDLER und FAÇON. Der vierte Typus wird durch eine totale Hemiatrophie einer Körperhälfte dargestellt. RAYMOND und SICARD berichten über ein praktisches Beispiel dieser Art. Wir sahen eine 50jährige Frau, bei der sich in den letzten Jahren, etwa seit Beginn der Menopause, ganz allmählich eine Hemiatrophia corporis sinistri eingestellt hatte, die am stärksten im linken Arm ausgeprägt war, aber auch die linke Gesichtshälfte, das linke Bein und den linken Rumpf betraf. Es handelte sich um eine Atrophie aller die betreffenden Körperteile zusammensetzenden Abschnitte. Nur an wenigen Stellen fanden sich sklerodermatische oder abnorm pigmentierte Partien. Es traten auch vasomotorische Störungen auf, Erblassen und Blauwerden der linken Körperhälfte. Fälle von solcher totalen Hemiatrophie sind ferner beschrieben worden von ORBINSON, KNAPP (Hemiatrophia totalis auf dem Boden der Sklerodermie) und MEYER. Bei dem letzteren war die Hemiatrophie kombiniert mit einer linksseitigen spastischen Hemiparese und einer Empfindungsstörung auf der linken Seite. In dem Falle von WARTENBERG begann die rechtsseitige Hemiatrophie im Alter von 10 Jahren, seit dem 18. Jahre traten rindenepileptische Krämpfe des linken Armes (bis 35 am Tage) auf, die zeitweise in allgemein epileptische übergingen. Ähnliches beschreibt BARKMAN. Sehr interessant sind die beiden von ČERNI beschriebenen Fälle von Hemiatrophia unilateralis totalis[1]. Im ersten Falle trat die Hemiatrophie im Verlaufe eines Jahres auf. Auf der erkrankten Hälfte bestand eine deutliche Störung der Schweißabsonderung. Außerdem klagte der Kranke über kurzdauernde Bewußtseinsverluste und Gedächtnisschwäche. Im zweiten Falle fanden sich neben der Hemiatrophie auf der erkrankten Seite intensiv pigmentierte Flecke auf der Haut, zum Teil mit sklerodermatischer Veränderung. Außerdem ist der Fall dadurch bemerkenswert, daß sich auf der erkrankten Zungenhälfte eine Geschmackshyperästhesie für alle Qualitäten nachweisen ließ. Bemerkenswert ist ferner die Beobachtung von STIEF, die er bei einer 60jährigen linkshändigen Kranken angestellt hat. Sie zeigte einen rechtsseitigen hochgradigen Gesichtsschwund, der sich später auf den rechten Hals, Schulter und untere Extremität ausbreitete. Sie starb in tiefer Demenz. Anatomisch fanden sich rechts Lungenspitzenverwachsungen mit der Pleura, schwere Veränderungen in den rechten Hals-Sympathicusganglien, Arteriosclerosis cerebri mit schweren Zirkulationsstörungen und zwar rechts Dilatation und Stase, links mehr eine Verengung der terminalen Gefäßgebiete; entsprechend diesen entgegengesetzten Zirkulationsstörungen differierten auch die durch diese bedingten Parenchymschädigungen. STIEF glaubt mit einer gewissen Wahrscheinlichkeit annehmen zu können, daß in der Pathogenese dieser Zirkulationsstörungen der Sympathicus eine wesentliche Rolle spielt und daß neben der Schädigung der contralateralen Hypothalamusgegend auch eine gleichzeitige homolaterale Sympathicusschädigung angenommen werden muß.

Im Anschluß an diese Fälle von Hemiatrophie des ganzen Körpers sei noch kurz auf diejenigen hingewiesen, bei denen die Atrophie sich nicht auf eine Seite erstreckte, sondern die obere Hälfte des Körpers einnahm. BARRAQUER hat als erster einen solchen Fall beschrieben. Es handelte sich um ein 25jähriges Mädchen. Mit 13 Jahren begann das Gesicht und der obere Teil der Brust abzumagern. Die Atrophie schritt immer weiter fort, betraf aber nur die obere Körperhälfte, das übrige blieb normal. Einen zweiten Fall dieser Art beschrieben PIC und GARDÈRE; schließlich hat SIMONS unter dem Namen Lipodystrophia progressiva ebenfalls eine solche Atrophie der oberen Körperhälfte beschrieben. Sie betraf ein ausgesprochen neuropathisches Individuum, bei dem ein völliger Fettschwund im Gesicht, am Rumpf und an den Armen bestand, während an dem Gesäß eine auffallende Fettvermehrung vorhanden war. Das Gesicht glich durchaus einem Totenkopf. Sklerodermatische Veränderungen an der Haut waren nicht vorhanden. SIMONS hat später unter Anführung weiterer eigener und fremder Beobachtungen die ganze Lehre von der Lipodystrophia progressiva ausführlich dargestellt. Das Leiden gehört offenbar nicht zur Sklerodermie, sondern stellt eine spezielle Form der Störung der Ernährung des Fettgewebes dar, auch weitere Beobachtungen haben keine Aufklärung über die Natur des Syndroms gebracht. Doch sind Fälle, wie sie z. B. von WOLFF und EHRENCLOU beobachtet sind, geeignet, auf diese Beziehungen einiges Licht zu werfen. Die Krankengeschichte ist kurz folgende[2]: 40jährige Frau, seit 8 Jahren zunehmende Abmagerung der linken Gesichtshälfte, seit 4 Jahren nervöse Übererregbarkeit mit Neigung zu depressiven Verstimmungen, seit 3 Jahren Gewichtszunahme von 120 auf 160 Pfund infolge massiger Fettablagerungen an Hüften und Beinen. Atrophie des Gesichtes, und zwar der Haut, Muskeln, Knochen, des Fettes links und der linken Zungenhälfte. Haut trocken, schuppend. Fett unregelmäßig verteilt, aber nirgends exzessiv abgelagert. Brust und Schultern klein. Weichteile ausgesprochen druckschmerzhaft. Die Verfasser sehen in der allgemeinen Gleichgewichtsstörung den Ausdruck krankhafter Veränderungen der trophischen Kontrolle in den höheren Abschnitten (Hirnstamm, Mittelhirn, 3. Ventrikel). (Siehe die eingehende Darstellung von NOTHMANN in diesem Handbuch.)

Der Beweis dafür, daß die Hemiatrophia faciei und auch die übrigen hier genannten Typen von der Sklerodermie im weiteren Sinne nicht abgetrennt werden können, wird nach CASSIRERS Auffassung durch die Fälle geführt,

---
[1] Ref. Zbl. Neur. Band 46, S. 597.
[2] Zit. nach Ref. STIEFLER: Z. Neur. 47.

in denen neben Erscheinungen der Hemiatrophia faciei solche ganz typischer Sklerodermie, teils am Gesicht selbst, teils am Körper vorhanden sind. Derartige Fälle sind zuerst von ROSENTHAL und EMMINGHAUS publiziert worden. In späterer Zeit ist die Reihe der hierher gehörigen Beobachtungen durch eine große Anzahl von Autoren vermehrt worden. CASSIRER hat mehrere derartige Fälle beobachtet, d. h. also Fälle von typischer Hemiatrophia faciei gesehen, bei denen außerdem am übrigen Körper sklerodermatische Veränderungen vorhanden waren. So beobachtete er, um nur ein Beispiel zu nennen, einen 44jährigen Mann mit einer linksseitigen typischen Hemiatrophie mit Ausfall der Schnurrbarthaare, Wimpern und Cilien; außerdem bestanden sklerodermatische Flecke in der Höhe der 6. und 7. Rippe und am Oberschenkel. Alle Veränderungen saßen auf der linken Seite, die linke Brustwarze war pigment- und haarlos. Das klinische Bild gestattete seines Erachtens demnach keine Abtrennung der Hemiatrophie von der Sklerodermie. Einen ähnlichen Fall beschreiben VOHWINKEL und ČERNI, der in seinen Fällen die Hemiatrophie pathogenetisch unabhängig von der Sklerodermie entstehen läßt und beide Erkrankungen gemeinsam auf einen pathologischen Prozeß in den höheren trophischen Zentren zurückführt.

Daß bei der Hemiatrophie mehr als sonst die Knochen betroffen werden, ist kein zur Abgrenzung ausreichendes Merkmal, besonders wenn wir bedenken, daß wir dasselbe bei manchen Fällen unzweifelhafter Sklerodermie an den verschiedensten Körperstellen finden können. Wenn diese Auffassung zu Recht besteht, so muß man, wie CASSIRER ausführt, für die Hemiatrophie dieselben pathogenetischen Bedingungen supponieren, wie für

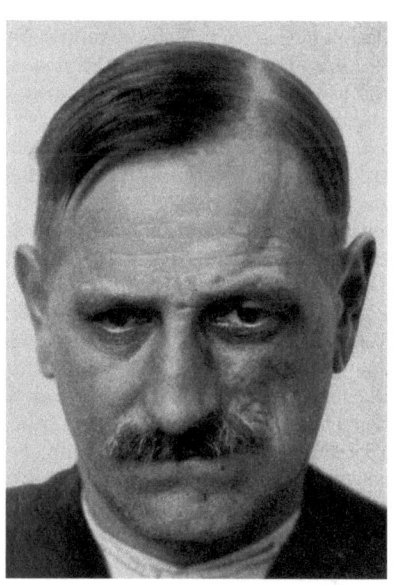

Abb. 13. Hemiatrophia faciei und Sklerodermie.

die Sklerodermie überhaupt. Die besondere Verteilung der Veränderung setzt naturgemäß eine besondere Lokalisation des krankmachenden Prozesses voraus. In diesem Sinne wären nach CASSIRER die oben mitgeteilten Erfahrungen zu verwerten, die teils an den Trigeminus, teils an den Halsstrang des Sympathicus, teils an noch zentraler gelegene Gebiete denken lassen, zumal der Prozeß naturgemäß nicht gleich lokalisiert zu sein braucht, wenn er nur eine und dieselbe Faserkategorie (vegetatives System) in der gleichen krankmachenden Weise angreift (OPPENHEIM, CASSIRER). Eine ganz ähnliche Auffassung vertritt KROLL, auf Grund eines von ihm beobachteten interessanten Falles, der große Ähnlichkeit mit der eben angeführten Kasuistik hat.

Die Frage nach den Beziehungen zwischen Hemiatrophia faciei und Sklerodermie wird auch von EHRMANN und BRÜNAUER kritisch behandelt. Sie äußern ihre Meinung dahin, daß die Fälle *reiner* Hemiatrophia faciei als eine Krankheitseinheit aufzufassen seien, die Fälle aber, in welchen bei mehr oder weniger halbseitigem Sitz sklerodermatischer Herde mit nachfolgenden Atrophien auch noch Stellen zu finden seien, an denen vorausgehende sklerodermatische Veränderungen nicht nachweisbar wären, als besondere klinische Erscheinungsformen der circumscripten Sklerodermie anzusehen seien, natürlich nur dann, wenn die sklerodermatischen Stellen alle Charaktere der umschriebenen Sklerodermie aufwiesen.

STIEFLER betont auf Grund seiner Beobachtung, bei der keinerlei Störungen des Halssympathicus nachzuweisen waren und die ursächliche Bedeutung einer traumatischen Einwirkung auf den Trigeminus gesichert erschien, daß die Schädigung von im Quintus verlaufenden trophischen Fasern *parasympathischen* Ursprungs für die Hemiatrophia faciei verantwortlich zu machen wäre.

L. R. MÜLLER sieht als Ursache der Hemiatrophia faciei einen chronischen Reizzustand trophischer Fasern des Halssympathicus, seiner Zentren oder seiner Ausläufer an.

Von den früheren Autoren ist eine ganze Reihe von Ansichten über die Pathogenese der Hemiatrophie vertreten worden. Für die eine Gruppe stellt sie das Prototyp einer Trophoneurose dar (ROMBERG, SAMUEL), für andere steht sie in direkter Abhängigkeit vom Trigeminus und wird durch eine Neuritis interstitialis proliferans hervorgerufen. Wieder andere sehen in ihr eine rein lokale Affektion, hervorgerufen durch einfachen primären Bindegewebsschwund mit erhaltenbleibenden elastischen Fasern und mit sekundärer Schädigung des unterliegenden Gewebes (LANDE, BITOT). Eine ähnliche Auffassung vertritt auch MÖBIUS. VIRCHOW und E. MENDEL haben zuerst unter Hinweis auf klinische und anatomische Erfahrungen die Ansicht geäußert, daß Affektionen des N. trigeminus für die trophischen Störungen verantwortlich zu machen seien. Eine ähnliche Auffassung hat auch JADASSOHN vertreten. Einen vermittelnden Standpunkt zwischen der Trigeminus- und der Sympathicustheorie hat JENDRASSIK eingenommen, der den Ort der Läsion an der Schädelbasis an der Stelle vermutet, wo der Plexus carotideus und das Ganglion Gasseri benachbart sind. In letzter Zeit tritt vor allem HANS CURSCHMANN für die Trigeminustheorie ein, indem er folgende theoretische Erwägung anstellt: gewisse Nerven (vor allem der N. medianus) beantworten ihre Alteration bisweilen ganz vorwiegend mit trophischen und vasomotorischen Störungen, denen gegenüber die motorischen und sensiblen Ausfalls- und Reizerscheinungen zurücktreten können. Analog diesem Verhalten erscheint es ihm durchaus plausibel, daß es gewisse (wohl nie grobe, oft chronische) Einwirkungen geben mag, die regelmäßig nur die trophischen Funktionen des Nervus trigeminus schädigen, ohne konstant zu gröberen sensiblen und motorischen Schädigungen desselben zu führen. Allerdings sei es wahrscheinlich, daß auch Störungen im Sympathicus den Prozeß verursachen könnten.

Der Vollständigkeit halber sei noch erwähnt, daß STIER die Erkrankung den Heredodegenerationen zuzählt, während F. BÖNHEIM auf Grund von zwei von ihm beobachteten Fällen ebenfalls von einer Heredodegeneration mit endokriner Mitbeteiligung (Hypophyse, Schilddrüse, Genitalorgane) spricht. Mit Recht bemerkt HANS CURSCHMANN, daß in den selten auftretenden endokrinen Symptomen nur koordinierte Teilerscheinungen einer degenerativen Anlage zu sehen seien.

Die bisher erhobenen *pathologisch-anatomischen* Befunde sind vorläufig noch nicht geeignet auf die pathogenetischen Fragen einiges Licht zu werfen. Anatomische Untersuchungen in sog. reinen Fällen von Hemiatrophia faciei sind bisher nur selten angestellt worden, von VIRCHOW-MENDEL und von LÖBL und WIESEL, aber gerade in dem Fall von MENDEL lag neben einer typischen linksseitigen Hemiatrophie auch eine Atrophie vor, die, an der Mittellinie des Rückens zwischen 4. und 7. Dorsalwirbel beginnend, über die Fossa infraspinata unter Beteiligung des Musculus infraspinatus bis zur Achselhöhle reichte und von hier aus, auf die Volarseite der linken oberen Extremität übergreifend, sich bis auf die Hand erstreckte. Es fand sich in sämtlichen Ästen des linken Trigeminus von seinem Ursprung bis zur Peripherie eine Neuritis interstitialis proliferans und dasselbe anatomische Bild im linken Radialis, dagegen keine Veränderungen im Facialis. Es ist also jedenfalls keine Rede von einer absoluten Beschränkung der Veränderungen auf die das Gesicht beherrschenden Nervenabschnitte. In dem Fall von LÖBL und WIESEL sind ähnliche Veränderungen im Trigeminus beschrieben worden, nämlich neuritische Erscheinungen vom Ganglion Gasseri bis in die peripheren Verzweigungen, von der auch die motorischen Äste nicht ausgenommen sind. Es ist uns aber zweifelhaft, ob der Fall von LÖBL und WIESEL überhaupt hierher zu rechnen ist oder ob er nicht vielmehr eine sog. symptomatische Hemiatrophie darstellt. Das Leiden hatte sich bei dieser Patientin angeblich im Laufe von 10 Monaten entwickelt, ist dann für den Rest der Lebenszeit, d. h. für 18 Jahre zum Stillstand gekommen. In der Krankengeschichte findet sich ferner die Angabe einer beiderseitigen reflektorischen Pupillenstarre, wie übrigens auch im Falle von LANGELAAN. Im anatomischen Befunde ist die außerordentlich hochgradige und schwere Affektion der Kaumuskulatur von Bedeutung, so daß die Vermutung nicht von der Hand zu weisen ist, daß es sich bei der Patientin um eine echte Neuritis des Nervus trigeminus gehandelt hat, vielleicht auf dem Boden der Lues, die im 22. Lebensjahre sich entwickelte, worauf naturgemäß in erster Linie die reflektorische Pupillenstarre zu beziehen ist. Damit würde der Fall dann aus der Reihe der unkomplizierten Fälle der Hemiatrophia faciei ausscheiden und wäre in eine Reihe zu stellen mit denjenigen Fällen von Hemiatrophie, die sich im Verlauf eines organischen Nervenleidens entwickeln. Ein von GRABS eingehend untersuchter Fall bot ein völlig negatives Sektionsergebnis. Gelegentlich wurden auch Veränderungen in den sympathischen Halsganglien gefunden (STAEMMLER u. a.).

Wir haben schon vorher (S. 331) von den Komplikationen der Hemiatrophia faciei mit anderen organischen Erkrankungen des Zentralnervensystems gesprochen und möchten im Anschluß an unsere Besprechung der sehr dürftigen pathologisch-anatomischen Beobachtungen zu diesem Thema noch einige Bemerkungen machen. Wie wir schon bei der Sklerodermie gesehen haben, sind auch die Erscheinungen von Hemiatrophia faciei nicht selten auf dem Boden der *Syringomyelie* beobachtet worden. Fälle dieser Art sind von GRAF, DÉJÉRINE und MIRALLIÉ, SCHLESINGER, CABANNES, LAMACQ u. a. mitgeteilt worden. Es sind das Fälle, in denen der syringomyelische Prozeß auf bulbopontine Abschnitte übergriff. Schädigungen solcher Abschnitte liegen auch in anderen Fällen symptomatischer Hemiatrophie vor, von denen wir erwähnen die bei der Tabes beobachteten von JOLLY und BASSI, bei der Paralyse von GRAFF. Ferner sahen PISSLING das Krankheitsbild bei einem Tumor der Dura, JOLLY bei multipler Sklerose, GRÄFE und SALOMON bei Lues, MURATOFF bei einem Echinococcus der hinteren Schädelgrube mit Übergreifen auf das Ganglion Gasseri sich entwickeln. ANDRÉ LÉRI sah folgenden Fall: die damals 32jährige Frau zeigte neben der Hemiatrophia faciei, dis sich fast ausschließlich auf das Unterhautfettgewebe bezog, eine Lähmung des 3.—7. Hirnnerven der gleichen Seite und leichte Parese des Arms der entgegengesetzten Seite. Er nimmt eine mesencephale Läsion an und glaubt, daß die Hemiatrophia faciei auf einer mesencephalen Störung des Sympathicus beruht. KIRSCHENBERG sah eine 28jährige Frau, bei der sich im Verlaufe eines Jahres ein allmählich zunehmender Schwund des subcutanen Fettgewebes, weniger der Haut und des Knochens des Gesichts entwickelte; außerdem fanden sich tonische Kontraktionen der Kaumuskeln und eine Hemihypästhesie und Hyperhydrosis rechts. Auch er nimmt an, daß es sich bei seinem Falle um eine symptomatische Hemiatrophia faciei handelt und bezieht die vasomotorischen Störungen auf einen zentralen Herd im Mesencephalon oberhalb der Trigeminuskerne. VIVADO nimmt in seinem Falle einen meningoencephalitischen Prozeß an mit dem Erfolge einer Schädigung der vegetativen Zentren: Es handelte sich um einen 28jährigen Mann, der im Alter von 6 Jahren eine vorübergehende Erkrankung der linken Gesichtshälfte aufwies. Kurz darauf erlitt er einen epileptischen Anfall. Nicht lange nachher trat eine langsame, schmerzlose Atrophie der linken Gesichtshälfte ein, die am Unterkieferwinkel mit einem im Zentrum depigmentierten, in der Peripherie dunklen Fleck begann. Die Atrophie erstreckte sich bald auch auf das Unterhautzellgewebe und den Knochen und trat allmählich auch an anderen Stellen des Gesichtes auf. Später ging sie auf den linken Arm und das Bein über. In der Folgezeit traten starke dauernde schmerzhafte Masseterkrämpfe links ein. Von Interesse ist ferner das gleichzeitig mit der Atrophie eintretende Ergrauen der Haare an den betroffenen Körperstellen. Hierher gehören auch die wichtigen Mitteilungen von POLLAK und MANKOWSKI.

Daß derartige Fälle geeignet sind, auch auf die Pathogenese der *reinen* Formen von Hemiatrophie ein Licht zu werfen, ist klar, wenn es auch zu weit geht, aus diesen immerhin vereinzelten Beobachtungen den Schluß zu ziehen, daß auch die *idiopathische* Form der Hemiatrophie auf anatomische Veränderungen gliomatöser Art in der Nachbarschaft des Ependyms (Hypothalmus) schließen läßt, wie das BRISSAUD, CALMETTE und PAGÈS, KOPCZINSKI u. a. wollen.

Der Hemiatrophia faciei bzw. der Hemiatrophia totalis steht die *Hemihypertrophia faciei* und *totalis* als Gegenstück gegenüber. Die Zahl der hierher gehörigen Beobachtungen ist nicht ganz klein. Obwohl MACKAY gewiß recht hat, wenn er eine exakte Scheidung zwischen den kongenitalen und den erworbenen Formen dieses Leidens nicht durchführen zu können glaubt, muß doch der Versuch einer Trennung dieser beiden Formen gemacht werden, weil ihre Pathogenese offenbar wesentlich verschieden ist. SABRAZÈS und CABANNES haben 17 Fälle von kongenitaler und 5 von erworbener halbseitiger Gesichtshypertrophie aus der Literatur zusammengestellt und eine eigene Beobachtung hinzugefügt. 40 Fälle sind in der Arbeit von GESELL gesammelt; die Erkrankung war auf die Geschlechter fast gleichmäßig verteilt. LENSTRUP beobachtete 8 Fälle von Hemihypertrophie, davon 6 Mädchen. In allen Fällen waren die Extremitäten befallen, in 6 Fällen die äußeren Genitalien, in 20 Fällen der Rumpf, in 3 Fällen das Gesicht und äußere Ohr, in einem Falle die Zunge. RUBASCHEW (zit. nach KROLL) hat aus der Literatur einschließlich seiner eigenen Beobachtungen 95 Fälle von totaler Hemihypertrophie, 14 Fälle von gekreuzter Hemihypertrophie, 43 Fälle von Hemihypertrophia faciei gesammelt. Der Hemihypertrophia cruciata hat KULKOW eine Studie gewidmet. Derartige Fälle sind beschrieben von KOSCHEWNIKOW (zit. nach KULKOW) (erworbene Hypertrophie der rechten Gesichtshälfte und der linken oberen und in geringerem Grade der unteren Extremität, die Umfangszunahme betrifft die weichen Gewebe und den Knochen), KUJASCHANSKY (linke Gesichtshälfte stärker als rechts, rechte Brustdrüse vorgewölbt, linke hängend, linke Extremitäten stärker als rechts), SLAUGHTER und EBERHARD (rechte Gesichtshälfte, rechter Arm, linkes Bein), KULKOW (rechts Hypertrophie des Arms, Schultergürtels, Hand, links Hypertrophie des Gesichts). Ähnliche Fälle sind von FORDYCE beschrieben. Recht selten scheinen Fälle wie derjenige von JANSEN und EIBRINK beobachtete: Hemihypertrophia dextra und Hemiatrophia sinistra. Sehr auffällig war in diesem Falle die bedeutende Vergrößerung der Zähne der rechten Seite mit Diastase derselben. Die Fälle von kongenitaler Hypertrophie sollen hier außer Betracht bleiben, wenigstens soweit es sich um stationäre Zustände handelt, die bei der Geburt abgeschlossen erscheinen. Beobachtungen von erworbener Hemihypertrophia faciei progressiva liegen vor von STILLING, BERGER, MONTGOMERY, DANA,

CASSIRER [1], HOFFMANN; TERRIEN-VEIL-CHEVANG (mit Buphthalmus); letzterer beschreibt 2 Fälle:

Bei dem 14jährigen Kinde wurde im 2. Lebensjahr angeblich im Anschluß an das Zahnen die rechte Seite des Gesichtes etwas dicker; erst in den letzten 2—3 Jahren hat die Zunahme stärkere Fortschritte gemacht; seit 2 Jahren besteht auf der rechten Oberlippe ein starkes Haarwachstum, die rechte Backe ist geschwollen, die rechte Nasenseite ist vergrößert, die Vergrößerung erstreckt sich bis zum unteren Augenwinkel und bis zum Kinn. Zunge und harter Gaumen zeigen eine stark vorgewölbte Schleimhaut, diese ist schwammig und verdickt. Die Hypertrophie läßt die Knochen frei; Sensibilität und Geschmacksvermögen sind intakt.

HOFFMANN erwähnt, daß in 3 Fällen dem Ausbruch des Leidens eine Verletzung oder Erkrankung der befallenen Seite vorausging (STILLING, BERGER, MONTGOMERY), in einem Falle von SCHIECK und dem eigenen von HOFFMANN ist eine Ursache nicht festzustellen. Aus der späteren Literatur sind noch die Fälle von MINOR und MACKAY zu erwähnen, ferner ein Fall von TSCHERBACK, bei dem es sich angeblich um eine Hemihypertrophia faciei, die durch Sklerodermie kompliziert war, handelte. Leider besitzen wir über den Fall keine ausführlichen Angaben, obwohl er natürlich von großer Bedeutung ist, indem er uns an die Beziehungen zwischen Sklerodermie und Hemiatrophia faciei erinnert.

Den Übergang von den kongenitalen zu den erworbenen Formen bilden diejenigen Fälle, in denen bei der Geburt schon eine geringe Hypertrophie an irgendeiner Stelle des Gesichts konstatiert wurde, in denen aber im weiteren Verlauf nicht eine Konstanz der Erscheinungen beobachtet wurde, sondern der Prozeß fortschritt. Hierher gehören die von STIER beobachteten Fälle, in denen nicht nur die Vergrößerung des kongenital schon abnorm großen Abschnittes des Gesichts allmählich fortschritt, sondern die Hypertrophie sich auf die übrigen Teile des Gesichts ausdehnte.

Fälle von erworbener *Hemihypertrophia totalis* sind von SCHULTE, MAC GREGOR, TILANUS, PIAZZA beschrieben worden. In dem Falle von PIAZZA handelte es sich um einen 8jährigen Knaben, der im Alter von 4 Jahren einen Typhus durchgemacht hatte; als er nach dieser Krankheit aus dem Bett aufstand, bemerkte man ein Hinken und einen Monat später fiel es auf, daß der rechte Oberschenkel dicker war. Die allmähliche Zunahme war dann weiterhin auch deutlich zahlenmäßig feststellbar; sie erstreckte sich auf die ganze rechte Körperhälfte, war aber im Bein dauernd erheblich größer als in den anderen Partien. An der inneren Fläche des rechten Knies fand sich ein Naevus.

Auch wir selbst haben einen derartigen Fall beobachten können.

Bei einer 28jährigen Frau, die bis dahin gesund war, traten neuralgische Schmerzen im ganzen Rücken, besonders in den Schulterblättern auf; aber es kamen unangenehme Empfindungen im rechten Arm dazu und dieser Arm nahm dann ganz allmählich an Umfang zu. Irgend eine Größenzunahme des rechten Beines wurde nicht bemerkt. Es handelt sich um ein leicht erregbares, ängstliches, schreckhaftes Individuum, das seit langem schon an Kopfschmerzen litt, leicht Herzklopfen hatte und bei dem bei der Untersuchung der rechte Ober- und Unterarm ganz erheblich dicker war als der linke; z. B. betrug der größte Umfang des rechten Oberarmes 34, des linken 29 cm. Auch im Längenwachstum bestand eine erhebliche Differenz zugunsten der rechten Seite, so daß auch die Knochen an der Größenzunahme beteiligt sein mußte, ebenso war die Muskulatur rechts erheblich stärker entwickelt. Sensibilität und Motilität waren vollkommen intakt. In einem weiteren Falle fand CASSIRER bei einem zur Zeit der Beobachtung 37jährigen Manne eine allmählich im Verlauf der Beobachtung noch fortschreitende rechtsseitige Hypertrophie, die 7 Jahre vorher angefangen hatte. Gleichzeitig traten unangenehme dumpfe Empfindungen im Gesicht auf.

In einer Reihe dieser Fälle scheint nur die Haut und das Unterhautgewebe stärker befallen zu sein, während in anderen auch die Knochen von der Affektion mitbetroffen sind (z. B. im Falle LARSEN).

---

[1] CASSIRER: OPPENHEIMs Lehrbuch, 3. Aufl., S. 2175.

Über eine Hypertrophie der Muskeln erfahren wir im ganzen wenig; aber in einigen Fällen, so auch in den eben genannten eigenen, ist zweifellos auch eine Hypertrophie der Muskeln zu konstatieren gewesen.

Daß in diesen Fällen, und zwar sowohl bei der kongenitalen als auch bei der erworbenen Hemihypertrophie meist die rechte Seite beteiligt ist, wurde bereits erwähnt. STIER fand in einer Zusammenstellung 75 rechtsseitige und 45 linksseitige Hypertrophien, GESELL von 40 Fällen 27 rechtsseitige, LENSTRUP von 8 Fällen 5 rechtsseitige Hypertrophien.

Die Hypertrophie ist häufig nicht gleichmäßig entwickelt. Am stärksten betroffen sind gewöhnlich die Knochen des Jochbogens und des Oberkiefers, wie auch aus den Röntgenbildern hervorgeht, und die Weichteile der Wangen- und Oberlippengegend.

In der Mehrzahl der Fälle ist die Zahnbildung abweichend, insofern als ihre Zahl oder Größe die der anderen Seite übertrifft, meist auch von einem verfrühten Durchbruch berichtet wird. Aber SCHIECK, STIER und andere fanden auch das Entgegengesetzte.

Ein frühzeitiges Haarwachstum auf der hypertrophischen Seite ist mehrfach berichtet worden; so von SCHIECK, HOFFMANN, STIER.

Bemerkenswert ist, daß die Mitbeteiligung der Zunge, die in sehr vielen Fällen von angeborener Hypertrophie nachweisbar ist, bei erworbenen Fällen niemals gefunden wurde. Wir geben eine instruktive, dem Werke von L. R. MÜLLER entnommene Abbildung wieder.

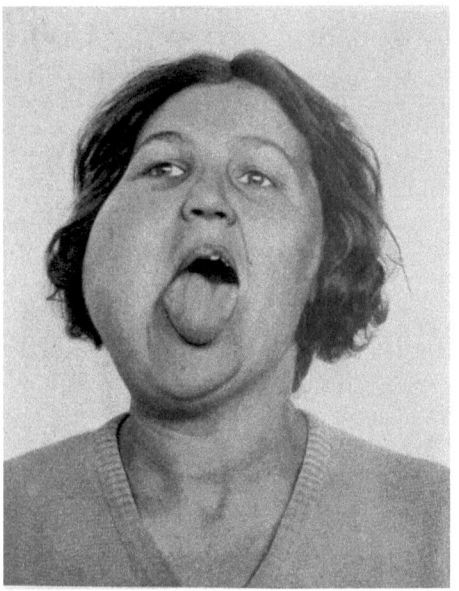

Abb. 14. Halbseitige Hypertrophie des Gesichts und der Zunge. (Medizinische Klinik Erlangen.)

Über die Pathogenese dieser Erkrankung können wir uns kurz fassen, indem wir im wesentlichen auf die Erörterungen bei der Besprechung der Sklerodermie hinweisen. LEWIN scheint der erste gewesen zu sein, der mit einiger Bestimmtheit die trophoneurotische Natur dieser Affektion behauptete, während andere diese Auffassung auf das energischste bekämpft haben und auch neuere Autoren von einer solchen Genese nichts wissen wollen.

In Übereinstimmung mit HOFFMANN, MACKAY, ZIEHEN glauben wir aber, daß wenigstens für eine große Reihe dieser Fälle, insbesondere für die später erworbenen progressiven, ein anderer Erklärungsmodus nicht möglich ist. Auch L. R. MÜLLER hat in dem abgebildeten Falle Schädigungen des Halssympathicus (HORNERsches Zeichen, vasomotorische Störungen) festgestellt, erklärt jedoch, daß uns vorläufig noch das Verständnis dafür fehlt, warum in einem Falle eine Atrophie, in anderen eine Hypertrophie des Fettpolsters entsteht.

HOFFMANN weist besonders auf das Vorkommen derartiger hypertrophischer Störungen bei gewissen organischen Erkrankungen des Nervensystems, vorzüglich bei der Syringomyelie und auch bei der Akromegalie hin und nimmt eine Störung der trophischen Zentren als Ursache dieser Veränderungen an. Wenn er freilich, indem er eine Affektion der periependymären grauen Substanz des Gehirns als Ursache dieses Leidens supponiert, diese Annahme noch weiter spezialisieren will, so geht er nach unserem Ermessen viel zu weit; wir glauben, daß man sich auch hier mit der Annahme bescheiden muß, daß die Störungen des Wachstums und der Nutrition auf einer Veränderung im Gebiet des vasomotorisch-sensiblen Systems beruhen, daß es aber nicht möglich ist, eine bestimmte Stelle dafür in Anspruch zu nehmen. Wir wollen daher auch die von STIER angegebene Möglichkeit, daß es sich um eine Erkrankung der subcorticalen Zentren handelt, nicht weiter diskutieren.

Es ist sehr wahrscheinlich, daß auch für einen Teil der *angeborenen* Fälle von Hemihypertrophie dieselben Entstehungsbedingungen vorliegen; dafür kann folgender Fall von ZIEHEN als Beispiel angeführt werden.

Es handelt sich um ein Mädchen, dessen Vater seit seinem 6. Jahre an multiplen Fibromen leidet. Es ist schwer geboren, sofort nach der Geburt soll das Gesicht schief, das linke Auge weit vorgerückt gewesen sein und offen gestanden haben. Die Gesichtsverbildung nahm mit den Jahren zu, es fand sich eine Schädelverbildung, die linke Orbita ist größer, die Weichteile des Gesichts sind links dicker, die Haut ist ungleichmäßig verdickt und zum Teil pigmentiert.

Die Begrenzung dieser Hemihypertrophie deckt sich durchaus mit dem Innervationsgebiet des Trigeminus. ZIEHEN nimmt als ihre Ursache eine im Uterus erfolgte Verletzung der großen Trigeminusäste am Ganglion Gasseri mit Beschädigung wesentlich nur der zutretenden vasomotorischen Fasern an. Auch hier scheint uns die Lokalisation zu weit getrieben zu sein, aber im Prinzip deckt sich sein Erklärungsversuch mit dem unseren.

CAGIATI, der eine gute Zusammenstellung der kongenitalen Hypertrophie gegeben hat, beschreibt ein Kind von 11 Monaten mit halbseitiger Hypertrophie; es findet sich eine Zunahme der Dicke der Haut auf der ganzen linken Körperseite und das Fettgewebe ist erheblich reicher entwickelt; das Skelet ist links stärker angelegt. Es besteht eine Hypertrophie der linken Herzspitze, Hypertrophie sämtlicher Blutgefäße, besonders die Media und Intima sind verdickt, eine größere Entwicklung der entsprechenden inneren Organe links. Eine Hypertrophie und Hyperplasie des Stützgewebes zwischen den Muskelbäuchen und an den peripheren Nerven ebenso wie in den Ganglien des Sympathicus liegt ferner vor. Nerven- und Muskelgewebe selbst sind ohne Veränderung; das Zentralnervensystem ist normal. Hier wird eine Störung des Mesenchyms in der ersten embryonalen Periode des intrauterinen Lebens angenommen, eine Störung, deren Abhängigkeit vom Nervensystem weder erweislich noch wahrscheinlich ist. Derartige Fälle sind in größerer Anzahl beschrieben worden, wie denn überhaupt die Zahl der angeborenen Fälle von Hypertrophie ähnlicher, d. h. offenbar nicht neurogener Genese erheblich größer ist als die der erworbenen (vergleiche auch die Arbeit von GESELL).

Verlauf und Prognose.

Man hat häufig versucht, die Sklerodermie in ihrem Verlauf in Stadien einzuteilen und hat danach unterschieden ein Stadium nervosum, das auch als Prodromalstadium bezeichnet wurde, ein Stadium oedematosum und ein Stadium indurativum und atrophicans. Die sog. Prodromalerscheinungen können auch ganz fehlen; sind sie vorhanden, beobachtet man in der Regel Störung des Allgemeinbefindens, Appetitlosigkeit, Magen-Darmbeschwerden, Parästhesien, Extremitätenschwäche, Schmerzen in den Gelenken. Im ganzen ist die Einteilung in Stadien schon darum nicht sehr wertvoll, weil an den verschiedenen Stellen des Körpers die Hautveränderungen sehr verschieden weit fortgeschritten zu sein pflegen. Man kann weiter zwischen akuten und chronischen Fällen unterscheiden. In der Mehrzahl der Fälle ist die Sklerodermie jedenfalls eine chronische Affektion, die jahre- und jahrzehntelang sich hinzieht. Fälle mit 30—40jähriger Krankheitsdauer sind vielfach beschrieben worden. Die Progression ist nicht immer eine stetige, es können sich lange Pausen von Stillstand einschieben; es können, während an anderen Stellen der Prozeß fortschreitet, hier und da Rückgänge sich vollziehen. Es kann eine Besserung auch dann sich noch einstellen, wenn schon das dritte Stadium, das der Induration, eingetreten ist. Aber im allgemeinen ist eine Besserung am ehesten beim akuten Verlauf und dann zu erwarten, wenn die lokale Affektion das ödematöse Stadium noch nicht überschritten hat. Auch die Haare können wieder nachwachsen, die übermäßige Pigmentation kann verschwinden, die Schweißsekretion wieder eintreten.

Für die bisweilen auftretenden akuten Verschlimmerungen hat man mancherlei Umstände verantwortlich gemacht, Traumen, Erschöpfungen nach Krankheiten; viele Kranke beschuldigen selbst schlechte Witterung, kaltes und nasses Wetter. Den chronischen Fällen stehen die mit *akutem* Verlauf gegenüber; auch dabei dauert es meist Wochen und Monate, ehe das vollständige Krankheitsbild vorliegt. EPSTEIN beschreibt z. B. einen Fall, bei dem die Sklerodermie ganz plötzlich begann: als das Kind an einem feuchten Nachmittag auf einer Wiese geschlafen hatte, entwickelte sich ein rasch vorübergehender fieberhafter Allgemeinzustand, an den sich die Ausbildung der Sklerodermie unmittelbar anschloß. MACCALLUM (zit. nach EHRMANN und BRÜNAUER) beschreibt Fälle, die außerordentlich stürmisch verlaufen und in kurzer Zeit zum Tode führen. Die akuten Fälle scheinen am ehesten bei Kindern sich zu entwickeln.

Es können bei allen Arten von Sklerodermie Besserungen und Heilungen vorkommen; das ist besonders der Fall bei den circumscripten Formen, die, wie EHRMANN und BRÜNAUER und andere Autoren betonen, fast immer teils spontan, teils unter Zuhilfenahme geeigneter therapeutischer Maßnahmen zur Ausheilung gelangen. Am wenigsten scheint bei der Sklerodaktylie die Tendenz dazu vorhanden zu sein. Aber Rückbildungen haben wir und andere auch dabei gesehen. Die Zahl der Heilungen geben LEWIN und HELLER im ganzen auf 16%, HERXHEIMER auf nur 8% an. Im allgemeinen scheint die Prognose bei Kindern eine bessere zu sein, indem die Zahl der Heilungen hier auf 30% steigt. Hier ist auch die Zahl der akuten Fälle, wie schon erwähnt, größer. Viel häufiger wurde über mehr oder minder weitgehende Besserung berichtet. Durch die Sklerodermie allein wird wohl nur selten der Tod herbeigeführt; immerhin ist das doch denkbar, wenn wir uns vergegenwärtigen, daß schwere Fälle von Sklerodermie von einer sehr erheblichen Kachexie begleitet zu sein pflegen und daß andererseits der sklerotische Prozeß wahrscheinlich auch auf lebenswichtige innere Organe übergreifen kann. Einige Male war es die besondere Lokalisation des Prozesses in der Haut, die den unglücklichen Ausgang herbeiführen half, wenn z. B. die Nahrungsaufnahme durch die Unmöglichkeit, den Kiefer zu öffnen, eine ungenügende wurde. Ein weiteres bemerkenswertes Symptom ist die Behinderung der Atmung, die Verwandlung des Thorax in einen festen Panzer, wie schon oben erwähnt ist. Oft aber tritt der Exitus ein im Verlauf interkurrenter Krankheiten, deren Aussichten durch eine schwere Sklerodermie naturgemäß ungünstig beeinflußt werden. Nach EHRMANN und BRÜNAUER gehen zahlreiche Kranke an Tuberkulose zugrunde, nach BROWN, O'LEARY und ADSON oft durch eine terminale Gefäßaffektion. Die circumscripten Formen der Sklerodermie können als solche natürlich niemals Todesursache werden.

Pathologische Anatomie.

Über die lokalen Veränderungen bei der Sklerodermie, insbesondere über die der Haut, liegen sehr zahlreiche Untersuchungen vor; von älteren Autoren nennen wir LEWIN, WOLTERS, DINKLER, v. NOTTHAFFT, KRYSZTALOWICZ, LUITHLEN, ALQUIER und TOUCHARD, von neueren in erster Linie EHRMANN und BRÜNAUER, ferner KOGOJ, GANS, H. HOFFMANN, E. I. KRAUS, BARKMAN, KROMPECHER.

Eine sehr sorgfältige kritische Darstellung der gefundenen Veränderungen findet sich bei EHRMANN und BRÜNAUER. Sie suchen in überzeugender Weise die

Differenzen in den Untersuchungsbefunden der einzelnen Autoren mit dem Hinweis auszugleichen, daß die Befunde, die durch verschiedene Untersucher in verschiedenen Stadien der Erkrankung an verschiedenen Fällen erhoben seien, notwendig differente Befunde ergeben müssen. Einzelheiten, die nur für den Dermatologen Interesse haben, sollen hier keine Erwähnung finden; wir verweisen vielmehr den Interessenten auf die grundlegende Arbeit von EHRMANN und BRÜNAUER.

Das *Stratum corneum* der Haut ist in vielen Fällen normal, zeigt jedenfalls keine erhebliche Alteration. Mangelhafte Verhornung kommt nur selten vor, häufiger ist eine Hyperkeratose mäßigen Grades beschrieben worden. EHRMANN und BRÜNAUER finden die Verdickung der Hornschichte in allen den Fällen, in denen die Papillarkörper nicht mehr erhalten sind und bezeichnen sie als eine Folge der Ernährungsstörungen, die durch die im Papillarkörper sich abspielenden Veränderungen bedingt sind. Das Rete Malpighi erscheint im atrophischen Stadium etwas verdünnt.

Die Hauptveränderungen betreffen das *Corium*. Je nach dem Stadium, in dem die Erkrankung sich befindet, findet man starke Abflachungen der homogenisierten und gequollenen papillären und subpapillären Schichten bis zum fast vollkommenen Schwund der Papillarkörper. Im spätesten Stadium verläuft die Epidermiscutisgrenze oft auf größeren Strecken als Wellenlinie, hin und wieder sieht man angedeutete Papillen (EHRMANN und BRÜNAUER). Das subcutane Gewebe und der Panniculus adiposus ist durch grobbalkiges Bindegewebe ersetzt, das späterhin eigentümliche Färbungsverhältnisse zeigt (EHRMANN und BRÜNAUER). Die Zellen des Bindegewebes sind verkleinert, ihre Zahl verringert; meist ist keine Spur von Protoplasma mehr sichtbar. Sehr strittig ist das Verhalten der elastischen Fasern. Die einen plädieren für ihre Vermehrung, andere für Verminderung, wieder andere für normales Verhalten. KOGOJ erklärt diese Widersprüche dahin, daß die Verminderung des Elastins nur eine scheinbare sei, indem die elastischen Fasern durch das gequollene Kollagen überlagert werden. In späteren Stadien der diffusen Sklerodermie komme es stellenweise zum Schwund der elastischen Fasern namentlich dort, wo die Sklerosierung perfekt sei. Das Kollagengewebe aller Schichten scheint in den späteren Stadien sklerosiert und homogenisiert, die Haarfollikel verschmälert und verdünnt, die Knäueldrüsen schwer verändert.

Über die *Pigmentation* liegen in neuerer Zeit Untersuchungen von BARKMAN, KOGOJ, E. I. KRAUS und EHRMANN und BRÜNAUER vor. Sie fanden die Epidermis, besonders das Stratum germinativum mitunter reich pigmentiert, mit Melanoblasten, die auch um das Blutgefäßnetz der Cutis, pigmententhaltend und vergrößert nachweisbar waren. Nach den meisten Angaben ist das Pigment auch im Corium vermehrt.

Ein sehr großes Interesse haben die Veränderungen in und an den *Gefäßen*, wegen der Rolle, die man ihnen für das Zustandekommen des Prozesses zugesprochen hat. Schon in der nächsten Umgebung der Gefäße pflegen die Veränderungen des Gewebes besonders stark akzentuiert zu sein. Die Erkrankung erstreckt sich von da aus auf alle 3 Häute anscheinend ziemlich gleichmäßig. Man hat den Eindruck, daß die Gefäßveränderungen von der Adventitia her nach innen vordringen, unter hauptsächlicher Proliferation der bindegewebigen Teile der Gefäßwand, das einen grobbalkigen Charakter annimmt. Allerdings tendieren auch die Muskelelemente und die Endothelien zur Proliferation. Nach EHRMANN und BRÜNAUER nimmt die Wucherung innerhalb der Gefäße, hauptsächlich der Arterien, nicht den zarten Charakter einer Endarteriitis an, sondern zeigt mehr eine grobbalkige Form. Oft ist das Gefäßlumen dadurch obliteriert. Das adventitiale Gewebe verschwindet schließlich ganz, so daß die Muscularis direkt an das umliegende Gewebe angrenzt. Die Lamina elastica kann hyalin entarten. Veränderungen der Blutgefäße und ihrer nächsten Umgebung sind selbst da vorhanden, wo das übrige Gewebe noch keine deutlichen Läsionen zeigt; andererseits kommen auch sklerodermatische Hautveränderungen da vor, wo die Gefäße noch nicht wesentlich erkrankt sind. TOUCHARD hebt hervor, daß die vasculären Veränderungen nicht die Ursache der Sklerose der umgebenden Partien sein können, da ein Parallelismus zwischen den beiden pathologischen Zuständen nicht vorhanden ist. In jüngster Zeit hat KROMPECHER der Erkrankung der kleinen Blutgefäße seine Aufmerksamkeit zugewendet und bezeichnet als Teleangiostenose stenosierende Intimabildungen, die an den kleinen Blutgefäßen auftreten und aus Elastoblasten und elastischen Membranen bestehen; als Elastofibrose bezeichnet er die allgemeine Vermehrung der elastischen Elemente, die außerhalb der Gefäßintima stattfindet. Bei der Untersuchung der Sklerodermie ergab sich ihm, daß dort eine Teleangiostenose und Elastofibrose vorhanden ist, wobei sich den Gefäßen entlang auch Rundzelleninfiltrate finden. Die Typizität dieses Befundes wird von G. B. GRUBER, der sich auf die KYRLEschen Befunde beruft, bestritten.

Auf die Lymphbahnen hat besonders UNNA geachtet. Er fand sie bei jeder diffusen Sklerodermie allesamt verengt. v. NOTTHAFFT und auch andere konnten diese Angaben nur zum Teil bestätigen. Ein sehr regelmäßiger Befund scheint die Hypertrophie der glatten Muskelfasern der Haut zu sein, die von vielen Autoren gesehen wurde. Die Nerven erwiesen sich meist als normal; nur eine Verdickung des Perineuriums wurde von vielen Autoren beobachtet; auch fanden sich gelegentlich degenerative Veränderungen. E. I. KRAUS fand z. B. sehr ausgeprägte degenerative Prozesse an den Markfasern, die zu ihrem Untergang geführt hatten. Im Interstitium waren Bindegewebs- und Fettgewebswucherungen zu erkennen. Eine Erkrankung der Gefäße der Nerven wurde auch beschrieben. Nach CASTELLINO und CARDI stellen die Veränderungen der Gefäßnerven einen regelmäßigen Befund dar.

Entsprechend der Tatsache, daß die Sklerodermie auch die tiefer liegenden Teile und die inneren Organe in Mitleidenschaft zieht, finden sich auch Veränderungen an den Sehnen, Gelenken, Muskeln und Knochen, an den inneren Organen, Leber, Lunge, Herz, Milz, endokrine Drüsen und am Nervensystem. Die großen Gefäße sind meist intakt; einige Male fand sich ein Atherom der Aorta und der Coronargefäße oder eine amyloide Degeneration sämtlicher Gefäße, einige Male eine Hypoplasie des Gefäßsystems. Die Veränderungen an den *Muskeln* bieten meist das Bild der Myositis interstitialis. LEREDDE und THOMAS, DINKLER, GOLDSCHMIDT, SCHULZ, v. NOTTHAFFT u. a. haben sie nachgewiesen. Die Muskelgefäße sind in ganz ähnlicher Weise wie die Gefäße der Haut schwer erkrankt (RAKE u. a.). Auch die Capillaren sind betroffen. Doch fand HEKTOEN auch wiederum ganz normale Gefäße inmitten schwerer Veränderungen der Zungenmuskulatur. Die Muskelfasern selbst sind wohl immer nur sekundär betroffen. RASMUSSEN beschrieb eine Verlötung der Intercostalmuskeln mit dem Periost der Rippen, weiter mit der Pleura. Verdichtung und Verdickung der Sehnen und Fascien sowie überhaupt der zwischen Haut, Muskeln und Knochen gelegenen Bindegewebspartien wurden ebenfalls festgestellt. Über Veränderungen von *Knochen* liegen auch eine Reihe von Untersuchungen vor. Nach den Röntgenbildern, von denen berichtet wurde, kann es keinem Zweifel unterliegen, daß die Knochen auch direkt am Prozeß beteiligt sind. Es kommt zu einer Einschmelzung der Compacta, die Knochenbälkchen der Spongiosa sind durch eindringendes Bindegewebe, bzw. die massenhaften Osteoclasten überall wie angenagt. Das Markgewebe war größtenteils nicht mehr zu erkennen, durch jugendliches Bindegewebe und Zellinfiltration ersetzt. Das Periost ist mit den umgebenden Weichteilen verwachsen, vom Knochen leicht abhebbar oder mit diesem durch junges, zellreiches Bindegewebe verbunden (EHRMANN und BRÜNAUER). Auch hier sind die Gefäße zum Teil schwer verändert. Ähnliche Veränderungen weisen die Gelenke auf. E. I. KRAUS findet allgemeine Osteoporose mit Bildung von Gallertmark.

Über Erkrankung der *inneren Organe* berichten SCHULZ, GOLDSCHMIDT, WESTPHAL, DINKLER, WOLTERS, JOPPICH, V. NOTTHAFFT, BRISSAUD, LEREDDE und THOMAS. Es scheint, als ob kein Organ von dem Prozeß verschont bliebe. Überall finden wir dasselbe Bild einer ödematösen Durchtränkung und Proliferation des Bindegewebes: zwischen den Alveolen der Lunge, zwischen den Acini der Leber, den Glomeruli der Niere, den Muskeltrabekeln des Herzens, der Pulpa, der Milz. Der Proliferation folgt die Atrophie und Kompressionen, Abschnürungen u. dgl. mehr schädigen sekundär das Parenchym. Überall sind auch die terminalen Gefäße an dem pathologischen Prozeß beteiligt. Arterien, Venen, Capillaren und auch das Lymphgefäßsystem werden ziemlich gleichmäßig befallen.

In den letzten Jahren hat sich die Untersuchung vielfach den endokrinen Drüsen zugewendet, nachdem schon seit vielen Jahren auf die Veränderungen der *Schilddrüse* geachtet worden ist. Anatomisch nachgewiesene Veränderungen finden wir schon bei SCOTT, SINGER, LEREDDE und THOMAS, HEKTOEN, UHLENHUTH, V. NOTTHAFFT. Vakuolenbildung, Kolloidverarmung, bzw. Entartung fanden BÉNARD und COULAUD, MATSUI, Kolloidstruma GORDON, PARHON, ISANOS und BRIESE, ENRICO, bindegewebige Entartung EHRMANN und BRÜNAUER, HORNOWSKI. E. I. KRAUS fand Atrophie im verbreiterten Zwischengewebe und hier und da Rundzelleninfiltrate, JEDLIČKA Vergrößerung und Verhärtung, Vermehrung des Bindegewebes, STRUKOV Hypertrophie. ROUX stellte Veränderungen an der *Hypophyse* fest, die jedoch von einzelnen Autoren als normal beschrieben wird (EHRMANN und BRÜNAUER). STRUKOV fand sie vergrößert, ein Überwiegen der basophilen Zellen fanden BÉNARD-COULAUD, eine Verminderung derselben MATSUI. E. I. KRAUS fand eine Vermehrung der Hauptzellen auf Kosten der chromaffinen und regressiven Veränderungen aller Zellformen. Atrophische Degeneration fand HORNOWSKI, Wucherung der ungranulierten Zellelemente auf Kosten der granulierten Zellen und Vermehrung des interfollikulären Gewebes JEDLIČKA. ENRICO fand die Neurohypophyse normal und zwischen vorderen und hinteren Anteilen kolloidale Cystenbildung. Im Falle PARHON, ISANOS und BRIESE fanden sich in der Hypophyse kleine protoplasmaarme Zellen, darunter auch einige eosinophile. Es bestand reichliche Vascularisation; in der Nachbarschaft des nervösen Lappens, der keine pigmentierten Zellen enthielt, Kolloidfollikel. Die *Parathyreoidea* fand JEDLIČKA normal, STRUKOW stellte eine Hypertrophie fest; E. I. KRAUS eine deutliche Vergrößerung mit den Anzeichen einer chronischen interstitiellen Parathyreoiditis, mit reichlicher Bindegewebs- und Gefäßwucherung und dichter lymphocytärer und plasmacellulärer Infiltration. Eine Fibrose des *Ovarium* sahen JEDLIČKA, GORDON, LHERMITTE und TRÉMOLIÈRE, STRUKOV, eine Atrophie HORNOWSKI, MATSUI, E. I. KRAUS u. a. Atrophische Hoden und interstitielle Orchitis fanden LONGCOPE und PARHON, ISANOS und BRIESE. Eine Atrophie der *Brustdrüsen* stellten LHERMITTE und TRÉMOLIÈRE und KREN fest. An den *Nebennieren* erhoben KRAUS, LHERMITTE und TRÉMOLIÈRE einen normalen Befund. Schwere Veränderungen sahen EHRMANN und BRÜNAUER, eine Vergrößerung BÉNARD-COULAUD, STRUKOV, MATSUI, Hypertrophie des chromaffinen Systems in den sympathischen Ganglienzellen und in den Nebennieren mit Verminderung der acidophilen Zellen HORNOWSKI, fleckige Lipoidvermehrung und Entzündung des periadrenalen Fettgewebes GORDON; Atrophie einer Nebenniere

LONGCOPE und MACCALLUM; Panarteriitis der Vasa vasorum der Suprarenalvenen, Totalnekrose beider Nebennieren JEDLIČKA, Zerstörung beider Nebennieren durch ein Hypernephrom BROOKS. Im Falle PARHON, ISANOS und BRIESE waren die Nebennieren klein und zeigten eine sehr ausgesprochene Sklerose, so daß jede Zelle von Bindegewebe eingeschlossen war; die Corticalis war arm an lipoiden Granulationen, die Zellen an Volumen verkleinert und in einigen Bezirken in Formen von Knötchen vereinigt. Die Befunde an den endokrinen Drüsen sind, wie sich aus dem vorherstehenden ergibt, teils uncharakteristisch, teils weichen sie in keiner Beziehung von den in den anderen Organen gefundenen ab.

Eine besondere Wertung verlangen die Veränderungen im *Nervensystem*. Auf die Veränderungen der Nerven wurde schon hingewiesen. Sie können selbstverständlich keine Bedeutung beanspruchen. Das Zentralnervensystem ist in einer Reihe von Fällen genau untersucht worden (DINKLER, CHIARI, VAN DER VELDE und WOLTERS, LEREDDE und THOMAS, V. NOTTHAFFT u. a.). Das Resultat war meist ein negatives. Nur wenige positive Befunde liegen vor. WESTPHAL fand an verschiedenen Stellen der Gehirnoberfläche knötchenartige Verdickung und Verhärtung der Windungen, auch in der Marksubstanz fanden sich, zum Teil ganz in der Mitte, ähnliche Herde. Der Autor erklärt, daß es sich um eine Lokalisation des sklerotischen Prozesses im Gehirn handle. EHRMANN und BRÜNAUER sahen Sklerosierung einiger Hirnwindungen. Ebenso wird man die Befunde von RAYMOND und ALQUIER auffassen müssen (mäßige Sklerose im Rückenmark). JAQUES und DE ST. GERMAIN fanden disseminierte myelitische Herde mit Höhlenbildung (Myélite cavitaire). STEVEN untersuchte einen Fall mit Hemiatrophia faciei et corporis dextra. Die mikroskopische Untersuchung des Rückenmarks ergab geringe, wenn auch unzweifelhafte Verminderung der Größe des rechten Vorderhorns. STEVEN ist der Ansicht, daß die Rückenmarksveränderungen die Sklerodermie hervorgerufen haben. Die Annahme, daß diese Veränderung des Rückenmarks nur eine Teilerscheinung der allgemeinen Hemiatrophie ist, hat offensichtlich mehr Wahrscheinlichkeit für sich. HERZOG fand cystische Bildungen im Bereich der hinteren Wurzel der Spinalganglien, in der bindegewebigen Wand leichte lymphocytäre Infiltrationen. HORNOWSKI sah Hypoplasie der Vorderhörner und Verminderung der Zellmenge in diesen und in den CLARKEschen Säulen. Im Falle von E. I. KRAUS fanden sich geringe degenerative und atrophische Veränderungen an den vorderen und hinteren Wurzeln und im Rückenmark in den Vorder- und Hinterhörnern, Schrumpfung vereinzelter Ganglienzellen und vakuoläre Degeneration einiger Ganglienzellen in den Vorderhörnern. KURÉ-YAMAGATA-KANEKO fanden die parasympathischen Zellen im Rückenmark und die entsprechenden Fasern in den hinteren Rückenmarkswurzeln unterentwickelt, an den parasympathischen Fasern in den Hautnerven Degeneration. STRUKOV fand eine starke Verdickung der harten Hirnhaut mit einer knöchernen Neubildung im Stirnteil. Keine Veränderungen am Nervensystem fanden MATSUI, GORDON, PARHON-ISANOS-BRIESE u. a.

Auch der Sympathicus ist mehrfach untersucht worden (HARLAY, DINKLER, V. NOTTHAFFT, LEREDDE-THOMAS, RAKE). BRÜNING fand einmal im exstirpierten Ganglion stellatum ausgesprochen entzündliche Veränderungen im Sinne einer lymphocytären Infiltration; später hat er niemals wieder in den sympathischen Ganglien krankhafte Veränderungen gesehen. RAKE fand die Ganglienzellen im Ganglion cervicale inferius anscheinend verringert, manche vergrößert, ohne feinere Struktur, manche wiederum klein geschrumpft; an den Blutgefäßen des Ganglion zeigte sich leichte Intimaproliferation. LERICHE-FONTAINE sahen an verschiedenen Sympathicusganglien teils gar keine Veränderungen, teils Bindegewebsnekrose, Entzündungsherde oder Degenerationserscheinungen an den Ganglienzellen. Angesichts dieser Befunde muß daher ausgesprochen werden, daß sich nichts Charakteristisches ergeben hat.

Pathogenese.

Die bisher publizierten Theorien über die Entstehung der Sklerodermie sind bereits im Jahre 1898 von VON NOTTHAFFT in vier Gruppen geteilt worden, die als *Schilddrüsentheorien, infektiöse Theorien vasculäre* und *neurotische Theorien* bezeichnet werden können. In Berücksichtigung der modernen Forschungsergebnisse wird man den Begriff ,,Schilddrüsentheorie" durch denjenigen der ,,endokrinen" Theorien zu erweitern haben und dabei der engen Beziehungen zwischen den endokrinen Drüsen und dem vegetativen System eingedenk bleiben müssen.

Die Erkrankung der *Schilddrüse* wird von einer großen Reihe von Autoren als Ursache der Sklerodermie angesehen. Die diese Auffassung stützenden klinischen und anatomischen Befunde wurden zum Teil bereits erwähnt. Besonders in Anspruch genommen für eine solche Auffassung wird das Vorkommen einer Kombination von Sklerodermie und BASEDOWscher Krankheit. LEUBE hat zuerst auf diese Kombination hingewiesen. Weitere Fälle wurden beschrieben von KAHLER, JEANSELME, SAINT MARIE, GRÜNFELD, RAYMOND, BEER, SATTLER, SINGER, KORNFELD, KRIEGER, MARINESCO und GOLDSTEIN, PARHON und CARAMAN und zahlreichen anderen Autoren. MORAWIECKA beschreibt die Kombination mit Osteomalacie und Basedow. Meist gesellten sich zu einem schon bestehenden Basedow allmählich die Erscheinungen der Sklerodermie. Nicht alle mitgeteilten Fälle halten einer strengeren Kritik stand. Es ist zu berücksichtigen, daß Abmagerung, Pigmentverschiebung, Schilddrüsenveränderungen und Irritabilität des Herzens auch der Sklerodermie als solcher zukommen, und daß auch ein gewisser Grad von Exophthalmus bei der Sklerodermie nichts Ungewöhnliches ist. Nicht nur bei der BASEDOWschen Krankheit, sondern auch fast bei allen anderen Schilddrüsenerkrankungen ist die Verbindung mit Sklerodermie beobachtet worden; bei Struma, bei Atrophie der Schilddrüse, bei Hypothyrrheoidismus, bei Syphilis der Schilddrüse, bei Hyperthyrrheoidismus. VALLERY und RADOT, LAMOTT und LITTLE haben Kranke gesehen, bei denen neben den sklerodermatischen Erscheinungen zuerst ein Basedow, später ein Myxödem bestand. Die Annahme der Anhänger der Schilddrüsentheorie geht dahin, daß durch die Schilddrüsenaffektion eine Dysthyrreoidie herbeigeführt werde, die die Hautveränderungen bedinge. Die ganze Theorie ist recht schwach fundiert, wie auch seinerzeit VON NOTTHAFFT hervorgehoben hat. Unter den vielen hundert Fällen von Sklerodermie, die in der Literatur bekannt geworden sind, gibt es kaum 70 dieser Kombination. Auch die gelegentliche, aber durchaus unregelmäßige und auch auf anderem Wege zu erklärende Wirksamkeit des Thyrrheoidins bei Sklerodermie ist ohne Beweiskraft. In den Fällen, in denen gewisse Beziehungen einer Erkrankung der Thyrrheoidea zu Sklerodermie vorhanden zu sein scheinen, ist mit der Möglichkeit einer auf gleichem Boden entwickelten koordinierten oder einer einfachen sekundären Schädigung der Schilddrüse zu rechnen. EHRMANN und BRÜNAUER machen darauf aufmerksam, daß in einer großen Anzahl von Fällen Erscheinungen von seiten der Tyrrheoidea fehlen und daß in Gegenden, in welchen Strumen häufig sind, doch kein gehäuftes Auftreten von Sklerodermie nachweisbar ist. Die gleiche Auffasssung vertritt JADASSOHN, der gleichzeitig darauf hinweist, daß es auch möglich sei, daß sklerodermatische Veränderungen der Schilddrüse von Einfluß auf die eigenartige Gestaltung des Krankheitsbildes sein könnten.

Noch weniger sicher ist die auf das Zusammenvorkommen von ADDISONscher Krankheit und Sklerodermie begründete Annahme von einer Erkrankung der Nebennieren als Ursache der Sklerodermie. Es ist zwar eine ganze Reihe von derartigen Fällen beschrieben worden, aber in den wenigsten hält die Diagnose Morbus Addisonii einer Kritik stand. ROSSBACH, WILLRICH, SCHULZ, BRISSAUD, NAUNYN, CHAUVET und CARLE, MENDEL, NOTHNAGEL, TSUCHIDA, LICHTWITZ, GOODHEART u. a. haben Fälle beschrieben, in denen sie die Vermutung oder die Überzeugung aussprachen, daß es sich um eine Kombination von Addison und Sklerodermie handele. EHRMANN und BRÜNAUER fügen noch Fälle von GERSON, ROESCH, THALMAN, SCHOLTZ hinzu, ferner Fälle von BOLTEN, CELASCO, H. HOFFMANN über Kranke mit auf eine Schwäche der Nebennieren hinweisenden Symptomen. Die Fälle JEDLICKA und BROOKS sind im anatomischen Teil bereits erwähnt, im Falle BROOKS fand sich eine Anämie und eine schwere Prostration, ferner eine braune Pigmentation der Haut des Gesichts und der Hände. Im Anschluß an den letzteren Fall äußern EHRMANN und BRÜNAUER die Ansicht, daß man angesichts eines solchen Befundes den Zusammenhang der Nebennierenläsion mit sklerodermatischen Veränderungen nicht von der Hand weisen könne. Man muß indessen das Bedenken äußern, daß viele der Erscheinungen des Addison der Sklerodermie als solcher zukommen, nicht nur die Pigmentverschiebungen und Schleimhautpigmentierungen, sondern auch die Kachexie. Derartige Befunde stellen Raritäten dar, so daß man doch wohl den Schluß ziehen kann, daß eine anatomisch sichergestellte Kombination von Sklerodermie und Addison zu den größten Seltenheiten gehört. Auch muß betont werden, daß in recht zahlreichen Fällen von Sklerodermie die anatomische Untersuchung der Nebennieren keinen pathologischen Befund ergeben hat (LICHTWITZ, KREN u. a.).

Einige Male wurde ein Zusammenvorkommen von Paralysis agitans mit Sklerodermie beschrieben (LUZZATO, PALMIERI, LUNDBORG, PANEGROSSI). LUZZATO hält das nicht für ein zufälliges Zusammentreffen, zumal die beiden Krankheiten sich im gleichen Maße entwickelten, sondern nimmt eine gemeinsame Ursache, und zwar wiederum offenbar eine Alteration einer endokrinen Drüse an. LUNDBORG hat ja an eine ähnliche Ätiologie schon bei der Paralysis agitans gedacht und in Rücksicht auf deren Kombination mit der Myoklonusepilepsie, für die er eine Funktionsstörung der Glandulae parathyrrheoideae zu vermuten geneigt ist, wäre damit auch für diese endokrinen Drüsen die Möglichkeit der Berücksichtigung gegeben. Der Fall von DUPRÉ und GUILLAIN, in dem Sklerodermie, Basedow und Tetanie zusammentreffen, könnte auch auf diese Spuren weisen, desgleichen der von MOEHLIG und DEPISCH beschriebene Fall von Sklerodaktylie und Tetanie.

NAEGELI weist auf das häufige Vorkommen von Sklerodermie und Calcinosis hin, das die Aufmerksamkeit auf die Thyreo-Parathyreoidea zu lenken geeignet ist. In diesem Zusammenhange sei wieder der Fälle gedacht, die nicht allzu häufig sind, in denen bei Sklerodermie eine Kataraktentwicklung beobachtet wurde, meist neben anderen endokrinen Störungen (SÉZARY, FAVORY und MARMON, SAINTON, MATHIEU-PINARD-FIEHRER). In jüngster Zeit gelang es SELYE, bei der Ratte durch Verabreichung von Epithelkörperchenextrakt unter gewissen Bedingungen eine Erkrankung zu erzeugen, die sowohl klinisch als auch morphologisch der Sklerodermie entspricht. Er rechnet die Sklerodermie in die Krankheitsgruppe der Hyperparathyreosen. Eine Bestätigung seiner Befunde steht vorläufig noch aus.

Nachdem von STRÜMPELL auf eine gewisse Gegensätzlichkeit im Symptomenbild der Sklerodermie und Akromegalie hingewiesen hatte (bei Akromegalie Hyperplasie von Haut und Knochen, bei Sklerodermie Schrumpfungsprozesse), hat man auch die Funktionsstörung der *Hypophyse* in den Bereich der Betrachtung gezogen. Roux und Lafond haben sich zu diesem Thema ausführlich geäußert, nachdem sie in ihren Fällen sklerotische Prozesse der Hypophyse festgestellt hatten, desgleichen Lereboullet. Weitere Untersuchungen haben jedoch diese Befunde nicht bestätigen können. Ehrmann und Brünauer haben in einigen Fällen radiologisch sichtbare Veränderungen des Türkensattels nachweisen können, desgleichen Arady, Armani, Kanno, Fuss, Büchler u. a. Andere Autoren fanden normale Verhältnisse (Russi). Im Falle von Arady bestand körperlicher und psychischer Infantilismus sowie doppelseitige Katarakt. Strunz sah bei einem $4^1/_2$jährigen Mädchen Sklerodermie und Progeria und führt das Bild auf eine Hyperfunktion des Hypophysenvorderlappens zurück. Blatt prüfte in 10 Fällen von Sklerodermie das endokrine und vegetative System und stellte regelmäßig eine Hypofunktion der Hypophyse fest. Untersuchung an 11 Sklerodermiefällen mittels des Abderhalden*schen Dialysierverfahrens* durch Kiess ergaben in 10 Fällen Abbau der Hypophyse. Der Abbau anderer Drüsen trat nicht mit derselben Regelmäßigkeit in Erscheinung. In diesem Zusammenhange erwähnen Ehrmann und Brünauer noch die Untersuchungen von Reines, der in 3 Fällen von diffuser Sklerodermie 3 mal Abbau der Schilddrüse und von Mesenterialdrüsengewebe feststellen konnte, während Nebennieren nur 2 mal, Hypophyse und Pankreas gar nicht abgebaut wurden. Ähnliche Resultate hatten Viehweger und Fuss. Leiner fand Abbau der Schilddrüse und Ovarien. H. Hoffmann betont, daß die Ausschläge bei Anwendung des Abderhalden*schen* Verfahrens so schwach seien, daß man aus diesen Versuchen keine bindenden Schlüsseziehen könne.

Eine Reihe von Autoren glaubt an einen Zusammenhang zwischen Sklerodermie und Störungen der *Keimdrüsen*. Sie weisen auf das Auftreten der Erkrankung im Anschluß an Störungen der Menstruation hin (Thiriol, Arndt, H. Hoffmann, Kren u. a.), bei Störungen der Ovarialtätigkeit (Mosenthin, Laignel-Lavastine, Matsui, Zadek u. a.); in anderen Fällen setzte die Störung mit der Schwangerschaft ein (Kogoj, Sequeira) oder entwickelte sich schubweise bei neuen Graviditäten (Studnicka, Stöckl u. a.). In einzelnen Fällen wurden pathologisch-anatomische Befunde an den Ovarien festgestellt (Ehrmann und Brünauer), die vielleicht als Teilerscheinung des Sklerosierungsprozesses zu deuten sind.

Covisa, Bejarano und Prieto berichten über einen Fall, der leichte Fettsucht, Menstruationsstörungen, männlichen Typus der Schambehaarung zeigte, im Falle von Petges und Roche traten die Erscheinungen im Anschluß an eine Uterusexstirpation mit Entfernung der Adnexe auf. Schwarz konstatierte eine Hypofunktion der Ovarien.

Zurückbleiben der körperlichen Entwicklung und Hodenhypoplasie sind wiederholt beobachtet worden (Heimann und Hatry, Werther u. a.).

In seltenen Fällen ist die Sklerodermie auch mit der *Thymusdrüse* in Zusammenhang gebracht worden (Hammer, Kumer).

Schon Touchard hat die Ansicht geäußert, daß die Sklerodermie nicht auf die Affektion einer einzigen endokrinen Drüse zu beziehen sei; in der Folgezeit haben sich eine große Reihe von Autoren diese Auffassung zu eigen gemacht. Bertelotti berichtet z. B. über Veränderungen der Schilddrüse und der Hypophyse, ebenso Enrico. Auch Haskovec und Basta betonen den Zusammenhang der Hautveränderungen mit denjenigen der Schilddrüse und anderer endokriner Drüsen; die günstigen Resultate mit der Thyreoidinbehandlung sprechen nach ihrer Ansicht für einen causalen Zusammenhang beider Veränderungen. Andererseits haben Sainton und Mamou über einen Fall von pluriglandulärer Insuffizienz mit Sklerodermie und Katarakt berichtet, bei dem bei Thyrosindarreichung Symptome des Hyperthyreoidismus auftraten. MILIAN und RIMÉ sprechen von einer Insuffizienz der Schilddrüse und Nebenniere, STRUKOV von einer Hyperfunktion der Schilddrüse und der Nebenniere und Ausfall der Ovarialfunktion. STROM weist auf das Zusammenvorkommen von Sklerodermie und Diabetes hin und nimmt Beziehungen zu einer Schilddrüsen- und Pankreasstörung an. Die Kombination von Störungen endokriner Drüsen, insbesondere auch von seiten der Sexualorgane, hat CASSIRER mehrfach beobachtet, ebenso MAŠKILEISSON, WOLF-VALLETTE.

Deutlicher noch weisen die Fälle auf eine *pluriglanduläre Insuffizienz* hin, welche STERLING unter dem Namen „Degeneratio genito-sclerodermica" zusammengefaßt hat, unter Aufzählung aller in der Literatur vorkommender einschlägiger Fälle, nachdem schon vorher VON NOORDEN diese Auffassung geäußert hatte. Seitdem ist wiederholt das pluriglanduläre Moment in den Vordergrund der Diskussion gestellt worden, unter anderen Autoren von BAU und PRUSSAKOWA. In seinen beiden Fällen waren neben dem eunuchoiden ein sklerodermatisches Syndrom ausgesprochen; er spricht von einem Späteunuchoidismus mit besonderer Affektion der Keim- und Schilddrüse und weist darauf hin, daß von dieser Kombination fast ausschließlich Frauen befallen werden[1].

Seine Beobachtung ist aus verschiedenen Gründen recht interessant. Die Kranke, eine neuropathisch schwer belastete Psychopathin, zeigte nach der Pubertät (Menarche mit 17 Jahren) ovarielle Hyperfunktion. Mit 40 Jahren wurde wegen klimakterischer Meteorrhagien die Röntgenkontraktion ausgeführt. Bald darnach traten endokrine Störungen in Erscheinung, und zwar nicht nur auf eine ovarielle Störung, sondern auch auf eine Schilddrüsen- und Nebennierendysfunktion hindeutend. Zwei Jahre nach der Kastration treten die sklerodermatischen Erscheinungen fast am ganzen Körper verstreut auf.

Auch STERLING hat in dieser Frage noch einmal das Wort ergriffen und einen lipodystrophischen und osteomalacischen Typus der genito-sklerodermatischen Degeneration aufgestellt. Er fand in seinen Fällen eine konstitutionelle Aplasie der inneren und äußeren Genitalien, Fehlen der Mehrzahl der sekundären Geschlechtscharaktere, Sklerodermie, Osteomalacie, Lipodystrophie (Erynnengesicht). An dieser Stelle mag der von ISOLA erwähnte Fall von Lues congenita und Infantilismus mit schwerer allgemeiner Dystrophie Erwähnung finden. Die Sklerodermie hat die Haut ergriffen und unter den endokrinen Drüsen jene ektodermalen Ursprungs, und zwar, wie der Autor bemerkt, in einer Intensität, die ihrer phylogenetischen Rangordnung parallel geht (schwere Entartung der Hoden, weniger schwere der Hypophyse und Schilddrüse). LONGCOPE berichtet über einen Fall von generalisierter, mit intensiver Pigmentation und Hypoglykämie einhergehender Sklerodermie, welcher bei der Obduktion Atrophie der einen Nebenniere, sowie eine interstitielle Orchitis aufwies[2].

---

[1] LHERMITTE und TRÉMOLIÈRES berichten über ein 19jähriges Mädchen mit Lungentuberkulose und hochgradiger Abmagerung. Während vom 13.—16. Jahre die Menses normal waren, trat plötzlich Amenorrhöe auf. Gleichzeitig Gefäßkrisen mit Erkalten und Weißwerden der Hände und Füße; nach diesen Anfällen erfolgte Cyanose und Vasodilatation. Allmählich trat eine Verbildung der Finger und Zehen auf, die von heftigen Gelenkschmerzen begleitet war. Erinnyengesicht, Beugekontraktur der Hände, Atrophie von Thenar und Hypothenar, entsprechend an den Füßen. Anatomisch Rückbildung der Ovarien und Brustdrüsen, Veränderung der Schilddrüsen und Nieren.

[2] Eine sehr merkwürdige Beobachtung machten FRITZSCHE und SCHOLL: Schwere neuropathische Belastung. Beginn des Leidens mit Gemütsstumpfheit, Gewichtsabnahme, Polyurie. Zunehmende Verkleinerung der Hände, Versiegen der früher abundanten Schweißsekretion, Schwellungen der Füße, Verdickung der Zehen und Fußrückenhaut und Geschwürsbildung. Trophische Störung der Nägel der Zehen. Zunahme des Kopfumfanges, vermehrter Fettansatz im Laufe der Zeit. Eintreten sklerodermatischer Veränderungen an Unterschenkeln und Füßen mit völligem Haarmangel und Sensibilitätsstörung. Fehlen der Axillesreflexe, Erweiterung der Sella turcica. Die Autoren fassen den Fall auf als Hydrocephalus acquisitus mit endokrinen Störungen auf der Basis des Alkoholismus.

Das vorliegende Material reicht unseres Erachtens nicht aus, eine *direkte* Abhängigkeit der Sklerodermie von der Erkrankung einer der endokrinen Drüsen plausibel zu machen, ein Schluß, dem sowohl FALTA wie ZONDEK zustimmen, deutet aber immerhin auf Beziehungen dieser Erkrankung zu pluriglandulären Störungen. Das gemeinsame Band, das diese verschiedenen Affektionen umschließt, scheint uns darin zu liegen, daß sie alle auf *Erkrankungen des vegetativen Systems* zu beziehen sind. In steigendem Maße haben die Arbeiten der letzten Jahre den Beweis der Wechselwirkung zwischen vegetativem Nervensystem und endokrinen Drüsen erbracht (s. zu diesem Thema L. R. MÜLLER: „Die Lebensnerven", und den Abschnitt im Handbuch der normalen und pathologischen Physiologie, Bd. 16. 1930). Dieser exakte Nachweis der Abhängigkeit des endokrinen Systems vom Nervensystem ist für die gesamte Pathologie der vasomotorisch-trophischen Erkrankungen, wie auch des Morbus Basedowii und Addisonii von fundamentaler Bedeutung und gerade er ist geeignet, die Koinzidenz von Symptomen dieser beiden Krankheiten unserem Verständnis näher zu bringen. Wenn wir z. B. annehmen, daß die Schilddrüsenerkrankung beim Basedow keine primäre Erkrankung ist, sondern nur ein in die Kette des pathologischen Geschehens eingeschobenes Glied darstellt, ihrerseits entstanden auf dem Boden einer Erkrankung des vegetativen Systems, so scheinen uns zunächst eine ganze Reihe von Tatsachen aus dem Gebiete des Morbus Basedowii selbst dem Verständnis näher gerückt, und außerdem das Zusammenvorkommen von Basedowsymptomen und sklerodermatischen Erscheinungen unter der Bedingung verständlich, daß wir der Sklerodermie eine ähnliche Pathogenese wie dem Basedow zuschreiben, daß wir ihre letzte Ursache in einer *Schädigung des vegetativen Systems* vermuten, die teils direkt, teils auf dem Wege der Veränderung der Sekretion der endokrinen Drüsen die Symptome des Leidens hervorruft. Um dieser Theorie, die eine Reihe von anderen Autoren ebenfalls vertritt, eine reale Basis zu verleihen, hat man in den letzten Jahren versucht, mittels der Untersuchungsmethodik des vegetativen Nervensystems der Beantwortung dieser Fragen näher zu kommen. Man hat ausgedehnte Funktionsprüfungen und Stoffwechseluntersuchungen nach allen Richtungen hin vorgenommen (H. HOFFMANN, SIROTA, MASKILEISSON, PETELIN, HILLMANN, ARADY, LONGCOPE, LORTAT und JACOB, PAUTRIER und BRUSSET, WALDORP und BASOMBRIO u. v. a.). H. HOFFMANN hat in mehreren Arbeiten über seine Resultate bei der pharmako-dynamischen Prüfung berichtet und folgendes festgestellt: eine krankhafte Veränderung *einer* endokrinen Drüse wurde nur vereinzelt, eine Erkrankung mehrerer mit Sicherheit überhaupt nicht gefunden. Dagegen erwies sich in allen Fällen (den diffusen und circumscripten) das sympathische System untererregbar (Blutzucker nach Adrenalin und allgemeine Adrenalinreaktion), das parasympathische übererregbar. Die Angaben von H. HOFFMANN werden im allgemeinen von STEPHAN ROTHMAN bestätigt. Es erübrigt sich, die zahlreich vorgenommenen pharmako-dynamischen Prüfungen, die zum Teil widersprechende Resultate geliefert haben, im einzelnen hier aufzuführen. Meistens wurde das sympathische Nervensystem als untererregbar, das parasympathische als übererregbar festgestellt. Andere Autoren (DEROTO u. a.) fanden wiederum normale Verhältnisse. Das gleiche gilt von den Stoffwechseluntersuchungen. Die Mehrzahl der Autoren fand eine Änderung des Grundumsatzes, in einer Reihe von Fällen wurde er jedoch normal gefunden (NAEGELI, GLASSER und LANZENBERG). Häufiger ist eine Erhöhung des Grundumsatzes notiert, besonders von französischen Autoren (LÉVY und ZORN, LORTAT-JACOB-FERNET-BUREAU, HUFSCHMIDT, ARADY, PARHON und CARAMAN, FLARER, MILIAN und PÉRIN, HOROVITZ). LORTAT und JACOB, LEGRAIN, H. HOFFMANN, ROTHMAN und LONGCOPE, HILLMANN u. a. hingegen fanden den Grundumsatz vermindert. PAUTRIER und BRUSSET fanden eine Herabsetzung oder Erhöhung von 40—60% und erwähnen, daß die Erhöhung häufiger vorkomme, als die Verminderung. Mit Recht weist jedoch STRANDBERG bei der Diskussion dieser Fälle darauf hin, daß Sklerodermie sowohl bei Hypo- wie bei Hyperthyreoidismus auftritt und die Störung des Grundumsatzes von dem Grade der Störung der Schilddrüsentätigkeit abhängig ist.

Wir haben bereits bei der Besprechung der Symptomatologie erwähnt, daß den Beobachtungen, bei denen Kalkablagerungen in den Geweben festgestellt worden sind, sich in den letzten Jahren das besondere Interesse der Autoren zugewendet hat (THIBIERGE-WEISSENBACH, BASCH u. a.). Diese Fragen sind ausführlich von O. NAEGELI diskutiert (Literatur). Eine Verminderung des Blutcalciumspiegels fanden WALDROP, BASOMBRIO, einen normalen Spiegel fanden KREBS und HARTMANN, THIÉBAUT, eine Vermehrung PULAY, sowie PAUTRIER, BRUSSET und ZORN, SANNICANDRO, DEVOTO. Zur Pathogenese dieser Erscheinung haben sich verschiedene Autoren geäußert (NAEGELI, DURHAM, LORTAT und JACOB, FERNET, BUREAU, DEVOTO), ohne eine Klärung zu bringen. DEVOTO z. B. deutet die Kalkablagerung und die Sklerodermie als den Ausdruck zweier verschiedener Prozesse, die beide ein und derselben auf eine Insuffizienz der Hypophyse zurückzuführenden Diathese ihre Entstehung verdanken. Eine Reihe von Autoren nimmt Beziehungen zu der Schilddrüse und Nebenschilddrüse an. Noch widersprechender sind die Angaben über die Blutzuckerwerte (LEWIN und KAHN, Hyperglykämie), desgleichen KAMBAYASHI-KIUCHI (zit. nach LUTZ), den N-Stickstoffwechsel, den Purinstoffwechsel und die Cholesterinämie.

Um unsere oben formulierte Auffassung weiter zu stützen, seien noch einige weitere Beobachtungen anderer Autoren angeführt: KLINGER beobachtete einen Fall von Sklerodermie, in dem die Erscheinungen des erhöhten Sympathicustonus dem Ausbruch der eigentlichen Sklerodermie vorangingen, indem sie dann während der Höhe der Erkrankung deutlich vorhanden waren und mit der Abheilung der Sklerodermie sich zurückbildeten. Über ähnliche Erfahrungen wie KLINGER berichtet REIMES, der 2 mal bei Sklerodermie neben Zuckerausscheidung eine mydriatische Substanz im Serum konstatieren konnte, und HESS und KÖNIGSTEIN. Bei einer diffusen Sklerodermie sahen sie in Attacken auftretende gegensätzliche Zustände vasomotorischer Störungen, auf der einen Seite Cyanose der distalen Partien der Extremitäten mit Kälte, Hyperästhesie und übermäßiger Trockenheit, wobei Pilocarpininjektionen versagten, auf der anderen Seite hellrote Verfärbung und Schweißausbruch. Im Zustand des Gefäßspasmus waltete ein depressiver Gemütsaffekt vor, nach Lösung des Krampfes griff eine mehr euphorische Stimmung Platz. Im ersten Stadium bestand neben der Unempfindlichkeit gegen Pilocarpin eine erhöhte Empfindlichkeit gegen Adrenalin, und zu dieser Zeit war im Serum eine Substanz nachweisbar, die die Froschaugenpupille erweiterte. Im zweiten Stadium wirkte Pilocarpin prompt und die mydriatische Substanz ließ sich nicht mehr nachweisen.

Die Annahme einer Alteration des Nervensystems als Ursache der Sklerodermie hat nun noch eine ganze Reihe anderer Momente für sich. Wir verweisen auf die häufige nervöse Belastung, die zahlreichen allgemein nervösen Erscheinungen, die wir bei den Sklerodermatikern finden, auf die Kombination mit allgemeiner funktioneller Übererregbarkeit. Wir erinnern daran, daß in einzelnen Fällen seelische Erschütterungen den unmittelbaren Anstoß zur Entwicklung des Leidens gegeben haben. Wir erinnern an die enge Verwandtschaft der Sklerodermie mit der RAYNAUDschen Krankheit, die wir auch als Erkrankung des vegetativen Systems auffassen.

Die Hypothese, daß die Sklerodermie eine nervöse Affektion sei, kann sich jedenfalls nicht auf den Nachweis einer Erkrankung des animalischen Nervensystems stützen. Die in dieser Hinsicht erhobenen pathologisch-anatomischen Befunde haben offensichtlich keine ursächliche Bedeutung. Die bisherigen Forschungen haben in dieser Beziehung keine Aufklärung gebracht. Unser Hauptaugenmerk ist auch hier wieder auf das vegetative System zu richten. Schon früher haben einige Autoren von einer Affektion des Sympathicus gesprochen, namentlich BRISSAUD diese Sympathicustheorie zu verteidigen gesucht. Seine Ausführungen verdienen, im Lichte der neueren Forschungsergebnisse betrachtet, wieder ernsthafte Beachtung. Unsere heutigen Erfahrungen und Anschauungen zwingen uns dazu, die Ursache der Sklerodermie in einer Alteration des vegetativen Nervensystems zu sehen, über deren Einzelheiten wir allerdings bisher nicht unterrichtet sind. Es ist selbstverständlich mit der Möglichkeit zu rechnen, daß verschiedene Teile des vegetativen Systems angegriffen sein können (SALKAN, PETELIN u. a.). Die nicht seltene Beschränkung auf ein einziges Nervengebiet könnte daran denken lassen, daß der Sitz der Krankheit wenigstens in diesen Fällen in einem peripheren Abschnitt des Systems zu suchen wäre; hierher würde dann auch nach CASSIRERs Ansicht die reine unkomplizierte Hemiatrophia faciei gehören. DORA GÖRING nimmt an, daß die Sklerodermie eine funktionelle, durch Reizzustände bedingte Erkrankung trophischer Nervenfasern ist, die dem Sympathicus angehören. HANS CURSCHMANN vertritt die Auffassung, daß die vegetativen Zentren im Gehirn und Rückenmark mit Einschluß des Grenzstranges erkrankt seien. Wenn neben den trophischen Zentren für die Haut und die subcutanen Gewebe auch die endokrinen Drüsen geschädigt seien, entstehe die Vereinigung von den Symptomen der pluriglandulären Insuffizienz mit den sklerodermatischen Dystrophien. SCALA spricht von einer ungenügenden Entwicklung aller ektodermalen Derivate, die sich am erheblichsten in den spinalen Zentren des Sympathicus und in den sympathischen Ganglien des Grenzstranges äußert („Ektodermopathia neurovegetativa").

Dieser Anschauung steht diejenige gegenüber, die annimmt, daß es sich bei der Sklerodermie um eine *Gefäßerkrankung* handelt (DINKLER, HOFFA, HERXHEIMER, E. I. KRAUS, KROMPECHER u. a.), und zwar um eine Erkrankung der terminalen Gefäße. Diese Hypothese kann sich auf die anatomischen Befunde stützen; wir haben ja gesehen, daß die terminalen Gefäße bei der Sklerodermie in weitestem Umfange erkrankt zu sein pflegen. Einige Autoren beziehen sich auf das Vorkommen von Teleangiektasien, auf die Erscheinungen abnormer Vasomotilität und auf Herzveränderungen. KROMPECHER bezeichnet die Teleangiostenose als morphologische Grundlage der Sklerodermie und findet außer derselben noch eine Elastofibrose, wobei sich den Gefäßen entlang auch Rundzelleninfiltrate finden. E. I. KRAUS faßt seine Ansicht über das Wesen der Sklerodermie dahin zusammen, „daß diese ebenso wie die RAYNAUDsche Krankheit ein Symptom einer Gefäßerkrankung ist, die in der Mehrzahl der Fälle in einer obliterierenden Arteriitis, in einem kleinen Teil der Fälle augenscheinlich in einer Angioneurose mit Angiospasmus der kleinen Arterien besteht. Erreicht die Gefäßveränderung (gleichviel ob durch Endarteriitis obliterans oder Angiospasmus bedingt) einen Grad, der die Ernährung des Gewebes unmöglich macht, so kommt es zu dem als RAYNAUDsche Gangrän bezeichneten Symptom. Ist die Gefäßveränderung weniger hochgradig, dann kommt es zu dem anderen Symptom der Sklerodermie, die je nach der Lokalisation und Ausdehnung der Gefäßstauung entweder teilweise oder diffus auftritt". Wir halten alle diese Behauptungen für unrichtig; die Einzelbeobachtung von KRAUS kann uns um so weniger überzeugen, als die

Untersuchung des Gehirns und des vegetativen Systems fehlt. Selbst da, wo die oben erwähnten Veränderungen gefunden worden sind, ist niemals der Nachweis geführt worden, daß die Gefäß- und Hautveränderungen in ihrer Ex- und Intensität einander parallel gingen. Es fehlt auch der Nachweis, daß die Gefäßveränderungen immer den übrigen Gewebsveränderungen vorausgehen, wenn sie auch bisweilen sicher sehr frühzeitig vorhanden waren. Es fehlt auch weiterhin selbst jeder ernsthafte Versuch des Nachweises, warum gerade diese Gefäßveränderungen die sklerodermatischen Erscheinungen hervorbringen sollen. Es gibt ganz wenige, ebenso verbreitete Gefäßalterationen bei der diffusen Arteriosklerose, die ganz ohne sklerodermatische Veränderungen zu produzieren verlaufen. Wenn wir uns die Verhältnisse an den Gefäßen ansehen, so verstehen wir, wie es da zu Stauungen, Blutaustritten, zu Pigmentbildungen, zu Ödemen und zu Nekrose kommen kann; aber die charakteristischen teils proliferierenden, teils regressiven sklerodermatischen Prozesse mit ihrem typischen Ausgang in bindegewebige Induration und Atrophie finden in der Gefäßalteration durchaus keine ausreichende Erklärung. Wir dürfen demgemäß in der Veränderung der Gefäße nur eine *Teilerscheinung* der Erkrankung, nicht ihre Grundlage sehen. Ein Teil der für die Gefäßtheorie eintretenden Autoren läßt übrigens die Möglichkeit offen, daß die Gefäßerkrankung letzten Endes doch wieder auf eine Läsion des Nervensystems zurückzuführen sei (von NOTTHAFFT, HERXHEIMER, SCHUBIGER, STERNTHAL, THIBIERGE).

Bei der Diskussion über die Pathogenese der Sclerodermia circumscripta erwähnen EHRMANN und BRÜNAUER, daß sie in 3 Fällen auffallende Störungen seitens des Verdauungskanals gefunden haben („gastro-intestinale Autointoxication"), wobei sie besonders auf das Auftreten von Erythemen aufmerksam machen, die der Sklerodermie vorausgehen oder auf ihrem Boden sich entwickeln und die durchaus den autotoxischen Erythemen gleichen. HOPPE-SEYLER rechnet auf Grund eines ganz vereinzelten Befundes die Sklerodermie zu den Infektionskrankheiten, GRASSET und ZAMBACCO sehen in ihr eine modifizierte Form der Lepra. Diesen auf vereinzelten Befunden und unzutreffenden Verallgemeinerungen aufgebauten Annahmen können wir nicht beipflichten. Daß gewisse exogene und endogene toxische Schädigungen gelegentlich den Anstoß zur Erkrankung abgeben können, wird dabei ohne Schwierigkeit konzediert werden können und ist bereits bei der Besprechung der Ätiologie berücksichtigt worden. SELLEI ist, wie schon erwähnt, der Auffassung, daß die Sklerodermie und die Sklerodaktylie (Akrosklerose) zwei voneinander verschiedene Krankheiten sind. Für die Ursachen der Sklerodermie macht er gewisse Fermentationsstörungen im Organismus und in der Haut verantwortlich. Er glaubt festgestellt zu haben, daß die Pankreasfermente, sowie die Fermente anderer Organe wie des Magens und Duodenums direkt auf die sklerodermischen Indurationen wirkten, indem diese, wenn auch langsam, erweichten und gänzlich resorbiert wurden.

BARKMAN diskutiert die Frage, ob man die Sklerodermie nicht auffassen könne als die Resultante einer angeborenen Veranlagung des Mesenchyms, in seiner Gesamtheit oder teilweise, eine Anlage, die auf verschiedene Ursachen hin, wie Infektion, Trauma, nervöse Gefäßschädigung im Mesenchym die charakteristischen Erscheinungen der Sklerodermie hervorruft. Man könnte nach BARKMAN in diesem Lichte die verschiedenen Theorien über die Pathogenese der Sklerodermie und die bei ihnen geltenden Faktoren betrachten als parallele Erscheinungen (vasculäre Prozesse) oder Folgeerscheinungen (endokrine Symptome) oder als bestimmende Faktoren (nervöser Einfluß auf dem Wege der vasculären Spasmen); wenn Reize auf ein von Geburt aus prädisponiertes Gewebe einwirken, reagiert dieses nach der spezifischen und besonderen Art, die die Sklerodermie charakterisiert (zit. nach Ref. STIEFLER: Z. Neur. 45). ISOLA betrachtet die Sklerodermie als einen abiotrophischen Prozeß, im Sinne einer Keimblattschädigung durch Syphilis der Vorfahren. DUBREUILH leugnet die Krankheitseinheit der Sklerodermie, die ein Symptom sei wie das Erythem.

Diagnose.

Die Diagnose der Sklerodermie ist in der Mehrzahl der Fälle leicht zu stellen. Wo einmal die charakteristische Veränderung der Haut ausgebildet ist, und sie ihre harte, pergamentartige, glatte, unverschiebliche und faltenlose Beschaffenheit angenommen hat, und wo nebenbei noch abnorme Pigmentierungen, Haarausfall, Asphyxie und Syncope locale das Bild vervollständigen, wird die Diagnose rasch und ohne Zaudern möglich sein. Selbst dann, wenn noch nirgends das atrophische Stadium erreicht ist, werden kaum diagnostische Zweifel sich erheben. Neben den genannten positiven Kennzeichen kommen als negative das Fehlen motorischer Ausfallserscheinungen, ebenso wie auch das Fehlen von Anästhesien scharf umschriebenen Charakters in Betracht. Auch Schmerzen fehlen oft, und wenn sie vorhanden sind, zeichnen sie sich ebenfalls durch ihre unbestimmte, diffuse, unsichere Verbreitung aus.

Gewisse Fälle von Sklerodermie zeigen große Ähnlichkeit mit den trophischen Störungen bei der *Syringomyelie*, besonders bei der Unterart, der MORVANschen Krankheit. Als sichere Unterscheidungsmerkmale gelten ausgesprochene Symptome von individualisierter degenerativer atrophischer Lähmung und von auf bestimmte spinale oder Wurzelgebiete beschränkter totaler oder dissoziierter Empfindungsstörung. Dazu kommen die spastischen Erscheinungen an den Beinen, die Urinbeschwerden, die oculopupillären Symptome. Immerhin bleiben ein paar Fälle übrig, in denen die Unterscheidung Schwierigkeiten machen kann. Dasselbe gilt für die Unterscheidung von Sklerodermie und *Lepra*. Neben der Herkunft der Kranken aus Lepragegenden, dem Nachweis der Bacillen, den Serumreaktionen, der typischen Verdickung der Nerven sind auch hier wieder die Sensibilitätsverhältnisse das entscheidende Moment, indem eine fleckweise, evtl. sogar dissoziierte Empfindungslähmung die Diagnose „Lepra" sicherstellt. Daß gelegentlich die Beantwortung dieser Fragen akut werden kann, beweist der Fall von HUDELO-RABUT, bei welchem irrtümlich zuerst die Diagnose „Lepra" während des 2jährigen Aufenthaltes der Kranken in Afrika gestellt wurde. Dabei handelte es sich, wie sich später herausstellte, um eine Sklerodaktylie mit trophischen Ulcera an den Fingern, Sklerodermie der unteren Vorderarme und des Gesichts. Außerdem fanden sich Pigmentflecke über Rumpf und Gliedmaßen verstreut. Auf die Differentialdiagnose sind in jüngster Zeit DENNEY-HOPKINS-JOHANSEN eingegangen. In den letzten Jahren ist die Frage von ACTON diskutiert worden, ob die Tropenkrankheit *Ainhum* eine Sklerodermie en bandes darstellt. Es finden sich bei ihr symmetrische palmare und plantare Hyperkeratosen, die sich auch auf das Dorsum erstrecken können. Typisch ist eine ausgesprochene Schnürfurche an den Zehen, die schließlich dazu führen kann, daß die Phalange allmählich abgeschnürt wird (spontane Amputation).

Für die übrigen organischen Nervenkrankheiten kann ein Zweifel kaum entstehen, vielleicht ausgenommen eine Erscheinung, die Glanzhaut *(glossy skin)* bei zentralen Nervenerkrankungen und nach peripheren Nervenverletzungen. Die glossy skin schildert O. FÖRSTER[1] derart, daß sie zumeist mit starken Schmerzen, Vasodilatation und mit gesteigerter Schweißsekretion verbunden ist. Sie ist fast nie auf das Endgebiet des verletzten Nerven

---

[1] O. FÖRSTER: Handbuch der Neurologie, Erg.-Bd. 2, S. 1496.

beschränkt, sondern nimmt oft, z. B. bei Medianus- oder Ulnarisläsion die ganze Volarfläche der Hand, oft die ganze Hand, oft auch die gegenüberliegende Hand mit ein.

Hier kommt natürlich nur die Verwechslung mit der Sklerodermie en bandes in Frage. KALISCHER ist auf die Differentialdiagnose zwischen beiden Erkrankungen eingegangen. Die trophische Störung erstreckt sich bei der glossy skin selten so weit in die Tiefe wie bei der Sklerodermie. Die Berücksichtigung der ätiologischen Momente ist natürlich von Wichtigkeit.

Es wurde schon früher darauf hingewiesen, daß sich wiederholt die Frage erhoben hat, ob neben der Sklerodermie noch ein *Morbus Addisonii* bestehe und wir haben schon betont, daß die Annahme einer Kombinatien beider Erkrankungen jedenfalls nur mit der größten Vorsicht gemacht werden darf (S. 350).

Einige Male ist die Abgrenzung der Sklerodermie, besonders im Stadium elevatum von dem *Myxödem* in Frage gezogen worden. Häufig wird ein Anlaß zu Verwechslungen nicht vorliegen; abgesehen von den Hautveränderungen wird der typische Geisteszustand von den an Myxödem Erkrankten, werden die zahlreichen wichtigen Begleitsymptome, die Störungen der genitalen Funktion, der Schweißsekretion usw. für die Diagnose bestimmend sein. Auf die BASEDOWsche Krankheit ist schon im Abschnitt „Pathogenese" eingegangen.

Das *angioneurotische Ödem* ist meist durch seine größere Flüchtigkeit ausgezeichnet. Falls es einmal längeren Bestand haben sollte, wird die Diagnose „Sklerodermie" fallen gelassen werden müssen, wenn nach Verlauf von Wochen und Monaten keine Induration bzw. Atrophie eintritt. Weitere diagnostische Schwierigkeiten im ödematösen Stadium der Sklerodermie dürften sich ergeben in der Abgrenzung gegenüber dem *Trophödem* (s. S. 394). Der weitere Verlauf wird im allgemeinen alsbald eine Entscheidung ermöglichen, da die schließlich resultierenden Veränderungen durchaus verschieden sind.

Häufig macht die Unterscheidung der Sklerodermie von den *idiopathischen Hautatrophien* Schwierigkeiten. Unter dieser Bezeichnung faßt man Symptomenbilder zusammen, die früher als Erythromelie (PICK), idiopathische diffuse Hautatrophie (BUCHWALD), Akrodermatitis (Dermatitis) atrophicans chronica progressiva (HERXHEIMER und HARTMANN), Dermatitis atrophicans diffusa progressiva (M. OPPENHEIM) beschrieben worden waren. FINGER und OPPENHEIM haben auf Grund der Literaturbefunde und eigener Beobachtungen das ganze Kapitel monographisch dargestellt. In jüngster Zeit hat M. OPPENHEIM nochmals im Handbuch der Haut- und Geschlechtskrankheiten, Bd. VIII, 2 im Abschnitt „Die eigentlichen entzündlichen Hautatrophien" zu diesen Fragen eingehend Stellung genommen, desgleichen an gleicher Stelle EHRMANN-BRÜNAUER. In bezug auf alle Einzelheiten, die überwiegend dermatologisches Interesse haben, sei auf diese Autoren verwiesen. Die Erkrankung beginnt meist mit der Bildung von Flecken, bei der HERXHEIMERschen Form mit teigig weichen Infiltraten, die alle Abstufungen vom hellsten Rot bis zum dunkelsten Blaurot zeigen können, die zuerst den Eindruck eines leicht entzündlichen Erythems oder einer passiven Hyperämie machen; sie vergrößern sich und fließen zusammen. Alsbald gesellt sich dazu ein weiteres bemerkenswertes Kennzeichen, eine abnorme Schlaffheit der Haut (Anetodermie), nachdem schon vorher gelegentlich über eigenartige Parästhesien geklagt worden ist. Es entsteht eine feine Fältelung ihrer oberflächlichen Schichten, die Haut erhält ein Aussehen wie Zigarettenpapier. Beim Aufheben einer Falte ist diese bei der Dermatitis atrophicans hart und knitterig, bei der Sklerodermie gerundet und weich; bei der Dermatitis atrophicans gleicht sich die Falte nur sehr langsam und zögernd aus infolge des Schwundes des elastischen Gewebes, bei der Sklerodermie gleich nach dem

Abheben, mit der Einschränkung, daß es sich nicht um ein seniles Individuum handelt (EHRMANN-BRÜNAUER). Die Oberfläche ist trocken, fettlos, es fehlt die Schweißbildung, die feinen Wollhärchen sind gering entwickelt. Unter der verdünnten Haut treten die tiefer gelegenen Bestandteile, besonders die Venen deutlich hervor. Die Affektion lokalisiert sich meist symmetrisch an den Extremitäten, befällt die Streckseiten regelmäßig intensiver als die Beugeseiten und geht nur selten auf den Rumpf über. Die Sensibilität ist objektiv nicht gestört. Wir haben Fälle dieser Art gesehen, in denen die Unterscheidung von der Sklerodermie große Schwierigkeiten machte, Fälle, in denen die Haut, namentlich am Unterschenkel und Fußrücken, wie das auch OPPENHEIM beschreibt, ziemlich straff gespannt, nur schwer faltbar und von auffallend gelbweißer Farbe war.

Die Beziehungen der Dermatitis atrophicans zu der Sklerodermie sind in den letzten Jahren Gegenstand lebhafter Diskussionen unter den Dermatologen gewesen. M. OPPENHEIM faßt seine sehr sorgfältigen kritischen Untersuchungen unter Berücksichtigung der Gesamtliteratur dahin zusammen, daß das Vorkommen echter Sklerodermie bei der Dermatitis atrophicans nicht erwiesen ist. Die gleiche Ansicht vertreten auch EHRMANN-BRÜNAUER und betonen, daß sie unter allen denjenigen Fällen, welche eine Kombination der beiden Erkrankungen darstellen sollten in kaum einem einzigen Fall die Überzeugung gewinnen konnten, daß wirklich eine Kombination beider Krankheiten bestand. Keinesfalls dürfe ohne eine eingehende histologische Untersuchung irgendein Fall als beweisend angesehen werden. Doch finden sich bis in die letzte Zeit hinein Autoren, welche in einzelnen Fällen die Annahme einer Kombination beider Erkrankungen vertreten oder jedenfalls für wahrscheinlich halten. (MAIRE und WORINGER, GOLOMB und FAJNGOLD, OSTROWSKI). PAUTRIER und ULLMO finden bei beiden Erkrankungen capillaroskopische Unterschiede, PAUTRIER und BRUSSET bei der Dermatitis atrophicans im Gegensatz zur Sklerodermie keine Störung des Grundumsatzes, ebensowenig wie im Kalkgehalt des Blutes.

Eine Abgrenzung von der Sklerodermie verlangt das *Sklerema neonatorum*. Wir sahen, daß echte Sklerodermie auch bei Säuglingen vorkommt. Die beiden Affektionen sind auch früher für identisch gehalten worden (THIRIAL u. a.). Jetzt faßt man unter dem Begriffe zwei verschiedene Hautveränderungen zusammen, welche bei Neugeborenen und Kindern in der ersten Lebenszeit auftreten: das Sklerema ödematosum (Sklerödem) und das Sklerema adiposum. Mehrfach ist auch eine Kombination beider Fälle beobachtet. Es handelt sich bei der ödematösen Form meist um Schwellungen der Füße, Waden, Oberschenkel, des Mons veneris, gelegentlich auch der oberen Extremitäten und der Augenlider, mit daraus sich ergebender Bewegungsbeschränkung. Auf Fingerdruck entsteht deutliche Dellenbildung; bei schweren Fällen ist die Haut prall elastisch. Die veränderten Hautpartien zeigen öfters eine rote oder livide Verfärbung, die später abblaßt. Im allgemeinen ist die Temperatur normal; nur bei Komplikationen stellt sich Fieber ein. In schweren Fällen tritt in wenigen Tagen der Tod ein; im allgemeinen wird eine Rückbildung der Erscheinungen beobachtet. Die pathogenetischen Theorien befriedigen vorläufig nicht; ätiologisch scheint die Kälteeinwirkung eine Rolle zu spielen.

Das Sklerema adiposum kann alle Körperteile befallen, welche ein deutliches Fettpolster besitzen, meist mit Ausnahme der Palmae und Plantae (EHRMANN-BRÜNAUER). Es handelt sich hier um eine diffuse Verhärtung der Haut, welche glatt und straff gespannt erscheint. Sie erscheint mit den unter ihr befindlichen Weichteilen wie fest verlötet; der Fingerdruck hinterläßt keine Delle; sie kann in Falten nicht abgehoben werden. Die Extremitäten erscheinen verdünnt, das Gesicht hat einen greisenhaften, starren Ausdruck. Aktive und passive Beweglichkeit sind eingeschränkt (EHRMANN-BRÜNAUER). Meist ist die Temperatur auffallend niedrig. Die Prognose ist im allgemeinen ungünstig. Die Unterscheidung der beiden Skleromformen verdanken wir LUITHLEN. Die Differenzen gegenüber der Sklerodermie liegen auf der Hand. Die letztere kommt, wenn auch sehr selten, bei Neugeborenen vor. Es fehlen aber hier durchaus die allgemeinen Störungen, Puls, Atmung und Temperatur sind normal. Auch gibt die im frühen Alter auftretende Sklerodermie eine günstige Prognose.

Als selbständiges Krankheitsbild beschreibt BUSCHKE das Skleroedema adultorum, welches er von der eigentlichen Sklerodermie vollkommen abtrennt. Diese Affektion stellt sich dar als eine Versteifung der tieferen Schichten der Cutis, der Tela subcutanea und wahrscheinlich zum Teil auch der Fascie und Muskulatur, welche ziemlich akut, anscheinend meist am Nacken beginnend, sich kontinuierlich auf das Gesicht, die Oberarme und mehr oder weniger weite Strecken des Rumpfes bis zum Abdomen fortsetzt. Die unteren Extremitäten können auch befallen sein. Diese eigenartige Veränderung der Haut tritt entweder unter voller sonstiger Gesundheit oder mit den Symptomen der Hinfälligkeit und Schwäche ein. Sie schließt sich am häufigsten anscheinend an eine vorausgegangene influenzaähnliche Affektion, auch an Scharlach und Parotitis an. Symptomatologisch ist hervorzuheben die absolute Schmerzlosigkeit; nur ein Gefühl von Spannung und Rigidität ist vorhanden. Durch die Starrheit der Haut wird die Beweglichkeit der unter der Haut gelegenen Gebilde mehr oder weniger beeinträchtigt (Atmung, Funktion der Extremitäten, Störung der Gesichtsmimik). Die Haut pflegt meist blaß zu sein (höchstens findet sich gelegentlich eine geringe Cyanose) und ist bei der Palpation in den oberen Schichten samtartig. Die Induration liegt in den tieferen Partien und ist so fest, daß eine Delle nicht eingedrückt werden kann und fast das Gefühl des Knorpels entsteht. Die Abgrenzung kann diffus oder scharf sein. Im allgemeinen lassen sich Hautfalten nicht abheben. Nennenswerte Sensibilitätsstörungen und Störungen der Talg- und Schweißsekretion sind nicht vorhanden; auch an den inneren Organen wurden Veränderungen nicht nachgewiesen. Die Affektion entsteht entweder ziemlich akut in Wochen, oder es dauert Monate, bis die Induration zum Abschluß gelangt ist und nicht mehr fortschreitet. Der weitere Verlauf ist durchaus gutartig; das Leiden dauert zwar Monate und Jahre, geht aber allmählich, ohne daß die Behandlung einen nennenswerten Einfluß zeigt, entweder restlos zurück oder es bleibt in geringem Umfange im Gesicht oder an den Extremitäten oder am Rumpfe die Induration zurück. Histologisch finden sich nur in den tieferen Teilen der Haut Veränderungen. Es besteht keine Hautatrophie, keine Pigmentierung, auch keine Depigmentierung.

Mit diesen Bemerkungen ist die Differentialdiagnose zwischen Sklerodermie und Sklerödem gegeben: während die Sklerodermie nach Monaten und Jahren in atrophische Zustände übergeht, und die charakteristischen Pigmentverschiebungen aufweist, zeigt das Sklerödem wie oben erwähnt weder Pigmentanomalien, noch oberflächliche Veränderungen der Epidermis und der oberen Coriumschichten. BUSCHKE selbst rechnet die Sklerodermie der Neugeborenen mit ihrer schnellen, den Körper überziehenden tiefen, harten Infiltration ohne entzündliche Symptome mit Ausgang in vollkommene Heilung mit Wahrscheinlichkeit dem Sklerödem zu.

Sehr schwierig kann die Unterscheidung zwischen chronischem *Gelenkrheumatismus* und Sklerodermie sein. Wie schon gesagt, kann der sklerodermatische Prozeß häufig zum großen Teil seinen Sitz in den Gelenken haben, auf der anderen Seite findet man bei arthritischen Affektionen Veränderungen der periartikulären Gewebe durch ödematöse Infiltration und ähnliche Vorgänge häufig genug, so daß es Fälle gibt, in denen eine sichere Unterscheidung unmöglich wird.

Ähnliche Beziehungen und differentialdiagnostische Schwierigkeiten können sich gelegentlich zwischen der Sklerodermie und der *Polymyositis subacuta* ergeben. Einen derartigen Fall hat OPPENHEIM beobachtet, den auch CASSIRER lange Zeit Gelegenheit hatte zu sehen. Während in den ersten Stadien an der Diagnose Dermatopolymyositis, die sich auch auf die Schleimhäute ausgedehnt hatte, kein Zweifel sein konnte, nahmen im weiteren Verlauf die Haut und die Muskeln eine solche Beschaffenheit an, daß man an die Diagnose einer Sklerodermie bzw. einer Myosklerose denken mußte. Eine starke Schmerzhaftigkeit der Muskulatur bestand allerdings dauernd. Und auf diesen Punkt wird wohl auch in Zukunft als wichtigstes Moment geachtet werden müssen, wenn auch nicht zu bezweifeln ist, daß eine starke Schmerzhaftigkeit der Muskeln auch bei myosklerotischen Prozessen gelegentlich vorkommt. Über eine ähnliche Beobachtung wie die OPPENHEIMs berichten ROSENTHAL und HOFFMANN [1]. KLINGMAN hat diesen Fragen vor kurzem seine Aufmerksamkeit zugewendet. Er beschreibt 12 Fälle von akuter und chronischer Dermatomyositis, die ätiologisch mit einer rheumatischen Erkrankung in Verbindung standen und nach Ablauf der entzündlichen Erscheinungen das Bild einer typischen Sklerodermie zeigten. Nach seiner Auffassung führen die Fälle von Dermatoneuromyositis mit Haut-, Muskel- und Nervenschädigung zu typischer Sklerodermie, während diejenigen, bei denen keine Nervenläsionen festzustellen sind, das Bild der Sklerodermie ohne trophische Störungen darbieten. Auch ALLAN weist auf dis Schwierigkeiten hin, die häufig der Diagnosenstellung entgegenstehen; FRIEDMANN und LANGMEAD (zit. nach EHRMANN-BRÜNAUER) sind der Ansicht, daß es sich bei beiden Erkrankungen um einen identischen Zustand handelt. Die Abgrenzung von äußerlich ähnlichen Krankheitsbildern, dem varicösen Symptomenkomplex und der Poikilodermie haben im wesentlichen nur dermatologisches Interesse.

Therapie.

Den nachfolgenden Ausführungen muß zunächst die betrübliche Tatsache vorangestellt werden, daß wir noch nicht im Besitze eines Mittels sind, mit dem wir die Krankheit wirksam zu beeinflussen vermögen. Gewiß sind Heilungen berichtet worden; aber wir wissen, daß die circumscripte Sklerodermie auch ohne jede Behandlung heilen kann, so daß Berichte über Heilungen durch bestimmte angewandte Mittel stets mit einer gewissen Skepsis zu bewerten sind (LEWIN, HELLER-HERXHEIMER u. a.). EHRMANN und BRÜNAUER bemerken, daß die diffuse Sklerodermie wohl Remissionen und Exacerbationen macht; eine wirkliche Spontanheilung haben sie jedoch im Laufe von 40 Jahren dermatologischer Tätigkeit nicht gesehen. H. CURSCHMANN macht darauf aufmerksam, daß die Therapie von der Pathogenese auszugehen habe. Man solle zunächst die pluri- und monoglandulären Störungen behandeln, von denen die ersten relativ am häufigsten seien. Zur Entscheidung der Frage, welche Organstörungen überwiegen, sei neben der einfachen klinischen Beobachtung heranzuziehen die Stoffwechseluntersuchung, insbesondere die Bestimmung des respiratorischen Grundumsatzes unter Hinzufügung der Prüfung der spezifisch dynamischen Einwirkung der Fleischkost auf den Grundumsatz.

Von den organo-therapeutischen Mitteln ist dem *Thyrrheoidin* die meiste Aufmerksamkeit geschenkt worden. Es wurde zuerst mit großer Zuversicht empfohlen, zumal es auch zu der von einigen Seiten aufgestellten Schilddrüsentheorie der Krankheit recht gut paßte. Es wurden glänzende Resultate berichtet, zuerst wohl von SINGER, der das Glück hatte, in seinem Fall von Sklerodermie kombiniert mit BASEDOWscher Krankheit beide Krankheiten unter dem Gebrauch dieses Mittels sich sehr wesentlich bessern zu sehen. Ähnliche Erfolge berichteten GRÜNFELD, STIEGLITZ und viele andere; aber in zahlreichen Fällen hat das Mittel vollkommen versagt, auch vielfach in den Fällen, in denen wir es angewendet haben. Über ähnliche Mißerfolge berichten VON NOORDEN, VON NOTTHAFFT, SCHOLZ und DÖBEL, SCHÄFFER, HERXHEIMER, HATOUSEK, STUDNIČKA und viele andere. ROUQES sah unter 80 Fällen in mehr als der Hälfte Erfolg und er rät, es in kleinen Dosen für Monate und Jahre zu geben. H. CURSCHMANN empfiehlt bei der Thyrrheoidinbehandlung mit der Dosierung sehr

---

[1] ROSENTHAL u. HOFFMANN: Z. Nervenheilk. 80.

vorsichtig vorzugehen und verabreicht zunächst 2mal täglich höchstens 0,05 Thyrrheoidin MERCK; nach 2 Wochen steigert er die Dosis langsam bis auf 3—4mal täglich 0,05 Thyrrheoidin. Bei Eintreten von Übelkeiten raten PAUTRIER und VORINGER und WHITEHOUSE die Behandlung abzubrechen (zit. nach EHRMANN und BRÜNAUER). Wichtig ist jedenfalls, wie bereits erwähnt, daß man vorher eine Grundsatzbestimmung ausführt und sich in seinen Maßnahmen von ihrem Ergebnis leiten läßt. Im allgemeinen wird man VON NOTTHAFFT Recht geben müssen, daß es nur insofern berechtigt ist, die erzielten Erfolge auf das Thyrrheoidin zu beziehen, als das Thyrrheoidin den allgemeinen Stoffwechsel stark beeinflußt und in dem einen oder anderen Falle dadurch auch eine günstige Wirkung auf die sklerodermatischen Hautpartien ausübt. Ein spezifisches Heilmittel ist es jedenfalls nicht, und die Behandlung bedarf unter allen Umständen sehr sorgfältiger Überwachung.

Von anderen Organpräparaten ist von UHLENHUTH Nebennierenextrakt versucht worden, ebenso von WINFIELD und MILLARD. SIROTA sah nach intracutanen Adrenalininjektionen eine Rückbildung der verhärteten Herde. HARVIER und LICHTNITZ sahen bei einer *ovariellen* Therapie mit Injektionen von Follikelextrakt rasche Rückbildung der Hauterscheinungen. SELLEI verordnet Pankreastabletten (0,25 Pankrin, Chemische Fabrik Richter, Pest, 8—9 pro die), außerdem Rohpankreas in der Suppe täglich auf nüchternen Magen, $1^1/_2$ Stunden später salzsaures Pepsin. Monatelang soll eine Diät mit wenig Fett und leicht verdaulichen Speisen innegehalten werden. Bei Raynaudsymptomen sei diese Therapie erfolglos. MICHAELIS hat einen schweren Fall von Sklerodermie und Myosklerose, der mit Raynaudsymptomen kompliziert war, unter dem Einfluß einer Insulinbehandlung sich ganz erheblich bessern sehen, nachdem alle vorher angewandten therapeutischen Versuche erfolglos geblieben waren; einen ähnlichen verblüffenden Erfolg mit der gleichen Therapie hat STEINER zu verzeichnen. SCHÖNGUT hat Padutin erfolgreich versucht. Mit einer Behandlung eines Extraktes von Mesenterialdrüsen vom Schaf (Coeliacin 0,3 1—2mal täglich) will SCHWERDT Besserung erzielt haben. Auch KÖLLE empfiehlt diese Behandlung.

In den letzten Jahren ist man dazu übergegangen, sich der pluriglandulären Therapie zu bedienen. FLETSCHER verwendete Schilddrüsenextrakt und Hypophysinpräparate im Gegensatz zu ACUNA ohne Erfolg; LEREBOULLET sowie BURGHI sahen von einer kombinierten Behandlung mit Schilddrüsen-, Hypophysin- und Nebennierenpräparaten Besserung der subjektiven Beschwerden und Zurückgehen der objektiven Erscheinungen. Unterbrechung der Behandlung führte zum Stillstand der Besserung. Auch wir haben mehrfach in schweren komplizierten und bis dahin stetig progredienten Fällen durch eine Behandlung mit verschiedenen Organextrakten (Thyrrheoidin, Ovoglandol, bzw. Thelygan und Hypophysin) in Kombination mit parenteraler Eiweißtherapie (Yatrencasein) auffällige Erfolge erzielt und dabei beobachten können, daß die Besserung bei Aufhören der Behandlung stillstand. Andere Autoren wandten Kombinationen von Schilddrüsen- und Ovarialpräparaten an. DEVOTO gibt ein Pluriglandol benanntes Präparat (Schilddrüse, Hypophyse, Thymus, Hämostasin). Andere Autoren können diese günstigen Erfolge mit Organpräparaten nicht bestätigen und EHRMANN und BRÜNAUER weisen mit Recht darauf hin, daß man bei der Beurteilung derartiger günstiger oder ungünstiger Behandlungsresultate immer bedenken müsse, daß es einerseits zeitweise Spontanremissionen namentlich in der warmen Jahreszeit gebe, und daß man andererseits niemals wisse, welche Substanzen in den kombinierten Präparaten wirksam seien. Von verschiedener Seite vorgenommene Implantationen von endokrinen Geweben sind erfolglos geblieben.

HAMMER[1] verwendete Röntgenreizbestrahlung der Thymus unter Abblendung der Schilddrüse. In einem Falle fand er einen günstigen Einfluß, ein zweiter Fall verhielt sich refraktär. Durch die Reizung der Thymus sollte eine endokrine Stoffwechselbalance eintreten, unter der von HAMMER gemachten Voraussetzung, daß es sich bei der Sklerodermie um eine Thyrrheotoxikose handelt. DONATH bestreitet diese Auffassung und führt den HAMMERschen Erfolg auf eine wohl unabsichtlich erfolgte Röntgenreizung der Schilddrüse zurück. Die Entfernung eines Epithelkörperchens soll nach LERICHE und JUNG günstig auf die Störung des Kalkstoffwechsels wirken. HEINISMAN und ČERNI haben 2 Fälle erfolgreich mit Röntgenbestrahlung der Schilddrüse und Hypophyse behandelt; andere Autoren bestrahlen die Thymus in Kombination mit diesen Drüsen. NOBL und GLASBERG empfehlen Diathermiebehandlung der Schilddrüse.

SCHÖNHOF hat die Wirbelsäulengegend bei diffuser Sklerodermie mit Röntgenstrahlen behandelt, ebenso VIGANO, letzterer mit folgender Technik (zit. Ref. STIEFLER, Z.N. 57, 348): S.E. (Distanz) 35 cm, Filter 0,5 Zn + 2 Al; $^1/_3$ DE (H.E.D.). Therapie jeden 8. Tag 7—8 Wochen lang. Mit dieser Methode hat ZUPPA bemerkenswerte Erfolge erzielt, während er bei Bestrahlung der Schilddrüse und der erkrankten Hautstellen nur sehr bescheidene Erfolge hatte. Sklerodermatische Hautpartien haben wiederholt von verschiedenen Autoren eine Röntgenbestrahlung erfahren, allerdings mit widersprechenden Erfolgen, z. B. konten MARBURG-SGALITZER die guten Erfahrungen anderer Autoren nicht bestätigen.

Die Quarzlichtbestrahlung ist in letzter Zeit wiederholt ausgeführt worden, meist als Unterstützung der pluriglandulären Therapie. ARMANI empfiehlt sie frühzeitig und bei Jugendlichen anzuwenden, JANICHEWSKI erwähnt, daß Kranke mit alten und schweren sklerodermatischen Veränderungen gegen diese Behandlung refraktär sind. Nach JANICHEWSKI soll die Bestrahlung mit einer Hanauer Lampe von 750 Kerzen Lichtstärke täglich im Beginn 5 Minuten lang, steigend bis 30 Minuten durchgeführt werden. LOUSTE, JUSTER und DAVID haben die gemeinsame Anwendung von Quarzlicht und Jodkaliumionisation mit Erfolg durchgeführt. Auch sonst wurde die Iontophorese hauptsächlich von französischen Autoren empfohlen. EHRMANN und BRÜNAUER haben diese Behandlung bereits 1888 durchgeführt und die Wirksamkeit der verschiedensten Substanzen konstatiert, vor allem des Jod.

MACKAY hat Radiumchlorid intravenös mit einer Anfangsdosis von 25 Mikrogramm und weitere Dosen von 10 Mikrogramm in Zwischenräumen von etwa 2 Wochen bis zu einer Gesamtmenge von 190—250 Mikrogramm injiziert. Es erfolgte allgemeine Besserung und eine partielle Absorption der verhärteten Gewebe. Ähnliches berichtet STUDNIČKA. Bei der umschriebenen Sklerodermie ist die Radiumbehandlung von ZOON, HERCZOG und WERTHER empfohlen worden (zit. nach EHRMANN-BRÜNAUER). EPSTEIN verwendet mit Erfolg Thorium-X-Salbe.

In allen möglichen Formen wurde der *elektrische* Strom angewendet. BROCQ u. a. erzielte glänzende Erfolge mit der Elektrolyse in Fällen, die bis dahin jeder Behandlung getrotzt und keine Zeichen einer spontanen Heilung gezeigt hatten. Andere benutzten den galvanischen Strom, andere wieder die Franklinisation. Hier und da wurde ein Erfolg gesehen, meist war auch diese Behandlung nutzlos. LEREDDE und THOMAS wandten elektrische Bäder an, mußten sie aber aufgeben, weil sich am Unterarm und an der Schulter Schorfe bildeten, die nur langsam verheilten. HUET und SICARD wollen durch Anwendung von Hochfrequenzströmen Erfolge erzielt haben; diese werden auch von anderen Autoren empfohlen.

---
[1] HAMMER: Münch. med. Wschr. **1921 II**, 1109.

Die *Massage* ist vielfach verwendet worden. Sie leistet unzweifelhaft nützliches, indem sie eine gewisse Geschmeidigkeit der Haut, wenigstens für einige Zeit aufrecht erhält und außerdem die Muskulatur stärkt und vor der Inaktivitätsatrophie bewahrt. LEWIN-HELLER machen andererseits darauf aufmerksam, daß sie durch Reizung der an und für sich entzündeten Gefäße wohl auch schaden könnte. Die Substanz, mit der massiert wird, trägt jedenfalls nichts zur Einwirkung bei. HELLER und FRANKE fanden Salicylvaselin und Resorbin wirkungslos. MOSLER empfiehlt Einreibungen mit Ichthyolvaselin, dazu Vollbäder mit 60 g Ichthyol und innerlich 0,1 Calcium-Sulfo-Ichthyol und sah davon einigen Erfolg. EHRMANN und BRÜNAUER berichten, daß bei der Behandlung umschriebener sklerodermatischer Flecken die Massage in nahezu allen Fällen sich erfolgreich auswirkte, wenn ihr jedes Mal eine Glühlichtbehandlung oder ein warmes Bad vorausgeschickt wurde. Sie machen darauf aufmerksam, daß das Massieren nicht ein ausdauerndes Streichen sein muß, sondern mehr ein Kneten zwischen den Fingern, bei bandförmigen Herden ein Dehnen. Auch andere Autoren haben mit dieser Therapie gute Erfolge erzielt. Vorsichtige Gymnastik vermag wohl in passenden Fällen einiges zu nützen.

Hydriatische Prozeduren wurden oft angewendet: warme Duschen (VIDAL, MOSLER), Dampfbäder, die verschiedenen natürlichen Bäder, besonders Moor- und Schwefelbäder, auch Radiumbäder und Radiumtrinkkuren wurden empfohlen. Heißluftbehandlung wurde zuerst von NEUMANN angewendet. Wir haben einige Male, namentlich in den Fällen von Sklerodaktylie, ebenso wie OPPENHEIM, von einer konsequenten Heißluftbehandlung recht gute Erfolge gesehen.

EHRMANN und BRÜNAUER berichten, daß in manchen ihrer Fälle Herde, die sich im erythematösen Stadium befanden, durch Alkoholumschläge nach SCHÄFER zum Verschwinden gebracht wurden, ohne daß es zur Induration gekommen sei.

Von den *internen* Mitteln sind neben den oben genannten vor allem Tonika zur Anwendung gekommen: Eisen, Arsen, Chinin, Strychnin. Die Beobachtung, daß die Allylsulfocarbanide (Fibrolysin, zuletzt von SEMINARIO und DANERI empfohlen, Thiosinamin) auf Narbengewebe erweichend einwirken, haben zuerst HEBRA dazu geführt, Injektionen von Thiosinamid zu versuchen; auch SCHOLZ und KAPOSI, sowie BRAMWELL empfehlen das Mittel, an dessen Stelle jetzt meist das Fibrolysin angewendet wird. Unsere eigenen Erfahrungen lauten durchaus nicht durchwegs günstig; aber wir raten doch zu Versuchen mit dem Mittel (jeden 2. Tag 0,3—0,5 ccm einer 15% alkoholischen Lösung subcutan). EHRMANN und BRÜNAUER ebenso wie SEGURA erwähnen, daß in einzelnen Fällen diese Injektionen von bedrohlichen Erscheinungen gefolgt sein können. HERZOG u. a. versuchten intravenöse Injektionen einer 10%igen Kochsalzlösung in einer Dosis von 10 ccm durchschnittlich 30 Injektionen: die cyanotische Haut wurde rötlich und wärmer, Schmerzen und Parästhesien ließen nach, Trockenheit und Pigmentierung besserten sich, auch reinigten sich die Geschwüre. Den Erfolg der Kochsalzinjektionen führt der Autor in erster Linie auf Beeinflussung der Kreislaufstörungen und der Vasomotilität zurück. Andere Autoren (SANNICANDRO) haben ähnlich gute Erfahrungen mit dieser Therapie gemacht. GAUCH, SOHIER und DE COURRÈGES wollen mit intravenösen Injektionen von Pilocarpinnitrat (5 mg) Erfolge gesehen haben, KEN KURÉ, HERZOG mit Pilocarpin.

Eine unspezifische Reiztherapie stellen die von KLINGMÜLLER u. a. empfohlenen Terpentininjektionen dar; andere Autoren empfehlen Caseosan und Milchinjektionen (STRANDBERG, zit. nach EHRMANN und BRÜNAUER). Salicylpräparate wurden zuerst von PHILIPPSON warm empfohlen. Die Resultate lauten widersprechend. BALLER und ERKES empfahlen Lebertran.

In einem Fall von EHRMANN und BRÜNAUER wurde neben Salol auch noch Massage, Gymnastik und Diätbehandlung ausgeführt. Unter dieser Therapie trat volle Heilung nach Monaten ein, nachdem die Erkrankung unter zahlreichen Nachschüben 10 Jahre angedauert hatte. BREITMANN wandte mit Erfolg Joddämpfe an.

Auch *chirurgische* Eingriffe sind gemacht worden. HOFFA excidierte eine streifenförmige sklerodermatische Stelle, angeblich weil aus der lokalisierten oft eine diffuse Sklerodermie wird. Wir schließen uns LEWIN und HELLER an, die diesen Eingriff als durchaus zwecklos bezeichnen. Neuerdings ist die Methode der *periarteriellen Sympathektomie* empfohlen worden. Diese ist schon vor langen Jahren von HIGIER bei gewissen vasomotorisch-trophischen Erkrankungen angegeben worden. In neuerer Zeit haben sie LERICHE in Frankreich und BRÜNING in Deutschland wieder in Anwendung gebracht, und zwar kommen im wesentlichen 3 Operationen in Frage: 1. die Durchschneidung der präganglionären Äste, der Rami communicantes, 2. die Entfernung von einem oder mehreren Ganglien, bzw. des Grenzstranges, 3. die eigentliche periarterielle Sypathektomie. Von dem von uns seit langem stets vertretenen Gedanken ausgehend, daß die Nervenreizung gegenüber der Nervenlähmung in der Pathogenese der vasomotorisch-trophischen Störungen eine überragende Rolle spielt, haben BRÜNING und FORSTER einen Fall von Sklerodermie in dieser Weise mit dem Endresultat der völligen Heilung behandelt. Bei der Nachuntersuchung des Falles, dessen Operation ein Jahr zurücklag, konnte BRÜNING feststellen, daß die früheren schmerzhaften Anfälle von Gefäßspasmen, die mit Kälte und Cyanose der Hand einhergingen, seit der Operation nicht ein einziges Mal wiedergekehrt waren. Hand und Finger waren bedeutend schlanker geworden, so daß die Konturen der Fingergelenke besser heraustraten. Die Beweglichkeit der Finger und die Gebrauchsfähigkeit der Hand hatten sich erheblich gebessert.

Wie bei der RAYNAUDschen Krankheit sind auch bei der Sklerodermie die Erfahrungen, die wir selbst mit der Sympathektomie gemacht haben, bzw. an von anderer Seite operierten Fällen gesehen haben, nicht besonders günstige. Soweit wir beurteilen können, scheint es sich meist um vorübergehende Erfolge zu handeln.

LERICHE und FONTAINE behandelten im ganzen 9 Fälle, davon 2 Fälle generalisierter Sklerodermie von denen der eine auch Erscheinungen von Sklerodaktylie zeigte und einige Fälle von Sklerodermie des Gesichts und der oberen Extremitäten. Sie hatten recht erfreuliche Erfolge zu verzeichnen, soweit es sich um Frühfälle handelte. In den Fällen, in denen die obere Extremität, der Hals und das Gesicht betroffen sind, verbinden sie mit dem Eingriff am cervicalen Grenzstrang eine peribrachiale Sympathektomie. Bei isolierter Sklerodermie beschränken sie sich auf die zuletzt erwähnte Operation. An den unteren Extremitäten wird entsprechend die perifemorale Sympathektomie bei örtlichen Schädigungen angewandt, Sympathektomie des lumbalen Grenzstranges mit perifemoraler Sympathektomie bei Schädigungen, die den Beckengürtel überschreiten. Bei eingetretener Mumifikation ist die Operation zwecklos. BREGMAN führte die Sympathektomie bei einem mit Sklerodermie kombinierten Fall von RAYNAUDscher Krankheit an der Arteria brachialis aus. Während der Operation trat ein starker Gefäßkrampf auf mit Exacerbation der Schmerzen, die sich alsbald besserten. Nach 6 Monaten war ein recht guter Erfolg zu verzeichnen. PERITZ hat in einem Falle von Sklerodermie und Sklerodaktylie des rechten Armes und der rechten Hand die Exstirpation des rechten Ganglion stellatum und eines Teiles des rechten Grenzstranges vornehmen lassen. Als Folgeerscheinung stellte er Abnahme der Sklerodermie und Hebung des Allgemeinzustandes fest. Die Besserung hielt ein halbes Jahr an; dann trat eine erhebliche Verschlimmerung ein, die Sklerodermie verbreitete sich über den ganzen Körper und der Zustand der rechten Extremität verschlimmerte sich erheblich. PERITZ rät, nur solche Fälle zu operieren, bei denen die Erkrankung viele Jahre stationär blieb. BRÜNING bestätigt, daß bei schweren Fällen von Sklerodermie die Sympathicusoperation versagt. SUTOVA operierte eine 28jährige Frau mit allgemeiner Sklerodermie: es wurde an der Aorta die Adventitia in einer Ausdehnung von 2—3 cm, an der Arteria iliaca von 6—7 cm entfernt. Es stellte sich eine weitgehende Besserung der Haut an den Armen und Beinen ein; sie wurde bedeutend weicher und die Schweißsekretion setzte ein. Nach 3 Wochen trat jedoch eine erneute Hautverdickung auf. Ein 7jähriger Knabe wurde wegen einer Sklerodermie an der inneren Fläche des rechten Schenkels an der Arteria iliaca communis und der Arteria poplitea operiert. Die Haut verlor ihre harte Konsistenz. Es wurde in diesem Falle eine Nachbehandlung mit ultravioletten Strahlen durchgeführt. Der Kranke wurde 3 Jahre beobachtet, ohne daß ein Fortschreiten der Erkrankung festzustellen war. ADSON, O'LEARY und BROWN haben die vasospastischen Typen der Sklerodermie mittels Resektion der sympathischen Ganglien und Trunci behandelt. Sie berichten über 16 Beobachtungen. Sie haben die Erfahrung gemacht, daß der Erfolg der Behandlung von dem jeweiligen Stadium der Sklerodermie abhängig ist. Am günstigsten liegen die Fälle, in denen die Gefäßstörungen der Entwicklung der Sklerodermie vorausgehen (MAYO-ADSON). KREIBICH (zit. nach EHRMANN und BRÜNAUER) hat in einem Falle von Sklerodaktylie eine wesentliche Besserung nach der Operation auftreten sehen. Diesen bedingten Erfolgen stehen eine Reihe Publikationen über Mißerfolge gegenüber (BOGDANOVIC, SCHÖNHOF, ORMSBY u. a.). Mit Recht bemerken EHRMANN und BRÜNAUER, daß angesichts der Tatsache, daß der Prozeß bei der diffusen Sklerodermie ein diffuser oder plurizentrischer ist, die Ablösung der Adventitia nur einen Einfluß auf das von dieser Arterie versorgte Gebiet ausüben kann. Auch H. CURSCHMANN drückt sich vorsichtig aus: bei einer partiellen Sklerodermie hat sich die periarterielle Sympathektomie anscheinend bisweilen bewährt.

Über die Therapie der Hemiatrophia faciei ist wenig zu sagen. Man hat ohne besonderen Erfolg die gleichen Medikamente wie bei der Sklerodermie angewendet. Die von manchen Autoren empfohlene Galvanisation haben andere wieder ohne jeden Erfolg ausgeführt. In einigen Fällen hat sich die kosmetische Behandlung (Paraffin, Ölvaselin) bewährt. MOSZKOVICZ verzeichnet ein zufriedenstellendes kosmetisches Resultat bei einem Kranken, bei welchem er einen Fettlappen vom Oberschenkel auf die Wange transplantiert hat, BØE wendet Ausdehnungsprothesen im Mund an, wobei Fettgewebe und Muskeln an Volumen zunahmen.

VII. Das akute umschriebene Ödem (QUINCKEsches Ödem).

Im Jahre 1882 beschrieb QUINCKE ein Krankheitsbild, das er folgendermaßen charakterisierte: „In der Haut und im Unterhautzellgewebe treten an umschriebenen Stellen ödematöse Schwellungen von 2—10 cm Durchmesser auf; am häufigsten werden die Extremitäten befallen, besonders in der Umgebung der Gelenke, aber auch Rumpf und Gesicht sind beteiligt; die Schwellungen scheinen nicht scharf abgegrenzt zu sein, die normale Hautfarbe ist nicht wesentlich verändert, bisweilen etwas blässer, andermal etwas röter als normal. Es besteht etwas Spannung und Jucken. Auch die Schleimhäute können gleichzeitig befallen sein, die Lippen, das Gaumensegel, der Pharynx und Larynx, die Darm- und Magenschleimhaut. Die Schwellungen entstehen und vergehen rasch, im Verlauf von Stunden, höchstens Tagen, aber rezidivieren sehr oft. Das Allgemeinbefinden pflegt wenig oder gar nicht gestört zu sein. Das Leiden zeigt nahe Beziehungen und Übergänge zur Urticaria." Im gleichen Jahre behandelte ein Schüler QUINCKEs, DINKELACKER, in seiner Dissertation die Affektion ausführlicher.

Bereits 10 Jahre vor der QUINCKEschen Publikation hat MILTON die gleiche Erkrankung als „Giant Urticaria" beschrieben und hat es auch klar ausgesprochen, daß seine Fälle sich auch von den schwersten Formen der Urticaria scharf unterscheiden. Noch früher haben STOLPERTUS 1778 und ERICHTON 1801 einschlägige Fälle mitgeteilt. Ferner beschrieb GRAVES die Affektion im Jahre 1848 exakt und schlagend. Von wichtigeren Arbeiten aus der späteren Zeit nennen wir die von BOERNER, JOSEPH, STRUEBING, SCHLESINGER, RAPIN, COLLINS. Auch QUINCKE selbst hat später noch einmal mit GROSS zusammen einen Beitrag zur Pathologie dieses Leidens geliefert. Endlich hat er zuletzt 1921 zusammenfassend über die Krankheit berichtet.

Die Nomenklatur der Krankheit ist eine außerordentlich verschiedenartige. Die einen betonen in ihrer Namensgebung die engen Beziehungen zur Urticaria. Ältere französische Autoren haben die ätiologischen Beziehungen besonders hervorgehoben und vom rheumatischen und arthritischen Ödem gesprochen. Das Umherziehen des Ödems über den ganzen Körper kommt in anderen Bezeichnungen zum Ausdruck. QUINCKE gab ihr den Namen „akutes umschriebenes Hautödem". 1917 hat dieser in einer Arbeit über Rheumatismus darauf hingewiesen, daß das herdförmige Auftreten dieser Schwellungen zeige, daß gegen den in den Körpersäften kreisenden Giftstoff nicht alle Teile der Haut gleich empfindlich sind, oder daß in bestimmten Regionen des Gewebes der Haut (oder der versorgenden Nerven) eine größere elektive Anziehung besteht, als an anderen. Bei demselben Individuum wurden in verschiedenen Anfällen oft die gleichen Hautstellen befallen, oder doch bevorzugt, z. B. beim Jodismus gewisse Stellen des Gesichts. QUINCKE vermutet, daß bei der akuten Myalgie in dem intermuskulären und intramuskulären Bindegewebe, manchmal auch bei rheumatischer Erkrankung der Gelenke und ihrer Adnexe ähnliche Vorgänge sich abspielen, wie auf der Haut bei Urticaria und dem akuten Ödem. Wie diese sind sie flüchtig, können wandern, zeigen eine Vorliebe für bestimmte Stellen.

Wir glauben, wenn wir, wie das nach den neueren Erfahrungen geschehen muß, statt Hautödem nur „Ödem" setzen, so haben wir einen genügend bezeichnenden und nichts präjudizierenden Namen. Auch QUINCKE hat in seiner letzten Publikation die Krankheit „akutes umschriebenes Ödem" bezeichnet. SCHLESINGER hat vorgeschlagen, alle die hierher gehörigen Affektionen als *Hydrops Hypostrophos* zu bezeichnen, doch hat diese Bezeichnung kein rechtes Bürgerrecht gewinnen können.

Ätiologie.

Das akute umschriebene Ödem ist keine seltene Erkrankung; es scheint bei Männern und Frauen ungefähr gleich häufig vorzukommen. Von 36 Fällen, die QUINCKE bis 1921 beobachtete, waren 18 Männer, 18 Frauen. Unter letzteren fand er mehr atypische und kompliziertere Fälle.

Die von der Krankheit befallenen Individuen stehen meist im 3. und 4. Lebensjahrzehnt. Das Durchschnittsalter ist etwa 26 Jahre, jedoch bleibt kein Lebensalter ganz davon verschont. DINKELACKER beschreibt einen Fall, in dem mit 3 Monaten die ersten Krankheitszeichen auftraten; WASON sah bei einem 3 Monate alten Kinde, dessen Bruder an ähnlichen Schwellungen litt, während 4 Wochen wiederholt umschriebene Anschwellungen an verschiedenen Körperteilen auftreten; das Kind erstickte an einem perakut einsetzenden umschriebenen Pharynx- und Epiglottisödem. Auch sonst finden sich in der neueren

Literatur ähnliche Beobachtungen. Wir selbst sahen ebenfalls einen Kranken mit sehr charakteristischen Symptomen, der angab, von frühester Kindheit an unter diesen Erscheinungen zu leiden. Andererseits haben wir eine 79jährige Frau gesehen, bei der das Leiden 10 Jahre vorher zum erstenmal aufgetreten war. RAVEN beschreibt eine 86jährige Frau, bei der plötzlich die rechte Zungenhälfte anschwoll; das Ödem war nach einem Tage verschwunden, ein ähnlicher Anfall kam später noch einmal wieder.

Die *Heredität* spielt in der Ätiologie dieser Krankheit eine große Rolle. Sie gehört zu denjenigen Leiden, die nicht selten den Mitgliedern einer Familie als stets recht unbequemes, den Lebensgenuß beeinträchtigendes Erbe für einen längeren oder kürzeren Abschnitt ihres Lebens mitgegeben ist. Es gibt sogar Familien, in denen ganz regelmäßig eine Reihe von Mitgliedern einer besonders gefährlichen Form dieses Leidens, dem Glottisödem, erliegen. Solche Beobachtungen verdanken wir QUINCKE und DINKELACKER, STRUEBING, SCHLESINGER, OSLER, DIEHL, BULLOCH[1], ENSOR, MENDEL, RAPIN u. v. a. H. W. SIEMENS hat über die spezielle Vererbungspathologie dieses Leidens gearbeitet. Er stellt fest, daß dominante Vererbung nur in einer Reihe von Fällen beobachtet worden ist, während in vielen anderen Fällen nichts von Erblichkeit zu konstatieren war. Das akute umschriebene Ödem konnte durch fünf Generationen verfolgt werden. In einem großen Stammbaum, der von OSLER publiziert ist, finden sich 20 Kranke gegenüber 15 Gesunden (darunter ein Konduktor). Überspringen kommt gelegentlich vor. ENSOR sah unter 80 Familienmitgliedern in 3 Generationen 33 von der Krankheit befallen werden, von denen 12 an Glottisödem starben. In der Familie MENDELs kamen wegen der gefährlichen Lokalisation am Kehldeckel sechs von den neun behafteten Personen infolge Erstickung ums Leben; ganz ähnlich die Familie, von der DEUTSCH berichtet. Gelegentlich einmal wurden nur die männlichen Mitglieder der Familie befallen; doch ist das keineswegs die Regel. In einer Reihe von Fällen wiederholt sich bei den einzelnen Mitgliedern das Krankheitsbild mit photographischer Treue, in anderen kommen Abweichungen vor, indem z. B. das Erbrechen, das bei dem einen Familienmitglied die Schwellungen begleitet, bei dem anderen fehlt. 1922 haben PHILLIPS und BARROWS auf Grund der bis dahin bekannten Fälle zusammenfassend und kritisch zur Frage der Erblichkeit des QUINCKEschen Ödems Stellung genommen. Sie stellten unter den Kindern der Behafteten in 31 Familien 168 Kranke zu 167 Gesunden fest; in 16 Fällen waren beide Eltern befallener Kinder gesund. In 10 dieser Fälle war der Großvater gleichfalls behaftet. DIEHL und RAPIN berichten über das Vorkommen anderer vasomotorisch-trophischer Neurosen und Symptome in solchen Ödemfamilien. Dahin rechnen sie auch das Auftreten von Migräne, Asthma und Urticaria, die auch in den Familien der Fälle PHILLIPS-BARROWS nachgewiesen wurden. SMITH untersuchte eine Familie von 94 Personen in 5 Generationen in bezug auf Vererbung der Allergie: 56,2% Personen waren allergisch, 4 litten an Asthma, 11 an Heufieber, 15 an vasomotorischer Rhinitis, 17 an Urticaria, 6 an QUINCKEschem Ödem, 14 an Ekzem. Mit diesen Ausführungen streifen wir bereits die Forschungsergebnisse, auf die wir bei der Besprechung der Pathogenese einzugehen haben werden, die zu dem Resultate geführt haben, daß in etwa 50% aller Fälle von Allergie die Disposition, allergisch zu werden, ererbt ist (STORM VAN LEEUWEN u. a.), und daß demnach bei Durchmusterung der Familiengeschichten an QUINCKEschem Ödem leidender Patienten sich öfters das Vorhandensein anderer allergischer Erkrankungen in Aszendenz und Familie nachweisen läßt.

---

[1] BULLOCH: Treasury of human inheritance **2**, 32 (1909).

Außer der direkten gleichartigen Vererbung kommt übrigens auch noch andere Belastung vor, wie Epilepsie, Chorea. Von sonstigen Diathesen wäre noch die *gichtische* zu erwähnen. Nach der Meinung von BOLTEN ist die gichtische Konstitution die notwendige Basis für das Auftreten des angioneurotischen Ödems, gerade in den Fällen, bei denen das hier behandelte Syndrom als eine kongenitale Affektion auftritt. Diesen Zusammenhang betonen auch HIS und LINDEMANN.

ROSENTHAL hat einen erbbiologischen Beitrag geliefert, in welchem er in einer Familie, deren Mitglieder Krankheitserscheinungen, die zum Kreise des „Arthritismus" gehören, darboten, bei 4 Mitgliedern Neigung zu flüchtigen Schwellungen im Gesicht, kombiniert mit rezidivierender Facialislähmung und Lingua plicata feststellte. Als Erklärung für diese Symptomentrias wird von ihm eine erhöhte Vulnerabilität der Gewebe des Gesichtsschädels auf Grund kongenitaler Entwicklungsanomalien angenommen. Seiner Auffassung nach kommt es infolge der verminderten Widerstandsfähigkeit der Gewebe bei diesen aus Arthritismusfamilien stammenden, mit einer „präexistenten Wetterempfindlichkeit" (I. BAUER) behafteten Persönlichkeiten unter Witterungseinfluß, besonders bei Abkühlung, zu den Facialislähmungen und flüchtigen Gesichtsödemen.

Daß bei einer Reihe von Fällen *Nahrungsmittelallergene* eine ätiologisch bedeutsame Rolle spielen, ist von einer Reihe von Autoren an der Hand überzeugender Beobachtungen sichergestellt worden. Allerdings müssen wir betonen, worauf auch H. CURSCHMANN aufmerksam macht, daß im ganzen der Einfluß der Aufnahme bestimmter Nahrungsmittel (in auffälligem Gegensatz zu den Verhältnissen bei der nahe verwandten Urticaria) relativ gering ist. QUINCKE und GROSS sahen das Ödem 60 Stunden nach Genuß von Austern und Champignons entstehen, FEER nach Fischsuppe mit Hummern und Langusten, KLINKART nach Erdbeeren und Trüffeln, BLAUSTEIN nach Ziegenmilch, TURETTINI nach Milch (PASTEUR, VALLERY-RADOT und HEIMANN sowie STORM VAN LEEUWEN), Brot, Mehl und Hühnerei, DUNLAP nach Buchweizen. Der Genuß von Schweinefleisch, Kalbfleisch, Fisch, rohem Pferdefleisch wird von PASTEUR und VALLERY-RADOT und HEIMANN, STORM VAN LEEUWEN, PHILLIPS, LESNÉ und M. LEVY als ätiologisch bedeutsam angegeben. In 2 Fällen von QUINCKE wirkte fleischreiche Kost begünstigend auf das Auftreten der Krankheit. Das gleiche wurde von manchem Kranken QUINCKES von der Stuhlträgheit behauptet. Auf die gastro-intestinale Autointoxikation als Ätiologie weisen auch STAEHELIN, LE CALVÉ, MORICHEU und BEAUCHANT, LAIGNEL-LAVASTINE u. a. hin. In gleichem Sinne ist auch das Auftreten des QUINCKEschen Ödems nach Einverleibung von gewissen *Arzneimitteln* zu bewerten. Hier scheinen Salicylpräparate gelegentlich eine bedeutsame Rolle zu spielen: Aspirin (PASTEUR, VALLERY-RADOT und HEIMANN), Salicylsäure (STORM VAN LEEUWEN), Atophan (STIEFLER), Sanocrysin (GÓMEZ). STORM VAN LEEUWEN und BORRIES berichten über das Auftreten des QUINCKEschen Ödems bei Kranken, die in zahnärztlicher Behandlung standen, bei denen einerseits Lysoform, andererseits Formol, im Falle BORRIES Novocain angewandt wurden. WAGNER sah die Erkrankung nach Morphingebrauch bei einem Kinde, JOLTRAM im Verlaufe der Entwöhnung bei einem Morphinisten auftreten. Auch Nikotinismus wurde einige Male (STEINER, VALOBRA) beschuldigt. MORAWITZ beobachtete mehrere Jahre hindurch einen Patienten, bei dem Tabakrauch als Allergen wirksam war. Der Patient bekam seine Schwellungen nicht nur, wenn er selbst rauchte, sondern auch wenn er sich in rauchigen Zimmern aufhielt. Neben der Überempfindlichkeit gegen Tabakrauch bestand eine wenn auch nur geringfügige Neigung auf Salicylsäure und Pferdeserum zu reagieren. NEUDA beobachtete einen Fall, bei dem eine akute Anschwellung an den Hoden auftrat, sobald der Kranke Grünzeug angefaßt hatte. In einem Falle von Anwendung von Chromsäure auf Granulationen im Trommelfell sah Lewin das Ödem auftreten; bei gleicher Anwendung hatte sich dasselbe Bild schon früher einmal gezeigt. Etwas komplizierter liegen die Verhältnisse bei der Empfindlichkeit vieler Kranker gegen Insektenstiche, die sich nicht nur dadurch dokumentiert, daß die durch den Stich hervorgerufenen Quaddeln besonders groß sind, sondern bisweilen dadurch, daß sich an die Schwellungen an der Stichstelle anderweitige Schwellungen anschließen.

Die „focal infection" scheint in einigen Fällen eine ätiologisch bedeutsame Rolle zu spielen: Turnbull beobachtete in 2 Fällen eines jahrelang bestehenden, alle 2—3 Wochen auftretenden angioneurotischen Ödems eine chronische Eiterung der Nasennebenhöhlen mit polypösen Wucherungen und eine chronische Entzündung der Tonsillen. Nach der Operation hörten die Anfälle auf. Muench beobachtete allergische Larynxödeme infolge entzündlicher Prozesse im Rachen, Weiss und Florentin im Anschluß an einen kleinen Absceß in der Vallecula. Toxine aus einem Entzündungsherd dürften in folgendem Falle Quinckes die Ursache gewesen sein: 28jähriger Patient erkrankt an Cholecystitis mit lokaler Schmerzhaftigkeit; kein Ikterus, ganz geringe Temperaturerhöhung. Am 5. Tage paroxysmale Schwellung der Augenlider, in den frühen Morgenstunden einsetzend, bald rechts, bald links; dabei örtlich Kopfschmerzen, gegen Abend schwindend (Nebenhöhlen frei). Leidet hartnäckig an Oxyuren; beschäftigt sich mit Darmparasiten. Die Ödeme dauern noch einige Zeit an, verschwinden erst, nachdem die chronisch entzündete Gallenblase exstirpiert ist. Auch Martinico berichtet über Fälle, die mit Ascaridiasis kompliziert waren. Menagh fand unter 260 Fällen von Quinckeschem Ödem und Urticaria in 48,8% Störungen seitens des Gallentraktes. Mussio-Fournier sah eine 43jährige Frau mit Hydatidencyste der Leber und gleichzeitiger Urticaria, Asthma und Quinckeschem Ödem.

Grete Stern sah eine 48jährige Frau mit Urticaria und schwerem Quinckeschem Ödem, das jeder Behandlung trotzte. Nach Entfernung einer Oberkieferprothese, die aus einer Kautschukplatte mit Porzellanzähnen bestand, verschwanden die Anfälle, um nach Wiederanlegen der Prothese wiederzukehren. Neumann sah das Krankheitsbild nach der zweiten Insulinkur auftreten, Hoke nach einer Alttuberkulininjektion.

Einige Male wurde chronischer Alkoholmißbrauch als Ursache der Krankheit beschuldigt (Joseph, Oppenheimer, Bircher, Diethelm). Mathieu und Sikora teilen eine Beobachtung mit, in der flüchtige Ödeme nach leichter Kohlenoxydvergiftung auftraten.

Die *Malaria* scheint mehrfach eine ätiologische Rolle gespielt zu haben; das ist besonders für die Fälle anzunehmen, in denen die Ödeme auf die Stunde genau regelmäßig wiederkehrten (Matas, Keefe). Tremolière und Schulmann berichten über eine Luica mit Neuralgien radikulären Ursprungs, bei der Ödeme aller 4 Extremitäten auftraten, welche nach einer Lumbalpunktion nach 36 Stunden schwanden. Loewenheim berichtet über ein urticarielles Ödem, das angeblich in Niederschlesien besonders häufig auftreten soll. Die Fälle sollen im Juli und August sich häufen und nur aus Gegenden, die tiefer im sumpfigen Terrain gelegen sind, stammen; vielleicht handelt es sich hier um die Anwesenheit von Klimaallergenen, auf die Storm van Leeuwen besonders aufmerksam gemacht hat, deren Anwesenheit nach seiner Auffassung von klimatischen Einflüssen abhängig sein soll; es soll sich hier fast ausschließlich um Zersetzungsprodukte von tierischen oder pflanzlichen Mikroorganismen handeln, welche in der Einatmungsluft in Häusern oder auch in der Außenluft schweben. Über ein gehäuftes Auftreten von Ödemen im Gefängnis in

Düsseldorf berichtet auch ESCHWEILER. Alle Arbeiter, die daran erkrankten, waren mit einer bestimmten Tätigkeit beschäftigt, die vielleicht einen toxischen Einfluß ausgeübt hat. ROSENBERGER hat das Ödem nach Naphthalineinatmung auftreten sehen.

Es gibt noch eine Reihe weiterer, die unmittelbare Entstehung der Ödeme begünstigender Momente. Wir rechnen hierher zunächst kleine *lokale Traumen*; so genügte mehrfach das feste Anfassen eines Gegenstandes, z. B. eines Beiles, um Ödeme hervorzurufen. HALSTEDT sah nach Radfahren enorme Schwellungen am Scrotum und Penis auftreten. Bei COURTADES trat der erste Anfall nach einem Stich ins Auge im 15. Lebensjahr auf. Seither hatte der Kranke immer wieder neue Anfälle, stets an Stellen, wo ein leichtes Trauma einwirkte, beim Gehen an den Füßen, beim Sitzen an den Glutaei, beim Arbeiten an den Händen. VAN ITERSON sah nach Tonsillotomie ein zum Exitus führendes Glottisödem entstehen. Erst später erfuhr man, daß bei dem Patienten auch sonst leichte Verwundungen stets starke Schwellungen bedingt hatten. Bei einem Kranken von TARP trat das Ödem nach einer Zahnextraktion auf. In einem Falle von QUINCKE wirkte operativer Blutverlust steigernd auf die Anfälle. OLKON sah sie nach operativer Entfernung der Prostata, VOELCKER nach Harnstauung auftreten.

Bei lokal einwirkenden *Traumen* kann anfangs wohl das Ödem auf den Ort des Traumas beschränkt bleiben, später aber auch an anderen Körperstellen erscheinen. Den Einfluß leichter lokaler Traumen sehen wir bei einer verwandten Affektion, der *Epidermolysis bullosa hereditaria*, besonders in den Vordergrund treten. Es ist auch eine Kombination beider Krankheitsbilder von WILHELM beschrieben worden.

Ätiologisch wirksam sind auch akute *körperliche Erschöpfungszustände*. Von besonderem Interesse sind thermische Schädlichkeiten. Kälteeinwirkungen in mannigfachen Formen und Variationen wurden oft als auslösendes Moment beschuldigt. Dahin gehört auch die Erscheinung, daß in nicht wenigen Fällen immer nur die von Kleidung nicht bedeckten Körperteile vom Ödem befallen wurden. Eine Kombination von thermischen und mechanischen Einwirkungen war bei einer unserer Patientinnen im Spiel, die einem Hagelwetter ausgesetzt war. Die Schwellungen traten nur an den Stellen auf, die von den Hagelkörnern getroffen worden waren. Auch in 2 Fällen der Kombination von flüchtigen Ödemen mit paroxysmaler Hämoglobinurie war die Entstehung bzw. Lokalisation auf Kältewirkung zurückzuführen.

Die *neuropathische Diathese* der an Ödemen leidenden Patienten wird nicht allein durch die hereditäre Belastung, von der wir schon gesprochen haben, sondern häufig auch durch nervöse Erscheinungen, die das Individuum selbst betreffen, dokumentiert. Es sind oft im ganzen erregbare, nervöse, ängstliche, in irgendeiner Beziehung neuropathische Personen, die von der Krankheit ergriffen werden. In manchen Fällen verweben sich die Symptome des akuten Ödems so eng mit den übrigen Symptomen der Neurose, daß man am besten nur von symptomatischen, flüchtigen Ödemen spricht. Recht häufig finden wir sie bei der Migräne. Hier kann das Ödem gelegentlich an Stelle eines Migräneanfalles auftreten (GAENSSLEN u. a.). Noch häufiger begleiten sie einfach die Migräne. Wir werden auf diesen Zusammenhang noch später zu sprechen kommen. Einmal sahen wir die Kombination von migraine ophtalmique, rezidivierender Oculomotoriuslähmung und angioneurotischem Ödem. Psychische Erschütterungen können einen Einfluß ausüben (QUINCKE, ALLESSANDRI, FLANDIN). Oft genug trat das Ödem zum erstenmal nach einer starken Erregung, nach einem großen Ärger, einem heftigen Schreck oder auch nach intensiver geistiger Anstrengung auf. Ein Beispiel: Ein Patient STEKELs, der an Platzangst litt, bekam flüchtige Schwellungen der Beine, wenn er über einen Platz ging. Tat er das in Begleitung eines Arztes, so blieben diese aus. Eine unserer Patientinnen bekam flüchtige Schwellungen in dem Moment, in dem sie dieselben bei ihrem Kinde auftreten sah. Ein Kuriosum ist eine Beobachtung von I. H. Schultz: 34jähriger Mann erlitt aus vollem Wohlbefinden eine isolierte Schwellung des Grundgliedes des Ringfingers der rechten Hand. Patient lebte in einer erotisch unbefriedigenden Ehe. Am Abend vor Auftreten der Schwellung war seine Frau auf 3 Wochen verreist; die Schwellung blieb diese 3 Wochen bestehen und verschwand am Tage der Rückkehr der Frau. Sie hinderte den Patienten, den Ehering zu tragen. Dufke behandelte eine 28jährige Frau, die eine Urticaria mit Hitzegefühl und Jucken bekam, sobald sie Samt und Seide berührte. Diese Erscheinungen traten aber auch, wenn auch in geringerem Grade auf, wenn ihr die Suggestion gegeben wurde, daß es sich um Seide handle. Slobodnik sah ein Quinckesches Ödem des Halses und Kehlkopfs bei einem vasoneurotischen Manne nach einer ihn stark erregenden Unterredung in Erscheinung treten, bei der er sich bemühte, seine Stimme zu dämpfen.

Über das Vorkommen von *organischen* Nervenkrankheiten im Zusammenhang mit unserem Ödem ist nur weniges bekannt. Schlesinger sah zweimal flüchtiges Ödem an den Extremitätenabschnitten, die auch sonst infolge eines extramedullären, das Rückenmark komprimierenden Tumors Veränderungen erlitten hatten. Das Ödem entwickelte sich schmerzlos in wenigen Minuten, ohne Hautrötung, um nach kürzerem oder längerem Bestand so rasch wie es gekommen zu verschwinden. Über einen ähnlichen Fall hatten früher schon Mathieu und Weil berichtet. Flüchtige Ödeme kommen ferner im Zusammenhang mit den Blitzschmerzen bei der Tabes dorsalis vor (Kuerbitz). Bolten sah die Kombination mit Tetanie, Lieben die Erkrankung im Anschluß an eine Grippe mit gleichzeitigem Einsetzen einer Chorea auftreten.

Will und Cooper sahen sie bei Hebephrenie und Amentia, Mannheimer bei Melancholikern, bei denen man ja Zirkulationsanomalien an den Extremitäten und, wie wir schon erwähnt haben, auch das Vorkommen von Asphyxie locale gar nicht so selten feststellen kann.

Die Erscheinungen der *Menstruation, Gravidität,* des *Puerperium* und *Klimakterium* müssen in manchen Fällen als krankheitsauslösende Ursachen bezeichnet werden. Boerner hat direkt menstruelle und klimakterische flüchtige Ödeme als eigene Erscheinungen beschrieben. Auch H. Curschmann steht dieser Auffassung nahe, indem er dem Quinckeschen Ödem das flüchtige Ödem gegenüberstellt, das bei Chlorotischen, Dysmenorrhoischen und Klimakterischen vorkommt. Er betrachtet es jedoch nicht als eine Krankheit sui generis, sondern als Teilerscheinung einer dysgenitalen Neurose; das klimakterische Ödem beschreibt er als eine nicht deutlich anfallsweise auftretende, relativ geringfügige, meist nicht scharf umschriebene Schwellung. Die Prädilektionsstellen sind die Hände und die vordere Hälfte der Unterarme, die fast stets symmetrisch befallen werden, selten treten die Schwellungen an Unterschenkeln und im Gesicht auf; sie rezidivieren meist zu bestimmten Tageszeiten, vor allem in den Morgenstunden, und ähneln der inkompletten Form des Myxödems.

Hier mag auch die Bemerkung eingeschaltet werden, daß beim Trophoedème Meige, von dem an anderer Stelle die Rede sein wird, wiederholt Beziehungen zum Generationsprozeß aufgedeckt worden sind (Moniz, Slatmann, Sainz de Aja). In den Fällen von Moniz war bei 2 Schwestern das Ödem im Gesicht lokalisiert; eine dritte Schwester litt an Quinckeschem Ödem. Das Trophödem war von akuten entzündlichen Schüben begleitet, die mit den Menses auftraten und nach der Verheiratung sistierten. Sehr instruktiv ist der von

SLATMANN beschriebene Fall: Bei einer 26jährigen Frau traten vor 5 Jahren in der Zeit zwischen den Menses Ödeme der oberen Gesichtshälfte auf, die zur Zeit der Menses exacerbierten, nach einem Jahre völlig schwanden. Sie traten wieder auf, als die ersten Menses nach der Lactation einsetzten und stellten sich seitdem periodisch zur Zeit der Menses ein. Außerdem litt die Kranke an vorübergehendem Ödem an den Unterkieferwinkeln, Pastosität der Stirnhaut und der Unterschenkel. Ähnliche Beobachtungen stammen von MAY. Diese Fälle sind in letzter Zeit von PASTEUR, VALLERY-RADOT und HEYMANN besprochen. Daß die Ödeme die Zeit der Menses bevorzugen, gelegentlich während der Zeit der Gravidität aussetzen, ähnlich wie es bei der Migräne oft der Fall ist, hat schon QUINCKE beobachtet. Andererseits sah BALLERINI 2 Fälle von vorübergehendem Ödem bei der Schwangerschaft sich einstellen. In dem einen Fall bestand es auch nach der Entbindung bei andauernder Amenorrhöe fort.

Auch die Ödeme bei *Morbus Basedowii* tragen unzweifelhaft den Charakter des akuten umschriebenen Ödems, sie dürfen dort, wo sie neben den übrigen Symptomen der BASEDOWschen Krankheit höchstens eine diesen gleichwertige Rolle spielen, nicht als selbständige Krankheit angesehen werden. Besonders häufig sind hier flüchtige, manchmal aber auch länger anhaltende Schwellungen an den Augenlidern. SCHLESINGER hat derartige Beobachtungen publiziert.

Symptomatologie.

Es sind zu unterscheiden: 1. die durch das Ödem der äußeren Haut hervorgebrachten Symptome, 2. die durch Beteiligung innerer Organe entstandenen Krankheitszeichen, von denen zum Teil auch noch der Augenschein lehrt, daß sie auf ein Ödem der Schleimhaut direkt zurückgeführt werden können, das sind die Schwellungen an den Schleimhäuten der Mund- und Rachenhöhle und des Kehlkopfeingangs, der Augenbindehaut, die Magen-Darmsymptome, die Symptome von seiten der tieferen Luftwege.

Hieran schließen sich die durch passagere Ergüsse in die Gelenke (Hydrops articulorum intermittens) oder Sehnenscheiden oder Muskeln hervorgerufenen Störungen, endlich Symptome von noch zweifelhafter Bedeutung, namentlich von seiten der Nieren (Polyurie, Albuminurie, Oligurie, Hämoglobinurie, Urobilinurie).

Eine Anzahl weiterer Symptome, besonders von seiten der nervösen Zentralorgane, ist genetisch unklar; es ist zweifelhaft, ob es sich um Lokal- oder um Allgemeinsymptome handelt, welch letztere jedoch gelegentlich sicher vorkommen.

Zu den typischen Fällen des akuten Ödems gesellen sich die Fälle, die nach einer oder der anderen Richtung vom Typus abweichen. Hierher gehören vor allem die Übergangsbilder zur Urticaria, die sehr häufig sind, ferner Fälle, in denen sich Anklänge an andere vasomotorisch-trophische Neurosen, an Akroparästhesien, RAYNAUDsche Krankheit, Sklerodermie, multiple neurotische Hautgangrän finden (s. oben).

Die Krankheit setzt meist akut, ohne Vorboten ein; gelegentlich finden sich als Prodromalsymptome ein geringeres oder stärkeres allgemeines Unbehagen, Mattigkeit, Frösteln, Temperatursteigerung, Appetitlosigkeit. Die Hautschwellungen sind umschrieben, von sehr wechselnder Größe, meist derb elastisch, von blasser, gelblicher Farbe, seltener ins Rosa oder Rötliche hinüberspielend. Sie entstehen rasch im Verlauf von Minuten und Stunden, um meist etwas länger, gelegentlich selbst tagelang im Stadium voller Entwicklung zu bleiben und dann sehr rasch wieder zurückzugehen. Wegen des langsamen Abklingens ist die Dauer des einzelnen Anfalls nicht genau bestimmbar. Die Schwellungen sind meist schmerzlos, jucken nicht oder nicht sehr stark und fallen nur durch ein Gefühl von Spannung lästig. Die Entstellungen der äußeren Form, die sie hervorrufen können, sind ganz erheblich, besonders störend dann, wenn sie das Gesicht betreffen. Die Größe der Schwellungen wechselt. Sie können erbsen- bis haselnußgroß sein oder ein andermal die Größe eines Handtellers annehmen. Der Durchmesser der erkrankten Hautstelle beträgt 2 bis 10 cm (QUINCKE). Oft schwillt sogar ein ganzer Körperteil, ein Unterarm, eine Hand oder beide (KOENIG), ein Unterschenkel an. Es wurden auch Schwellungen des ganzen Körpers beobachtet, besonders in dem merkwürdigen Fall von DIETHELM. In dem von PANOFSKY und STAEMMLER beobachteten Falle traten mit $1^{1}/_{2}$ Jahren zum ersten Male bis 3 Tage lang dauernde Schwellungen am ganzen Körper auf, die sich im Laufe des Lebens wiederholten. Das Mädchen starb an Glottisödem; die Mutter hatte das gleiche Ende gefunden.

Die Schwellungen scheinen meist in der Haut und im Unterhautbindegewebe zu sitzen. Die Konsistenz steht in der Mitte zwischen fest und weich. MILTON trifft das richtige, wenn er sie mit der des kontrahierten Biceps vergleicht. Fingerdruck bleibt nicht, wie bei vielen anderen Ödemen, lange bestehen, sondern es besteht entweder gar keine oder nur eine kurze Zeit anhaltende Eindrückbarkeit. Die Temperatur der Schwellungen wird der Farbe meist parallel gehen. Mit der Röte pflegt sich auch Hitze einzustellen und damit zugleich auch meist heftiger Juckreiz. Auf diese Weise entsteht dann das Bild der typischen Urticaria, zu der die Übergänge durchaus fließende sind.

Sehr selten wurde beobachtet, daß heftigere Schmerzen dem Auftreten der Schwellungen vorausgingen. Objektive Sensibilitätsstörungen fehlen stets. Die einmalige Schwellung hinterläßt wohl niemals ein Residuum. Die Teile bleiben unverändert, nur in wenigen Fällen schilfert die Haut später ab. Auch bei steter Wiederholung des Ödems an derselben Stelle kommt es in der Regel nicht zu einer dauernden Veränderung der betreffenden Teile. Doch wurden davon abweichende Fälle beobachtet. Namentlich an den Augenlidern scheinen häufig dauernde Veränderungen vorzukommen, bisweilen selbst schon nach wenigen Anfällen, gelegentlich mit HORNERschem Syndrom (IVANOFF). ASAI sah ein sojabohnengroßes Ödem in der Conjunctiva bulbi unter leichter Hyperämie, das 5 Stunden dauerte, als Begleiterscheinung des QUINCKEschen Ödems auftreten. Vor einiger Zeit hat RADIMSKA-JANDOVA unter dem Titel ,,Dauerform des QUINCKEschen Ödems" einen Fall beschrieben, bei dem nach wiederholtem Auftreten von Ödem im Gesicht, besonders im Bereich der Augenlider, Infiltration und Induration der betroffenen Teile zurückblieb. Chinin brachte bedeutende Besserung. Einen ähnlichen Fall haben auch wir beobachtet. SCHALIT berichtet über 3 Beobachtungen von angioneurotischem Ödem der Kaumuskulatur mit nachfolgender Hypertrophie. RIEHL sah einmal Bildung kleiner Blasen an den ödematösen Partien, dasselbe lehren FORSSBERG, FUERSTNER, BITTORF, RUMPEL und eigene Beobachtungen. Einige Male wurde ein geringer Blutaustritt beobachtet (SCHLESINGER, ORMEROD, LOVETT, TREUMANN). Stärkere Hautblutungen im Verein mit flüchtigen Ödemen wurden auch sonst noch mehrfach gesehen. Wir betreten damit das Gebiet der *Purpura toxica* (SCHÖNLEIN-HENOCH). Es ist eine ganze Anzahl von Beobachtungen von Purpura berichtet worden, in deren Verlauf akute flüchtige Ödeme von der bekannten Beschaffenheit mehr oder minder ephemer vorkamen. KÄMMERER, der in seiner Monographie der Purpura ein besonderes Kapitel gewidmet hat, rechnet diese zu den allergischen Krankheiten, wodurch ätiologisch verwandtschaftliche Beziehungen mit gewissen Formen des QUINCKEschen Ödems hergestellt würden. KREIBICH beschreibt einen Fall von QUINCKEschem Ödem mit Ausgang in nekrotisierende Entzündung und Atrophie, bei WILLAN endet in einem Falle eine Anzahl der Purpuraflecken in Gangrän, ebenso in einem von KUHN mitgeteilten, aber recht komplizierten und schwer zu beurteilenden Fall.

Von sekretorischen Symptomen wird wenig berichtet; Hyperhidrosis wurde gelegentlich gesehen (WHITING, LAUDON, VALOBRA).

Die Schwellungen können an den verschiedensten Körperteilen sitzen, kaum ein Körperteil ist ganz immun dagegen; am seltensten scheint die behaarte Kopfhaut befallen zu werden.

Die Lokalisation ist sicher bisweilen von äußeren Bedingungen abhängig. Auf die Einwirkung der Kälte haben wir schon hingewiesen, ebenso auf die von Traumen. Eine Bevorzugung der Akra ist nicht zu beobachten. Die Schwellungen sind auch recht selten symmetrisch. Die Verteilung der Ödeme in der

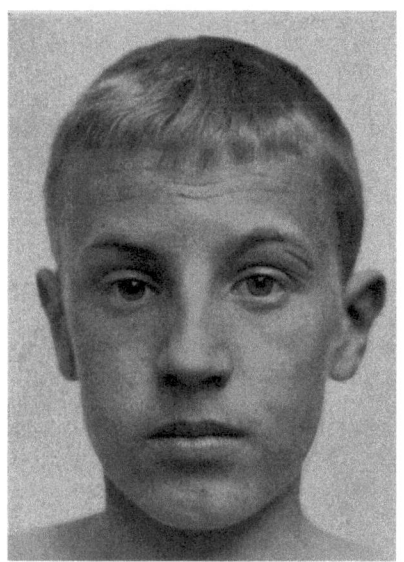 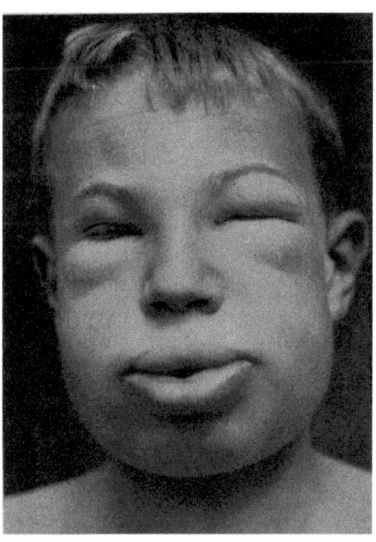

Abb. 15. Patient mit QUINCKESchem Ödem vor dem Anfall. 14 Jahre alt.   Abb. 16. Derselbe Patient während des Ödemanfalles.
(Aus DE QUERVAIN: Spez. chirurg. Diagnostik. 9. Aufl. 1931).

Haut läßt weder Beziehungen zu den peripheren Nerven, noch zu spinalen oder radikulären Segmenten, noch auch zu bestimmten Gefäßterritorien erkennen.

Es steht fest, daß die Stelle, an der das Ödem aus irgendwelchen Gründen zuerst aufgetreten ist, auch für die späteren Anfälle ein Locus minoris resistentiae bleibt. Aus diesen stets gleich lokalisierten Ödemen hat man besondere Affektionen gemacht. Mit Unrecht. Bisweilen sitzen die Schwellungen in den tieferen Teilen, näher den Knochen, unter unveränderter Haut, wie in den Fällen von FÉRÉOL, QUINCKE, GROSS, HERZ, LUBLINSKI, STERN. Häufig sitzen die Ödeme periartikulär. SCHLESINGER hat zuerst den Verdacht ausgesprochen, daß auch die intermittierende Form der Parotisanschwellung in das Gebiet der flüchtigen Ödeme hineingehöre. Ein Fall, den FREUDENTHAL beschrieben hat, ist in der Tat so zu deuten, ebenso TALLEYs Fall, der als angioneurotisches Ödem der Speicheldrüsen mitgeteilt wird. Wir selbst haben viele Jahre eine Patientin beobachtet, bei der sich Parotisschwellungen erst auf der einen, dann auf der anderen Seite anfallsweise einstellten, mit großen Schmerzen und leichten Fiebersteigerungen, die anfänglich als Mumps angesehen wurden.

Allmählich bildeten sich die geschwollenen Drüsen nicht mehr zur Norm zurück, aber die Intensität der Parotisschwellungen wechselte noch fortwährend. Daneben besteht auch eine Schwellung der Glandulae sublingualis und submaxillaris, also ein mit der Mikuliczschen Krankheit übereinstimmender Symptomenkomplex, wie wir ihn auch gelegentlich einmal in einem Falle von Sklerodaktylie gesehen haben. Neuda beobachtete anfallsweise auftretende Schwellungen der Submaxillargegend und der Lippen, der Epiglottis und angrenzenden Teile des Kehlkopfes bei einem Kranken. In einem Falle von Blaustein waren befallen: Lippen, Wangen, Augenlider, Parotis, Penis, Scrotum, Perineum; den Anfällen gingen heftiges Jucken und Brennen, sowie Schwindel, Übelkeit und Erbrechen voraus. Dabei stellte sich vollständige Anurie ein, die als Folge eines Ödems der Ureteren und des Nierenbeckens gedeutet wurde. Die Anfälle dauerten wenige Stunden bis zu 4 Tagen.

Unter der Bezeichnung *Pseudolipom* hat man zum Teil Zustände beschrieben, die auch in diesem Zusammenhang Erwähnung verdienen und hierher gehören. Namentlich französische Autoren haben Schwellungen in den Supraclaviculargruben beobachtet und beschrieben, die zweifellos als flüchtige Ödeme zu deuten sind. Wir sahen eine Frau, die seit 2 Jahren unter intermittierenden Anschwellungen der Brüste litt, die mit geringen Schmerzen einhergingen und nach einigen Stunden wieder verschwanden. Auch hier wird es sich gewiß um flüchtige Ödeme gehandelt haben.

Häufig werden die Schleimhäute der Mund- und Rachenhöhle und des Kehlkopfeingangs befallen, nach Collins in 21% der Fälle. Es kann die Wangenschleimhaut, die Schleimhaut des Zahnfleisches, die Zunge, die Mandeln, der Gaumen, der ganze Pharynx befallen sein. Die Zunge kann zur Hälfte oder ganz anschwellen, so daß sie die ganze Mundhöhle ausfüllt und ein ernsthaftes Atmungshindernis bietet. Halstedt beschreibt einen solchen Fall genauer; er sah eine gelblichweiße, durchsichtige Schwellung der rechten Rachenseite, des vorderen und hinteren Gaumenbogens, des rechten Velum, der Uvula, während Tonsillen, Zunge und Kehlkopfeingang frei blieben. Auch die Nasenschleimhaut kann befallen werden. Am wichtigsten ist die Schwellung des Kehlkopfeingangs wegen der schweren und beängstigenden Symptome, die aus ihr resultieren. In einigen dieser Fälle war eine laryngoskopische Untersuchung möglich; es fand sich ein starkes Ödem der Epiglottis und der aryepiglottischen Falten, eine sehr voluminöse, leicht durchscheinende, graurot gefärbte, zitternde, gallertartige Schwellung. Die Uvula hängt in manchen Fällen sackartig in den Kehlkopfeingang. In einigen Fällen konnte auch eine anatomische Untersuchung der betreffenden Teile vorgenommen werden, die die laryngoskopischen Ergebnisse eines hochgradigen Ödems der Epiglottis und des Aditus laryngis bestätigte, während die Schwellungen im Kehlkopf, in der Luftröhre und an den echten Stimmbändern geringer waren. Selbstverständlich machen diese Ödeme von vornherein sehr starke subjektive Beschwerden, Schluckbeschwerden und Atemnot. Diese steigern sich gewöhnlich sehr rasch zu beträchtlicher Höhe. Die Atemnot wird ganz außerordentlich hochgradig. In einer Reihe von Fällen konnte nur die Tracheotomie, die auch wiederholt bei demselben Patienten ausgeführt werden mußte, einen unglücklichen Ausgang verhüten, in anderen Fällen trat wirklich der Exitus ein, zuweilen mit furchtbarer Schnelligkeit (s. unten). In der Mehrzahl der Fälle sind die Ödeme freilich meist doch von kürzerer Dauer, so daß, obwohl bedrohliche Symptome eintreten, eine ernste Gefahr sich nicht herausbildet. Eine hochgradige Schwellung kann im Laufe einer halben Stunde entstehen und spurlos wieder verschwinden.

Mehrfach ist auch eine Schwellung der Nasenschleimhaut beobachtet worden. Daß auch zahlreiche Fälle von sog. vasomotorischem Schnupfen hierher gehören, ist uns nicht zweifelhaft. Die Kombination mit anders lokalisierten flüchtigen Ödemen beweist diesen Zusammenhang.

Daß weiter auch die tieferen Luftwege befallen werden können, lehren mehrfache Beispiele. Auch bei dem akuten Larynxödem ist die Trachea gelegentlich mitbeteiligt gewesen. SCHLESINGER wies auf die Möglichkeit hin, daß manche Formen von Asthma nervosum hierher zu rechnen sind. Andere Autoren (RAPIN, SOLIS-COHEN, PACKARD, STAEHELIN, KÖNIG) haben später ähnliche Fälle beschrieben. Wir werden auf diesen Zusammenhang noch zu sprechen kommen; ebenso auf die sehr nahen Beziehungen zum sog. Heuschnupfen, wofür wiederum RAPIN eine ganze Reihe von recht instruktiven Beispielen bringt. In einzelnen Fällen bildet das paroxysmale Lungenödem eine Teilerscheinung der flüchtigen Ödeme. JAMIESON, MUELLER und eine sehr interessante Beobachtung von QUINCKE und GROSS, sowie von FEER lehren das. Bronchitis fibrinosa mit Asthma als Teilerscheinung sah SCHORER. Auch der von GROSS, FUCHS und ADLER beschriebene rezidivierende Exophthalmus gehört hierher. Über diesen Zusammenhang hat in den letzten Jahren MEYER-HÜRLIMANN berichtet. Er beschreibt eine umschriebene Schwellung des Gesichts, Ohres und Unterschenkels mit subperiostaler Exsudation, ferner eine Schwellung an mehreren Rippen, des weichen Gaumens, des Pharynx, ein akutes Lungenödem, heftige explosive Diarrhöen und schließlich einen in kürzester Zeit auftretenden und rasch wieder verschwindenden Exophthalmus bald des linken, bald des rechten Auges bei einem Kranken. Die Dauer der Anfälle schwankte zwischen 1—14 Tagen. Die Ursache für die letzte Erscheinung sieht er in einer Lymphansammlung im Bulbus, aber auch des ganzen Fettgewebes, der Orbita und der Muskeln des Bulbus. Diese Beobachtung sichert die Zusammengehörigkeit zwischen dem akuten Exophthalmus und dem QUINCKEschen Ödem.

Sicher sind gewisse intermittierend auftretende *Magen-Darm*-Erscheinungen zur Symptomatologie der QUINCKEschen Krankheit zu rechnen. Ihr Zusammenhang mit dem flüchtigen Ödem wurde schon früh erkannt. Die Erfahrungen der sog. Urticaria interna hatten von vornherein darauf hingewiesen. Schon QUINCKE und DINKELACKER sahen und deuteten derartige Störungen richtig; unter den späteren Autoren haben sich besonders eingehend STRUEBING und RAPIN mit ihnen beschäftigt. Aber auch zahlreiche andere Autoren haben Beispiele beigebracht. COLLINS berechnete, daß in 34% der Fälle von akutem flüchtigem Ödem Magen-Darmerscheinungen aufgetreten sind. In den leichteren Fällen finden sich nur mehr oder minder intensive Schmerzen in der Magengegend, verbunden mit einem Spannungsgefühl und Appetitlosigkeit. Der Schmerz kann eine außerordentlich hohe Intensität erreichen. RAPIN spricht von einer Migraine abdominelle, andere Autoren von „crises solaires" (LAUBRY, BROSSE und VAN BOGAERT, VALLERY-RADOT-PASTEUR-BLAMOUTIER). Bei weiterer Entwicklung kommt es zu Brechneigung, schließlich zu wirklichem Erbrechen. Anfangs wird Mageninhalt erbrochen, später werden reichliche wässerige Mengen herausbefördert. In diesen schwersten Fällen haben wir ganz dasselbe Bild wie bei den gastrischen Krisen der Tabes vor uns. Bei einer Kranken von LANDWEHR glich der Anfall einer Gallensteinkolik. In den Fällen von MACDONALD und BUENDIA wurde einmal eine Cholecystitis, ein anderes Mal eine Appendicitis vorgetäuscht.

Bisweilen leiten die Intestinalerscheinungen die QUINCKEsche Krankheit ein (EHRENWALL und GERHARTZ), bisweilen stehen die Magensymptome ganz im Vordergrund, während die übrigen Erscheinungen des flüchtigen Ödems keine wesentliche Rolle spielen. Von da aus gibt es Übergänge aller möglichen Art bis zu den Fällen, in denen die Magenbeschwerden nur ganz episodisch die

Ödeme begleiten. Es gibt auch Fälle, am häufigsten sind es familiäre, in denen schwere Symptome von seiten des Magens sich zu solchen von seiten der Atmungsorgane gesellen. In einem Falle von NEUDA war das QUINCKEsche Ödem mit periodischem Erbrechen und akuter circumscripter Schwellung der Harnblase kompliziert (ähnlich der erwähnte Fall von BLAUSTEIN).

In einem Falle von STRUEBING ergab die Untersuchung des Erbrochenen, daß es aus Schleim und einigen mikroskopisch nachweisbaren Epithelien der Magenschleimhaut bestand. QUINCKE und GROSS fanden einen erheblichen Eiweißgehalt in der erbrochenen Flüssigkeit, die stark alkalisch reagierte. In einem Falle von MORRIS wurde beim Ausspülen durch die Magensonde gelegentlich ein Stückchen Schleimhaut herausbefördert; es fand sich ein sehr hochgradiges Ödem, die Lymphräume waren bedeutend erweitert, die Zellen durch weite Räume getrennt, die Bindegewebsfasern auseinandergedrängt.

Mit den Magenbeschwerden zusammen, seltener ohne diese, treten auch Darmerscheinungen auf: heftige kolikartige Schmerzen, Meteorismus, Empfindlichkeit des Abdomen und profuse Diarrhöen, die von den gewöhnlichen Zeichen solcher Zufälle, heftigem, brennenden Durst, Verminderung der Harnmenge, großer Erschöpfung begleitet sein können. Mehrfach wird von intestinalen Hämorrhagien, die bei derartigen Anfällen sich einstellten, berichtet.

In einem Fall von angioneurotischem Ödem wurde gelegentlich eines schweren Kolikanfalles eine Eröffnung des Abdomen vorgenommen. Es fand sich dabei eine durch Kontraktion bedingte Verdickung des unteren Abschnittes der Wand des Ileum (HARRINGTON), also ein enterospastischer Zustand, wie er auch sonst bei Ileus nervosus gelegentlich vorkommt. In diesem Zusammenhange sei der folgende von QUINCKE beobachtete Fall zitiert:

Frau H., 35 Jahre alt. Leidet an zeitweise auftretenden Schwellungen an Beinen, Leib, Händen und Gesicht seit ihrem 12. Jahr (möglicherweise schon in den Kinderjahren). Erst seit der Verheiratung mit einem Arzt sei die Sache genauer beobachtet. Am schlimmsten sei es in der Schwangerschaft gewesen. Bald danach Arsenikkur längere Zeit, danach habe sie 50 Pfund verloren. Seitdem trete die Krankheit in gelinderer Form auf. Die Anfälle von Schwellung dauern oft wochenlang. Sie muß dann liegen. Manchmal wurden die Anfälle durch Erregung veranlaßt. Verdauungsstörungen seien ohne Bedeutung. Die Schwellungen betreffen das Gesicht in toto, gewöhnlich dabei auch die Hände und den Leib ringsum in der Höhe des Epigastriums „wie ein Wasserkissen". Manchmal bestänDen kolossale Wasserausscheidungen durch den Darm, manchmal Darmkrämpfe, so daß man die harten Stellen fühlen könne. Auch an Colitis membranacea habe sie gelitten. Die Gelenke seien nie befallen gewesen. In der Familie kamen ähnliche Zustände nicht vor.

Zwei Kranke von SCHORER, die innerhalb weniger Tage Gewichtszunahmen von vielen Kilogrammen und Oligurie darboten, zeigten an Intensität wechselnde, die ganze Körperoberfläche befallende Hautödeme. Er sah gastrointestinale Erscheinungen in Gestalt heftiger, rezidivierender Koliken, Durchfälle, die explosionsartig enorme Stuhl- und Schleimmassen zutage förderten. Im Falle NOVOA SANTOS bestand bei universellem neurotischen Ödem ein Hydrops abdominalis intermittens. Andere Kranke zeigten Hautblutungen, Albuminurie, Hämaturie. STAEHELIN dagegen sah 3 Fälle von QUINCKEschem Ödem, bei denen diese Anfälle deutlich mit Obstipation einhergingen (zit. nach LUTZ). DE GROOT jr. sah periodische Anschwellung von Vagina und Brüsten als Manifestation des QUINCKEschen Ödems. Überhaupt sind die Genitalien oft Sitz der circumscripten Ödeme: Penis, Skrotum, Vagina.

Eine seltene Lokalisation stellte eine von SCHLESINGER beobachtete intermittierende Anschwellung der *Sehnenscheiden* dar (Hydrops hypostrophos tendovaginarum). Die Anfälle begannen unter heftigen Parästhesien, zeigten zur Zeit der Menses Verschlimmerung und zessierten während der Gravidität. Die Anschwellung der Sehnenscheiden wird öfters durch schmerzhafte Beugekontrakturen der Finger eingeleitet, die wir auch mehrfach in Fällen gesehen haben, wo sich ein periarticuläres Ödem bildete. Paroxysmale Schwellungen von Schleimbeuteln und Sehnenscheidenhygrome zeigt auch der von QUINCKE beobachtete folgende Fall:

39jährige Frau. Seit 4 Jahren öfters stenokardische Anfälle bei Nierenschrumpfung, Hypertonie und Herzhypertrophie; bei salzloser Kost und häufig wiederholten Aderlässen etwas Besserung des Befindens. Daneben besteht seit etwa einem Jahre an den Beugern des rechten Unterarmes ein halbtaubeneigroßes Sehnenscheidenhygrom, das mit Einsetzen der Menses unter Spannungsgefühl für deren Dauer anschwillt, dann wieder abschwillt. Derselbe Vorgang vollzieht sich an Schleimbeuteln, die oberhalb des inneren und äußeren Condylus humeri, über dem inneren Kopf des rechten Deltamuskels und vor dem rechten Ligamentum patellae als flache, fluktuierende Beutel fühlbar sind, aber sonst keine Beschwerden machen. Umschriebene Hautödeme traten nicht auf.

Flüchtige Ödeme der *Muskeln* haben wir wiederholt beobachten können. Sie sind meist von heftigen Schmerzen begleitet. Die Muskeln fühlen sich dann deutlich teigig infiltriert, verdickt, geschwollen an. Ihre passive Beweglichkeit ist behindert. In einem derartigen Falle, den wir sahen, traten dabei gelegentlich Fiebersteigerungen auf. ERNA BALL beschrieb einen in unserer Poliklinik beobachteten Fall von Kieferklemme, die durch akutes umschriebenes Ödem hervorgerufen war. Es trat eine anfallsweise Schwellung in der rechten Gesichtshälfte stets während der Menstruation auf. Während des Anfalls konnte die Patientin den Mund nur wenig öffnen; in der anfallsfreien Zeit blieb eine geringe Schwellung bestehen, so daß die Patientin den Mund nie normal öffnen konnte. Der Sitz des Ödems war der rechte Musculus temporalis und masseter. Die Kieferklemme war auf das Ödem des Musculus masseter zurückzuführen.

QUINCKE äußert die Vermutung, daß auch manchen *Neuralgien* akute umschriebene Ödeme im Bindegewebe des Nervenstammes zugrundeliegen dürften; er beschreibt einen Fall, der an einer Neuralgie in mehreren Ästen des Lumbalplexus litt, welche ausgezeichnet war durch ihre jahrzehntelange Wiederkehr, gewöhnlich auf bestimmte Anlässe und häufig nach einem gewissen Typus bei vollkommen beschwerdefreien Intervallen. Es konnten seiner Ansicht nach nicht anatomische Schäden, sondern nur flüchtige Veränderungen im Gebiet des Lumbalplexus dieser Neuralgie zugrunde liegen. Er vermutet ein akutes umschriebenes Ödem. Neuralgiforme Schmerzen ähnlicher Art auf dem ganzen Körper herumwandernd, bisweilen von großer Heftigkeit, so daß sie geradezu an die lanzinierenden Schmerzen der Tabiker erinnern, habe ich (CASSIRER) öfter in Fällen einer konstitutionellen Labilität des vegetativen Systems beobachtet. Die Begleiterscheinungen machten es auch mir wahrscheinlich, daß es sich auch da um flüchtige Ödeme in den Nervenscheiden, evtl. auch in den Muskeln handelte. MACKAY führt eine Neuritis des Nervus ulnaris bei einem Kranken mit QUINCKEschem Ödem auf diese Ätiologie zurück.

Wässerige *Ergüsse* in den *Gelenken* können eine Teilerscheinung der QUINCKE-schen Krankheit darstellen. SCHLESINGER hat in dieser Frage wiederholt das Wort genommen und selbst 15 Fälle, darunter nur zwei Männer, beobachtet. Er macht darauf aufmerksam, daß häufig in den gleichen Familien andere Affektionen mit neurovasculärer Disposition, Labilität des Gefäß- und Nervensystems mit Beziehungen zu anaphylaktischen Vorgängen (LOVÉN) beschrieben sind. Er berichtet über Fälle, in denen die intermittierenden Gelenkschwellungen bei mehreren Mitgliedern einer Familie in zwei Zweigen derselben auftritt, der Hydrops gelegentlich vom angioneurotischen Ödem begleitet ist, dessen Lokalisation sehr oft derjenigen entspricht, die meist beim QUINCKEschen Ödem beobachtet wird. Zwei Mitglieder der Familie leiden an Hämophilie. Auch FRENKEL-TISSOT (zit. nach SIEMENS) haben eine Familie beschrieben, in der die Erkrankung bei der Mutter und drei von ihren Kindern aufgetreten ist.

Es sind über 100 Fälle beschrieben worden; meist wurden nervöse Individuen befallen. Zwei Kranke von SCHLESINGER litten an manisch-depressivem Irresein. Ohne veranlassendes Moment tritt eine Schwellung eines oder mehrerer Gelenke auf, die nach mehrtägigem, höchstens mehrwöchentlichem Bestand verschwindet und nach längerer oder kürzerer Zeit wiederkommt. Die Anfälle kehren oft in regelmäßigem Typus wieder, so daß nach SCHLESINGER die Kranken oft wochenlang vorher wissen, wann der Anfall zu erwarten ist. Gelegentlich stellen sich vorher oder während des Anfalles Parästhesien und neuralgiforme Schmerzen im Bereiche von Hüfte und Oberschenkel ein. Die Haut über den Gelenken ist blaß, manchmal leicht ödematös, die Gelenke sind nicht druckschmerzhaft. In nicht weniger als 94% der Fälle waren ein oder beide Kniegelenke betroffen, nur zweimal war das Kniegelenk gar nicht befallen. PLETZER und HOMEN sahen die Affektion bei Basedow, FÉRÉ bei Epilepsie. Zuweilen sind nicht nur die Gelenke, sondern auch die Weichteile um diese herum befallen. Aber die Ödeme finden sich gelegentlich auch an anderen Stellen, am Gesäß, im Gesicht (eigene Beobachtung). KAMP beschrieb einen wechselweise in beiden Knien auftretenden Fall von Hydrops, der seit Jahren, früher alle 9, jetzt alle 4 Tage, sich bildete. Jede Therapie war machtlos. MENDEL berichtet von einer Frau, die an einem stets zur Zeit der Menses wiederkehrenden Hydrops beider Kniegelenke litt, was auch BENDA schon beobachtet hatte. BURCHARD sah einen Fall, bei dem Gelenkschwellungen und Asthmaanfälle abwechselten. Bei einem Patienten OPPENHEIMs bildete ein periodisch in regelmäßigen Intervallen auftretender Oberschenkelschmerz anscheinend ein Äquivalent des früheren Hydrops. Gelegentliche Gelenkschwellungen im Laufe der QUINCKEschen Krankheit haben wir wiederholt gesehen. In einem Falle von PULAWSKI trat im Anschluß an einen Typhus Hydrops articulorum intermittens beider Knie auf. Als Prodromalsymptome bemerkte der Kranke unangenehme Sensationen in der Wirbelsäule und in den unteren Extremitäten.

In einem Falle fand SCHLESINGER als Röntgenbefund geringe Gelenkveränderungen mit schwachem Osteophytbelag an einigen Rändern der Gelenkfläche. SCHLESINGER (und ebenso RHEINDORF) glaubt, daß hormonale Vorgänge im Sinne einer Funktionsanomalie (Unterfunktion der Ovarien) eine Rolle spielen müssen und hat bei Frauen durch subcutane Darreichung von Placentarextrakt gute Erfolge erzielt. Er empfiehlt, wenigstens bei Frauen, die von diesem Leiden befallen sind, die vorübergehende Sterilisierung durch Röntgenstrahlen in Erwägung zu ziehen.

OPPENHEIM hat zuerst die Vermutung ausgesprochen, daß sich auch eine Opticusaffektion als Teilerscheinung des QUINCKEschen Ödems entwickeln kann. Er hat 2mal eine *Neuritis optica* bei Personen entstehen sehen, bei denen eine ausgesprochene Neigung zu vasomotorischen Störungen vorlag und jede andere Grundlage und Ätiologie fehlte. HANDWERK hat genauer einen Fall beschrieben, bei dem eine kurzdauernde Schwellung der Sehnervenpapillen eines Auges neben anderen akuten Ödemen zu beobachten war. Es traten plötzlich Lichterscheinungen vor dem rechten Auge auf, denen alsbald eine Herabsetzung der Sehschärfe des Auges folgte. Auch QUINCKE berichtet über einen solchen Fall. OPPENHEIM machte weiterhin darauf aufmerksam, daß in einzelnen seiner Fälle von MENIÈREschem Syndrom die Symptome auf einer vasomotorischen Störung dieses Ursprunges zu beruhen schienen. Drei Fälle von angioneurotischem Ödem mit MENIÈRE hat kürzlich DEDERDING beobachtet. Eine Verbindung von MENIÈREschen Symptomen und echten angioneurotischen Schwellungen haben wir an unserem Material und in der Literatur bisher allerdings nicht feststellen können. An der Möglichkeit derartiger Entstehungen zweifeln wir aber nicht. OPPENHEIM beobachtete ferner in 2 Fällen bei neurotischen

Individuen eine *rezidivierende Iritis*, die ihn in der Art des Auftretens sehr an das Bild des Hydrops intermittens erinnerte. Auch MORICHAU-BEAUCHANT und LANDRY beobachteten einen ähnlichen Fall.

Zu erwähnen sind ferner Anomalien der *Harnentleerung*: Oligurie, die vielleicht sekundäre Bedeutung hatte, bei intensivem Erbrechen, Polyurie bzw. der Wechsel beider Erscheinungen, wie in einem Falle von DIETHELM. Auch von einer passageren Albuminurie wird berichtet. Sehr interessant ist das Vorkommen einer paroxysmalen *Hämoglobinurie*, die JOSEPH u. a. sahen. NEUDA konnte in 5 Fällen von QUINCKEscher Krankheit folgende drei Kardinalsymptome feststellen, die sich für den Anfall als charakteristisch erwiesen: eine palpatorisch und perkutorisch nachweisbare Milzschwellung, exquisite Urobilinurie, evtl. Albuminurie, Eigentümlichkeiten des Blutbildes, wie Anstieg des Hämoglobingehaltes und des Färbeindex unmittelbar vor dem Anfall und im Anfall. Er deutet diese Befunde im Sinne einer Hämolyse, die den Anfall charakterisiert. Der gleiche Autor sah auch eine circumscripte Schwellung der Harnblase als Ausdruck der QUINCKEschen Krankheit.

Kardiale Symptome sind nicht häufig. SCHLESINGER führt paroxysmale Tachykardie an, ebenso SOLIS-COHEN. Von einer im Anfall sich einstellenden Herzerweiterung und dem Auftreten eines systolischen Geräusches an der Herzbasis berichten MÜLLER-DIETHELM in ihrem sehr eigentümlichen Fall, bei dem die Ödeme sich über die ganze Körperfläche ausdehnten und damit im Zusammenhang außerordentliche Schwankungen des Körpergewichts vorkamen, indem das Körpergewicht zunächst im Beginn des Anfalls von 65 auf 72 kg stieg, um dann im Verlauf von 9 Tagen wieder auf 65 kg abzusinken. Damit verbanden sich außerordentlich intensive Temperatursteigerungen bis auf 40,1°, Erhöhung der Pulsfrequenz und schwere Allgemeinerscheinungen. Über starke Körpergewichtsschwankungen berichtet auch MENDEL.

Allgemeine cerebrale Symptome sind mehrfach beobachtet worden: Mattigkeit, Schläfrigkeit, ja ausgeprägte Schlafsucht und Kopfschmerzen (ULLMANN, STRÜBING, SCHLESINGER, DINKELACKER, RAPIN, FOURNIER-MUSSIO-GARRA, OLIARO, VAN BOGAERT), psychische Veränderungen, Verstimmung, Reizbarkeit. Den höchsten Grad erreichten diese in einer von ULLMANN mitgeteilten Beobachtung, bei der neben ödematösen Schwellungen an der Haut plötzlich Erscheinungen von Hirndruck, Pulsverlangsamung, Bewußtseinsverlust, Atmungsstillstand und allgemeine Krämpfe auftraten. Der Autor glaubt die Krämpfe auf meningeale Schwellungen in der Art der Meningitis serosa zurückführen zu können. Ein ähnlicher Fall von RAD ist nicht ganz eindeutig. BECK führt in seiner obenerwähnten Selbstbeobachtung das zweimalige Auftreten von völliger Bewußtlosigkeit während des Anfallstadiums auf Ödem der Hirnhäute zurück. HAHN berichtet von einem 12jährigen Kinde, das im Verlauf eines Typhus eine 6 Tage anhaltende komplette motorische Aphasie bekam, mit leichter Parese des rechten Facialis. Besserung erfolgte allmählich im Verlauf einiger Tage. Gleichzeitig damit bestand eine Urticaria gigantea am rechten Unterarm, an der linken Wange, am nächsten Tage Schwellungen am linken Unterarm und den Oberschenkeln. Die Flüchtigkeit der Aphasie und ihre Koinzidenz mit flüchtigen Hautschwellungen läßt die Annahme einer durch später rasch resorbierte Ödeme entstandenen Aphasie hier durchaus plausibel erscheinen. KENNEDY sah einen in mittlerem Lebensalter stehenden Kranken, der im Laufe eines Jahres vier Anfälle von passagerer Hemiplegie darbot, die zweimal von kompletter motorischer Aphasie begleitet waren; mit den Erscheinungen von seiten des Nervensystems setzte auch eine Urticaria ein. Nach 36 Stunden verschwanden alle Erscheinungen. Patient litt 10 Jahre lang, bevor die Hemiplegie auftrat, wiederholt an Attacken von QUINCKEschem

Ödem des weichen Gaumens, der Lippen, der Wangen, gelegentlich auch der Arme und des Rumpfes. Außerdem beobachtete er einen 28jährigen Kranken, dessen Mutter an Urticaria litt, der in der Kindheit an Asthma und QUINCKEschem Ödem litt. In den letzten Jahren traten während der Anfälle passagere Hirnsymptome auf: Schläfrigkeit, Kopfschmerzen, Sehstörung. Einmal stellte sich 14 Tage lang eine Blindheit des rechten Auges ein. Im schwersten Anfall zeigte er doppelseitige Taubheit, Aphonie, Gaumensegel- und Zungenparese, Sehstörung, Sphincterenlähmung mit langsamer Rückbildung. Im Anfall Entrundung und trägere Pupillenreaktion. GORDINIER berichtet über einen jungen Mann mit Asthmaanfällen und einer 10 Tage dauernden Aphasie mit Hemiplegie und JACKSONschen Anfällen. In einem Fall von SEPP lokalisierten sich die Ödeme außer an der Hand noch innerhalb der Schädelhöhle, wodurch Migräne hervorgerufen wurde, welche einmal von Ophthalmoplegie infolge der Kompression des Abducens und des Oculomotorius begleitet wurde. Er weist darauf hin, daß auch Fälle von rezidivierender Oculomotoriuslähmung ebensolcher Genese sein können. Einen ähnlichen Fall hat CASSIRER auch einmal beschrieben. MELKERSSON sah eine rezidivierende Facialislähmung: es handelte sich um einen 35jährigen Mann, der an dieser Erkrankung vom 3.—18. Jahre litt. Nach dem 18. Jahre wurde die Lähmung stationär. Während der ganzen Zeit und auch später fanden sich QUINCKEsche Ödeme der Lippen; zuletzt blieb die Schwellung an der Oberlippe konstant. Einen ähnlichen Fall habe ich bei einem jungen Mädchen beobachtet. Auch ROSENTHAL hat solche Beobachtungen gemacht.

Sehr interessant ist das Vorkommen von angioneurotischen Ödemen bei myasthenischer Paralyse (DILLER, eigene Beobachtung). In unserem Falle waren die typischen myasthenischen Erscheinungen eng mit denen des flüchtigen Ödems verknüpft, beide spielten sich im wesentlichen in derselben Gegend ab und gingen auch einigermaßen miteinander parallel.

FULTON und BAILEY beobachteten ein 15jähriges Mädchen, das nach einem fieberhaften Rheumatismus Auftreten von Durst, vorzeitiges Auftreten der Menses, Fettsucht, Schlafsucht, Sehschwäche, periodische Extremitätenschwäche, QUINCKEsches Ödem, Kopfschmerzen, Opticusatrophie darbot. Er faßt in diesem Falle das angioneurotische Ödem als Anzeichen dafür auf, daß der 3. Ventrikel ergriffen ist. STERTING hat Fälle von periodischer Lähmung mit QUINCKE kombiniert gesehen, in denen sämtliche, oder nur die unteren Extremitäten affiziert waren. Er vermutet, daß das Ödem die ganze Rückenmarksubstanz in Mitleidenschaft ziehen könne.

Über die Beziehungen zwischen *Migräne* und QUINCKEschem Ödem hat zuletzt QUINCKE selbst sich geäußert: unter 36 seiner Fälle litten 7 an anfallsweise auftretendem Kopfschmerz, meist in einer als Migräne anzusprechenden Form. Zeitliche Beziehungen zwischen den Anfällen des akuten, umschriebenen Ödems und der Migräne bestanden nur in einigen Fällen. In einem Fall habitueller Migräne zeigten sich äußerlich sichtbare Schwellungen an Schläfen und Augen als Begleit- bzw. Einleitungssymptome des Anfalls erst im Alter von etwa 50 Jahren. Sie betrafen Augenlider, Stirn, Nase und Unterkiefergegend, wahrscheinlich auch das Zellgewebe der Orbita und der seitlichen Nackengegend, dann des Halses. Später traten solche Schwellungen flüchtig, auch ohne Migräneanfall auf. QUINCKE ist der Ansicht, daß der zeitliche Ablauf der Anfälle es hier gewiß nahe legen würde, in den Hirnhäuten ähnliche Vorgänge wie an der äußeren Haut zu vermuten. Es erscheint QUINCKE daher die übrigens auch sonst vielfach vertretene Annahme einer Hemicrania meningooedematosa ebenso berechtigt, wie die der vasomotorischen Hemikranien; auch die Halbseitigkeit, oft mit genauer Abgrenzung bis zur Mittellinie, trifft, wie er hervorhebt, beim akuten Ödem häufiger zu als bei den reinen Gefäßneurosen. Als Sitz des Ödems nimmt er für die rein neuralgischen Formen die harte Hirnhaut an, was uns sehr unwahrscheinlich erscheint, während bei den Fällen mit Symptomen seitens der Augen, der Motilität, der Sensibilität und der Sprache auch ein umschriebenes Ödem der Pia vorliegen dürfte. Dem Einwande, daß nur ein kleiner Bruchteil der Migränekranken sichtbare, akute, umschriebene Ödeme aufweist und daß eine zeitliche Koinzidenz des Migräneanfalles mit solchen selten sei, begegnet er mit dem Hinweis, daß auch die Erkrankungen anderer tief gelegener Organe, die man als akutes umschriebenes Ödem deutet, durchaus nicht immer zeitlich mit Hautschwellungen zusammenfallen. Die ganze Frage erscheint aber noch keineswegs spruchreif. In den zahlreichen Fällen von Meningitis serosa acuta, die wir zu Gesicht bekommen haben, ist uns der Nachweis von angioneurotischen Ödemen anderen Sitzes niemals gelungen. Andererseits waren in einigen wenigen Fällen unseres Beobachtungskreises die Erscheinungen der Meningitis serosa so flüchtiger Art, daß man in der Tat an ein flüchtiges Ödem der Hirnhäute denken konnte.

BOLTEN verficht die Behauptung, daß zwischen dem angioneurotischen Ödem und der genuinen Epilepsie Beziehungen bestehen, in dem er die Epilepsie als ein angioneurotisches Ödem der Großhirnrinde auffaßt. Für diese Auffassung macht er folgende Gründe geltend: 1. die Kombination von Epilepsie mit anderen exsudativen Symptomen und zahlreichen vasomotorisch-trophischen Erscheinungen; 2. das Vorhandensein pathologisch-anatomischer Veränderungen in den endokrinen Drüsen; 3. das Auftreten von epileptischen Anfällen nach ausgedehnten Strumektomien; 4. die mit Organotherapie erreichten Erfolge. Er stellt sich vor, daß durch den pathologischen Stoffwechsel bei der genuinen Epilepsie, der träge sein soll, sich intermediäre, sauere Stoffwechselprodukte anhäufen, die zu einer Azidose führen; daraus resultieren lokales Ödem der Hirnrinde, erhöhter Hirndruck und infolgedessen der Anfall. Mit Recht steht DUSSER DE BARENNE diesen Ausführungen kritisch gegenüber [1].

Daß manche Fälle von Epilepsie dem Kreise der allergischen Krankheiten zuzurechnen sind, nimmt auch STORM VAN LEEUWEN an; er läßt jedoch in seiner Monographie die Beziehung von Migräne, Epilepsie, QUINCKES Ödem zur Allergie mit Rücksicht darauf, daß dabei die Verhältnisse noch schwer zu übersehen sind, außer Betracht, wenn er auch die Tatsache zugibt, daß eine Allergie manchmal Anfälle von Migräne und Epilepsie verursachen kann. FERET beschrieb flüchtige Ödeme bei Epileptikern und KENNEDY berichtet über ein 2jähriges Mädchen mit heftigen Urticariaanfällen. Einem solchen Schub ging einmal ein Anfall voraus, bei dem das Kind mehrmals am Tage laut aufschrie und an den Kopf faßte. Später trat in Verbindung mit Urticaria eine Reihe epileptischer Anfälle auf.

Daß gelegentlich Fieber beobachtet wird, wurde schon betont. Der erwähnte Fall von DIETHELM zeigt die höchste Temperatursteigerung. Bei einer unserer Patientinnen wurden in mehreren Stadien ihres Leidens Fieberanstiege bis zu 39^0 beobachtet. Nicht selten finden wir allgemeine Erytheme, die dem Auftreten der Ödeme vorausgehen (WILLS, COOPER, YARIAN, OSLER, DINKELACKER, SCHLESINGER u. a.), im Falle PESOPOULOS hohes Fieber mit Hautblutungen.

Die Stoffwechseluntersuchungen bei QUINCKESCHEM Ödem (HRYNIEWIECKI, SCHULTZER, LINDNER, ROUSSEL u. a.) haben keine eindeutigen Resultate ergeben; DESAUX-GUILLAUMIN stellen Hypocalcämie fest und führen sie auf eine Störung der Nebenschilddrüse zurück. Das gleiche gilt von den pharmakologischen Prüfungen, die von verschiedener Seite angestellt worden sind (Literatur bei TÖRÖK). Erwähnung verdient jedoch die von einer Reihe von

---

[1] Zit. nach DUSSER DE BARRENNE: Zbl. Neur. 40, 924 (1925).

Autoren festgestellte Eosinophilie (NAEGELI, KÄMMERER). GÄNSSLER fand bis zu 20% Eosinophilie, die höchsten Werte 6—8 Tage nach dem Auftreten des Ödems.
 Es gibt Fälle, in denen sich die Krankheit über die ganze Lebensdauer des Individuums hinweg erstreckt. STRÜBING kannte einen Fall, in dem vom 26. bis 70. Lebensjahr Anfälle auftraten und Ähnliches ist gar nicht selten beobachtet worden. Das Intervall zwischen den einzelnen Anfällen variiert sehr. Es gibt Beobachtungen, wo sie ein sehr seltenes Vorkommnis darstellen. SALLES notierte sie im Verlauf von 25 Jahren nur 4mal. Sie können alle paar Monate erscheinen oder jeden Monat. Dann halten sie sich oft an den Termin der Menses. Es gibt Fälle, wo sie Jahre hintereinander immer mehrmals im Monat auftraten. MILTON sah seit Jahren nie eine Woche ohne Anfall vorübergehen. Meist kamen sie sogar jeden 2. Tag. Auch tägliches Auftreten wird beobachtet, andererseits kann es bei einem einzigen Anfall sein Bewenden haben (QUINCKE). Eine Patientin PARKERS hatte seit 2 Jahren täglich an irgendeiner Stelle der Haut oder der Luftwege eine Schwellung.
 Manchmal stellen sich die Anfälle stets zur bestimmten Zeit ein oder in sehr regelmäßigen Intervallen.
 In manchen Fällen kombinieren sich die Erscheinungen der QUINCKEschen Krankheit, soweit wir sie bisher geschildert haben, mit *anderen vasomotorischen* und *vasomotorisch-trophischen Symptomen* zu komplizierteren Krankheitsbildern, die sich einer ganz bestimmten und sicheren Klassifikation entziehen und Übergangsformen darstellen, wie sie auch sonst auf unserem Gebiete so überaus häufig sind. Einen solchen Fall haben kürzlich VALLERY-RADOT, PASTEUR und BLAMOUTIER publiziert. Am nächsten steht die QUINCKEsche Krankheit unzweifelhaft der *Urticaria*, von der sie überhaupt nicht vollkommen zu trennen ist. So macht QUINCKE in seiner letzten Abhandlung darauf aufmerksam, daß vier seiner Kranken, die an typischer Urticaria litten, später mit Anfällen von akutem umschriebenem Ödem erkrankten und daß in der Familie von Ödemkranken Urticariafälle vorkommen. Er erwähnt, daß solche Mischformen bei Hunden nicht selten vorkommen; so beobachtete er sie bei einem jungen Foxterrier. Am engsten sind die Beziehungen zu der sog. Urticaria gigantea. Wenn im allgemeinen die Urticariaquaddeln durch Röte, Jucken, Hitze, die des flüchtigen Ödems durch Blässe, Kühle, Fehlen von subjektiven Störungen ausgezeichnet sind, so gibt es doch die mannigfaltigsten Übergänge der einzelnen Schwellungen, und es kommt zum Auftreten von Schwellungen sehr verschiedener Art bei demselben Individuum. Einschlägige Fälle sind vor nicht langer Zeit von STROUSE berichtet worden. Ein Fall betrifft einen 56jährigen Mann, in dessen Familie Heufieber, Diabetes, Gicht, Migräne und Fettsucht heimisch waren. Er bekam wiederholt Attacken von generalisierter Urticaria, zeigte zeitweise Ödeme der Lider und Lippen. Die Erscheinungen waren vom Fleischgehalt der Nahrung abhängig. Im Harn war das Indikan vermehrt. Die Behandlung erfolgte mit proteinfreier Diät, Joghurt und Hinterlappenhypophysenextrakt und brachte Heilung, die nunmehr 8 Jahre andauert.
 TÖRÖK handelt das QUINCKEsche Ödem in dem Abschnitte „Urticaria" ab, indem er von Fällen spricht, in welchen *ausschließlich* die großen Anschwellungen auftreten; es handle sich bei beiden tatsächlich um denselben krankhaften Prozeß, „wie das relativ häufige Zusammentreffen von typischen Quaddeln und größeren ödematösen Anschwellungen an Stellen mit lockerem Unterhautbindegewebe (Augenlider, äußere Genitalien und Ohrläppchen usw.), das Alternieren von Quaddelausbrüchen und ödematösen Schwellungen in demselben Falle bzw. bei Mitgliedern derselben Familie, die Ähnlichkeit der Symptome von seiten innerer Organe und der Lokalisation an Schleimhäuten und anderen Organen, die Identität der pathologisch-anatomischen Veränderungen der Haut

und die Ätiologie zur Genüge beweisen." PASTEUR-VALLERY-RADOT und HEIMANN trennen die Urticaria vom QUINCKEschen Ödem ab, ohne die nahen verwandtschaftlichen Beziehungen zu verkennen.

Ein besonderes Interesse beansprucht die von ASSMANN und E. RUHEMANN bei der Besprechung der RAYNAUDschen Krankheit bereits erwähnte Beobachtung, bei der außer dem QUINCKEschen Ödem und einem Hydrops articulorum intermittens Migräne, multiple angiospastische Zustände und RAYNAUD-Symptome aufgetreten sind. Die genannten Autoren fassen die Krankheitserscheinungen als verschieden hohe Reizgrade *einer* Krankheitseinheit auf, der angioneurotischen exsudativen Diathese. Sehr merkwürdig ist infolge der Vielseitigkeit der allergischen Erscheinungen der Fall, den VAUGHAN-WARREN-HAWKE beschrieben haben. Im Zeitraum von wenigen Jahren sahen sie bei dem Kranken im Anschluß an Tomaten- und Eiergenuß die folgenden Symptome auftreten: Anfälle von rechtsseitigem Abdominalschmerz, der klinisch eine akute Appendicitis vortäuschte, anhaltenden Husten mit Symptomen einer chronischen Sinusitis, röntgenologisch Pleuraverdickungen und tuberkuloseverdächtige Lungenherde, die aber sämtlich allmählich von selbst verschwanden; Hydrarthrose an den verschiedensten Gelenken, Anfälle ausgesprochener Erythromelalgie, mehrere Anfälle von ausgesprochenem Menière mit peripheren vasomotorischen Erscheinungen, Parästhesien in den Armen, doppelseitige Ulnarislähmung, Nierenkoliken, schwerer Meningismus mit partieller Blindheit, Verschluß der Urethra, Anfälle von Blasentenesmen; die meisten Erscheinungen schwanden prompt nach Adrenalininjektionen. Die Erscheinungen an den inneren Organen waren meist mit Hautsymptomen verbunden.

Vielfach haben wir flüchtige Schwellungen typischer Ausprägung zusammen mit den typischen Symptomen von *Akroparästhesien* gesehen. Wir sind Fällen begegnet, die bald das Bild der Urticaria, bald des flüchtigen Ödems, bald der Akroparästhesien boten.

Nicht selten finden sich wie in dem Falle von ASSMANN Beziehungen zur RAYNAUDschen Krankheit. Daß Unregelmäßigkeiten in der Blutverteilung der Haut öfter beobachtet wurden, ist schon erwähnt worden. Ausgeprägte RAYNAUDsche Symptome, wie Syncope locale und Asphyxie locale, sind seltener, aber JOSEPH, STARR, WIDOWITZ, CALMAN, SCHLESINGER u. a. haben solche Fälle erwähnt. Wir selbst haben in den letzten Jahren eine Reihe von Kranken beobachtet, bei denen die Symptome der RAYNAUDschen Krankheit in ihrer klassischen Form vorhanden waren, bei denen aber auch ganz charakteristische flüchtige Ödeme auftraten. Wir sahen z. B. einen Fall, bei dem auf der einen Seite RAYNAUDsche Symptome in voller Intensität ausgeprägt waren, allerdings zeigten sich die trophischen Störungen weniger in der Form nekrotischer Veränderungen, als in der einer dauernden Schwellung der Weichteile; auf der anderen Seite standen zahlreiche Erscheinungen des flüchtigen Ödems, Hautschwellungen, Schwellungen der Muskeln, Ergüsse in die Gelenke, symmetrische Schwellungen der Mundspeicheldrüsen und Fieberattacken. In einem weiteren komplizierten Falle dieser Art fanden sich teils Symptome der RAYNAUDschen Krankheit teils der Erythromelalgie neben den Erscheinungen der flüchtigen Schwellungen. Die ersteren traten in Form ausgesprochener vasomotorischer und sensibler Reizerscheinungen an den gipfelnden Teilen der Hände und Füße, in Synkope, Hyperämie, Asphyxie zutage. PARKES WEBER sah einen 38jährigen Mann, der zunächst intermittierendes Hinken des rechten Beines mit zeitweiligem vasomotorischen Störungen an Händen und Füßen zeigte. Später trat unter heftigen Schmerzen eine cyanotische Verfärbung des Fußes mit Geschwürsbildung ein; ungefähr $1/2$ Jahr danach stellten sich Anfälle von Urticaria und angioneurotischem Ödem ein. ETTINGER beschreibt einen sehr komplizierten

Fall von flüchtigen Ödemen und multipler Hautgangrän. SCHLESINGER hat die Kombination von Erythromelalgiesymptomen und flüchtigen Ödemen erwähnt, doch ist der Fall nicht eindeutig.

Ebenso findet MAY Beziehungen zur Erythromelalgie, außerdem zur Arthritis und Tetanie. Es handelte sich um eine 53jährige Frau mit leicht myxödematösem Habitus und symmetrischer chronischer Schwellung der submaxillaren Drüsen und der Parotis, die in der Kindheit an einem häufig rezidivierenden Gesichtsödem mit Schwellung der Lider litt, das in der Jugend deutliche Beziehungen zur Menstruation zeigte. 16 Jahre später traten Anfälle von schmerzhaftem Ödem der oberen Extremitäten, verbunden mit tetanischen Beugekrämpfen in den Vorderarmen auf. Einige Monate später schmerzhafte Parästhesien in den Beinen; nach einer Pause von 8 Jahren Anfälle von Rötung und ödematöser Schwellung beider Beine. Abgesehen davon seit einigen Jahren Arthritis deformans an den 4. und 5. Fingern beider Hände. Wa.R. positiv. SIMONS sah erythematöse und ödematöse Schwellungen periodisch auftreten.

Eine andere Kombination stellt das von WILHELM zuerst beobachtete Zusammenvorkommen von flüchtigen Ödemen und Epidermolysis bullosa dar.

Als hereditäre Neigung zur Blasenbildung stellte GOLDSCHEIDER 1882 Fälle aus einer Familie vor, bei deren Mitgliedern auf das geringste Trauma hin an den betroffenen Stellen Blasen auftraten. Derartige Fälle sind später von einer ganzen Reihe von Autoren — wir nennen VALLENTIN, KÖBNER, JOSEPH, BETTMANN, STÜHMER, MASCHKILLEISSON, HACHEZ, JENNY, FUHS, HOFMANN, CURTIUS und STREMPEL, SCHOCH, H. MÜLLER u. a. — beschrieben worden. Eine eingehende Darstellung der Erkrankung stammt aus der Feder von RIECKE, die auch die Gesamtliteratur enthält. Um die Erforschung dieser Erkrankung, speziell ihrer Vererbungspathologie, hat sich besonders H. W. SIEMENS verdient gemacht. Wir folgen im wesentlichen der von ihm gegebenen Darstellung. Die abnorme Neigung schon auf ganz unbedeutende Hautreize mechanischer oder toxischer Natur mit Blasenbildung zu reagieren, kann hochgradig erblich bedingt sein. Die einzelnen Blasen heilen entweder folgenlos ab, während sich immer neue bilden (Epidermolysis mechanica simplex), oder sie können Atrophien, Epidermiscysten und Nageldystrophien zurücklassen (Epidermolysis mechanica dystrophica). Die Blasenbildung erfolgt bei den erstgenannten Fällen überwiegend oberflächlich, bei den letztgenannten tief zwischen Epidermis und Cutis. Indessen hat FUHS beobachtet, daß Übergänge und ein Nebeneinandervorkommen von oberflächlicher zu tieferer Blasenbildung bei beiden Formen nachzuweisen ist, so daß er der Ansicht ist, daß verwertbare gesetzmäßige Beziehungen nicht vorliegen. SIEMENS, dem sich auch MASCHKILLEISSON und andere Autoren anschließen, trennt die beiden Gruppen auch erbbiologisch scharf voneinander. Er fand bei der Bullosis mechanica simplex in 16 Familien ein Verhältnis von 177 Kranken zu 158 gesunden Geschwistern. Die Vererbung konnte durch sieben Generationen verfolgt werden. Er fand ferner, daß gelegentlich ein Überspringen von Generationen vorkommt, möglicherweise etwas häufiger bei Weibern. Er betrachtet die einfache Epidermolysis in der Mehrzahl der Fälle als eine dominante Idiodermatose mit in engen Grenzen gehaltenen Manifestationsunregelmäßigkeiten. Die Bullosis mechanica dystrophica dagegen findet sich nur selten in mehreren Generationen einer Familie. SIEMENS fand 20 Geschwisterfälle und sechsmal elterliche Blutsverwandtschaft und nimmt eine überwiegend recessive Erbanlage an.

Auch MASCHKILLEISSON ist der Ansicht, daß es sich bei beiden Formen um dem Wesen nach insofern verschiedene Erkrankungen handelt, als sie zwar angeboren, aber nicht durch die gleichen Störungen des Keimplasmas bedingt sind. Er betont, daß sichere Fälle von gleichzeitigen Erkrankungen an beiden

Formen bei Gliedern einer Familie bisher nicht bekannt sind. Ätiologisch nimmt er eine angeborene Minderwertigkeit des elastischen Gewebes an.

Zu der dystrophischen Form gehören als Unterabteilung die von HOFMANN beschriebenen Fälle von Bullosis mechanica dystrophica mutilans, die ebenfalls recessiv auftritt und narbige Kontrakturen der Finger mit Ankylosen und Verkürzungen der Endphalangen zeigt. Hierher gehört auch die von JENNY beschriebene Form, die SIEMENS als Bullosis mechanica letalis sive maligna bezeichnet. Es handelte sich um sieben Kinder aus fünf Geschwisterschaften, die zwei Familienkreisen der gleichen Gegend angehören. Vier Eltern waren blutsverwandt. Bei den befallenen Kindern war die Neigung zur Blasenbildung von Geburt an eine so starke, daß ausnahmslos nach Wochen und Monaten der Tod eintrat. In diesen Fällen konnte sowohl experimentell als auch nach der Lokalisation die mechanische Genese der Hautblasen, der Nagelveränderungen und der Schleimhautulcerationen aufgedeckt werden. Der Stammbaum, der bis ins 17. Jahrhundert verfolgt werden konnte, ließ recessive Vererbung erkennen, wie sie SIEMENS für die dystrophische Form postuliert hat.

Eine ähnliche Familie hat H. MILLER beschrieben. Es handelt sich um vier von derselben Mutter stammende Kinder, die entweder schon mit Blasenbildungen am ganzen Körper und erheblichen Epidermisdefekten geboren wurden, oder solche am ersten und zweiten Tage nach der Geburt zeigten. Alle Kinder starben bald nach der Geburt. Die Mutter der Kinder ist die Tochter der Schwester des Mannes, eines Arztes, der trotz genauester Erhebungen sonst keine hereditäre Belastung aufdecken konnte.

In dem von MENDES DA COSTA beschriebenen Fall von Epidermolysis bullosa dystrophica, der klinisch ein sehr atypisches Bild zeigte und auch mit Hypotrichosis verbunden war, zeigte sich ebenfalls eine recessiv geschlechtsgebundene Vererbung. In dieser Familie waren sieben Vettern befallen, die vier verschiedenen Geschwisterschaften angehörten und deren Mütter Schwestern waren.

Eine recht interessante Beobachtung publizieren CURTIUS und STREMPEL, die in einer Familie ein gleichzeitiges Vorkommen von RECKLINGHAUSENscher Krankheit und Epidermolysis bullosa traumatica hereditaria dystrophica gesehen haben. Die an Epidermolysis bullosa dystrophica leidende Kranke zeugte mit einem an familiärer RECKLINGHAUSENscher Krankheit leidenden Manne sechs Kinder, von denen ein Knabe nur an Epidermolysis bullosa dystrophica, ein anderer nur an RECKLINGHAUSENscher Krankheit, vier Kinder an beiden Krankheiten litten. Bei einzelnen Mitgliedern der Familie fand sich eine Scapula scaphoidea.

Im einzelnen ist zu erwähnen, daß sich häufig bei der Bullosis mechanica eine Hyperhydrosis palmaris und plantaris findet, gelegentlich eine Alopecia congenita. Die Blasen treten besonders während der heißen Jahreszeit auf und bilden sich an allen Stellen, an denen die Haut einer mechanischen Reizung ausgesetzt ist. Vereinzelt wurden sie auch auf Schleimhäuten beobachtet. Ein plötzliches starkes Trauma, Schlag, Quetschung, ruft keine Blasenbildung hervor, sondern nur die gewöhnlichen geringen traumatischen Schädigungen, das Tragen der Kleider, Strumpfbänder, der Schuhe, die gewöhnlichen Beschäftigungen des Lebens. An den betroffenen Stellen entsteht zunächst ein roter juckender Fleck, auf dem sich unter fortgesetztem Jucken und Brennen eine kleine, erbsen- bis nußgroße, klare, prall gefüllte Blase bildet. Die Blasen werden dann trübe, platzen, es resultiert eine nässende Fläche, die nach 2 Tagen eintrocknet. Bei der einfachen Form bleiben Narben nicht zurück, auch keine Pigmentierungen.

Bei der zweiten Gruppe, der Bullosis dystrophica, wird häufig eine besondere Lokalisation angegeben, und oft ist auch eine gewisse Symmetrie vorhanden. In einigen Fällen sind es besonders die Extremitäten: Hände und Füße, und zwar besonders die Streckseite, die Gelenke, Ellenbogen und Knie, die befallen werden. Außer der Prädilektion für gewisse Stellen und der Symmetrie sind weitere Unterscheidungsmerkmale, die den Blaseneruptionen folgenden, weitgehenden Hautveränderungen. Es kommt zu Pigmentierungen, zu Narbenbildungen, zur Atrophie der Haut und sehr häufig zu Veränderungen der Nägel. HELLER erklärt diese durch einen der Blasenbildung analogen Prozeß in der Nagelmatrix, dessen Folge eine Schädigung des Nagelwachstums ist. Die Nägel können schon bei der Geburt fehlen oder bald danach ausfallen, wechseln mehrmals, um schließlich ganz oder teilweise auszufallen, oder sie sind verdickt, grau, verkrümmt oder in einzelne Schichten gespalten abblätternd oder klauenartig deformiert, glanzlos. BETTMANN hat an der Haut von Kranken mit Epidermolysis bullosa beider Formen capillaroskopische Untersuchungen angestellt und findet äußerst zarte unregelmäßig angeordnete kleine Gefäße; auch bei Abheilung kehrt der normale Gefäßtypus nicht zurück. Außerdem fielen ihre Abweichungen vom typischen Leistenbild der Haut bis zum völligen Fehlen der Papillarleisten auf. Er spricht — für die dystrophische Form wenigstens — die Vermutung aus, daß es sich um eine Anomalie handelt, bei der eine Störung im Sinne einer anatomischen Mißbildung des Gefäßabschnittes vorliegen könne. SKALETZ stellt Lymphocytose fest.

Es scheint uns, als ob die Affektion pathogenetische Beziehungen zum flüchtigen Ödem hat. Es ist nämlich sehr wahrscheinlich, daß ihre Ursache in einer abnormen Irritabilität oder Durchlässigkeit der Gefäße zu suchen ist, die auf einer mangelhaften oder fehlerhaften Entwicklung des Gefäßsystems beruht. Die Kombination von flüchtigen Ödemen und Epidermolysis bullosa wurde in dem schon erwähnten Falle von WILHELM konstatiert. Allerdings handelte es sich um eine nicht hereditäre Form. Bemerkenswert ist es noch, daß der Kranke von WILHELM an schweren nervösen Diarrhöen litt, ein Symptomenbild, das an die inneren Symptome bei dem flüchtigen Ödem erinnert, das wir auch sonst bei Vasoneurotikern häufig genug zu sehen bekommen. Auf Grund seiner Beobachtungen an drei interessanten Fällen, davon zwei Brüdern, nimmt er als Grundursache eine schwere Störung der Schilddrüse und davon vielleicht abhängig der Nebennierenfunktion an, ohne jedoch für diese Ansicht genügende Beweise zu bringen. Noch weniger gestützt ist freilich die Annahme, daß die spinalen grauen Zentren der eigentliche Sitz der Erkrankung sein sollen. Daß auch sonst Beziehungen zu vasomotorischen Erkrankungen bestehen, beweisen die Beobachtungen von LINSER und ferner von STÜHMER. Ersterer fand bei Epidermolysis in einigen Fällen eine abnorme vasomotorische Reizbarkeit im Sinne RAYNAUDscher Krankheit, STÜHMER vasomotorische Störungen im Sinne einer Akroasphyxie, Cutis marmorata, Dermographie, Urticaria. Und auch hier wird es nicht immer möglich sein, die Entscheidung darüber zu treffen, ob eine Kombination zweier Krankheitsbilder oder Misch- oder Übergangsformen vorliegen.

Prognose.

Das bedrohlichste Symptom bilden die Glottisödeme. Durch diese Erscheinungen ist in einer ganzen Reihe von Fällen das Leben schwer gefährdet und in einer erheblichen Anzahl in der Tat der Exitus herbeigeführt worden. Die ersten beiden derartigen Beobachtungen sind von METTLER beschrieben worden. Seitdem sind noch eine große Reihe von Fällen, die diesen unglücklichen Ausgang nahmen, publiziert worden. In einzelnen Familien (ENSOR, FRITZ, WHITING, MENDEL, HLAVÁČEK) starben eine ganze Reihe von Mitgliedern regelmäßig an Glottisödem. Bei diesen unglücklich ausgehenden Fällen handelt es sich meist um familiäre. Der Tod kann außerordentlich rasch eintreten, so daß zu der sonst lebensrettenden Tracheotomie keine Zeit mehr ist. Einzelne Patienten wurden, wie schon erwähnt, mehrfach tracheotomiert, einzelne wurden dauernd gezwungen, eine Kanüle zu tragen. Daß auch das angioneurotische Lungenödem gelegentlich zum Exitus führen kann, ist nicht zu bezweifeln, doch liegt ein solcher Fall in der Literatur bisher nicht vor. Zu denken ist auch daran, daß schwere Gehirnerscheinungen nach Art der von ULLMANN berichteten einen letalen Ausgang herbeiführen können.

Ungünstig ist die Prognose quoad restitutionem. Es kommen sehr lange Intermissionen vor, von 10 und 15 Jahren, aber die Neigung zu steten Rezidiven ist doch sehr groß. Eine Tendenz zu allmählichen spontanen Besserungen mit zunehmendem Alter läßt sich in manchen Fällen nicht verkennen. Doch zieht sich das Leiden bisweilen durch das ganze Leben hin, ohne in der übergroßen Zahl der Fälle die Lebensdauer abzukürzen.

Pathogenese.

Das am meisten in die Augen fallende Symptom der QUINCKEschen Krankheit sind die *Ödeme*, die auch sonst in der Symptomatologie der vasomotorisch-trophischen Neurosen im allgemeinen eine erhebliche Rolle spielen.

Als Ödem bezeichnet man bekanntlich die Flüssigkeitsansammlung in den Geweben, die durch eine abnorm starke, kürzere oder längere Zeit dauernde Durchtränkung der Gewebe mit der den Blutgefäßen entstammenden Lymphe entsteht. Den für uns nicht in Betracht kommenden Formen des Stauungsödems, des kachektischen oder hydrämischen und des entzündlichen Ödems steht das neurotische Ödem gegenüber, mit dem allein wir es hier zu tun haben. Was die Frage seiner Entstehung betrifft, so sind über die Lymphbildung im allgemeinen im großen und ganzen zwei Hypothesen aufgestellt worden: das eine ist die Filtrations-, das andere die Sekretionshypothese. Die Filtrationshypothese besagt, daß die Lymphe ein Filtrat der Blutflüssigkeit ist (LUDWIG und seine Schule). Demgegenüber gipfelt HEIDENHAINs Ansicht in dem Satz, daß bei der Lymphbildung unter normalen Zirkulationsverhältnissen die Filtration keine Rolle spielt; vielmehr glaubt er, daß die Capillarzellen als sezernierende Elemente bei der Lymphbildung beteiligt sind. Aber selbst bei Annahme der ersten Hypothese können wir nicht der Ansicht beipflichten, daß die Ödeme immer eine Folge vasomotorischer Störungen sind; denn in vielen Fällen sehen wir gar nichts von solchen vasomotorischen Störungen und in anderen Fällen fehlt es an jedem Parallelismus zwischen ihnen und den Ödemen.

Diese Fragen haben vor einigen Jahren durch C. ÖHME eine kritische Bearbeitung erfahren; er weist darauf hin, daß die klinische Beweisführung der neurogenen Pathogenese bei den mannigfaltigen Bildern eine verschiedene Sicherheit hat und daß in der Mehrzahl der Fälle die anatomische oder funktionelle nachgewiesene oder auf Grund allgemeiner Erwägungen mehr deduzierte Bedeutung der Nervenläsion nur die Rolle eines unterstützenden Momentes hat. Aus seinen Ausführungen geht hervor, daß unsere Kenntnisse noch sehr lückenhafte sind, so daß sich ein Eingehen auf die zur Zeit zur Diskussion stehenden Theorien an dieser Stelle erübrigt.

Ein experimenteller Nachweis für den Einfluß der Nerven auf die Lymphbildung ist jedenfalls bisher nicht erbracht worden. KÄMMERER weist auf den Zusammenhang des QUINCKEschen Ödems mit bestimmten anderen Gefäßalterationen hin, ihre unmittelbare Abhängigkeit von den vasomotorischen Zuständen, und denkt daher in erster Linie an Capillarschädigungen, an eine erhöhte Durchlässigkeit der Gefäßepithelien und in zweiter Linie an eine Schädigung und damit erhöhte Quellungsbereitschaft der Gewebe. Allergisch-anaphylaktische Genese würde nach seiner Ansicht ebenfalls in diesem Sinne sprechen. Eine ähnliche Rolle weist Török bei der Urticaria der Permeabilität der Gefäßwände zu.

Was nun die Ursache der Reizung betrifft, die letzten Endes als wirksam für die Ödembildung in Frage kommt, so scheint uns die klinische Beobachtung auf zwei Möglichkeiten hinzuweisen und die Veranlassung zur Zweiteilung der im Rahmen der Quinckeschen Krankheit beobachteten Erscheinungen zu geben.

Wir rechnen in die erste Gruppe die Fälle, die auf toxischem, autotoxischem oder infektiösem Wege entstehen, akut einsetzen und akut verlaufen, wie eine Intoxikation oder Infektion, keine Neigung zu Rezidiven haben oder doch nur insoweit, als sie immer wieder durch dieselbe toxische Schädlichkeit ausgelöst werden. Dieser Gruppe hat man in den letzten Jahren ein besonderes Interesse entgegengebracht, seitdem man erkannt hat, daß mit ihr Krankheitszustände innerlich zusammenhängen, deren enge pathogenetische Verwandtschaft bisher unbekannt war. Es handelt sich um die Zusammengehörigkeit von Migräne, Asthma, Heufieber, Urticaria, Ekzem, Serumkrankheit, angioneurotischem Ödem und bestimmten gastrointestinalen Störungen. Diese Lehre, von amerikanischen und englischen Autoren in der Hauptsache begründet (Crowder, Wolff-Eisner, Walker, Ramirez, Rackemann, Sterling, Coke, Freemann, Hurst, Rolleston, Auld, Widal u. a.) hat im Laufe der Jahrzehnte vielfache Erweiterungen, Einschränkungen und Umgestaltungen erfahren (Coca, Doerr, Kämmerer, Storm van Leeuwen), ohne daß es bisher gelungen ist, für die Pathogenese des Quinckeschen Ödems allgemeingültige Gesetze aufzustellen. Andererseits unterliegt es keinem Zweifel, daß in einer Reihe von Einzelfällen das Quinckesche Ödem als Überempfindlichkeit gegenüber bestimmten Allergenen gedeutet werden muß. Der gesamte Komplex hierhergehöriger Fragen hat durch Storm van Leeuwen und Kämmerer eine monographische Bearbeitung erfahren; diese Autoren nehmen zu den gegenwärtig diskutierten Anschauungen über Allergie, Idiosynkrasie, Anaphylaxie und ihre Beziehungen zueinander Stellung. Diese Erörterungen greifen jedoch weit über die Interessensphäre der Neurologen hinaus, so daß es ausreicht, an dieser Stelle die Fragen anzudeuten und auf die einschlägige Literatur hinzuweisen. Eskuchen und später W. Misch haben in Sammelreferaten dieses Gebiet bearbeitet. Wir legen unserer Darstellung im wesentlichen das Referat Eskuchen zugrunde.

Das Gemeinsame aller dieser Ordnungsversuche liegt darin, daß hier von einem einheitlichen *ätiologischen Momente,* der *Proteinintoxikation,* ausgegangen wird. Die Krankheitsgruppe wird demnach jene der Proteinintoxikationen oder der Proteinüberempfindlichkeitskrankheiten genannt; Eskuchen schlägt jedoch aus verschiedenen Gründen die Bezeichnung „*toxische Idiopathien*" vor, weil sie weniger einschränkend ist und dafür etwas Wesentliches betont. Diese toxischen Idiopathien sind der Ausdruck einer spezifischen Proteinüberempfindlichkeit bei konstitutionell disponierten Individuen. Vererbt und angeboren wird in der Regel nicht eine *spezifische* Überempfindlichkeit, sondern die Neigung zur Sensibilisierung überhaupt. Die *latente* Überempfindlichkeit kann durch einmalige, wiederholte oder dauernde Proteinintoxikation *manifest* werden.

Gleichartigen und in gleicher Weise aufgenommenen Proteinen können verschiedenartige klinische Symptome entsprechen. Häufig ist die Überempfindlichkeit keine. *isolierte* (durch *ein* Protein bedingte), sondern eine *polygene,* woraus verwickelte Kombination resultieren können. Von großer Bedeutung für die Frage der Pathogenese des angioneurotischen Ödems erscheinen in diesem Zusammenhange noch eine Reihe von Arbeiten; auf die folgende soll noch in Kürze hingewiesen werden. Phillips berichtet über interessante Tierexperimente, die er an Hunden vorgenommen hat, bei denen das angioneurotische

Ödem dem menschlichen sehr ähnlich ist. Er hat bei diesen Hunden angioneurotisches Ödem unter dem klinischen Bilde des Ekzems, der Urticaria und des Asthmas gesehen; eine 5 Monate alte Bulldogge erhielt zum ersten Male Schweinefleisch; kurz darauf erfolgte Erbrechen, teilweise blutige Durchfälle, sehr heftiges Kratzen, Entwicklung eines Ödems der Haut, das nach 48 Stunden verschwunden war. Sie war später frei von Anfällen bei schweinefleischfreier Ernährung. 1 Jahr später zeigte sie deutliche Reaktion bei Applikation von Schweinefleischprotein auf die geritzte Haut. Unter den Vorfahren und Geschwistern des Hundes waren niemals auf Überempfindlichkeit beruhende Erkrankungen beobachtet worden. Ein anderer Hund litt regelmäßig nach dem Genuß von frischem oder konserviertem Fisch an plötzlich auftretenden Ödemen am Kopf, Rippen und Zunge, welche nach 24—48 Stunden verschwanden. Von den Nachkommen starb eines an Eklampsie, eines litt an Asthma bzw. später an Erythema exsudativum multiforme. Die Hautproben verliefen bei dem Hunde negativ, nachdem er 5 Jahre keinen Fisch bekommen und seine Empfindlichkeit gegen Ernährung mit Fisch verloren hatte. Im Anschluß daran berichtet PHILLIPS auch beim Menschen über einen Fall von angioneurotischem Ödem des Gesichts und der Lippen bei Überempfindlichkeit gegenüber Schweinefleischeiweiß, die auch durch intracutane Injektionen festgestellt war.

Wir werden demnach für die Mehrzahl der Fälle, welche der oben erwähnten Gruppe angehören, annehmen müssen, daß bei *disponierten* Individuen durch Proteine der Lymphgefäßeapparat im weiteren Sinne gereizt wird und auf dem Wege der erhöhten Lymphsekretion oder der erhöhten Durchlässigkeit der Gefäße oder auch der erhöhten Aufsaugungsfähigkeit des umliegenden Gewebes das Ödem hervorgebracht wird, meist unter gleichzeitigem Auftreten vasomotorischer und sensibler Phänomene. Dieser Reiz wirkt hier entweder direkt oder auf dem Wege peripherer oder zentraler Apparate. Bei manchen Individuen handelt es sich um eine angeborene Überempfindlichkeit (Allergie), bei anderen um die Neigung, gegen fremde Proteine empfindlich zu werden (Anaphylaxie). Meist ist die Aufnahme von Nahrung, gegen welche der Patient überempfindlich ist, das auslösende Moment, experimentell wurde das Krankheitsbild aber auch durch subcutane Injektionen von Proteinen aus Flachssamen und verschiedenen Pollenarten hervorgerufen.

Auch KÄMMERER erachtet es keineswegs für unbegründet, daß Nahrungsmittelallergie und autotoxische Shockgifte den Symptomenkomplex auslösen können, hält es aber für wahrscheinlich, daß auch bakterielle Antigene und Infektionen Bedeutung haben können, z. B. Nebenhöhleneiterungen.

Daß bei einer erheblichen Anzahl angioneurotischer Ödeme jedoch allergische Vorgänge keine nachweisbare Rolle spielen, muß als feststehend angesehen werden, wenn auch STORM VAN LEEUWEN selber das Vorkommen von QUINCKEschen Ödemen ausschließlich bei allergischen Fällen beobachtet hat.

In der zweiten heredofamiliären oder konstitutionell neuropathischen Gruppe, die natürlich von der ersten nicht ganz scharf zu trennen ist, wirkt der Reiz auf dem Wege nervöser Übertragung, die die nervösen Zentren und Bahnen des Lymphgefäß- und Vasomotorenapparates benutzt und dann wie in der ersten Gruppe in derselben Weise die flüchtigen Ödeme schafft. An die, wie uns allerdings scheinen will, nicht gerade naheliegende Möglichkeit, daß durch die primäre nervöse Erregung toxische Stoffe gebildet werden, die dann in völlig gleicher Weise wirken, wie bei der ersten Gruppe, muß noch gedacht werden. Worin die für die zweite Gruppe zu supponierende Empfindlichkeit des Nervensystems besteht, ist im einzelnen nicht mit Sicherheit zu sagen. Auch hier kommt, wie in der ganzen Gruppe, die Instabilität des vegetativen

Systems als konstitutionelle oder erworbene Grundlage in Frage. Anhaltspunkte für die Annahme einer solchen gesteigerten Empfindlichkeit dieses Systems finden wir häufig genug; aber es gelingt nicht, hier so wenig wie in den anderen Symptomenbildern, mehr als diese allgemeine Diathese nachzuweisen. Insbesondere ist das Vorliegen sympathicotroper oder vagotroper Erscheinungsreihen einwandfrei nicht nachgewiesen worden. BOLTEN glaubt auf experimentell-therapeutischem Wege festgestellt zu haben, daß das angioneurotische Ödem die Folge der Sympathicushypotonie sei; seine Schlüsse sind keineswegs bindend. Er gibt Schilddrüsen- und Nebennierenextrakt in der Idee, daß die Sympathicushypotonie Hypothyreoidismus zur Folge habe und daß damit eine Verzögerung in den zahlreichen fermentativen Prozessen des intermediären Stoffwechsels einträte. Dabei entstehende Toxine seien offenbar geeignet, Ödeme hervorzurufen. Seine therapeutischen Erfolge sind die Hauptstütze dieser Anschauung. Aber sie sind weder eindeutig, noch konstant. Wir kommen damit nicht weiter als bis zu der Annahme des Vorliegens einer hereditären oder erworbenen Instabilität des vegetativen Systems, in gleicher Weise, wie wir das in den früheren Kapiteln der RAYNAUDschen Krankheit und Sklerodermie auseinandergesetzt haben. Die Beziehungen zwischen dieser Labilität und etwaigen Störungen von endokrinen Drüsen, die man auch für das flüchtige Ödem als primäre Ursachen in Anspruch zu nehmen die Neigung hat, sind hier noch ganz ungeklärte. Positive Anhaltspunkte sind hier spärlicher noch als bei den früher genannten Affektionen; es bleiben eigentlich nur die flüchtigen Ödeme bei Basedow beachtenswert. Der Vollständigkeit halber möge jedoch erwähnt werden, daß eine Reihe von Autoren enge pathogenetische Beziehungen zwischen den endokrinen Drüsen und dem Auftreten des QUINCKEschen Ödems und des Trophödems annimmt: CASTELLINO und PENDE: Trophödem mit myxödematösem Habitus, MAY: Tetanie und Myxödem, CERVENKA: Hyperthyreoidismus. Auf die Beziehungen zu den Generationsphasen des Weibes ist bereits eingegangen worden. CASTELLINO und PENDE nehmen als Ursache des QUINCKEschen Ödems eine Thyreodystrophie plus Keimdrüsenerkrankung an, PARHON und STOCKER glauben, daß die Voraussetzung zum Auftreten des Trophödems immer eine Störung im Blutdrüsenapparat, das auslösende Moment eine nervöse Beeinflussung der pathologischen Lymphbildung sei[1]. In jüngster Zeit vertreten PASTEUR-VALLERY-RADOT und V. HEIMANN die Anschauung, daß ein Teil der Erkrankungen auf eine Störung des endokrinen Systems zurückzuführen sei, möglicherweise auf eine Sensibilisierung durch ein endokrines Hormon.

Diagnose.

Die Diagnose macht in allen typischen Fällen keine Schwierigkeiten. Selbstverständlich wird man zunächst darauf bedacht sein müssen, Ödeme, die im Verlauf von Herzkrankheiten und Nierenkrankheiten, von Kachexien, Nährschäden, Schilddrüsenerkrankungen entstehen, auszuschließen. Daß die Unterscheidung von der Urticaria nicht immer möglich ist, wurde betont. Ebenso sind die Zusammenhänge und die sich daraus ergebenden differentialdiagnostischen Schwierigkeiten gegenüber den vasomotorisch-trophischen Erkrankungen anderer Art bereits erwähnt. Und ebenso wurde bereits gesagt, daß diese flüchtigen Schwellungen in manchen Fällen nicht den Wert eines eigenen Krankheitsbildes haben, sondern nur als symptomatische Züge, im Verlauf eines anderen Leidens, wie der Migräne, des Basedow, der Neuralgie, der Tabes, gelegentlich auch der Gliosis und bei Kompressionserkrankungen des Rückenmarkes vorkommen. Neurotische Ödeme bei Syringomyelie sind zuerst von

---

[1] Zit. nach FALTA: Die Erkrankungen der Blutdrüsen. Berlin: Julius Springer 1928.

REMAK beschrieben worden; sie wurden aber bisher im ganzen nur recht selten gesehen (GNESDA, SCHLESINGER, FÜRSTNER, ZACHER). Nach SCHLESINGERS Angaben dauern sie meist längere Zeit, vergehen nur selten schon nach mehreren Tagen. Die Ödeme betreffen nicht nur die Haut, sondern auch die tiefen Gebilde. Wiederholt wurde das Zusammentreffen mit einer Arthropathie gesehen. Jedenfalls entstehen sie fast regelmäßig nur da, wo sonst Zeichen einer organischen Veränderung des Nervensystems in Form von Sensibilitätsstörungen und Motilitätsstörungen vorliegen. Diese ermöglichen die Diagnose.

Eines der Hauptkennzeichen der hier beschriebenen Ödeme ist ihre *Flüchtigkeit*. Nur sehr selten kommen Schwellungen dieser Art im Rahmen der QUINCKEschen Krankheit vor, die nicht rasch entstehen, sondern allmählich über bestimmte Teile des Körpers fortkriechen. Wo aber überhaupt keine Spur eines paroxysmalen Auftretens vorhanden ist, haben wir nicht mehr die Berechtigung, von der QUINCKESCHEN Krankheit zu sprechen.

Solche *chronisch-neuropathischen* Ödeme treten entweder als selbständige Krankheitsform auf oder als Symptome anderer Nervenkrankheiten.

Symptomatische Ödeme dieser Art finden wir z. B. auch bei Hemiplegien, oft zusammen mit anderen vasomotorischen Störungen; ferner bei der Hysterie in der Form des Oedème blanc und Oedème bleu, auch hier meist zusammen mit anderen hysterischen Symptomen, mit Lähmungen, Kontrakturen und Anästhesien. Das Ödem ist meist einseitig und singulär, aber es kommt auch eine Generalisierung bzw. eine Dissemination der Ödeme vor. Es kann plötzlich erscheinen und verschwinden, ist aber meist von langer Dauer.

Wenn wir erwägen, daß die QUINCKESCHE Affektion oft genug neuropathische Individuen betrifft, so müssen wir auch mit der Möglichkeit einer Kombination von Hysterie und echten QUINCKEschen Ödemen rechnen. BABINSKI leugnet auf Grund seiner neueren Anschauungen die Existenz hysterischer Ödeme vollkommen. Er sieht in ihnen entweder Artefakte oder bestreitet ihren hysterischen Charakter. In einer Reihe derartiger Fälle wurde in der Tat auch nachgewiesen, daß es sich um Kunstprodukte handelte (GLORIEUX, MEIGE). CLAUDE fand auf der anderen Seite in einem Fall, der als hysterisches Ödem angesehen wurde, als Ursache des Ödems des Handrückens eine Tuberkulose der Sehnenscheide. HEUYER berichtet, daß seit der Diskussion über diese Fragen, die im Jahre 1908 in der Société de neurologie stattgefunden hat, kein einziger Fall eines sicheren hysterischen Ödems beschrieben worden ist; er zitiert die Auffassung von CLOVIS VINCENT, nach der mechanische Ödeme sich im Laufe einer hysterischen Lähmung entwickeln können, ebenso wie Paresen und ein gewisser Grad von Hypertonie als Folgeerscheinung der Lage dauernder Akinese eines herabhängenden Gliedes. Diese Symptome verschwinden in dem Augenblick, in dem das Glied wieder seine normale Beweglichkeit ausführt. Zu allen diesen Fragen hat F. KEHRER eingehend kritisch Stellung genommen. Wir verweisen auf das Kapitel ,,Spezielle Symptomatologie der Hysterie und Neurasthenie" (dieses Handbuch, Erg.-Bd. 1, S. 176f.). An dieser Stelle finden sich auch hierhergehörige Betrachtungen über das traumatische Sklerödem, die nicht noch einmal rekapituliert zu werden brauchen. Ob diese Erfahrungen aber ausreichen, um die Möglichkeit einer hysterischen Genese der Ödeme für *alle* Fälle abzulehnen, scheint uns doch noch nicht gänzlich klargestellt. Rechnet man mit der Existenz hysterischer Ödeme, so wird für die Unterscheidung vom QUINCKESCHEN Ödem die lange Dauer, die Kombination mit anderen massiven hysterischen Symptomen (Paresen, Kontrakturen), eventuell der direkte Nachweis der psychogenen Entstehung und Beeinflussung zugunsten der Annahme einer Hysterie zu verwerten sein, aber es werden auch bei sorgfältiger Analyse Zweifel übrigbleiben.

Es gibt in der Literatur Fälle, und wir haben auch eigene derartige Beobachtungen anstellen können, in denen *allmählich* Ödeme sich entwickelten, für deren Entstehung einer der gewöhnlichen Ursachen nicht gefunden werden konnte, und die sich dadurch und auch durch das Vorhandensein anderer nervöser Symptome als neuropathische Ödeme zu demonstrieren schienen. Es gibt also *chronische neuropathische Ödeme*, die zum Teil einen segmentären Typus innehalten und daher von DEBOVE als Oedème segmentaire, in ähnlicher Weise auch von VIGOUROUX u. a. beschrieben wurden.

Hierher gehören dann vor allem die Fälle, die in der englischen Literatur unter dem Namen "an undescribed variety of hereditary oedema" zuerst von MILROY, in der französischen von MEIGE als «Trophoedème chronique héréditaire» beschrieben wurden. Weitere Beiträge sind später von RAPIN, MABILLE, LANNOIS, VALOBRA, AYALA u. v. a. geliefert worden. In Deutschland fand das Leiden merkwürdig wenig Beachtung, eine etwas ausführlichere Schilderung erfolgte erst 1913 in einer Dissertation von HENNING, eine eingehende Darstellung in CASSIRERS Monographie. Später haben BOKS, VAN VLIET, RIETTI, PARKES, WEBER, GOLDSCHLAG, SUSINI, CID, MILROY, MEMMESHEIMER u. a. weitere Kasuistik geliefert.

MEIGE hat drei Gruppen unterschieden: isolierte Fälle, heredofamiliale Fälle und kongenitale. Die Familiarität ist oft sehr ausgesprochen. MEIGE berichtete vor kurzem über Katamnesen, die er bei 8 Mitgliedern der gleichen Familie in fünf Generationen erhoben hat, welche um das Jahr 1900 von ihm beschrieben wurden. Das Trophödem zeigt im Laufe der Generationen Neigung zur Abschwächung, verträgt sich mit guter Allgemeingesundheit. HOPE und FRENCH konnten in fünf Generationen von 42 Mitgliedern 13 affiziert sehen, TOBIESEN berichtet von 4 Fällen in drei Generationen, NONNE sah in seinen 7 hierher zu rechnenden Fällen in drei Generationen acht Personen befallen werden. 1928 hat MILROY wieder über sorgfältige genealogische Untersuchungen berichtet und dabei festgestellt, daß die Ehe mit normalen Personen das Ödem in günstigem Sinne beeinflußt, daß es jedoch nie ganz aus einer Familie verschwindet. Bisweilen lag nicht eine homologe, sondern eine anderweitige neuropathische Belastung vor. Nach SIEMENS folgt die Erkrankung in der Regel dem Gesetze der unregelmäßig dominanten Vererbung. In der Aszendenz fanden sich sonst noch Epilepsie, chronische Chorea usw. (HOPE und FRENCH); diese Angabe konnte MILROY jedoch nicht bestätigen. Das Leiden ist meist kongenital, häufig entstehen die ersten Erscheinungen erst um die Pubertät, zwischen dem 15. und 25. Jahr; späterer Beginn ist selten. MILROY fand unter den Mitgliedern der von ihm beschriebenen Familie vier Betroffene im Alter zwischen 66 und 82 Jahren.

Während das MILROYsche Krankheitsbild zweifellos ein scharf umschriebenes Krankheitsbild darstellt, ist das bei den von MEIGE beschriebenen Krankheitsbildern nicht der Fall. WIRZ hat dieser Frage seine Aufmerksamkeit geschenkt und festgestellt, daß die wenigsten von den als Morbus MEIGE beschriebenen Fällen etwas mit der MILROYschen Krankheit zu tun haben; es sind meist nicht vererbte, im späteren Lebensalter aufgetretene Fälle unklarer Ätiologie oder zweifelsfreie Fälle von echter Elephantiasis mit Fieber und örtlichen Entzündungen. MEMMESHEIMER glaubt, daß es sich bei einem Teil der Fälle um eine endokrin bedingte Dystrophie handelt.

Es handelt sich stets um ein *weißes, hartes, elastisches* Ödem, das sich *schmerzlos* entwickelt. Der Fingerdruck hinterläßt entweder gar keinen oder nur einen unbedeutenden Eindruck. Die Färbung der Haut ist im allgemeinen normal. Es kommt aber auch eine leichte hellrosa oder violette Färbung vor. Die Haut ist in Falten nicht abhebbar. Sie erscheint häufig etwas verdickt, mit der Unterlage etwas fester verwachsen als unter normalen Bedingungen. Bei Punktion des Ödems entleert sich eine milchartige Flüssigkeit, die an Lymphe erinnert (MONIZ u. a.). Das Röntgenbild zeigte in einigen Fällen Dickenabnahme des Femur (MONIZ); im Falle von GOLDSCHLAG deckte die Röntgenaufnahme ein Bild auf, das der von LÉRI beschriebenen Melorheostose glich (enorme Hyperostose). Einen ähnlichen Befund erhebt ZAROSCHY. Das Ödem verwischt die Konturen der davon befallenen Körperabschnitte. Die Zunahme des Umfanges kann eine ganz erhebliche sein. In einem Falle von PARHON und FLORIAN maß die rechte Wade 30, die linke 46 cm. Durch Gehen und Stehen wird oft noch eine weitere Umfangszunahme erzielt, die im Liegen dann wieder verschwindet.

In der Mehrzahl der Fälle befällt das Ödem die unteren Extremitäten, bald ein Bein, bald beide; es kann sich auf die distalen Abschnitte beschränken, kann aber auch die ganze Extremität in Anspruch nehmen. Doch sahen PARHON und CAZACOU auch eine isolierte symmetrische Anschwellung beider Oberschenkel. Die oberen Extremitäten werden viel seltener befallen. Aber es kommt doch auch eine Beteiligung eines Armes oder beider Arme vor (RAPIN, ETIENNE, BEUTTER, ACHARD, RAMOND, AMYOT u. a.). In einem Falle von FOLLET und in dem von HERTOGHE und von EGAS MONIZ, sowie von RICHARDS-DIKINSON war das Gesicht mitaffiziert. Die Diagnose dieser Fälle ist aber nicht ganz sicher. Im Falle von BOKS bestand auch ein Ödem des Scrotum; die mikroskopische Untersuchung der Scrotalhaut ergab stark erweiterte Lymphräume. Von 24 Personen zweier Generationen waren hier 6 betroffen. Häufig ist das Zusammentreffen von Trophödem mit Spina bifida. Es ist von ANDRÉ LÉRI die Ansicht ausgesprochen worden, daß vielleicht in manchen Fällen von Trophödem der Beine die Spina bifida die Ursache des Trophödem infolge des Zuges an den Nerven der Cauda equina oder infolge Kompression des Rückenmarkes und seiner Wurzeln sein könnte. Vielleicht sei auch die Spina bifida lediglich der Zeuge für meningomedulläre, radikuläre Veränderungen, die fast immer die Spina bifida begleiten und das Trophödem erzeugen. Die Nervenläsion wirke insbesondere auf die Innervation der Lymphgefäße und verursache eine lymphatische Stase. Zur Begründung seiner Ansicht bringt er einige Fälle, die die Kombination von Trophödem und Spina bifida illustrieren. Gemeinsam mit NOEL PÉRON berichtet er über einen Fall, bei dem die Operation deutliche Veränderungen rungen der Cauda equina aufdeckte. In einem Falle von DELHAYE fand sich neben der Spina bifida occulta ein Naevus im Gebiete der Dermatome von S 1 und S 2. Das Ödem war sichtbar auf der rechten Körperseite in S 2. Bei dem Knaben, über den JAROSCHY berichtet, fand sich außer der Spina bifida occulta ein in seiner Stärke variierender Kniegelenkerguß. LORTAT-JACOB beschreibt einen Fall, der mit kongenitaler Hüftgelenkluxation kompliziert war; PRYNTON ein kongenitales Ödem bei Mutter und Tochter, die beide an angeborenem Herzfehler litten.

Die Begrenzung der Schwellung des Trophödems ist eine gliedsegmentäre, wie die französischen Autoren sagen. Wir können uns aber nur dahin aussprechen, daß entweder die Füße, oder die Füße und die Unterschenkel, oder die ganze Extremität befallen werden, bzw. die entsprechenden Teile an den oberen Extremitäten, daß die Begrenzung sich also im wesentlichen nach den einzelnen Gliedabschnitten richtet.

Eines der Hauptkennzeichen ist die allmähliche, langsame, progressive Entstehung des Ödems, das sich aus unmerklichen Anfängen langsam entwickelt, so daß es Jahre bis zu seiner höchsten Ausdehnung braucht. In einem Falle eigener Beobachtung fanden sich an dem ödematösen Bein auch Zeichen vasomotorischer Störungen, eine vasomotorische Labilität, ein häufiger Farbenwechsel, bedingt durch Unzulänglichkeit der regulatorischen, vasomotorischen Reflexe. Die Beziehungen zu dem flüchtigen Ödem waren in unserem Falle dadurch gegeben, daß die Patientin gelegentlich früher an flüchtigen Ödemen gelitten hatte, und daß auch ihre Schwester an solchen erkrankt gewesen ist. In anderen Fällen gaben sich derartige Relationen dadurch kund, daß die Progression der Entwicklung zunächst keine stetige war, daß vielmehr erhebliche Schwankungen im Fortschreiten des Leidens festgestellt werden konnten, oder sich das Leiden sogar aus einzelnen Attacken heraus entwickelte. Bisweilen sind diese Attacken von Fieber, von zeitweiligen Schmerzen, die auch in unserem Fall zu registrieren waren, begleitet. Die Schübe können sich selbst auch erst im weiteren Verlauf des Leidens einmal einstellen, nachdem zu Anfang der Fortschritt des Leidens ein ganz allmählicher gewesen ist. Eine interessante in diesen Rahmen gehörende Beobachtung hat MELLI publiziert: Es handelte sich um einen 68jährigen Mann, dessen Erkrankung mit allgemeiner Muskelschwäche und diffusen Schmerzen begann; allmählich breiteten sich Ödeme an beiden Armen, Hals, Gesicht, oberer Thoraxgegend und später am Larynx, Pharynx und — ein ganz ungewöhnliches Vorkommnis — am Oesophagus aus. Die Ödeme bildeten sich nach einigen Tagen etwas zurück, wurden dann aber stationär. MELLI sieht in dem Charakter und Verlauf des Ödems, das zwischen der QUINCKEschen und MEIGEschen Form steht, einen Beweis für die Einheitlichkeit beider Erkrankungen, denen er eine nervöse Pathogenese zuschreibt.

VALOBRA beobachtete folgendes: Eine junge, nicht hysterische Frau, bekam im Anschluß an eine intestinale Vergiftung die Erscheinungen der QUINCKEschen Krankheit. Die Ödeme wiederholten sich und betrafen besonders die rechte Hand. Die Kranke wird gesund, die Ödeme verschwinden; aber die rechte Hand bietet dauernd das Bild einer Art von chronischem persistierendem Trophödem. Wir haben auch hier also den Übergang des QUINCKEschen Ödems in das chronische Ödem in der ausgesprochensten Form vor uns. Es erinnert das an die Fälle, von denen schon oben die Rede gewesen ist, bei denen sich allmählich unter dem Einfluß dauernder, d. h. an derselben Stelle immer wieder eintretender flüchtiger Schwellungen gewisse Veränderungen der Haut ganz allmählich herausbilden, wie das z. B beim flüchtigen Lidödem häufig der Fall ist. Auch im einzelnen erinnern die Schwellungen in ihrer Art oft ganz an die flüchtigen Schwellungen und weichen von dem gewöhnlichen Typus des Trophödems ab, indem gelegentlich das Ödem nicht so hart, nicht so weiß und nicht so elastisch ist, wie sonst beim Trophödem.

VALOBRA hat sich demgemäß auch dahin ausgesprochen, daß Urticaria, QUINCKEsche Krankheit und Trophödem nur verschiedene Grade derselben Affektion sind, die unter dem Einfluß derselben ätiologischen Faktoren je nach der Dauer sich in verschiedener Weise äußert. Bei der nahen Beziehung zwischen Trophödem und QUINCKEscher Krankheit verweisen wir in der Hauptsache auf das bei der Besprechung der Pathogenese der letztgenannten Affektion Gesagte. Es sei nur kurz darauf hingewiesen, daß MEIGE unter Hinweis auf den segmentären Charakter eine Läsion des Nervensystems, CALVÉ, GARNIER und HUGUENIN eine Dystrophie des peripheren Sympathicus, MONIZ einen Einfluß der Geschlechtsdrüsen und der ihnen koordinierten endokrinen Drüsen annehmen. RIETTI denkt an Hypothyreoidismus und Hypopituitarismus, an pathogenetische Beziehungen zum sympathischen System, speziell zum Vasomotorenzentrum, sowie an Stoffwechselstörungen des Wasserhaushaltes und des Salzstoffwechsels. Eine ähnliche Auffassung vertritt GOLDSCHLAG. So berichtet OSMAN, der drei Fälle von MILROYscher Erkrankung in zwei Generationen derselben Familie sah, daß er in mehreren Fällen Wasserretention in den Geweben und Alkaliverminderung im Blute nachgewiesen habe und macht darauf aufmerksam, daß durch Alkalibehandlung die Ödeme zum Schwinden gebracht werden können. MILROY selbst führt in einer jüngst erschienenen Arbeit das Trophödem auf vasomotorische Einflüsse zurück, auf der Basis einer Funktionsstörung der endokrinen Drüsen, vor allem der Schilddrüse; eine wichtige Rolle spielen kolloidale Veränderungen im Körper, Störung der Viscosität und des Dispersionsvermögens und des normalen Verhältnisses zwischen Serumalbumin und Serumglobulin. MCGUIRE, JOHNSON und ZEECK sahen eine Kombination des Leidens mit Dystrophia adiposogenitalis. PARKES WEBER nimmt eine chronische Lymphangitis mit Obstruktion im Lymphgefäßapparat, sowie Entwicklungshemmungen der Arterien bei kongenitalen Aneurysmen an. Die Diagnose wird sich auf den Nachweis der Heredität und die segmentäre Verteilung der chronisch verlaufenden Erkrankung zu stützen haben.

Vom *stabilen Ödem* ist die Unterscheidung der flüchtigen Ödeme meist nicht schwierig. Die Anamnese (wiederholte Erysipele) und die Persistenz der Ödeme, die dabei noch immer großen Schwankungen unterliegen, machen die Differentialdiagnose leicht. Doch haben wir einen Fall gesehen, bei dem sich Schwierigkeiten der Deutung ergaben, weil nach bestimmten Angaben der Mutter des 10jährigen Jungen die früheren Attacken in einer auf psychische Traumen hin einsetzenden Schwellung einer Gesichtshälfte bestanden, die anfänglich ganz zurückging, während allmählich immer noch unter anfallweiser Steigerung eine dauernde Schwellung sich entwickelte.

Die Differentialdiagnose gegenüber dem *Erythema multiforme* kommt vorzüglich für die der Urticaria nahestehenden Formen in Betracht. Doch unterscheiden sich die Efflorescenzen dieser Affektion durch ihre größere Beständigkeit und ihre Lokalisation (meist symmetrisch auf Hand und Fußrücken, evtl. auf der Streckseite in der Gegend der Ellbogen und Kniegelenke).

Auch vom *Erythema nodosum* ist die Unterscheidung meist nicht schwierig. Die anfangs blassen später intensiv roten oder livide Knoten von derber Konsistenz befallen zunächst nur Unterschenkel und Fußrücken, erst bei größerer Zahl Oberschenkel, Vorderarme und Oberarme, am seltensten Rumpf und Gesicht. Sie sind oft spontan, mehr auf Druck schmerzhaft, verschwinden in wenigen Tagen, indem sie in charakteristischer Weise die Farbenveränderungen sich resorbierender Blutextravasate zeigen; meist sind erhebliche Allgemeinerscheinungen vorhanden.

Sehr große diagnostische Schwierigkeiten können sich ergeben, wenn die Hauptsymptome in den Hintergrund treten und nur die inneren Symptome auf dem Plan erscheinen, Brechanfälle, Larynxödeme und ähnliches. Man wird in diesen Fällen mit der Diagnose recht vorsichtig sein und Wert auf das Vorkommen anderweitiger Begleiterscheinungen ödematöser oder vasomotorischer Natur legen müssen.

Therapie.

Die Behandlung des akuten umschriebenen Ödems führt nur selten zu einem vollen Erfolg. Die schon erwähnte Tatsache, daß es ein ganzes Leben lang immer wieder mit neuen Anfällen erscheinen kann, weist darauf hin, daß wir stete Rezidive durch unsere Mittel nicht verhindern können, und selbst die bescheidenere Aufgabe, den einzelnen Anfall zu mildern und abzukürzen, können wir oft genug nicht erfüllen.

Überall dort, wo das Ödem in innigem Zusammenhang mit einer Grundkrankheit auftritt, werden wir versuchen, dort Änderung zu schaffen, den schlechten Allgemeinzustand unserer Kranken durch Diät und andere Mittel bessern, die Behandlung der allgemeinen Neurose an erste Stelle setzen, wenn Symptomenbild und Verlauf der Krankheit uns einen Zusammenhang annehmen lassen.

In geeigneten Fällen wird man neben psychotherapeutischen Maßnahmen eine Behandlung mit Organpräparaten versuchen dürfen; entscheidende Erfolge hat man jedoch von denselben — es wurden Thyreoidin, Nebenschilddrüsenpräparate (SELLEI, SUCHER, WARFIELD, letzterer täglich 15 Einheiten Parathyreoideaextrakt COLLIP) und Nebennierenextrakt verwendet — nicht gesehen. Bei den flüchtigen Ödemen, die im Zusammenhang mit Generationsvorgängen beobachtet werden, wird die Darreichung von Ovaria, Thyrosin (MATUSIS und ROJTMAN, PASTEUR VALLERY-RADOT und HEIMANN) empfohlen. Empfohlen wird auch das Ephedrin (BROWN), das in seiner pharmakologischen Wirkung dem Adrenalin vergleichbar ist; bei Ödemen der Lider empfiehlt BOHUMICZKY Einträufeln von Suprarenin.

Handelt es sich um Ödeme, die auf die oben abgehandelten toxischen Idiopathien zu beziehen sind, so wird man die therapeutischen Maßnahmen anwenden, die sich bei Proteinüberempfindlichen eine Hebung der allgemeinen Widerstandsfähigkeit zum Ziele setzen. Den größten Wert wird man auf die Fernhaltung bzw. Entfernung der schädigenden Substanzen zu legen haben. Sind jedoch die schädigenden Proteinkörper Nahrungsmittel des täglichen Lebens, dürfte man oft auf Schwierigkeiten stoßen; immerhin sind eine Reihe von Fällen bekannt geworden, in denen bei Vermeidung des Allergie verursachenden Nahrungsmittels (Schweinefleisch, Fisch) Heilung eingetreten ist (PHILLIPS). Bei Berufsüberempfindlichkeiten (Mehlstaub, Holzstaub) bleibt unter Umständen nur der Berufswechsel übrig. Wenn Bakterienproteine die Ursache der Erkrankung sind, so müssen sie aus dem Körper entfernt werden (Nebenhöhlen, Tonsillen, Zähne). Trotz gelegentlicher guter Resultate ist jedoch die Prophylaxe nicht immer durchzuführen. In diesen Fällen ist die *desensibilisierende Behandlung* angezeigt, auf deren Technik hier nicht im einzelnen eingegangen werden kann. Man unterscheidet bekanntlich eine digestive, cutane, subcutane, lokale Desensibilisierung.

ESKUCHEN hat die Methoden des Desensibilisationsbehandlung zusammengestellt. Sie gestaltet sich bei den toxischen Idiopathien im Prinzip folgendermaßen: Nachdem mit Hilfe der Anamnese, der klinischen Untersuchung und der Cutanreaktion festgestellt worden ist, welchem Protein gegenüber Überempfindlichkeit besteht, wird dem Körper dieses Protein in minimaler, unschädlicher Menge zugeführt; ganz allmählich wird die Dosis des Giftes gesteigert, bis schließlich ein so hoher Grad der Immunität, d. h. eine so erhebliche Herabsetzung der Empfindlichkeit erzielt worden ist, daß der Patient auch bei Kontakt mit großen, früher zu schweren Attacken führenden Mengen des schädlichen Proteins mit keinerlei Symptomen mehr reagiert: Zustand der Antianaphylaxie oder der Desensibilisation. Je nachdem es sich um Bakterienproteine oder um alimentäre, Tierhaare- oder Pollenproteinintoxikation handelt, werden verschiedene Wege der Desensibilisation eingeschlagen, die im einzelnen zu schildern zu weit führen würde. Es ist aber zu bemerken, daß die Desensibilisation rasch wieder zurückgeht, so daß alljährlich wieder von neuem desensibilisiert werden muß. Die Resultate der Desensibilisation scheinen beim QUINCKESchen Ödem im ganzen nicht besonders günstige zu sein, wenn auch vereinzelt über sehr gute Erfolge berichtet wird. WATKINS empfiehlt zu diesem Zwecke die WALKERSSche Scarifikationsmethode. Von 184 auf Proteinüberempfindlichkeit beruhenden Fällen ergaben 55% eine positive Hautreaktion, davon zeigten wiederum 60% multiple Überempfindlichkeit. Bei Nahrungsmittelüberempfindlichkeit wurde die Desensibilisierung auch auf diesem Wege durchgeführt.

PAGNIEZ und PASTEUR-VALLERY-RADOT geben ihren Patienten 1 Stunde vor Einnahme derjenigen Mahlzeit, durch welche sie sensibilisiert zu werden pflegen, 0,5 g Pepton. Sie wollen mit dieser Behandlung, welche einige Wochen fortgesetzt wird, beim QUINCKEschen Ödem gute Erfolge gesehen haben. Auch BROWN empfiehlt konzentrierte Peptonlösung subcutan (2mal wöchentlich je 1 ccm) oder Peptonum siccum innerlich. CHARVÁT empfiehlt intracutane Darreichung von Peptoni puri 0,05, Natrium chloratum 0,005, Aqua dest. 1,0 ad ampullam und will mit dieser Behandlung drei refraktäre Fälle geheilt haben.

Verschiedentlich ist auch die *Eigenserumbehandlung* empfohlen worden. ESKUCHEN sah von ihr in der Regel keinen Erfolg (einmalige größere Dosis 5—10 ccm intravenös), mehrere Male einen schnell vorübergehenden, je einmal verschwand eine quälende Urticaria dauernd. ACHARD und FLAUDIN wandten subcutane Reinjektionen mit 0,5—2 ccm Serum an; Resultate: 2 Urticariafälle mit 3 bzw. 14 Injektionen geheilt, ein QUINCKEsches Ödem nach 3 Serien zu 3—6 Injektionen gleichfalls geheilt. Von anderer Seite werden nichtspezifische Behandlung mit Pferdeserum, ferner durch Injektionen von sterilisierter Vollmilch (BROWN) empfohlen. VALLERY-RADOT-PASTEUR-BLAMOUTIER wollen durch wiederholte Injektionen von konzentriertem Schweinemilzextrakt erhebliche Besserungen erzielt haben, KRETZ durch Darreichung von Parathyreoideaextrakt.

Der Alkohol ist zu verbieten. Sehr wichtig ist die Regelung der Darmtätigkeit. In dieser Beziehung wurden mehrfache Erfolge von Badekuren (Kissingen) gesehen. Auch die Anwendung von sog. Darmdesinfizientien (Menthol, Salol, Campher) ist da indiziert. Auch die Hefe ist versucht worden. Die Diät soll meist eine lakto-vegetabile sein.

In den wenigen Fällen, in denen das Ödem als larvierte Malaria aufzufassen war, schien Chinin ohne Erfolg zu sein, dagegen wirkte Arsen günstig.

Von Massage und Elektrizität ist nicht viel zu erwarten; auch der vorsichtig angewendete Versuch mit Röntgenbestrahlung mißlang uns in einem Falle. Hochgebirgsklima schien uns meist günstig zu wirken.

Von inneren Mitteln werden das Strychnin und das Arsen empfohlen. Letzteres haben wir viel verwendet, wie uns schien, relativ oft mit Erfolg, in Form von subcutaner Injektion. Auch Chinin in kleineren Dosen längere Zeit gebraucht, scheint uns günstig einzuwirken. DINKELACKER sah guten Erfolg von Atropin in subcutaner Injektion. Ein Versuch damit ist anzuraten. H. CURSCHMANN hat gute Resultate mit Darreichung von Kalk erzielt; die gleiche Erfahrung haben auch andere Autoren gemacht, z. B. LAIGNEL-LAVASTINE, GERLACH und WASFIELD (3mal täglich 0,5 Calcium lacticum).

Die einzelne Schwellung wird nur selten Gegenstand der Behandlung sein. Sie kann wohl entstellen, aber Gefahren bringt sie doch eigentlich nur bei Sitz im Larynxeingang, wo dann in der Tat ein rasches chirurgisches Handeln (Scarifikationen, Tracheotomie) nötig wird.

Besonders quälend können die Magensymptome werden; sie erwiesen sich mehrmals gegen jede Behandlung ebenso refraktär, wie die gastrischen Krisen bei der Tabes. In schwersten Fällen brachte nur Morphium Erleichterung. Gegen das Jucken und Brennen, das auch bei flüchtigem Ödem sehr heftig sein kann, wird Bromocollsalbe oder Euguform empfohlen.

Gegen die periodische Gelenkschwellung hat PULAWSKI Autoserotherapie, Bettruhe, Galvanisation, Arsen und Psychotherapie angewendet, so daß er nicht angeben kann, durch welchen Faktor die Besserung des Zustandes erfolgt ist. Die Therapie des *Trophödems* ist eine undankbare. RIETTI hat Afenilinjektionen angewendet, HERTOGHE u. a. empfehlen Schilddrüsendarreichung, Eierstock- und kombinierte Präparate. LE CALVÉ schlägt periarterielle Sympathektomie, unseres Erachtens ohne hinreichende Begründung vor; SUSINI hat eine Operation ausgeführt, die das Zellgewebe, die Fascie und das harte infiltrierte Venengeflecht ausräumt. Bandagen empfehlen SUSINI und PARKES WEBER.

Literatur.
Allgemeines.

Assmann, H.: Über periphere Gefäßstörungen im jugendlichen und mittleren Lebensalter. Klin. Wschr. **1929 II**, 1342.
Bloch, Br.: Hautkrankheiten und Stoffwechsel. Wien. med. Wschr. **1925 II**, 2751. — Brüning, F.: Eine neue Erklärung für die Entstehung und Heilung trophischer Geschwüre nach Nervendehnung. Zbl. Chir. **1920**, Nr 48, 1433. — Zur Frage der Entstehung und Heilung trophischer Geschwüre nach Nervendurchschneidung. Zbl. Chir. **1921**, Nr 23. — Die trophische Funktion der sympathischen Nerven. Klin. Wschr. **1923 I**, 67. — Drei Jahre periarterielle Sympathektomie. Dtsch. med. Wschr. **1925 II**, 1516—1518.
Cassirer, R.: Die vasomotorisch-trophischen Neurosen. Berlin: S. Karger 1912. (Gesamtliteratur.) — Cassirer, R. u. R. Hirschfeld: Vasomotorisch-trophische Erkrankungen. Spezielle Pathologie und Therapie innerer Krankheiten von F. Kraus u. Th. Brugsch, Bd. 10, Teil 3. 1924. (Literatur.) — Curschmann, Hans: Vasomotorische und trophische Neurosen. (Neurotisches Ödem, Erythromelalgie.) Münch. med. Wschr. **1924 I**, 985—987. — Vasomotorische und trophische Erkrankungen. Handbuch der inneren Medizin von Mohr und Staehelin. Berlin: Julius Springer 1926.
Demel, R.: Die Leistungen der periarteriellen Sympathektomie und ihr verwandte Verfahren bei Erkrankungen der Gliedmaßen. Arch. klin. Chir. **160**, 179 (1930).
Edens, E.: Die Krankheiten des Herzens und der Gefäße, S. 703. Berlin: Julius Springer 1929.
Flandin, Ch.: Les réactions cutanées d'origine émotive. Bull. Soc. méd. Hôp. Paris **42**, No 26, 1264—1267 (1926). — Flothow, P. G.: Diagnostic and therapeutic injections of the sympathetic nerves. Amer. J. Surg., N. s. **14**, 591—604, 625 (1931). — Foerster, O.: Die Symptomatologie der Schußverletzungen der peripheren Nerven. Handbuch der Neurologie. Berlin: Julius Springer 1929.
Gans, Oskar: Histologie der Hautkrankheiten. Berlin: Julius Springer 1925. — Gonzalez-Aguilar, I.: Die Sympathicuschirurgie bei peripheren Gefäßaffektionen. Rev. cir. Barcelona **2**, 85—121 (1931). — Gruber, G. B.: Gefäßstörung und Gangrän. Z. Kreislaufforsch. **23**, 537 (1931).
Hahn: Die Chirurgie des vegetativen Nervensystems. Bruns' Beitr. **134**, H. 3. 321—335 (1925). — Heine, I.: Über ein eigenartiges Krankheitsbild von diffuser Sklerosis der Haut und innerer Organe. Virchows Arch. **262**, 351 (1926). — Heller: Die Krankheiten der Nägel. Handbuch der Haut- und Geschlechtskrankheiten, Bd. 13, Teil II, S. 230. Berlin: Julius Springer 1927. — Herzog, E.: Histopathologische Veränderungen im Sympathicus und deren Bedeutung. Verh. Ges. österr. Nervenärzte, 18. Jverlg **1928**. — Heuyer, G.: Troubles trophiques. Nouveau traité de Médecine. Tome 21. Paris: Masson & Cie. — Higier, H.: Über Angiospasmen, ihre diagnostische und pathogenetische Bedeutung bei Gehirnkrankheiten. Warszaw. Czas. lek. **7**, 801, 821, 846 (1930).
Inclan, José Luis: Die periarterielle Sympathektomie. Rev. españ. Cir. y Urol. **10**, 479—497 (1928). — Ipsen, Johs.: Über Sympathicuschirurgie, besonders die periarterielle Sympathektomie. Bibl. Laeg. (dän.) **119**, Juni-H., 457—475, und französische Zusammenfassung 1927, S. 575—578.
Jacobi, W. u. G. Magnus: Über das Ödem der Hirnhäute. Erg. Path. II **21**, 562—610 (1926).
Kahane: Elektrodiagnostik und Elektrotherapie. Wien u. Berlin: Urban & Schwarzenberg 1922. — Karplus, J. P.: Trophische, vasomotorische und sekretorische Störungen. Wien. med. Wschr. **1927 I**, 279. — Kaunitz, J.: Chronic endemic ergotism, its relation to the vasomotor and trophic diseases. Arch. int. Med. **47**, 548 (1931). — Koelsch: Gewerbliche Angioneurosen. Opera collecta **1929**, 470. — Kosmadis, W.: Die Temperatur der Haut und ihre Bedeutung bei der Behandlung verschiedener Hautkrankheiten. Med. Mysl' (russ.) **3**, 6 (1925). — Kroll, J. M.: Die neuropathologischen Syndrome. Berlin: Julius Springer 1929. — Kümmell jr., Hermann: Beobachtungen und Erfahrungen an 52 Sympathektomien. Zbl. Chir. **50**, Nr 38, 1434—1439 (1923). — Kyrle, J.: Vorlesungen über Histo-Biologie der menschlichen Haut und ihrer Erkrankungen. Wien u. Berlin: Julius Springer 1925.
Laignel Lavastine: Anatomie pathologique des systèmes sympathiques. Progrès méd. **52**, 49 (1924). — Laqueur: Die Praxis der physikalischen Therapie. Berlin: Julius Springer 1926. — Lehmann, Walter: Die Dauererfolge der periarteriellen Sympathektomie. Bruns' Beitr. **143**, H. 2. 320—329 (1928). — Grundzüge der Neurochirurgie. Dresden: Theodor Steinkopff 1930. — Leriche, R.: Résultats de la chirurgie de douleur. Presse méd. **35**, 561 (1927). — Lutz, W.: Stoffwechsel und Haut. Handbuch der Haut- und Geschlechtskrankheiten Bd. 3. Berlin: Julius Springer 1929.
Marburg, O. u. M. Sgalitzer: Die Röntgenbehandlung der Nervenkrankheiten. Wien u. Berlin: Urban & Schwarzenberg 1930. — Mayr, Julius: Über Psychogenese von Hautkrankheiten. Zbl. Hautkrkh. **23**, 1 (1927). — Mindlin, S. u. D. Cernjavskaja: Material

zur Frage der Anwendung der Hautcapillaroskopie bei innerer Pathologie. Med. Mysl' (russ.) **5**, 14 (1929). — MÜLLER, O.: Die Capillaren der menschlichen Körperoberfläche. Stuttgart: Ferdinand Enke 1922.
NAEGELI u. FELLNER: Haut und Klimakterium. Endokrinol. **8**, 81 (1931).
PARISOT et CORNIL: Troubles vasomoteurs in Nouveaux traités de Médecine, H. 21. Paris: Masson & Cie. 1927. — POLLAND, R.: Über hämatogene, neurogene und psychogene Hautaffektionen. Dermat. Z. **53**, 468 (1928).
SACK, W. TH.: Zur Methode der Erforschung psychogener Dermatosen. Arch. f. Dermat. **154**, 410 (1928). — SIBLEY, W. KNOWSLEY: The uses of diathermy in dermatology. Urologic Rev. **25**, H. 9, 513. — SIEMENS, H. W.: Die Vererbung in der Ätiologie der Hautkrankheiten. Handbuch der Haut- und Geschlechtskrankheiten, Bd. 3. Berlin: Julius Springer 1929. — SLESINGER, E. G.: Periarterial sympathectomy. Practitioner **119**, No 1, 49—55 (1927).
TAMBURRI, T.: Sulle poliendocrino simpatosi. Riforma med. **1930 I**, 83.
WOHLWILL, F.: Zur pathologischen Anatomie des peripheren Sympathicus. Verh. Ges. dtsch. Nervenärzte, 18. Febr. **1928**.

Raynaudsche Krankheit.

ADSON, ALFRED W.: Surgical relief of RAYNAUDs disease and other vascular disturbances by sympathetic ganglionectomy and perivascular neurectomy. Ann. Clin. med. **5**, Nr 2, 161—167 (1926). ADSON, A. and G. BROWN: RAYNAUDs disease of the upper extremities. J. amer. med. Assoc. **92**, 444—449 (1929). — The treatement of RAYNAUDs disease by resection of the upper thoracic and lumbar sympathetic ganglia and truncs. Surg. etc. **4**, 577 (1929). — ADSON, ALFRED W. and GEORGE E. BROWN: Treatment of RAYNAUDs disease by lumbar ramisection and ganglion ectomy and perivascular sympathetic neurectomy of the common iliacs. J. amer. med. Assoc. **84**, Nr 25, 1908—1910 (1925). — ALESSANDRI, ROBERTO: RAYNAUDs disease and tromboangiitic gangrene of the upper extremities treated by resection of the sympathetic ganglia and trunc. Amer. J. Surg. **14**, 68 (1931). — ALLEN, EDGAR, V. and GEORGE E. BROWN: Erroneous diagnosis of RAYNAUDs disease in obliterative vascular disease (Thromboangiitis obliterans). I. Vasomotor disturbances simulating RAYNAUDs disease. — Amer. J. med. Sci. **174**, Nr 3, 319—329 (1927). II. Thromboangiitis obliterans of the lower extremities with pulsating pedal arteries. Amer. J. med. Sci. **174**, Nr 3, 329—337 (1927). — RAYNAUDs disease affecting men. Ann. int. Med. **5**, 1384—1386 (1932). — ALURRALDE, MARIANO y BENJAMIN B. SPOTA: RAYNAUDscher Symptomkomplex. Rev. argent. Neur. etc. **3**, 234—241 (1928). — AMABILINO, R.: Syndrome del Raynaud. Pisani **50**, 47 (1930). — APPELBAUM, S. J. and MACY L. LERNER: RAYNAUDs disease with ocular complications. Amer. J. Ophthalm. **9**, Nr 8, 569—573 (1926). — ASSMANN, H.: Über periphere Gefäßstörungen im jugendlichen und mittleren Lebensalter. Klin. Wschr. **1929 II**, 1342.
BAILEY, H.: The treatment of RAYNAUDs disease by peri-arterical sympathectomy. Brit. J. Surg. **16**, 61, 166 (1928). — BAJPAYEE, A.: A case of RAYNAUDs disease. Indian med. Gaz. **64**, 692 (1929). — BARBER, LEWELLYS F.: Two patients suffering from RAYNAUDs disease. Discussion of medical and surgical treatment with comments upon the present status of surgery of the vegetative nervous system. Internat. Clin. XXXV. s. 4, 72—82 (1925). — BARMWATER, KNUD: Über symmetrische (RAYNAUDsche) Gangrän bei Neugeborenen. Wien. klin. Wschr. 1928 I, 320—322. — BECK, ALBERT: Résultats du traitement chirurgical de la meladie de RAYNAUD. Strasbourg méd. **85**, No 3, 69—82; No 6, 106—122; No 9, 141—150 (1927). — BEJARANO, J.: Ein Fall von RAYNAUDscher Krankheit bei Lues congenita. Progr. Clinica **1924**, No 154, 679—683. — BENEDEK, LADISLAUS: RAYNAUDscher Symptomenkomplex bei Halsrippe. Dtsch. Z. Nervenheilk. **82**, H. 3/4, 217—223 (1924). — BENNETT, T. IZOEL and E. P. POULTON: RAYNAUDs disease associated with cancer of the stomac. Amer. J. med. Sci. **176**, 654—657 (1928). — BERNARD, L. et L. PELLISSIER: Maladie de RAYNAUD et tuberculose. Bull. Soc. méd. Hôp. Paris **45**, 393 (1929). — BLOCH, ERNST: RAYNAUDsche Krankheit und Hypophyse. Klin. Wschr. **1927 I**, 457—459. — BOGAERT, LUDO VAN et R. DELBEKE: Acromégalie et syndrome de RAYNAUD. J. de Neur. **25**, No 8, 511—519 (1925). — BOGGON, R. HODGSON: Removal of the stellate ganglion in RAYNAUDs disease. Proc. roy. Soc. med. **24**, 984 (1931). — BOMBI, G.: Sindrome di RAYNAUD da settima costa cervicale. Policlinico **1929 II**, 1508. — BORAK, J.: Zur Pathogenese und Therapie der RAYNAUDschen Krankheit. Z. Neur. **111**, H. 1/2, 1—16 (1927). — Über die Knochenveränderungen bei der RAYNAUDschen Krankheit. Fortschr. Röntgenstr. **36**, H. 3, 609—615 (1927). — Die Röntgenbehandlung der RAYNAUDschen Krankheit. Wien. med. Wschr. **1929 I**, 536. — BORGHESAN, E.: Considerazioni su di un caso di sindrome di Raynaud con turbe labirintiche. Valsalva **7**, 98 (1931). — BOROWSKY, M.: Zur Frage über die Pathogenese der RAYNAUDschen Krankheit. Dtsch. Z. Nervenheilk. **114**, 232 (1930). — BRAEUCKER W.: Die Anatomie und Chirurgie der vegetativen Nervensystems. Verh. Ges dtsch. Nervenärzte, 18. Jverslg **1928**. — Die Behandlung der RAYNAUDschen Krankheit. Chirurg **3**, 756 (1931). — Arch. klin. Chir. **167**, Kongreßber., 807 (1931). — BRANDESS, THEO: Symmetrische

Gangrän beider Füße bei febrilem Abort und gleichzeitiger Synergendarreichung. Zbl. Gynäk. **52**, Nr 10, 620—622 (1928). — BREGMAN, L. E.: Operation von LERICHE bei Sklerodermie mit Morbus Raynaud. Warszaw. Czas. lek. 1, Nr 7, 267—269 (1924). — BROOKE, CH.: RAYNAUDs phenomen treated by physical measures. Physik. Ther. **47**, 215—225 (1929). — BROWN, G.: Observations on the surface capillaries in man following cervicothoracic sympathetic ganglionectomy. J. clin. Invest. **9**, 115 (1930). — BROWN, GEORGE E.: Three cases of vascular diseases affecting the feet. (Thromboangiitis obliterans, RAYNAUDs disease and erythromelalgia. Med Clin. N. Amer. **8**, Nr 4, 1189—1202 (1925). — The skin capillaries in RAYNAUDs disease. Arch. int. Med. **35**, Nr 1, 56—73 (1925). — BÜCHLER, PAL: Fall von RAYNAUDscher Erkrankung und Sklerodermie kompliziert mit polyglandulärer Erkrankung. Orv. Het. (ung.) **68**, Nr 51, 906—908 (1924). — BYWATER, H.: RAYNAUDs disease with paroxysmal hemoglobinuria. Lancet **1930 II**, 632.

CALHOUN, F. Phinizy: Cyanosis retinae, occuring in a case of erythromelalgia which terminated in RAYNAUDs disease. Contrib. to Ophthalm. **1926**, 29—33. — CAPONE-BREGS, P.: Pseudo-sindrome di Raynaud unilaterale da costala supranumeraria. Policlinico, sez. prat., **1929 II**, 1281. — CARP, L.: The association of RAYNAUDs disease with cerebral symptoms. Arch. Surg. **22**, 409 (1931). — CASTANA, V.: Forma anomala du morbo di Raynaud in un lattante. Pediatria **31**, H. 24, 1305—1316 (1923). — CATTANEO, DONATO: Morbo di Raynaud e cataratta. Arch. Ottalm. **38**, 684—702 (1931). — CHAUFFARD: La maladie de RAYNAUD. J. des Prat. **38**, No 7, 97—100 (1924). — CLAUDE, H. et J. TINEL: Syndrome de Raynaud d'origine émotive Guérison par opothérapie hypophysaire et ovarienne. Bull. Soc. méd. Hôp. Paris **41**, No 13, 570—590 (1925). — CRICHLOW, RICHARD S.: Treatment of RAYNAUDs disease by negative pressure. New Orleans med. J. **78**, Nr 8, 511—515 (1926). — CUNNINGHAM, W. F.: RAYNAUDs disease. A pathologic entity. Reporting a case following Leriche operation. N. Y. State J. Med. **26**, Nr 23, 972—974 (1926).

DAHMEN, O.: Über Akroasphyxia chronica, RAYNAUDsche Krankheit und Sklerodermie. Dermat. Wschr. **1926 I**, 737—742. — DAL MASO, PIETRO: Contributo allo studio clinico del morbo di RAYNAUD. Policlinico, sez. prat. **33**, H. 17, 581—585 (1926). — DAUNIC et LAURENTIER: Syndrome de RAYNAUD et lésions de la parotide. Contribution à l'étude des endocrinides syphilitiques. Ann. de Dermat. **4**, No 12, 721—732 (1923). — DÁVALOS, M.: Das Acetylcholin bei RAYNAUDschem Syndrom. Rev. Especial. méd. **5**, 1838 (1930). — DAVIS, LOYAL and ALLEN B. KANAVEL: Sympathectomy in RAYNAUDs disease, erythromelalgia and other vascular diseases of the extremities. Surg etc. **42**, Nr 6, 729—742 (1926). — D'ANTONA, L.: Disturbi trofici e vasomotori Raynaud-simili associati a poliglobulia splenomegalica. Arch. Sci. med. **53**, 84 (1929). — DEMEL, R.: Die Leistungen der periart. Sympathektomie und ihr verwandter Erfahrungen usw. Arch. klin. Chir. **160**, 179 (1930). — DU BOSE, F.: Thérapeutic paravertebral alcohol block. Observations of its effect following its use in RAYNAUDs disease. Amer. J. Surg., N. s. **11**, 497 (1931). — DUERDOTH: Schwerer Fall von RAYNAUDscher Krankheit, durch Witterungseinflüsse ausgelöst. Ärztl. Sachverst.ztg **34**, Nr 10, 149 (1928). — DUPÉRIÉ, R.: Le syndrom de RAYNAUD chez le nourrisson. Paris méd. **14**, No 38, 222—224 (1924). — DURANTE, LUIGI: Simpatectomia periarteriosa sulle arterie periferiche degli arti nelle simdromi di RAYNAUD. Arch. ital. Chir. **17**, H. 5, 552—564 (1927).

ERIKSSON, J.: Ein Fall von Morbus Raynaud. Hygiea (Stockh.) **88**, H. 7, 273—279 (1926).

FAY, TEMPLE: Partial unilateral thoracic ganglionectomy for RAYNAUDs disease with bilateral improvement. Arch. of Neur. **24**, 416 (1930). — FEILING, A.: Peripheral neuritis, followed by RAYNAUDs disease with gangrene: Results of sympathectomy. Proc. roy. Soc. Med. **21**, Nr 2, sect. neur., 11—12 (1927). — FERNANDEZ, SANZ: Zum RAYNAUDschen Symptomenbild. Med. ibera **18**, Nr 335, 313—315 (1924). — FLANDIN, POUMEAU-DELILLE-VAN BOGAERT: Un cas de causalgie avec syndrome de RAYNAUD et erythromelalgie posttraumatique. Bull. Soc. méd. Hôp. Paris **47**, 1293 (1931). — FORNERO, ARTURO: Ein Fall von RAYNAUDscher Krankheit (Dysendokrinismus) während der Prämenopause, Opotherapie und Genesung. Wien. med. Wschr. **1925 II**, 2270—2271. — FRICK, F.: Beitrag zur Klinik der Angioneurosen. Ein Fall von Akroparästhesie, symmetrischer Gangrän (Raynaud), Sklerodaktylie und Scleroderma diffusum. Acta dermato-vener. (Stockh.) **5**, H. 3, 449—465 (1924). — FRIEDENWALD, JULIUS and WILLIAM S. LOVE jr.: RAYNAUDs disease complicated with gastric ulcer. J. amer. med. Assoc. **85**, Nr 2, 83—85 (1925). — FULTON, JOHN F.: Vasomotor and reflex sequelae of unilateral cervical and lumbar ramisectomy in a case of RAYNAUDs disease with observations on tonus. Ann. Surg. **88**, 827—841 (1928).

GALLAVARDIN, L. et P. P. RAVAULT: Sur une forme particulière de cyanose permanente des extrémités, non paroxystique, distincte de la maladie de RAYNAUD et compliquée de gangrène parcellaire. Lyon méd. **138**, No 27, 3—7 (1926). — GAUCH, SOHIER et DE COURRÈGES: Deux cas de sclérodermie dont l'un avec maladie de RAYNAUD. Bull. Soc. franç. Dermat. **36**, 78 (1929). — GENNES, L. DE et P. ISAAC-GEORGES: Sur un cas de syndrome de RAYNAUD avec gangrène symétique des extrémités. Bull. méd. Soc. Hôp. Paris **42**, No 9,

353—358 (1926). — GERBIS: Bleigangrän oder RAYNAUDsche Krankheit. Ärztl. Sachverst.ztg **36**, 161 (1930). — GERBIS, H., A. GROS, F. MEYER-BRODNITZ u. I. ROBINSON: Die Verhütung von Gesundheitsschädigungen durch Anklopfmaschinen. Berlin: Julius Springer 1931. — GERNEZ, L.: Troubles nerveux et vasculaires (syndrome de RAYNAUD) par ostéochondromatose du coude. Rev. d'Orthop. **18**, 330 (1931). — GIROUX, R. et N. KISTHINIOS: Les extraits pancréatiques désinsulinés dans le traitement de la maladie de RAYNAUD. Bull. méd. **1931 I**, 140—141. — GOUGEROT, P. BLUM et J. ZHA: Syndrome de RAYNAUD unilatérale localisé aux 3. et 4. doigts projectile dans le bras. Bull. Soc. franç. Dermat. **38**, 199 (1931). — GOUGEROT et BURNIER: Maladie de RAYNAUD. Etat sclérodermiforme de la face, lipomatose des membres, télangectiasies etc. Bull. Soc. franç. Dermat. **35**, 803—804 (1928). — Maladie de RAYNAUD, état sclérodermiforme de la face. Hôp. S. Louis **1**, 180 (1928). — GOUGEROT, H. et JEAN MEYER: Maladie de RAYNAUD et sclérodactylie pseudolipomatose (ou état myxoedémateux) de la face et des mains etc. Arch. dermato-syph. Hôp. St. Louis **2**, 660 (1930). — GOUIN, J. et A. BIENVENUE: Résultat de la radiothérapie fonctionelle sympathique dans les érythrocyanosis surmalléolaires et troubles associés et dans l'hypophysie et la maladie de RAYNAUD. Bull. Soc. franç. Dermat. **38**, 924 (1918). — GRAHAM, DOUGLAS: Massage in RAYNAUDs disease (dry gangrene). Med. Tim. **53**, Nr 2, 44—47 (1925). — GRUSZECKA, ANNA: Ein Fall von RAYNAUDscher Krankheit, kompliziert durch zahlreiche exsudative Prozesse, und Myositis acuta. Neur. polska **8**, H. 2, 143—146 (1925). — GRENET, HENRI et ISAAC-GEORGES: De l'importance des lésions artérielles dans la pathogénie du syndrome de RAYNAUD. Ann. Méd. **20**, No 1, 27—35 (1926). — Etude histol. des artérioles cutanées dans trois cas de syndrome de RAYNAUD. Bull. Soc. méd. Hôp. Paris **42**, No 4, 151—153 (1926). — L'exploration oscillométrique des artères des membres au cours du syndrome de RAYNAUD. Presse méd. **34**, No 29, 449—451 (1926).

Handbuch der Haut- und Geschlechtskrankheiten. Herausgeg. von J. JADASSOHN, Bd. 6, Teil 2. — HEITZ, JEAN et P.-L. VIOLLE: Du temps de résorption de la boule d'oedème intra-dermique dans les troubles locaux de la circulation (artérites oblitérantes des membre syndrome de RAYNAUD, troubles vaso-moteurs). C. r. Soc. Biol. Paris **96**, No 16, 1283—1286 (1927). — HOLSCLAW, FLORENCE N. and IEWYE A. BOOTLI: Report of a case of symmetrical gangrene following excessive dose of pituitrin. Arch. of Pediatr. **42**, Nr 1, 64—67 (1925).

IMPERIALE, C.: Di un caso di gangrena simmetrica delle estrimità consecutiva a tifo addominale. Riforma méd. **44**, No 10, 242—244 (1928). — ISAAC-GEORGES, P.: Deux cas de syndrome de RAYNAUD apparus à la suite de congestion pulmonaire grippale. Bull. Soc. méd. Hôp. Paris **43**, No 30, 1423—1425 (1927). — IWAI, SAISHIRO und NIN MEISAL: Etiology of RAYNAUDs disease. Jap. med. World **5**, Nr 5, 119—121 (1925). — Ursache der RAYNAUDschen Krankheit. Verh. jap. Ges. inn. Med. **1926**, 7. — Etiology of RAYNAUDs disease. Jap. med. World **6**, Nr 12, 345—347 (1926).

JAUSION, LARTIGUE et CERVAIS: Acrodermatite staphylococcique et maladie de RAYNAUD. Bull. Soc. franç. Dermat. **38**, 624 (1931).

KERR, WILLIAM: RAYNAUDs disease, recent experimental studies. California Med. **34**, 91 (1931). — KIAER, SVEN: Thromboangiitis obliterans Bürger. Acta orthop. scand. **2**, 103 (1931). — KLAPPENBACH, W.: Zwei Fälle von Sklerodermie mit RAYNAUDschem Symptomenkomplex. Diss. Frankfurt a. M. 1917. — KOCH: Die Klinik der peripheren Zirkulationsstörungen und Gangräne der Extremitäten. Bratislav. lék. Listy **9**, 784 (1929). — KOLODNY, A.: RAYNAUDs disease in the upper extremities. J. amer. med. Assoc. **95**, 1020 (1930). — KOPF, HANS: Hypophyse und RAYNAUDsche Krankheit. Münch. med. Wschr. **1925 II**, 940. — KRAETZER, A.: RAYNAUDs disease associated with chronic arsenical retention. J. amer. med. Assoc. **94**, 1035 (1930). — KRAUS, ERIK: Zur Pathogenese der diffusen Sklerose. Zugleich ein Beitrag zur Pathogenese der Epithelkörperchen. Virchows Arch. **253**, 710 (1924).

LANDAU, ANASTAZY u. RÓŻA HERMAN: Ein durch Symptome der RAYNAUDschen Krankheit komplizierter Fall von Acrocyanosis chronica, über das Verhalten des Gasaustausches und des Kreislaufsystems. Warszaw. Czas. lek. **8**, 1107—1112, 1138—1140 (1931). — LANDIS, E.: Micro-injection studies of capillary blood pressure in RAYNAUDs disease. Heart **15**, 247 (1930). — LANGERON et DESBONNETS: Côte cervicale avec troubles vasculaires graves et gangrène de la main. Bull. Soc. nat. Chir. Paris **57**, 704 (1931). — LAPINSKY, MIHAJLO, N.: Ein Beitrag zur Frage des Vasomotorenspieles in peripheren Gefäßen infolge von Störungen in den Bauchorganen. Lyečn. Vijesn. (serbokroat.) **44**, H. 3, 109—135; H. 4, 171—195 (1922). — LASSILA, W.: Die Ätiologie des Auftretens der RAYNAUDschen Krankheit bei Kindern. Duodecim (Helsingfors) **46**, 435 (1930). — LAWSON, ROBERT S.: RAYNAUDs disease. Proc. roy. Soc. Med. **21**, 1850 (1928). — LEHRNBECHER, A.: Über Calcinosis interstitialis und ihre Beziehungen zur RAYNAUDschen Krankheit. Bruns' Beitr. **142**, H. 2, 380—397 (1928). — LERICHE, R. et R. FONTAINE: Section des rameaux communicants cervicaux inférieurs et du premier dorsal suivie de sympathectomie péri-humérale, dans un cas de maladie de RAYNAUD; résultats immediats. Strasbourg méd. **83**, No 6,

205—207 (1925). — LEWIS, THOMAS: Experiments relating to the peripheral mechanisme involved in spasmodic arrest of the circulation of the fingers, a variety of RAYNAUDs disease. Heart 15, 7 (1929). — LEWIS, THOMAS and EUGEN LANDIS: Some physiological effects of sympathetic ganglionectomy in the human being and its effect in a case of RAYNAUDs malady. Heart 15, 151 (1930). — Further observations upon a variety of RAYNAUDs disease with special reference to arteriolar defects and to scleroderma. Heart 15, 329 (1931). — LIVINGSTON, W. K.: Occlusive disease of arteries of the lower extremities. W. J. Surg. etc. 39, 173 (1931). — LOESSL, JOHANN: Über einen Fall von RAYNAUDschem Symptomenkomplex verursachender Halsrippe. Dtsch. Z. Chir. 196, H. 4/5, 346—352 (1926). — LORTAT-JACOB et BOUTELIER: Angiomes multiples d'apparition tardive chez une malade présentant un syndrome de RAYNAUD et une slero. fruste. Bull. Soc. franç. Dermat. 32, No 2, 46—48 (1925). — LOUBIERE, MAURICIO: Heilung eines 15 Jahre bestehenden Raynaud. Prensa méd. argent. 14, 900—901 (1928).

MARCUS, HENRI: RAYNAUDsche Krankheit und Infektion. Diskussionsbemerkungen. 16. Jverslg Ges. dtsch. Nervenärzte Düsseldorf 1926. — MARCUS, HERBERT: Ein Fall von RAYNAUDschem Symptomenkomplex mit Sympathicusaffektion bei hereditärer Syphilis. Sv. Läkartidn. 22, Nr 30, 856—864 (1925). — MARGOLIN, G. S.: Tetanie und RAYNAUDsche Krankheit. Klin. Wschr. 1926 I, 148. — MARQUÉZY, R., A. HÉRAUX et BAGUETTE: Gangrène disséminée de la peau à prédominance digitale chez un nourrisson de cinq semaines. Bull. soc. Pédiatr. Paris 28, 343 (1930). — MARTINEZ, J.: Un cas de maladie de Maurice Raynaud. Ann Mal. vénér. 24, 864 (1929). — MARTINEZ, VARGAS: Zum Studium der RAYNAUDschen Krankheit. Med. Niñ. 31, 257 (1930). — MAURIAC, PIERRE et FERD. PIÉCHAUD: La maladie de RAYNAUD. La pathogénie. Bull. méd. 36, No 6, 159—162 (1924). — MESCHEDE, HERMANN: Zur Frage der juvenilen Gangrän und periarteriellen Sympathektomie nach LERICHE. Wien. klin. Wschr. 1929 II, 1138—1140. — MESSING, ZYGMUNT: Ein Fall von Morbus Raynaud durch Insulin geheilt. Now. lek. (poln.) 39, H. 21. 1—3 (1927). — MIRENGHI, N.: Ricerche sulla vasoregolazione cutanea nel morbo di RAYNAUD. Boll. Soc. ital Dermat. 1931, H. 4, 167. — MONAHAN, JAMES JOHN: RAYNAUDs disease. Limitations of the classical picture as a guide to diagnosis; report of a case showing extensive bone involvement. Amer. J. med. Sci. 171, Nr 3, 346—358 (1926). — MONDIO, ENRICO: Contributo clinico allo studio della malattie di RAYNAUD. Il Manicomio 37, No 3, 281—290 (1924). — MONIER-VINARD, DELHERM et HENRY BEAU: La radiothérapie dans la maladie de RAYNAUD. Gaz. Hôp. 1929 I, 389. — Bull. Soc. Radiol. méd. France 17, 69 (1929). — MORTON, JOHN and W. MERLE SCOTT: Some angiospassic Syndroms in the extremities. Ann. Surg. 94, 839 (1931). — Methods for estimating the degree of sympathetic vasoconstriction in peripheral vascular diseases. New England J. med. 204, 955 (1931). — MUMFORD, P. B.: Two cases of RAYNAUDs syndrome presenting unusual factures. Brit. J. Dermat. 37, Nr 10, 414—417 (1925).

NICOLAS, J., J. LACASSEYNE et F. ROUSSEL: Sur un cas de maladie de RAYNAUD. Bull. Soc. franç. Dermat. 36, No 4, 351—353 (1929). — NOBÉCOURT: Syndromes de MAURICE RAYNAUD et de WEIR-MITCHELL chez les enfants. Progrès méd. 52, No 11, 165—170 (1924).

OPPEL, W. A.: Die RAYNAUDsche Krankheit als Hyperadrenalinaemia. Arch. klin. Chir. 149, H. 2, 301—330 (1928).

PALLASSE, I. DECHAUME et ARNAUD: Lésions de la chaîne sympathique dans la maladie de RAYNAUD. Lyon méd. 1931 II, 117. — PANCRAZIO, F.: Sul morbo di RAYNAUD. Atti Soc. med.-chir. Padova ecc. 8, 119 (1931). — PAULINY-TÓTH: RAYNAUDsche Gangrän. Bratislav. lék. Listy 2, 258 (1929). — PFAB, BRUNO u. OTTO HOCHE: Untersuchungen mit dem Capillarmikroskop bei chirurgischen Gefäßerkrankungen. Mitt. Grenzgeb. Med. u. Chir. 38, H. 1, 123—131 (1924). — POLAK, EMERICH: Klinische und experimentelle Betrachtungen über periarterielle Sympathektomie. Acta chir. scand (Stockh.) 60, H. 6, 541—572 (1926). — POLLAK, F.: Zur Frage der cerebralen Trophik. Arch. f. Psychiatr. 89, 788 (1930).

RIEDER: Dauerheilung RAYNAUDscher Krankheit nach Entfernung des Ganglion stellatum? Arch. klin. Chir. 157, Kongreßber., 165 (1929). — RIEDER, W.: Klinik und Pathologie der RAYNAUDschen Erkrankung, zugleich ein Beitrag zur Frage der Capillarfunktion und der Autonomie der peripheren Gefäßnetze. Arch. klin. Chir. 159, 1 (1930). — RONZINI, M.: Sopra un caso di gangrena spontanea del piede tipo Raynaud e suo tratamento. Policlinico, sez. prat., 34, No 47 (1927). — ROYLE, NORMAN D.: Sympathetic truncsection: A new operation for RAYNAUDs disease and spastic paralysis of the upper limb. Med. J. Austral. 1928 II, 436—439. — RUBASCHOW, S.: Einige Erfahrungen bei periarterieller Sympathektomie. Zbl. Chir. 55, Nr 12, 727—728 (1928). — RUBÁŠZEV, S.: Die theoretische Begründung der periarteriellen Sympathektomie. Nov. Chir. (russ.) 1925, Nr 6, 767—777 (1925). — RUD, EINAR: Ein Fall RAYNAUDscher Krankheit mit Nebenniereninsuffizienz. Hosp.tid. (dän.) 70, Nr 2, 45—50, Nr 4, 73—80 (1927).

SANNICANDRO: Sclerodermia a striscie con infiltrati cutanée nodulari e sclerodattilia con syndrome di RAYNAUD. Arch. ital. Dermat. 6, 468 (1931). — SANNICANDRO, GIUSEPPE: Sindromi di RAYNAUD e di WEIR-MITCHELL ed ipofisi. Endocrinologia 3, H. 1, 79—90 (1928). — SHINKLE, CLYDE E.: A case of RAYNAUDs disease involving the feet, the left retina and the heart wall. J. amer. med. Assoc. **83**, Nr 5, 355—356 (1924). — SIMON, A.: Über Kupferschädigungen und die Beziehungen zum RAYNAUDschen Symptomenkomplex. Arch. Gewerbepath. **2**, 71 (1931). — SIMPSON, S. LEVY, G. BROWN and A. ADSON: RAYNAUDs disease. Arch. of Neur. **26**, 687 (1931). — SLAUGHTER, WILLIAM H.: Symmetrical gangrene of malarial origin. J. amer. med. Assoc. **86**, Nr 21, 1607—1611 (1926). — SPURLING, R. GLEN, FRANKLIN JELSMA and JAMES B. ROGERS: Observations in RAYNAUDs disease, With histopathologic studies. Surg. etc. **54**, 584—593 (1932). — STAEMMLER: Zur pathologischen Anatomie des sympathischen Nervensystems. Dtsch. med. Wschr. **1924 I**, 457; **1925 I**, 603. — STEPHENS, G.: The basic bloodpressure in RAYNAUDs disease. Brit. med. J. **1930**, Nr 3633, 284. — STRADIN, P.: Über vasokonstriktorische Substanzen im Blute bei Gangraena spontanea und Claudicatio intermittens. Dtsch. Z. Chir. **189**, H. 4/6, 269—278 (1925). — SZARKA, VILMA: Ein interessanter Fall von RAYNAUDscher Krankheit. Kinderärztl. Prax. **2**, 445 (1931).

TAKATS, G. DE: The differentiation of organic and spastic vascular occlusions. Ann. Surg. **94**, 321 (1931). — TELFORD and STOPFORD: The vascular complications of cervical rib. Brit. J. Surg. **18**, 557 (1931). — THURZÓ, EUGEN u. EUGEN ORSÓS: Ein Fall von Halsrippe mit symptomatischer RAYNAUDscher Krankheit. Dtsch. Z. Nervenheilk. **104**, 297—307 (1928). — THURZÓ, JENÖ u. JENÖ ORSÓS: Halsrippe mit konsekutiver RAYNAUDscher Erkrankung. Orv. Hetil. (ung.) **72**, Nr 17, 466—470 (1928). — TOKARSKI, KAROL: Ein Fall von symmetrischer Hautgangrän am Arme. Polska Gaz. lek. **4**, Nr 46, 977—978 (1925). — TOENNIS, W.: Über eine seltene Form der Gangrän an den Fingern. Münch. med. Wschr. **1927 II**, 1671. — TÖRÖK, LAJOS: Über den Entstehungsmechanismus der Hautcyanose bei Akrocyanose, Cutis marmorata, Rosacea, Hautatrophie und RAYNAUDscher Erkrankung. Gyogyászat (ung.) **66**, Nr 51/52, 1146—1148 (1925). — TOLOSA, COLOMER: RAYNAUDsche Krankheit und paroxysmale Hämoglobinurie. Arch. f. Neurobiol. **9**, 273 (1929). — Über den Wert der Capillaroskopie bei der Diagnose der RAYNAUDschen Krankheit und anderer trophisch-vasomotorischer Neurosen. Rev. med. Barcelona **12**, 440 (1929). — RAYNAUDsche Krankheit und Frosterythem. Ecos. españ. Dermat. **6**, 87 (1930). — Sur quelque cas d'endartérite oblitérante simulant la maladie de RAYNAUD. J. de Neur. **30**, 880 (1930). — TRAMBUSTI, BRUNO: Contributo alla conoscenza delle gangrene simmetriche della cute nell' infanzia. Rev. Clin. pediatr. **25**, H. 6, 390—409 (1927). — TRINCAS, M.: La anastomosi arterio-venosa nel morbo di RAYNAUD. Riforma med. **1931 I**, 203.

ULLRICH, O.: Über familiäre „symmetrische Gangrän" mit Beginn in der Neugeburtsperiode. Z. Kinderheilk. **42**, H. 3/4, 272—285 (1926).

VENTURA, JUNCA, R.: RAYNAUDscher Symptomenkomplex (Erblues und lokale Leukopenie). Rev. méd. Chile **59**, 613 (1931). — VILLARET, MAURICE et L. JUSTIN-BESANÇON: Syndrome de RAYNAUD: Etude des pressions veineuses et capillaires. Action de l'histamine et de l'acétylcholine. Bull. Soc. méd. Hôp. Paris **42**, No 11, 465—472 (1926). — VONCKEN: Quelques cas de sympathectomie périartérielle. J. de Chir. et Ann. Soc. belge Chir. **1927**, No 5/6, 133—140.

WEDROW, N.: Die RAYNAUDsche Krankheit und Pigmentdystrophien in Verbindung mit Lupus erythematodes. Russk. Vestn. Dermat. **3**, Nr 7, 613—614 (1925). — WEISSENBACH, VIGNAL et GUILLAUMIN: Concrétions calcaires sous-cutanées des doigts, associées à une acrocyanose permanentex avec accès d'acrocyanose parosystique (syndrome de RAYNAUD). Bull. Soc. franç. Dermat. **36**, 910—927, 1007—1015 (1929).

ZELLER, O.: Die präsenile Gangrän der Extremitäten. RAYNAUDsche Krankheit und Erythromelalgie. Jkurse ärztl. Fortbildg **19**, 36—53 (1928).

Akroasphyxia chronica. Akrocyanose.

AIELLO, G.: Contributo casistico allo studio dell'acrocyanosi e della sclerodermia. Osp. magg. **18**, 443 (1930).

BEDARIDA, NINO: Acroasfissia iperestesica da arterite e flebite produtiva. Arch. ital. Chir. **17**, 639 (1927). — BEJLIN, I.: Über die pathologische Bedeutung der Akroasphyxie. Med.-biol. Ž. (russ.) **5**, H. 2. 129 (1929). — BETTMANN, S.: Stauungsbefunde im Gefäßendabschnitt der Haut. Arch. f. Dermat. **157**, 105 (1929). — BOAS, E.: The capillaries of the extremities in acrocyanosis. J. amer. med. Assoc. **79**, 1404 (1922). — BORAK, I.: Ein neues Behandlungsverfahren akroangioneurotischer Affektionen. Klin. Wschr. **1926 II**, 1830.

CLAUDE, H. et H. BARUK: L'acrocyanose orthostatique, sa valeur dans la catatonie. C. r. Soc. Biol. Paris **107**, 702 (1931). — COMBY, JULES: L'acrocyanose permanente des jeunes sujets. Arch. Méd. Enf. **31**, 645 (1928). — CROCQ, J.: L'acrocyanose. J. de Neur. **21**, 201 (1921).

DAHMEN, O.: Über Akroasphyxia chronica, RAYNAUDsche Krankheit und Sklerodermie. Dermat. Wschr. **1926 I**, 737. — D'ANTONA, L.: Acroasfissia cronica e poliglobulia. Atti Accad. Fisiocritici Siena **3**, 500 (1929).

FLARER, F.: Le acrodermatosi in relazione coi disturbi circolatori. Acrodermatosi in rapporto all'apparato circolatorio. Giorn. ital. Dermat. **73**, 542—636 (1932).
GALENKO, W.: Ein Fall von Polyneuritis und Acroasphyxia localis. Med. Mysl' (russ.) **3**, 30 (1926). — GRAÇOSKI et CL. HURMUZACHE: Un cas de livedo reticularis et acrocyanose. Bull. Soc. pediatr. Jaşi **1**, 3 (1930).
HAY, K.: Case of acrocyanosis. Proc. roy. Soc. Med. **20**, 3, 195 (1927).
JASO, E. u. M. TERCERO: Die Capillarresistenz in einem Fall von Akrocyanose. Arch. españ. Pediatr. **16**, 65—71 (1932).
KLINGMÜLLER, V. and O. DITTRICH: Perniosis oder Erythrocyanosis. Arch. of Dermat. **22**, 615 (1930). — KREINDLER, A. u. H. ELIAS: Zur Klinik und Pathogenese der juvenilen Akrocyanose. Z. Kinderheilk. **50**, 608 (1931).
LAYANI, F.: Les Acrocyanoses. Paris: Masson et Cie 1929. — LEDOUX, E.: Un cas d'acrocyanose traité et considerablement amélioré par la sympatectomie humérale. Lyon chir. **21**, 182 (1924). — LEREBOULLET, P.: Hypophyse et dystrophies infantiles. J. méd. franç. **11**, 321 (1922). — LEWIS, THOMAS and EUGEN LANDIS: Observations upon the vascular mechanism in acrocyanosis. Heart **15**, 229 (1930). — LEYSER, E.: Zur Pathogenese der akralen Haut- und Nervenerkrankungen. Mschr. Psychiatr. **60**, 117 (1925).
MARAÑÓN, G.: Über die hypogenitale Hand (= Akrocyanose). Siglo méd. **68**, 672 (1921). — MARINESCO, G., KREINDLER u. BRUCH: Einige vasculäre und capillaroskopische Angaben bei Akrocyanosis. Rev. Stiint. med. (rum.) **18**, 731 (1929). — MATHEZ, A.: Une forme particulière d'acrocyanose combinée avec des troubles moteurs des doigts. Rev. méd. Suisse rom. **48**, 1 (1928). — MATHEZ, J. A.: Note complémentaire à propos d'une forme particulière d'acrocyanose combinée à des trobles moteurs. Rev. méd. Suisse rom. **48**, 1022 (1928). — MAY, C., et DREYFUS-SÉÉ: Un cas d'acrocyanose d'origine thermique. Bull. Soc. méd. Hôp. Paris **43**, 340 (1917).
NARDELLI, L.: Eritema indurato Bazin e acrocianosi. Giorn. ital. Dermat. **67**, H. 1, 83 (1926).
OBREGIA et URECHIA: Un cas d'acroasphyxie chronique. Encéphale **16**, 240 (1921).
PARISOT et CORNIL: L'Acrocyanose. Nouveau Traité de Médecin, Tome 21. — PIERINI: Akrocyanosis. Semana méd. **1931 I**, 478. — PINELES, F.: Über die endokrinen Beziehungen der Akrocyanose. Endokrinol. **5**, 227 (1929).
ROCH: L'acropathologie. Rev. méd. Suisse rom. **41**, 3 (1921). — ROTHFELD, J.: Vasomotorisch-trophische Extremitätenstörungen durch Kälte und Unfälle. Polska Gaz. lek. **2**, 145 (1923).
SANNICANDRO, G.: I disturbi provocati di circolo nello studio delle acrodermatosi. Giorn. ital. Dermat. **73**, 654—669 (1932).
THOMAS, E.: L'acrocyanose dans la période scolaire. Schweiz. Rdsch. Med. **21**, 193 (1921). — TÖRÖK, L.: Über den Entstehungsmechanismus der Hautcyanose bei Akrocyanose, Cutis marmorata, Rosacea, Hautatrophie und RAYNAUDsche Erkrankung. Gyógyászat (ung.) **66**, Nr 51/52, 1146 (1925). — TÖRÖK, L. u. E. RAJKA: Über das Verhalten der Blutgefäße der Haut auf lokale Gefäßnervencyanose und erweiternde Einwirkungen bei der Akrocyanose und bei der Cyanose nach Umschnüren des Armes. Klin. Wschr. **1915 II**, 1642. — TORREVELLA, MARIO: Un caso di acrocianosi intermittente in bambino eredoluetico. Pediatria **30**, 1081 (1922).
VILLARET, M. u. FR. SAINT GIRONS: L'acrocyanose des jeunes femmes. Arch. Méd. Enf. **32**, 79 (1929).
WEBER, F., PARKES: Case of acrocyanosis. Proc. roy. Soc. Med. **19**, 70 (1926).

Erythromelalgie. Akrodynie.

ACHARD, CH.: Erythromélalgie. Bull. méd. **40**, No 3, 69—72 (1926).
BALBI, E.: Sopra un caso di eritromelalgia. Arch. ital. Dermat. **1**, H. 6, 604 (1926). — BIKELES, G. u. RADONICIC: Ein Fall von Erythromelalgie mit spontaner Gangrän. Wien. klin. Wschr. **1915 I**, 816. — BING, ROBERT: Über traumatische Erythromelalgie und Erythroprosopalgie. Nervenarzt **3**, 506 (1930). — BRANDENBURG: Umfrage über die periarterielle Sympathektomie. Med. Klin. **1924 I**, 532. — BROWN, G.: Three cases of vascular diseases affecting the feet. Med. Clin. N. Amer. **8**, 1189 (1925). — BROWN, GEORGE E.: Erythromelalgia and other disturbances of the extremities accompanied by vasodilatation and burning. Amer. J. med. Sci. **183**, 468—485 (1932). — BRÜNING, F. u. F. FORSTER: Die periarterielle Sympathektomie in der Behandlung der vasomotorisch-trophischen Neurosen. Zbl. Chir. **49**, 913 (1922).
CALHOUN, F. PHINIZY: Cyanosis retinae, occuring in a case of eryhtromelalgia which terminated in RAYNAUDs disease. Contribut. to ophthalm. Sci., Jacbison birthday-Bd., p. 29—33. 1926. — CASSIRER, R.: Vasbmotorisch-trophische Neurosen, 2. Aufl. Berlin 1912 (hier Literatur bis 1912 zu finden). — Die vaomotorisch-trophischen Neurosen in M. LEWANDOWSKYs Handbuch der Neurologie. Berlin: Julius Springer 1914 (hier Literatur bis 1914 zu finden). — Fall von Erythromelalgie. Berl. Ges. Psychiatrie u. Nervenheilk.,

Jan. 1915. — CASSIRER, R. u. R. HIRSCHFELD: Vasomotorisch-trophische Erkrankungen. KRAUS-BRUSGCH' Spezielle Pathologie und Therapie innerer Krankheiten. Wien u. Berlin: Urban & Schwarzenberg 1924. — CLARKE, I. TERTIUS: The treatment of erythromelalgia by injections of antimony. J. trop. Med. **26**, 285 (1923). — CURSCHMANN, HANS: Vasomotorische und trophische Neurosen. Münch. med. Wschr. **1924 II**, 985. — Vasomotorische und trophische Erkrankungen. Handbuch der inneren Medizin von MOHR und STAEHELIN, Bd. 5, 2. Teil. 1926.
DAVIS, LOYAL and ALLAN B. KANAVEL: Sympathectomy in RAYNAUDs disease, erythromelalgia and other vascular diseases of the extrensitus. Surg. etc. **42**, Nr 6, 729—742 (1926). — DU BOIS: Un cas d'erythromélalgie. Schweiz. med. Wschr. **1923 I**, 631. — DUMAS, A. et CHEVALIER: Erythromélalgie dans un cas de tabes avec impotence des membres inférieurs. Lyon. méd. **135**, 676 (1925).
FEER, EMIL: Die FEERsche Krankheit. Handbuch der Kinderheilkunde, 4. Aufl., Bd. 2, S. 528. 1931. — FOSSIER: Erythromelalgie. N. Y. med. J. a. med. Rec. **47**, 1238 (1913).
GANS, A.: Gutartige Anfälle von Erythromelalgie bei einem 8jährigen Kinde. Nederl. Tijdschr. Geneesk. **69**, 1915 (1925). — GRAVES, A.: Erythromelalgia. Amer. J. Surg., N. s. **12**, 40 (1931). — GRJASEV, F.: Ein Fall einer kombinierten Erkrankung an Erythromelalgie und Polycythämie. Russk. Klin. **11**, 28 (1929). — GSTREIN, H. u. R. SINGER: Polyglobulie mit dem Symptomenkomplex einer Erythromelalgie. Zbl. inn. Med. **39**, 423 (1918).
HARE, D.: Erythromelalgie secundary to arteriosclerosis. Proc. roy. Soc. Med. **21**, 23 (1927). — HELLER, J.: Die Krankheiten der Nägel. Handbuch der Haut- und Geschlechtskrankheiten, Bd. 13, 2. Teil. 1927. — HORIUCHI, S.: Über die Erythemelalgie und die Vagotonie. Acta dermato-vener. (Stockh.) **4**, 311 (1922). — HVAL, EINAR: Erythromelalgie cum polyglobulia megalosplenica. Lues. Norsk. Mag. Laegevidensk. **89**, 31 (1928).
JIRASEK, I.: Erythromelalgie. Rev. Neur. (tschech.) **21**, 101 (1924).
KAPPIS: Die Chirurgie des Sympatshicu. Erg. inn. Med. **25**, 562 (1924). — KELLY, S.: Erythromelalgiea causalgia and allied conditions. J. of Neur. **3**, 55 (1922). — KLAUDER: Thermalgia. Arch. of Dermat. **14**, Nr 5, 612 (1926). — KOENIGSTEIN: Haut-, Muskel-, Knochenatrophie einer Extremität bei gleichzeitiger Erythromelalgie und Hyperglobulie. Wien. dermat. Ges. 25. Okt. 1923. Ref. Zbl. Hautkrkh. **11**, 286. (1923). — KRAEGER, F.: Ein Fall von Erythromelalgie bei Polycythämie. Inaug.-Diss. Freiburg i. B. 1915. — KRUGLOW, A.: Über Erythromelalgie. Vrač. Delo (russ.) **12**, 1481 (1929). — KUNSTMANN: Zur Frage der Erythromelalgie. Dermat. Wschr. **1920 I**, 745.
LAEWEN, A.: Über Nervenreizung bei Amputation. Amputationsneuromen, Angiospasmen, Erythromelalgie, seniler Gangrän und Ulcus cruris. Bruns' Beitr. **133**, 405 (1925). — LAIGNEL-LAVASTINE: Erythromelalgie. J. de Pract. **37**, 755 (1923). — LERICHE, R.: Some researches on the periarterial sympathatics. Ann. of Surg. **74**, 385 (1921).
MAY, ETIENNE: Syndromes vasomoteurs intermédiares a l'érythromelalgie et a la maladie de QUINCKE. Associations de tétanie et de rhumatisme chronique. Bull. Soc. méd. Hôp. Paris **40**, 575 (1924). — MAY, E. et P. HILLEMAND: Deux cas d'érythromélalgie chez des syph ilitiques. Bull. Soc. méd. Hôp. Paris **39**, 1024 (1923). — MAYESIMA: Ein durch die FÖRSTERsche Operation erfolgreich behandelter Fall von Erythromelalgie. Dtsch. Z. Chir. **122**, 81 (1913). — MENDEL, K.: Intermittierendes Hinken. Differentialdiagnose gegen Erythromelalgie. Zbl. Neur. **27**, 85 (1922). — MEYER, E.: Erythromelalgie (Fall von SCHIRMACHER). Vereinsbeilage der Med. Wschr. — MUMFORD, P.: A case of monolateral erythromelalgia of apparently hysterical origin. Brit. J. Dermat. **41**, 478 (1929).
NIEKAU: Erg. inn. Med. **1922**, 522. — NIELSEN, LARS: Erythromelalgie nach Suicidversuch mit Gyngeren. Münch. med. Wschr. **1928 I**, 736. — NOBÉCOURT: Syndromes de MAURICE RAYNAUD et de WEIR-MITCHELL chez les enfants. Progrès méd. **52**, 165 (1924). — NOVEA SANTOS, R.: Erythromelalgia anaesthetica und Acroerythrosis paraesthetica mit erythromelalgischen Krisen. Ann. de Neur. **2**, 171 (1921).
PADILLA, T.: Der endokrine Faktor in der Pathogenese des WEIR-MITCHELLschen Symptomen komplexes der Erythromelalgie. Semana méd. **28**, 117 (1921). — PARISOT et CORNIL: L'Erythromelalgie. Nouveau Traité de Medicine, Tome 21. — PARRISIUS: Dtsch. Z. Nervenheilk. **72**. — PRINCI, P.: Erythromelalgie di WEIR-MITCHELL. Fol. med. (Napoli) **8**, 532 (1922).
RADONIČIČ, K.: Kombination von Erythromelalgie mit RAYNAUDscher Krankheit. Ges. inn. Med. **3**, 12 (1914). — RAPOPORT, L.: Erythromelalgie. Diss. Basel 1931. — ROBERTS, STEWART: Scleroderma associated with Erythromelalgie and Myxedema. Med. Clin. N. amer. **12**, 1429 (1929). — ROCAZ, CH.: L'acrodynie infantile. (Literatur.) Paris: G. Doin & Cie. 1932.
SAINTON, P. et PAUL VÉRAN: Erythromelalgie et syndrome de Basedow. Gaz. Hôp. **101**, 997 (1928). — SAITO, M.: Über die chirurgische Behandlung der Erythromelalgie. Mitt. Grenzgeb. Med. u. Chir. **41**, 203 (1929). — SCHIRMACHER: Zur Kenntnis der Erythromelalgie. Arch. f. Psychiatr. **53**, 1 (1914). — SCHLESINGER, H.: Vasomotorisch-trophische

Neurosen. Wien. med. Wschr. **1924** II, 1165. — SMITH, ALLAN: Erythromelagia consequent to hemiplegia. Med. J. a. Rec. **133** (581 (1931). — SPIELMEYER, W.: Zur Klinik und Anatomie der Nervenschußverletzungen. Berlin: Julius Springer 1915. — STALKER, JAMES: Erythromelalgie treated with colloidal calcium. Brit. med. J. **1923**, Nr 3287, 1261.

TSUJI, KWANJI: Ein Fall von Erythromelalgie mit Polycythämie und BENCE-JONESscher Albuminurie. Acta Scholae med. Kioto **12**, 259 (1929).

VEDEL, PUECH et CHARDONNEAU: Crises d'angiospasme avec érythromélalgie et manifestations angineuses d'origine névraxitique probable. Bull. Soc. Sci. Méd. et biol. Montpellier **8**, 77 (1927).

WEBER, F. PARKES: Erythromelalgia—libre symptoms with high blood-pressure. Proc. roy. Soc. Med. **25**, 403—404 (1932). — WEBER, PARKES: Spurious Erythromelalgia. Brit. J. Dermat. **27** (6) (1915). — The significance of erythromelalgia in cases of intermittant claudication of the lower extremities. Lancet **1922** I, 176.

ZADEK: Erythromelalgie bei Polycythaemia vera. Berl. klin. Wschr. **1918** II, 1193. — ZELLER, O.: Die präsenile Gangrän der Extremitäten. RAYNAUDsche Krankheit und Erythromelalgis. Jkurse ärztl. Fortbildg **19**, 36 (1928). — ZIERL: Einfluß des vegetativen Nervensystems auf die Haut in L. R. MÜLLERs Die Lebensnerven. 2. Auflage des „Vegetativen Nervensystems". Berlin: Julius Springer 1924.

Akroparästhesien.

BALLERINI, G.: Sulla genesi di alcune forme di acroparaestesia. Fol. gynaec. (Genova) **14**, 1 (1921). — BOLTEN, G. C.: Die vasomotorische Neurose NOTHNAGELs (Akroparästhesie). Dtsch. Z. Nervenheilk. **70**, 256 (1921). — BORAK, I.: Über den Ursprung der Akroparästhesien. Endokrinol. **5**, 9—28 (1930).

GROTJAHN, M.: Untersuchungen bei Anklopfern in der Schuhindustrie. Arch. Gewerbepath. **1**, 687 (1931).

HAHN, J.: Zur Ätiologie der vasoconstrictorischen Akroparästhesien Mikrocapillarbeobachtungen. Zbl. inn. Med. **44**, 465 (1923). — HEISSEN, F.: Zur Klinik der einfachen Akroparästhesien. Klin. Wschr. **1922** II, 2473.

KAHN, W.: New studies on acroparästhesia and its relation to the eye. J. nerv. Dis. **60**, 350 (1924).

POGORELSKY, B.: Vasoconstrictorenneurose der Extremitäten (SCHULTZEsche Akroparästhesien). Semana méd. **34**, 392 (1927).

ROCH, M.: L'acropathologie. Rev. méd. Suisse rom. **41**, 3 (1921). — ROSLING, E.: Ein Fall von ADDISON-BIERMERscher Krankheit mit Glossitis und Akroparästhesien als Initialsymptomen, aber ohne manifeste Anämie. Acta med. scand. (Stockh.) **71**, 467 (1929).

STRAUS, E. u. E. GUTTMANN: Die nosologische Stellung der Akroparästhesien. 15. Jverslg Ges. dtsch. Nervenärzte, 5. Sept. 1925.

Multiple neurotische Hautgangrän.

BIANCALANI, A.: Alterazioni cutanei e disturbi nervosi per avvelenamento acuto da gas illuminante. Arch. di Antrop. crimin. **50**, 1423 (1930). — BOLTEN, G. C.: Ein Fall von „hysterischer" Gangrän. Nederl. Tijdschr. Geneesk. **65** II, 1570 (1921). — Über die hysterische Gangrän. Mschr. Psychiatr. **51**, 1 (1922). — BONNET, L. M.: Gangrène cutanée primitive ou essentielle. Lyon méd. **1928** II, 181—185. — BULLE, E. u. W. HAASE: Mediane disseminierte Hautnekrosen durch vasomotorische Neurosen bei einer Hysterika. Münch. med. Wschr. **1927** II, 1498.

CASAZZA, R.: Diffuse lesioni cutaneo in isteriche. Giorn. ital. Dermat. **70**, 1281 (1929).

FINKELSTEIN, HERMANN: Über eine Beobachtung von multipler Hautgangrän. Dermat. Wschr. **1932** I, 405—409. — FREY, K.: Multiple neurotische Hautgangrän. Schweiz. Arch. Neur. **20**, 170 (1927).

MUCHA, JADASSOHNs Handbuch der Haut- und Geschlechtskrankheiten, Bd 4, 2.

PICK, ERWIN: Hautgeschwüre bei funktioneller Anästhesie. Dermat. Wschr. **1922** I, 177.

SACK, W.: Zur Kasuistik und Problematik psychogener Dermatosen. Nervenarzt **2**, 86—96 (1929). — STOKES, J. and VAUGHN GARNER: The diagnosis of selfinflicted lesions of the skin. J. amer. med. Assoc. **93**, 438 (1929).

WERTHER: Die psychogenen Dermatosen. Z. ärztl. Fortbildg **26**, 341 (1929).

Sklerodermie, Sklerodaktylie.

ACTON, HUGHES, AINHUM, a band Scleroderma. Indian. J. med. Res. **15**, 1085 (1928). — ACUÑA, MAMERTO u. JOSÉ MARIA MACERA: Allgemeine progressive Sklerodermie. Semana méd. **31**, 1114 (1924). — ADSON, ALFRED W., PAUL A. O'LEARY and GEORGE E. BROWN: Surgical treatment of vasospastic types of scleroderma by resection of sympathetic ganglia and trunks. Ann. int. Med. **4**, 555—568 (1930). — AIELLO, GIUSEPPE: Contributo casistico allo studio dell'acrocianosi e della sclerodermia. Osp. magg. **18**, 443—448 (1930). —

AKOBDSZANJANZ, G.: Ein Fall von Sklerose mit fleckweiser Atrophie und Kalkablagerungen in der Haut. Russk. Vestn. Dermat. **3**, 2 (1925). — ALJAVDIN, A.: Zur Kasuistik der subcutanen Knotenbildungen bei atrophischer Akrodermatitis mit Sklerosis. Russk. Vestn. Dermat. **4**, 726 (1926). — ALLAN, W.: Dermatomyositis or scleroderma? Arch. of Dermat. **19**, 265 (1929). — ARADY, KALMAN v.: Über einige seltenere Symptome der Sklerodermie. Z. klin. Med. **106**, 406 (1927). — ARMANI, LUDOVICO: Alcuni aspetti radiologici della sclerodermia. Arch. di Radiol. **3**, 576 (1927). — Note terapeutiche sulla sclerodermia. Giorn. Clin. med. **8**, 220 (1927). — ARONSTAM, NOAH E.: Scleroderma following trauma with complete recovery. Report of a case. Urologic Rev. **33**, 812—814 (1929). — ARTOM, MARIO e PIEO FORNARA: Particolari aspetti della sclerodermia localizzata nell'infanzia. Arch. ital. Dermat. **3**, 25 (1927).

BALBAN: Sclerodermia diffusa et circumscripta. Zbl. Hautkrkh. **41**, 290, 291 (1932). — BARKMAN, ÅKE: Parmi les théories pathogéniques les plus en vogue à l'heure actuelle en est-il une qui explique avec précision l'origine de la Sclerodermia? Uppsala Läk. för. Forh. **31**, 463 (1926). — BARTHÉLEMY, R.: Sclérodermie généralisée et traumatisme. Arch. Dermato-syph. Hôp. St. Louis **1**, 617—626 (1929). — BAU-PRUSSAK, S.: La dégénérescence génito-sclérodermique. Revue neur. **33**, 316 (1926). — BERTACCINI, G.: Sclerodermia e atrofia a chiazze in soggetto ipo-sviluppato. Interessante reperto istologico. Il Dermosifilogr. **5**, 229—244 (1930). — BERTIN, E.: Les rapports de la syphilis et de la sclérodermie. Ann. de Dermat. **7**, 175 (1926). — BLATT, O.: Klinische Beiträge zur Frage der Atrophodermien. Dermat. Wschr. **1929 I**, 190. — BORY, L.: Un cas de morphée cervicale associée à une maladie de RAYNAUD. Bull. franç. Dermat. **36**, 952, 1007 (1929). — BREGMAN, L. E.: Operation von LERICHE bei Sklerodermie mit Morbus RAYNAUD. Warszaw. Czas. lek. **1**, 267 (1924). — BROWN, H.: The aetiology of alopecia areata and its relationship to vitiligo and possibly scleroderma. Brit. J. Dermat. **41**, 299 (1929). — BROWN, GEORGE E. and PAUL A. O'LEARY: Skin capillaries in scleroderma. Arch. int. Med. **36**, 73 (1925). — BROWN, GEORGE, E., PAUL A. O'LEARY and ALFRED W. ADSON: Diagnostic and physiologic studies in certain forms of scleroderma. Ann. int. Med. **4**, 531—554 (1930).— BRUNSCHWEILER, H. et O. L. FOREL: A propos d'un cas de sclérodermie. Schweiz. Arch. Neur. **22**, 313 (1928). — BRUUSGAARD, E.: Über Hautkrankheiten bei Stoffwechselstörungen und endokrinen Leiden mit besonderer Berücksichtigung der Pathogenese der Sklerodermie. Med. Rev. **65**, 618 (1927). — Ein Fall von universeller Sklerodermie mit ausgebreiteten Kalkablagerungen in dem cutanen Gewebe. Dermat. Z. **53**, 80 (1928). — BÜCHLER, PÁL: Fall von RAYNAUDscher Krankheit und Sklerodermie, kompliziert mit polyglandulärer Erkrankung. Orv. Hetil. (ung.) **68**, 906 (1924). — BUSCHKE, A.: Verringerung bzw. Mangel an freier Salzsäure bei Sklerodermie. Dermat. Wschr. **1927 II**, 1077.

CARO-PATON, T.: Sclérodactylie et Raynaud. Actas dermo-syfiliogr. **23**, 661 (1931). — CAROL, W. u. F. VAN DER ZAUDE: Adiponecrosis subcutanea neonatorum (sog. Sklerodermie). Acta dermato-vener. (Stockh.) **7**, 180 (1926). — CELASCO, JUAN: Zu einem Fall von Sklerodermie mit Sklerodaktylie. Semana méd. **32**, 1522 (1925). — ČERKES, A.: Pathogenese und Therapie der Sklerodermie. Sovrem. Psichonevr. (russ.) **3**, 183 (1924). — COVISA, J. S., J. BEJANARO u. J. PRIETO: Zum Studium der Sklerodermie. Actas dermo-sifiliogr. **19**, 121 (1927). — CROSTI, AGOSTINO: Herpes zoster in sclerodermia generalizzata. Giorn. ital. Dermat. **68**, 37 (1927). — A proposito de un caso de sclerodermia generalizzata progressiva. Giorn. ital. Dermat. **68**, 1097 (1917). — ČUMAKOV, N.: Ein Fall von Sklerodermie mit histologischen Untersuchungen. Russk. Vestn. Dermat. **5**, 226 (1927). — CURSCHMANN, H.: Zur Behandlung der Sklerodermie. Ther. Gegenw. **67**, 249 (1926).

DAHMEN, O.: Über Acroasphyxie chronica, RAYNAUDsche Krankheit und Sklerodermie. Dermat. Wschr. **82**, 737 (1926). — DANILEWSKAJA, E. u. G. MARKOV: Ein Fall von einseitiger punktförmiger Sklerodermie mit Hautödem derselben Körperhälfte. Med. Mysl' (russ.) **3**, 52 (1925). — DELHERM, MOREL-KAHN et COUPUT: Sclérodermie et lésions osseuses. Bull. Soc. méd. France **13**, 110 (1925). — DENNEY, HOPKINS, JOHANSEN: Sclerodermalike lesions in lepers. South. med. J. **23**, 1003 (1930). — DEVOTO, A.: Sopra un caso de sclerodattilia. Giorn. ital. Dermat. **66**, 1071 (1925). — Sopra un caso di sclerodermia generalizzata con turbe del metabolismo calcico e insuff. ipofisaria. Boll. Sez. reg. Soc. ital. Dermat. **4**, 238 (1931). — DISS et FR. WORINGER: Les fausses sclérodermies des nourrissons. Bull. Soc. franç. Dermat. **36**, No 7, 960—972, 1007—1015 (1929). — DOWLING, G. B.: Superficial scleroderma. Proc. roy. Soc. Med. **25**, 1326 (1932). — DUBREUILH, W.: A propos de la sclérodermie. Bull. Soc. franç. Dermat. **36**, No 7, 891—892, 1007—1015 (1929). — DURHAM, R.: A case of scleroderma with extensive subcutaneous periarticular and vascular calcification. Ann. of chir. Med. **5**, 679 (1927). — Scleroderma and Calcinosis. Arch. int. Med. **42**, 467 (1928).

EDEIKEN, L.: Scleroderma with sclerodactylia. Amer. J. Roentgenol. **22**, 42 (1929). — EGUCHI, H.: Über Katarakt bei pluriglandulärem Infantilismus mit Sklerodermie. Acta Soc. ophthalm. jap. **35**, 167 (1931). — EHRMANN, F.: Demonstration von Präparaten von diffuser Sklerodermie. Arch. f. Dermat. **151**, 428 (1926). — Über Sklerodermie. Dermat. Z.

53, 164 (1928). — EHRMANN, S. u. R. BRÜNAUER: Sklerodermie. Handbuch der Haut- und Geschlechtskrankheiten, Bd. 8. Teil 2, S. 717. **1931**. — ENRICO, CESARE: Contributo alla patogenesi della sclerodermia. Policlinico **33**, 1493 (1926). — FÉNYES, I.: Sklerodermie mit elektrischem Befund. Berl. Ges. Psychiatr., **14**. Jan. **1929**. — FESSLER, A. u. R. POHL: Stenosierender Prozeß des Oesophagus bei Sklerodermie. Dermat. Z. **63**, 164—169 (1932). — FILLIÉ: Ein Fall von lokalisierter Sklerodermie mit einseitigem Gewebsschwund in den Extremitäten. Med. Klin. **1930 II**, 1789, 1790. — FISCHL, R.: Zur Sklerodermiefrage. Arch. Kinderheilk. **92**, 237 (1931). — FLARER, F.: Considerazioni eziopatogenetiche terapeutiche su cinque casi di sclerodermia. Giorn. ital. Dermat. **70**, 1107 (1929). — FREUND, E.: Su un caso di sclerodermia «en bande». Giorn. ital. Dermat. **71**, 1053—1063 (1930). — FICK, F.: Beitrag zur Klinik der Angioneurosen. Ein Fall von Akroparästhesie, symmetrischer Gangrän (Raynaud), Sklerodaktylie und Sclerema diffusum. Acta dermato-vener. (Stockh.) **5**, 443 (1924). — FRITZSCHE, G. u. K. SCHOLL: Ein bemerkenswerter Fall von trophischer Neurose. Mitteldtsch. Ärztebl. **1925**, Nr 17, 2—4 (1925).

GADRAT, J.: Sclérodermie acrostatique et calcémie. Bull. Soc. franç. Dermat. **39**, 741—742 (1932). — GATÉ, I. et I. CHARPY: Sclérodermie progressive du visage et du cou avec sclérodactylie. Bull. Soc. franç. Dermat. **38**, 480 (1931). — GAUCH, SOHIER et DE COURRÈGES: Deux cas de sclérod. dont l'un avec maladie de RAYNAUD. Bull. Soc. franç. Dermat. **36**, 48 (1929). — GAZIA, HOR.: Ein Fall von Sklerodermie des Neugeborenen. Arch. lat.-amer. Pediatr. **20**, 720 (1926). — GLASSER et LANZENBERG: Sclérodermie des membres supérieurs de la nuque et de la face chez une jeune fille. Bull. Soc. franç. Dermat. **36**, No 7, 900—902, 1007—1015 (1929). — GOLDSMITH, W.: A case of clinical morphoea with tuberculous histology. Brit. J. Dermat. **41**, 226 (1929). — GOLOMB, I. u. L. FAJNGOLD: Zur Frage der zwischen Atrophia cutis idiopathica und Sklerodermie bestehenden Beziehungen. Russk. Vestn. Dermat. **7**, 736 (1929). — GOLŠMID, K.: Über die Ätiologie der Sklerodermie. Venerol. (russ.) **1927**, Nr 8, 708, 713. — GORDON, HAROLD: Diffuse scleroderma, with a case report and autopsy findings. Ann. int. Med. **2**, 1309 (1929). — GOTTESMAN, JULIUS: Gangrene of finger due to scleroderma. J. amer. med. Assoc. **83**, Nr 15, 1162 (1924). — GOUGEROT, H. et BURNIER: Mal de RAYNAUD, état sclérodermiforme de la face etc. Arch. dermato-syph. Hôp. St. Louis **1**, 180 (1929). — Sclérodermie en bandes et sclérodermie en plaques sans infiltrats. Bull. Soc. franç. Dermat. **38**, 758 (1931). — GOUGEROT, H., CARTEAUD et J. WEIL: Sclérodermie en plaques, en gouttes, en gouttelettes (on pointillée). Forme de transition vers le lichen. Bull. Soc. franç. Dermat. **37**, No 2, 267—268 (1930). — GOUGEROT, H. et JEAN MAYER: Maladie de RAYNAUD. Etat sclérodermiforme des doigts. Aspects myxoedémateux et pseudo-lipomatose. Télangiectasie multiples, placards erythémato-squameuse plantaires. Bull. Soc. franç. Dermat. **36**, No 8, 1030—1032 (1929). — GOUGEROT, H., PÉRIN et FILLIOL: Sclérodermie en plaques du cou et du cuir chevelu avec pigmentation maculeuse. Arch. dermato-syph. Hôp. St. Louis **1**, 627—629 (1929). — GOUGEROT, H. et PAUL VIGNE: Atrophies cutanées de types multiples chez un même malade. Sclérodermie, morphées en gouttes, dermite atrophiante diffuse avec atrophie musculaire correspondante, atrophies maculeuses cyaniques (anétodermie?). Arch. dermato-syph. Hôp. St. Louis **1**, 630—634 (1929). — GRIVEAUD: Erythromélie de PICK et sclérodermie. Bull. Soc. franç. Dermat. **37**, No 1, 24—26 (1930). — GROEDEL, FRANZ M. u. GEORG HUBERT: Ein Fall von Sklerodermie nach Unfall. Wien. klin. Wschr. **1925 I**, 409. — GUILLAIN, GEORGES et J. CELICE: Sur un cas de Tabes avec sclérodermie. Bull. Soc. méd. Hôp. Paris **40**, 1661 (1924).

HAELST, A. VAN, et DELCROIX: Descriptions cliniques et radiologiques d'un cas d'hypertrophie congénital du membre inférieur chez une fillette de 4 ans. Le Scalpel **1930 II**, 1002. — HALDIN-DAVIS, H.: Sclerodermia and thyroid tumour. Brit. J. Dermat. **44**, 29—33 (1932). — HARVIER, P. et A. LICHTNITZ: Traitement par la folliculine d'un cas de sclerod. Paris méd. **1928 II**, 43. — HEIMANN-HATRY, WALTER: Zur Ätiologie der Sklerodermie. Universelle Sklerodermie bei hypophysärem Zwergwuchs. Med. Klin. **1925 II**, 1082. — HEINISMAN, J. u. W. CZERNY: Zur Frage der Röntgentherapie bei Sklerodermie. Dtsch. med. Wschr. **53**, 358 (1927). — HERZOG, FRANZ: Über die Behandlung der Sklerodermie mit intravenöser Injektion von Kochsalzlösung. Med. Klin. **1926 II**, 1178. — HILLMANN, H. J.: Beitrag zur Kenntnis der Sklerodermie. Diss. Hamburg 1930. — HINCKY, LANZENBERG et ZORN: Sclérodermie à plaques multiples pigmentées. Bull. Soc. franç. Dermat. **37**, No 7, 786—789 (1930). — HOFFMANN, HEINRICH: Untersuchungen über endokrine Störungen bei Hautkrankheiten, insbesondere Sklerodermie und Acrodermatitis atrophicans. Klin. Wschr. **1925 I**, 978. — Untersuchungen über endokrine Störungen bei Hautkrankheiten, insbesondere Sklerose und Akrodermatitis. Acta dermato-vener. (Stockh.) **6**, 423 (1926). — HUDELO et RABUT: Deux cas de sclérodermies progressives. (Diagnostic différentiel avec la lèpre.) Bull. Soc. franç. Dermat. **36**, No 7, 899—900, 1007—1015 (1929). — A propos des sclérodermies partielles. Bull. Soc. franç. Dermat. **36**, No 7, 938, 939, 1007—1015 (1929). — HUFSCHMITT: Quatre cas de sclérodermie. Bull. Soc. franç. Dermat. **36**, No 7, 892—899, 1007 bis 1015 (1929).

Isola, Domenico: Distrofia generalizzata, sclerodermia in adolescente affecto da gravi fenomeni patologici di ordine endocrino. Arch. di Biol. **3**, 57 (1926). — Distrofia generalizzata, sclerodermia in adolescente affetto da gravi fenomeni patologici di ordine endocrino. Note Psichiatr. **13**, 397 (1925).
Jaffé, Kaete: Zwei Fälle von Sklero-Poikilodermie. Arch. f. Dermat. **159**, 257—268 (1930). — Janichewski: Traitement de la sclérodermie par les rayons ultraviolets. Presse méd. **33**, 863 (1925). — Jeanselme et Burnier: Sclérodermie en plaques avec dyschromie pigmentaire symétrique. Bull. Soc. franç. Dermat. **33**, 704 (1926). — Jedlička, V.: Sklerodermie und innere Sekretion. Česka Dermat. **8**, 57, 92 (1927). — Jordan, Arthur: Sklerodermie und Syphilis. Dermat. Z. **53**, 327 (1928).
Kanno, E.: Über Sklerodermie. Jap. J. Dermat. **25**, 903 (1925). — Keilmann, Klaus: Sklerodermie im Säuglingsalter. Bemerkung zur Arbeit von Dr. Walter Kuczszka. Arch. f. Dermat. **148**, 1 (1924). — Klingmann, Walter O.: Dermatoneuromyositis resulting in sclerodermia. Arch. of Neur. **24**, 1187—1198 (1930). — Kogoj, Fr.: Über Atrophodermien und Sklerodermien. Acta dermato-vener. (Stockh.) **7**, 63 (1926). — Krasnowa, P. u. L. Erlich: Zur Kasuistik der sog. Sklerodermie des Säuglings. Klin. det. Bol. (russ.) **2**, 86 (1928). — Kraus, Alfred: Beitrag zur Klinik und Anatomie der Sklerodermie im Kindesalter. Med. Klin. **21**, 921 (1925). — Kraus, Erik Joh.: Zur Pathogenese der diffusen Sklerose. Zugleich ein Beitrag zur Pathologie der Epithelkörperchen. Virchows Arch. **253**, 710 (1924). — Krebs, E., E. Hartmann et F. Thiébaut: Un cas familial de syndrome de sclérodermie avec cataracte, troubles endocriniens et neuro-végétatifs associés. Revue neur. **37** I, 606—618 (1930). — Addendum à notre communication, sur un cas familial de syndrome de sclérodermie avec cataracte, troubles endocriniens et neurovégétatifs associés. Revue neur. **37** II, 121—125 (1930).
Laennec-Delarne: Les sclérodermies. Gaz. Hôp. mil. **100**, 109 (1927). — Lechelle, P.: H. Baruk et D. Douady: Association de sclérodermie et de maladie de Dupuytren chez un spécifique. Bull. Sci. méd. Hôp. Paris **43**, 622 (1927). — Leiner: 4jähriges Mädchen mit bandförmiger Sklerodermie im atrophischen Stadium. Mitt. Ges. inn. Med. Wien **25**, 102 (1925). — Lereboullet: Hypophyse und dystrophies infantiles. J. Méd. franç. **11**, 321 (1922). Lereboullet, P. et M. Lelong: Concrétions calcaires multiples de la peau avec sclérodermie localisée chez la mère et la fille. Bull. Soc. Pédiatr. Paris **28**, 53—58 (1930). — Léri, André et R. Barthélemy: Sclérodermie progressive chez une syphilitique. Bons effets du traitement bismutique. Bull. Soc. franç. Dermat. **31**, 186 (1924). — Léri, André, R. Barthélemy et Alice Linossier: Sclérodermie et syphilis. Bull. Soc. méd. Hôp. Paris **41**, 324 (1925). — Leriche, René et René Fontaine: Résultats un peu éloignés des interventions sur le sympathique dans la sclérodermie. Rev. de Chir. **65**, 285 (1927). — Les lésions des ganglions sympathiques dans la sclérodermie. Bull. Soc. franç. Dermat. **36**, No 7, 982—987, 1007—1015 (1929). — Le traitement chirurgical de la sclérodermie par les interventions sur le sympathique. Bull. Soc. franç. Dermat. **36**, 995 (1929). — Leriche, R. et A. Jung: Résultats de trois opérations parathyroïdiennes dans la sclérodermie. Bull. Soc. franç. Dermat. **38**, No 8, 1265—1276 (1931). — Lévy, Georges: Sclérodermie en bande du cuir chevelu. Bull. Soc. franç. Dermat. **34**, 297 (1927). — Lévy, Georges et Zorn: Sclérodactylie «sans atteinte des mains». Bull. Soc. franç. Dermat. **36**, No 7, 888—891, 1007—1015 (1929). — Lévy-Franckel et E. Förster: Le rôle des perturbations du système nerveux sympathique et des glandes endocrines dans la pathogénie des affections cutanées. Rev. franç. Dermat. **2**, 277 (1926). — Lhermitte, Jean et Gabrielle Lévy: Sclérodactylie mutilante, amyotrophie, troubles vaso-moteurs trophiques et sensitifs du membre supérieur consécutif à un traumatisme direct de la main datant de 30 ans. Revue neur. **37** I, 621—631 (1930). — Lhermitte, J. et F. Trémolières: Sclérodermie atrophique généralisée avec syndrome ovaro-mammaire d'origine tuberculeuse (Syndrome génito-sclérodermique de Sterling). Rev. Méd. **47**, 202—220 (1930). — Liebner, Ernst: Ein Fall von Sklerodermie mit Syphilis. Dermat. Wschr. **83**, 1195 (1926). — Loewenberg, Richard D.: Zur angeborenen diffusen Sklerodermie. Dermat. Wschr. **1924** I, 893. — Longcope, Warfield: Hypoglycemia in scleroderma. J. amer. med. Assoc. **90**, 1 (1928). — Lorenzo, R.: Sklerodermie in Streifen, Kalkinfiltration, Knochengewebe vortäuschend. Rev. Soc. méd. argent. **39**, 251 (1926). — Lortat-Jacob et Boutelier: Angiomes multiples d'apparition tardive chez une malade présentant un syndrome de Raynaud et une sclérodermie fruste. Bull. Soc. franç. Dermat. **32**, 46 (1925). — Lortat-Jacob, Fernet et Y. Bureau: Atrophie cutanée avec sclérodermie, mélanodermie et concrétions calcaires. Bull. Soc. franç. Dermat. **36**, 256 (1929). — Atrophie cutanée avec sclérodermie mélanodermie et concrétions calcaires (hypercalcémie et augmentation du métabolisme basal.) Bull. Soc. franç. Dermat. **36**, No 7, 902—906, 1007—1015 (1929). — Sclérodermie avec goitre et augmentation du métabolisme basale. Bull. Soc. franç. Dermat. **36**, No 7, 906—909, 1007—1015 (1929). — Lortat-Jacob et P. Legrain: Sclérodermie et syphilis. Progrès méd. **52**, No 6, 79—81 (1924). — Louste, Juster et David: Sclérodermie en plaques très améliorée par un traitement combiné de rayons ultra-violets et d'ionisation indurée.

Bull. Soc. franç. Dermat. **34**, 322 (1927). — LOUSTE, JUSTER et MICHELET: Sclérodermie familiale. Bull. Soc. franç. Dermat. **36**, 440 (1929). — LOUSTE et RACINE: Sclérodermie progressive à évolution rapide. Bull. Soc. franç. Dermat. **39**, 675, 676 (1932). MACCALLUM, W.: Acute diffusa scleroderma. Trans. Assoc. amer. Physicians **41**, 190 (1926). — MACKAY, H.: Scleroderma and its treatment by radium. Canad. med. Assoc. J. **16**, 142 (1926). — MAIRE et FR. WORINGER: Association d'une dermatite chronique atrophiante au début avec une sclérodermie généralisée aux 4 membres. Bull. Soc. franç. Dermat. **26**, No 7, 780—783, 809—815 (1929). — MALOSSI, C.: Sulla patogenesi della sclerodermia. Arch. ital. Dermat. **7**, 103—131 (1931). — MANKROSKIJ, B.: Über die neurotische Entstehung der Sklerodermie. Sovrem. Psichonerv. (russ.) **4**, 255 (1927). — MARCUS, M. u. H. VOLLMER: Trophoneurotische Hypertrophie einer Extremität durch verkalkten Senkungsabsceß. Z. Kinderheilk. **51**, 127 (1931). — MAŠKILEISSON, W.: Zur Kasuistik der diffusen symmetrischen Sklerodermie und Sklerodermie mit Sklerodaktylie. Venerol. (russ.) **1926**, 917. — MATRAS, AUGUST: Über Veränderungen in der Muskulatur bei diffuser Sklerodermie der oberen Extremität, amputiert wegen eines bullösen und gangräneszierenden Erysipels. Dermat. Wschr. **1932 I**, 829—834. — MATSUI, SUTEHACHIRO: Über die Pathologie und Pathogenese von Sclerodermia universalis. Mitt. med. Fak. Tokyo **31**, H. 1, 55—116 (1924). — MÉSZÁROS, K.: Capillarmikroskopische Beobachtungen bei Sklerodermie. Acta med. scand. (Stockh.) **72**, 241 (1929). — Capillar-mikroskopische Untersuchungen bei Sklerodermie. Orv. Hetil. (ung.) **1929 I**, 60—63. — MGEBROV, M. u. L. BRODSKIJ: Zur Frage der Sclerodermia alba guttata superficialis. Trudy odessk. dermato-venerol. Inst. **1**, 159 (1927). — MICHAELIS, O.: Influence spécialement remarquable de l'insuline dans un cas de sclérodermie totale. Acta dermato-vener. (Stockholm) **10**, 491—502 (1929). — MILIAN, PÉRIN et HOROWITZ: Sclérodermie calcaire. Bull. Soc. franç. Dermat. **37**. No 4, 475—479; No 5, 551, 552 (1930). — MILIAN et RIMÉ: Erythème scléro-oedemateux avec myopathie et myasthénie. Bull. Soc. franç. Dermat. **32**, 470 (1926). — MOEHLIG, R.: Clinic on endocrinopathies. Ann. clin. Med. **5**, 247 (1926). — MONIER-VINARD et BARBOT: Sclerodermia et cataracte. Syndrome familial. Bull. Soc. méd. Hôp. Paris **44**, 708 (1928). — MORAWIECKA, J.: Un cas de maladie de Basedow associée à la sclérodermie et à l'osteomalacie. Revue neur. **35**, 217 (1928). — MURRAY-WILL: Scleroderma and Syphilis. Brit. J. Dermat. **39**, 201 (1927).

NAEGELI: A propos des sclérodermies. Bull. Soc. franç. Dermat. **36**, No 7, 883—888, 1007—1015 (1929).

O'LEARY, PAUL A. and RUBEN NOMLAND: A clinical study of 103 cases of scleroderma. Amer J. med. Sci. **180**, 95—112 (1930). — OLIVER, E. LAWRENCE: Generalized scleroderma in children. Report of three cases and review of the literature. Arch. of Dermat. **25**, 72—88 (1932). — OPPENHEIM, MORITZ: Atrophien. Handbuch der Haut- und Geschlechtskrankheiten, Bd. 8, Teil 2, S. 500. 1931. — ORLOF, P.: Sclerodermia diffusa. Russk. Vestn. Dermat. **3**, 608 (1925). — OSTROWSKI, ST.: Bestehen Grundlagen für die Einreihung der Dermatitis chronica atrophicans und der Sklerodermie in eine Gruppe? Przegl. dermat. (poln.) **24**, 296 (1929).

PAISSEAU, G., H. SCHAEFFER et SCHERBER: Sclérodermie généralisée avec lésions osseuses et arthropathies. Arch. Méd. Enf. **33**, 407—415 (1930). — PARHON, C. I., M. ISANOS et MARIE BRIESE: Note anatomo-clinique sur un cas de sclérodermie. Bull. Soc. roum. Neur. etc. **4**, No 4, 1—11 (1930). — PARHON, C. et ZOE CARAMAN: Association de la sclérodermie au syndrome de Basedow. Arch. gen. di Neur. **8**, 69 (1927). — PATRICK, H.: A case of scleroderma. J. Neur. **17**, 560 (1927). — PAUTRIER, L.-M.: Sclérodermie à évolution rapide, en plaques multiples. Importance des lésions vasculaires initiales et tardives dans l'étude de la sclérodermie. Bull. Soc. franç. Dermat. **36**, No 7, 928—938, 1007—1015 (1929). — Les rapports de la dermatite chronique atrophiante de l'anétodermie et de la sclérodermie. L'étude des troubles du métabolisme du tissu conjonctif. Bull. Soc. franç. Dermat. **36**, No 7, 973—978, 1007—1015 (1929). — PAUTRIER, L.-M. et J. BRUSSET: Le métabolisme basal dans les atrophies cutanées et dans les sclérodermies. Bull. Soc. franç. Dermat. **36**, No 7, 987—991, 1007—1015 (1929). — PAUTRIER, L.-M. et GEORGES LÉVY: L'anatomie pathologique des sclérodermies. Bull. Soc. franç. Dermat. **36**, No 7, 978—982, 1007—1015 (1929). — PAUTRIER, L.-M. et A. ULLMO: Note sur la capillaroscopie de la dermatite chronique atrophiante et de la sclérodermie. Bull. Soc. franç. Dermat. **36**, No 7, 776—780, 809—815 (1929). — PAUTRIER, L.-M. et ZORN: La calcémie dans les atrophies cutanées et dans les sclérodermies. Bull. Soc. franç. Dermat. **36**, No 7, 991—993, 1007—1015 (1929). — PAYENNEVILLE et CAILLIAN: Un cas de sclérodermie en bande avec «white spot disease». Bull. Soc. franç. Dermat. **36**, No 7, 939—941, 1007—1015 (1929). — PER, M.: Note rel. à un cas de sclérodermie superfic. circonscr. en plaques. Acta dermato-vener. (Stockh.) **9**, 155 (1928). — PERITZ, Sklerodermie (Demonstration). Berl. Ges. Psychiatr. u. Nervenkrkh., 9. Febr. u. 9. März 1925. Ref. Z. Neur. **41**, 347 (1925). — PERNET, J.: Über einen Fall von Sklerodermie mit Hautverkalkung. Arch. f. Dermat. **152**, 337 (1926). — PETELIN, S.: Sklerodermie und ihre Pathogenese. Fortschr. Med. **46**, 789 (1928). — PETGES, G.: Un cas d'hémisclérodermie alterne de la face du tronc et des membres chez un hérédo-syphilitique. Bull. Soc. franç. Dermat. **36**, No 7, 880—883, 1007—1015 (1929). — PETGES, G., LECOULANT et DELAS: Syndrome de RAYNAUD associé à une sclérodactylie. Amélioration par des alternances de traitement endocrinien et par l'acétylcholine. Bull. Soc. franç. Dermat. **36**, No 7, 877—880, 1007—1015 (1929). — PETGES, G. et J. ROCHE: Sclérodermie postopératoire (hystérectomie totale). Bull. Soc. franç. Dermat. **36**, No 7, 972, 973, 1007—1015 (1929). — PEYRI, JAQUES et M. CHARLES CARDENAL: Sur la »monocytose« et les »botryomycomes« apparus dans un cas de sclérodactylie. Bull. Soc. franç. Dermat. **36**, No 7, 953—960, 1007—1015 (1929). — POUSSEPP, L. et J. RIVES: Un cas de sclérodactylie accompagné de sclérodermie »en bande«. Ann. Méd. **19**, 19 (1926). — PRAKKEN, J. R.: Etwas über die Bedeutung des Calciums bei der Sklerodermie. Nederl. Tijdschr. Geneesk. **1932**, 2617—2623.

RAKE, G.: On the pathology and pathogenesis of scleroderma. Bull. Hopkins Hosp. **48**, 212 (1931). — RAMAZOTTI, VIRGINIO: Patogenesie terapia della sclerodermia. Giorn. ital. Mal. vener. pelle **64**, 57 (1923). Zit. nach MARBURG. — ROBERTS, STEWART R.: Scleroderma associated with symptoms of Erythromelalgia and myxedema. Med. Clin. N. Amer. **12**, 1429 (1929). — ROEDERER, J.: Sclérodermie en bande du front. Bull. Soc. franç. Dermat. **34**, 284 (1927). — Un cas de sclérodermie en plaques guéri par l'opothérapie pluriglandulaire. Bull. Soc. franç. Dermat. **36**, No 7, 993, 994, 1007—1015 (1929). — ROTHMANN, ST.: Über endokrine Störungen bei Sklerodermie. Klin. Wschr. **1925 II**, 1691. — ROTNES, P.: Ein Fall von Melanodermie mit sklerodermatischen und atrophischen Veränderungen. Forh. nord. dermat. For. (dän.) **1929**, 116. — ROWE, ALLEN W. and FRANCIS H. McCRUDDEN: Metabolism observations in scleroderma. Brit. med. J. **190**, Nr 4, 121—123 (1924). — ROXBURGH, A.: The aetiology of alopecia areata and its relation to vitiligo and scleroderma. Brit. J. Dermat. **41**, 351 (1929). — RUSSI, F.: Contributo clinico alto studio della sclerodermia. Gazz. Osp. **46**, 221 (1925).

SAINTON, P. et H. MAMOU: Hyperthyroidisme provoqué par le thyroxine synthétique chez un malade atteint d'un syndrome pluriglandulaire avec sclérodermie et cataracte. Bull. Soc. méd. Hôp. Paris **43**, 1685 (1927). — SALKAN, D.: Pathogenese der Sklerodermie. Vrač. Delo (russ.) **9**, 407 (1926). — SANNICANDRO, G.: Contributo alla conoszenza della sclerodermia etc. Arch. ital. Dermat. **4**, 427 (1929). — SCALA, G.: La patogenesi della sclerodermia. Fol. med. (Napoli) **14**, 7 (1928). — SCHÖNGUT, ERNÖ: Hormonale Beeinflussung und neues Heilverfahren bei Sklerodermie und endokriner Polyarthritis. Gyógyászat (ung.) **1931 II**, 762—763. — SCHWARZ, P.: Sklerodermie und Röntgenkastration. Schweiz. med. Wschr. **1926 I**, 276. — SCOLARI, E.: La sclerodattilia e la sclerodermia diffusa con speciale riguardo alle turbe vasomotorie. Loro rapporti con il morbo di RAYNAUD. Giorn. ital. Dermat. **72**, 1477—1524 (1931); **73**, 669—688 (1932). — SEALE, EVERETT: Endocrin aspects of scleroderma; Report of a case with endocrin dysfunction. South. med. J. **22**, 85 (1929). — SELLEI, JOSEF: Die Behandlung der Sklerodermie mit Pankreasfermenten. Med. Klin. **1930 II**, 1859, 1860. — Fermenttherapie der Sklerodermie. Münch. med. Wschr. **1930 II**, 2220, 2221. — Skleroderma und Dermatitis atrophicans cutis. Börgyógy. Szemle (ung.) **8**, 231 (1930). — Die Akrosklerosis (Sklerodaktylie) und deren Symptomenkomplex nebst neueren Untersuchungen bei Sklerodermie. Arch. f. Dermat. **1931**, 343. — Akrosclerosis (Sklerodaktylie, progressive Sklerodermie). Zbl. Hautkrkh. **41**, 296 (1932). — Die Akrosklerose (früher Sklerodaktylie, progressive Sklerodermie). Orv. Hetil. (ung.) **1932**, 677—679. — Zur Klinik und Therapie der Sklerodaktylie, progressive Sklerodermie (Akrosklerose). Dermat. Z. **64**, 138—146 (1932). — SELYE, HANS: A condition simulating human scleroderma in rats injected with parathyroid hormone. J. amer. med. Assoc. **99**, 108 (1932). — Die Sklerodermie und ihre Entstehungsweise. Virchows Arch. **286**, 96 (1932). — SEMINARIO, C. u. M. DANERI: Zwei Fälle von Fibrolysinbehandlung allgemeiner Sklerodermie. Rev. argent. dermato-siph. **14**, 48 (1931). — SÉZARY, A.: Sympathiques et pigmentation cutanée. Revue neur. **33**, 1070 (1926). — SÉZARY, A., A. FAVORY et H. MAMOU: Syndrome tardif de sclérodermie avec cataracte associé à des troubles endocriniens. Bull. Soc. méd. Hôp. Paris **46**, 358—363 (1930). — SIROTA, L.: Über zwei klinisch beobachtete Sklerodermfälle. Dermat. Wschr. **81**, 1228 (1925). — SPILLMANN, L. et I. L. CRÉHANGE: Un cas de sclérodermie en plaques du thorax et de l'avant-bras. Bull. Soc. franç. Dermat. **38**, 1074 (1931). — STEINER, G.: Die Insulintherapie der vasomotorischen Hautneurosen. Gyógyászat. (ung.) **1928 II**, 1504. — STEINITZ, HERMANN u. ANNELIESE CASPER-FÜRSTENHEIM: Abortivform von STILLscher Krankheit mit Sklerodermie. Med. Klin. **1930 I**, 700—702. — STERLING: Der lipodystrophische und der osteomalazische Typus der genitosklerodermischen Degeneration. Polska Gaz. lek. **7**, 99 (1928). — STÖCKL, E.: Sklerodaktylie und Gravidität. Ginek. polska **6**, 1035 (1927). — STOYE, W.: Ein Beitrag zur Ätiologie der STILLschen Krankheit und der herdförmigen Sklerodermie. Z. Kinderheilk. **41**, 538 (1926). — STROM, AXEL: Sklerodermie und Diabetes. Norsk Mag. Laegevidensk. **89**, 671 (1928). — STRUKOV, A.: Zur Frage der pathologischen Anatomie und Pathogenese der diffusen Sklerodermie. Vrač. Delo (russ.) **12**, 880—882 (1929). — STRUNZ, F.: Ein Fall von Progeria, beginnend mit ausgedehnter Sklerodermie. Z. Kinderheilk. **47**, 401

(1929). — STUDNIČKA, B.: Diffuse Sklerodermie, behandelt mit Thyreoidin und Radiumemanation. Rev. Neur. (tschech.) **23**, 334 (1926). — ŠUTOVA, T.: Zur Frage der Sklerodermie. Ž. Nevropat. (russ.) **20**, 491 (1927).
THIBIERGE, L. SPILLMANN et WEISSENBACH: Sclérodermie et granulations calcaires sous-cutanées. Bull. Soc. franç. Dermat. **32**, 58 (1925). — TOLOSA, COLOMER E.: Über den Wert der Capillaroskopie bei der Diagnose der Raynaud- und anderer vasomotorisch-trophischen Neurosen. Rev. méd. Barcelona **12**, 440 (1929). — TOMMASI, L.: Sclerodermia generalizzata e distioridismo postencephalitico. Giorn. ital. Dermat. **68**, 282 (1927). — Atrofia idiopatica generalizzata della cuto con discromia et sclerodermia. Giorn. ital. Dermat. **69**, 663 (1928). — TOWAINE et RIMÉ: Vitiligo et sclérodermie en bandes chez une hérédo-syphilitique. Bull. Soc. franç. Dermat. **39**, No 5, 567—570 (1932). — TREMOLIÈRES, F., J. LHERMITTE, A. TARDIEUES et A. CARTEAUD: Sclérodermie atrophique généralisée avec syndrome ovaro-mammaire d'origine tuberculeuse. Bull. Soc. méd. Hôp. Paris **45**, 938 (1929).
VALLERY-RADOT, PASTEUR, P. HILLEMAND et B. CHOMEREAU-LAMOTTE: Maladie de BASEDOW, myxoedème, sclérod. généralisée, avec état sclérodermique du voile du palais. Bull. Soc. méd. Hôp. Paris **42**, 1149 (1926). — VEROTTI, ITALO: Über einen Fall von bandförmiger Sklerodermie und Zosternarben. Dermat. Wschr. **1924 II**, 1250. — VIGANO, E.: Sclerodermia e radioterapia. Commun. 16. Riun. Soc. Lit. Dermat. Roma, 18./20. Dez. 1919. Zit. nach MARBURG. — VOHWINKEL, K. H.: Zur Pathogenese der Sklerodermie. Arch. f. Dermat. **158**, 28 (1929). — VUL, I.: Über Pathogenese der Sklerodermie. Sovrem. Psichonevr. (russ.) **7**, 169 (1928).
WALDORP, C. und G. BASOMBRIO: Endokrinosympathische Studien bei Sklerodermie und Ichtyosis. Semana méd. **33**, 1351 (1926). — WEBER, F. PARKES and O. B. BODE: Scleroderma and myasthenia gravis. Proc. roy. Soc. Med. **25**, 966 (1932). — WEISSENBACH, R.: Concrétions calcaires de la sclérodermie ou sclérodermie calcaire. Bull. Soc. franç. Dermat. **38**, 808 (1931). — WEISSENBACH, R., E. VIGNAL et CH. GUILLAUMIN: Concrétions calcaires sous-cutanées des doigts, associées à une acrocyanose permanente avec accès d'acrocyanose paroxystique. Bull. Soc. franç. Dermat. **36**, 910, 1007 (1929). — WEISSENBACH, R.-J., GEORGES BASCH et MARIANNE BASCH: Essai critique sur la pathogénie des concrétions calcaires des sclérodermies (syndrome de THIBIERGE-WEISSENBACH) et des syndromes voisins. Ann. Méd. **31**, 504—529 (1932). — WENNBERG: Ein Fall von Sklerodermie bei hohem Körpergewicht. Ecos españ. Dermat. **6**, 339—343 (1930). — WIGLEY, J. E. M.: Scleroderma. Proc. roy. Soc. Med. **23**, 159, 160 (1929). — WOLF, MAURICE et A. VALLETTE: Goutte calcaire et sclérodermie dans leurs rapports avec le métabolisme du calcium. Rev. Méd. **43**, 1121 (1926).
ZEHRER, H.: Ein Fall von symmetrischer universeller Sklerodermie. Arch. f. Psychiatr. **88**, 455 (1929). — ZUPPA, ARMANDO: Radioterapia e sclerodermia. Arch. di Radiol. **5**, 967—975 (1929).

Hemiatrophia, Hemihypertrophia faciei.

ANDREWS: Scleroderma and facial hemiatrophy. Arch. of Dermat. **12**, 914 (1925). — ARCHAMBAULT, LA SALLE and NELSON K. FROMM: Progressive facial hemiatrophy. Report of three cases. Arch. of Neur. **27**, 529—584 (1932). — AWGUSCHEWITSCH, P.: Elephantiasis des oberen Augenlides, Hemihypertrophia faciei und Hydrophthalmus etc. Klin. Mbl. Augenheilk. **83**, 91 (1929).
BEN, F.: Hemiatrophia faciei und Sklerodermie. Dermat. Wschr. **1926 II**. — BERNSTEIN, EUGEN: Hemiatrophia alternans facialis progressiva mit halbseitiger Alopecia, Pigmentverschiebung und Hautatrophie. Dermat. Wschr. **1930 I**, 235—237. — BOARDMAN: Total hemiatrophy with scleroderma. Ref. Zbl. Hautkrkh. **24**, 263 (1927). — BÖNHEIM, E.: Zahnextraktion, periphere Facialislähmung, Hemiatrophia facialis progressiva. Dtsch. Mschr. Zahnheilk. **45**, 353 (1927). — BOGAERT, VAN et J. HELSMOORTEL: Syndrome paratrigéminal du sympathique oculaire. J. Neur. **27**, 222 (1927). — BOROWSKIJ, M.: Ein Fall von Hemiatrophia faciei progressiva mit halbseitiger Hypoplasie des Rachens und Kehlkopfs. Sovrem. Psichonevr. (russ.) **1**, 121 (1925). — BORY, LOUIS: Un cas d'hémiatrophie faciale progressive avec sclérodermie partielle du cuir chevelu. Bull. Soc. franç. Dermat. **36**, No 7, 863—865, 877 (1929). — BOST, CRAWFORD: Progressive facial hemiatrophy. Arch. Pediatr. **44**, 497 (1927). — BUDINA, R.: Zur Frage über die Pathogenese der Hemiatrophia faciei und der Heterochromia der Iris. Sovrem. Psichonevr. (russ.) **11**, 316 (1930).
ČERNI, L.: Zur Frage der Klinik und Pathogenese der Hemiatrophia faciei. Ukraïn. med. Visti **1925**, Nr 5/6, 63. — Zwei Fälle von Hemiatrophia unilateralis totalis. Sovrem. Psichonevr. (russ.) **3**, 494 (1926). — CHASANOW, M.: Beiträge zur Ätiologie der Hemiatrophie des Gesichts. Z. Neur. **140**, 473—485 (1932). — CORDS, R.: Strichförmige Gesichtsatrophie und Auge. Ber. dtsch. ophthlam. Ges. **1929**, 53—59.
DARDANI, REMO: Per un caso di emi-ipertrofia congenita. Pediatr. riv. **37**, 535 (1929). — DOHI, S.: A case of hemiatrophia facialis. Jap. J. of Dermat. **25**, 15 (1925).

Fordyce, A.: Hemihypertrophia alterna. Arch. Dis. Childh. **3**, 300 (1928).
Gesell: Hemihypertrophy and twinning. Amer. J. med. Sci. **173**, 542 (1927). — Grütz, O.: Die Sklerodermia guttata follicularis mit halbseitiger Gesichts- und Körperatrophie und endokrinen Krankheitssymptomen. Dermat. Z. **53**, 227 (1928).
Jansen, G. A. H. Eibrink: Zur Frage der Hemihypertrophia dextra und Hemiatrophia sinistra. Tijdschr. Tandheelk. (holl.) **35**, 131 (1928). — Jossmann: Hemiatrophia faciei. Berl. Ges. Psychiatr. u. Nervenkrkh., 11. Nov. 1929.
Kirschenberg, E.: Ein Fall von Hemiatrophia facialis progressiva mit zentraler Genese. Fol. neuropath. eston. **5**, 94 (1926). — Kitaigorodskaja, O.: Angeborene Hypertrophie im Kindesalter. Jb. Kinderheilk. **125**, 38 (1929). — Knjažanskij: Hemihypertrophia totalis. Sovrem. Psichonevr. (russ.) **3**, 414 (1926). — Koschewnikow, A. M.: Hemiatrophia cruciata und Hemihypertrophia cruciata. Gross. Mer. Enzykl. (russ.) **6** (1929). Zit. nach Kulkow. — Krotoska, Marja: Ein Fall von Hemihypertrophia cruciata bei einem 3jährigen Kinde. Pediatr. polska **8**, 305 (1928). — Kul'kov, R.: Hemihypertrophia cruciata. Sovrem. Psichonevr. **11**, 60—66 (1930). — Kulkow, A.: Hemihypertrophia cruciata. Z. Neur. **122**, 525 (1929).
Lauber, H.: Ein Fall von Hemiatrophia facialis progressiva mit Beteiligung des Auges. Z. Augenheilk. **57**, 492 (1925). — Lenstrup, E.: Eight cases of hemi-hypertrophy. Acta paediatr. (Stockh.) **6**, 205 (1926). — Léri, A.: Sur la dissociation du réflexe oculo-cardiaque et des épreuves pharmacologiques dans l'exploration sympathique. Revue neur. **33**, 1092 (1926). — Léri, André et Jean Weill: Phenomène de Marcus Gunn congénital et héréditaire etc. Bull. Soc. méd. Hôp. Paris **45**, 875 (1929). — List, C. F.: Atrophie des subcutanen Fettgewebes eines Beines bei einem Kinde. Berl. Ges. Psychiatr. 6. Mai 1929. — Löwenberg: Hemiatrophia und halbseitige Sklerodermie. Zbl. Hautkrkh. **16**, 19 (1925).
Mankowski, B.: Zur Pathogenese der Hemiatrophia facialis. Arch. f. Psychiatr. **78**, 572 (1926). — Manthey, P.: Hemiatrophia faciei nach Strumektomie. Z. Neur. **114**, 192 (1928). — Marinesco, G., A. Kreindler et E. Façon: Sur la pathogénie de l'hémiatrophie faciale. Bull. Sect. sci. Acad. roum. **14**, 155—166 (1931). — Mayers, L.: Hemihypertrophia. Surg. etc. **43**, 746 (1926). — Mezzatesta, F.: Emiatrofia facciale e disturbi visivi. Riv. otol. ecc. **4**, 315 (1927). — Moszkowicz, Ludwig: Fettplastik bei Hemiatrophia faciei. Med. Klin. **1930 II**, 1478.
Nemlicher, L. J. u. B. J. Rappoport: Hemiatrophie des Gesichts und des Körpers mit idiopathischen Hautprozessen kombiniert. Vrač. Delo (russ.) **8**, 270 (1925). — Noica, D. et A. Vicol: Un cas de hémiatrophie faciale droite. Bull. Soc. méd. Hôp. Bukarest, **6**, 96 (1924).
Petrillo, Luis et Juan Oreggia: Hemiatrophia facialis. Arch. lat.-amer. Pediatr. **21**, 696 (1927). — Pollak, Franz: Zur Frage der cerebralen Trophik. Arch. f. Psychiatr. **89**, 788—801 (1930). — Ein eigenartiger Fall von einseitiger Hemiatrophie und seine Beziehungen zum vegetativen Nervensystem. Arch. f. Dermat. **159**, 188—193 (1930). — Popova, N.: Pathologie und Therapie der Hemiatrophia faciei et corporis. Sovrem. Psichonevr. (russ.) **4**, 475 (1927).
Ratner, F.: Über einen Fall von Hemiatrophia cruciata progressiva. Dtsch. Z. Nervenheilk. **97**, 304 (1927). — Roederer et Klein: Bull. Soc. Pédiatr. Paris **25**, No 8/9 (1927). Zit. nach Kulkow.
Smirnitsbuj, J.: Zur Pathogenese der Hemiatrophia faciei. Ž. Nevropat. (russ.) **12**, 599—604 (1929). — Sorsby, Arnold and Marcelli Shaw: The refraction in cases of congenital torticollis associated with hemiatrophy of the face. Brit. J. Ophthalm. **16**, 222—225 (1932). — Stief, Sándor u. Tanka, Dezsö: Seltener Fall von Hemiatrophia faciei. Orv. Hetil. (ung.) **69**, 459 (1925). — Stiefler: Ein Fall von posttraumatischer Hemiatrophia faciei progressiva im vorgeschrittenen Alter, nebst Bemerkungen zur Pathogenese. Z. Neur. **88**, 305 (1924). — Surat, W.: Über einseitige Störung der Gesichtstrophik (Hemiatrophia faciei). Mschr. Psychiatr. **77**, 202 (1930).
Terrien, Veil, Chavany: Hémihypertrophie faciale et buphthalmie. Bull. Soc. Ophtalm. Paris **3**, 131 (1931). — Tobias, Norman: Congenital hemiatropy associated with linear naevus. Arch. of Pediatr. **45**, 673 (1928). — Trepte, Gertr.: Hemiatrophia totalis und Sympathicusoperation. Berl. Ges. Psychiatr., 6. Mai 1929. — Hemiatrophia totalis mit Sklerodermie und Sympathicusoperation. Z. Neur. **124**, 809—819 (1930). — Trömner: Hemihypertrophia und Hemiatrophia faciei. Ärztl. Ver. Hamburg, 25. Jan. 1927. Ref. Zbl. Neur. **46**.
Vazquez, Rodr.: Ein Fall von Hemiatrophie des Gesichts. Pediatr. españ. **16**, 135 (1927). — Vivado, A.: Über einen Fall von Hemiatrophie sympathischer Herkunft. Rev. méd. Chile **56**, 1066 (1928). — Voljfsohn, N.: Zur Klinik der Hemiatropie des Gesichts. Med. Mysl' (russ.) **5**, 89 (1929).
Wartenberg, R.: Zur Klinik und Pathologie der Hemiatrophia faciei progressiva. Arch. f. Psychiatr. **74**, 602 (1925). — Wolff, H. G.: Progressive facial hemiatrophy. Arch. of Otolaryng. **7**, 580 (1928). — J. nerv. Dis. **69**, 140 (1929). — Wolff, H. G. and A. Ehrenclou:

Trophic disorders of central origin. Report of a case of progressive facial hemiatrophy, associated with a Lipodystrophy. J. amer. med. Assoc. **88**, 991 (1927).

Angioneurotisches Ödem. Epidermolysis bullosa.

ASAI, J.: Eine interessante Form von rezidivierendem circumscriptem Ödem der Conjunctiva bulbi sinistra bei einer Kranken mit chronischer Pyelitis und paroxysmaler Tachykardie. Acta dermat. (Kioto) **9**, H. 4. 393—399, und deutsche Zusammenfassung 1927, S. 399—400.
BASSET, A., Y. HAGUENAU et GAUTHRON: Trophoedème du membre inférieur. Revue neur. **37 I**, 258 (1930). — BETTMANN: Abnormer Aufbau des Gefäßendabschnitts und seine capillarmikroskopische Kontrolle. Arch. f. Dermat. **159**, 140 (1929). — BLAUSTEIN, N.: Angioneurotic edema of entire genito-urinary system. J. of Urol. **16**, Nr 5, 379—390 (1926). — BOGART, A.: The surgical significance of intestinal angion. edema. Ann. Surg. **61**, 324 (1915). — BOHUMICZKY, ENDRÉ: Tonogen in der Therapie des angioneuritischen Ödems. Gyôgyászat (ung.) **67**, Nr 41, 922—924 (1927). — BOLTEN, G.: Myxödem, angioneurotische Ödeme, Kachexia strumipriva und Epilepsie. Mschr. Psychiatr. **78**, 253 (1931). — BOLTEN, G. C.: Die Genese und Behandlung der exsudativen Paroxysmen. Nederl. Mschr. Geneesk. **12**, Nr 10, 518—561 (1924). — Über Genese und Behandlung der exsudativen Paroxysmen (QUINCKEsche Krankheit, Migräne, Asthma usw.). Abh. Neur. usw. **1925**, H. 31, 1—110 (1925). — Zwei besondere Fälle von flüchtigem Ödem. Geneesk. gids. **3**, H. 12, 273—277 (1925). — BORAK, J.: Ein neues Behandlungsverfahren akroangioneurotischer Affektionen. Klin. Wschr. **1926 II**, 1830. — BORRIES, G.: Zur Klinik des idiopathischen Larynxödems. Otologia (Fukuoka) **3**, 671. — BRAEUKER, W.: Das traumatische Ödem. Mschr. Unfallheilk. **38**, 241 (1931). — BROWN, GRAFTON: The treatment of urticaria and angioneur. edema. Ann. int. Med. **3**, 591 (1929). — BUNGENBERG DE JONG, W. J. H.: Ein Fall von QUINCKEschem Ödem des Larynx. Nederl. Tijdschr. Geneesk. **1928 II**, 5226.
CALLENBERG, J.: Über das Verhältnis der Urticaria chronica periodica zum Serumkalkspiegel bei ovarieller Dysfunktion. Klin. Wschr. **1924 I**, 533, 534. — CANALE, PIERO: Contributo allo studio degli edemi nervosi, Sopra un caso di emiedema dell'arte superiore destro da probabile lesione del simpatico cervicale. Riv. klin. med. **29**, 699—721 (1928). — CAPECCHI, EGISTO: Sindrome rara di edema di QUINCKE. Valsalva **2**, H. 3. 103—112 (1926). — CASAUBON, ALFREDO u. ANGEL PEPA: Chronisches Trophödem Meige. Arch. latino-amer. Paediatr. **16**, 810 (1922). — ČASOVNIKOV, R.: Ein Fall von chronischem neuropathischem Gesichtsödem als Komplikation des QUINCKEschen Ödems. Trudy tomsk. med. Inst. **1**, 61—68 u. deutsche Zusammenfassung, 1931. S. 68. — CERVENKA, JOSEF: QUINCKEsches Ödem. Sborn. lék. (tschech.) **24 I**, H. 1/6, 402—405 (1923). — CHALLIOL, VIKTOR: Klinische Mitteilung über zwei nicht gewöhnliche Fälle des Morbus Quincke. Dtsch. Z. Nervenheilk. **85**, H. 1/2, 13—20 (1925). — CHARVÁT, J.: Behandlung des Asthma bronchiale, der Migräne und des QUINCKEschen Ödems mit Peptoninjektionen. Čas. lék. česk. **1930 I**, 669. — CID, JOSÉ M.: Chronisches Trophödem. Rev. méd. del Rosario **17**, No 11, 618—622 (1927). — CURTIUS, F. u. R. STREMPEL: Gleichzeitiges Vorkommen von Morbus Recklinghausen und Epidermis bullosa traumatica hereditaria dystrophica in einer Familie. Dermat. Z. **51**, H. 6, 401—416 (1928).
DEDERDING, D.: Drei Fälle von Morbus Menière in Verbindung mit QUINCKES Ödem. Arch. Ohr- usw. Heilk. **1926**, 121 (1930). — DELHAYE, A.: Meige trophöedema bei Spina bifida occulta. Vlaamsch. geneesk. Tijdschr. **5**, 688 (1924). — DEUTSCH, EMIL: Ein Fall von familiär auftretendem QUINCKEschem Ödem der oberen Luftwege. Z. Hals- usw. Heilk. **21**, 148—155 (1928). — DEVOTO, A.: Epidermolisi bollosa. Relat. 27. Riun. soz. ital. dermat., p. 1. 1931. — DITTRICH: QUINCKEsches Ödem mit annulärem Exanthem. Zbl. Hautkrkh. **41**, 666 (1932). — DOERR, R.: Die Idiosynkrasien. Naturwiss. **12**, H. 47, 1018—1031 (1924). — DRYSDALE, H. H.: Acute circumscribed edema (QUINCKE). J. amer. med. Assoc. **89**, Nr 17, 1390—1393 (1927). — DUFKE, FRANZ: Zur psychischen Urticaria. Dermat. Wschr. **82**, Nr 21, 705—708 (1926). — DUKE, W. W.: Urticaria caused specifically by the action of physical agents. J. amer. med. Assoc. **83**, Nr 1, 3—9 (1924). — DUNLAP, H. and WILLIS S. LEMON: The hereditary type of angioneurotic edema. Amer. J. med. Sci. **177**, 259 (1929).
EBBECKE: Capillarerweiterung, Urticaria und Shock. Klin. Wschr. **1923 II**, 1725—1727. EISELT: Anaphylaxie und Neurologie. Rev. neuropsychopath. **20**, No 3, 81—84; No 4, 115—118; No 5, 152—155 (1923). — ELLIS, W. B.: Two cases of congenital edema. Proc. roy. Soc. Med. **25**, 956, 957 (1932). — EVANS, E.: Three cases of congenital edema (MILLROYs disease) in two generations of the same family. Proc. roy. Soc. med. **23**, 1585 (1930). — EZICKSON, WILLIAM J.: Angioneurotic edema of penis and scrotum. J. amer. med. Assoc. **87**, Nr 8, 561, 562 (1926).
FEER, W.: QUINCKEsches Ödem, primär in der Lunge. Schweiz. med. Wschr. **1913 I**, 186. — FINDER: Handbuch von DENKER u. KAHLER, Bd. 3. 1928. — FLIEDERBAUM: Untersuchungen über den Einfluß des autonomen Nervensystems und der endokrinen Drüsen

auf die Ödembereitschaft der Haut. Z. exper. Med. **76**, 659 (1931). — FRENKL, H.: Ein Fall von Epidermolysis bullosa dystrophicans mit tödlichem Ausgang. Pedjatr. polska **10**, 306 (1930). — FUHS, H.: Über Epidermolysis bullosa traumatica hereditaria (KÖBNER). Arch. f. Dermat. **153**, H. 1, 157—168 (1927). — FULTON, I. u. PERCIVAL BAILEY: Neuer Beitrag über Tumoren des 3. Ventrikels. Ihr Zusammenvorkommen mit dem RECKLINGHAUSENschen Symptomenkomplex und dem QUINCKEschen Ödem. Arch. argent. Neur. **5**, 3 (1930).
GALANT, JOHANN SUSMANN: Überempfindlichkeitsneurosen. Psychiatr.-neur. Wschr. **1925 I**, 31—35. — GARNIER, M. et RENÉ HUGUENIN: Un cas de trophoedème acquis. Bull. Soc. méd. Hôp. Paris **39**, 1192 (1923). — GERLACH, FRIEDRICH: Zur Therapie des angioneurotischen Ödems. Md. Klin. **1923 II**, 1198, 1199. — GOLDSCHLAG, F.: Über eine Kombination von Trophödem Meige mit Melorheostose Léri. Dermat. Wschr. **1929 II**, 1761. — GÓMEZ, F.: Angioneurotisches Ödem im Verlauf der Goldbehandlung. Semana méd. **1930 II**, 1060. — GORDON, ALFRED: Segmental trophic edema of cerebral origin. J. nerv. Dis. **66**, Nr 4, 381—389 (1927). — GRANT, R. T.: On the urticarial reaction and its physiological meaning. Brit. J. Dermat. **38**, Nr 11, 425—430 (1926). — GRIMM: Überempfindlichkeit gegen Kautschuk als Ursache von Urticaria und QUINCKESches Ödem. Bemerkungen zu der Mitteilung von GRETE STERN. Klin. Wschr. **1927 II**, 1479. — GROOT jr., J. DE: Eine eigenartige Lokalisation angioneurotischen Ödems bei der Frau. Nederl. Tijdschr. Verloskde **29**, H. 4, 387—391 (1924).
HACHEZ, EDUARD: Über Epidermolysis bullosa hereditaria dystrophica. Dermat. Z. **37**, 153 (1922). — HAJOS, W.: Vasculäre Überempfindlichkeitskrankheiten der Haut. Klin. Wschr. **1930 II**, 1618. — HEITZ, JEAN et P.-L. VIOLLE: Du temps de résorption de la boule d'oedème intra-dermique dans les troubles locaux de la circulation. C. r. Soc. Biol. Paris **96**, No 16, 1283—1286 (1927). — HLAVÁČEK, VLADIMIR: Familiäres QUINCKE-Ödem des Kehlkopfes. Čas. lék. česk. **1932**, 784—787. — HOFMANN, EDMUND: Über den Erbgang bei Epidermolysis bullosa, hereditaria. Arch. Rassenbiol. **18**, H. 4. 353—368 (1926). — HOKE, EDMUND: Seltene Vorkommnisse im Verlaufe der diagnostischen und therapeutischen Anwendung des Tuberkulins. (Herpes zoster; QUINCKESches Ödem. Periodontitis; Urticaria; Purpura; Polyneuritis; Phrenicusdruckpunkte; anaphylaktischer Shock.) Z. Tbk. **38**, 346—348 (1923). — HRYNIEWIECKI, STANISLAW: Zur Ursache des QUINCKEschen Ödems. Polska Gaz. lek. **2**, Nr 47, 777 (1923).
IVANOFF, S.: Ein Fall von Angioneurose in der Supraorbitalgegend. Klin. Mbl. Augenheilk. **75**, Sept.-Okt.-H., 388—398 (1925).
JANCSÓ, MIKLÓS u. MIKLÓS JANCSÓ jr.: Der angioneurotische Symptomenkomplex infolge Veneninjektionen. Orv. Hetil. (ung.) **1928 II**, 1123—1128. — JAROSCHY, WILHELM: Chronisches Trophödem und Spina bifida occulta. Bruns' Beitr. **152**, 632—644 (1931). — JENNY, ED.: Über eine letal verlaufende Form von Epidermolysis bullosa hereditaria beim Säugling. Z. Kinderheilk. **43**, H. 1/2, 138—148 (1927). — JOLTRAIN, E.: Les urticaires. Paris: G. Doin & Cie. 1930. — JOLTRAIN, E., D. MORAT et JAQUES LEY: Urticaire géante observée chez un morphinomane à chaque tentative de sevage. Presse méd. **35**, No 90, 1361—1363 (1927).
KÄLLMARK, F.: Rezidivierendes flüchtiges Glottisödem (QUINCKE). Hygiea (Stockh.) **86**, H. 22, 801—804 (1924). — KÄMMERER, HUGO: Über allergische Konstitution und primäre spezifische Allergie (Idiosynkrasien, Urticaria, QUINCKESches Ödem etc.). Münch. med. Wschr. **1924 I**, 459—462. — Zur Klinik der allergischen Krankheiten. Med. Klin. **1930 II**, 1175. — KENNEDY, FOSTER: Cerebral symptoms induced by angioneurotic edema. Arch. of Neur. **15**, Nr 1, 28—33 (1926). — KOENIG, PAUL: Ein Fall von QUINCKESchem Ödem des Kehlkopfes mit tödlichem Ausgang. Z. Laryng. usw. **13**, H. 1, 76—82 (1924). — KRIJNEN, I.: Zur Epidermolysis bullosa traumatica hereditaria dystrophica. Arch. f. Dermat. **164**, 61 (1931).
LAIGNEL-LAVASTINE: Syndromes sympathiques sous-cutaneés. Le Scalpel **76**, No 52, 1481—1485 (1923). — LAUBRY, BROSSE, VAN BONGAERT: Oedème angioneurotique et crises solaires. Bull. Soc. méd. Hôp. Paris **47**, 378 (1931). — LAVAL, F. et A. VIÉLA: La localisation laryngée du syndrome de QUINCKE. Otol. internat. **13**, 93 (929). — LEHNER, EMMERICH: Anaphylaktischer Shock, hervorgerufen durch intracutane Aolaninjektion bei einem mit Urticaria behafteten Individuum. Wien. med. Wschr. **1923 II**, 1566—1571. — LEOPOLD, JÉROME and ROGATZ: Unilateral edema. Amer. J. Dis. childr. **39**, 1045 (1930). — LÉRI, A. et NOEL PÉRON: Le „syndrome" trophoedème; trophoedème nerveuse, trophoedème lymphatique. Bull. Soc. méd. Hôp. Paris **39**, 1834 (1924). — LESNÉ et DREYFUS: L'anaphylaxie alimentaire. J. Méd. franç. 15. Jan. **1913**. — LESNÉ et M. LÉVY: Accidents anaphylactiques (maladie de QUINCKE) survenus à la suite d'ingestion de viande crue de cheval. Soc. de Pédiatrie, 8. Juli 1924. — LIEBEN: Über die Ursache des QUINCKEschen Ödems. Dtsch. med. Wschr. **1919 II**, 1919. — LINDBER, KAJ.: Beitrag zur Kenntnis des Purinstoffwechsels, Beobachtungen bei einem Fall von Urticaria mit flüchtigem Ödem. Finska Läk.sällsk. Hdl. **67**, Nr 11, 943—972 (1925). — LOEB, L.: Die Peptonbehandlung

bei allergischen Krankheiten. Fortschr. Ther. **6**, 167 (1930). — LOUSTE et GADAUD: Epidermolyse bulleuse. Bull. Soc. franç. Dermat. **38**, 1141 (1931). — LUNEDEI, A.: A propos. di un caso di edema di QUINCKE con iperemia emicongiungtivale bilat e di un caso di emiurticaria. Riv. otol. ecc. **6**, 289 (1929). MACDONALD, J. u. B. BUENDIA: Die Visceralkrisen der angioneurotischen Ödeme. Siglo méd. **74**, No 3704, 554, 555 (1924). — MACKAY, W.: Peripheral neuritis as a complication of angioneurotic oedema. Description of a case. Lancet **1932 I**, 777, 778. — MACLEOD, I.: A case of aquired epidermolysis bullosa. Brit. J. Dermat. **43**, 420 (1931). — MARCOZZI: Epidermolisi bollosa distrofica con ematoporfinuria ed alteratione endocrinosimpatica. Arch. ital. Dermat. **4**, 555 (1929). — MARIOTTI, E.: Epidermolisi bollosa ered. Riforma med. **1929 II**, 1690. — MARTINICO, GIULIO: Ascaridiasis e sindrome di QUINCKE. Gazz. Osp. **48**, No 24, 556—558 (1927). — MASCHKILLEISSON, L. N.: Beiträge zur Kenntnis der dystrophischen Form der Epidermyolysis bullosa hereditaria. Acta dermato-vener. (Stockh.) **9**, 274—301 (1928). — MATUSIS, I. u. R. ROJTMAN: Zur Frage der Ätiologie des Oedema Quincke. Odessk. med. **3**, 681 (1928). — MAXWELL, L. A. IVAN: Modern views of asthma, hay fever and allied disorders such a Urticaria, angio-neurotic oedema and serum sickness. Med. J. Austral. **2**, Nr 19, 483—491 (1923). — MAY, ETIENNE: Syndrome vaso-moteur intermédiaire à l'érythromélalgie et à la maladie de QUINCKE. Association de tétanie et de rheumatisme chronique. Bull. Soc. méd. Hôp. Paris **40**, No 14, 575—579 (1924). — McGUIRE, JOHNSON and PEARL ZEEBI: Pathogenesis of chronic hereditary edema of extremities (MILROYS disease). J. amer. med. Assoc. **98**, 870—873 (1932). — MELKERSSON, E.: Ein Fall von rezidivierender Facialisparese im Zusammenhang mit angioneurotischem Ödem. Hygiea (Stockh.) **90**, 737—741 (1928). — MELLI, G.: Edema angioneurotico di QUINCKE e trofoedema cronico di Meige. Minerva med. **1930 I**, 723. — MEMMESHEIMER: Trophoedème Meige. Dermat. Z. **55**, 23. — MENAGH, FRANK R.: The etiology and results of treatment in angioneurotic edema and urticaria. J. amer. med. Assoc. **90**, Nr 9, 668—671 (1928). — MICHAIL, D.: Angeborenes angioneurotisches, mit germinativer Displasie und larviertem Hyperthyreoidismus kombiniertes Lidödem. Z. Augenheilk. **73**, 337 (1931). — MILLER, T. u. O. PEPPER: Metabolism studies of angion. edema. Arch. int. Med. **17**, 551 (1917). — MILLET, ROSCOE: Heat sensitivness, angioneurotic edema, purpura and ulcers of the leg following bilateral femoral thrombophlebitis. Med. Clin. N. Amer. **15**, 237 (1931). — MILROY, W. F.: Chronic hereditary edema: MILROYs disease. J. amer. med. Assoc. **91**, 1172—1175 (1928). — MISCH, WALTER: Diagnostik und Therapie der allergischen Erkrankungen. (Asthma, Ekzem, Urticaria, QUINCKEsches Ödem, Migräne.) Dtsch. med. Wschr. **1926 I**, 781—784. — MONIZ, EDGAR: Sur le trophoedème chronique de Meige. Revue neur. **28**, 1086 (1921). — MORAWITZ, P.: Zur Ätiologie und Therapie der angioneurotischen Ödeme (QUINCKE). Fortschr. Ther. **2**, H. 13, 417—420 (1926). — MÜHLPFORDT, H.: Generalisierte Urticaria nach Wespenstich. Dtsch. med. Wschr. **1929 I**, 106. — MÜLLER, H.: Über Epidermolysis bullosa. Z. Kinderheilk. **48**, 339 (1929). — MÜNCH, W.: Das allergische Larynxödem usw. Passow-Schaefers Beitr. **28**, 18 (1930). — MUSSIO-FOURNIER, J. C. et C. SEVANE: Asthme, oedème de QUINCKE et kyste hydatique du foie. Bull. Soc. méd. Hôp. Paris **43**, No 9, 327—329 (1927).

NAPP, V.: Über einen Fall von Epidermolysis bullosa dystrophicans hereditaria tarda Dermat. Z. **59**, 103 (1930). — NEUMANN, ALFRED: Ein Fall von QUINCKEschem Ödem nach Insulin. Wien. med. Wschr. **1928 II**, 1363, 1364. — NOICA, D. et N. PARVULESCO: Un cas d'oedème aigu de la face. Rev. neur. **35 I**, No 5, 686—690 (1928).

OEHME, KURT: Grundzüge der Ödempathogenese mit besonderer Berücksichtigung der neueren Arbeiten dargestellt. Erg. inn. Med. **30**, 1—84 (1926). — OLKON, D. M.: QUINCKES edema and the prostrate gland. Illinois med. J. **54**, 217, 218 (1928).

PANOFSKY u. STAEMMLER: Zur pathologischen Anatomie des QUINCKEschen Ödems. Dermat. Wschr. **1924 I**, 469—481. — PASTEUR, VALLERY-RADOT et V. HEIMANN: Hypersensibilités spécifiques dans les affections cutanées. Paris: Masson & Cie 1930. — PELOQUIN et A. JUNG: Un cas d'oedème d'origine vasomotrice traité par le sympatectomie. Gaz. hôp. **1929 II**, 1267. — PEREIRA, A.: Ein Fall von Trophödem. Siglo méd. **72**, 721 (1923). — PESOPOULOS, SPIRO: Ein Fall von mit hohem Fieber und Hautblutungen einhergehendem QUINCKEschem Ödem. Münch. med. Wschr. **1932 I**, 541, 542. — PHILLIPS, JAMES MCILVAINE and BARROWS WILLIAM MORTON: Heredity of angioneurotic edema based on a review of the literature. Genetics **7**, Nr 6, 573—582 (1922).

RAESCHKE: Bemerkungen zum traumatischen chronischen Ödem. Klin. Wschr. **1927 II**, 1763. — RHEINDORF, GÜNTHER: Über zwei Fälle von Hydrops articulorum intermittens SCHLESINGER. Münch. med. Wschr. **1932 I**, 749, 750. — RICHARDS jr., DICKINSON, W.: Chronic familial edema, affecting all extremities, a variant of MILROYs disease. Med. Clin. N. Amer. **15**, 1369—1382 (1932). — RIECKE: Epidermolysis bullosa. Handbuch der Haut- und Geschlechtskrankheiten. Bd. 7, Teil 2, S. 222. Berlin: Julius Springer 1931. — ROSENTHAL, C.: Klinisch erbbiologischer Beitrag zur Konstitutionspathologie. Gemeinsames Auftreten von rezidivierender familiärer Facialislähmung, angioneurotischem Gesichtsödem und Lingua plicata in Arthritismusfamilien. Z. Neur. **131**, 475 (1931). — ROUSSEL, I.:

Chron. urticaria, a thyro- adrenal syndrom. South. med. J. **22**, 668 (1929). — ROWE, ALLAN W. and FRANCIS H. McCRUDDEN: Metabolism observations in a case of urticaria scripta. Boston med. J. **191**, Nr 2, 60, 61 (1924). — RUHEMANN, ERNST: Beitrag zur Pathologie der angioneurotischen exsudativen Diathese. Z. Neur. **115**, 443—477 (1928).

SÁINZ DE AJA, E. ALVAREZ: Anaphylaxien in Form des QUINCKEschen Ödems nach Medikamenten. Actas dermo-sifiliogr. **15**, No 3, 120—124 (1923). — Chronisches symmetrisches Ödem. Typus Meige. Actas dermo-sifilogr. **20**, No 1, 31—34 (1927). — Urticaria pigmentosa, akutes QUINCKESches Ödem und Neurodermitis geheilt durch Schilddrüseneierstocktherapie. Actas dermo-sifiliogr. **22**, 473 (1930). — SCHAEFER, H.: Generalisierte Urticaria nach Wespenstich. Dtsch. med. Wschr. **1929 II**, 1368. — SCHALIT, A.: Angioneurotische Ödeme im Bereich des Gesichtsschädels, vergesellschaftet mit Hypertrophie der Kaumuskulatur. Z. Stomat. **28**, 637 (1930). — SCHLESINGER, H.: Über den Hydrops articulorum intermittens und seine familiäre Form. Wien. klin. Wschr. **1926 I**, 68. — Neue therapeutische Versuche beim Hydrops artic. intermittens. Wien. klin. Wschr. **1929 I**, 832. — SCHOCH, A.: Beiträge zur Kenntnis der Epidermolysis bullosa hereditaria (KÖBNER). Acta dermatovener. (Stockh.) **9**, 169 (1928). — SCHORER, G.: Das angioneurotische Ödem (QUINCKE) mit ungewöhnlichen Begleiterscheinungen. Schweiz. med. Wschr. **1925 I**, 340—346. — SCHREUS, H.: Wesen und Therapie der Urticaria. Dermatologia (Budapest) **2**, 335 (1928). — SCHUBIGER: Zur Vererbung des angioneurotischen Kehlkopfödems. Ges. schweiz. Hals-, Nasen-Ohrenärzte. Ref. Zbl. Hals- usw. Heilk. **3**. — SCHULTZ, J. H.: Zur Psychologie des angioneurotischen Ödems. Med. Klin. **1926 I**, 576, 577. — SCHULTZER, POUL: Serumkalkbestimmungen bei QUINCKES Ödem. Hosp.tid. (dän.) **68**, Nr 13, 308—310 (1925). — SELLEI, JÓZSEF: Die Heilung der chronischen Urticaria mit Parathyreoideainjektionen. Gyógyászat (ung.) **68**, Nr 21, 484, 485 (1928). — SEQUEIRA, J.: Case of epidermolysis bullosa with epidermal cystes. Proc. roy. Soc. Med. **14**, 19 (1921). — SIEMENS, H. W.: Literarisch-statistische Untersuchungen über die einfache und dystrophische Form der sog. Epidermolysis. Arch. f. Dermat. **143**, 390 (1923). — SIMON, A.: Ein Fall von traumatischem Ödem der Hand. Ärztl. Sachverst.ztg **36**, 227 (1930). — SIMONS, EDWIN: Angioneurotic edema. Minnesota med. **12**, 343 (1929). — SLATMANN, A. F.: Ein Fall von Trophoedema chronicum faciei in seinen Beziehungen zu der Menstruation. Zbl. Gynäk. **51**, Nr 36, 2279—2282 (1927). — SLOBODNIK, M.: Ein seltener Fall von angioneur. Ödem des Halses und des Kopfes. Z. Laryng. usw. **17**, 380 (1929). — SMITH, ABIGAIL ELIOT: Occurence of hypersensitiveness or allergy in five generations of one family. Arch. int. Med. **41**, Nr 4, 472—481 (1928). — SOMALO, MARCOS: Die Behandlung der QUINCKEschen Krankheit. Semana méd. **1929 II**, 987. — SPIEGEL, E. A. u. H. KUBO: Anaphylaxie und Nervensystem. Z. exper. Med. **38**, H. 4/6, 458—477 (1923). — SPITZY, HANS: Periodische angioneurotische Gelenkaffektionen. Erkrkgn Beweggsappar. **1924**, H. 1, 5. — STELWAGON, A.: On diseases of the skin. Philadelphia: Saunders 1916. — STERN, GRETE: Überempfindlichkeit gegen Kautschuk als Ursache von Urticaria und QUINCKEschem Ödem. Klin. Wschr. **1927 I**, 1096, 1097. — STERNBERG, H.: Über klinisch ungeklärte Todesfälle von laryngologischem Interesse. Mschr. Ohrenheilk. **1920**, 673. — STERLING, WLADYSLAW: Die Rolle des angioneurotischen Ödems für die Pathogenese der periodischen Lähmung. Warszaw. Czas. lek. **3**, Nr 3, 122—125 (1926). — STOLZ, CH.: Angioneurotic edema. Urologic Rev. **33**, 232 (1929). — STORM VAN LEEUWEN, W.: Überempfindlichkeitskrankheiten (Asthma bronchiale, Urticaria, Migräne, Epilepsie usw.). Naturwiss. **11**, H. 30, 660—665 (1923). — A possible explanation for certain cases of hypersensitiveness to drugs in men. J. of Pharmacol. **24**, Nr 1, 25—32 (1924). — Etiologie et Therapie de l'asthme et des maladies connexes (Urticaire, oedème de QUINCKE, Migraine etc.). J. Physiol. et Path. gén. **23**, No 1, 57—69 (1925).— Allergische Krankheiten, 2. Aufl. Berlin: Julius Springer 1928. — SUCHER, A.: Über eigenartige Wirkungen von Parathyreoideapräparaten. Wien. klin. Wschr. **1929 II**, 1504. — SUSINI, MIGUEL u. ALFREDO CASAUBON: Chirurgische Resultate beim chronischen Trophoödem (Meige). Rev. Especial. méd. **1**, Nr 3, 474—497 (1926).

TESONE, P.: Angioneurotisches Ödem von Pharynx und Larynx. Rev. Especial. méd. **5**, 1097 (1930). — THOMAS, E.: Un cas de trophoedème causé par le spina bifida occulta. Rev. méd. Suisse rom. **51**, 307 (1931). — TÖRÖK: Handbuch der Haut- und Geschlechtskrankheiten, herausgeg. von J. JADASSOHN, Bd. 6. Berlin: Julius Springer 1928. — TÖRÖK, L. u. E. RAJKA: Beitrag zur Pathogenese der Hyperämie und des Ödems bei der Urticaria und der akuten Entzündung der Haut. Arch. f. Dermat. **147**, H. 3, 559—580 (1924). — Klin. Wschr. **1924 II**, 1539—1540. — TUBETTINI: Maladie de QUINCKE par sensibilisation tardive au pain et aux autres farineux. Soc. Méd. Hôp., 19. Mai 1922.

VALLERY-RADOT, PASTEUR et BLAMOUTIER: Essai de traitement de l'urticaire, de l'oedème de QUINCKE par un extrait splénique de porc. Bull. Soc. méd. Hôp. Paris **46**, 1666 (1930). — Un cas mortel de la maladie de QUINCKE avec crises douloureuses abdominales accompagniés de spasmes vasculaires. Bull. Soc. méd. Hôp. Paris III **47**, 459 (1931). — VAUGHAN, WARREN and E. K. HAWKE: Angioneurotic edema with some unusualmanifestations. J. Allergy **2**, 125 (1931).

WARFIELD, LOUIS M.: Chronic urticaria and angioneurotic edema. Internat, Clin. XLI. s. 4, 99—105 (1931). — WASON, ISABEL M.: Angioneurotic edema. Report of a case with necropsy findings. J. amer. med. Assoc. 86, Nr 18, 1332, 1333 (1926). — WATKINS, R. M.: The practical application of protein sensibilisation. Surg. Clin. N. Amer. 4, Nr 4, 1033—1039 (1924). — WEBER, F. PARKES: A note on the nature of the Milroy-Nonne disease. Brit. J. Childr. Dis. 26, 204 (1929). — Thromboangiitis obliterans of lower limbs with attacks of urticaria and angioneurotic edema. Proc. roy. Soc. Med. 24, 1355 (1931). — WEISS-FLORENTIN, WALTHER: Über einen Fall von Oedema fugax des Larynx und Pharynx. Z. Hals- usw. Heilk. 21, 614—622 (1928). — WIRZ, FRANZ: Die Entstehung der urticariellen Quaddeln und ihre Beziehungen zum Gefäßsystem. Arch. f. Dermat. 146, H. 2, 153—228 (1924). — Elephantiasis. Handbuch der Haut- und Geschlechtskrankheiten, Bd. 8, Teil 2, S. 924. 1931. — WISE: Epidermolysis bullosa acquisita. Arch. of Dermat. 3, 92 (1921).

Nachtrag.

RAYNAUDsche Krankheit.

ALLEN, EDGAR and GEORGE BROWN: RAYNAUD's disease affecting men. Ann. int. Med. 5, 1384—1386 (1932). — RAYNAUD's disease. A clinical study of one hundred and forty-seven cases. J. amer. med. Assoc. 99, 1472—1478 (1932). — RAYNAUD's disease: A critical review of minimal requisites for diagnosis. Amer. J. med. Sci. 183, 187—200 (1932).

BENATT, A. u. L. HÖNIGHAUS: Der Einfluß natürlicher kohlensaurer Soolbäder auf die subpapillären Venenplexus der Haut. Z. klin. Med. 126, 202—229 (1933).

CRAIG, MC K., WINCHELL and J. W. KERNOHAN: The surgical removal and histological studies of sympathetic ganglia in RAYNAUD's disease etc. Surg. etc. 56, 767—778 (1933).

FREY, E. K.: Über ein neues inneres Sekret des Pankreas, das Kreislaufshormon Kallikrein, und seine therapeutische Bedeutung. Dtsch. Z. Chir. 233, 481—516 (1931).

GAGEL, O. u. J. W. WATTS: Zur Pathogenese der RAYNAUDschen Gangrän. Z. klin. Med. 122, 110—117 (1932). — GALLOIS, J. et D. ROUTIER: Un cas de maladie de RAYNAUD avec périartérite rétinienne. Bull. Soc. Ophtalm. Paris 1, 32—34 (1934).

JASIEŃSKI, J.: Morbus RAYNAUD, operativ nach der Methode LERICHES geheilt. Polska Gaz. lek. 12, 774—776 (1933).

LANDAU, A. et R. HERMAN: Acrocyanose chronique compliqué d'un syndrome de maladie de RAYNAUD. Arch. Mal. Coeur. 26, 560—578 (1933). — LERICHE, R. et R. FONTAINE: Résultats du traitement chirurgical de la maladie de RAYNAUD. Presse méd. 1933 I, 233—236. Sur la nature de la maladie de RAYNAUD. Presse méd. 1932 II, 1921—1925. — Troubles trophiques et nécrotiques singuliers des doigts comme premiers signes d'une leucémie. Faux syndrome de RAYNAUD. Presse méd. 1932 II, 1941—1942.

MAYO, W. J. and A. W. ADSON: RAYNAUD's disease, thrombo-angitis obliterans and scleroderma etc. Ann. Surg. 96, 771—786 (1932). — MIRENGHI, U.: Ricerche sulla vasoregolazione cutanea nel morbo di RAYNAUD. Il Dermosifilogr. 7, 225—236 (1932). — MUCHA, V.: Die RAYNAUDsche Krankheit. Handbuch der Haut- und Geschlechtskrankheiten. Berlin: Julius Springer 1928.

PARISOT et CORNIL: Troubles vaso-moteurs. Nouv. Traité Méd. 21 (1927).

RICHET fils, CH., MARCEL SOURDEL et A. MEYER-HEINE: Syndrome de RAYNAUD consécutif à une hématémèse. Bull. Soc. méd. Hôp. Paris III. s. 50, 993—997 (1934). — ROGER, H., SEDAN, ARNAUD et AYMES: Spasmes vasculaires rétiniens intenses chez un angio-spasmodique (syndrome de RAYNAUD et spasmes sylviens) mort subite. Rev. d'Otol. etc. 11, 210—212 (1933).

SCHWARZKOPF, ARTHUR: Die Behandlung RAYNAUDscher Krankheit mit dem gefäßerweiternden Hormon Padutin. Ther. Gegenw. 72, 382—383 (1931). — STOLKIND, E.: RAYNAUD's disease, sclerodermia, telangiectases, paroxysmal eye troubles and paralysis agitans. Proc. roy. Soc. Med. 25, 399—400 (1932).

Akroasphyxia chronica.

ANDRÉ-THOMAS: Hémiacrocyanose. Revue neur. 40 I, 685—692 (1933).

BARBIER: Discussion sur les acrocyanoses. C. r. Congr. franç. Méd. 1933, 117—120.

COMEL, M.: Sulle sindromi ischemiche e asfittiche delle estremità Acrocianosi e acrorigosi. Giorn. ital. Dermat. 73, 1595—1611 (1932).

DE JONG: Le syndrome vasc. dans la démence précoce. Thèse de Paris 1931. — DUMAS, A.: Rôle du choc hémoclasique dans les crises syncopales ou gestives des extrémités. C. r. Congr. franç. Méd. 1933, 134—140.

FRENKEL-TISSOT: Arch. Rassenbiol. 15, 337.

GLÉNARD, ROGER: Un cas d'acrocyanose avec ptoses viscérales l'origine hypophysaire probable. C. r. franç. Méd. 1933, 174—177.

JACQUELIN, A. et J. BERTRAND: Acrocyanose et asthme. C. r. Congr. franç. Méd. **1933**, 155—159. — JACQUELIN, ANDRÉ et H. BONNET: Acrocyanose et terrain morphologique. C. r. Congr. franç. Méd. **1933**, 152—154. — JOLTRAIN, E.: Hémoclasie et troubles périphériques. C. r. Congr. franç. Méd. **1933**, 141—149.
LAIGNEL-LAVASTINE: Cuti-réaction à l'histamine dans l'acrocyanose. C. r. Congr. franç. Méd. **1933**, 150—151. — LEVY-FRANKEL et JUSTER: Le rôle du syst. endocrin. dans la pathol. de certains tr. trophiques cutanés. Presse méd., 28. Juli **1893**.
MARANON, G.: Acrocyanose et glandes génitales. C. r. franç. Méd. **1933**, 160—173. — MARTINET: Sur l'hyposphyxie. Presse méd. **1912**. — MAY, ÉTIENNE, J. LAGADE et F. LAYANI: Étude interférométrique de l'acrocyanose essentielle. C. r. Soc. Biol. Paris **110**, 1185—1186 (1932).
ROCH: Les lois de l'hydraulique et les troubles circulatoires des extrémités. C. r. Congr. franç. Méd. **1933**, 120—121. — ROUSSY-MOSINGER: À propos des acrocyanoses. C. r. Congr. franç. Méd. **1933**, 109—116.
STRANDBERG, J.: Haut und innere Sekretion. Handbuch der Haut- und Geschlechtskrankheiten. Berlin: Julius Springer 1929.
VILLARET, MAURICE, L. JUSTIN-BESANÇON et RENÉ CACHERA: Contribution à l'étude des troubles vasculaires périphériques au cours des perturbations de la sécrétion ovarienne. Nutrition (Paris) **2**, 281—287 (1932). — VINCENT et CURTIS: Effets du I. post Hypo. s. circulat. Endocrinol., Nov. **1926**.
ZIMMERN, A. et R. BRUNET: Agents physiques dans les acrocyanoses. C. r. Congr. franç. Méd. **1933**, 178—181.

Erythromelalgie.

BROWN, GEORGE E.: Erythromelalgia and other disturbances of the extremities etc. Amer. J. med. Sci. **183**, 468—485 (1932).
CEDERBERG †, ARMAS: Über die Erythromelalgie und ihr Verhältnis zur Bothriocephalusinfektion. Duodecim (Helsingfors) **49**, 1011—1020 (1933).
HOSHINA, K.: Two cases of erythromelalgia. Acta dermat. (Kioto) **22**, 153 (1933).
JSHIDA, IWAO: Erythromelalgie bei einem 10jährigen Mädchen mit Sympathicotonie. Orient. J. Dis. Infants **10**, 39—40 (1931).
KAKU, T.: Zur Behandlung der Erythromelalgie mit Eigenblutinjektionen. Arch. jap. Chir. **10**, 916—933 (1933).
LEWIS, THOMAS: Clinical observations and experiments relating to burning pain in the extremities, and so-called „erythromelalgia" in particular. Clin. Sci. **1**, 175—211 (1933).
SELTER, PAUL: Von „Akrodynie" bis „Encephalitis vegetativa", die Geschichte einer Krankheit. Erg. inn. Med. **46**, 315—349 (1934).
WEBER, F. PARKES: Erythromelalgia-like symptoms with high blood pressure. Proc. roy. Soc. Med. **25**, 403 (1932).

Akroparästhesien.

JELLIFFE, SMITH ELY: Acroparesthesia and Quinidine. J. nerv. Dis. **79**, 631—651 (1934).
SAMAJA, RUBINO: Su di un caso di acroparestecia. Policlinico, sez. prat. 1934, 1321—24.
URECHIA, C. I.-RETEZEANU: Le calcium sanguin dans un cas d'acroparesthésie. Arch. internat. Neur. **52 I**, 329—331 (1933).

Multiple neurotische Hautgangrän.

BODE, H.-G.: Ein Beitrag zur Kenntnis der multiplen (neurotischen) Hautgangrän. Arch. f. Dermat. **168**, 274—295 (1933).
LÖHE u. H. ROSENFELD: Multiple Hautgangrän bei Periarteriitis nodosa. Ein Beitrag zur Kenntnis der multiplen neurotischen Hautgangrän und der Hautveränderungen bei Periarteriitis nodosa. Dermat. Z. **61**, 299—320 (1931).
VERCELLINO, LUIGI: Su particolari manifestazioni cutanee in soggetto isterico. Il Dermosifilogr. **7**, 77—87 (1932).

Sklerodermie.

AJMAR, FRANCO: Asportazione dei gangli stellato ed intermedio del simpatico cervicale di destra in un caso di sclerodermia. Arch. Soc. ital. Chir. **1933**, 992—997. — ANSELMINO, KARL: Über Sklerodermie und Schwangerschaft. Z. Geburtsh. **103**, 60—66 (1932).
BARBER, H. W.: Scleroderma with atrophy of the subcutaneous tissue and muscle. Proc. roy. Soc. Med. **25**, 1545—1546 (1932). — BARSONY, TH.: Antagonismus zwischen den Krankheitszeichen bei Akromegalie und jenen bei Akromikrie (Sklerodaktylie). Wien. klin. Wschr. **1933** I, 750. — BASCH, G., R. LEIBOVICI, A. DURUPT, M. BASCH: Sclérodermie avec concrétions calcaires associée à une atrophie cutanée. Bull. Soc. Méd. Paris, III. s. **50**, 516—521 (1934). — BERNUTH, F. v.: Über Sklerodermie, Osteopoikilie und Kalkgicht

im Kindesalter. Z. Kinderheilk. **54**, 103, 116 (1932). — BOHN-NAGEOTTE: Nouveaux cas d'acrodermatite atrophiante avec sclérodermie. Bull. Soc. franç. Dermat. **40**, No 7, 1309—1312 (1933). — BREITMANN, M.: Über die Behandlung der Hautkrankheiten, besonders der Sklerodermie, mit Joddämpfen. Dermat. Wschr. **1932 II**, 1678—1680. — BROCK, G.: Dermatomyositis and diffuse scleroderma. Arch. of Dermat. **30**, 227—240 (1934). COMEL, M.: Studi clinici sugli stati sclerodermici. Giorn. ital. Dermat. **75**, 855—902 (1934). — CORDIVIOLA, LUIS: Ödematöse Sklerodermie HARDY. Rev. argent. Dermat. **15**, 49—60 (1931). — COURTOIS, A. et Y. ANDRÉ: Sclérodermie généralisée au cours d'un syndrome de démence précoce. Ann. méd.-psychol. **91 II**, 47—51 (1933). — CRAIG, WINCHELL McK. and JAMES W. KERNOHAN: The surgical removal and histological studies of sympathetic ganglia in RAYNAUD's disease and scleroderma. Surg. etc. **56**, 767—778 (1933).

DUVOIR, L. et J. SAINTON: Sclérodermie généralisée à évolution ascendente subaiguë. Bull. Soc. franç. Dermat. **41**, No 6, 919—922 (1934).

EDEL, K.: Betrachtungen über die Pathogenese der Sklerodermie. Nederl. Tijdschr. Geneesk. **1933**, 2817—2822. — EPSTEIN, STEFAN: Zur Behandlung von Sklerodermie und Akrodermatitis atrophicans mit Thorium X. Arch. f. Dermat. **167**, 533—542 (1933).

FESSLER, A. u. R. POHL: Stenosierender Prozeß des Oesophagus bei Sklerodermie. Dermat. Z. **63**, 164—169 (1932). — FLARER, F.: Le acrodermatosi in relazine coi disturbi circulatori. Giorn. ital. Dermat. **73**, 542, 636 (1932). — FOLLMANN, JENÖ u. BELA BALLÓ: Beiträge zu den klinischen Untersuchungen und zur pathologischen Histologie der endokrinen Drüsen bei Sklerodermie. Dermat. Wschr. **1933 II**, 1779—1788.

GADRIN, J.: Sclérodermie acrostatique et calcémie. Bull. Soc. franç. Dermat. **39**, 741—742 (1932). — GOUGEROT: Sclérodermies atypiques. Bull. Soc. franç. Dermat. **39**, No 9, 1667—1669 (1932). — GRAY, A. M. H.: Scleroderma in a tuberculous subject. Proc. roy. Soc. Med. **25**, 667—668 (1933). — GUARINI, CARLO: L'indagine radiologica dello scheletro degli sclerodermici. Arch. di Radiol. **9**, 7—56 (1933).

HALBERTSMA, TJ.: Über Sklerödem, Sclerema adiposum und diffuse Sklerodermie. Mschr. Kindergeneesk. **3**, 263—276 (1934). — HERCOG, PAUL: Die Behandlung der Sklerodermie mit Pilocarpin. Wien. klin. Wschr. **1933 II**, 1041.

KURÉ, KEN, KENJI YAMAGATA u. YOSHITOMO KANKO: Pathogenese der Sklerodermie und Spinalparasympathicus. Klin. Wschr. **1932 II**, 1415—1418.

LAEDERICH, L., H. MAMOU et H. BEAUCHESNE: Sclérodermie bronzée cachectisante. Bull. Soc. méd. Hôp. Paris **48**, 1652—1656 (1932). — LERICHE, R. et ADOLPHE JUNG: Le chlorure d'ammonium dans la thérapeutique de la sclérodermie. Presse méd. **1933 II**, 1041. — LIVIERATOS, S. G. u. P. A. TSELIOS: Ein Fall von universeller Sklerodermie und Sklerodaktylie. Wien. klin. Wschr. **1932 II**, 1440, 1442.

MATHIEU, PAUL, MARCEL PINARD et A. FIEHRER: Sclérodermie avec concrétions calcaires sous-cutanées etc. Bull. méd. Paris, III. s. **48**, 1644—1646 (1932). — MATRAS, A.: Über Veränderungen in der Muskulatur bei diffuser Sklerodermie der oberen Extremität Dermat. Wschr. **1932 I**, 829—834. — MAURIAC, PIERRE, G. PETGES et P. BROUSTET: Syndrome complexe associé de sclérodermie progr., acrocyanose, syndrome de RAYNAUD etc. C. r. Congr. franç. Méd. **1933**, 128—133. — MAYO, WILLIAM J. and ALFRED WADSON: RAYNAUD's disease, thromboangiitis obliterans ans scleroderma. Ann. Surg. **96**, 771—786 (1932). — MICHAELIS, O.: Beiträge zur Sklerodermie und Akrosklerose. Münch. med. Wschr. **1932 II**, 2121. — MILBRADT, W.: Atypische diffuse Sklerodermie mit OSLERschem Syndrom und Laberstörung. Dermat. Wschr. **1934 II**, 973—979. — MOULONGUET, P.: Sclérodermie avec concrétions calcaires associée à un adénome parathyroidien. Bull. Soc. natur. Chir. Paris **57**, 1529—1531 (1931).

PASINI, A.: Sclerodermia e metabolismo del calcio. Giorn. ital. Dermat. **75**, 195—202 (1934). — PAUTRIER, L. M.: Sclérodermies chéloides et calcémie. Presse méd. **1933 I**, 345—347. — De la sclérodermie à la dermatite chronique atrophiante. Presse méd. **1933 II**, 1706—1707. — PAUTRIER, L.-M. et LEPINAY: Sclérodermie en plaques et vitiligo. Bull. Soc. franç. Dermat. **39**, No 9, 1466—1469 (1932). — PERUTZ, A.: Zur Frage der Calcinosis bei Sklerodermie. Dermat. Wschr. **1932 I**, 189—193. — PRAKKEN, J. R.: Etwas über die Bedeutung des Calciums bei der Sklerodermie. Nederl. Tijdschr. Geneesk. **1932**, 2617—2623.

RENNEDY, ROGER: Calcinosis and scleroderma. J. of Pediatr. **1**, 667—673 (1932). — ROEDERER, CARLE et JEAN HALLÉ: Myosclérose généralisée. Bull. Soc. Pédiatr. Paris. **31**, 163—169 (1933).

SCARPA, ANGELO: Un caso di sclerodermia emilaterale. Arch. ital. Dermat. **8**, 385—414 (1932). — SCHÖNGUT, ERNÖ: Hormonale Beeinflussung und neues Heilverfahren bei Sklerodermie etc. Gyógyászat (ung.) **1931 II**, 762—763. — SCOLARI, F.: La sclerodattilia e la sclerodermia diffusa con speciale riguardo alle turbe vasomotorie. Giorn. ital. Dermat. **72**, 1477—1524 (1931). — La sclerodattilia e la sclerodermia con speciale riguardo alle turbe vasomotorie. Giorn. ital. Dermat. **73**, 669—688 (1932). — SELLEI, J.: Pankreastherapie bei Sklerodermie. Orv. Hetil. (ung.) **1931 I**, 13. — Zur Klinik und Therapie der

Sklerodaktylie. Dermat. Z. **64**, 138—146 (1932). — Beiträge zur Sklerodermie und Akrosklerose. Münch. med. Wschr. **1932** II, 1625—1629. — Akrosklerosis. Zbl. Hautkrkh. **41**, 296 (1932). — SELLEI, JOSEF: Zur Akrosklerose. Wien. klin. Wschr. **1933** II, 1359. — Beiträge zur Sklerodermie und Akrosklerose. Münch. med. Wschr. **1933** I, 314—315. — Sklerodermie und Schleimhaut. Arch. f. Dermat. **170**, 464—466 (1934). — SELYE, H.: Die Sklerodermie und ihre Entstehungsweise. Virchows Arch. **286**, 91—115 (1932). — A condition simulating human scleroderma in rats injected with parathyroid hormone. J. amer. med. Assoc. **99**, 108 (1932). — SÉZARY, A. et A. HOROWITZ: Le traitement de la sclérodermie par l'hémocrinothérapie. ovarienne. Bull. Soc. franç. Dermat. **41**, No 1, 68—71 (1934). — SIEMENS, H. W.: Die Vererbung in der Ätiologie der Hautkrankheiten. Handbuch der Haut- und Geschlechtskrankheiten. Berlin: Julius Springer 1929. — STEINER, KARL: Ein rudimentärer Fall von Sklerodermie und Kalkgicht. Arch. f. Dermat. **169**, 142—148 (1933). — STOLKIND, E.: RAYNAUD's disease, sclerodermia, telangiectases etc. Proc. roy. Soc. Med. **25**, 399—400 (1932).

TOURAINE, A., CH. GUILLAUMIN et W. AUBRUN: Sclérodermie avec concretions calcaires. Bul.. Soc. franç. Dermat. **41**, No 4, 662—669 (1934). — TOURAINE et RIMÉ: Vitiligo et sclérodermie en bandes chez une hérédo-syphilitique. Bull. Soc. franç. Dermat. **1932**, No 5, 567—570.

WEBER, F. PARKES and O. BODE: Sclerodermia and myasthenia gravis. Proc. roy. Soc. Med. **25**, 966 (1932). — WEILL, JEAN et ROGER MAIRE: Rétraction de l'aponévrose palmaire et sclérodermie. Paris méd. **1934** I, 263—268. — WEISSENBACH, R. J., G. BASCH et M. BASCH: Essai critique sur la pathogénie des concrétions calcaires des sclérodermies. Ann. Méd. **1932**, 504—529. — Les formes cliniques du syndrome de THIBIERGE-WEISSENBACH: Concrétions calcaires des sclérodermies. Ann. de Dermat. **4**, 1—27, 125—149 (1933). — WEISSENBACH, R. I., I. GATELLIER et A. DURUPT: Sclérodermie progressive et parathyroidectomie. Bull. Soc. franç. Dermat. **40**, No 8, 1439—1448 (1933).

YAMAGATA, KENJI: Über die Pathogenese der Sklerodermie und ihre Pilocarpinbehandlung. Mitt. med. Ges. Tokyo **46**, 1535—1575 (1932).

Hemiatrophia faciei.

ARCHAMBAULT, LA SALLE and NELSON K. FROMM: Progressive facial hemiatrophy. Arch. of Neur. **27**, 529—584 (1932).

BOE, HILMAR: Ein Fall von Hemiatrophia faciei progressiva mit einer Expansionsprothese in der Mundhöhle behandelt. Med. Rev. **50**, 212 (1933). — A case of hemiatrophia facialis progressiva treated with expansion Prothesis of the mouth. Acta psychiatr. (Københ.) **9**, 1—27 (1934). — BRÜCKNER, STAN. u. ERICH OBSTÄNDER: Über einen Fall von sogenannter Hemiatrophia faciei. Psychiatr.-neur. Wschr. **1932** I, 448—451.

CAMPBELL, D.: Ein Fall von Hemihypertrophie des Gesichts. Fortschr. Röntgenstr. **47**, 198—202 (1933). — CHASANOW, M.: Beiträge zur Ätiologie der Hemiatrophie des Gesichts. Z. Neur. **140**, 473—485 (1932).

ESAU: Die angeborene Hemihypertrophia des Körpers. Med. Klin. **1931** II, 1861—1863.

FABER, KNUD: Hemiatropia faciei. Vitiligo-Myxoedema. Ugeskr. Laeg. (dän.) **1933**, 1207—1211. — Facial hemiatrophy-vitiligo-Myxoedema. Acta med. scand. (Stockh.) **82**, 419—432 (1934). — FLINT, GORDON: Case of partial atrophy of right side of face. Trans. ophthalm. Soc. U. Kingd. **52**, 308—309 (1933).

GILLIES, H.: Hemiatrophy of the face (unilateral lipodystrophy). Proc. roy. Soc. Med. **27**, 642—643 (1934). — GUILLAIN, GEORGES et P. R. BIZE: Hémihypertrophie du corps, de type congénital, total et pur, associée à un dolichocôlon. Revue neur. **41**, 76—84 (1934).

LARSEN, ERIK: Examination of the sympathetic innervation of a case of hemihypertrophy. Acta psychiatr. (Københ.) **7**, 339—342 (1932).

MOLLARET, PIERRE: Contribution à l'étude clinique et étiologique de l'hémiatrophie faciale progressive. Revue neur. **39** II, 463, 474 (1932).

PICK, WILLY: Sclérodermie en coup de sabre mit osteoporotischer Zone im Stirnbein oder Hemiatrophia faciei? Arch. f. Dermat. **167**, 543—549 (1933).

SHOJI, Y.: Eine unbemerkte halbseitige Gesichtshypertrophie. Acta Soc. ophthalm. jap. **37**, 1312—1316 (1933). — SLOANE, P.: Facial hemiatrophy. Arch. of Neur. **30**, 693—694 (1933). — SORSBY, A. and MARCELLI SHAW: The refraction in cases of congenital torticollis associated with hemiatrophy of the face. Brit. J. Ophthalm. **16**, 222—225 (1932). — STERNBERG: Über eine besondere Form der Hemiatrophia faciei. Arch. f. Psychiatr. **99**, 815—816 (1933). — STIEF, A.: Über einen Fall von Hemiatrophie des Gesichts mit Sektionsbefund. Z. Neur. **147**, 573—593 (1933). — STIEFLER, GEORG: Über die Hemiatrophia faciei progressiva bilateralis. Jb. Psychiatr. **51**, 277—292 (1934).

TRUFFI, G.: Emiatrofia facciale sinistra con sclerodermia circoscritta. Il Dermosifilogr. **8**, 90—99 (1933).

Vassilevskij, M.: Ein Fall von progressiver Hemiatrophie des Gesichts, Schultergürtels und der Hand. Sovet. Nevropat. **2**, H. 7, 78 (1933). — Vinar, Josef: Hemiatropia faciei. Čas. lék. česk. **1934**, 865—867.
Wakefield, E. G. and Edgar A. Hines jr.: Congenital hemihypertrophy. Amer. J. med. Sci. **185**, 493—500 (1933).
Zass, R.: Exophthalmus und Enophthalmus alternans im Zusammenhang mit Morbus Basedowii und Hemiatrophia sinistra. Sovet. Vestn. Oftalm. **4**, 480—482 (1934).

Angioneurotisches Ödem.

Abbott, W.: Periodic edema of hand with seven day cycle. J. amer. med. Assoc. **100**, 1328—1329 (1933). — Amyot, Roma: Trophoedème de Meige ou maladie de Milroy. Un. méd. Canada. **62**, 911—919 (1933). — Assmann: Angioneurotische exsudative Diathese. Dtsch. med. Wschr. **1932 II**, 1275—1279.
Bazan, F. u. Herta Otte: Chronisches Trophödem nach Meige. Arch. argent. Pediatr. **4**, 727—737 (1933). — Becker, S.: Dermatoses associated with neurocirculatory instability. Arch. of Dermat. **25**, 655—682 (1932). — Bogaert, Ludo van: Symptômes oculaires et cérébello-vestibulaires dans l'oedème angioneurotique de Quincke. Rev. d'Otol. etc. **12**, 321—327 (1934). — Boucher, Romeo: Un cas de maladie de Milroy. Un. méd. Canada **61**, 1287—1293 (1932). — Braeucker, W.: Klinische Untersuchungen über den Kreislauf beim traumatischen Ödem der Extremitäten. Z. Kreislaufforsch. **24**, 601—612 (1932).
Carnevalis: Idrope intermittente del ginocchio. Chir. Org. Movim. **20**, 233—239 (1934). — Časovnikov, R.: Ein Fall von chronisch-neuropathischem Gesichtsödem als Komplikation des Quinckeschen Ödems. Trudy tomsk. med. Inst. **1**, 61—68 (1931). — Cerutti, P.: Contributo allo studio dell' epidermolisi bollosa. Giorn. ital. Dermat. **74**, 335—375 (1933). — Cole, Julia and H.-M. Korns: Visceral manifestations of angioneurotic oedema. J. Allergy **5**, 347—356 (1934). — Cornil, M.: Deux cas d'oedèmes des membres inférieurs. Ann. Méd. phys. et physiobiol. **25**, 1—3 (1932). — Curschmann, H.: Über klimakterisches Ödem. Med. Klin. **1933 II**, 1270—1271.
Desaux, A. et Ch. O. Guillaumin: Recherches interférométriques faites avec un opzime parathyroidien au cours de deux cas d'oedème de Quincke. Bull. Soc. franç. Dermat. **40**, 1359—1362 (1933). — Dittrich: Quinckesches Ödem mit annulärem Exanthem. Zbl. Hautkrkh. **41**, 666 (1932). — Dorst, Stanley F. and Ethel Hopphan: Angioneurotic edema. J. Labor. a. clin. Med. **18**, 7—11 (1932). — Driak, F.: Ein Fall von persistierendem Ödem der Oberlippe. Z. Stomat. **29**, 1241—1243 (1931).
Ellis, R.: Two cases of congenital oedema. Proc. roy. Soc. Med. **25**, 956—957 (1932). — Enderle, Erna Stantien: Persistent angioneurotic edema. J. Allergy **3**, 583—585 (1932).
Faber, H. and H. Lusignan: Hereditary elephantiasis etc. Amer. J. Dis. Childr. **46**, 816—825 (1933). — Fournier, J. C. Mussio et A. Garra: Troubles neurologiques produits par l'oedème de Quincke. Revue neur. **39 I**, 1444—1447 (1932). — Frank, Philip: A case of giant urticaria cured by tonsillectomy. Urologic Rev. **37**, 185—186 (1933).
Gay, Prieto J.: Zur Pathogenese der Epidermolysis bullosa dystrophica. Actas dermosifiliogr. **24**, 178—189 (1931). — Gjessing, H. Chr.: Der angioneurotische Symptomenkomplex während der Arsenobenzolbehandlung. Acta dermato-vener. (Stockh.) **15**, 59—68 (1934).
Herrmann: Zur Behandlung des Quinckeschen Kehlkopfödems. Arch. Ohr. usw. Heilk. **134**, 173—176 (1933). — Heuyer: Troubles trophiques. Nouv. Traité Méd. **21** (1927). — Hlváček, V.: Familiäres Quincke-Ödem des Kehlkopf. Čas. lék. česk. **1932**, 784—787. — Horsch, K.: Über eine elephantiastische Form von neuropathischem Ödem. Brun's Beitr. **159**, 515—526 (1934).
Jaroschy, W.: Chronisches Trophoedem und Spina bifida occulta. Bruns' Beitr. **152**, 632—644 (1931). — Joltrain: A propos des oedèmes circonscrits. Maladie de Quincke. Bull. Acad. Méd. Belg., V. s. **13**, 154—165 (1933).
Kretz, J.: Zur Behandlung vasoneurotischer Ödeme mit Parathyreoidextrakt. Wien. med. Wschr. **1932 I**, 1256—1258.
Lennon, W.: Angioneurotic oedema. Lancet **1933 II**, 739—740. — Leven: Zur Kenntnis des Trophoedem Meige-Milroy. Dermat. Wschr. **1931 I**, 777—783. — Lovén, K.: Zwei Fälle von Hydrops intermittens genus. Acta. chir. scand. (Stockh.) **73**, 181—202 (1933).
Mackay, W.: Peripheral neuritis as a complication of angioneurotic oedema. Lancet **1932 I**, 777—778. — McGuire, Johnson and Pearl Zeek: Pathogenesis of chronic hereditary edema of extremities. J. amer. med. Assoc. **98**, 870—873 (1932). — Meige, H.: Complément à l'histoire clinique d'une famille atteinte de trophoedème héréditaire. Revue neur. **40 I**, 70—71 (1933). — Milian, G.: Maladie de Quincke et syphilis. Rev. franç. Dermat. **10**, 157 (1934). — Myers, C.: Milroy's disease. Proc. roy. Soc. Med. **25**, 795—796 (1932).

Nouhuys, F. van: Ein Fall von Quinckeschem Ödem. Nederl. Tijdschr. Geneesk. **1934**, 659—661. — Novoa, Santos R.: Ein seltener Fall von ,,Hydrops abdominalis intermittens" mit gleichzeitigem universellem neurotischem Ödem. Zbl. inn. Med. **1932**, 1271—1276.

Oddy, H.: Oedema, Milroy type. Proc. roy. Soc. Med. **27**, 640—641 (1934). — Oliaro, Tomaso: Über cerebrale Symptome bei Quinckeschem angioneurotischem Ödem. Klin. Wschr. **1933 II**, 1185—1186.

Pesopoulos, Spiro: Ein Fall von mit hohem Fieber und Hautblutungen einhergehendem Quinckeschem Ödem. Münch. med. Wschr. **1932 I**, 541—542. — Petráček, E.: Meige-Milroysche Krankheit. Česká Dermat. **12**, 285—290 (1931). — Pierini, L.: Epidermolysis bullosa dystrophica. Rev. argent. Dermat. **15**, 20—52 (1932). — Polano, M. K.: Der Kochsalzstoffwechsel bei Kranken mit Epidermolysis bullosa dystrophica. Nederl. Tijdschr. Geneesk. **1932**, 4207—4210.

Rheindorf, G.: Über zwei Fälle von Hydrops articulorum intermittens. Münch. med. Wschr. **1932 I**, 749—750. — Richards jr., W. Dickinson: Chronic familial edema affecting all extremities. Med. Clin. N. Amer. **15**, 1369—1382 (1932). — Rubaltelli, E.: Edema angioneurotico di Quincke da sostanze medicamentose. Valsalva **9**, 158—169 (1933).

Scarpa, A.: Sopra un caso di epidermolisi bollosa distrofica. Giorn. ital. Dermat. **74**, 67—83 (1933). — Sellei, J.: Die Behandlung der chronischen alimentären Urticaria, des Quinckeschen Ödems in der täglichen Praxis. Dermat. Wschr. **1931 II**, 1963—1967. — Sieben, H.: Bakterielle Toxine als ätiologisches Moment des angioneurotischen Ödems. Med. Klin. **1933 I**, 678—679. — Skaletz, H.: Ein Fall von Epidermolysis bullosa hereditaria. Jb. Kinderheilk. **139**, 193—199 (1933).

Vernieuwe: Les oedèmes angio-neurotiques. Bull. Acad. Méd. Belg., V. s. **13**, 141—153 (1933). — Rev. de Laryng. etc. **54**, 903—916 (1933). — Voelcker, F.: Quinckesches Ödem, durch Harnstauung verursacht. Dtsch. Z. Chir. **234**, 815—816 (1931). — Vogl, A.: Zur Frage der Zusammenhänge zwischen Hydrops articulorum intermittens und Ovarialfunktion. Wien. klin. Wschr. **1932 II**, 1344—1346.

Warfield, L.: Chronic urticaria and angioneurotic edema. Internat. Clin., IV. s. **41**, 99—105 (1931). — Weber, F. Parkes: Orthostatic oedema of the dorsum of both feet of the Nonne and Milroy type. Proc. roy. Soc. Med. **25**, 801 (1932). — Persistent oedema of both legs. Proc. roy. Soc. Med. **26**, 51 (1932). — Weber, Parkes: Persistent oedema of the right lower limb. Proc. roy. Soc. Med. **26**, 53—54 (1932). — Weber, Parkes and E. Schwarz: Erythroderma with oedema. Brit. J. Dermat. **44**, 187—192 (1932). — Welti, Max: Dermatite bulleuse chez un nevropathe. Ann. de Dermat. **3**, 40—49 (1932).

Zoon, J. u. C. P. Penning: Zur Epidermolysis bullosa hereditaria dystrophica. Dermat. Z. **67**, 244—252 (1933).

Die neurasthenische Reaktion.

Von ERNST BRAUN-Kiel.

Mit 2 Abbildungen.

I. Pathogenese.

Einleitung. Als der Amerikaner BEARD im Jahre 1880 die Nervenschwäche als typische amerikanische Erkrankung beschrieb, begann er damit die Entwicklung des modernen Neurastheniebegriffs. Neurasthenie, meinte BEARD, sei die Folge der überraschend schnell entwickelten Zivilisation, wie sie das Charakteristikum des damaligen Amerika war, und ihre Grundlage eine Unterernährung des Nervengewebes, dessen Funktionskraft den ungeheuer gestiegenen Anforderungen nicht mehr gewachsen sei und in zunehmendem Maße der Erschöpfung anheimfalle. Diese Verarmung an Nervenkraft äußere sich in Reflexreizungen, an denen vornehmlich Sympathicus und Vasomotoren beteiligt seien, Symptomen rein funktioneller Natur also, deren Abgrenzung von organisch bedingten Schädigungen BEARD viel Mühe zuwandte.

Wenn BEARD so den größten Wert auf die *exogene* Entstehung der Neurasthenie legte und ihrer konstitutionellen Unterlegung nur gelegentlich Erwähnung tat, betonte bald nach ihm MÖBIUS um so schärfer die ererbte Grundlage dessen, was er die „Nervosität" nannte und mit übergroßer Reizbarkeit und Schwäche des Nervensystems umschrieb. Exogene Schädigungen waren nach MÖBIUS als Ursache nervöser Störungen nur insoweit wirksam, als ihre Stärke in besonders ungünstigem Verhältnis zur individuell verschiedenen angeborenen nervösen Widerstandskraft stand. Es mochte wohl vorkommen, daß ungewöhnlich schwere Schädigungen auch gesunde Menschen nervös machten; in weitaus den meisten Fällen aber war es die durch die Konstitution gegebene Bereitschaft, die nervöse Diathese, die zum Versagen auch gegenüber relativ leichten, unter Umständen sogar alltäglichen und physiologischen Reizen führte.

Damit näherte sich MÖBIUS Begriffen, die schon 30 Jahre vor ihm der Franzose BOUCHUT in seinem Etat nerveux und im Nervosisme bemerkenswert klar herausgearbeitet hatte. Auf der anderen Seite gab er damit MARTIUS und STILLER eines ihrer Stichworte, als sie im Anfang unseres Jahrhunderts die Konstitution und die Funktion gegenüber der rein pathologisch-anatomischen Forschungsrichtung ihrer Zeit auszuspielen begannen. Beiden wurde die Nervosität als konstitutionell bedingte reine Funktionsstörung ein wichtiger Bestandteil ihres Lehrgebäudes, den sie von verschiedenen Gesichtspunkten — MARTIUS von dem der konstitutionellen Überempfindlichkeit der Hirnrinde, STILLER von dem des Habitus asthenicus aus — in ihre Vorstellungen einzufügen suchten. Von hier aus führte der Weg weiter über die Partialkonstitutionen von MARTIUS zu den Organneurosen, zu den „vegetativ Stigmatisierten" v. BERGMANNs und endlich zu dem, was wir heute die endogene (ASCHAFFENBURG) oder konstitutionelle (BUMKE) Nervosität nennen.

Konstitutionelle Nervosität ist die angeborene, ererbte Bereitschaft zu ungewöhnlich starken oder ungewöhnlich langdauernden Funktionsabweichungen rein quantitativer Art. Diese Funktionsabweichungen äußern sich in den somatischen und psychischen Reaktionen des Organismus auf die Reize, die durch das Leben und seine Anforderungen auf körperlichem und seelischem Gebiet gesetzt werden.

Die konstitutionelle Nervosität hat also neben dem somatischen auch ein psychologisches Gesicht, und gerade dieses hat eigentlich im Mittelpunkt der Forschung der letzten Jahrzehnte gestanden. MÖBIUS und BEARD hatten psychologische Gesichtspunkte nur insoweit berücksichtigt, als es sich um klinische Symptombeschreibung und allgemein-psychologische Erwägungen über die Zusammenhänge zwischen Nervosität und Zivilisation, Beruf, Geschlecht usw. handelte; demgegenüber waren es die Franzosen, die um die gleiche Zeit ihr Augenmerk auf die feinere individuelle psychologische Struktur des Nervösen und seiner Reaktionen richteten. Namen wie der CHARCOTS oder JANETS — der die Nervosität bezeichnenderweise Psychasthenie nannte — kennzeichnen das Programm dieser Forschungsrichtung, deren unmittelbare Nachfolge später von der Psychoanalyse und der Individualpsychologie angetreten wurde. Gegenüber diesen mehr auf dogmatischer Theorie und spekulativer Hypothese beruhenden Einsichten der sog. Tiefenpsychologie blieb die Klinik — und hier naturgemäß in erster Linie die Psychiatrie — dem rein empirischen Bemühen treu, die klinische Psychologie der nervösen Persönlichkeit, ihrer Reaktionen und Entwicklungen mehr und mehr zu vertiefen, ihre einzelnen Typen und Spielarten immer plastischer herauszuarbeiten und ihre Grenzen gegenüber anderen Kreisen funktionell-nervöser, zumal rein psychogener Erscheinungsformen, wie der Hypochondrie oder Hysterie (ERB, JOLLY, WOLLENBERG) abzustecken.

Uns Heutigen, für die der Kampf um die Grenzen der Krankheitseinheiten überhaupt mehr und mehr an Interesse verliert, scheint freilich der Aufwand an Kraft und Zeit, der an diesen Streit um die Selbständigkeit der Nervosität und um ihre Begrenzung gesetzt wurde, schier übertrieben. Wir glauben zu wissen — HOCHE und zumal BUMKE haben es immer wieder ausgesprochen —, daß im Bereich der abnormen Persönlichkeiten und der ungewöhnlichen, rein funktionellen Reaktionen das Suchen nach festen Grenzen grundsätzlich der Wirklichkeit nicht gerecht zu werden vermag. Es ist auch bei der konstitutionellen Nervosität so: Ihre Grenzen sowohl zur normalen als auch zur psychopathischen Persönlichkeitsanlage sind grundsätzlich fließende, und gerade die Formenkreise der hysterischen und hypochondrischen Reaktion, aber auch die anderer psychopathologischer Erscheinungsformen werden von ihr weithin überschnitten. Der konstitutionell Nervöse ist, von solchen Gesichtspunkten aus gesehen, zu einer Spielart der psychopathischen Persönlichkeiten geworden, deren wesentliches, obligates Kennzeichen die somatische Unterlegung ihrer Erscheinungsbilder in Gestalt der nervösen Funktionslabilität körperlicher Organe und Organsysteme ist.

Neurasthenische Reaktion. Wir sind auf die Begriffsentwicklung der konstitutionellen Nervosität eingangs unserer Ausführungen über die neurasthenische Reaktion (n. R.) deshalb etwas näher eingegangen, weil beide Begriffe neben- und miteinander entstanden sind und ihre grundsätzlichen Unterschiede erst seit dem Kriege herausgearbeitet wurden. Wenn die konstitutionelle Nervosität mehr auf dem Boden der MÖBIUSschen Anschauungen von der endogenen und ererbten nervösen Beschaffenheit erwuchs, umfaßt die n. R. jene namentlich von BEARD diskutierten Fälle, in denen vornehmlich oder allein durch *exogene* Schädigungen ein nervöses Zustandsbild hervorgerufen wird. Dabei bleibt die Konstitution, auf die die nervösmachende Schädigung trifft, grundsätzlich außer Betracht; grundsätzlich ist — um einen auf die Hysterie gemünzten Ausdruck HOCHES zu variieren — *jeder* Mensch neurastheniefähig. Daran ändert nichts, daß — die Verhältnisse liegen hier ähnlich wie im Gebiet der hysterischen Reaktion — der konstitutionell Nervöse einer nervösmachenden Schädigung natürlich besonders leicht unterliegt. Auch der Robuste, nervös Gesunde kann eine n. R. bekommen; dann nämlich, wenn die nervösmachende Schädigung stark genug ist, um seine nervöse Widerstandskraft zu überwinden.

Damit verschieben sich die Fragestellungen, die im Gebiet der konstitutionellen Nervosität mehr den konstitutionellen Grundlagen der Persönlichkeit und ihrer psychologischen und psychopathologischen Beschaffenheit und Entwicklung gelten, für die n. R. mehr nach dem Biologischen i. e. S. Die Fragen nach Stärke und Art der schädigenden Noxe, ihrer Wirkungsweise, ihren Angriffspunkten, den biologischen Vorgängen, die beim Zusammentreffen zwischen Schädigung und Funktionsgetriebe des Organismus endlich zum neurasthenischen Syndrom führen, nach diesem selbst in seinen verschiedenen Abwandlungen, das sind die Kernprobleme der n. R. Demgegenüber treten die Fragen nach der konstitutionellen Unterlegung, nach der psychologischen Verarbeitung der Reaktion und ihren sozialen Auswirkungen mehr in den Hintergrund.

Bevor wir uns jedoch diesen Fragestellungen im einzelnen nähern, wird der Versuch zu machen sein, den Begriff der n. R. genauer zu definieren und seinen Geltungsbereich abzugrenzen. Wir nennen n. R. *eine Störung nervöser Funktionen, die durch exogene, zu Übermüdung und Erschöpfung der Funktionskraft führende Schädigung verursacht ist, sich klinisch in einem nervösen Syndrom mit der besonderen Note der Reizbarkeit und Schwäche äußert und in reinen Fällen zu schnellem Ausgleich neigt.* Der Ausdruck „exogen" ist dabei in seiner allgemeinsten Bedeutung gemeint; er hat, wie wir noch genauer sehen werden, neben dem stets vorhandenen somatisch-biologischen sehr oft auch psychologischen Sinn. Die besondere Note der Erschöpfung hebt die Reaktion in ätiologischer und pathogenetischer Beziehung von Erscheinungsformen ähnlicher Symptomatologie ab, auf die bei Besprechung der Grenzen des Begriffs näher einzugehen sein wird. Auf die Art der Funktionsstörung und die mutmaßliche Auswahl der Funktionen, die von ihr betroffen werden, werden wir ebenfalls noch zurückkommen müssen. Wenn wir das neurasthenische Syndrom zunächst mit dem rein klinisch gemeinten Begriff der reizbaren Schwäche umschreiben, so folgen wir damit einer althergebrachten, schon von Möbius eingeführten Formulierung, die die eindrucksvollsten Symptome der n. R. recht gut umschreibt. Wir werden zu zeigen haben, wie weit es klinischen und physiologischen Bemühungen seit Möbius gelungen ist, diesen Begriff zu vertiefen.

Dem Wesen nach steht die n. R. also den exogenen Reaktionsformen nahe, wie sie Bonhoeffer beschrieben hat, ja sie ist vielleicht sogar selbst, wie Stertz des näheren ausgeführt und begründet hat, die leichteste Form der exogenen Reaktionen. Bonhoeffer selbst führt namentlich die emotionell-hyperästhetischen Schwächezustände, die das Rekonvaleszenzstadium nach Infektionskrankheiten häufig charakterisieren und im wesentlichen neurasthenischen Zuständen gleichen, unter den exogenen, also durch Intoxikation, Infektion, allgemeine oder lokalisierte Hirnschädigungen usw. verursachten psychisch-nervösen Störungen an. Neurasthenische Zustandsbilder sind seitdem bei zahlreichen Infektionen und Vergiftungen beschrieben worden; ein Überblick, wie ihn Leschke letzthin über die wichtigsten Vergiftungen gab, hat namentlich bei den chronisch wirksamen Metallvergiftungen auf Schritt und Tritt mit neurasthenischen Bildern zu tun; schon das Infektionsprodrom, das einleitende Stadium der Infektionskrankheit bis zum Beginn der spezifischen Symptome trägt oft neurasthenischen Charakter (Braun), und Stertz findet unter seinen Typhusrekonvaleszenten bis zu 60%, die unter neurasthenischen Erscheinungen leiden. Des weiteren kennt man neurasthenische, oder wie man aus klinisch-systematischen Gründen vorsichtiger zu sagen pflegt, pseudoneurasthenische Syndrome im Rahmen der verschiedensten groborganischen Hirnerkrankungen, der Paralyse, der Arteriosklerose, des Alkoholismus, des Hirntumors usw. Kurz, alle jene exogenen Schädigungen, die von BONHOEFFER als Ursachen der symptomatischen Psychosen genannt werden, sind auch imstande, neurasthenische Syndrome hervorzurufen.

Das kann natürlich kein Zufall sein und es legt den Gedanken nahe, der Entstehung dieser neurasthenischen und pseudoneurasthenischen Zustände ähnliche Vorgänge zugrunde zu legen, wie sie BONHOEFFER für die symptomatischen Psychosen gefordert hat. BONHOEFFER folgerte bekanntlich aus den unspezifischen, allen Hirnschädigungen in ziemlich unterschiedsloser Weise zugeordneten Formen der exogenen Reaktionstypen, daß zwischen ätiologischem Faktor und symptomatischer Geistesstörung noch ätiologische Zwischenglieder eingeschaltet seien, unter denen er sich unspezifisch toxisch wirkende Stoffwechselstörungen dachte. Etwas ähnliches mag für die exogenen neurasthenischen und pseudoneurasthenischen Bilder gelten. Allerdings liegen hier die Verhältnisse insofern anders und vielleicht einfacher, als es sich nicht wie dort um großenteils wohl abgesetzte, ausgesprochen qualitative und heteronome psychische Störungen, sondern um grundsätzlich rein quantitative, homonome Verschiebungen normaler Funktionen handelt. Es wäre also denkbar, daß mindestens *ein* ätiologisches Zwischenglied, eben jenes, das gerade die symptomatische *Psychose* verursacht und von KLEIST bekanntlich in einem konstitutionellen Moment gesehen wird, bei den n. R. wegfiele. Vielleicht greifen hier die toxischen Vorgänge unmittelbarer am Substrat an als bei den symptomatischen Psychosen i. e. S.

Was nun die n. R. i. e. S., die durch Erschöpfung erworbene neurasthenische Funktionsschwäche angeht, so wird man sie in erster Linie in nähere Beziehung zu jenen exogenen Reaktionen bringen müssen, die durch chronische Toxikose entstanden sind. Man wird also mit anderen Worten vor der Frage stehen, ob man die Erschöpfung als einen Vorgang auffassen kann oder muß, der zu toxischen — oder den toxischen ähnlichen — Wirkungen führt. Hier werden uns die Erfahrungen von Nutzen sein, die die Physiologie über die Stoffwechselvorgänge und nervösen Regulationsverschiebungen bei der Ermüdung, Erschöpfung und Erholung, dem Schlaf-Wach-Rhythmus und ähnlichen, die Ausgabe, Wiederherstellung und Erhaltung der Funktionskräfte besorgenden Funktionsabläufen gemacht hat.

Erschöpfung und Übermüdung. Wir schließen uns der Darstellung VERWORNs an, wenn wir zunächst am Stoffwechselgetriebe mit HERING eine Phase der Assimilation und eine Phase der Dissimilation unterscheiden. Dissimilation ist dabei der Zerfall bestimmter, Leben und Funktion der Zelle repräsentierender Eiweißmoleküle, der in erhöhtem Maße bei stärkerer Reizung, also erhöhter Zelltätigkeit auftritt und schließlich zur Ausscheidung der Zerfallsprodukte, der Stoffwechselschlacken führt. Assimilation ist demgegenüber der Aufbau dieser selben, von VERWORN „Biogene" genannten Eiweißmoleküle aus den dem Organismus zugeführten Nahrungsstoffen, unter denen der Sauerstoff eine besonders wichtige Rolle spielt. Es leuchtet ohne weiteres ein, daß der Phase der Dissimilation die Zelltätigkeit, der der Assimilation die Ruhe entspricht. Oder, um das Problem gleich auf das Gebiet der nervösen Regulationen hinüberzuleiten: Die Phase des Aufbaues $\varkappa\alpha\tau'\dot{\varepsilon}\xi o\chi\dot{\eta}\nu$ ist der Schlaf, die des Zerfalls in der Tätigkeit das Wachen.

Beide Phasen lösen einander ab. Sie haben — um es teleologisch auszudrücken — die Aufgabe, einerseits die Kräfte bereitzustellen, deren der Organismus zur Selbsterhaltung und Selbstentfaltung gegenüber der Umwelt im Wachsein bedarf, andererseits im Schlaf verbrauchte Kräfte zu ersetzen und Zerfallsprodukte auszuscheiden. Sie tun das vermöge einer „inneren

Selbststeuerung des Stoffwechsels" (HERING), deren Regulationsabläufe wir im vegetativen System KRAUSscher Prägung, also den aufs mannigfachste ineinander verwobenen und aufeinander abgestimmten vegetativen Funktionen von der Grenzmembrandurchlässigkeit bis hinauf zur Zwischenhirnsteuerung zu suchen haben[1]. Das vegetative System schafft also, indem es durch Selbststeuerung über antinome Phasen zum Stoffwechselgleichgewicht strebt, die Vorbedingungen für die animalischen[2] Funktionen des Organismus. Den Phasen des Aufbaus und Zerfalls werden — das läßt sich am deutlichsten wiederum von der Schlaf-Wachfunktion ablesen — Funktionsänderungen oder, wie man seit EPPINGER und HESS gern sagt, Tonusverschiebungen im vegetativen System entsprechen. *Störungen* des Stoffwechselgleichgewichts zwischen Assimilation und Dissimilation, des „Biotonus", wie VERWORN diesen Quotienten nennt, werden zugleich zu Störungen der vegetativen Funktionen führen, die durch Veränderung der regulierenden Impulse den Versuch machen müssen, das Funktionsgleichgewicht wieder herzustellen.

Um diesen Störungen näher nachgehen zu können, müssen wir mit VERWORN noch zwei neue Begriffe einführen, die „Ermüdung" und die „Erschöpfung". Wenn die Dissimilation bis zu einem gewissen Grade fortgeschritten ist, wenn also die in der Assimilationsphase aufgebauten Biogene zum Teil zerfallen und zu Stoffwechselschlacken geworden sind, tritt Ermüdung ein, d. h. der Organismus — wiederum spielt hier das vegetative System die entscheidende Rolle — wird zur Ruhe und endlich zum Schlaf gedrängt, die zum Wiederaufbau nötig sind. Mosso hat am Muskel gezeigt, daß diese „Arbeitslähmung" (VERWORN) bis zu völliger Leistungsunfähigkeit zunehmen kann; sie kann behoben oder wenigstens gebessert werden, wenn der Muskel mit Kochsalzlösung durchspült (RANKE zit. nach VERWORN) oder unter Sauerstoffzutritt der Ruhe überlassen wird (HERMANN, JOTEYKO zit. nach VERWORN). Es sind also offenbar die Stoffwechselschlacken, toxisch wirkende sog. Ermüdungsstoffe — am bekanntesten sind die Kenotoxine WEICHARDTs —, die Arbeitslähmung und Ermüdung hervorrufen. Unter gleichen Gesetzen stehen, wie sich experimentell erweisen läßt, die Ganglienzellen des Nervensystems, aber auch der gesamte Organismus, dessen Ruhe- und Schlafbedürfnis von den im Blute kreisenden Ermüdungsstoffen abhängt. In den Ablauf der Schlaf-Wachfunktion sind außerdem noch nervöse regulierende Instanzen eingeschaltet, als deren höchste man graue Massen am Boden des III. Ventrikels anzusehen pflegt.

Wird dem Bedürfnis nach Ruhe oder Schlaf stattgegeben, so tritt *Erholung* ein, d. h. die Stoffwechseltoxine werden beseitigt, und es findet ein Aufbau statt, aus dessen Kräften die neue Tätigkeitsphase des Muskels, der Ganglienzelle oder des Organismus bestritten werden kann. Geschieht das nicht oder nicht in ausreichendem Maße, wie z. B. bei schweren Infektionen oder in Kriegszeiten, so setzt der Körper zunächst seine Reserven ein (A. PICK).

Diese Reservekräfte entnimmt er nach GOLDSCHEIDERs Ansicht wahrscheinlich Reservedepots von Sauerstoff und Nährstoffen, die nach VERWORN höchstwahrscheinlich in den Zellkernen zu suchen sind. Als weitere Reserven bei fortgesetztem Überwiegen der Dissimilationsphase dient das Zellmaterial gewisser Gewebsarten, die, wie z. B. das Fett- und Muskelgewebe, zugunsten lebenswichtiger Organe wie des Herzens und des Zentralnervensystems eingeschmolzen werden können. Wenn aber alle Reservedepots entleert sind, oder jedenfalls

---

[1] Für die Darstellung des vegetativen Systems, die im Rahmen dieser Arbeit einen zu großen Raum einnehmen würde, verweisen wir auf die zusammenfassenden Darstellungen von KRAUS, L. R. MÜLLER und seinen Mitarbeitern, und im BERGMANN-BETHEschen Handbuch.
[2] Wir gebrauchen hier die Gegensätze vegetativ und animalisch im Sinne von KRAUS.

— was sehr viel früher der Fall sein dürfte — nicht mehr genügend Aufbaumaterial geliefert werden kann, um das Stoffwechselgleichgewicht gegenüber der gesteigerten Dissimilation aufrecht zu erhalten, tritt *Erschöpfung* ein. Ermüdung i. e. S. ist also nach VERWORN Überlastung mit toxisch wirkenden Stoffwechselschlacken, Übermüdung die Steigerung des Ermüdungsvorgangs über die Grenze der Norm hinaus, Erschöpfung Mangel an Assimilationsmaterial.

Beides, Übermüdung und Erschöpfung, tritt natürlich im praktischen Einzelfall meist gemeinsam auf. Dabei scheint es aber, daß gerade das Nervensystem — oder doch das nervöse Substrat der Neurasthenie — relativ unabhängig vom Mangel an Nährstoffen ist. Wenigstens findet man immer wieder extrem abgemagerte Menschen ohne Neurasthenie und umgekehrt schwer „nervös Erschöpfte" bei gutem oder doch ausreichendem Ernährungszustand; schon BEARD ist es aufgefallen, daß ein großer Teil seiner Neurastheniker „fett und munter, robust und kraftstrotzend" aussah, ja sogar fetter werden konnte, obwohl das Befinden sich verschlechterte. Man wird annehmen müssen, daß die Übermüdung, also die toxische Schädigung des Funktionssubstrats durch Stoffwechselschlacken, die Hauptursache der n. R. ist; deshalb haben wir auch oben bei dem Versuch, die n. R. zu definieren, die Übermüdung in den Vordergrund gerückt.

Die Funktion, die dem lebendigen Organismus als geeignetstes, ja schließlich einziges Mittel zum Ausgleich von Ermüdung und Übermüdung gegeben ist, ist der Schlaf, der Hand in Hand mit einer dem Vagotonischen zuneigenden Tonusumstellung im vegetativen System die Stoffwechselreinigung und die Auffüllung der Kraftdepots, den Wiederaufbau der Biogene, am schnellsten und vollkommensten besorgt. Schlafmangel, der die Erholung des Nervensystems nach Ermüdung und Übermüdung verhindert, muß also, so können wir von vornherein aus theoretischen Erwägungen heraus vermuten, eine der Hauptursachen der n. R. sein. Demgegenüber wird die reine Erschöpfung der Körperkräfte nur eine nebensächliche Rolle spielen[1]. Um es etwas epigrammatisch auszudrücken: Nicht der Hunger macht neurasthenisch, sondern die Schlaflosigkeit.

Krankhafte Überempfindlichkeit. An dieser Stelle wird nun zu fragen sein, wie denn Ermüdung und Übermüdung im einzelnen auf das Nervensystem wirken; wie kann man sich insbesondere das Entstehen der eigentümlichen neurasthenischen Schwäche und Reizbarkeit als Effekt der Übermüdungstoxikose vorstellen? Hier werden wir gut tun, zunächst den Gedankengängen zu folgen, die GOLDSCHEIDER beim Studium der „krankhaften Überempfindlichkeit" entwickelt hat. GOLDSCHEIDER stützt sich neben der VERWORNschen Lehre vom Aufbau und Zerfall der Biogene namentlich auf die von Zoologen und Physiologen — unter anderem wiederum von VERWORN — aufgebaute Lehre von der Reizbarkeit der lebendigen Zelle und den Reizwirkungen. Jede Zelltätigkeit, in VERWORNs Sinn also jeder Dissimilationsvorgang am Biogen, wird durch Reize verursacht. Besonders starke Reize steigern die Dissimilation und damit sekundär die den Stoffwechselausgleich herbeiführende Assimilation. GOLDSCHEIDER schließt aus anderen Erfahrungen, z. B. im Gebiet der Muskelphysiologie und der Immunbiologie, daß gesetzmäßig die Assimilation mit einem funktionellen und materiellen Überschuß arbeitet. Er glaubt ferner, daß „bei besonders tiefgehender Aufsplitterung der Atomkomplexe eigenartige Modifikationen der Biogenmoleküle von besonders labiler Beschaffenheit" gebildet würden. Der Grad der Reiz-

---

[1] Eine Unterscheidung, die freilich im praktischen Einzelfall bedeutungslos zu sein pflegt, weil Unterernährung, Schlafmangel und psychische Alteration selten oder nie voneinander getrennt werden können. Man denke etwa an die BONHOEFFERschen kriegsgefangenen Serben.

barkeit einer Zelle oder eines Zellkomplexes bemißt sich nach dem Grade der Zerfallsbereitschaft der Biogene. Besonders labile Biogene würden also gegenüber Reizen von gleicher Art besonders leicht zersetzlich sein. Mit anderen Worten: Ist durch verstärkte Dissimilation eine überschüssige, von GOLDSCHEIDER „kumulative" genannte Assimilation eingetreten, so besteht eine erhöhte Reizbarkeit des geschädigten Funktionssubstrats. Diese Erregbarkeitssteigerung kann eine zeitlich begrenzte sein, kann aber auch für längere Dauer fixiert werden, wenn die Zellen stärker geschädigt sind oder wenn die Reize immer wiederkehren. Von hier aus läuft nun eine gerade Linie zur krankhaften Übererregbarkeit, einer „Erniedrigung der Neuronschwelle", wie sie ein Charakteristikum der n. R. ist.

Diese Lehre GOLDSCHEIDERs von der Entstehung einer besonderen Erregbarkeit durch immer wiederholte Reize erinnert an die namentlich von russischen Autoren ausgebaute Lehre PAWLOWs von den bedingten Reflexen. Allerdings beziehen sich die GOLDSCHEIDERschen Betrachtungen gewissermaßen auf die tiefste somatische Schicht, die der Zellen und ihrer Funktionen, während PAWLOWs Bemühungen einer wesentlich höheren Schicht gelten, deren Erscheinungsformen ja zum großen Teil schon sehr komplexe und höchst differenzierte, hochwertige nervöse Apparate darstellen. Auch hier finden wir aber eine durch immer wiederholte oder sehr starke Reize bewirkte Umstimmung und Übererregbarkeit nervöser Mechanismen. Wenn wir auch gegenüber der namentlich von seinen Schülern geübten Überspannung der PAWLOWschen Lehre[1], die schließlich in der Seele nichts anderes mehr sieht als eine Reflexmaschine, sehr zurückhaltend bleiben werden, so werden wir uns ihrer manchmal angesichts gewisser Phobien, eingeschliffener Reflexmechanismen und Organbereitschaften mit Nutzen erinnern können. Gerade bei gewissen Störungen der Schlaffunktion, auf deren besondere Wichtigkeit im Rahmen der n. R. wir bereits hingewiesen haben, mögen bedingte Reflexe eine sehr wesentliche Rolle spielen.

Reizbare Schwäche. Wenn solche physiologischen Erfahrungen und Theorien den Zugang zum Verständnis der neurasthenischen *Reizbarkeit* — einer Reizbarkeit der *Funktion* — bahnen, so läßt sich das Symptom der neurasthenischen *Schwäche* — einer Schwäche der *Leistung* — direkt aus der Übermüdung und Erschöpfung des nervösen Funktionssubstrats entwickeln. Die lähmende Wirkung toxischer Stoffwechselprodukte einerseits und die Erschöpfung der Reservedepots andererseits verhindern die Entstehung vollwertiger Biogene. Die Folgen sind Schwäche und vorzeitige Ermüdbarkeit ihrer Tätigkeit.

Beide, die durch übermäßige Reizung erworbene Reizbarkeit und die Schwäche der Ermüdung und Erschöpfung, treten nun im neurasthenischen Syndrom nebeneinander auf. Die Lähmung der Übermüdung gleicht also nicht, wie man an sich vermuten könnte, die übermäßige Erregbarkeit durch Reize aus. Beide Anomalien der Funktion scheinen sich vielmehr gewissermaßen unabhängig voneinander zu entwickeln. Man kann sich, wenn man den GOLDSCHEIDERschen Gedanken von der Entstehung besonders labiler, zu schnellem Zerfall geneigter Biogene festhält, die Dinge so vorstellen, daß bei übermäßiger Inanspruchnahme des nervösen Funktionssubstrats zunächst hauptsächlich oder ausschließlich diese nicht vollwertige Abart der Biogene gebildet wird, deren Funktionskraft eben vermöge ihres schnellen, schon bei geringsten Reizen einsetzenden Zerfalls, besonders schwach und zugleich schnell ermüdbar ist. Die Minderwertigkeit dieser Ersatzbiogene würde sich also sowohl in der überschnellen Auslösbarkeit des Zerfalls als auch in seinem besonders schnellen Ablauf äußern.

Im übrigen findet man diese Kombination von Schwäche und Reizbarkeit nach übermäßiger Beanspruchung der Funktion auf mannigfachen Gebieten

---

[1] Eine zusammenfassende Darstellung gibt ISCHLONDSKY.

der Pathophysiologie. Man kann, wenn man mit MOSSO und GOLDSCHEIDER einen teleologischen Gesichtspunkt einführt, darin Schutzregulationen des Organismus sehen, die weiterer übermäßiger Inanspruchnahme eines Funktionssubstrats vorbeugen sollen. Das ist ohne weiteres einleuchtend bei der einfachen Ermüdung, die durch Lähmung des Funktionssubstrats zur Untätigkeit und endlich zum Schlafe zwingt oder zu zwingen sucht. Das Übermaß an Reizbarkeit dagegen, das neben Schwäche und Ermüdbarkeit das Kennzeichen der Übermüdung und Erschöpfung ist, wird man unter anderem [1] als Verfeinerung des Signalapparats auffassen können, der den Organismus möglichst frühzeitig vor Gefahren warnt und ihre Vermeidung herbeizuführen sucht.

Daß unter Umständen erhöhte Reizbarkeit zur Vermeidung von Reizen führt, sieht man auf einem mehr psychologischen Gebiet beim Neurasthenischen, der, soweit es ihm möglich ist, jeden stärkeren Reiz flieht und z. B. dem Zusammensein mit Menschen, starken Sinneseindrücken, Affekterregungen usw. auszuweichen sucht. Wenn er das sehr viel früher getan hätte, würde er möglicherweise die n. R. überhaupt vermieden haben, aber Pflichtbewußtsein, Ehrgeiz, Kampf um die Existenz und ähnliche Faktoren der Zivilisation, denen er unterliegt, haben ihn dazu gezwungen, die Zeichen der Erschöpfung so lange als möglich zu übersehen. Im Gegensatz zum Primitiven, der unangenehme Reize unbeschwert von Verantwortungsgefühl und Streben nach höheren Zielen vermeidet und damit der Entstehung der krankhaften Reizbarkeit vorbeugt, entwickelt sich beim Zivilisierten ein Circulus vitiosus, der den Erfolg des natürlichen Schutzmechanismus zu Schanden macht: Die übergroße Reizbarkeit führt mit Fortgang der Reizungen zu immer schnellerem Zerfall der Biogene und immer stärkerem Verbrauch der Funktionskraft, die schließlich infolge Mangels an Aufbaumaterial und fehlender Erholung in immer unzulänglicherem Grade ersetzt wird. Je unzulänglicher die Ersatzbiogene sind, desto größer ist wiederum ihre Reizbarkeit usw.

Theoretisch müßte eine derartige dauernd fortgesetzte Überanstrengung des nervösen Funktionssubstrats ohne Erholung und ohne Zufuhr von Aufbaustoffen endlich zu völliger Erschöpfung und damit zu Funktionsunfähigkeit, ja schließlich zum Tode führen [2]. Bei sehr komplizierter Versuchsanordnung läßt sich im Tierexperiment tatsächlich zeigen, daß völlige Unerregbarkeit des Nervengewebes auf diese Weise zu erreichen ist (VERWORN). Dazu gehört aber die Absperrung des wichtigsten Aufbaustoffes, des Sauerstoffs, etwas, was im Experiment durch Ersatz des Blutes durch eine isotonische Kochsalzlösung erreicht werden kann, beim lebendigen Menschen aber natürlich nicht vorkommt. Beim Menschen kann die Erschöpfung i. e. S. also nur mäßige Grade erreichen, und auch die Ermüdung pflegt selbst unter ungünstigsten Umständen immer wieder bis zu einem gewissen Grade dadurch ausgeglichen zu werden, daß sich der Schlaf gegen alle Willensanspannung und äußeren Hindernisse endlich doch durchsetzt. Man schläft schließlich selbst im Trommelfeuer in höchster Lebensgefahr ein, und ich erinnere mich aus dem Kriege, bei großer Erschöpfung selbst im Marschieren und Reiten zeitweise in einen Halbschlaf verfallen zu sein. Das alles genügt freilich nicht, um das Nervensystem vor Schädigungen durch Überanstrengung völlig zu schützen. Bevor es aber zu den schwersten Graden der irreparablen Lähmung kommen kann, pflegen die Funktionsstörungen, die durch Schwäche und Reizbarkeit verursacht werden, längst zu sozialer Unbrauchbarkeit und Unerträglichkeit, zum Ausscheiden aus dem schädigenden Milieu

---
[1] Daß damit die Bedeutung der Reizbarkeitssteigerung nicht erschöpft ist, geht aus der GOLDSCHEIDERschen Darstellung hervor.
[2] Natürlich gehört der Erschöpfungstod infolge Versagens des Herzens nicht hierher, wo es sich allein um die Erschöpfung des Nervensystems handelt.

und damit zur Erholung geführt zu haben. Das, was wir also am Krankenbett als neurasthenische Reaktion zu Gesicht bekommen, bildet immer nur ein bestimmtes, leichtes oder mittelschweres, grundsätzlich der Reparation zugängliches Stadium der Übermüdung und Erschöpfung des Funktionssubstrats.

Das Funktionssubstrat. Wir wollen den Versuch machen, noch einen weiteren Gesichtspunkt einzuführen, der zum Verständnis der n. R. und ihrer Symptomatologie von Nutzen sein mag. Wir haben im vorhergehenden mehrfach von dem *Funktionssubstrat* gesprochen, dessen Schädigung durch übermäßige Inanspruchnahme wir der n. R. zugrunde legten, und meinten damit die Zellen oder Zellverbände, deren Stoffwechselstörungen zu den Funktionsänderungen führen, die für die n. R. charakteristisch sind.

Daß diese Stoffwechselstörungen, soweit sie unmittelbar zum neurasthenischen Symptom führen, im Zentralnervensystem wirksam werden, wird angesichts des psychisch-nervösen Charakters der Symptome kaum eines Beweises bedürfen. Wir werden dabei aber einmal im Auge behalten müssen, daß wir bei der Entwicklung der Pathogenese der n. R. zum Teil von rein körperlichen Vorgängen — Stoffwechselverschiebungen, Intoxikationen usw. — ausgehen mußten, die erst sekundär zu toxischen Wirkungen auf das Nervensystem führen. Wir werden ferner nicht vergessen dürfen, daß man gerade im Gebiet der sog. funktionellen nervös-psychischen Störungen, dessen Grenzen zum Normalen ja fließende sind, immer wieder auf ein unlösbares Ineinandergreifen körperlicher und psychisch-nervöser Funktionen stößt, deren hierarchisch geordnete, wechselseitig aufeinander abgestimmte Abläufe im Zusammenwirken die Persönlichkeit in ihrer unteilbaren, lebendigen Ganzheit repräsentieren. Seelische Vorgänge können unmittelbar zu körperlichen führen — wir wissen das seit langem, obwohl wir uns vielleicht immer noch keine genügende Vorstellung vom Ausmaß dieser Zusammenhänge zu machen pflegen. Körperliche Vorgänge aber können umgekehrt einen Einfluß auf den Ablauf psychisch-nervöser Funktionen ausüben.

Das gilt zunächst für die Norm, wobei wir in diesem Zusammenhang ganz davon absehen können, daß wir uns ja überhaupt keinen psychisch-nervösen Funktionsablauf ohne Unterlegung durch körperliche Funktionen vorstellen können, sondern nur an die seelischen Rückwirkungen bestimmter somatischer Organe, des Herzens, der Drüsen mit innerer Sekretion usw. und ihrer Funktionen denken wollen. Am deutlichsten aber werden solche Korrelationen dann, wenn somatische Funktionsverschiebungen stärkerer Art über die Norm hinaus zu psychisch-nervösen Störungen führen, wie sie gerade im Bereich der endokrinen Erkrankungen, z. B. beim Basedow, bei der Menstruation, beim Klimakterium usw. am bekanntesten sind. Hier muß also die zunächst rein körperliche Drüsenstörung einen sekundären, psychische Funktionen störenden Einfluß ausüben, deren Wirkungsfeld man nicht wohl anderenorts als im Zentralnervensystem suchen muß[1].

Derartige innersekretorisch bedingte Syndrome allgemein-nervöser Art haben nun insofern nähere Beziehungen zur n. R., als sie den Erscheinungsformen neurasthenischer und konstitutionell-nervöser Herkunft klinisch sehr nahe stehen, so nahe, daß beide Syndromarten rein symptomatologisch oft nicht voneinander zu unterscheiden sind. Auch bei der n. R. muß man also die Möglichkeit einer Beteiligung innersekretorischer oder überhaupt körperlicher Faktoren an der Pathogenese in Betracht ziehen. Dem entspricht, daß z. B. BUMKE nachdrücklich auf die innere Sekretion als pathogenetisches Moment im Rahmen der Neurasthenie hinweist, und daß auch sonst immer wieder Versuche auftauchen, bestimmte innersekretorische Anomalien für die Nervosität oder die n. R.

---

[1] Vgl. dazu die zahlreichen Arbeiten über die Zusammenhänge der inneren Sekretion mit psychischen Störungen. EWALD hat diese Probleme zusammenfassend dargestellt.

verantwortlich zu machen. So bringt etwa SZONDI die Nebennieren, KLOTZ die Hypophyse, W. JAENSCH die Schilddrüse mit nervösen Erscheinungen in Verbindung, und auch jene leichtesten Fälle inkompleter Thyreotoxikosen[1] von den Formes frustes CHARCOTs, dem Thyreoidismus CHVOSTECKs bis zum Basedowoid R. STERNs mögen hier zu erwähnen sein. Allerdings wird sich in allen diesen Fällen schwerlich erweisen lassen, wie weit es sich hier um konstitutionelle, also der konstitutionellen Nervosität nahestehende, wie weit um exogene, im Rahmen der neurasthenischen Reaktion von außen her verursachte Anomalien handelt. Ähnlich steht es mit Stoffwechselstörungen, deren Beurteilung und Verwertung, wie WUTH gelegentlich hervorhebt, im Bereich der Neurasthenie an und für sich besonders zweifelhaft ist, und die wohl stets — soweit sie bisher untersucht worden sind — eher Hinweise auf konstitutionelle Eigentümlichkeiten geben. Um nur einige der Untersuchungen der letzten Zeit zu nennen, so fanden BECHER bei Neuropathen Indican und Urobilinogen im Urin vermehrt, WALINSKI Herabsetzung der Alkalireserve im Blut, JANUSCHKE einen Sauerstoffmangel der Gewebe, WILDER ebenso wie SZONDI starke Schwankungen der alimentären Blutzuckerkurve, CAMERON allgemeine Labilität des Stoffwechsels, EXNER zahlreiche Abweichungen von den Normalkurven des Sauerstoffverbrauchs usw.

So unsicher also unsere bisherigen Kenntnisse über die grundlegenden körperlichen Störungen der n. R. auch sind — wir werden auf andere mehr symptomatologisch aufzufassende noch zurückkommen —, so viel steht doch fest, daß die Neurasthenie verursachende Schädigung nicht — oder jedenfalls nicht ausschließlich — am Großhirn angreift, wie noch z. B. MARTIUS meinte, wenn er die Neurasthenie auf eine Überempfindlichkeit der sensiblen Hirnrinde zurückführen wollte. Im Bereich der n. R. und wohl überhaupt in dem der sog. funktionellen psychisch-nervösen Störungen muß die Frage nach der Lokalisation — sofern man hier von Lokalisation überhaupt reden will — vielmehr grundsätzlich anders gestellt werden. Nicht die Schädigung eines umschriebenen Hirnbezirks allein, wie man sie bis vor kurzem etwa für die motorische Aphasie annahm, kann für die n. R. verantwortlich gemacht werden. Es muß sich dabei vielmehr um sehr viel umfassendere Störungen handeln, die sowohl somatische als auch zugleich seelische Funktionen in ihren Bereich ziehen und — wie wir noch genauer sehen werden — sowohl vom Körperlichen als auch vom Psychischen her wirksam werden können.

Ist es möglich, sich ein — wenigstens vorläufiges — Bild des körperlich-seelischen Funktionssubstrates zu machen, das von der n. R. vornehmlich oder ausschließlich befallen wird? Wir müssen hier, um dieser Fragestellung nachzugehen, auf Vorstellungen zurückgreifen, die wir uns über die sog. ,,vitale Person" gebildet haben[2], die übrigens ihren Ausgang von der klinischen Beobachtung des Nervösen und des Neurasthenischen nahmen, wenn sie auch im weiteren Ausbau zu umfassenderen Betrachtungen gelangten. Unter vitalen Eigenschaften verstanden wir dort dynamisch gedachte, körpernahe Funktionen der tiefsten seelischen Schicht, die untereinander in engen gegenseitigen Beziehungen stehen und als relativ abgeschlossenes Ganzes innerhalb der Person — eben als ,,vitale Person" — einen relativ selbständigen Funktionsbetrieb aufrecht erhalten. Als klinisch wichtigste Funktionen in diesem Sinn betrachteten wir des genaueren den vitalen Antrieb, die vitale Stimmung, die vitale

---
[1] Daß umgekehrt Schreck und wohl auch Erschöpfung gelegentlich eine echte BASEDOWsche Krankheit hervorrufen oder wenigstens manifest machen können, ist seit langem bekannt (FRIEDEMANN und KOHNSTAMM). Basedow und Basedowoid werden denn auch gelegentlich unter den Symptomen der n. R. aufgeführt (KEHRER, GIERLICH u. a.).
[2] BRAUN: Die vitale Person. Leipzig 1933.

Reizempfänglichkeit und den Schlaf. Diese vitalen Eigenschaften, die an der Grenze zwischen Körper und Seele eingefügt sind, empfangen Impulse von beiden Seiten und greifen sowohl in die psychischen als auch in die somatischen Funktionen ein. Ihre Aufgabe ist dabei im Funktionsplan des Organismus die Regulation und Erhaltung eines an die Anforderungen des Lebens angepaßten Funktionsgleichgewichts — Schlaf-Wachen —, die Bereitstellung von Funktionskräften — Antrieb —, die Registrierung von exogenen und endogenen Reizen — Reizempfänglichkeit und Stimmung. Sie unterlegen alle psychischen Funktionen, die ohne sie gar nicht zum Ablauf kommen könnten; ihre — angeborene oder erworbene — Beschaffenheit bestimmt maßgeblich Art und Leistungsfähigkeit der Persönlichkeit.

Diese vitalen Eigenschaften der Persönlichkeit sind es unseres Erachtens, die bei der n. R. in erster Linie geschädigt werden. Schlafstörungen, Antriebsschwäche, Verstimmung und Reizbarkeit sind die psychischen Grundsymptome der n. R., über deren Auswirkung im Psychischen wir unten Genaueres hören werden. Es wird zu fragen sein, wie man sich das biologische Substrat dieser von der Neurasthenie geschädigten „vitalen Person" vorstellen kann und wie die stets vorhandenen körperlichen Regulationsstörungen der n. R., wie Herz-Gefäßstörungen, Blutdruckherabsetzung, Impotenz, Appetitlosigkeit, Schmerzen usw.[1] damit in Zusammenhang zu bringen sind.

Was diese letzteren angeht, so fällt zunächst auf, daß sie sich größtenteils auf dem Gebiete von Organen abspielen, deren Funktionen unmittelbar dem vegetativen Nervensystem unterstehen. KRAUS hat bekanntlich den Begriff des „vegetativen Systems" geprägt, das die miteinander in enger Funktionskorrelation stehenden Regulationssysteme der Drüsen mit innerer Sekretion und des vegetativen Nervensystems umfaßt, die ihrerseits wieder in unmittelbaren Beziehungen zum Ionenhaushalt, zur Grenzmembrandurchlässigkeit usw. stehen. Es besteht also ein einziges, riesiges, hierarchisch geordnetes System von ineinandergreifenden und aufeinander abgestimmten Funktionen, das praktisch von der Funktion der einzelnen Körperzelle bis hinauf zur höchsten bisher bekannten Regulationsinstanz des vegetativen Systems, dem Zwischen-Mittelhirn (KARPLUS und KREIDL u. a.), reicht. Dieses System beherrscht den gesamten Stoffwechsel des Organismus im Sinne des immer wieder erstrebten Gleichgewichts gegenüber den Anforderungen, die die animalischen Funktionen in ihrer Wechselwirkung mit den Einwirkungen der Außenwelt und dem Eigenleben des Organismus — Wachstum, Gewebeersatz, Geschlechtszellenproduktion usw. — stellen. Dieses Gleichgewicht wird in antagonistischem Zusammenarbeiten — Sympathicus und Parasympathicus — des vegetativen Systems erreicht, während übergeordnete Kontroll- und Regulationsinstanzen der Medulla oblongata und des Hirnstamms in mehrfacher Sicherung (LESCHKE) den ordnungsmäßigen Ablauf der nervös-endokrin gesteuerten Funktionen gewährleisten. Jede Störung eines seiner Glieder, z. B. einer endokrinen Drüse, übt vermöge der innigen funktionellen Verbundenheit des ganzen Systems Wirkungen auf andere, unter Umständen fernliegende Glieder und die übergeordneten Regulationsinstanzen aus. Je peripherer die Störung ansetzt, je leichter sie ist, desto eher wird ihr Ausgleich gelingen, ohne daß die höchsten Regulationsfunktionen in Mitleidenschaft gezogen werden. Je schwerer die Störung, je zentraler ihr Sitz, desto mehr werden Zwischen- und Mittelhirn gezwungen sein, bei der Wiederherstellung des Gleichgewichts mitzuarbeiten, desto ausgedehnter und allgemeiner werden auch die Rückwirkungen seiner Funktionsstörung auf das ganze System sein.

---

[1] Einzelheiten siehe weiter unten.

Wir sind uns bewußt, daß diese Darstellung des Funktionsablaufs im vegetativen System in vielem noch hypothetisch bleiben muß und — vor allem mit dem Ziele klinischer Brauchbarkeit — die Dinge sehr viel einfacher sieht, als sie in Wirklichkeit liegen mögen. Immerhin finden wir in der Literatur, soweit wir sehen, keine Tatsachen, die ernsthaft gegen solche Auffassung des vegetativen Funktionsablaufs sprechen. Andererseits ergibt sich so die Möglichkeit, manche Erscheinungen normaler und pathologischer Art von einem neuen Gesichtspunkt aus zu sehen. Wir müssen dieserhalb, da der Rahmen dieses Beitrags eine breitere Erörterung nicht erlaubt, auf unsere monographische Darstellung verweisen.

Das, was in diesem Zusammenhang noch wichtig ist, sind nun die Beziehungen des vegetativen Systems und namentlich seiner obersten Instanz im Zwischen-Mittelhirn zur sog. ,,vitalen Person". Hier begegnen wir Gedankengängen von REICHARDT, KLEIST, KÜPPERS, EWALD u. a., die von sehr verschiedenen Standpunkten aus dem Hirnstamm sowohl als der inneren Sekretion nahe Beziehungen zum Antrieb und zur Stimmung beilegen. Man wird ferner nach den Erfahrungen, die namentlich mit der Encephalitis epidemica in den letzten $1^1/_2$ Jahrzehnten vielfach gemacht worden sind, wohl mit Sicherheit annehmen dürfen, daß ein höchstes regulierendes Schlaf-Wach-Zentrum in den grauen Massen am Übergang vom Zwischen- zum Mittelhirn zu suchen ist (ECONOMO, PETTE u.a.). Diese Tatsachen zusammen mit anderen Überlegungen anatomischer, physiologischer und phylogenetischer Art — für deren Einzelheiten wir wiederum auf unsere ausführliche Arbeit verweisen müssen —, bestimmen uns, dem Zwischen-Mittelhirn im Rahmen der ,,vitalen Person" eine besonders wichtige Stellung einzuräumen. Wir stellen uns vor, daß zwar die Zellen des Körpers, die Organe mit ihrer endokrin-vegetativen Regulierung die breite, kraftspendende Grundlage der ,,vitalen Person" sind, daß aber im Zwischen-Mittelhirn die ordnende Zusammenfassung geschieht, vielleicht auch die Umwandlung der rein körperlichen Funktionskräfte in halbwegs psychische, wie es Antrieb, Stimmung, Reizempfänglichkeit und Schlaf-Wachen sind, stattfindet. Andererseits halten wir es mit STERTZ für möglich, daß hier die Umschaltstelle zu suchen ist, in der rein psychische Impulse, z. B. Affekte, in körperliches Geschehen, z. B. Änderungen der Herzaktion, übergeführt werden. Das Zwischen-Mittelhirn ist also unserer Anschauung nach der Mittler zwischen körperlichem und psychischem Geschehen. Es hat neben der Möglichkeit direkter Einwirkung auf die einzelnen durch das Vegetativum gesteuerten Organfunktionen als weitere allgemein auf den gesamten Organismus wirkende Regulationsmöglichkeit den Einfluß auf die vitalen Qualitäten zur Verfügung. Senkung des Antriebs und der Stimmung bewirken Ruhe des Organismus, Erhöhung der Reizempfänglichkeit und Verstimmung Ablassen von schädlichem Tun, und der Schlaf ist schließlich der unentbehrliche, umfassende Ausgleicher, der vermittels einer Umstellung des gesamten Stoffwechselgetriebes die angegebenen vitalen Kräfte wieder ersetzt und damit ein neues aktionsfähiges Gleichgewicht schafft. Die ,,vitale Person" ist also als weitere, schon halbwegs psychische Regulationsinstanz dem vegetativen System, der KRAUSschen ,,Tiefenperson", unmittelbar angeschlossen.

Schädigungen, die an irgendeiner Stelle das vegetative System treffen, werden, wenn sie nur stark genug sind, um bis zum Zwischen-Mittelhirn hinauf Funktionsänderungen zu bewirken, allermeist auch zu Veränderungen innerhalb der ,,vitalen Person" führen. Je nach Ursache und Angriffspunkt mögen solche vitalen Funktionsverschiebungen anders aussehen. Man gelangt auf diese Weise zu einer Reihe von ,,vitalen Syndromen", die charakterisiert sind durch das Ineinandergreifen von körperlichen, insbesondere vegetativen

Funktionsverschiebungen und von Störungen psychischer Art, die sich auf solche der „vitalen Person" zurückführen lassen. Als solche vitalen Syndrome sind sehr bekannt gewisse innersekretorisch bedingte Störungen wie die BASEDOWsche Krankheit, der Eunuchoidismus, das Klimakterium, ferner chronische Vergiftungen, wie der Morphinismus, das STERTZsche Zwischenhirnsyndrom und manche andere mehr. Unter anderen gehören unseres Erachtens zu diesen vitalen Syndromen auch die konstitutionelle Nervosität und die n. R.

Jede Tätigkeit des Organismus im Wachsein, psychische wie körperliche, bedarf, um überhaupt vor sich gehen zu können, der vitalen Kräfte, die von der Gesamtheit der Zellfunktionen geschaffen und vom vegetativen Geschehen bereitgestellt werden. Kraftausgabe führt also im vegetativen System zu Gleichgewichtsschwankungen, die durch seine regulierenden Funktionen wieder ausgeglichen werden müssen, indem neue, während der Ruhe und des Schlafs gesammelte, vitale Kräfte eingesetzt werden. Bei länger fortgesetzter Tätigkeit wird ein Augenblick erreicht, in dem die in der Ruhephase gesammelten Kräfte schließlich ausgegeben sind; statt dessen haben sich im Stoffwechselkreislauf die Dissimilationsprodukte — Ermüdungsgifte — so erheblich vermehrt, daß nunmehr ihre lähmende Wirkung beginnt: Es tritt Müdigkeit ein, die Schlaf-Wach-Funktion drängt zur Vollziehung der vegetativen Gesamtumstellung, die endlich, wenn sie nicht durch Willensimpulse oder äußere Reize gehindert wird, im Schlafe stattfindet. Wird sie aber gehindert, so kann der Organismus seine Tätigkeit dennoch weiter ausüben, indem er nunmehr seine Reservekräfte einsetzt. Daß diese Reservekräfte keineswegs gering sind, haben wir im Kriege erfahren, in dem wir immer wieder mit Erstaunen die ungeheuren psychischen und körperlichen Leistungen selbst schwächlicher Individuen beobachteten (BONHOEFFER, NONNE, BUMKE u. a.).

Über die physiologischen Vorstellungen, die man sich von diesen Vorgängen der Ermüdung, Übermüdung und Erschöpfung machen kann, haben wir oben gesprochen. Es ist kein Zweifel, daß hierbei dem vegetativen System, wie wir es oben geschildert haben, besondere Anstrengungen zugemutet werden müssen. Namentlich die Schlaf-Wachfunktion wird dabei am physiologischen Ablauf behindert, sie ist nicht mehr imstande, die immer mehr angehäuften giftigen Dissimilationsprodukte zu beseitigen und dem Organismus die periodische Ruhe zu geben, deren er zur Wiederherstellung seiner Kräfte bedarf. Der Mangel an Funktionskräften führt zu Schwächung und Unzulänglichkeit aller psychischen und körperlichen Tätigkeit, aber auch zu immer schwererem Versagen der vegetativen Funktionen und ihrer Regulationen, die durch übermäßige Inanspruchnahme hervorgerufene „krankhafte Überempfindlichkeit" (GOLDSCHEIDER) zu immer größerer Erregbarkeit und Ermüdbarkeit des Gesamtorganismus, namentlich aber seines vegetativen Regulators. Schließlich kommt es durch immer weiter fortgesetzte Inanspruchnahme einerseits und immer weiter fortschreitende Unzulänglichkeit der vegetativen Funktionen andererseits zu einem Circulus vitiosus mit schwereren nicht mehr ohne weiteres ausgleichbaren Regulationsstörungen im vegetativen System; falsche Funktionsgewohnheiten schleifen sich ein, die Überempfindlichkeit wird eine Dauererscheinung; durch die vegetativen Regulationsstörungen werden endlich im Körperlichen die bekannten nervösen Funktionsunregelmäßigkeiten, z. B. am Herz-Gefäßsystem, im Psychischen die charakteristische neurasthenische Veränderung der „vitalen Person", Antriebsschwäche, Schlafstörungen, Verstimmung und reizbare Schwäche mit ihren sekundären Wirkungen auf höhere psychische Schichten, Willen, Gedächtnis, Affekte, Triebe usw. hervorgerufen.

Es mag heute noch nicht möglich sein, sich über das, was wir flüchtig skizziert haben, hinaus Vorstellungen über den Ort des Angriffs der neurasthenischen

Schädigung und die Einzelheiten ihres Ablaufs zu machen. Wenn man der Meinung ist, daß es sich beim Vegetativum um ein in sich bis zu einem gewissen Grade geschlossenes System von aufeinander abgestimmten Funktionen handelt, kann es schließlich auch relativ gleichgültig sein, ob der Ansatzpunkt der Störung peripher bei den Organzellen oder bei ihrem vegetativ-innersekretorischen Regulationsapparat oder am Zwischen-Mittelhirn selbst gesucht werden muß. Genug, daß jede Schädigung, sie möge angreifen wo sie wolle, vermöge ihrer engen Korrelation auf *alle* Glieder des Systems wirken kann, und daß namentlich die höchste Instanz, das Zwischen-Mittelhirn stets durch Regulationsstörungen an diesen Vorgängen beteiligt ist.

Wenn wir dem Zwischen-Mittelhirn dabei eine besonders wichtige Rolle zuschreiben, so deswegen, weil, soweit unsere Kenntnisse bisher reichen, von hier aus das gleichzeitige Auftreten körperlicher und psychischer Symptome am einleuchtendsten erklärt werden kann, dann aber auch, weil es diese zentrale Regulationsstelle ist, die vermöge ihrer Mittlerrolle zwischen Körper und Seele unmittelbar sowohl körperlichen als auch psychischen Schädigungen in gleicher Weise ausgesetzt ist. Übermäßige Inanspruchnahme des Systems, die schließlich zu neurasthenischen Störungen führt, kann nämlich, wie wir noch genauer sehen werden, nicht nur durch körperliche Erschöpfung, sondern erst recht durch psychische, zumal affektive Anforderungen überstarker Art herbeigeführt werden. Als Beispiel eines plötzlichen, sehr heftigen Stoßes, der vom Psychischen aus die „vitale Person" und ihr Funktionssubstrat treffen kann, haben wir a. a. O. den Schreck beschrieben. Es ist kein Zufall, wenn dem Schreck, der neben psychischen bekanntlich auch körperliche Störungen hervorbringt, in der n. R. erhebliche pathogenetische Wirksamkeit zugeschrieben wird (BIRNBAUM, GAUPP, HAUPTMANN u. a.).

Es versteht sich von selbst, daß die Beschaffenheit des vegetativen Systems, seine Widerstandsfähigkeit gegenüber schädlichen Einwirkungen, die Kraft und Funktionssicherheit seiner Regulierungen, konstitutionellen Bedingungen unterliegen und daher von Hause aus sehr verschieden sein können. Jemand, dessen vegetative Regulierungen angeborener- und ererbtermaßen schwächlich und unsicher sind, wird naturgemäß Schädigungen, die gerade dieses Regulationssystem treffen, leichter unterliegen, als jemand, der von vornherein über „stählerne" Nerven verfügt. · Mit anderen Worten: Der konstitutionell Nervöse, wie wir den Menschen mit *angeborener* reizbarer Schwäche der vegetativnervösen Regulierungsfunktionen nennen, wird einer n. R. schon dann erliegen, wenn die psychischen oder körperlichen Schädigungen vom Robusten noch kaum registriert oder jedenfalls mit Leichtigkeit überwunden werden. Es ist kein Zufall, wenn wir im klinischen Alltagsbetrieb immer wieder eine n. R. statt in die grundsätzlich zu erwartende Genesung in die chronischen Funktionsstörungen der konstitutionellen Nervosität übergehen sehen. Es ist eben bei beiden das gleiche Funktionssubstrat, das einmal konstitutionell minderwertig ist und zum andern von der exogenen neurasthenisch machenden Schädigung getroffen wird.

Wir wollen an dieser Stelle die theoretischen Erörterungen über das Wesen der n. R. abbrechen, obwohl wir manche Fragestellungen, die sich namentlich aus unserer Anschauung vom Funktionssubstrat der n. R. ergeben, noch nicht berührt haben. Das trifft vor allem auf die sog. pseudoneurasthenischen Erscheinungen zu, wie sie z. B. bei beginnender Arteriosklerose, als Einleitungsphase des Hirntumors, als Folgezustände nach Hirntraumen, bei gewissen innersekretorischen Störungen und als postinfektiöse Schwächezustände bekannt sind. Wir möchten glauben, daß sich diese Erscheinungen in befriedigender Weise in den Rahmen unserer oben dargelegten Anschauungen einfügen lassen würden, wollen aber hier davon absehen, unsere Darstellung auf die pseudoneurasthenischen Zustände, die traditionsgemäß nicht mehr zur n. R. i. e. S. gerechnet werden, auszudehnen.

Wir haben die theoretischen Erörterungen über das Wesen der n. R. überhaupt namentlich deswegen etwas länger ausgesponnen, weil uns hier sehr viel mehr als im rein Klinisch-symptomatischen die eigentliche heutige Problematik der n. R. zu liegen scheint. Mehr und mehr setzt sich, wie wir glauben, im Gebiet der sog. funktionellen psychisch-nervösen Störungen der Gedanke durch, daß nur von ihrer biologischen Unterlegung aus — unbeschadet aller Psychologie — ein befriedigendes Verständnis dieser Erscheinungen gewonnen werden kann. Das hat z. B. BUMKE von jeher betont, das klingt immer wieder aus den zusammenfassenden Darstellungen im Handbuch der Psychiatrie — STERTZ nimmt z. B. gerade für die n. R. eine Beteiligung des Hirnstamms an — und ergibt sich endlich aus den Bemühungen SZONDIs und anderer Autoren, die die innere Sekretion in den Vordergrund ihrer Forschungen stellen. Hinter allen solchen Bemühungen steht der moderne Gedanke von der Einheit der menschlichen Persönlichkeit, der in körperlichen und psychischen Gegebenheiten keine Gegensätze, sondern einander ergänzende und über Bindeglieder von halbwegs körperlicher, halbwegs psychischer Beschaffenheit unmerklich ineinander übergehende Glieder eines unteilbaren Ganzen sieht.

II. Klinische Stellung und Ätiologie.

Indem wir uns nunmehr den klinischen Problemen der n. R. zuwenden, wird es zunächst unsere Aufgabe sein, eine Abgrenzung der n. R. gegenüber der Norm und gegenüber anderen klinischen Begriffen zu versuchen. Man begegnet überall im Gebiet der funktionellen nervösen Störungen bestimmten grundsätzlichen Schwierigkeiten, wenn es sich um die Umgrenzung einer einzelnen Erscheinungsform, sei es einer Reaktion, eines Persönlichkeitstyps oder einer Organneurose, handelt. Sie liegen in den fließenden Übergängen, die jede dieser Formen mit der Norm sowohl als auch mit benachbarten Erscheinungen verbinden (HOCHE, BUMKE). „..... eines wird bleiben", meint BUMKE gelegentlich, „auch eine zukünftige Psychiatrie wird auf starre Grenzlinien innerhalb dieses Gebietes verzichten und sich auf die Aufstellung typischer Konstitutionen und Reaktionen beschränken".

Die reine neurasthenische Reaktion. Auch bei der neurasthenischen Reaktion bestehen keine festen Grenzen, auch hier werden wir gut tun, uns einer typologischen Gliederung zu bedienen. Im Mittelpunkt unserer Betrachtung würde dann der Typ der *reinen n. R.* stehen, der nach der einen Seite mit nur einigermaßen willkürlich festsetzbarer Grenze in die Norm, nach einer anderen mit vollkommen fließenden Grenzen in die konstitutionelle Nervosität, nach einer dritten in Mischformen, wie sie durch die sog. pseudoneurasthenischen Erscheinungen repräsentiert werden, übergeht [1].

Die reine Form der n. R. entsteht bei Gesunden, nervös Robusten durch körperliche und — namentlich — psychische Erschöpfung als spezifische Ursache (BIRNBAUM); sie geht grundsätzlich in Heilung über. Es versteht sich, daß diese Fälle wenigstens zu normalen Zeiten recht selten sind (BONHOEFFER). Sie mögen im Kriege häufiger gewesen sein, obwohl hier wohl ihre Reinheit durch die Vielseitigkeit der Kriegsätiologie mit ihrem Nebeneinander von Aufregungen, Schreckerlebnissen, Infektionen und Intoxikationen beeinträchtigt wurde. Im Frieden sind es namentlich Menschen, die unter der Peitsche des Ehrgeizes

---

[1] CIMBAL hat im Kriege eine ähnliche Einteilung zwischen „reiner" und „komplizierter" Neurasthenie vorgeschlagen.

oder Erwerbstriebs sich einem Übermaß von schlafkürzender, verantwortungsvoller, mit Konkurrenz und ständiger psychischer Höchstspannung verbundener Tätigkeit unterziehen, die neurasthenisch werden. Oder solche, die einem langdauernden, Aufregungen und Sorgen bringenden Kampf um die bedrohte Existenz unterliegen, dessen Ängste und Depressionen sie bis in den Schlaf verfolgen. Bei beiden Gruppen mögen aber Intoxikationen durch Genußmittel — Alkohol, Nicotin, Kaffee — als Hilfsursache eine Rolle spielen; bei beiden sind es vornehmlich psychische, und zwar affektive Schädigungen, die zur Erschöpfung des Funktionssubstrats und damit zur neurasthenischen Regulationsstörung führen; bei beiden ist ferner der Schlafentzug, der die einzige wirksame Erholungsmöglichkeit ausschaltet, ein wichtiges — vielleicht das wichtigste — pathogenetische Moment. Demgegenüber spielt die einfache körperliche Erschöpfung für sich allein ebensowenig eine Rolle wie die reine, von Affekten nicht überladene geistige ,,Überarbeitung" (BUMKE), sofern beides durch ausreichenden Schlaf wieder ausgeglichen werden kann.

Wenn man vom Normalen her kommt, wird man aus praktischen Gründen gut tun, die Grenzen dieses Begriffs der n. R. nicht allzu weit zu ziehen. Jener Zustand der Übermüdung, den wohl jeder nach besonders großer körperlicher Anstrengung, besonders ausgedehnter nächtlicher geistiger Arbeit oder nach einer Gesellschaft, die gegen Morgen mit reichlichem Kaffeegenuß geendet hat, kennt, mag sich mit seiner Schlafstörung und Verstimmung, seinem Herzklopfen und seinen unangenehmen Sensationen zwar dem Wesen nach nicht von der n. R. unterscheiden, da ja Übermüdung von Erschöpfung nicht zu trennen ist (BONHOEFFER). Niemand aber wird diese leichtesten, durch den Schlaf einer Nacht wieder ausgleichbaren Störungen als n. R. bezeichnen.

Erst da, wo nervöse Regulationsstörungen eine gewisse Dauerhaftigkeit bekommen, wo sie trotz Schlafes von einer oder mehreren Nächten — sofern sie es dazu überhaupt kommen lassen — nicht verschwinden, pflegen wir von einer n. R. zu sprechen. Auch dann ist der Augenblick, in dem man beginnen will, nervöse Unregelmäßigkeiten als n. R. zu bezeichnen, bis zu einem gewissen Grade der Willkür überlassen. Praktisch bedeutet das allerdings keine allzu große Schwierigkeit, da der Arzt die n. R. im allgemeinen erst dann zu Gesicht bekommt, wenn sie voll ausgebildet ist.

Grenzen zur konstitutionellen Nervosität. Anders liegen die Dinge, wenn es sich um die Abgrenzung gegenüber Erscheinungsformen funktionell-nervöser Art, die wir oben als der n. R. benachbart erwähnt haben, handelt. Da ist zunächst die konstitutionelle Nervosität; ihr gegenüber ist eine klinische Grenzsetzung überhaupt so gut wie unmöglich. Von der klassischen Form der rein exogenen n. R. bis zur schweren konstitutionellen Nervosität, deren Erscheinungen wesentlich von der *endogenen* Regulationsschwäche bestimmt werden, läuft eine ununterbrochene Reihe von Übergangsfällen. Deshalb handelt es sich bei differentialdiagnostischen Bemühungen fast regelmäßig nicht um die einfache alternative Fragestellung: Nervosität *oder* n. R.?, sondern darum, wieweit endogene, wieweit exogene Strukturanteile das Zustandsbild bestimmen. Wenn man will, wird man den Großteil mindestens der *akuten* nervösen Erscheinungen der klinischen und poliklinischen Praxis als n. R. auffassen können; denn exogene Schädigungen körperlicher oder psychischer Art pflegen mit großer Regelmäßigkeit in den anamnestischen Angaben der Nervösen eine Rolle zu spielen. Aus dem Verhältnis oder Mißverhältnis zwischen Schädigung und Reaktion wird man allerdings zumeist von vornherein auf besondere, mehr oder minder starke Disposition im Sinne der konstitutionellen Nervosität schließen müssen. Dann aber, wenn die nervösen Erscheinungen nicht wie erwartet abklingen, wenn mehr und mehr endogene Mechanismen die führende Rolle im Zustandsbild übernehmen, wenn insbesondere hypochondrische, hysterische oder „nervöse" (ADLER) Entwicklungen einsetzen — auf andere differentialdiagnostische Kriterien kommen wir noch zurück —, wird man in zunehmendem Maße und schließlich allein in der endogenen Anlage und ihrer eigengesetzlichen Entwicklung die Grundlage der Störungen suchen müssen (BONHOEFFER).

Es mag zwischen nervöser Anlage und n. R. mannigfache Beziehungen geben. Es mag oft so sein, daß ein alltägliches Ereignis, ein kleiner Schreck im Straßenverkehr, ein kurzer Zwist mit dem Nachbarn oder eine etwas unbequeme Arbeit am Anfang langdauernder nervöser Beschwerden stehen. Dann hat die harmlose Schädigung — sofern man von einer solchen überhaupt sprechen will — offenbar eine Veranlagung getroffen, die aus irgendeinem innergesetzlichen Grunde reif zur Manifestation nach außen war; sie hat nicht mehr als pathogenetisches, sondern nur als auslösendes Moment den leichten Anstoß gegeben, der noch nötig war, um einen zum Ablauf bereiten Mechanismus in Bewegung zu setzen. Solche Fälle sind Legion; HORN hat einige von ihnen beschrieben, in denen — zweifellos zu Unrecht — von hohen Versorgungsbehörden Dienst- oder Berufsbeschädigung anerkannt wurde.

Im ganzen tut man in diagnostischer Hinsicht schon aus prognostischer Vorsicht gut, auch gegenüber der konstitutionellen Nervosität das Gebiet der n. R. möglichst einzuschränken. Selbst im Kriege wies die Mehrzahl der neurasthenisch Erkrankten psychopathische und nervöse Belastung auf (BONHOEFFER, NONNE u. a.). Insbesondere wird man nicht etwa daraus, daß bis zu der differentialdiagnostisch schwierigen nervösen Phase keine nervösen Erscheinungen bestanden haben — oder angeblich bestanden haben sollen —, den Schluß ziehen wollen, daß eine Veranlagung überhaupt keine Rolle spiele. Es ist sehr wohl möglich, daß eine latente Veranlagung, auch bei bis dahin überaus leistungsfähigen und anscheinend nervös robusten Menschen, durch eine erste schwere n. R. gewissermaßen mobilisiert wird, um von da an für lange Zeit nicht mehr zur Ruhe zu kommen. Wenn man unseren Meinungen über Pathogenese und Substrat der n. R. folgt, wird man hier unschwer den ersten Stoß erkennen, der ein an sich nicht sehr widerstandsfähiges, den landläufigen Anforderungen aber gerade noch gewachsenes, vegetativ-vitales Regulationssystem versagen und von nun an für lange Zeit nicht mehr ins Gleichgewicht kommen läßt.

Ich gebe als Beispiel einen Fall: [1]

Fall 1. O. L., Kellner, geb. 88. Mütterlicherseits mit verschiedenen Psychosen belastet. Selbst von Haus aus gesund, in der Schule und als aktiver Soldat besonders ehrgeizig und leistungsfähig. Im Kriege Unterseebootssteuermann, ungewöhnlich zuverlässig und tüchtig, nie nervös. 1915 schwere, aufregende Kriegsfahrt, bringt nach Ausfall der Offiziere das Boot selbständig in 10tägiger Fahrt bei fast völligem Schlafentzug in den Hafen. Unmittelbar nach der Landung erste neurasthenische Symptome, aus denen sich eine schwere n. R. entwickelt. Nach 4wöchiger Lazarettbehandlung geheilt, wieder U-Bootsdienst. 1917 nach ähnlicher, obwohl nicht so schwieriger Situation neue n. R. Seitdem nicht wieder ganz gesund, Garnisondienst, 1919 mit K.D.B.-Rente entlassen. Im Frieden auf der Werft, später Kellner. Stets etwas nervös, bei Konflikten, Berufsschwierigkeiten, stärkerer Anspannung usw. stärkere nervöse Beschwerden, öfter arbeitsunfähig, Erholungskuren. Als Kellner manchmal viel Alkohol. 1929 ungünstige soziale Lage, aufreibende Tätigkeit im Nachtcafé mit viel Alkohol. — Kopfdruck in Schläfen und Nacken, ermüdbar, Schlaflosigkeit, allgemeines Schwächegefühl, mißmutige, gedrückte Stimmung, innere Unruhe, reizbar, leicht aufgeregt, zittert und schwitzt dann, hat Herzklopfen. Überempfindlichkeit gegenüber Geräuschen. Impotenz bei erhaltener Libido. Ticartiges Zucken im Gesicht, Tachykardie, Dermographismus, lebhafte Reflexe, Fingertremor. Nach mehrwöchiger Behandlung gebessert entlassen.

Bei dem zwar erblich belasteten, aber bis zum 27. Lebensjahr anscheinend völlig gesunden, nervös robusten, besonders leistungsfähigen Mann hat schwere körperlich-seelische Schädigung zunächst zu einer typischen, nach einigen Wochen

---

[1] den ich schon in der „vitalen Person" als Fall 5 ausführlicher veröffentlicht habe,

überwundenen n. R. geführt; sie wiederholt sich, diesmal schon leichter auslösbar, 2 Jahre später, läßt jetzt aber eine dauernde Schädigung in Gestalt leichter, bei geringen exogenen Schädigungen exacerbierender, nervöser Regulationsstörungen zurück. Eine Dauerbereitschaft zu nervösen Reaktionen, die bis zum 30. Lebensjahr verborgen geblieben war, ist jetzt manifest geworden, und wenn auch neurastheniemachende Schädigungen bei schwereren Störungsphasen in der letzten Zeit mitwirken mögen: das Schwergewicht der Störungen ist entschieden nach dem Endogenen hin verschoben worden.

Fälle wie diesen mag HELLPACH im Auge haben, wenn er vor einer allzu schematischen günstigen Prognose bei der n. R. warnt. Manche Neurastheniker, meint er, seien nach Abklingen der akuten Reaktion „doch nicht mehr die Alten". Praktisch sind solche Erfahrungen natürlich vor allem bei der Begutachtung von Wichtigkeit. Man wird akute, schwere, neurasthenische Erscheinungen, zumal dann, wenn sie sich auf umschriebene, überdurchschnittlich schwere Schädigungen zurückführen lassen, ohne weiteres als Dienst-, Berufs- oder Arbeitsschädigung anerkennen können. Entwickelt sich aber aus diesem akuten Stadium ein chronisches, ohne daß neue Schädigungen dafür verantwortlich gemacht werden können, treten insbesondere stärkere psychologische Verarbeitung und gewisse Prädilektionssymptome der konstitutionellen Nervosität auf, dann wird man der zunehmenden Bedeutung konstitutioneller Momente auch im Gutachten Rechnung tragen müssen. Der Zeitpunkt, in dem man zu solche differentialdiagnostischen Erwägungen gestellt wird, mag je nach Lage des Falles, Schwere und Dauer der schädigenden Einwirkung sehr unterschiedlich sein. Nach unseren Erfahrungen entscheidet sich diese Frage bei sonst günstiger — therapeutischer usw. — Lage des Falles spätestens 4—6 Monate nach Beginn der n. R. Setzt sich freilich der Neurasthenische, bevor die Rekonvaleszenz, also ein besonders neurasthenie-empfängliches Stadium, beendet ist, neuen Schädigungen aus, so wird ein echter Rückfall möglich sein; ja, es ist denkbar, daß sich bei immer neuen Schädigungen eine Kette von n. R. über Jahre hinzieht, ohne daß eine angeborene Bereitschaft im Sinne der konstitutionellen Nervosität dabei eine Rolle zu spielen braucht.

Fall 2. M. E., geb. 78, Krankenschwester. Vater und Bruder Diabetiker. Sonst keine erbliche Belastung. Von Haus aus sehr gesund und leistungsfähig, nie nervös. Kurze, kinderlose Ehe. Danach mit 23 Jahren Krankenschwester. 1915 Oberschwester in einem türkischen Kriegslazarett. Pflegte unter ungünstigsten Verhältnissen bei sehr großen Anstrengungen, Entbehrungen und Gefahren jahrelang schwer Seuchenkranke. Nachweislich beste Leistungen. Seit 1917 Schwester in Erholungsheimen und Feldlazaretten in Palästina. Auch hier schwere Anstrengungen und Entbehrungen in tropischem Klima, trotzdem niemals versagt. Juli 18 ruhrähnlicher Darmkatarrh. Wegen Personalmangels erst nach 4 Wochen Heimatsurlaub; wegen Truppenverschiebungen sehr erschwerte Heimreise, wochenlange Aufenthalte in unzivilisierten Orten, erst 4 Wochen später in Deutschland. In Kissingen Heilung des Darmkatarrhs, mehrfache, schließlich erfolgreiche Bandwurmkuren. Noch anämisch und „erholungsbedürftig" entlassen. Mehr und mehr treten jetzt neurasthenische Symptome in den Vordergrund. Ständige Müdigkeit und Kraftlosigkeit bei Schlaflosigkeit, überempfindlich, menschenscheu, grundlose Depressionen und Tränenausbrüche. April 19 gebessert; aber jetzt tritt ein Unterleibsleiden (Lageveränderung) hinzu, wegen dessen sie sich in gynäkologischer Behandlung geben muß; außerdem im Sommer 1919 heftiger Rückfall des Darmkatarrhs. Versorgungszeugnis vom Januar 1920 erkennt Neurasthenie als K.D.B. an. Seit September 1920 wieder in der Krankenpflege tätig. April 1921 wieder Rückfall des Darmkatarrhs mit neuer Verschlimmerung der neurasthenischen Beschwerden. Seit Ende 1921 wieder Krankenpflege. 1922 Abfindung der Rente; Blutarmut und Nervenschwäche nicht mehr nachweisbar. Mehrere Anträge auf Heilverfahren in den nächsten Jahren abgelehnt. Indessen Verlust des Vermögens, Stellungslosigkeit, schwierige wirtschaftliche Situation. Dazu Klimakterium mit starken Beschwerden. 1926—1930 in Amerika in Stellung. Dort Anfang 1928 an — zunächst nicht erkannter perniziöser Anämie mit langsam fortschreitender funikulärer Myelose erkrankt. 1930 völliger Zusammenbruch zugleich mit fieberhafter Grippe. Rücktransport nach Deutschland, Erkennung und Behandlung der organischen Störungen. 1932 Begutachtung:

Anämie und funikuläre Myelose nur noch in — allerdings charakteristischen — Resten nachzuweisen. Klagen über Schwächegefühl, innere Ruhelosigkeit bei starker Ruhebedürftigkeit, Erregbarkeit und Reizbarkeit, schlechte Stimmung, emotionelle Schwäche, Schlafstörungen; bei Aufregung und Anstrengung Herzklopfen und dumpfer Kopfdruck. Die Augenklinik (Geheimrat HEINE) führt eine Schwäche des äußeren Augenmuskelapparates auf Neurasthenie zurück. Die Klagen werden durch den objektiven Befund größtenteils bestätigt. Ungewöhnlich starke, explosive Affektäußerungen und Tränenausbrüche bei kleinem Anlaß. Einschläge von Verbitterung und Rentenkampfstellung, leichte hypochondrische Einstellung.

Fälle wie dieser, in denen man trotz intensiven Bemühens letzte Zweifel an der Grundlage der nervösen Erscheinungen nicht beseitigen kann, begegnen einem gerade in der Gutachtertätigkeit [1] relativ häufig. Immerhin scheint uns bei der Krankenschwester, wenigstens für die Jahre 1918—1921, der Hauptakzent auf den exogenen Reaktionen zu liegen, von denen eine der anderen folgte, bevor die vorhergehende schon völlig abgeklungen war. Gerade das Rekonvaleszenzstadium, in dem Regulationsstörungen eben erst halbwegs überwunden und jederzeit zu neuem Ausbruch bereit sind, ist — das ist auch therapeutisch von Wichtigkeit — neuen, auch verhältnismäßig leichten Schädigungen gegenüber besonders gefährdet. Man mag sich schließlich an die „Einschleifung" von Fehlfunktionen erinnern, jenen Vorgang, dem KRETSCHMER auf einem nicht allzu weit abliegenden psychopathologischen Gebiete eine besondere Wirksamkeit zugesprochen hat. In ähnlichem Sinne mag durch eine einmalige neurasthenische Regulationsstörung die Bereitschaft zu weiteren erworben werden und vielleicht für lange Zeit erhalten bleiben. Gerade bei Fällen wie dem geschilderten, für die ungewöhnliche Leistungs- und Widerstandsfähigkeit bis zur ersten neurasthenischen Reaktion geradezu charakteristisch ist, bei denen erst ausnahmsweise schwere und langdauernde Schädigungen zum neurasthenischen Erliegen geführt haben, fällt die Annahme einer angeborenen Veranlagung besonders schwer. Andererseits taucht natürlich die Frage auf, weshalb denn gerade hier die n. R. nicht recht zur Ausheilung kommt, auch nachdem die Reihe der Schädigungen endlich für Jahre abgerissen ist, und weshalb schließlich noch nach einem Jahrzehnt verhältnismäßig geringfügige Schädigungen wie leichte BIERMERsche Krankheit und Grippe zu neuem neurasthenischem Zusammenbruch führen. In solchen Fällen wird man schließlich doch resignieren müssen. Zweifellos gibt es nicht nur akute, sondern auch chronische nervöse Zustände, in denen sich endogene und exogene Komponenten auf keine Weise sicher voneinander trennen lassen.

Körperliche Krankheiten und Schädigungen als Ursachen. Wir wollen damit das Gebiet der Differentialdiagnose und der Abgrenzung der n. R. von der konstitutionellen Nervosität verlassen, um zu einem benachbarten überzugehen, das wir im Fall 2 schon gestreift haben. Während wir bisher nur von der Erschöpfungsätiologie der n. R. sprachen, haben wir hier die n. R. aus Schädigungen entstehen sehen, bei denen neben der Erschöpfung körperliche Erkrankungen, eine Infektion, ein gynäkologisches Leiden, eine Blutkrankheit die maßgebliche Rolle spielen. Natürlich gehen körperliche Krankheiten, namentlich soweit sie chronisch und mit starkem Verbrauch der Körperkräfte und ihres Zellsubstrates verbunden sind, mit Erschöpfung einher. Chronischer Schmerz muß schließlich zur krankhaften Reizbarkeit führen, die Blut- oder Herzkrankheit die Sauerstoffversorgung ungenügend machen oder das Frauenleiden zu innersekretorischen Verschiebungen Anlaß geben. Mannigfache Wege mögen von körperlichen Erkrankungen her

---

[1] Wir gehen im übrigen im Rahmen dieser Arbeit auf das Problem der Begutachtung funktionell-nervöser Störungen grundsätzlich nicht näher ein und verweisen dafür auf das einschlägige Kapitel dieses Handbuches, ferner auf die Arbeiten von REICHARDT, STIER, HOCHE, v. WEIZSÄCKER, RIESE und die Verhandlungen über die Unfallneurose im Reichsarbeitsministerium vom Jahre 1929.

über Stoffwechsel und innere Sekretion zu den Regulationsstörungen führen, die der n. R. zugrunde liegen. Bei der fieberhaften Infektionskrankheit aber kommt noch etwas besonderes dazu: Die Vergiftung. Wie immer man sich den Vorgang der Intoxikation durch Infektionserreger oder ihre Toxine vorstellen mag, das vegetative System wird jedenfalls sehr frühzeitig und sehr ausgiebig dabei in Mitleidenschaft gezogen. Schon das Infektionsprodrom zeigt — wir haben andernorts darauf hingewiesen — ein „vitales Syndrom", d. h. eine Verkopplung von vegetativen Symptomen — Herzklopfen, Schweißausbrüche, Kopfweh, Frösteln — mit vitalen Störungen — Antriebsschwäche, Verstimmung, Schlafstörung, Reizbarkeit. Das Fieber, das ja von den Physiologen als Ausdruck einer Regulationsstörung des Wärmehaushalts — KREHL z. B. nimmt als Funktionssubstrat dieser Regulation das Gebiet des Tuber cinereum an — aufgefaßt wird (ISENSCHMIDT, FREUND), ist eine bis zu einem gewissen Grade charakteristische Begleiterscheinung der Allgemeininfektion, die ihrerseits wieder mit heftiger Alteration des vegetativen Systems einhergeht. Während des ganzen Kampfes des Organismus mit dem Infektionserreger steht also das vegetative System mit seinen Regulationen gewissermaßen in vorderster Front; es wird von den Toxinen in erster Linie geschädigt und zugleich zu heftigster Gegenaktion aufgepeitscht. Es ist nicht weiter sonderbar, wenn es schließlich in erschöpftem und überempfindlichem Zustand zurückbleibt, und seine Regulationen unter Umständen noch auf lange hinaus neurasthenische Unsicherheit zeigen. Wie lange das der Fall ist, hängt wiederum von Schwere, Art und Dauer der Infektion einerseits und dem — angeborenen oder erworbenen — Zustand des vegetativen Systems andererseits ab.

Erschöpfung und Vergiftung lassen sich also bei der Infektionskrankheit im allgemeinen nicht auseinanderhalten. Daß überhaupt toxische Vorgänge an der Pathogenese beteiligt sind, ergibt sich am ehesten bei jenen leichten kurzdauernden Infektionen, die — wie manche Grippeanfälle — kaum zu Fieber, vielleicht nicht einmal zu Bettlägerigkeit führen und dennoch ein ausgesprochenes neurasthenisches Syndrom hinterlassen.

Eindeutiger liegen jene Fälle, in denen übermäßiger Gebrauch von Genußmitteln, Alkohol, Kaffee, Tee, Nicotin, Morphium, zu neurasthenischen Zuständen führt. Auch hier mag zwar der Schlafentzug, der etwa mit dem Alkoholmißbrauch aus äußeren Gründen verbunden zu sein pflegt, von Kaffee, Tee, Nicotin aber künstlich erzeugt wird, eine pathogenetische Hilfsrolle spielen. Daß aber die Hauptschädigung toxischer Art sein muß, geht schon aus der prompten Wirkung dieser Mittel auf das vegetativ-vitale System hervor. Diese Wirkungen sind es ja gerade, wegen deren diese „Stimmungsgifte" immer wieder gesucht werden.

Im praktischen Einzelfall wird es allermeist so liegen, daß in der Ätiologie der n. R. sowohl vergiftende als auch erschöpfende Momente zu finden sind[1]. Das hat sich besonders im Kriege erwiesen, der uns ja ein sehr großes Erfahrungsmaterial gebracht hat. In vielen Fällen ist es eben nicht eine einzige starke Wurzel, etwa schwere Infektion oder extreme Überanstrengung, aus der die n. R. erwächst, sondern es sind zahlreiche schwächere und schwächste, die erst im Zusammenwirken stark genug werden, um die vegetativ-vitale Regulationsstörung hervorzurufen. Schon aus praktischen Gründen wird es deshalb nicht tunlich

---

[1] Einzig und allein die infektiöse Intoxikation für alle nervösen Symptome verantwortlich zu machen, wie PÄSSLER es neuerdings will, heißt meines Erachtens wiederum die toxische Ätiologie einseitig überwerten. Gewiß mag PÄSSLER, indem er auf die toxische, neurastheniemachende Wirkung chronischer Tonsillitiden, Alveolarpyorrhöen und Zahnwurzelkrankheiten hinweist, damit einen Sonderfall der Neurasthenieentwicklung treffen. Allzu häufig scheinen mir diese Fälle aber nicht zu sein.

sein, die toxisch verursachte von der Erschöpfungsneurasthenie zu trennen. Die Mehrzahl der Autoren (BUMKE, STERTZ) — denen wir uns anschließen wollen — folgt denn auch dem Modus, die toxisch verursachten nervösen Störungen mit in die n. R. einzubeziehen, und wenn z. B. HAUPTMANN die n. R. nur auf die Fälle beschränken will, in denen aktive Überanstrengung zu nervösen Symptomen führt, dann scheint uns das — wir schließen uns hier STERTZ an — eine allzu enge Begriffsfassung, die der praktischen Wirklichkeit nicht ganz gerecht wird.

Zur echten n. R. gehören demnach auch die hyperästhetisch-emotionellen Schwächezustände, die BONHOEFFER als Folgezustände nach symptomatischen Psychosen zuerst beschrieben hat, und die ja auch nach unkomplizierten Infektionskrankheiten etwas Häufiges sind.

Anders oder wenigstens praktisch einfacher liegen die Dinge dann, wenn neurasthenische Zustände im Rahmen und auf der Grundlage andersartiger, funktioneller oder organischer, somatischer oder cerebraler Krankheiten auftreten. Hier sind zunächst die innersekretorisch bedingten nervösen Störungen zu nennen. Wir haben oben schon gelegentlich ausgeführt, daß wir die Beteiligung des Endokriniums an der n. R. für wahrscheinlich halten müssen, sei es, daß innersekretorische Verschiebungen im Sinne des prädisponierenden Moments wirksam werden, sei es, daß das endokrine Drüsensystem von der exogenen Noxe direkt oder auf dem Umwege über seine vegetativen Korrelationen angegriffen wird. Hier handelt es sich nun um umschriebene und bis zu einem gewissen Grade spezifische Störungen, deren Grund oder doch wenigstens ausschlaggebende Ursache im Versagen einer *bestimmten* Drüse gesucht wird. Es ist üblich und entspricht wohl auch den klinischen Erfordernissen, daß diese i. e. S. innersekretorisch bedingten nervösen Zustände, etwa die BASEDOWsche Krankheit oder das Klimakterium, von der n. R. getrennt werden, obwohl es auch hier Übergangs- und Mischfälle geben mag, bei denen die differentialdiagnostische Entscheidung mehr der Willkür anheimgestellt ist.

Ähnlich liegen die Verhältnisse in bezug auf die sogenannten **pseudoneurasthenischen Erscheinungen,** jene nervösen Erscheinungen also, die als Einleitungssyndrom der Arteriosklerose (RAECKE, PICK, BUMKE), der Lues cerebri und progressiven Paralyse (BOSTROEM), des Hirntumors, mancher anderen organischen Hirnerkrankung, als Folgezustand nach Hirnverletzungen (PFEIFER, FRIEDMANN) usw. auftreten. STERTZ, der eine ziemlich weite Fassung des Neurastheniebegriffs bevorzugt, ist geneigt, auch sie zu den echten n. R. zu rechnen, während z. B. BUMKE sie bei ihren Grundkrankheiten abhandelt, obwohl auch er innere Beziehungen dieser exogenen Reaktionsformen zur n. R. für möglich hält. Vielleicht wird eine zukünftige Zeit imstande sein, solchen Meinungen exaktere Grundlagen zu geben, als wir sie heute haben. Gerade Vorstellungen, wie wir sie über die pathogenetische Beteiligung des vegetativen Systems mit seinen cerebralen Regulationen für die n. R. entwickelt haben, werden hier vielleicht als Arbeitshypothese von Nutzen sein.

Solche Bemühungen, die auf eine den neurasthenischen und pseudoneurasthenischen Erscheinungen gemeinsame pathogenetische Grundlage abzielen, ändern natürlich nichts an der Tatsache, daß klinisch die jeweils verschiedene organische Grundkrankheit durchaus im Mittelpunkt aller diagnostischen und therapeutischen Maßnahmen stehen muß. Dabei wird bei der Arteriosklerose der beginnenden Gefäßerkrankung (BINSWANGER und SCHAXEL), bei der Lues der allgemeinen oder lokalen infektiösen Schädigung des Hirns und seiner Häute (BOSTROEM), beim Tumor dem Hirndruck und der Hirnschwellung (REDLICH, REICHARDT, PFEIFER), bei Verletzungen und Erschütterungen der

Schädigung des Gesamthirns, der Zirkulationsstörung, der toxischen Gewebsdegeneration, den Druckverschiebungen (POPPELREUTER, HORN, GOLDSTEIN, WINDSCHEID, FRIEDMANN) und dem Narbenzug (FÖRSTER, SCHWAB, HAUPTMANN) besonderer Wert beizulegen sein.

Die Differentialdiagnostik innerhalb dieses Grenzgebiets stellt bekanntlich an Verantwortungsbewußtsein und Gründlichkeit des Untersuchers oft sehr hohe Anforderungen. Dabei kann das Symptombild selbst noch lange Zeit rein neurasthenisch bleiben, wenn die einstweilen symptomlose Entwicklung der organischen Grundkrankheit schon begonnen hat. In solchen Fällen können Anamnese und Begleitumstände der Erkrankung Hinweise auf eine organische Grundlage enthalten. Wenn neurasthenische Beschwerden zum ersten Male im 5. oder 6. Lebensjahrzehnt auftreten, wenn unerträglicher, nächtlich exacerbierender Kopfschmerz das erste und konstanteste Symptom ist, wenn eine sorgfältige, namentlich auch nach psychogenen Schädigungen forschende Anamnese keinen hinreichend verständlichen Grund für die n. R. und auch keine konstitutionelle Bereitschaft im Sinne der Nervosität aufdeckt, endlich aber auch, wenn neurasthenische Beschwerden beim nicht oder nicht erheblich Disponierten der Therapie über Monate hin trotzen, dann wird der Verdacht auf organische Grundlagen des Zustands auftauchen und entsprechende diagnostische und therapeutische Bemühungen fordern. Selbstverständlich ist man dabei besser allzu vorsichtig als allzu schnell beruhigt. Auch ein konstitutionell Nervöser kann an einem Hirntumor, auch der Herzneurotiker — obwohl nicht übermäßig häufig (FINKELNBURG) — an Arteriosklerose erkranken; und selbst dann, wenn die n. R. an sich symptomatologisch und pathogenetisch genügend gesichert scheint, darf damit das Vorhandensein organisch-cerebraler Hilfsursachen noch nicht als völlig ausgeschlossen gelten. Wir geben einen Fall als Beispiel solcher Schwierigkeiten:

Fall 3. M. M., geb. 95, Redakteur. Keine erbliche Belastung bekannt. Von Haus aus gesund, robust, besonders strebsam und arbeitskräftig. Buchdrucker und Schriftsetzer gelernt. 1915—1918 im Krieg, leicht verwundet, sonst keinerlei Krankheit. Nach dem Krieg ungewöhnlich angestrengt tätig, 16—19 Arbeitsstunden täglich als Schriftsetzer, nebenbei Weiterbildung zum Redakteur. Ende 1918 schwere fieberhafte Grippe mit starkem Schlafbedürfnis. Noch nicht erholt wieder im Beruf tätig. Anfang 1919 heftige Kopfschmerzen, tags erträglich, nachts heftiger und schlafstörend, in 3wöchigen Perioden mit monatelangen Pausen auftretend. Trotzdem sehr angestrengt als politischer Redakteur unter einem ungeduldigen, höchste Anforderungen stellenden Chef tätig. 1924 Grippe mit Fieber, Schlaflosigkeit und Kopfschmerzen, im Anschluß daran neuralgische Schmerzen in beiden Beinen. Seit dieser Krankheit Verstärkung der nervösen Beschwerden. 1928 im Anschluß an besonders heftige Kopfschmerzen vorübergehend Doppelbilder mit Schwäche der Muskulatur des linken Auges. Zugleich besonders unruhiger und kurzer Schlaf. Nach 4 Wochen ambulanter Behandlung ist die Augenmuskelstörung behoben, der nervöse Zustand wieder gebessert. — Seit Anfang 1932 wieder Verstärkung der nervösen Beschwerden. Anhaltende heftige Schmerzen in linker Schläfe und linker Stirn, etwas geringere im Hinterkopf und Nacken. Schwindelgefühl, Augenflimmern — aber keine Doppelbilder —, Schwanken beim Gehen, zumal in der Müdigkeit, fühlte sich einmal nach links hinten gezogen, so daß er fast gestürzt wäre. Eingewiesen im April 1932 aus der Medizinischen Klinik mit folgendem Bericht: Von seiten der Augen liegen beiderseits besonders links eine leichte Gesichtsfeldeinschränkung, eine geringe Atrophie des linken N. opticus und leichte Stauung der Venen, eine geringe Schwäche des linken Oculomotorius, leichte Anisokorie und Herabsetzung der Pupillenreaktionen vor. Die Augenklinik vermute einen entzündlichen Prozeß links vor dem Chiasma. Der Liquorbefund sei bis auf einen (im Liegen gemessenen) Lumbaldruck von 300 mm negativ. Luesreaktionen im Blut und Liquor negativ. Die Klinik vermute Tumor oder Meningitis serosa, halte aber auch Encephalitisfolgen für möglich. — Bei der ersten poliklinischen Untersuchung klagte M., abgesehen von den erwähnten körperlichen Beschwerden, über Schlaflosigkeit mit Zusammenfahren im Schlaf, allgemeine Übererregbarkeit mit Zittern, Herzklopfen, Schweißausbruch und Zunahme der Schmerzen bei Aufregung, mißmutige, grüblerische, zeitweise exacerbierende Verstimmung, müde Gleichgültigkeit und Antriebsschwäche. Die Untersuchung ergab außer sehr lebhaften Sehnenreflexen und leichtem Finger- und

Zungenzittern eine leichte Unsicherheit beim Finger-Nasen-Versuch links und vielleicht eine leichte Adiadochokinese links. — Wir vermuteten, daß außer der durch Infektion, Erschöpfung und übermäßige seelische Spannung verursachten n. R. ein organischer Krankheitskern dem Zustand zugrunde liege, wobei die Druckerhöhung und die leichten neurologischen Symptome am ehesten auf einen Tumor, die Vorgeschichte mit ihren Grippeanfällen und den vorübergehenden Doppelbildern und der Augenbefund auf einen encephalitischen Prozeß hinzuweisen schienen. — Eine Nachuntersuchung im Mai 1932 ergab das gleiche unklare Bild. — Ende Mai 1932 wurde M., nachdem ein aufregender, erschöpfender und schlafraubender Wahlkampf seinen neurasthenischen Zustand weiter verschlimmert hatte, zur Behandlung aufgenommen. Mehrfache eingehende neurologische Untersuchungen überzeugten uns schließlich, daß die leichten neurologischen Störungen, soweit sie überhaupt noch nachweisbar waren, nicht sicher zu verwerten waren; allerdings blieb der Augenbefund bestehen. M. war überaus ruhe- und einsamkeitsbedürftig und blieb das auch noch lange, nachdem die schweren Schlafstörungen, die zunächst das Bild beherrschten, in relativ kurzer Zeit überwunden waren. Auch die Verstimmungen, die auf kleinste Anlässe hin, oft aber auch ohne jeden erkennbaren Grund eintreten konnten, dauerten noch an, als die körperlichen Beschwerden, z. B. das Kopfweh, längst verschwunden waren. Unter sehr aktiver Behandlung, die u. a. mit gutem Erfolg die unspezifische Reizkörpertherapie in Gestalt von Milchinjektionen verwandte, trat nach einigen Monaten rasch fortschreitende Besserung mit Gewichtszunahme, Fortfall der körperlichen Beschwerden, gutem Schlaf, zunehmender psychischer Frische und guter, gleichmäßiger Stimmung ein. Anfang September 1932 wurde M. beschwerdefrei entlassen.

Es ist in diesem komplizierten Fall bis zuletzt unklar geblieben, ob der n. R., deren Entstehung durch Schlafentzug, Erschöpfung, Aufregung und Infektion an sich genügend begründet scheint, nicht doch ein organischer Hirnprozeß wenigstens als Hilfsursache mit zugrunde gelegen hat. Das mag am ehesten ein entzündlicher Vorgang gewesen sein, der vielleicht mit einer Meningitis serosa einherging und als Restsymptom den Augenbefund hinterlassen hat. Man mag daraus, daß die n. R. zu völligem Abklingen gekommen ist und daß die — von Anfang an nicht sehr sicheren — neurologischen Symptome völlig zurückgetreten sind, schließen, daß dieser organische Prozeß, welcher Art immer er sei, ebenfalls wenigstens vorläufig zur Ruhe gekommen ist. Man sieht aber aus solchen Fällen, wie innig sich neurasthenische und organisch-cerebrale Symptome miteinander mischen können, welche diagnostischen Schwierigkeiten dabei erwachsen können, und wieviel Vorsicht auch dann noch am Platze ist, wenn die Diagnose der n. R. an sich in Vorgeschichte und Symptombild ausreichend begründet erscheint.

Die psychischen Ursachen. Wir verlassen damit das Grenzgebiet zwischen der reinen n. R. und den sog. pseudoneurasthenischen Erscheinungen organischer Genese, um noch eine letzte Grenzsetzung zu versuchen, die gegenüber den sog. psychogenen Reaktionen. Psychogene Reaktionen — wir lehnen uns einer früher von uns gegebenen Definition an — sind jene ungewöhnlichen, aber im großen und ganzen in Entstehung und Äußerungsform verständlichen Reaktionen, die durch die emotionale Wirkung psychischer Erlebnisse verursacht werden. Wir haben schon kurz darauf hingewiesen, daß psychische Erlebnisse, insbesondere solche emotionellen Charakters, n. R. herbeiführen können, ja, daß die psychische Schädigung als Ursache wenigstens zu gewöhnlichen Zeiten sogar sehr häufig und als Hilfsursache fast immer anzutreffen ist. Dennoch ist die n. R. keine psychogene Reaktion im allgemein üblichen Sinne des Wortes.

STERTZ hat, wie uns scheint, das wesentliche Unterschiedsmerkmal hervorgehoben, indem er darauf hinweist, daß bei der psychogenen Reaktion ursächliches Erlebnis und Inhalt der Reaktion in verständlichem Zusammenhang stehen, während das bei der n. R. grundsätzlich nicht der Fall ist. Das deprimierende Erlebnis etwa führt verständlicherweise zu trauriger Verstimmung, die den wesentlichen Inhalt der depressiven Reaktion bildet, die explosive, die paranoide Reaktion bleibt wenigstens in ihrem Strukturkern „Erlebnis-Reaktion" einfühlbar. Anders die n. R. Hier handelt es sich um einen rein kausalen

Zusammenhang im JASPERSschen Sinn, einen wesentlich körperlichen Symptomenkomplex, der in gleicher unspezifischer Weise durch körperliche sowohl wie psychische Schädigungen verursacht werden kann. Kopfschmerzen, Schlaflosigkeit, ein Fingertremor, eine emotionelle Schwäche, die durch Verantwortungsdruck oder langdauernde seelische Spannung erzeugt sind, bleiben dem psychologischen Einfühlungsvermögen schließlich ebenso unzugänglich wie der Mitralfehler nach Gelenkrheumatismus. Gewiß gibt es auch im Rahmen der psychogenen Reaktionen körperliche Symptome der verschiedensten Art[1], aber sie bleiben, wenn man von den hysterischen Reaktions- und Persönlichkeitsformen absieht — die ja aber gerade in dieser Beziehung noch recht wenig „entlarvt" (HOCHE) sind —, relativ bedeutungslose Begleiterscheinungen, während das Geschehen der psychogenen Reaktion selbst psychologischen Gesetzen gehorcht und sich ausschließlich im Psychischen abspielt. Hier liegen also grundsätzliche Unterschiede zwischen der n. R. und den psychogenen Reaktionen, und wenn KRAEPELIN noch 1915 die n. R. unter den „psychogenen Erkrankungen" abhandelt — übrigens verfahren noch alle großen Lehrbücher ähnlich, indem sie die n. R. bei den psychopathischen und degenerativen Erscheinungsformen unterbringen —, so dürfte die weitere Entwicklung des Neurastheniebegriffs ihn trotz gelegentlicher Psychogenese mehr und mehr den exogenen Reaktionen annähern. Wir haben oben bereits darüber gesprochen.

Es wird zu fragen sein, wie man sich eine derartige uneinfühlbare, rein kausalen Gesetzen unterliegende Wirkung psychischer Erlebnisse auf halbwegs körperliche Funktionen, wie es die vegetativ-vitalen Regulationen sind, vorstellen soll. Wir werden auch hier das Moment der Erschöpfung in den Vordergrund stellen müssen und zunächst zu fragen haben, von welcher Art und Wirkungsweise psychische Erlebnisse sein müssen, wenn sie durch übermäßige Inanspruchnahme des Funktionssubstrats die oben näher charakterisierte neurasthenische Regulationsstörung herbeiführen sollen. Wir haben schon gelegentlich darauf hingewiesen, daß es nicht so sehr das Erlebnis als solches als vielmehr seine emotive Wirkung auf den Einzelnen ist, die zu neurasthenischen Erscheinungen führen kann, genau so übrigens, wie es allein Affektwirkungen sind, die sog. psychogene Reaktionen verursachen. Man weiß seit langem (E. WEBER 1910), daß seelische, zumal affektive Vorgänge Regulationsänderungen im körperlichen, insbesondere im vegetativen System, ganz besonders aber im Vasomotorium (KÜPPERS) hervorbringen. Experimentalpsychologische Untersuchungen (WEINBERG) und klinische Beobachtung (KNAUER und BILLIGHEIMER, HORN u. a.), die Physiologie (HESS) und die von HEYER und den Russen ausgebaute Reflexlehre PAWLOWS haben auf diesem Gebiete eine große Reihe von Einzelkenntnissen gewonnen, die v. WYSS letzthin monographisch zusammengefaßt und durch eigene Erfahrungen vermehrt hat.

Jede Emotion — soviel wollen wir diesem großen Sondergebiet entnehmen, ohne auf seine Einzelheiten eingehen zu können — läßt also Veränderungen im vegetativen System entstehen; sie sind am eingehendsten beim Schreck studiert, als dessen Folge KNAUER und BILLIGHEIMER vor allem einen „chokartigen Zusammenbruch des Vasomotoriums" neben zahlreichen anderen vegetativen Regulationsstörungen, Herzbeschleunigung, Arrhythmie, Veränderungen der Pupillenweite, abnormem Schwitzen, Blasenschwäche, trophischen Störungen der Nägel und Haare usw. nennen. Das sind also Symptome, die gerade in dieser Kombination wieder aufs Nachdrücklichste auf die regulativen Funktionen des Zwischenhirns hinweisen, deren Bedeutung für das vegetative System wir seit KARPLUS und KREIDL kennen. Wir selbst haben gelegentlich — nicht

---
[1] Wir verweisen auf die entsprechenden Kapitel in BUMKES Handbuch der Geisteskrankheiten.

zuletzt aus solchen Erfahrungen heraus — den Schreck als Beispiel eines reflexähnlichen Vorgangs dargestellt, der sich innerhalb der vitalen Schicht der Persönlichkeit — bei deren biologischer Unterlegung wir dem Zwischen-Mittelhirn eine wichtige Rolle zuwiesen — zwischen Reizempfang und Antrieb abspielt.

Ein schwerer Affektstoß wie der Schreck führt also zu sehr erheblichen akuten Regulationsstörungen im vegetativen, vor allem dem sympathischen System; sie mögen wohl einmal so schwer sein, daß vor Schreck der Tod eintritt, obwohl einwandfreie Fälle dieser Art nicht bekannt sind (KNAUER und BILLIGHEIMER). Demgegenüber wirken die emotiven Schädigungen, die zu den sehr viel weniger stürmischen, dafür aber um so hartnäckigeren Symptomen der n. R. führen, nicht in einmaligem schwerem Stoß wie der Schreck, sondern in lang hingezogener, zermürbender Minierarbeit; die Stöße, die hier das vegetative Regulationssystem treffen, mögen jeder für sich relativ leicht sein, aber sie wiederholen sich in unmittelbarer Folge so lange bis die Reservekräfte erschöpft sind, bis ein regulatorischer Ausgleich nicht mehr möglich ist und endlich ein letzter Stoß — der z. B. ein mehr oder minder gelinder Schreck sein mag — genügt, um die bis dahin mit letzter Willensanspannung verdeckte Regulationsstörung manifest zu machen.

Das gilt etwa für die emotiven Schädigungen des Krieges, bei denen Schreckerlebnisse, die Aufregungen des Kampfes, die dauernde Erwartungsspannung des Schützengrabendaseins, die Angst[1] des wehrlosen Beschossenwerdens einander ablösen. Wenn man dazu noch die Sorge um Familie und Beruf in der Heimat, die von HELLPACH unseres Erachtens über Gebühr in den Vordergrund gestellten Reibungen zwischen Vorgesetzten und Untergebenen und — zumal bei Offizieren — den Druck der Verantwortung, unbefriedigten Ehrgeiz, die im Laufe der Zeit immer schmerzlicher werdenden kulturellen und geistigen Entbehrungen nimmt, dann mögen damit noch immer nicht *alle* neurasthenisch machenden psychischen Kriegsschädigungen erfaßt sein. Im ganzen vereinen sich also — und das trifft auch für die Fälle des Friedens zum großen Teil zu — chronische, langhin wirkende affektive Belastungen mit immer wiederholten Emotionsstößen. Jede dieser emotionellen Alterationen für sich mag — wenigstens vom nervös Robusten — ohne Schwierigkeiten und nervöse Nachteile ertragen werden. Erst ihre Häufung, ihre unablässige Wiederholung oder ihre überlange Dauer führen endlich zum Versagen der Widerstandskraft, oder, um es in unserem Sinne mehr biologisch auszudrücken, zur Erschöpfung und damit zu Störungen und Verschiebungen im Regulationsgetriebe des vegetativ-vitalen Systems, wie wir sie im einleitenden Kapitel des Näheren charakterisiert haben. Hier scheint uns also, wenn wir der von uns skizzierten Arbeitshypothese folgen, das Bindeglied zu liegen, das den psychogen und den somatogen entstandenen neurasthenischen Symptomen gemeinsam ist: in der durch Erschöpfung entstandenen Regulationsstörung des vegetativ-vitalen Systems.

---

[1] Es fällt mir beim neuerlichen Studium der Kriegsliteratur — die übrigens in den Referaten von BIRNBAUM mustergültig zusammengefaßt ist — auf, wie wenig Wert der Angst als neurastheniefördernder Emotion beigelegt wird, obwohl ihre besonders starke Wirksamkeit auf körperliche Funktionen seit langem bekannt ist. Dabei scheint mir die dauernde, je nach den äußeren Umständen fast stets leise fühlbare, oft aber heftig anschwellende Angst (zu dieser vgl. KIERKEGAARD, HOCHE, KAHN, MISCH u. MISCH-FRANKL) die eindrucksvollste Emotion zu sein, die der Frontsoldat in diesem Kriege erlebte. Ich erinnere mich, daß Offiziere von Infanterieformationen, unter denen gewiß „Helden" waren, sich das oft gegenseitig eingestanden; ja, wir pflegten, wenn jemand behauptete, von Angst ganz frei zu sein, seinem Vermögen oder auch seinem Willen zur Selbstbeobachtung gewisse Zweifel entgegenzubringen. Das Heldentum dieses Krieges bestand nicht so sehr im Draufgängertum als vielmehr in der immer wiederholten Überwindung der Angst zugunsten der Pflichterfüllung. Ich bin davon überzeugt, daß dieser ständige heimliche Kampf mit der Angst die nervenzermürbendste Schädigung dieses Krieges gewesen ist.

Ähnliches gilt nun für die psychogenen n. Rn. der Friedenszeit, von denen wir charakteristische Typen schon eingangs dieses Kapitels erwähnt haben. Aber es liegt in der Natur der Dinge, daß hier die langhingezogenen, durch ihren unabwendbaren Druck zermürbenden seelischen Ursachen weitaus gegenüber den chokartig wirkenden Erlebnissen überwiegen. Gewiß mögen beim Börsenspekulanten oder beim ehrgeizigen Politiker auch Aufregungen, plötzliche schwere Enttäuschungen und Beängstigungen in das Ursachenbündel ihrer n. R. mit eingehen; gewiß mögen in den sehr seltenen Fällen von Verkehrs-, Explosions- oder Erdbebenkatastrophen (BAELZ, STIERLIN, HORN, BRUCHANSKY, BRUSSILOWSKI, BALABAN) schwere Schreckemotionen [1] vorkommen; aber die Mehrzahl der Fälle, die Heimatneurasthenie (HELLPACH) der Kriegerfrauen, die in jahrelanger ängstlicher Spannung um das Schicksal ihrer Männer, in Sorgen um die Existenz der Familie leben, die Neurasthenie des Kaufmanns, der in monate- und jahrelangem Kampf mit der Wirtschaftskrise seine Kräfte erschöpft, des debilen Studenten, der seiner intellektuellen Unzulänglichkeit die Fertigkeiten abzuringen sucht, die das drohend heranrückende Examen von ihm fordern wird (BUMKE), der berufstätigen Frau, die einer Verantwortung erliegt, der sie aus biologischen und psychologischen Gründen nicht gewachsen ist — um nur einige typische immer wiederkehrende Konstellationen zu nennen —, sie alle entstehen nicht so sehr aus einem plötzlichen Schlage, sondern aus der Erschöpfung durch die überlange und überstarke Anspannung der affektiven Funktionen und vegetativ-vitalen Regulationen.

„Die Emotion ist von der Erschöpfung nicht zu trennen", hat BONHOEFFER im Kriege einmal gesagt, um die unlösliche Verflechtung körperlicher und psychischer Wurzeln der n. R. zu kennzeichnen. Vielleicht können wir heute über diese Formulierung schon hinausgehen; wir können vermuten, daß auch die Emotion — wenn sie nämlich stark genug ist und lange genug dauert — eine Erschöpfung macht, die der rein körperlichen in ihren Äußerungen und vielleicht ihrem Wesen, zum mindesten aber in dem von ihr betroffenen Funktionssubstrat gleicht. Daran liegt es, wenn man im klinischen Bilde körperliche nervöse Erschöpfungswirkungen von den emotionell gesetzten nicht trennen kann.

Dazu kommt allerdings, daß die Bedingungen, unter denen eine n. R. zustande kommt, fast stets so gestaltet sind, daß körperliche und psychische Schäden notwendigerweise Hand in Hand gehen. Wir haben auf den Circulus vitiosus, in den z. B. Schlafentzug und psychische Schädigung zum Nachteil der Erholungsmöglichkeit zu geraten pflegen, schon hingewiesen. Ähnlich geht es mit zahlreichen anderen körperlichen Schäden, die neurasthenisierenden Konstellationen eigen zu sein pflegen und oft untrennbar mit den emotionellen Noxen verquickt sind. Daß im Kriege in jedem einzelnen Fall neben den psychischen Schädigungen körperliche Überanstrengung, Entkräftung, Schlafentzug, Unterernährung, Infektionen, Intoxikationen und Mißbrauch von Genußmitteln — unter denen HELLPACH dem Nicotin (KÜLBS, SIEBELT) besondere Bedeutung beimißt — eine unter Umständen maßgebliche Rolle spielten, ist selbstverständlich. Auch bei den Fällen des Friedens aber sind neben seelischen Momenten oft auch körperliche im Spiele; vor allem ist es der Schlafentzug, der auch hier wieder von besonders ungünstiger Wirkung ist, er mag nun durch übermäßige Arbeitslast, übertriebene gesellschaftliche Verpflichtungen (BUMKE) oder durch Sorgen, Erwartung (ISSERLIN) und Aufregungen entstanden sein; dazu kommen auch hier oft narkotisierende oder aufpeitschende Genußmittel, von denen namentlich Kaffee, Nicotin und Tee ihrerseits wieder schlafstörende Wirkungen entfalten.

---

[1] Die übrigens im allgemeinen mehr zu hysteriformen als zu neurasthenischen Reaktionen zu führen pflegen,

Demgegenüber pflegt man heute gewissen sexuellen Entgleisungen, die früher (LÖWENFELD) als *körperliche*, nervösmachende Schädigung aufgefaßt wurden, nur mehr psychologische Wirkungen zuzusprechen, soweit sie überhaupt noch im Rahmen der n. R. diskutiert werden. Das gilt — namentlich seit ERBS autoritativem Auftreten (zit. nach KRONFELD) — für die Onanie, bei der der ständige niederlagenreiche Kampf des Willens mit dem beschämenden Trieb, hypochondrische Erwartungen und Ängste die emotionelle Schädigung herbeiführen (KRONFELD, KAHN). Ähnliches gilt wohl auch für den Coitus interruptus, dessen Nachteile KRONFELD weniger in körperlichen Vorgängen als vielmehr in der Angst sucht, die ja oft mit sexuellen Fehlhandlungen auf eine nicht weiter erklärbare Weise verbunden ist (FREUD). KRONFELD denkt dabei an moralische und religiöse Hemmungen, deren Übertreibung sich durch Angst rächen soll. Die Brücke, die REICH demgegenüber vom Somatischen zum Psychischen zu schlagen versucht, indem er die Angst als psychisches Korrelat einer durch unabgebaute toxische Hormon- und Stoffwechselprodukte verursachten ständigen Erregung des vegetativen Systems auffaßt, scheint uns nicht sehr tragfähig zu sein.

Um noch einmal auf die Grenzen zwischen psychogener und emotionell verursachter n. R. zurückzukommen, so erscheinen sie trotz der erwähnten grundsätzlichen Unterschiede häufig verwischt. Daran sind weniger sog. „fließende Übergänge" als vielmehr Mischformen Schuld, die auf mannigfache Weise entstehen können. Einmal kann die Emotion nicht nur eine neurasthenische, sondern zugleich eine psychogene Reaktion herbeiführen, neben der somatischen also zugleich eine psychologische Wirkung entfalten. Das gilt etwa für die neurasthenische Depression, die AWTOKRATOW im russisch-japanischen Krieg beschrieb und die WOLLENBERG u. a. im Weltkrieg in ähnlicher Form beobachteten. Ebendahin gehört ein Teil der nervösen Depressionen BUMKES und die neurasthenische Melancholie FRIEDMANNS. Neben den neurasthenischen Symptomen stehen dabei je nach der Färbung des emotionellen Erlebnisses bald die reine depressive Verstimmung, bald die Reproduktion von Schreck- oder Angsterlebnissen (WOLLENBERG) im Vordergrund. Je mehr diese psychogenen Symptome in den Vordergrund treten, desto mehr nähern sich die Krankheitsbilder den echten psychogenen Reaktionen, die ja ihrerseits häufig von exogenen oder endogenen nervösen Symptomen begleitet werden. Es kann auch so liegen, daß die n. R. bei entsprechender psychopathischer Veranlagung Anlaß und Gegenstand einer psychogenen Verarbeitung wird; dann kommt es z. B. zu hypochondrischen oder hysterischen Entwicklungen oder zu psychogenen Fixierungen einzelner nervöser Symptome oder des ganzen Syndroms. Es ist kein Zweifel, daß die neurasthenische Schwächung der körperlichen und psychischen Widerstandskraft psychogene Reaktionen, sofern sie anlagemäßig bereitliegen, in erheblichem Maße begünstigt. Immer aber sind psychogene Zutaten — das ist bei Begutachtungsfragen von besonderer Wichtigkeit — Hinweise auf eine abnorme konstitutionelle Beschaffenheit des Reaktionsträgers. Bei der reinen n. R., die den Robusten getroffen hat, kommen sie nicht vor (NONNE, BONHOEFFER u. a.).

Der Versuch, die klinischen Beziehungen der n. R. zu ihren Nachbargebieten durch Abschreiten ihrer Grenzen zu klären — er sollte zugleich einen Überblick über die Ursachenreihe bringen —, soll hiermit abgebrochen werden. Wir stellen rückblickend noch einmal fest: Um das Kerngebiet der „reinen" n. R., die durch körperlich-seelische Erschöpfung erworben wird und den anlagemäßig Robusten nach Art einer exogenen Reaktion trifft, gruppieren sich Formen, die teils von der konstitutionellen Grundlage (Nervosität, Psychopathie), teils von der Ätiologie (Infektion, Intoxikation, organische Hirnerkrankung) her ihre besondere

Färbung erhalten. Übergangs- und Mischformen sind an den Grenzen des Gebietes überaus häufig; ununterbrochene Typenreihen laufen von der reinen n. R. zu allen Nachbargebieten.

Neurasthenische Reaktion ein vitales Syndrom. Der neurasthenische Symptomenkomplex wird so, wenn man seine klinische Verbreitung überblickt, zu einem Syndrom HOCHEscher Prägung, das in grundsätzlich immer gleicher Form von den verschiedensten Ursachen ausgelöst werden und im Rahmen der verschiedensten Formenkreise auftreten kann. An seinem Zusammentreffen mit psychogenen Erscheinungen haben wir ferner zu zeigen versucht, wie verschiedenartig seine Funktion im Strukturaufbau des Einzelfalls sein kann. Daß endlich dieses neurasthenische Syndrom weiterhin eingefügt ist in die große Reihe der „vitalen Syndrome" mit ihrer charakteristischen Pathogenese und ihrer in großen Umrissen einheitlichen Symptomverteilung, haben wir an anderer Stelle des näheren ausgeführt.

Biologische und soziale Hilfsursachen. Es bleibt noch übrig, einen Blick auf gewisse Momente biologischer und sozialer Natur zu werfen, die als prädisponierende Hilfsursachen von einigem Belang sein mögen. Ich halte mich dabei an einen statistischen Überblick, den ich aus den 108 Fällen von n. R. gewonnen habe, die in den vier Jahrgängen 1928—31 in der Kieler Klinik beobachtet wurden.

Die Fälle wurden so ermittelt, daß ich außer den mit „n. R." bezeichneten Krankengeschichten aus denen der „konstitutionell Nervösen" diejenigen heraussuchte, in denen eine einigermaßen umschriebene und belangreiche Schädigung als unmittelbar auslösende Ursache der nervösen Beschwerden notiert wurde. Postinfektiöse Schwächezustände wurden mit einbezogen. Nur bei 15 von diesen 108 Fällen wurde keinerlei konstitutionelle Belastung festgestellt. Bei den übrigen lagen in der Familie oder in der eigenen Vorgeschichte schon mehr oder minder schwere nervöse Manifestationen vor.

Wir geben zunächst eine Kurve, die das Lebensalter der Träger n. R. bei der Aufnahme in die Klinik darstellt.

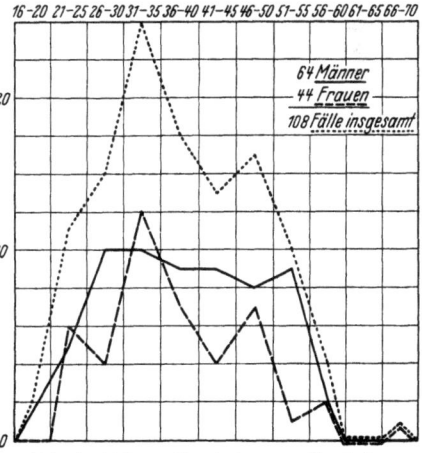

Abb. 1. Lebensalter bei neurasthenischer Reaktion.

Die Kurve der Frauen zeigt gewisse Schönheitsfehler, die wohl aus der geringen Zahl der Fälle zu erklären sind. Beide Geschlechter verhalten sich im übrigen ungefähr gleich; aber die Kurve der Frauen scheint im ganzen etwas früher abzufallen als die der Männer, zeigt dafür aber eine prononciertere Zacke im Rückbildungsalter. Die durch Addition aller Fälle gewonnene dritte Kurve gibt dann einen klareren Überblick über das Verhältnis der Morbidität zum Lebensalter[1]. Hier zeigt sich zunächst, daß das Lebensalter zwischen 31 und 35 Jahren am meisten gefährdet ist. Das mag damit zusammenhängen, daß in diesem Alter durchschnittlich die berufliche Selbständigkeit mit ihrer stärkeren Verantwortlichkeit erworben wird; wenigstens mehren sich um diese Zeit unter meinen Fällen — männlichen wie weiblichen — die Angaben über

---

[1] Gewonnen an dem Material der Klinik einer mittleren Stadt mit starker Arbeiterbevölkerung und erheblichem agrarischen Hinterland, einem Material, das also in mancher Beziehung von den Sprechstundenbesuchern einer Großstadt oder den Insassen eines Landkrankenhauses unterschieden ist.

berufliche Schwierigkeiten, Geschäftssorgen, gerichtliche Konflikte und ähnliches. Im Kriege scheint das, wie HELLPACH berichtet, anders gewesen zu sein: gerade die jungen Kriegsfreiwilligen erkrankten besonders häufig an Neurasthenie. Es mag sein, daß die seelische und körperliche Überlastung, die der Krieg mit sich brachte, gerade den noch weichen, der Anstrengungen, Gefahren und Entbehrungen ungewohnten Jugendlichen besonders gefährlich war, während die Jugend unter Friedensverhältnissen von Verantwortung und Existenzsorgen noch nicht so belastet sein mag wie die Älteren. An der gemeinsamen Kurve fällt des weiteren eine Zacke auf, die zwischen dem 46. und 50. Lebensjahr den steilen Abfall unterbricht. Ich scheue mich, sie als reines Zufallsprodukt der allzu kleinen Zahl anzusehen, weil sie sich bei beiden Geschlechtern, und zwar charakteristischerweise bei den Frauen sehr viel stärker und ein Jahrfünft früher als bei den Männern, findet. Ich halte es für wahrscheinlicher, daß sie auf das Rückbildungsalter zurückzuführen ist, dessen biologische und psychologische Schwächung der neurasthenischen Schädigung Vorschub leistet (STERTZ).

Unter den Frauen finden sich in dieser Altersstufe auffallend viele, die in gehobenen Berufen verantwortlich und angestrengt tätig sind, etwa Eisenbahnsekretäre, Telegraphenassistenten und ähnliches. Unter den Männern zwischen 51 und 55 Jahren fallen einige früh gealterte leitende Beamte von Werften und Behörden auf, die der an sich nicht vermehrten Verantwortung und Arbeit nicht mehr recht gewachsen gewesen waren. Daß es gerade der Verantwortungsdruck gehobener oder selbständiger Arbeit ist, der die Gefahr der n. R. in besonderem Grade heraufbeschwört, ist eine alte Erfahrung. Vor 30 Jahren fanden schon LEUBUSCHER und BIBROWICZ, daß unter den gelernten Arbeitern die Neurasthenie ungleich häufiger sei als unter den ungelernten. Auch gewisse Kriegserfahrungen gehören hierher. HELLPACH z. B., der bei Soldaten und Offizieren die Zahl der Hysteriefälle mit der der n. R. verglich, fand, daß die Offiziere in höherem Prozentsatz an n. R. erkrankten als die Mannschaften, bei denen wiederum die Hysterie sehr viel häufiger war.

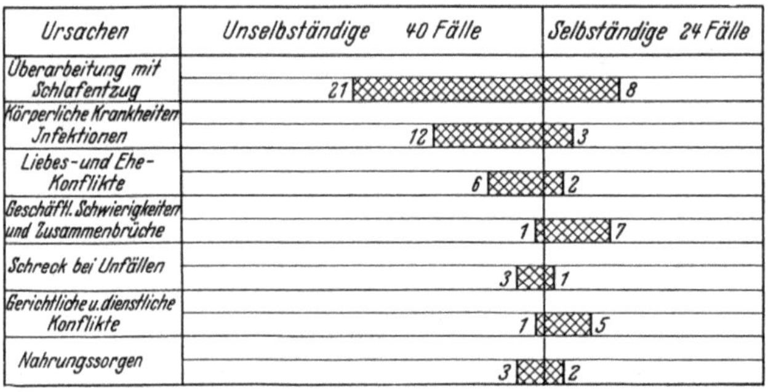

Ursachen	Unselbständige 40 Fälle	Selbständige 24 Fälle
Überarbeitung mit Schlafentzug	21	8
Körperliche Krankheiten Infektionen	12	3
Liebes- und Ehe-Konflikte	6	2
Geschäftl. Schwierigkeiten und Zusammenbrüche	1	7
Schreck bei Unfällen	3	1
Gerichtliche u. dienstliche Konflikte	1	5
Nahrungssorgen	3	2

Abb. 2. Ursachen bei neurasthenischer Reaktion.

Ich gebe in Abb. 2 eine Tabelle, die die 64 neurasthenischen Männer meines Materials erfaßt. Sie sind aufgeteilt in solche — 24 —, die in selbständigen Berufen verantwortlich tätig sind, eine Gruppe, die etwa vom Werkmeister und selbständigen Kaufmann an aufwärts die höheren sozialen Stufen umfaßt; ihnen gegenüber steht eine Gruppe von 40 Unselbständigen, in der Hauptsache gelernten und ungelernten Arbeitern. Es ist auffällig, daß — im Gegensatz zu HELLPACHs Kriegsmaterial — die „Offiziere" in meinem Material so sehr in der Minderzahl geblieben sind. Das ist aber zum Teil sicher ein Fehler, der aus den besonderen klinischen Verhältnissen erwächst. Meine poliklinischen Ziffern z. B. — auf die ich hier nicht weiter eingehen will — sehen, schon durch die vielen neurasthenischen Studenten, ganz anders aus und in einer Praxis elegans der Großstadt würde sich das Zahlenverhältnis zweifellos umgekehrt verhalten. Man geht als selbständiger, pflicht- und verantwortungsbewußter Mann nicht gern seiner Nerven wegen in eine öffentliche Klinik, man sucht sich so lange wie möglich selbst zu helfen, begnügt sich mit ambulanter ärztlicher Beratung oder geht schlimmstenfalls in ein Sanatorium.

Die Tabelle gibt zugleich einen Überblick über die Ursachen der n. R. und ihre Verteilung auf die beiden Gruppen. Unselbständige sind danach durch Überarbeit mit Schlafentzug mehr gefährdet als Selbständige. Ich finde unter ihnen namentlich Kellner, Kaffeehausmusiker, einen Nachtportier, Monteure, Lokomotivbeamte und Chauffeure mit übermäßigem Nachtdienst. Ebenso scheinen Infektionen und andere körperliche Erkrankungen die Unselbständigen mehr mit n. R. zu bedrohen als die Selbständigen. Auch das dürfte aber weniger auf inneren, d. h. biologischen Gründen als vielmehr auf den sozialen und sonstigen äußeren Bedingungen beruhen, deren Einfluß die beiden Gruppen unterliegen. Den Selbständigen halten seine beruflichen Interessen oder sein schärferes Gesundheitsgewissen davon ab, derartige, z. B. postinfektiöse, Schwächezustände zum Gegenstand klinischer Fürsorge zu machen, er ist auch mehr als der Unselbständige in der Lage, das Ausmaß seiner Tätigkeit seinem schonungsbedürftigen Zustand anzupassen, weil er nicht dem üblen Schematismus einer bürokratischen Krankenfürsorge unterliegt, die nur die Extreme: Arbeitsunfähigkeit oder völlige Leistungsfähigkeit, aber keine Zwischenstufen zwischen beiden kennt. Unter diesen Fällen finden sich neben postinfektiösen Schwächezuständen mehrere solche, die durch langdauernde schmerzhafte Krankheiten, z. B. Amputationsstümpfe, mehrfach wiederholte Bauchoperationen u. ä. zu neurasthenischen Störungen gekommen sind; es ist bemerkenswert, daß über die Hälfte gerade dieser Fälle keine Belastung im Sinne der konstitutionellen Nervosität erkennen läßt. Daß geschäftliche Schwierigkeiten und Zusammenbrüche ebenso wie gerichtliche und dienstliche Konflikte vornehmlich die Selbständigen treffen, bedarf keines Kommentars. Die restlichen Ursachen verteilen sich auf beide Gruppen einigermaßen gleichmäßig.

Unter den 44 Frauen befinden sich 7, bei denen n. R. nach schweren Geburten (2), nach Abort (4) oder nach überlangem Stillen der Kinder (1) eingetreten sind. In 30 Fällen handelt es sich um berufliche Konflikte, Überanstrengung und Nachtarbeit, in den übrigen 7 Fällen um Liebes- und Ehekonflikte (4) und körperliche Krankheiten (3). Die besondere berufliche Gefährdung der Frau tritt auch hier wieder hervor.

Die Krankheit unserer Zeit. Damit gewinnen wir wieder den Anschluß an einen Gedanken, den schon BEARD und MÖBIUS ihren bahnbrechenden Arbeiten über Nervosität zugrunde gelegt hatten: den Gedanken der Abhängigkeit der neurasthenischen Erscheinungen von den Schädigungen der modernen Zivilisation. Zwar hat der Krieg mit seinen ungeheuren Leistungen zur Genüge erwiesen, daß von einer „nervösen Entartung" unseres Volkes nicht die Rede sein kann (BUMKE); die Gefahr der Entartung droht vielmehr, wie J. LANGE nachgewiesen hat, von einer ganz andern Seite her, nämlich von der allmählichen Verschlechterung unserer Erbmasse. Aber das Schlagwort von der „Krankheit unserer Zeit" hat auch heute noch — oder vielmehr heute erst recht — seine Bedeutung. Gegenüber den Schädigungen unserer heutigen Zivilisation, angefangen von der einseitigen Überlastung des Schulkindes über die Lösung ganzer Volksschichten von jeder Bindung und Hingabe an außermaterielle Ziele bis zur Hetze eines ungehemmten Konkurrenzkampfes auf der einen Seite und der Arbeitslosigkeit von Millionen andererseits, gegenüber diesen Schädigungen mögen die der friedlichen achtziger Jahre ein Kinderspiel gewesen sein. His hat schon vor dem Kriege in sehr ernster Mahnung auf diese Gefahren der „Überkultur" hingewiesen, und HELLPACH meinte kurz vor Kriegsschluß, daß nach dem Kriege die Bekämpfung der Neurasthenie eine wichtige Aufgabe sein würde. Wir haben leider nach dem Kriege zuviel anderes zu tun gehabt, als daß wir diesem Wunsche HELLPACHs hätten nachkommen können. Der verlorene Krieg, der Zusammenbruch unseres Volkes, seine politische und soziale Zerrissenheit seither, Inflation, Wirtschaftskrise und Verelendung, sie alle haben im Gegenteil das Ihre getan, um die Zahl der Neurasthenischen zu vermehren. Nicht mehr der hochzivilisierte Großstädter allein, der im Lärm und Stank seiner Straßen, in der Gehetztheit der Überarbeit und des betäubenden Genusses seine Nerven aufreibt, erkrankt jetzt an neurasthenischen Erscheinungen; auch der Bauer, der trotz schwerer Mühe sein Erbe schwinden sieht, der Arbeitslose, der sich und seine Familie nicht mehr aus eigenen Kräften zu erhalten vermag, der Beamte, der infolge des Abbaus von Kollegen übermäßige Arbeit und Verantwortung zu tragen hat, die Frau, von der berufliche Leistungen verlangt werden, denen sie ihrer Natur nach nicht gewachsen ist, sie alle unterliegen in zunehmender Zahl der neurasthenischen Erschöpfung. ANTONI hat am Material der Kieler Nervenklinik nachgewiesen, daß unter der ländlichen Bevölkerung die Nervosität — und damit auch die neurasthenische Reaktion — heute relativ häufiger ist als in der städtischen, daß Kopfarbeiter, bei denen nach MOEBIUS die „Nervosität zu Hause" sein sollte, relativ seltener mit nervösen Erscheinungen beobachtet wurden als Handarbeiter. Es mag mancherlei Ursachen geben, die diesen überraschenden Verhältnissen zugrunde liegen. Eins jedenfalls scheinen solche Erfahrungen zu bestätigen: die Nervosität ist mehr denn je eine Krankheit unserer Zeit. Sie beschränkt sich nicht mehr auf jene hochzivilisierte Oberschicht, an der MOEBIUS und BEARD einst ihre Beobachtungen anstellten. Sie ist im ganzen Volke heimisch geworden [1].

III. Symptomatologie, Ausgänge und Behandlung.

Randsymptome. Nachdem wir bereits in den vorhergehenden Abschnitten gelegentlich auf die Symptomatologie der n. R. eingegangen sind, können wir uns jetzt darauf beschränken, das neurasthenische Syndrom als Ganzes zu charakterisieren, um dann einzelne seltenere Symptome in Kürze zu besprechen. Im vollausgebildeten neurasthenischen Syndrom vereinen sich regelmäßig körperliche mit seelischen Symptomen. Fälle, in denen sich dieses Ineinandergreifen somatischer und psychischer Störungen nicht aufweisen läßt, gehören unseres Erachtens nicht zur n. R.; wir würden es vorziehen, rein psychische Syndrome zu den psychogenen Reaktionen zu zählen, während rein körperliche, auch dann, wenn sie denen der n. R. ähneln oder gleichen, stets den Verdacht auf eine larvierte Organerkrankung [2] erwecken, oder allenfalls den sehr seltenen Fällen von Nervosität ohne psychische Alterationen zuzuweisen sind, die KRETSCHMER gelegentlich erwähnt. Die körperlichen Symptome sind grundsätzlich rein funktionell-nervöser Natur. Wenn Organbefunde erhoben werden, die anatomische Läsionen voraussetzen, dann handelt es sich unseres Erachtens

---

[1] *Zusatz bei der Korrektur.* Es bedarf wohl kaum der Feststellung, daß diese Sätze *vor* dem Jahre 1933 geschrieben wurden. Die nationalsozialistische Staatsführung hat inzwischen manche Übel jener fast schon historisch gewordenen Zeit an der Wurzel angepackt und ist damit zum besten Arzt vieler Nervöser geworden. Die Nachwirkungen jener Schäden sind aber selbstverständlich nicht von heut auf morgen zu beheben, und insofern gilt das, was in diesem Absatz gesagt wurde, auch heute noch.

[2] Vgl. die Anschauungen v. BERGMANNs über den „Abbau der Organneurose".

um — bei den oft komplizierten Schädigungen gewiß nicht verwunderliche — Nebenbefunde anderer Ätiologie, die mit der n. R. nichts zu tun haben. Das dürfte z. B. für die von NONNE und MANN bei neurasthenischen Kriegsteilnehmern beschriebenen Polyneuritiden gelten. Auch die Herzerweiterung mit akzessorischen Geräuschen, die BRUGSCH bei erschöpften Kriegsneurasthenischen fand, scheint uns mehr der Erschöpfung durch rein somatisch-mechanische Überbelastung des Organs als der n. R. zugeschrieben werden zu müssen. Die charakteristische körperliche Störung der n. R. ist demgegenüber die nervöse Regulationsstörung der Organfunktionen. Die vitale Regulationsstörung, die allgemeine reizbare Schwäche — eine Reizbarkeit der Funktion bei Schwäche der Leistung — ist das Achsensyndrom, der obligate Kern der neurasthenischen Symptomatologie, um den herum sich eine Reihe von jeweils verschiedenen, akzessorischen Randsymptomen gruppiert. Die übermäßige Inanspruchnahme eines bestimmten Organs oder Organabschnitts, etwa der Beinmuskulatur, mag zur hochgradigen lokalen Ermüdung mit Ermüdungstremor, Muskelwogen (GIERLICH), Überregbarkeit des Muskelgewebes (MAYERHOFER), unter Umständen sogar mit Areflexie (SCHARNKE und HAESELER) führen. Das ist aber noch keineswegs eine n. R., sondern eine einfache lokale Erschöpfungserscheinung. Wohl aber ist es möglich und sogar natürlich relativ häufig, daß derartige umschriebene Erschöpfungssymptome in den Rahmen einer n. R. eingefügt sind, und als Randsymptome das an sich einförmige Bild der zentralen Regulationsstörung pathoplastisch ausgestalten. Daß dabei die Erschöpfung des Einzelorgans die zentrale Regulationsstörung begünstigt, ist ebenso selbstverständlich wie das Umgekehrte, daß nämlich die neurasthenische Regulationsstörung, die ja die vitale Kraft des gesamten Organismus herabsetzt, der Erschöpfung des peripheren Einzelorgans Vorschub leistet.

Auf dem Boden solcher Funktionsbeziehungen besorgen dann konstitutive und konstellative Momente in wechselseitigem Wirken die Auswahl des Organs oder Organsystems, dessen neurasthenische Funktionsschwäche sich im Einzelfall besonders heraushebt. Wenn sich bei der reinen n. R. die Regulationsstörung in erster Linie auf das Herzgefäßsystem (BRUGSCH u. a.) bezieht, dann mag das in vielen Fällen daran liegen, daß das Vasomotorium mehr als alle anderen Organe von der körperlich-seelischen Erschöpfung in Mitleidenschaft gezogen wird. In manchen anderen Fällen aber wird die angeborene Funktionsunsicherheit und Schwäche, die konstitutionelle Minderwertigkeit des Organs, diese Auswahl unterstützen oder erst ermöglichen. Wenn der RITTERSHAUSSche Offizier nach stundenlangem Bedienen des Telefons im Gefecht Pseudoakoasmen bekam, dann wird man diese Symptomwahl auf die besondere Konstellation des Falles zurückführen müssen. Wenn aber KEHRERS Patienten das neurasthenische Nystagmoid zeigten, dann sind es in erster Linie konstitutionelle Momente, die dieser seltenen Anomalie zugrunde liegen.

Die **vegetativ-nervöse Regulationsstörung** selbst wirkt sich dabei — ebenso wie übrigens bei der konstitutionellen Nervosität — keineswegs in ein und demselben — etwa vagotonischen oder sympathicotonischen — Sinne aus. Vielmehr können — ganz abgesehen von der Unterschiedlichkeit der Fälle untereinander — auch im Einzelfalle nebeneinander sowohl sympathicotonische als auch vagotonische Symptome, also z. B. neben der Tachykardie Neigung zum Schwitzen usw. stehen. Gerade solche Erfahrungen — die ja auf dem Gebiet der endogenen Funktionsstörungen des vegetativen Systems gang und gäbe sind und die v. BERGMANN bekanntlich zu dem Begriff der „Vegetativ Stigmatisierten" geführt haben — in Zusammenhang mit der Verteilung der Funktionsstörungen auf mannigfache Gebiete gaben uns ja Veranlassung, an die Beteiligung sehr hoher diencephaler Regulationsinstanzen zu denken.

Der klinische Ausdruck solcher vegetativer Regulationsstörungen ist neben der vegetativen Tonusverschiebung die reizbare Schwäche der Organfunktionen, die auf geringste Reize im Übermaß anspricht, um nach kurzer, schwächlicher Tätigkeit vorzeitig zu versagen. In sinngemäßer Anwendung kann man, wenn man will, schon hier von einer Störung der Reizempfänglichkeit, der Stimmung und des Antriebs sprechen, von Qualitäten also, die wir ,,vitale" nannten und im allgemeinen mehr auf psychische Vorgänge bezogen wissen wollten. Wenn das Auge des Neurasthenikers den Lichteinfall schmerzlich empfindet, dann ist seine Reizempfänglichkeit offenbar erhöht, und wenn es nach geringer Anstrengung ermüdet, dann hält seine Funktionskraft, deren psychisches Korrelat der Antrieb ist, nicht lange genug vor, und beides mag aus einer ,,Verstimmung" der vegetativen Vorgänge erwachsen, die den Tonus seiner Funktionen unterlegen.

Solche Beziehungen, die auf körperlichem Gebiet naturgemäß mehr die Kennzeichen kausal verknüpfter, biologischer Funktionszusammenhänge tragen, gewinnen, wenn man ihnen auf dem Gebiet der psychischen Neurastheniesymptome nachgeht, ein psychologisches, ,,verständliches" Gesicht. Auch hier sind es offenbar die grundlegenden, die psychische Funktionskraft spendenden, ,,vitalen" Schichten der Seele, auf deren Schädigung sich alle psychischen Symptome der n. R. zurückführen lassen. Wenn jemand konzentrationsunfähig oder initiativelos ist, dann reicht offenbar seine vitale Funktionskraft, sein Antrieb, nicht aus, um die an sich ungeschädigten Apparate des Denkens und Willens ordnungsmäßig in Betrieb zu setzen. Wenn er bei geringstem Anlaß zornig aufbraust oder in Tränen ausbricht, dann besteht eine ,,krankhafte Überempfindlichkeit" (GOLDSCHEIDER) der Reizempfänglichkeit, der er andererseits Rechnung zu tragen sucht, wenn er sich von der Umgebung zurückzieht, alles Laute und Grelle zu meiden sucht und jeder Gemütsbewegung ausweicht. Wenn man dazu noch die moros-depressive Verstimmung und die Störungen der Schlaf-Wach-Funktion nimmt, dann ist das psychische Bild der n. R. bereits in groben Zügen umrissen.

Um zunächst bei den **körperlichen Symptomen** der n. R. zu bleiben, so wollen wir hier die allgemein bekannten Auswirkungen der vegetativen Regulationsstörungen nur kurz streifen. Es sind das die zahlreichen vago-sympathicotonischen Funktionsunregelmäßigkeiten und reizbaren Schwächen der verschiedensten Organe, wie sie vom konstitutionell Nervösen, vegetativ Stigmatisierten häufig beschrieben und auch in diesem Handbuch an anderen Stellen ausführlich behandelt worden sind. Wir wollen hier vielmehr nur eine Reihe von selteneren Symptomen aufzählen, die im Rahmen der neurasthenischen Erscheinungen besprochen zu werden pflegen. Manche von ihnen sind Randsymptome in unserem Sinne, besitzen also nur bestimmte Häufigkeitsbeziehungen zur n. R. Andere mögen einzelnen, besonders häufigen zentralen Regulationsstörungen entsprechen. Festzuhalten ist, daß keins dieser Einzelsymptome pathognostischen Wert besitzt. Erst der Überblick über den Gesamtbestand der Symptome kann diagnostisch entscheidend sein (GAUPP). Unentbehrlich für die Diagnose ist die umfassende vegetativ-vitale Regulationsstörung mit ihren körperlichen und psychischen Symptomen.

Wir beginnen mit den Sinnesorganen und wenden uns zunächst dem Auge zu. Die neueste handbuchmäßige Darstellung (WEBER und RUNGE) betont, daß es sich bei den nervösen Erscheinungen am Auge allermeist um vorgebildete, also der konstitutionellen Nervosität angehörende oder sonstige angeborene Anomalien handle, die durch neurasthenisierende Erlebnisse nur gesteigert würden. Das gilt z. B. für die kongenitale ein- oder doppelseitige Ptosis, von der ich mehrere Fälle kenne, die sich in der Müdigkeit oder Erschöpfung verstärken. Das gilt weiter vom nervösen Nystagmoid, dem asthenischen Typ des Nystagmus, bei dem sich nach KEHRERS Meinung die Reizerscheinungen der nervösen Erschöpfung auf die Blickwender ausdehnen; meistens bestehen daneben andere Störungen am Sehapparat, die die Disposition zum neurasthenischen Nystagmoid verstärken. Auch der Nystagmus der Grubenarbeiter ist nach Meinung WEBERS und RUNGES wahrscheinlich auf Ermüdungserscheinungen zurückzuführen. OHM analysiert die Ätiologie des Augenzitterns der Bergleute genauer, er findet äußere und innere Ursachen und nennt als erstere die Grubengase, die Grubenbeleuchtung, die Flözhöhe und die Tiefe der Grube, unter den letzteren Augenerkrankungen anderer Art, Alkoholismus und besondere konstitutionelle Disposition.

Auch über Asthenopie wird von Neurasthenischen gelegentlich geklagt. Es handelt sich dann wohl um eine funktionelle rasche Ermüdbarkeit der Akkommodation, die übrigens häufig mit Kopfweh und Lichtscheu einhergeht (WEBER und RUNGE).

Als Ermüdungssymptom des Sehorgans werden ferner flüchtige Ringskotome aufgefaßt, die bei Menschen gefunden wurden, die lange Zeit, z. B. als Flieger oder Ballonabwehrkanoniere (ZADE), besonders starker Blendung ausgesetzt waren. Es handelt sich nach GELB und GOLDSTEIN um eine abnorm schnell eintretende, von außen nach innen fortschreitende Ermüdbarkeit der Sehsubstanz, die das Gesichtsfeld von der Peripherie her zunehmend vernebelt erscheinen läßt. In den Fällen von GELB und GOLDSTEIN bestanden allerdings Hirnverletzungen, die von den Autoren als Grundlage der Störung herangezogen wurden. In ähnlicher Richtung bewegen sich die FÖRSTER-WILBRANDSchen Untersuchungen, die bei der Ermüdung eine zunächst schneller, dann langsamer zunehmende Einengung des Gesichtsfeldes feststellten (KÖLLMER). Die Übergänge vom Physiologischen zum Pathologischen sind hier natürlich fließend. Eine Nachprüfung dieser Untersuchungen unter dem Gesichtspunkt der verfeinerten psychiatrischen Diagnostik erscheint wünschenswert.

Seit jeher pflegt man ferner dem Lidflattern bei geschlossenen Augen (ROSENBACH) als einem nervösen Stigma besondere pathognostische Bedeutung zuzumessen. KEHRER will das Symptom als rein asthenisch nur bei festem Lidschluß und nach Ausschluß aller rein psychisch verursachten Lidbewegungen anerkennen. Zuverlässiger, obwohl praktisch schwerer erkennbar sind gewisse Symptome, die BUMKE am Auge selbst festgestellt hat. Er findet bei Ermüdeten und bei Neurasthenikern die galvanische Lichtempfindlichkeit etwas gesteigert bei sehr viel stärkerer Verminderung der galvanischen Reflexempfindlichkeit. An den Pupillen findet er Erweiterung bei vermehrter Pupillenunruhe. KEHRER macht auf die — soweit ich sehe nur in einzelnen Fällen feststellbare — Verkürzung der Lichtreflexbewegung der Pupille bei Neurasthenikern aufmerksam. Auch Pupillendifferenzen (KNAUER und BILLIGHEIMER) und schneller Wechsel der Pupillenweite (WEBER und RUNGE) lassen sich gelegentlich feststellen. Sie beruhen wohl auf der besonderen neurasthenischen Labilität des sympathischen Systems.

Endlich ist aus dem Kriege mehrfach über optische Sinnestäuschungen in Erschöpfungszuständen berichtet worden. WOLLENBERGS Gewährsleute sahen z. B. weiße Häuser am Straßenrand, feindliche Kavallerie, ein niedergehendes Luftschiff, alles in „eigentümlich fließender Bewegung". Auch die „Engel von Mons", die den erschöpft zurückflutenden Engländern erschienen und von Tausenden gesehen wurden, gehören hierher. Solche Pseudohallluzinationen oder Illusionen werden ihrem Inhalt nach natürlich vom Psychischen, dem Kriegserlebnis, bestimmt; der biologische Boden, der sie trägt, ist aber die neurasthenische Überempfindlichkeit, von deren experimentellem Nachweis wir oben sprachen.

Auch auf *akustischem Gebiet* gibt es solche Pseudohalluzinationen. Wir erwähnten schon den RITTERSHAUSSchen Offizier. WOLLENBERG berichtet von Glockenläuten, das in Zuständen hochgradiger Erschöpfung gehört wurde. LEIDLER und LOEWY suchen gewisse statosensorische Täuschungen mit der Erschöpfung des Neurasthenischen zu erklären, die die genaue optische und sensible Kontrolle der Körperlage und der Eigenbewegungen behindre. Demgegenüber muß der eigentliche nervöse Schwindel, über den Neurasthenische anfallsweise oder bei bestimmten Lageveränderungen klagen, mehr auf vasovegetative Schwankungen zurückgeführt werden, wenn auch in sehr vielen Fällen eine Übererregbarkeit des Vestibularisapparats hinzukommt, die übrigens experimentell durch calorische Minimalreize nachgewiesen werden kann (LEIDLER und LOEWY).

Besonders charakteristisch für die n. R. sind dann gewisse Ermüdungssymptome der Hörfähigkeit, die von HAMMERSCHLAG (zit. nach LEIDLER und LOEWY) zuerst beschrieben, später von ALBRECHT weiter erforscht worden sind. Es handelt sich dabei um ein vorzeitiges Ermüden gegenüber Gehörsreizen, das man z. B. mittels der Stimmgabel feststellen kann. Der Ton der Stimmgabel wird zwar bis zum Ausklingen gehört, aber doch nur dann, wenn die Stimmgabel von Zeit zu Zeit für einige Sekunden vom Ohr entfernt und damit dem Gehör eine kurze Ruhepause gegönnt wird. ALBRECHT fand neben dem frühen Verklingen ein intermittierendes gesteigertes Wiederhören des Tons. MAUTHNER stellte daneben bei Neurasthenischen eine Verkürzung der Hörweite für Flüstersprache fest. Kombiniert mit solcher ,,Vertäubung" (KÜMMEL) findet sich oft eine besondere Übererregbarkeit des Vestibularisapparats, die sich bei gewöhnlicher Labyrinthprüfung, ja manchmal schon bei tiefem Einatmen (ALEXANDER und BRAUN) in Schwindel, Übelkeit, Erbrechen, Pulsveränderung, Erröten und Erblassen äußert.

Gegenüber dieser Schwäche der Leistung äußert sich die Übererregbarkeit der Funktion am Ohr in der bekannten Hyperakusis, die Geräusche von gewöhnlicher Stärke als unangenehm, ja schmerzhaft empfinden läßt (MAUTHNER). Sie entspricht der Überempfindlichkeit anderer Sinnesorgane, des Auges, des Geruchs und der Körperfühlsphäre. Ebenso wie am Auge, an dem vom Neurasthenischen oft über Flimmern und Mouches volantes geklagt wird, kommen auch am Ohr des Neurasthenischen subjektive Ohrgeräusche in besonders quälender — oder doch so empfundener — Form ohne jeden organischen Befund vor. LEIDLER und LOEWY stellen fest, daß es gerade Fälle mit starker Beteiligung des vasovegetativen Systems sind, die über diese Beschwerden besonders lebhaft klagen. Es ist möglich, daß hier innere Zusammenhänge bestehen. Auf der anderen Seite wird man bedenken müssen, daß vom Psychischen her, durch mangelnde Willensspannung und Konzentrationsfähigkeit — die ja auch den Gesunden über mancherlei kleine Mißempfindungen hinwegsetzen müssen — beim Neurasthenischen alle diese subjektiven Empfindungen besonders ungünstig beeinflußt werden.

Das gilt nun ebenso für die zahlreichen *Schmerzen* und *Mißempfindungen*, die in den verschiedensten Körpergegenden auftreten, oft unbestimmt und flüchtig, oft hartnäckig an umschriebener Stelle verweilend. Am bekanntesten ist hier der neurasthenische Kopfschmerz, der bald als dumpfer diffuser Druck, bald als stechender oder wühlender Schmerz beschrieben und bald in die Stirn — oft auch isoliert in die Augen — bald in den Kopf oder die Schläfen lokalisiert wird. Hier werden vasomotorische Vorgänge in erster Linie zur Erklärung herangezogen werden müssen. Anders liegt es vielleicht bei den neuralgiformen (STERTZ) Schmerzen, die sich gelegentlich dem Gebiet bestimmter peripherer Nerven einzufügen scheinen und möglicherweise, wie KEHRER meint, einer

Dauerreizung sensibler Nerven entsprechen. BRUGSCH hat sogar flüchtige Hautgefühlsstörungen dabei festgestellt, und die neurasthenischen Polyneuritiden von NONNE und MANN habe ich bereits erwähnt. Natürlich wird man aber bei dem vielverschlungenen Wurzelwerk gerade der Kriegsneurasthenien niemals die Mitwirkung rheumatischer oder anderer Noxen bei solchen neuritischen oder neuritoiden Erscheinungen ausschließen können. STERTZ z. B. steht der neurasthenischen, also kenotoxischen Genese dieser Schmerzen skeptisch gegenüber und denkt mehr an ein zentrales, also wohl auf das Großhirn zu beziehendes Zustandekommen der Sensationen.

Am *Muskelapparat* werden zahlreiche Phänomene als mehr oder minder charakteristisch für die n. R. beschrieben. An erster Stelle rangiert hier der neurasthenische Tremor, das myoneurasthenische Zittern, das an den Händen, der Zunge und anderen Muskelgebieten dann eintritt, wenn ungewöhnliche Stellungen eingenommen, z. B. die Zunge herausgestreckt oder die Finger gespreizt werden. GIERLICH meint, daß das feinschlägige Vibrieren mehr für die nervöse Veranlagung spreche, während man bei akuter nervöser Erschöpfung mehr grobschlägige Exkursionen sehe. Besonders eindrucksvoll wird die Erscheinung durch das sog. QUINQUAUDsche Phänomen, das Krepitieren, das man fühlt, wenn man die Handfläche gegen die gespreizten Finger des Untersuchten legt (KEHRER). Zittern ist das „physiologische Dissoziationsphänomen des Motoriums schlechthin" (KEHRER). Es ist an sich keineswegs krankhaft, sondern wird erst dann abnormes Symptom, wenn es ohne oder bei geringstem Anlaß mit ungewöhnlicher Stärke und Dauer auftritt. Es kann auch beim gleichen Menschen durch die verschiedensten Ursachen hervorgerufen werden. Differentialdiagnostisch wichtig gegenüber dem neurasthenischen Zittern ist vor allem der Nicotintremor, dann der alkoholische Tremor, endlich — zumal bei alternden Patienten — das Zittern der beginnenden extrapyramidalen Schädigung arteriosklerotischer oder anderer Herkunft. Über die Erblichkeit des Zitterns mit ihren verschiedenen genealogischen Beziehungen haben sich MINOR und namentlich KEHRER in eingehenden Studien geäußert.

Dem neurasthenischen Zittern nahe mag jene leichte von Neurasthenischen gelegentlich geklagte koordinatorische Störung stehen (BRUGSCH), die feinere Hantierungen und Zielbewegungen beeinträchtigt und z. B. das Schreiben, das Zeichnen und die Ausübung von Instrumentalmusik stören kann.

Als charakteristisches muskuläres Symptom der n. R. wird von GIERLICH die Steigerung der direkten mechanischen Muskelerregbarkeit angegeben. Auch MAYERHOFER betrachtet die Dellen- und Wulstbildung der quergestreiften Muskeln bei leichtem Beklopfen als Symptom der Erschöpfung. Freilich ist, wie KEHRER bemerkt, das Symptom keineswegs charakteristisch für neurasthenische Zustände. Ich selbst habe es bei einer großen Reihe von Schizophrenen gesehen, vorzüglich allerdings solchen, die abstiniert hatten und in ihrem Allgemeinzustand sehr heruntergekommen waren. Einer Übererregbarkeit der Muskulatur mag auch das Muskelwogen und -flimmern entsprechen, das OPPENHEIM zumal bei leichter Kälteeinwirkung sah. Auch das ist aber zweifellos nicht charakteristisch für die n. R.

Entsprechend der Übererregbarkeit des „erschöpften Nervmuskelpräparats" (CURSCHMANN, zit. nach KEHRER) pflegen die *Reflexe* der Gliedmaßen übermäßig lebhaft zu sein. Auch die Hautreflexe beteiligen sich gelegentlich an dieser Steigerung, die sich an sich von der organisch bedingten in nichts unterscheidet (KEHRER). KEHRER macht darauf aufmerksam, daß die neurasthenische Reflexerhöhung den besten Boden für die willkürliche Reflexverstärkung bilde, in der KRETSCHMER bekanntlich eins der Hauptphänomene der Hysterie sieht. Auch über Abschwächung der Reflexe wird gelegentlich berichtet (v. Hösslin, Gierlich, Cimbal); sie ist aber zweifellos sehr selten (Gierlich), so selten, daß ich selbst sie — und namentlich die von Gierlich angegebene Ungleichheit der Achilles- und Bauchdeckenreflexe — nur mit größter Vorsicht als neurasthenische Zeichen verwerten möchte (s. dazu Guttmann).

Alle diese körperlichen Zeichen, die dem Kranken selbst zum guten Teil gar nicht zu Bewußtsein kommen und oft erst durch besondere Untersuchungsmaßnahmen aufgedeckt werden müssen, treten nun an klinischer Bedeutung hinter den Störungen zurück, die man gewohnheitsmäßig auf das vegetative System i. e. S. bezieht. Dabei wollen wir an dieser Stelle dahingestellt sein lassen, wie weit etwa die aufgezählten körperlichen Symptome der reizbaren Schwäche — etwa der Muskulatur oder der Sinnesorgane — von Funktionsstörungen des vegetativen Systems abhängig sind. Wenn man mit Kraus, L. R. Müller u. a. der Meinung ist, daß das vegetative System in der Krausschen Fassung den Funktionstonus der animalen Funktionen vorbereitet, erhält und wiederherstellt, wird man die Möglichkeit gelten lassen, daß manches von dem, was sich als reizbare Schwäche peripherer animaler Organe äußert, von zentralen Regulationsstörungen im vegetativen System verursacht wird. Freilich sind solche Vermutungen einstweilen nicht viel mehr als Fragestellungen. Die zahlreichen Arbeiten, die sich z. B. mit der vegetativen Unterlegung des Muskeltonus befassen, haben noch nicht zu unbestrittenen Resultaten geführt (Regelsberger in L. R. Müller). Wir müssen für diese Fragen wie überhaupt für die Probleme des vegetativen Systems im einzelnen wiederum auf die zusammenfassenden Darstellungen von L. R. Müller und seinen Mitarbeitern, von Leschke u. a. verweisen.

Demgegenüber sind die nunmehr zu schildernden Funktionsstörungen innerer Organe mit sehr viel größerer Sicherheit auf vegetative Regulationsschwankungen zurückzuführen. Ganz im Vordergrunde des Bildes stehen hier die kardiovasculären Störungen, die neben den üblichen nervösen vagosympathicotonischen Funktionsabweichungen gewisse für die Erschöpfungsneurasthenie charakteristische Besonderheiten zeigen. Wir verdanken ihre Kenntnis in erster Linie einer Kriegsarbeit von Brugsch, deren Resultat später mehrfach (Cimbal, Knauer und Billigheimer, Horn u. a.) nachgeprüft und bestätigt wurde. Brugsch fand in seinen Fällen erschöpfter Frontsoldaten eine Erweiterung des Herzens nach links mit akzessorischen Geräuschen, Herabsetzung des Blutdrucks, schlecht gefüllte Arterien, kleinen Puls, Beschleunigung oder — seltener — Verlangsamung der Herzaktion, Herzsensationen und Vasomotorenschwäche. Dem Kranken selbst kommen davon am unangenehmsten die Herzsensationen zu Bewußtsein, Unregelmäßigkeiten der Herzaktion, paukendes Herzklopfen, das namentlich nach dem Essen, nach kleinen Anstrengungen oder beim Hinlegen auftritt (Hellpach) und durch seine Atembeklemmungen und die pulssynchronen, subjektiv wahrgenommenen Geräusche das Einschlafen behindern kann. Daß Schwindel, Kopfweh und manches andere neurasthenische Symptom als sekundäre Folgeerscheinung der kardiovasculären Störung aufzufassen sind, haben wir schon erwähnt. Dem gegenüber mißt Kehrer den Innervationsstörungen der peripheren Gefäßnerven, in erster Linie also den verschiedenen Spielarten des Dermographismus (Goldscheider und Hahn) mehr die Bedeutung eines konstitutionellen Stigmas bei. Dasselbe trifft nach J. H. Schultz für die auf experimentellem Wege zu erzeugenden Änderungen der Pulsfrequenz zu, also für die durch Druck auf den Augapfel (Aschner) oder tiefes Bücken (Erben) hervorgerufene Pulsverlangsamung, die Änderung der Pulsfrequenz bei Druck auf die Herzspitze (Braun und Fuchs) und die respiratorische Arrhythmie. Ebenso sieht Bumke in dem lästigen

Klopfen der peripheren Arterien, soweit es nicht etwa durch organische Veränderungen bedingt ist, ein Zeichen der konstitutionellen Nervosität.

HORN hat im Kriege den Versuch gemacht, den „*Schreckneurosen*" im Rahmen der nervösen Funktionsstörungen eine klinische Sonderstellung zuzuweisen. Wenn er dabei den kardiovasculären Symptomenkomplex mit Blutdruckerhöhung — KNAUER und BILLIGHEIMER finden dem gegenüber den systolischen Blutdruck bei Schreckneurosen nicht erhöht, den diastolischen sogar beträchtlich erniedrigt — als besonderes Charakteristikum in den Vordergrund stellt, stehe ich dem ebenso wie KEHRER zweifelnd gegenüber. Der „chokartige Zusammenbruch des Vasomotorentonus", der — wenigstens theoretisch — unter Umständen sogar zum „Sterben vor Schreck" führen könnte (KNAUER und BILLIGHEIMER), mag als unmittelbare Schreckfolge vorkommen und dann bis zu einem gewissen Grade spezifisch sein. Im Rahmen der n. R. nach Schreck — über deren Geltungsbereich wir oben gesprochen haben — unterscheiden sich die vasomotorischen Symptome kaum von denen anderer n. Rn. Bezeichnender — allerdings sehr selten gefunden — sind die trophischen Symptome an Nägeln und Haaren, vor allem das — unter Umständen halbseitige — Ergrauen und das Ausfallen der Haare (KNAUER und BILLIGHEIMER).

Andere von den genannten Bearbeitern der „Schreckneurose" angeführte Symptome können wiederum im vegetativen Symptombild *aller* n. Rn. auftreten: Abnormes Schwitzen, abnormes Erröten, Appetitlosigkeit, Durchfall, Verstopfung, Atemnot (CIMBAL), Menstruations- und Potenzstörungen, Blasenschwäche, alles das sind die Zeichen der allgemeinen vegetativen Regulationsstörung, wie sie den Kern des neurasthenischen Syndroms bildet. Über gewisse Stoffwechselbefunde und ihre Beziehungen zur n. R. haben wir im Kapitel über die pathophysiologischen Grundlagen schon gesprochen; ebenso haben wir dort schon die Beziehungen zu gewissen innersekretorischen Störungen, zumal zum BASEDOW und seinen Miniaturformen bereits berührt.

Es erübrigt nunmehr, noch auf die **psychischen Symptome** der n. R. kurz einzugehen. Wir haben bereits darauf hingewiesen, daß sie unseres Erachtens sämtlich auf die Störungen der vitalen Qualitäten, Antrieb, Stimmung, Reizempfänglichkeit und Schlaf-Wach-Funktion zurückgeführt werden können, daß aber diese Qualitäten in innigstem funktionellem Konnex untereinander stehen, so daß keine von ihnen in stärkerem Grade alteriert werden kann, ohne daß zugleich alle anderen, die gesamte „vitale Person", dabei beteiligt würden. Wenn wir sie jede für sich betrachten, so geschieht das in dem Bewußtsein, daß wir damit der Darstellung zuliebe etwas im Grunde Naturwidriges tun. Es ist immer wieder ein und dasselbe im Grunde unzerreißbare funktionelle Geschehen, zu dem wir — allerdings von verschiedenen Ausgangspunkten aus — gelangen; die einzelnen vitalen Eigenschaften, die wir dabei streifen werden, sind nicht mehr als verschiedene Facetten ein und desselben Ganzheitsgeschehens.

Dem Körperlichen am nächsten steht von diesen Funktionen der *Schlaf*, der bei der n. R. so gut wie regelmäßig gestört ist. Wenn man sich dessen erinnert, was wir über die pathogenetische Rolle der Schlaf-Wach-Funktion eingangs gesagt haben, über ihre hervorragende Bedeutung innerhalb des vitalen Funktionsablaufs als Trägerin der Assimilationsphase und ihre besondere Zugänglichkeit gegenüber den verschiedenen körperlichen und seelischen Ursachen der n. R., dann wird man von vornherein annehmen können, daß gerade *ihre* Schädigung besonders stark sein muß. Gerade hier entwickelt sich ja häufig der besonders ungünstige Circulus vitiosus zwischen fortgesetzter Schädigung und zunehmender Erschöpfung, der oben geschildert wurde. Reine Erschöpfung, die noch nicht zu schwereren und dauernden Regulationsstörungen geführt hat, äußert sich naturgemäß zunächst nur in starkem Schlafhunger, dem der Erschöpfte manchmal auch unter den ungünstigsten Umständen erliegt [1]. Berichte aus dem Kriege (BONHOEFFER, STELZNER, GAUPP u. a.) beschreiben sehr anschaulich den eigentümlichen Eindruck, den man erhielt, wenn man in einen Saal mit frisch eingelieferten, erschöpften Frontsoldaten kam: Sie schliefen sämtlich Tag und Nacht, unter Umständen mehrere Tage lang. Die meisten von ihnen waren nach wenigen derartig verbrachten Tagen wieder in Ordnung (BONHOEFFER). Einige aber behielten über diese Tage hinaus neurasthenische Regulationsstörungen zurück.

Unter diesen Störungen befinden sich nun regelmäßig solche des Schlafs. Der Neurasthenische klagt über Störungen des Einschlafens — das häufig von schlagartigem Zusammenfahren unterbrochen wird — sowohl als namentlich über Erwachen und Nicht-mehr-einschlafen-können nach kurzem Tiefschlaf. Der Schlaf ist ungleichmäßig, oft sehr leicht, von schreckhaften und ängstlichen Träumen — Reproduktion von Kriegserlebnissen (BONHOEFFER, WOLLENBERG) — beeinträchtigt oder durch minimale Sinnesreize unterbrechbar, oft aber auch, zumal gegen Morgen, besonders tief. Allerhand Sensationen, Herzklopfen, Schwitzen, Hautjucken, Heiß- und Kaltwerden, lassen den Kranken nicht zur Ruhe kommen. Das Erwachen bringt demgemäß nicht die gewöhnliche Erquickung; Müdigkeit, Antriebslosigkeit, benommener Kopf, schlechte Stimmung ziehen sich über den Tag hin. Das alles hängt nicht so sehr wie bei den konstitutionell Nervösen und psychogenen Reaktionen von psychischen Einflüssen ab, die Schlafstörung des — rein — Neurasthenischen nähert sich vielmehr den organischen Schlafstörungen, sie macht den Eindruck der von seelischen Vorgängen relativ unabhängigen biologischen Regulationsstörung.

Der Schlaf ist die Phase der Assimilation, in der die vitalen Triebkräfte bereitgestellt werden, deren der Organismus zum Betrieb der animalischen Funktionen in der Wachphase bedarf. Störungen der Assimilation, wie sie u. a. durch die neurasthenische Beeinträchtigung des Schlafes verursacht werden, müssen natürlich in erster Linie ungünstige Rückwirkungen auf die Produktion und Bereitstellung des vitalen *Antriebs* ausüben. Der Zustrom der Kräfte, von denen alle auf die Außenwelt gerichteten Handlungen und Funktionen der Gesamtpersönlichkeit getragen werden, wird spärlicher, ungleichmäßiger und weniger dauerhaft, als er es beim Gesunden mit ausreichend langem und tiefem Schlaf ist. Beim Neurasthenischen kommt hinzu, daß die Antriebsfunktion durch die vorhergehende übermäßige Inanspruchnahme sowieso erschöpft und in ihren Regulationen gestört ist.

Der Neurasthenische sitzt also — soweit er überhaupt aus dem Bett zu bringen ist — matt und schlaff herum, er muß ungewöhnliche Willenskräfte aufwenden, um alltägliche Verrichtungen, das Aufstehen, die Morgentoilette, das Essen, eine allereinfachste Unterhaltung, zu vollbringen. Sein Antrieb reicht vielleicht gerade hin, um einen Spaziergang zu unternehmen, ein Gesellschaftsspiel, eine leichte Lektüre zu beginnen. Aber nach kurzer Betätigung ist alle Kraft wieder erloschen, der Spaziergänger todmüde, der Leser nicht mehr imstande, sich auf die Lektüre zu konzentrieren. Die Unterhaltung versiegt nach wenigen Minuten, weil dem Neurasthenischen die Gedanken ausgehen oder weil er auch die einfachsten nicht mehr zu formulieren vermag. Infolge seiner Konzentrationsunfähigkeit ist er auch nicht mehr in der Lage, etwas zu behalten; er vergißt von Augenblick zu Augenblick, was er erlebt hat, Namen und Ziffern entfallen ihm, Verabredungen und Vorsätze werden nicht eingehalten, teils, weil sie vergessen sind, teils, weil die Willenskraft und Entschlußfähigkeit, die die Ausführung fordert, nicht aufgebracht werden. Auch die von

---

[1] Vgl. unsere Ausführungen im Abschnitt über die Ätiologie.

umschriebenen Trieben, etwa dem Sexualtrieb, getragenen Handlungen und Strebungen zeigen die gleiche Schwächlichkeit und Ermüdbarkeit; auch die Triebe werden also offenbar durch das Versiegen des Antriebs ihrer besten Kraft beraubt. So gewinnt die Gesamtpersönlichkeit des Neurasthenischen ein eigentümlich konturloses, weichliches und willensschwaches Aussehen. Der energische, mutige Offizier, der optimistische, unternehmende Kaufmann, der selbstbewußte und verantwortungsfrohe Beamte, sie alle sind im neurasthenischen Zustand mit seiner Schwunglosigkeit und trübseligen Schlaffheit kaum wiederzuerkennen.

Dazu kommt nun, daß auch die *Stimmung* des Neurasthenischen regelmäßig in erheblichem Grade beeinträchtigt ist. Es handelt sich dabei zunächst um eine Verschiebung der Grundstimmung ins Dysphorische, Unbehagliche, Unzufriedene und Pessimistische. Dies ist die eigentliche neurasthenische, vitalen Regulationsstörungen entspringende „Verstimmung". Je nach der Persönlichkeitsartung und dem Augenblicksanlaß treten weitere Züge hinzu, die das Bild modifizieren. Der Weichere, zu depressiven Reaktionen Geneigte, zeigt depressive Phasen und weinerlich-wehleidige Insuffizienzgefühle, der Härtere, Ungeduldige, vertieft im vergeblichen Kampf des unzulänglichen Willens mit der Antriebslosigkeit und den körperlichen Beschwerden seine Dysphorie bis zur Gereiztheit und gelegentlichen Zornausbrüchen, die dann vielleicht nicht so sehr der Umgebung und ihren Reizen als vielmehr ihm selbst und seiner eigenen Kraftlosigkeit gelten. Querulatorische, paranoide, hypochondrische oder hysterische Elemente mögen weiter vorübergehend das Bild färben; sie entwachsen regelmäßig der besonderen Persönlichkeitsanlage. Treten sie beherrschend in den Vordergrund oder überdauern sie die eigentliche n. R., so handelt es sich um selbständige, besonderer psychopathischer Anlage entspringende Entwicklungen, die nicht mehr der n. R. zugerechnet werden dürfen (BONHOEFFER, NONNE, GAUPP, HELLPACH u. a.).

Mit diesen Störungen der Stimmung sind nun untrennbar solche der *Reizempfänglichkeit* verbunden. Wir haben sie auf dem Gebiete des Körperlichen und der Sinnesorgane bereits kennengelernt. Sie spielen im Bereich der psychischen Funktionen eine womöglich noch größere, jedenfalls vom Kranken und namentlich seiner Umgebung besonders unangenehm empfundene Rolle. Der Neurasthenische ist ungewöhnlich empfindlich und leicht aufgebracht. Kleine Störungen seiner Gewohnheiten, ein mißverstandenes Wort, ein harmloses Versehen der Angehörigen führen zu unverhältnismäßig starken Affektstößen. Zornexplosionen, heftige Vertiefung der Mißstimmung, Tränenausbrüche sind die erste Folge dieser neurasthenischen „Reizsamkeit" — ein Ausdruck NIETZSCHES, den HELLPACH in die Fachliteratur eingeführt hat. An sie schließen sich naturgemäß weitere Konflikte mit der Umgebung an, die ihrerseits wiederum zu neuen Reizen Anlaß geben, womit dann ein besonders peinigender Circulus vitiosus eröffnet ist. Ähnliches zeigt sich hinsichtlich anderer Affekte. Bei jeder albernen Sentimentalität in Theater oder Kino, beim Aufzählen seiner Beschwerden, beim Hören melodiöser und süßer Musik übermannt den Neurasthenischen peinliche Rührseligkeit (WOLLENBERG), Tränen des Mitleids mit sich selbst kommen ihm in die Augen, wenn er sich alter Erlebnisse erinnert, und vor Schluchzen kann er nicht weitersprechen, so sehr er sich bemüht, seine Affektinkontinenz zu unterdrücken. Dabei zeigt sich auch hier die charakteristische Verknüpfung von Reizbarkeit der Funktion mit Schwäche der Leistung: Es sind gerade die Nichtswürdigkeiten und Nadelstiche des Alltags, die zum ununterdrückbaren Affektschwall führen, während alle Erlebnisse höheren seelischen Niveaus, die dem Gesunden allein einer leidenschaftlichen und kraftvollen affektiven Hingabe würdig erschienen wären, vom neurasthenisch

Gewordenen mit einer ihm selbst unbegreiflichen Teilnahmlosigkeit betrachtet werden. Da der Neurasthenische das Beschämende und Persönlichkeitsfremde dieses Zustands selbst schmerzlich empfindet und unter seiner Reizsamkeit selbst heftig leidet, sucht er schließlich alles zu meiden, was ihm „auf die Nerven fallen" könnte, er zieht sich von aller Geselligkeit zurück, er gibt — was andererseits ja auch seiner Antriebsschwäche entspricht — den Besuch von Theater und Konzerten auf, er sucht auch innerhalb der Familie nach Möglichkeit die Einsamkeit und wird so mehr und mehr zum erlebnis- und menschenscheuen Einzelgänger.

Auch diese Alteration der Reizempfänglichkeit macht beim Neurasthenischen den Eindruck einer von psychologischer Mobilisierung relativ unabhängigen, der Persönlichkeit — im Gegensatz z. B. zum Psychopathen und Nervösen — fremden, mehr biologisch bedingten Störung. Sie wird charakteristischerweise am deutlichsten da, wo schwerere organische Prozesse, eine Infektionskrankheit, die Arteriosklerose, eine grobe Hirnerkrankung, dem Zustand zugrunde liegen. Hier finden sich Übergänge zur organischen Affektinkontinenz, bei der die Ausdrucksmechanismen, beispielsweise der Tränenfluß, plötzlich in Gang geraten, obwohl eine entsprechende Affektregung fehlt. Auch rein Neurasthenische, zumal Frauen, klagen gelegentlich darüber, daß ihnen plötzlich, während der Arbeit, Tränen in die Augen kommen, ohne daß sie eigentlich wissen, weshalb. In unmittelbare Nachbarschaft dieser Erscheinungen mögen jene Kontrastreaktionen gehören, über die KLEIST aus dem Kriege berichtete: Offiziere, die schwer erschöpft aus langdauernden verlustreichen Kämpfen kamen, konnten während der Unterhaltung ein ihnen selbst unangemessen und peinlich erscheinendes Lachen nicht unterdrücken, mit dem sie vom Tode der Kameraden und den furchtbaren Erlebnissen berichteten.

Ich will die kurze Schilderung der neurasthenischen Symptomatologie hier abbrechen und nur noch darauf hinweisen, daß je nach der Ätiologie und der Grundkrankheit das eine oder andere Symptom in den Vordergrund treten kann, oder gewisse Besonderheiten des Syndroms einen Hinweis auf die Grundkrankheit geben können. Im postinfektiösen Zustand wird das etwa der hyperästhetisch-emotionelle Schwächezustand BONHOEFFERS sein, bei der beginnenden Arteriosklerose ist die Kombination von Schlafstörung, Kopfweh, Schwindel, Reizsamkeit und Merkfähigkeitsstörung besonders charakteristisch, die groborganische Hirnerkrankung pflegt relativ frühzeitig eine den Klagen widersprechende Stumpfheit und Euphorie zu bringen usw. Aber das alles ist nicht sehr zuverlässig. Wichtig ist, in jedem Falle daran zu denken, daß körperliche Erkrankungen die Grundlage der n. R. bilden können, und danach Anamnese und Untersuchung einzurichten.

Was die **Prognose** der neurasthenischen Reaktion angeht, so ist sie — wenigstens bei der reinen n. R. — ausgesprochen gut. CIMBAL, der allerdings schwer erschöpfte Kriegsfälle im Auge hat, meint, daß die gröbsten Erscheinungen nach 8—10 Tagen überwunden seien. Das mag für die akuten Erschöpfungssymptome gelten, nicht aber für die eigentliche neurasthenische Regulationsstörung, die Wochen und Monate zu ihrem Ausgleich braucht (GAUPP). STERTZ z. B. findet bei seinen posttyphösen Neurasthenischen eine Durchschnittsdauer der reinen n. R. von 6—8 Wochen. Dabei haben jene Fälle, die durch rein körperliche Erschöpfung geschädigt sind, eine bessere Prognose als die psychisch entstandenen (NONNE); das mag damit zusammenhängen, daß sich psychische Schädigungen sehr viel weniger leicht eliminieren lassen als körperliche.

Prognostisch sehr viel ungünstiger liegen natürlich die Fälle, in denen die n. R. auf eine psychopathische oder nervöse Veranlagung trifft oder nur symptomatologischen Wert im Rahmen andersartiger, z. B. cerebraler,

Krankheitsprozesse hat. Die Prognose der symptomatischen n. R. fällt mit der ihrer Grundkrankheit zusammen. Die der konstitutionell unterlegten, auf deren differential-diagnostische Besonderheiten wir schon mehrfach hingewiesen haben, bedarf noch einer kurzen Besprechung.

Psychogene Entwicklungen. Der körperlich-seelische Schwächezustand der n. R., dessen Entstehung einerseits, wie wir geschildert haben, durch konstitutionelle Faktoren, insbesondere die endogene Nervosität, begünstigt wird, bildet andererseits einen Zustand vitaler Widerstandsschwäche, einen „Status minoris resistentiae", der körperlichen wie seelischen Schädigungen und Krankheitsbereitschaften Vorschub leistet. Auf körperlichem Gebiet mag sich das unter Umständen in einer erhöhten Empfänglichkeit und herabgesetzten Widerstandskraft gegen Infektionen äußern (BIRNBAUM). Auf seelischem besteht vor allem die Gefahr der psychogenen Reaktion, die zur Fixierung, Verstärkung und Weiterentwicklung der neurasthenischen Symptome führen kann.

Auch hier spielt — wie überhaupt bei den psychogenen Reaktionen — die besondere Disposition des Individuums für Entstehung und Form der Reaktion die ausschlaggebende Rolle. Der neurasthenische Symptomenkomplex ist in vielen Fällen nichts anderes als eine Gelegenheitsursache, deren sich die psychogene Reaktion als eines willkommenen Vehikels bedient. Sie würde auch andere Krankheiten oder Erlebnisse dazu gebrauchen können, eine Verletzung etwa oder einen Granatschreck. Die n. R. freilich leistet ihr insofern besonderen Vorschub, als sie vermöge der vitalen Schwächung, die sie setzt, das „Gesundheitsgewissen" (KOHNSTAMM) entkräftet und willensmäßige Hemmungen beiseite räumt, die sonst der psychogenen Reaktion im Wege stehen würden.

Psychogene Reaktionen werden verursacht und geformt von starken affektiven Triebkräften, die zu ungewöhnlichen (BRAUN) oder abnormen (SCHNEIDER) körperlich-seelischen Entäußerungen Anlaß geben. Angst, Begehren und Traurigkeit sind die Affekte, die im Zusammenhang mit der n. R. in erster Linie entstehen können; sie führen zu charakteristischen Weiterentwicklungen des neurasthenischen Zustandsbildes, wobei je länger desto mehr die neurasthenischen Symptome hinter dem psychogenen Syndrom zurücktreten, um schließlich nur mehr gelegentlich als Ausdrucksmaterial von ihm benutzt zu werden.

Die Bereitschaft zu ängstlicher Verstimmung wurde schon bei Besprechung der Einzelsymptome hervorgehoben. Sie mag mannigfache Wurzeln haben, körperliche sowohl — z. B. die Herzangst — als auch seelische, wie sie etwa durch die Nachwirkung von Schreck- und Angsterlebnissen gegeben sind. Vor allem aber ist es das „hypochondrische Denken" (JAHRREISS), das an die zahlreichen körperlichen Mißempfindungen anknüpft, von der Angst um Gesundheit, Leben, Berufsfähigkeit und Zukunft getragen der ängstlichen Verstimmung Inhalt gibt und beim anlagemäßig Disponierten zur hypochondrischen Reaktion und Entwicklung führen kann.

Schon hierbei pflegen depressive Einschläge das Bild der Reaktion zu vervollständigen. In manchen Fällen aber treten die depressiven Züge, aus dem Schmerz über die eigene Leistungsunfähigkeit, die Unterbrechung des gewohnten Daseins mit seiner Arbeit und seinen Genüssen, aus der Angst vor der Zukunft und ähnlichem entstanden, stärker und reiner hervor. Hierher mag wohl ein Teil der von AWTOKRATOW, FRIEDMANN u. a. erwähnten neurasthenischen Depressionen gehören. Gerade Menschen, die bis zum Beginn der n. R. gewohnt waren, über ihre vitalen Kräfte nach Belieben zu verfügen, leiden unter dem Bewußtsein ihrer Schwäche, die sie oft als etwas Erniedrigendes und Beschämendes empfinden, besonders stark. Hier sind dann Einschläge von Ungeduld, Gereiztheit und Nörgelei nichts Seltenes.

In das Gebiet der hysterischen Reaktion führen dann jene Entwicklungen, deren tragender und symptomgestaltender Affekt der Wunsch ist, aus dem neurasthenischen Syndrom irgendeinen Vorteil, im Kriege die Rücksendung in die Heimat, im Frieden Pensionierung, Badekur, ärztliche Behandlung oder Exkulpierung vor Gericht, herauszuschlagen. Daß im Kriege solche Reaktionen besonders häufig waren (STERTZ, GAUPP u. a.), entspricht der eigenartigen Konstellation, die sowohl neurasthenische als auch hysterische Reaktionen in ungewöhnlichem Grade begünstigte. Aber auch im Frieden sind die hysterischen Ausschmückungen und Weiterentwicklungen der n. R. nicht selten, so daß man jedenfalls gut tut, bei jeder n. R. von vornherein mit der Möglichkeit hysterischer Zutaten zu rechnen und ihr vorzubeugen. Übrigens besitzen gerade die hysterisch-neurasthenischen Entwicklungen des Friedens oft ein kompliziertes ätiologisches Wurzelwerk. Neben dem Begehren nach irgendeinem Vorteil finden sich hier oft hypochondrische und depressive Vorstellungen, ehrliches Insuffizienzgefühl und — gerade in der heutigen Wirtschaftssituation — nur zu wohl begründete Sorgen und Ängste. Zwischen abortiven, flüchtigen und schwersten, von ihrer neurasthenischen Grundlage völlig gelösten Formen finden sich alle möglichen Übergänge, ebenso wie Übergangs- und Mischformen zwischen hypochondrischen, hysterischen und depressiven Entwicklungen etwas Gewöhnliches sind.

Wir brauchen an dieser Stelle auf Einzelheiten dieser psychogenen Entwicklungen nicht weiter einzugehen und verweisen dafür auf die entsprechenden Darstellungen der Literatur (BUMKE, REICHARD, HAUPTMANN, BRAUN u. a.). Die Prognose dieser auf der n. R. aufgebauten psychogenen Reaktionen ist natürlich unvergleichlich schlechter als die der reinen n. R. Sie hängt in erster Linie von der Konstellation ab, die der Reaktion und ihren emotionalen Triebkräften Vorschub geleistet hat. Nicht mehr die biologischen Gesetze, denen die n. R. unterliegt, sind für den Ausgang maßgebend, sondern die psychologischen Normen, denen die psychogene Reaktion gehorcht. Dabei werden die depressiven Reaktionen in ihrem Ablauf relativ am engsten an den Verlauf der n. R. gebunden sein: Mit der Rückkehr der vitalen Spannkraft und dem Schwinden der Mißempfindungen heben sich Stimmung, Wohlbefinden und Genesungshoffnung. Freilich handelt es sich bei den n. R. mit stärkerem depressivem Einschlag oft gerade um ältere Menschen, bei denen durch Rückbildung oder beginnende Arteriosklerose die Prognose der neurasthenischen Regulationsstörung schon an und für sich getrübt wird. Demgegenüber neigen sowohl hypochondrische als auch hysterische Reaktionen mehr zur Loslösung von der neurasthenischen Grundlage; sie folgen dementsprechend auch im Verlauf und Ausgang ihren eigenen Gesetzen und verlangen unter anderem auch therapeutisch grundsätzlich andere Maßnahmen.

Die **Therapie** der reinen neurasthenischen Reaktion ist denkbar einfach, wenn es möglich ist, die ursächlichen Schädigungen zu beseitigen. Wenn der körperlich-seelisch erschöpfte Frontsoldat aus der Feuerlinie herausgezogen wird und Gelegenheit hat, ausgiebig zu schlafen und sich bei leidlicher Pflege auszuruhen, bleibt dem Arzt meist nichts anderes zu tun übrig, als mit Geduld den natürlichen Heilungsprozeß abzuwarten und ihn allenfalls durch Unterdrückung einzelner Symptome, durch Herbeiführung ausreichenden Schlafs, durch Sorge für genügende, in ihrem Ausmaß dem jeweiligen Kräftezustand angepaßte Bewegung in frischer Luft — Sauerstoffzufuhr — zu unterstützen. Will man — z. B. in der Rekonvaleszenz nach Infektionskrankheiten — etwas Übriges tun, so kommen Kräftigungsmittel wie Promonta, Tonica, Arsenpräparate — besser subcutan zu geben, um die Magenfunktion zu schonen —, wohl auch appetitanregende Mittel in Betracht. Besonders gut bewährt sich oft, zumal bei sonnenlosem Winterwetter, eine vorsichtige Höhensonnenbestrahlung. Sind die gröberen Beschwerden, vor allem die Schlafstörung, behoben, so tut ein Aufenthalt im Mittelgebirge, zumal im Winter, vorzügliche Dienste. Genaue Dosierung von sportlicher und geistiger Betätigung wird dabei zunächst noch zu empfehlen sein. Ein gut angepaßter, zwischen Erholung und Arbeit, geistiger und körperlicher Betätigung genau abwägender, autoritativ vorgeschriebener Tagesplan nützt manchem Neurasthenischen, der vermöge seiner Willensschwächung zur Einhaltung einer vernünftigen Lebensführung nicht imstande ist. Es empfiehlt sich sehr, zumal bei körperlich kräftigen Individuen, Gymnastik, besonders Atemgymnastik (HEYER), Sport und Arbeit in freier Luft (EXNER), abhärtende hydrotherapeutische Maßnahmen in diesen Tagesplan einzubauen. Demgegenüber ist der Gebrauch von Reizmitteln, zu dem der Neurasthenische gern neigt, so weit als möglich einzuschränken. Die Gefahr liegt hier nicht so sehr beim Alkohol, der dem Neurasthenischen meist nicht bekommt und deshalb garnicht oder nur in harmlosen Dosen genossen zu werden pflegt, als vielmehr beim Kaffee, Tee und Nicotin — ganz zu schweigen vom Morphium und Cocain, dessen Mißbrauch wohl vom neurasthenischen Zustand begünstigt wird, dann aber natürlich besondere, eingreifende Maßnahmen erfordert. Kaffee und Tee, die schlafstörend und herzerregend wirken, müssen gemieden werden; einen guten Ersatz für den Tee bietet der brasilianische reizstoffarme Mate. Schwieriger liegen die Dinge beim Nicotin (HEINZ, MÜLLER, KÜLBS), dessen brüskes Absetzen die Willenskraft des Neurasthenischen oft übersteigt und durch sein Mißlingen ungünstige psychische Rückwirkungen hat. Ich pflege deshalb den Nicotingebrauch nur möglichst weit einzuschränken und die Zigarette durch die Zigarre, die schwere Zigarre durch die nicotinarme zu ersetzen.

Im ganzen tut man der reinen n. R. gegenüber gut, die medikamentöse Therapie möglichst einzuschränken und dafür die diätetischen und allgemein kräftigenden Maßnahmen, wie sie oben skizziert wurden, in den Vordergrund zu schieben. Wenn man, wie z. B. gegenüber der Schlafstörung, im Anfang gezwungen sein sollte, sich leichter Schlafmittel — die schweren Barbitursäurepräparate sind meist zu entbehren — zu bedienen, dann soll man sie so bald als möglich wieder absetzen. Man hüte sich vor Polypragmasie, die dem Neurasthenischen nur das Gefühl gibt, schwer erkrankt zu sein. Die zahllosen, von Fabriken, Apotheken und Charlatanen lancierten Mittel gegen die „Neurasthenie" sind allesamt entbehrlich. Wichtig ist es dagegen, den einmal festgelegten Heilplan konsequent durchzuführen und den Neurasthenischen fest in der Hand zu behalten, ihn immer wieder abzulenken, angemessen zu beschäftigen, ihn vor Grübelei und dem ungünstigen Einfluß gewisser Mitpatienten zu behüten[1].

Hier liegt überhaupt die Aufgabe, die der Psychotherapie gegenüber der n. R. in erster Linie zufällt: In der Verhütung und Bekämpfung der psychogenen Überlagerung des neurasthenischen Symptomenkomplexes, insbesondere also der hypochondrischen und hysterischen Entwicklung. Gerade die hypochondrische Reaktion bietet, wenn sie frühzeitig genug angegriffen wird, dem psychotherapeutischen Vorgehen ein dankbares Feld. BUMKE hat vor einigen Jahren darauf hingewiesen, welche schweren „iatrogenen" Schädigungen durch passive oder

---

[1] Ich pflege aus diesen Gründen auch die viel geübte planlose Verschickung des Neurasthenischen in x-beliebige Bäder, Sanatorien oder Erholungsheime zu widerraten, wenn ich nicht sicher bin, daß psychologische Fehler der angedeuteten Art vermieden werden. Wenn der Neurasthenische neben einer meist sehr umfangreichen medikamentösen Behandlung den größten Teil des Tages sich selbst bzw. den Hysterikern, Hypochondern und Nervösen überlassen bleibt, die in solchen Heilstätten zusammenzuströmen pflegen, kann für ihn nichts Gutes daraus erwachsen.

aktive Fehler des Arztes hier verursacht werden können. Dabei ist niemand so sehr durch hypochondrische Vorstellungen gefährdet wie der Neurasthenische, der — ob er es nun eingesteht oder nicht — oft nur seiner Krankheitsbefürchtungen halber zum Arzt kommt; niemand ist aber auch, wenn es gelingt, ihn von der Gegenstandslosigkeit seiner Ängste zu überzeugen, dankbarer und erleichterter. Man sollte daher niemals unterlassen, den Neurasthenischen autoritativ der Harmlosigkeit seiner Beschwerden zu versichern, etwas, was natürlich nur nach sorgfältiger Untersuchung geschehen kann. Oft genügt diese einmalige Versicherung, in hartnäckigeren Fällen wird man bei jeder Beratung von neuem den Kampf gegen die Krankheitsbefürchtungen des Neurasthenischen aufnehmen müssen. Einzelne Fälle freilich, deren Entwicklung durch schwere konstitutionelle Abnormität bestimmt ist, spotten jeder psychotherapeutischen Bemühung bis es gelungen ist, die körperlichen Symptome zu beseitigen oder bis die hypochondrische Entwicklung, ihren inneren Gesetzen folgend, von selbst abklingt.

Ähnliches gilt sinngemäß für die hysterische Überlagerung der n. R. Auch hier ist das wichtigste die Prophylaxe (EYRICH), also der Schutz des Neurasthenischen vor der Ansteckung und die frühzeitige Aufklärung über die harmlose und kurzdauernde Art der Störungen, die dem Neurasthenischen möglichst wenig Zweifel über die Aussichtslosigkeit etwaiger hysterischer Bestrebungen läßt. Kommt es dennoch zu manifesten hysterischen Symptomen, so bleibt nichts anderes übrig, als ihnen so energisch als möglich entgegenzutreten, auch wenn die Behandlung der neurasthenischen Symptome demgegenüber vernachlässigt werden müßte.

Wir brauchen auf diese therapeutischen Fragen, die jedem Arzt geläufig sind, der mit funktionellen psychisch-nervösen Störungen zu tun hat, nicht näher einzugehen. Auch jene pseudoneurasthenischen Symptome, die auf der Grundlage andersartiger organischer Krankheiten erwachsen und deren Behandlung mit der der jeweiligen Grundkrankheit zusammenfällt, bedürfen an dieser Stelle keiner Besprechung mehr.

Wenn die n. R., wie wir darzulegen versuchten, die Folge exogener Schädigungen ist, dann wird der prophylaktischen Abwehr dieser Schäden besondere Bedeutung beizulegen sein. In dieser Hinsicht sind sowohl dem Einzelnen — zumal dem Gefährdeten, konstitutionell Nervösen — als auch der Allgemeinheit Aufgaben gestellt, denen in neuerer Zeit mehr und mehr Verständnis entgegengebracht zu werden scheint. Sie fallen vornehmlich in den Rahmen einer körperlich-seelischen Hygiene, um die sich in Deutschland namentlich R. SOMMER verdient gemacht hat. Gewisse gesunde Tendenzen unserer Zeit, zumal unserer Jugend, ihre Liebe zu Sport und Naturnaheit, zur Pflege des Körpers in Enthaltsamkeit und Übung kommen solchen Bestrebungen aufs erfreulichste entgegen. Es wird Aufgabe der Führer jeden Ranges sein, hier Maß und Ziel zu finden und bewußt das schöne Gleichmaß zwischen Leib und Seele, Tätigkeit und Ruhe, Arbeit und Genuß zu erstreben, das den besten Schutz gegenüber der n. R. bietet. Den staatlichen Organen sind dabei in Belehrung, Aufsicht und gesetzlichen Schutzmaßnahmen besondere Aufgaben zugemessen. Mit am wichtigsten wird natürlich immer die Kleinarbeit des Arztes sein, der in Schule, Haus und Beruf manchen Schädigungen vorbeugen kann.

Es ist nicht einzusehen, warum es schließlich nicht gelingen sollte, die n. R., wenn auch natürlich nicht zu beseitigen, so doch ganz erheblich einzudämmen. Freilich: Krieg, Revolution und Krisen bieten keine günstigen Bedingungen dafür. Einmal aber — so können wir hoffen — wird eine Generation kommen, der die Nervosität nicht mehr „die Krankheit unserer Zeit" ist.

Literatur.

ADLER, A.: Studie über Minderwertigkeit von Organen. Wien 1907. — Über den nervösen Charakter. Wiesbaden 1912. — AIGINGER, J.: Die Phosphaturie, ein Indikator einer konstitutionellen Komponente von Neurosen. Ref. Zbl. Neur. **61**, 505 (1931). — ALBRECHT, TH.: Otologischer Beitrag zur objektiven Begründung neurasthenischer und verwandter Zustände. Münch. med. Wschr. **1919** I, 988. — ALLERS, R.: Über neurotische Schlafstörungen. Dtsch. med. Wschr. **1928** I, 817. — Zur Kenntnis der psychotherapeutischen Beeinflußbarkeit menstrualer Störungen. Allg. ärztl. Z. Psychother. **1** (1928). — ANTONI: Zur Frage der konstitutionellen Nervosität und der neurasthenischen Reaktion. Inaug.-Diss. Kiel 1933. — ARNDT: Neurasthenie. Wien-Leipzig 1885. — ATZLER, E.: Körper und Arbeit. Handbuch der Arbeitsphysiologie. Leipzig 1927. — AWTOKRATOW, P. M.: Die Geisteskranken im russischen Heere während des japanischen Krieges. Allg. Z. Psychiatr. **64** (1907).

BACK, E.: Über Emotionslähmung. Allg. Z. Psychiatr. **58** (1901). — BALABAN, N.: Neurosen und Psychosen als Folgezustände des Erdbebens in der Krim im Jahre 1927. Z. Neur. **119** (1929). — BAUER, J.: Der jetzige Stand der Lehre von der Ermüdung und deren Beseitigung. Dtsch. med. Wschr. **1922** I, 868. — Konstitutionelle Disposition zu inneren Krankheiten, 3. Aufl. Berlin 1924. — Die endokrin Stigmatisierten. Dtsch. med. Wschr. **1932** I, 439. — BAUER, J. u. P. SCHILDER: Über einige psychophysiologische Mechanismen funktioneller Neurosen. Dtsch. Z. Nervenheilk. **64** (1919). — BEARD, G. M.: Die Nervenschwäche, 3. Aufl. Leipzig 1889. — BECHER, E.: Über das Vorkommen von Hyperindicanurie und Hyperurobilinogenurie bei Neuropathen. Zbl. inn. Med. **1930**, 287. — BENJAMIN, E.: Grundlagen und Entwicklungsgeschichte der kindlichen Neurose. Leipzig 1930. — BERGMANN, G. v.: Zum Abbau der ,,Organneurosen" als Folge interner Diagnostik. Dtsch. med. Wschr. **1927** I. — Die vegetativ Stigmatisierten. Z. klin. Med. **108** (1928). — Die ,,vegetativ Stigmatisierten". Med. Klin. **1928** I, 844. — Psychophysische Vorgänge im Bereiche der Klinik. Dtsch. med. Wschr. **1930** II, 1684. — BERGMANN, V. u. BILLIGHEIMER: Das vegetative Nervensystem und seine Störungen. MOHR u. STAEHELINS Handbuch der inneren Medizin, Bd. 5, Teil 2. Berlin 1926. — BERLIT, B.: Erblichkeitsuntersuchungen bei Psychopathen. Z. Neurol. **134** (1931). — BIERNACKI: Zur Ätiologie der funktionellen Neurosen. Neur. Zbl. **17**, Nr 6 (1898). — BILLIGHEIMER, E.: Regulationsmechanismus des vegetativen Nervensystems. Klin. Wschr. **1931** I, 686. — BINSWANGER, O.: Pathologie und Therapie der Neurasthenie. Jena 1896. — Zur Pathogenese der Organneurosen. Dtsch. med. Wschr. **1928** II, 1403. — BINSWANGER, O. u. J. SCHAXEL: Beiträge zur normalen und pathologischen Anatomie der Arterien des Gehirns. Arch. f. Psychiatr. **58** (1917). — BIRNBAUM, K.: Kriegsneurosen und -psychosen auf Grund der gegenwärtigen Kriegsbeobachtungen. Z. Neurol. Ref. **11**, 321; **12**, 1, 317; **13**, 457; **14**, 193, 313; **16**, 1; **18**, 1. — BLEULER, E.: Physisch und psychisch in der Pathologie. Z. Neurol. **30** (1915). — Lehrbuch der Psychiatrie, 4. Aufl. Berlin 1923. — BLUM, K.: Über die Abhängigkeit psychischer und nervöser Störungen von atmosphärischen Einflüssen. Arch. f. Psychiatr. **96** (1932). — BOENHEIM, C.: Über den Tic im Kindesalter. Klin. Wschr. **1930** II, 2005. — BONHOEFFER, K.: Die Psychosen im Gefolge von akuten Infektionen, Allgemeinerkrankungen und inneren Erkrankungen. ASCHAFFENBURGs Handbuch der Psychiatrie, Spezieller Teil, Abt. 3. Leipzig u. Wien 1912. — Erfahrungen aus dem Kriege über die Ätiologie psychopathologischer Zustände mit besonderer Berücksichtigung der Erschöpfung und Emotion. Allg. Z. Psychiatr. **73** (1917). — Die exogenen Reaktionstypen. Arch. f. Psychiatr. **58** (1917). — BORCHARDT, L.: Klinische Konstitutionslehre. Berlin u. Wien 1930. — Über Konstitution und Konstitutionsstörungen, ihre Beziehungen zur Psychologie und Psychopathologie. Z. Neur. **125** (1930). — BRAUN, E.: Psychogene Reaktionen. BUMKES Handbuch der Geisteskrankheiten, Bd. 5. Berlin 1928. — Die vitale Person. Leipzig 1933. — BRAUN, L.: Herz und Psyche. Leipzig u. Wien 1926. — BRUCHANSKI, N.: Die psychischen Reaktionen auf das Erdbeben in der Krim. Z. Neur. **116** (1928). — BRUGSCH, TH.: Erschöpfung bei Kriegsteilnehmern. Z. ärztl. Fortbildg **12** (1915). — BRUSSILOWSKI, L.: Beeinflussung der neuropsychischen Sphäre durch das Erdbeben in der Krim 1927. — Z. Neur. **116** (1928). — BUMKE, O.: Die Pupillenstörungen bei Geistes- und Nervenkrankheiten, 2. Aufl. Jena 1911. — Kultur und Entartung, 2. Aufl. Berlin 1922. — Der Arzt als Ursache seelischer Störungen. Dtsch. med. Wschr. **1925** I, 3. — Psychopathische Reaktionen und Konstitutionen. MOHR u. STAEHELINS Handbuch der inneren Medizin, Bd. 5, Teil 2. Berlin 1926. — Die Revision der Neurosenfrage. Ref. Dtsch. Z. Nervenheilk. **88** (1926). — Lehrbuch der Geisteskrankheiten, 3. Aufl. München 1929.

CASSIRER, R.: Die vasomotorisch-trophischen Neurosen. Berlin 1912. — CIMBAL, W.: Die seelischen und nervösen Erkrankungen. Neur. Zbl. **34**, 411 (1915). — Die Zweck- und Abwehrneurosen als sozialpsychologische Entwicklungsformen der Nervosität. Z. Neur. **37** (1917). — Die Neurosen des Lebenskampfes. Berlin-Wien 1931. — CRAMER, A.: Die Neurasthenie. LEWANDOWSKYs Handbuch der Neurologie, Bd. 5. Berlin 1914. — CURSCHMANN, H.:

Über die Behandlung leichter Thyreotoxikosen. Fortschr. Ther. **6** (1930). — CURTIUS, F.: Organminderwertigkeit und Erbanlage. Klin. Wschr. **11**, 177 (1932).
DAIBER, G.: Über das Verhalten des Blutbildes bei Geistes- und Nervenkrankheiten. Arch. f. Psychiatr. **76** (1926). — DATTNER, B.: Analysen zur Somatogenese der Neurosen. Klin. Wschr. **1929**, 554. — DOCIADES, L.: Konstitutionelle Schwäche des kardiovasculären Systems im Kindesalter. Erg. inn. Med. **35** (1929). — DREIKURS, R.: Zum Problem der Neurasthenie. Internat. Z. Individ.psychol. **9** (1931). — Das nervöse Symptom. Wien u. Leipzig 1932. — DRESEL, K.: Erkrankungen des vegetativen Nervensystems. Aus Spezielle Pathologie und Therapie innerer Krankheiten. Herausgeg. von F. KRAUS u. TH. BRUGSCH, Bd. 10, Teil 3. — DRESEL, K. u. F. HIMMELWEIT: Vegetatives System und Person. Aus Biologie der Person. Herausgeg. von BRUGSCH u. LEWY, Bd. 3. 1930. —
EBBECKE, U.: Physiologie des Schlafes. BETHE u. BERGMANNs Handbuch der normalen und pathologischen Physiologie, Bd. 17. Berlin 1926. — ENKE, W.: Unfallneurose und Konstitution. Allg. ärztl. Z. Psychother. **2** (1929). — ENTRES, J. L.: Vererbung, Keimschädigung. Handbuch der Geisteskrankheiten. Herausgeg. von BUMKE, Bd. 1. Berlin 1928. — EPPINGER, H. u. HESS: Zur Pathologie des vegetativen Nervensystems. Z. klin. Med. **67, 68** (1909). — Die Vagotonie. Berlin 1910. — EXNER, R.: Luftbad-Bewegungstherapie der Neurotiker. Psychiatr.-neur. Wschr. **1928**, 531, 544. — Sauerstoffverbrauch bei Neurosen. Z. Neur. **119** (1929).
FAHRENKAMP, K.: Psychosomatische Beziehungen beim Herzkranken. Nervenarzt **5** (1929). — FALTA, W.: Die Erkrankungen der Blutdrüsen, 2. Aufl. Wien u. Berlin 1928. — FEINBERG, N.: PAWLOW und die moderne Psychophysiologie. Nervenarzt **1** (1928). — FEUDEL, H.: Die vegetative Neurose als kausaler Faktor in der Genese körperlicher und seelischer Erkrankungen. Frankfurt a. M. 1927. — FINKELNBURG, R.: Über die Bedeutung nervöser Herzgefäßstörungen für die Entstehung von Arteriosklerose. Dtsch. Z. Nervenheilk. **60** (1918). — FLATAU, G.: Neue Anschauungen über die Neurosen und ihr Einfluß auf die Therapie. Abh. Psychother. **1928**, H. 7. — FORSTER, E.: Tagesfragen. Mschr. Psychiatr. **74** (1929). — FRIEDMANN, M.: Über eine besondere schwere Form von Folgezuständen nach Gehirnerschütterung, und über den vasomotorischen Symptomenkomplex bei derselben im allgemeinen. Arch. f. Psychiatr. **23** (1892). — Über einen weiteren Fall von nervösen Folgezuständen nach Gehirnerschütterung mit Sektionsbefund. Dtsch. Z. Nervenheilk. **11** (1897). — Über neurasthenische Melancholie. Mschr. Psychiatr. **15** (1904). — FRIEDMANN, M. u. O. KOHNSTAMM: Zur Pathogenese und Psychotherapie bei BASEDOWscher Krankheit. Z. Neurol. **23** (1914).
GAUPP, R.: Kriegsneurosen. Z. Neur. **34** (1916). — Neurosen und Kriegsverletzungen. 8. Jverslg Ges. dtsch. Nervenärzte München, 22.—23. Sept. 1916. Dtsch. Z. Nervenheilk. **56** (1917). — Schreckneurosen und Neurasthenie. SCHJERNINGs Handbuch der ärztlichen Erfahrungen im Weltkrieg. Leipzig 1922. — GEBBING, M.: Die Erbanlage bei Neurotikern. Dtsch. Z. Nervenheilk. **125** (1932). — GELB, A. u. K. GOLDSTEIN: Über Gesichtsfeldbefunde bei abnormer „Ermüdbarkeit" des Auges (sog. „Ringskotome"). Graefes Arch. **109** (1922). — GIERLICH: Neuere Untersuchungen über die objektiven Krankheitszeichen der Neurotiker. Med. Klin. **1918 I**, 983. — GOLDSCHEIDER, A.: Über die krankhafte Überempfindlichkeit und ihre Behandlung. Leipzig 1919. — Die Neurosenfrage. Dtsch. med. Wschr. **1927 II**, 1207, 1250. — Die Neurosenfrage. Z. ärztl. Fortbildg **25**, 373 (1928). — Energetik und Circulus vitiosus. Dtsch. med. Wschr. **1932 I**, 879, 919. — GOLDSCHEIDER, A. u. H. HAHN: Über Dermographien. Dtsch. med. Wschr. **1925 I**, 424, 465, 508. — GOLDSTEIN, K.: Über körperliche Störungen bei Hirnverletzten. 2. Mitt. Münch. med. Wschr. **1918 I**, 65. — Zum Problem der Angst. Allg. ärztl. Z. Psychother. **2** (1929). — GRAFE, E.: Die pathologische Physiologie des Gesamtstoff- und Kraftwechsels bei der Ernährung des Menschen. München 1923. — GRAFE, E. u. L. MAYER: Über den Einfluß der Affekte auf den Gesamtstoffwechsel. Z. Neur. **86** (1923). — GREVING, R.: Die zentralen Anteile des vegetativen Nervensystems. Handbuch der mikroskopischen Anatomie des Menschen. Herausgeg. von MÖLLENDORFF. Berlin 1928. — Die Bedeutung der vegetativen Zentren für die Klinik. Klin. Wschr. **10**, 676 (1931). — GUTTMANN, E.: Zur Kasuistik und Pathogenese des Reflexverlustes bei funktionellen Erkrankungen. Z. Neur. **115** (1928).
HANSE, M.: Über die akute Kommotionspsychose und die Bedeutung der Hirnschütterung für anderweitige psychische Störungen. Arch. f. Psychiatr. **76** (1926). — HANSEN, K.: Zur Theorie der Symptombildung in der Neurose. Nervenarzt **1** (1928). — HAUPTMANN, A.: Kriegsneurosen und traumatische Neurose. Mschr. Psychiatr. **39** (1916). — Neurasthenische und hysterische Äußerungen und Konstitutionen. CURSCHMANN u. KRAMERs Lehrbuch der Nervenkrankheiten. Berlin 1925. — HEINZ, R.: Über die Giftigkeit des Tabakrauches, insbesondere des Zigarettenrauches. Dtsch. med. Wschr. **1923 I**, 318. — HELLER, TH.: Über Psychasthenie. Z. Kinderforsch. **39** (1931). — HELLPACH, W.: Nervosität und Kultur. Berlin 1902. — Therapeutische Differenzierung der Kriegsnervenkranken. Med. Klin. **13**, 1259 (1917). — Die Kriegsneurasthenie. Z. Neur. **45** (1919). — HESS, W. R.: Über die Wechselwirkungen zwischen psychischen und vegetativen Funktionen. Neurologische und

psychiatrische Abhandlungen, H. 2. Zürich 1925. — Die Funktionen des vegetativen Nervensystems. Klin. Wschr. **1930 I**, 1009. — HEYER, G. R.: Seelische Führung durch Gymnastik. Nervenarzt 1 (1928). — HEYER, G. R. u. K. BÜGLER: Möglichkeiten und Grenzen der Psychotherapie bei Organneurosen. Dtsch. Z. Nervenheilk. 98 (1927). — HIRSCHBERG, N.: Fleckfieber und Nervensystem. Berlin 1932. — HIS, W.: Medizin und Überkultur. Dtsch. med. Wschr. **1908 I**, 625. — PAUL FÜRBRINGER und das Hauptwerk seines Lebens. Dtsch. med. Wschr. **1931 I**, 591. — HOCHE, A.: Über die nach elektrischen Entladungen auftretenden Neurosen. Ärztl. Sachverst.ztg **1901**, 371. — Pathologie und Therapie der Angstzustände. Ref. Dtsch. Z. Nervenheilk. 41 (1911). — Schlaflosigkeit. Dtsch. med. Wschr. **1922 I**, 389. — Einige Grenzbestimmungen. Dtsch. Z. Nervenheilk. **100** (1927). — Die Wechseljahre des Mannes. Berlin 1928. — HOESSLIN, R. v.: Über den Verlust der Schmerzreflexe bei funktionellen Nervenkrankheiten. Münch. med. Wschr. **55**, 2597 (1908). — Über Lymphocytose bei Asthenikern und Neuropathen und deren klinische Bedeutung. Münch. med. Wschr. **1913 II**, 1129, 1206. — HOFF, H.: Die psychische Beeinflussung der Organfunktion. Wien. med. Wschr. **1929**, 932. — HOFF, H. u. P. WERMER: Über psychovegetative Schaltungen und ihre Beeinflussung. Klin. Wschr. **1928 I**, 346. — HOFFERBERT, A.: Untersuchungen über das weiße Blutbild bei gesunden und neurasthenischen Individuen. Berl. klin. Wschr. **1921 II**. 1326. — HOMBURGER, A.: Psychopathologie des Kindesalters. Berlin 1926. — HORN, P.: Über Schreckneurosen in klinischer und unfallrechtlicher Beziehung. Dtsch. Z. Nervenheilk. **53** (1915). — Über Symptomatologie und Prognose der cerebralen Kommotionsneurosen. Z. Neurol. 34 (1916). — BASEDOWsche Krankheit und Schreckeinwirkung. Ärztl. Sachverst.ztg **1932**, 295.

ISENSCHMID, R.: Physiologie der Wärmeregulation. BETHE-BERGMANNs Handbuch der normalen und pathologischen Physiologie, Bd. 17. — ISSERLIN, M.: Die Erwartungsneurose. Münch. med. Wschr. **1908 II**, 1427. — ISCHLONDSKY, N. E.: Der bedingte Reflex. Berlin u. Wien 1930. — IWANOW-SMOLENSKY, A.: Über pathophysiologische Grundmechanismen der Psychoneurosen. Schweiz. Arch. Neur. **22** (1928).

JACOBI, E.: Psychogene Spontanblutungen der Haut. Arch. f. Psychiatr. 88 (1929). — Die Psychosen und Psychoneurosen in der Involution des Mannes. Arch. f. Psychiatr. **93** (1931). — JAENSCH, E.: Grundformen menschlichen Seins. Berlin 1929. — JAHN, D.: Funktionsstörungen des Stoffwechsels als Ursache klinischer Zeichen der Asthenie. Klin. Wschr. **1931 II**, 2116. — JAHRREISS,W.: Das hypochondrische Denken. Arch. f. Psychiatr. **92** (1930). — JANOWSKI, W.: Pseudoneurasthenische Lungentuberkulose. Ref. Zbl. Nervenheilk. 54 (1931). — JANUSCHKE, H.: Neurasthenie, Angst und Kreislaufapparat. Wien. med. Wschr. **1929**, 1479. — JULIUSBURGER, O. u. W. LEIBBRAND: Beitrag zur Neurosenlehre. Mschr. Psychiatr. **75** (1930).

KAGLIN, E.: Die Hypertoniekrankheiten. Berlin 1930. — KAHN, E.: Bemerkungen zur Frage der Organminderwertigkeit. Nervenarzt 1 (1928). — KEHRER, F.: Psychogene Störungen des Auges und des Gehörs. Arch. f. Psychiatr. 58 (1917). — Über Hypochondrie. Allg. ärztl. Z. Psychother. 2 (1919). — Spezielle Symptomatologie der Hysterie und der Neurasthenie. LEWANDOWSKYs Handbuch der Neurologie, Erg.-Bd., Teil 1. Berlin 1923. — Über das erbliche Zittern und die Bedeutung von Langlebigkeit, Kinderreichtum und Zwillingsgeburten in Sippen mit heredodegenerativen Nervenleiden. Dtsch. Z. Nervenheilk. 114 (1930). — KELLER, H.: Das nervöse Kind in der Schule. Z. Kinderforsch. **35** (1929). — KIERKEGAARD, S.: Der Begriff der Angst. Jena 1923. — KLOTZ, R.: Über Insuffizienz von Hypophyse und Adrenalsystem, ein Beitrag zur Entstehung von Neurasthenie und Neurosen. Endokrinol. 4 (1929). — Die Atonie der Capillaren als organische Grundlage von Neurasthenie und Neurosen. Z. Kreislaufforsch. 21 (1929). — Die organischen Grundlagen der Neurasthenie. Dresden u. Leipzig 1930. — KNAUER, A.: Über den Einfluß normaler Seelenvorgänge auf den arteriellen Blutdruck. Z. Neurol. 30 (1915). — KNAUER, A. u. E. BILLIGHEIMER: Über organische und funktionelle Störungen des vegetativen Nervensystems unter besonderer Berücksichtigung der Schreckneurosen. Z. Neurol. 50 (1919). — KOCH, J. L. A.: Die psychopathischen Minderwertigkeiten. Ravensburg 1891. — KÖLLNER, H.: Die Untersuchung des indirekten Sehens. AXENFELD u. ELSCHNIGS Handbuch der gesamten Augenheilkunde. Die Untersuchungsmethoden. Bd. 3. Berlin 1925. — KOLLARITS, J.: Über positiven Schmerz und negative Lust bei Neurasthenie und bei Schopenhauer. Z. Neur. 29 (1915). — Das momentane Interesse bei nervösen und nicht nervösen Menschen. J. Psychol. u. Neur. 21 (1915). — Über Widersprüche des Gefühlslebens bei nervösen und nicht nervösen Menschen und über Ertragen des Leidens. Z. Neurol. **33** (1916). — Unterbrechungs- und Abbrechungsgefühle bei nervösen und nicht nervösen Menschen. Z. Neurol. **60** (1920). — KOWALEWSKY, P. J.: Zur Lehre vom Wesen der Neurasthenie. Zbl. Nervenheilk., N. F. 1, 241, 294. — KRAEPELIN, E.: Psychiatrie, 8. Aufl., Bd. 4. Leipzig 1915. — KRAEPELIN, E. u. J. LANGE: Psychiatrie. 9. Aufl., Bd. 2. Leipzig 1927. — KRAFFT-EBING, v.: Psychopathia sexualis, 12. Aufl. Stuttgart 1903. — KRAUS, F.: Ermüdung als Maß der Konstitution. Bibl. med. DI. H. 3. Kassel 1897. — Über konstitutionelle Schwäche des Herzens. Dtsch. med. Wschr. **1917 II**, 1153. — Allgemeine und spezielle Pathologie der Person. Besonderer Teil, I. Tiefenperson. Leipzig 1926. — Über das Neuroseproblem. Klin. Wschr. 1927 I, 537. — KREHL, L.: Entstehung, Erkennung und Behandlung innerer Krankheiten, Bd. 1. Pathologische Physiologie. Leipzig 1931. — KRETSCHMER, E.: Der Stand der psychiatrischen Konstitutionsforschung. Jkurse ärztl. Fortbildg 18 (1927). — Störungen des Gefühlslebens, Temperamente. BUMKES Handbuch der Geisteskrankheiten, Bd. 1. 1928. — KROETZ, CH.: Vegetative Neuroregulation. Klin. Wschr. 1931 I, 673. — KRONFELD, A.: Sexualpsychopathologie. ASCHAFFENBURGS Handbuch der Psychiatrie, 7. Abt. Leipzig u. Wien 1923. — Über psychische Impotenz. Nervenarzt 2, 521 (1929). — Die Lehre der genitalen Neurosen in ihrer Entwicklung seit P. FÜRBRINGER. Dtsch. med. Wschr. 1931 I, 567. — KÜLBS, F.: Zur Symptomatologie des Tabakabusus. Z. klin. Med. 99 (1924). — Über Tabakschäden. Ther. Gegenw. 1928, 11. — KÜNKEL, F.: Einführung in die Charakterkunde auf individualpsychologischer Grundlage, 2. Aufl. Leipzig 1928. — KÜPPERS, E.: Puls. Blutdruck. Vasomotorische Störungen. Blutverteilung. BUMKES Handbuch der Geisteskrankheiten, Bd. 3. Berlin 1928. — KUGLER, E.: Neurosis hypophysaria deconcentrationis. Wien. klin. Wschr. 1924, 1191. — KUNZ, M.: Zur grundsätzlichen Kritik der Individualpsychologie ADLERS. Z. Neurol. 116 (1928).

LANGE, J.: Zur Messung der persönlichen Grundeigenschaften. Kraepelins Psychol. Arb. 8 (1923). — Die Frage der geistigen Entartung in ihrer Beziehung zur Irrenfürsorge. Arch. Rassenbiol. 20 (1928). — LEIDLER, R. u. P. LOEWY: Beteiligung der Cochlea und des Labyrinths bei den Neurosen. ALEXANDER und MARBURGS Handbuch der Neurologie des Ohres. Berlin u. Wien 1926. — LESCHKE, E.: Fortschritte in der Erkennung und Behandlung der wichtigsten Vergiftungen (Chronische Quecksilbervergiftung). Münch. med. Wschr. 1931 II, 1909. — Erkrankungen des vegetativen Nervensystems. Leipzig 1931. — LEUBUSCHER, P. u. W. BIBROWICZ: Die Neurasthenie in Arbeiterkreisen. Dtsch. med. Wschr. 1905 I, 820. — LEYRER, E.: Das Neurosenproblem vom lebenswissenschaftlichen Standpunkt aus. Berlin 1927. — LIPPMANN, A.: Seltenere Tabakschäden. Klin. Wschr. 1931 I, 169. — LÖWENFELD, L.: Sexualleben und Nervenleiden. Wiesbaden 1906. — LÖWENSTEIN, K. u. K. MENDEL: Hirnschädigungen durch elektrische Einwirkung. Dtsch. Z. Nervenheilk. 125 (1932).

MANN, L.: Über Polyneuritis als Begleiterscheinung nervöser Erschöpfungszustände im Kriege. Neur. Zbl. 34, 150 (1915). — MARTIUS, F.: Pathogenese innerer Krankheiten, 3. Heft. Funktionelle Neurosen. Leipzig: Franz Deuticke 1903. — MATHES, P.: Der Infantilismus, die Asthenie und deren Beziehungen zum Nervensystem. Berlin 1912. — MAUTHNER, O.: Über Hörstörungen bei den Neurosen vom neurasthenischen Typus. Med. Klin. 1918 II, 1227. — Über einige psychogene bzw. psychogen-organische Symptome im Bereich des Kehlkopfes und Rachens, der Nase und des Gehörorgans. Mschr. Ohrenheilk. 62 (1928). — MAYER, A.: Psyche und kleine Gynäkologie. Z. ärztl. Fortbildg 28 (1931). — MAYERHOFER: Über das Muskelphänomen der Soldaten, das ist die mechanische Übererregbarkeit der quergestreiften Muskulatur als Symptom der Erschöpfung. Med. Klin. 1916 I. — McDOUGALL, W.: Psychopathologie funktioneller Störungen. Herausge. von H. PRINZHORN. Leipzig 1931. — MENDEL, K.: Klimakterium virile. Neur. Zbl. 1910, 1124. — MEYER, M.: Zur klinischen Bedeutung und nosologischen Stellung des vorzeitigen Alterns (Frühverbrauch). Nervenarzt 3 (1930). — MEYER, S.: Springender und schnellender Patellarreflex bei Neurosen. Neur. Zbl. 30 (1911). — MINOR, L.: Über das erbliche Zittern. Z. Neurol. 99 (1925). — MISCH, W. u. K. MISCH-FRANKL: Die vegetative Genese der neurotischen Angst und ihre medikamentöse Beseitigung. Nervenarzt 5, 415 (1932). — MÖBIUS, P. J.: Über nervöse Familien. Allg. Z. Psychiatr. 40 (1884). — Die Nervosität, 3. Aufl. Leipzig 1906. — MÜLLER, F. C.: Handbuch der Neurasthenie. Leipzig 1893. — MÜLLER, E. F. u. W. F. PETERSEN: Krankheitsbereitschaft und vegetatives Nervensystem. Münch. med. Wschr. 1928 II, 2127. — MÜLLER, L. R.: Lebensnerven und Lebenstriebe, 3. Aufl. Berlin 1931.

NEUBÜRGER, K.: Über zentrale traumatische Hirnerweichung und verwandte Prozesse. Dtsch. Z. gerichtl. Med. 14 (1930). — NONNE, M.: Über zwei durch zeitweiliges Fehlen der Patellarreflexe ausgezeichnete Fälle von Hysterie. Dtsch. Z. Nervenheilk. 24 (1903); 25 (1904). — Syphilis und Nervensystem, 3. Aufl. Berlin 1915. — Über Polyneuritis gemischter Nerven bei neurasthenischen Kriegsteilnehmern. Dtsch. Z. Nervenheilk. 53 (1915). — Neurosen und Kriegsverletzungen. 8. Jverslg Ges. dtsch. Nervenärzte München, 22.—23. Sept. 1916. Dtsch. Z. Nervenheilk. 56 (1917).

OHM, J.: Das Augenzittern der Bergleute. ALEXANDER u. MARBURGS Handbuch der Neurologie des Ohres. Berlin-Wien 1926. — OPPENHEIM, H.: Pathologie und Therapie der nervösen Angstzustände. Ref. Dtsch. Z. Nervenheilk. 41 (1911). — Zur Lehre von den neurovasculären Erkrankungen. Dtsch. Z. Nervenheilk. 41 (1911). — Die Neurosen und Kriegsverletzungen. Neur. Zbl. 34 (1915). — Neurosen nach Kriegsverletzungen. 8. Jverslg Ges. dtsch. Nervenärzte München, 22.—23. Sept. 1916. Dtsch. Z. Nervenheilk. 56 (1917). — Lehrbuch der Nervenkrankheiten, 7. Aufl. Berlin 1923.

PÄSSLER, H.: Über Beziehungen zwischen Erkrankungen des Nervensystems und unspezifischen chronischen Infektionsherden. Dtsch. Z. Nervenheilk. 126 (1922). —

PAHL: Gefäßkrisen. Leipzig 1905. — PANSE, F.: Über Schädigungen des Nervensystems durch Blitzschlag. Mschr. Psychiatr. **59** (1925). — Die Schädigungen des Nervensystems durch technische Elektrizität. Berlin 1930. — PAWLOW, J. P.: Die höchste Nerventätigkeit (das Verhalten) von Tieren. München 1926. — Physiologische Studien über die typischen Erscheinungen des Nervensystems und der Reflexe. Ref. Zbl. Neur. **51** (1929). — PERITZ, G.: Die Spasmophilie der Erwachsenen. Z. klin. Med. **77** (1913). — Über den Herzkrampf im Rahmen der Spasmophilie. Z. Neur. **102** (1926). — PETRUSCHKY, J.: Neurasthenia peripherica localis. Z. Tbk. **53** (1929). — PFAUNDLER, M.: Was nennen wir Konstitution, Konstitutionsanomalie und Konstitutionskrankheit? Klin. Wschr. **1922 I**, 817. — PFEIFER, B.: Psychosen bei Hirntumoren. BUMKES Handbuch der Geisteskrankheiten, Bd. 7. Berlin 1928. — Die psychischen Störungen nach Hirnverletzungen. BUMKES Handbuch der Geisteskrankheiten, Bd. 7. 1929. — PICK, A.: Der Krieg und die Reservekräfte des Nervensystems. Halle 1916. — PONGS: Der Einfluß tiefer Atmung auf den Herzrhythmus. Berlin 1923. — POPPELREUTER, W.: Die psychischen Schädigungen durch Kopfschuß im Kriege 1914/17, Bd. 2. Leipzig 1918. — POTOTZKY, C.: Die klinischen Ergebnisse der Capillaroskopie bei neuropathischen und geistesschwachen Kindern. Mschr. Psychiatr. **69** (1928).

RAECKE: Die Frühsymptome der arteriosklerotischen Gehirnerkrankung. Arch. f. Psychiatr. **50** (1913). — RAIMANN, E.: Fortschritte der Neurosenlehre. Wien. med. Wschr. **1927 II**, 1247, 1430, 1463. — REGELSBERGER: Über das Zustandekommen des Schlafes. Dtsch. med. Wschr. **1927 II**, 1847. — REICHARDT, M.: Lehrbuch der Unfallbegutachtung, 2. Aufl. Jena 1921. — Allgemeine und spezielle Psychiatrie, 3. Aufl. Jena 1923. — Hirnstamm und Psychiatrie. Mschr. Psychiatr. **68** (1928). — Über die sog. Neurosen. Dtsch. med. Wschr. **1930**, Nr 20/22. — RÖPER, E.: Heilerfolge bei Neurasthenie. Mschr. Psychiatr. **30** (1911). — ROMINGER, E.: Vegetative Diathese im Kindesalter. Arch. Kinderheilk. **89** (1930). — ROSENFELD, M.: Über die Beziehungen der vasomotorischen Neurose zu funktionellen Psychosen. Arch. f. Psychiatr. **46** (1910). — Über Kriegsneurosen, ihre Prognose und Behandlung. Arch. f. Psychiatr. **57** (1917). — Die vegetative Neurose in ihren Beziehungen zu psychischen Störungen. Mschr. Psychiatr. **60** (1926). — ROTHMANN, H.: Diagnose und Behandlung von vegetativen Neurosen. Z. ärztl. Fortbildg **28** (1931).

SCHAPIRO, B.: Neuere Gesichtspunkte zur Pathogenese und Therapie der verschiedenen Ejaculatio-praecox-Formen. Z. Sex.wiss. **18** (1931). — SCHARNKE u. HAESELER: Psycho- und neurologische Untersuchungen an trainierenden Wettkämpfern. Sitzgsber. Ges. Naturwiss. Marburg, Febr. 1925, Nr 2. — SCHILDER, P.: Der gegenwärtige Stand der Neurosenlehre. Klin. Wschr. **1927 I**, 49. — SCHINDLER, R.: Die Behandlung der Psychoneurosen des Verdauungstrakts. Arch. Verdgskrkh. **44** (1928). — SCHMIDT, R.: Zur Klinik der Basedowschen Erkrankung und thyreogener Krankheitszustände überhaupt. Münch. med. Wschr. **1931 I**, 983, 1044. — SCHMITZ, A. H.: Über die psychopathologischen Symptome bei der Bleivergiftung und ihre Bedeutung für den Gutachter. Dtsch. Z. gerichtl. Med. **19** (1932). — SCHNEIDER, K.: Die psychopathischen Persönlichkeiten, 2. Aufl. Leipzig u. Wien 1928. — SCHRÖDER, P.: Stimmungen und Verstimmungen. Leipzig 1930. — SCHULTZ, J. H.: Über psychologische Leistungsprüfungen an nervösen Kriegsteilnehmern. Z. Neur. **63** (1921). — Psychotherapie des Schlafmangels. Dtsch. med. Wschr. **1926 I**, 229. — Die konstitutionelle Nervosität. BUMKES Handbuch der Geisteskrankheiten. Berlin 1928. — Beruf und Nervosität. Allg. ärztl. Z. Psychother. **2** (1929). — Die Grundtypen des psychologischen Aufbaus sog. Organneurosen. Dtsch. med. Wschr. **57**, 219 (1931). — SCHULTZ-HENCKE, H.: Schicksal und Neurose. Versuch einer Neurosenlehre vom Bewußtsein aus. Jena 1931. — SCHULTZE, F.: Noch einmal über Neurosen und Psychosen nach Unfällen nebst Bemerkungen über Neurosen überhaupt. Dtsch. Z. Nervenheilk. **117/119** (1931). — SCHUSTER, P.: Die Neurasthenie. Z. ärztl. Fortbildg **25**, 143, 172 (1928). — SCHWAB, O.: Encephalographie, Liquorpassage und Liquorresorptionsprüfungen im Dienste der Beobachtung von sog. Commotionsneurosen. Z. Neurol. **102** (1926). — SEITZ, L.: Die chemisch-physikalischen Veränderungen in der Schwangerschaft in ihren Beziehungen zu neuralen und seelischen Störungen während der Gestationsperiode. Z. Neurol. **131** (1930). — Die Störungen der Lebensnerven in der Schwangerschaft (Schwangerschaftsvegetosen und Neurovegetosen). Arch. Gynäk. **145** (1931). Ref. Zbl. Neurol. **60**, 486 (1931). — SEMERAU-SIEMIANOWSKI, M.: Kardiovasculäre Neurosen auf Basis von Keimdrüseninsuffizienz. Med. Klin. **1927 II**, 1962, 1997. — SIEBELT: Tabakmißbrauch in ursächlichem Zusammenhange mit Kriegsneurosen, vor allem des Herzens. Med. Klin. **1917 II**, 68. — SIMSON, T.: Psychische und psychologische Reaktionen Erwachsener und Kinder bei Erdbeben. Z. Neurol. **118** (1928). — SIOLI, F.: Das Nervensystem bei Diabetes und Nierenkrankheiten. Münch. med. Wschr. **1932 I**, 941. — SOMMER, R.: Psychotherapie und psychische Hygiene. Allg. ärztl. Z. Psychother. **1**, 6, 129 (1928). — SPERLING, O.: Testversuche bei akuten nervösen Erschöpfungszuständen. Med. Klin. **1931**. — SPIEGEL, E. A.: Der Tonus der Skelettmuskulatur. Berlin 1927. — Der zentrale Aufbau des vegetativen Nervensystems. Klin. Wschr. **1930 II**. — STEIN, F. W.: Hypotonia nervosa, ein konstitutionelles Krankheitsbild. Med. Klin. **1929 I**, 180. — STEINER: Neurologisches und Psychiatrisches im Kriegslazarett. Z. Neur. **30** (1915). —

STELZNER, H.: Erschöpfungspsychosen bei Kriegsteilnehmern mit besonderer Berücksichtigung der Dämmerzustände. Arch. f. Psychiatr. **57** (1917). — STERTZ, G.: Typhus und Nervensystem. Berlin 1917. — Über die Senkung des Persönlichkeitsniveaus als funktionelle Störung und als Defektsymptom. Mschr. Psychiatr. **68** (1928). — Die neurasthenische Reaktion. BUMKES Handbuch der Geisteskrankheiten, Bd. 5. Berlin 1928. — STIEFLER, G.: Über Psychosen und Neurosen im Kriege, I. u. II. Jb. Psychiatr. **37/38** (1917). — STIER, E.: Neurasthenie. Aus: Spezielle Pathologie und Therapie innerer Krankheiten. Herausgeg. von KRAUS u. BRUGSCH, X, 1924. — STIERLIN, E.: Über psychoneuropathische Folgezustände bei den Überlebenden der Katastrophe von Courrières am 10. März 1906. Mschr. Psychiatr. **25**, Erg.-Bd. (1909). — Nervöse und psychische Störungen nach Katastrophen. Dtsch. med. Wschr. **1911 II**, 2028. — Nervöse Störungen nach Katastrophen. Dtsch. med. Wschr. **1911**. — STILLER, B.: Die asthenische Konstitutionskrankheit. Stuttgart 1907. — Grundzüge der Asthenie. Stuttgart 1916. — STÖWSAND, W.: Über die vegetativen Neurosen. Dtsch. med. Wschr. **1928 II**, 1416. — SZONDI, L.: Die Revision der Neurastheniefrage. Leipzig: Rudolf Novak & Co. 1930.

TANDLER, J.: Konstitution und Rassenhygiene. Z. angew. Anat. **1913**. — THIELE, R.: Kreislaufstörungen und Psychosen. Allg. Z. Psychiatr. **92** (1930). — TRAUTMANN, E.: Klinische Untersuchungen zu einer topischen Diagnostik des Kopfschmerzes. Z. Nervenheilk. **110** (1929).

„Unfall- (Kriegs-) Neurose", Die. Vorträge und Erörterungen gelegentlich eines Lehrgangs für Versorgungsärzte im Reichsarbeitsministerium vom 6.—8. März 1929. Berlin: Reimar Hobbing 1929.

VERWORN, M.: Allgemeine Physiologie, 5. Aufl. Jena 1909. — VOGEL, P.: Zur Symptomatologie und Klinik des Schwindels. Nervenarzt 5, 169 (1932). — VOGT, C.: Einige Ergebnisse unserer Neurosenforschung. Naturwiss. **9** (1921).

WALINSKI, F.: Alkalireserven im Blut bei Neurasthenie und organischen Nervenkrankheiten. Dtsch. med. Wschr. **1930 I**, 520. — WEBER, E.: Über die körperlichen Äußerungen psychischer Zustände. Jena 1910. — Der Einfluß psychischer Vorgänge auf den Körper, insbesondere auf das Blutverteilung. Berlin 1910. — WEBER, L. W. u. W. WEBER: Störungen und Veränderungen des Sehapparates bei Psychosen und Neurosen. SCHIECK u. BRÜCKNERs Kurzes Handbuch der Ophthalmologie, Bd. 6. Berlin 1931. — WEILER, K.: Organisch, funktionell, psychogen? Münch. med. Wschr. **1928 I**, 815. — WEINBERG, A. A.: Psyche und unwillkürliches Nervensystem. Z. Neurol. **85** (1923). — WEIZSÄCKER, V. v.: Soziale Krankheit und soziale Gesundheit. Berlin 1930. — WEXBERG, E.: Individualpsychologie. Eine systematische Darstellung. Leipzig 1928. — ALFRED ADLERs Lehre von der Organminderwertigkeit in ihrer Bedeutung für die innere Medizin. Allg. ärztl. Z. Psychother. **1**, 202 (1928). — WIEG-WICKENTHAL, K.: Über pseudohysteroneurasthenische Zustandsbilder. Wien. med. Wschr. **1928 I**, 944. — WILDER, J.: Probleme des Zuckerstoffwechsels in der Neurologie und Psychiatrie. Zbl. Neurol. **56**, 1 (1930). — WINDSCHEID: Über Hirnerschütterung. Dtsch. med. Wschr. **1910 I**, 8. — WITTKOWER, E.: Über affektivsomatische Veränderungen. Klin. Wschr. **1928 II**, 2193; **1929 I**, 1082; **1930 II**, 1296; **1931 II**, 1811. — WOHLWILL, F.: Über funktionell bedingtes Fehlen der Patellarreflexe. Neur. Zbl. **28**, 567 (1909). — WOLLENBERG, R.: Nervöse Erkrankungen bei Kriegsteilnehmern. Münch. med. Wschr. **1914 II**, 2181. — WYSS, W. H. v.: Körperlich-seelische Zusammenhänge in Gesundheit und Krankheit. Leipzig 1931.

ZIEGLER, K.: Klinische Bedeutung einiger Wurmparasiten des Darmes, besonders der Ascaridiasis. Med. Klin. **1917 II**, 1031. — Betrachtungen zur Pathophysiologie des vegetativen Nervensystems. Dtsch. med. Wschr. **1931 I**, 437, 489. — ZUCKER, K.: Über eine charakteristische Unterform der vegetativen Neurose. Dtsch. Z. Nervenheilk. **101** (1928). — ZWEIG, H.: Das Schlafproblem. Zbl. Neur. **55**, 353 (1930).

Die sog. Organneurosen.
Von WALTHER JAHRREISS-Köln.

Schon die Titelfassung dieses Beitrags weist darauf hin, daß hier vorsichtig zu schwierigen Fragen Stellung genommen werden soll, und daß manches Ergebnis und manche Folgerung fragwürdig sind und in der Schwebe bleiben müssen. Der Kern, um den es geht, ist die „Psychogenese körperlicher Störungen", d. h. ihre seelische Verursachung, oder doch wenigstens ihr seelischer Werdegang. Von hier aus hat sich das ärztliche Denken besonders im letzten Jahrzehnt erneut und breit der Diskussion um das Leib-Seele-Problem zugewandt und hat sich bemüht, in Wechselwirkung mit psychologischen und philosophischen Ergebnissen und Meinungen die körperlich-seelischen Abläufe in ihrer lebendigen Einheit zu begreifen, als „Organismus" etwa oder als „Person". Es ist verständlich, daß solche forschende und denkende Hinwendung zu einer „organismischen Biologie" in allen medizinischen Disziplinen anregend wirken mußte, und daß gerade die Fragen nach Aufbau und Behandlung sog. funktioneller Betriebsstörungen eine gewisse Klärung erfuhren. Eine Fülle von Arbeiten hat hier vor allem hervorgerufen der Einbruch psychologischer, besonders sog. tiefenpsychologischer Betrachtungsweisen mit ihrem Fahnden nach verständlichen Zusammenhängen zwischen individueller Lebensgeschichte und Krankheitserscheinung; mit ihrer symbolischen Deutung der Symptome oder deren finaler Auslegung als sinnvolle und tendenziöse Haltungen und Handlungen.

Im Ausgleich dazu sind von der somatologischen Betrachtungsweise her die Klinik, Physiologie und Pathologie des vegetativen Nervensystems und der endokrinen Vorgänge gefördert worden, und diese Förderung hat dazu beigetragen, das Übermaß psychopathologischer Konstruktionen und Verallgemeinerungen um die sog. Organneurosen abzubauen.

I. Psychophysische Korrelationen.
1. Begriffe und Begrenzungen.

Es wäre zu wünschen, daß dieser Abbau auch vor dem Namen „Neurose" nicht halt zu machen brauchte. Bereits 1925, auf der Jahresversammlung Deutscher Nervenärzte in Kassel wurde diese Forderung von REDLICH und von BUMKE[1] erhoben.

REDLICH empfiehlt statt von Neurosen von einer Gruppe der Neuropathien zu sprechen und BUMKE bekennt, daß ihm während seines Referates der Begriff Neurose unter den Händen zerronnen sei in diejenigen der nervösen Reaktionen und Konstitutionen, der Psychopathien und funktionellen Psychosen. Allgemein wird heute begrifflich die neurotische Störung der organischen gegenübergestellt, wobei als dritter Begriff die funktionelle Störung der neurotischen bald nebenbald übergeordnet oder auch einfach gleichbedeutend mit ihr gebraucht wird.

---
[1] In beiden Referaten über die Revision der Neurosenfrage kurzer geschichtlicher Überblick über die Entwicklung des Begriffes Neurose seit seinem Aufkommen Ende des 18. Jahrhunderts durch den Schotten CULLEN. Vgl. auch hierzu und zum folgenden den Artikel „Neurosen" von KEHRER in BIRNBAUMS Handwörterbuch.

BUMKE hat in dem genannten Referat dargelegt, wie „die geschichtliche Entwicklung aus dem ursprünglich rein somatologisch gedachten Begriff (sc. Neurose) schließlich einen in der Hauptsache psychologischen gemacht" hat[1]. In dieser Betonung des „Psychologischen" der Neurosen, d. h. ihrer seelischen „Entstehung" liegt eine Möglichkeit begründet, die große Gruppe der funktionellen Erkrankungen aufzuteilen in solche, bei denen die seelische und in solche, bei denen die körperliche Herkunft überwiegt (H. F. HOFFMANN). Daß sich bei dieser Zerlegung ein gemeinsames Mittelstück finden muß, bedarf keiner besonderen Begründung[2].

Für die Definition aller funktionellen Erkrankungen — im Gegensatz zu den organischen — wird gefordert, daß ihnen keine krankhaften anatomischen Veränderungen zugrunde liegen, und daß es sich klinisch um regelmäßig reversible Störungen handelt.

Es erscheint notwendig, jedem Einzelfall gegenüber diese begriffliche Schärfe anzuwenden. Nur so wird es möglich sein, Sowohl- als auch -Verschwommenheiten auszumerzen und den Strukturwert abzuschätzen, der grob organisch bedingten Erscheinungen, „rein" organischen Labilitäten körperlicher Funktionen, und wirklich oder scheinbar seelischen Reaktionen oder seelisch bedingten körperlichen Betriebsstörungen in dem Gesamt eines Krankheitsbildes zukommt. Gerade die moderne Beschäftigung mit dem Neurosenproblem sollte — man möchte es wenigstens wünschen — auch dem Vertreter somatischer Disziplinen gezeigt haben, wie auch-notwendig die psychologische Betrachtungsweise ist, und wie förderlich sie über die wissenschaftliche Ergründung und diagnostische Deutung hinaus in therapeutischer Beziehung sein kann[3].

Man muß sich nur dabei immer gegenwärtig halten, daß auch hinter den funktionellen Neurosen „somatische Veränderungen gesucht werden müssen, man mag sie sich dynamisch oder chemisch denken" (BUMKE).

Auf eine wichtige und gebräuchliche Begriffstrennung innerhalb des Neurosengebietes ist nunmehr einzugehen, nämlich auf die Scheidung in *Psychoneurosen* und *Organneurosen*. Es wurde ja schon erwähnt, welche sehr unterschiedlichen Krankheitsbilder und Verläufe unter dem Begriff der Psychoneurosen zusammengefaßt erscheinen: Neuropathien, psychopathische Reaktionen und Entwicklungen, ja selbst funktionelle Psychosen. Wenn man den Rahmen so weit spannt, ist freilich kaum einzusehen, warum die „Organneurosen" nicht auch in ihm aufgehen sollen. Eine begriffliche Trennung scheint erst dann einigermaßen begründet zu sein, wenn man die Psychoneurosen den Psychosen gegenüberstellt[4]. Dann zeigt sich, daß die Erscheinungen der *Psychoneurosen* — vorwiegend — seelischer, diejenigen der Organneurosen aber — vorwiegend — körperlicher Art sind. Wir sprechen von Organneurosen dann, wenn sich die seelisch entscheidend mitverursachten funktionellen Störungen scheinbar isoliert im Bereich einzelner Körperorgane oder Organsysteme abspielen. Diese

---

[1] Nicht der gleichen Meinung war REDLICH, der noch auf derselben Tagung unter den Neurosen abhandelt „Neuropathien organischen Gepräges" und darunter rechnet: Epilepsie, Migräne, MENIÈREschen Schwindel.
[2] Von einer Warte aus, die mehr das Einende betont, ist BUMKE zuzustimmen, wenn er meint: „Innerhalb des funktionellen Gebietes müssen wir .... auf ein starres Krankheitssystem grundsätzlich .... verzichten."
[3] Es wäre freilich gut, wenn der Internist, der Gynäkologe usw. durchweg an vorsichtige psychiatrische Berater kämen, und wenn wiederum der Psychiater und „Psychotherapeut" mit den Vertretern der Körpermedizin engste Fühlung behielte.
[4] Ein sowohl quantitativer wie sozialer Maßstab findet sich in Definitionen, wie sie etwa KEHRER gibt. „Innerhalb der funktionellen Krankheitszustände grenzt man heutzutage diejenigen als Neurosen ab, welche mehr vorübergehender Natur sind und nicht die sozialen Folgen der Geisteskrankheiten haben."

Beschränkung auf bestimmte „Ausdrucksmittel des Seelischen" also trennt die sog. Organneurosen von den Psychoneurosen im engeren Sinne.

v. MONAKOW-MOURGUE etwa sprechen geradezu von *Isolierungsphänomenen* im Bereich des organo-vegetativen Systems, „die manchmal für organische Affektionen gehalten werden können". An dieser Sonderstellung der Organneurosen soll hier — wie uns scheint mit zureichender Begründung — festgehalten werden, um so mehr als ihnen nicht nur erscheinungsmäßig, sondern auch pathogenetisch bestimmte Eigentümlichkeiten zukommen, auf die später eingegangen werden soll. Daß die Grenzen nach den nervösen Konstitutionen, aber auch nach den Psychoneurosen i. e. S. etwa gewissen hypochondrischen und hysterischen Reaktionen immer wieder überschritten werden müssen, versteht sich bei der Künstlichkeit aller solcher Einteilungen im Großgebiet der Psychoneurosen von selbst. Wir stimmen SIEBECK zu, wenn er meint, man kann nicht alles Funktionelle, alles Psychogene neurotisch nennen, sondern nur dann, wenn ganz besondere typische psychische Zusammenhänge zu krankhaften Erscheinungen führen. Ganz ähnlich drückt sich SCHILDER aus, wenn er sich auch begrifflich weniger festlegt: „Wir sprechen von Organneurosen erst dann, wenn durch die neurotische Einstellung des Individuums in der Funktion eines Organs wesentliche Änderungen eingetreten sind."

In den letzten Jahren hat sich I. H. SCHULTZ wiederholt um eine Gruppierung, der Neurosen bemüht. Er verläßt dabei die herkömmlichere Ordnungsform nach psychologisch-symptomatischen Gesichtspunkten, zugunsten einer Einteilung, die sich mehr nach dem Aufbau der Neurosen zu richten sucht. Dabei soll die Rangordnung der Neurosen von „gleichsam äußerlichen und körperhaften Produkten über das Gebiet der allgemeinen Psychogenie bis zur höchsten Problematik des abnormen Charakters gegeben sein". In der folgenden Tabelle[1] werden die entscheidenden Gesichtspunkte dieser Gruppierung einigermaßen deutlich:

I. Fremdneurosen (überwiegend exogen) allopsychischer Konflikt.
II. Randneurosen (überwiegend physiogen) physiopsychischer Konflikt.
III. Schichtneurosen (überwiegend psychogen) endopsychischer Konflikt.
IV. Kernneurosen (überwiegend charakterogen) autopsychischer Konflikt.

Auf eine Stellungnahme zu dieser „Konfliktstopographie" der Neurosen kann hier verzichtet werden.

Wichtig ist für die vorliegende Arbeit vor allem das Gebiet der sog. Randneurosen, in denen der Konfliktstoff in der Auseinandersetzung mit der eigenen Körperlichkeit liegt; „ein erheblicher Teil der Organneurosen würde hier seinen Platz finden". Die Entstehung dieser Randneurosen erscheint I. H. SCHULTZ vorwiegend physiogen, wobei er freilich auf das Doppelgesicht gerade dieser auch seelisch bedingten Betriebsstörungen hinzuweisen nicht vergißt. Er meint, daß hier die Physis als Neutralphänomen eine psychische und physische Erfassung zuläßt.

Diese Doppelgründigkeit der Entwicklung, des Verlaufes, der „Heilung" organneurotischer Symptome verleiht ihnen die oben gekennzeichnete Sonderstellung und die Ausweitung der diagnostischen Bemühungen im Einzelfall über ein *Entweder:* seelisch *oder* somatisch hinaus zu einem: wieviel seelisch *und* wieviel somatisch.

Es ist ja bekannt, wie sehr diese Bemühungen um eine Gesamtschau seelischleiblicher Beziehungen, Entsprechungen und Abhängigkeiten allerorts in die medizinischen Abhandlungen einbezogen sind. Ich erinnere nur an Arbeiten über das Problem der Durchflechtung organischer und hysterischer Erscheinungen

---

[1] Aus „Seelische Krankenbehandlung" von I. H. SCHULTZ, S. 241. Jena 1930.

und über die scheinbar hysterische Prägung organisch bedingter cerebraler Leistungsausfälle und kompensierender Neuleistungen [1].

Ihren besonderen Wert besitzen derlei Betrachtungen auf dem Gebiet der vegetativen Funktionsstörungen, aber sie bedeuten auch eine Versuchung und Gefahr. Leibseelische Korrelationen sind hier schon in der Norm evident; und der körperliche Ausdruck gewisser Affekte ist sprichwörtlich seit alters. Experimentelle Untersuchungen haben Möglichkeit und Umfang einer psychischen Beeinflussung des vegetativen Nervensystems in der Norm eindringlich dargetan. Auf der anderen Seite hat die verfeinerte somatische Diagnostik den Umfang anscheinend seelisch bedingter Störungen von Organfunktionen eingeengt, indem es ihr gelang, den Bereich der organischen, jedenfalls *nicht* psychischen Verursachung erscheinungsmäßig gleicher Vorgänge aufzudecken. Diese pathogenetische Vielfältigkeit, die in der Neigung des vegetativen Nervensystems liegt, auf verschiedenartige Reize mit der gleichen Krankheitsäußerung zu antworten [2] (polygenetisches Verhalten) (H. CURSCHMANN), muß die tatsächliche Begrenzung der sog. Organneurosen nach dem jeweiligen Stand unserer Kenntnisse verschieden ausfallen lassen. Von hier aus wird immer wieder der Überschuß an psychopathologischer Dichtung revidiert. Davon aber bleibt unangetastet die Fragestellung, ob und in welcher Weise organneurotische Reaktionen in dem hier gemeinten Sinne einer entscheidenden seelischen Mitverursachung sich vollziehen, sowie die grundsätzliche Forderung nach psychologischer und somatologischer Betrachtungsweise, und nach möglicher Klärung der jeweiligen Wertigkeit und zeitlichen Folge bekannter einzelner Glieder innerhalb der Ursachenkette. Es wird sich dann für die Organneurosen in der Regel mit überzeugender Wahrscheinlichkeit dartun lassen, daß es sich bei ihnen um ein sehr vielschichtiges Geschehen handelt, bei dem das jeweilige „Organ" infolge der innigen Korrelationen zwischen „Lebensnerven" — innerer Sekretion — und seelischem Verhalten nur im Mittelpunkt steht.

Insoweit ist die Bezeichnung „Organneurose" unzulänglich und ohne nähere begriffliche Begrenzung sogar ein „irreführendes Stichwort" (I. H. SCHULTZ). Dennoch erscheint es aussichtslos, „für ihren Tod zu plädieren" [3]. Ich halte es auch nicht für nennenswert besser von „allgemeinen Affektneurosen" *(Alkan)* oder von einer „Psychogenie krankhafter Funktionsabläufe" zu reden und glaube nicht, daß es sich einbürgern würde, wenn man im Anschluß an HANSEN von „ideagenen" oder eingebildeten krankhaften Funktionsabläufen, oder ideagenen (eingebildeten krankhaften) „Ausdrucksbewegungen des vegetativen Nervensystems" spräche.

2. Die seelische Beeinflussung des vegetativen Nervensystems in der Norm und im Experiment.

a) Physiologische Vorbemerkungen.

Für die Darstellung des schwierigen und in entscheidenden Punkten noch umstrittenen Gebietes einer Anatomie und Funktion des vegetativen Nerven-

---

[1] Eine ausgezeichnete kritische Stellungnahme hierzu und zu den einschlägigen Arbeiten von GOLDSTEIN, PÖTZL, H, BÜRGER, JOH. LANGE usw. findet sich bei ERICH GUTTMANN „*Organische Krankheitsbilder hysterischen Gepräges*" in den Fortschr. Neur. 4, 82 f. (1932).
[2] 1. „Scheinbar ganz spontan, bzw. ex causa ignota; 2. durch endokrine Einflüsse; 3. anaphylaktogen; 4. durch klimatische und analoge Faktoren; 5. durch grob körperliche Anomalien, Defekte u. dgl.; 6. aber auch rein psychogen." H. CURSCHMANN.)
[3] BUMKE meint Referat 1925 von der Bezeichnung Neurose: Da es eingeführt ist, wage ich freilich auch nicht für seinen Tod zu plädieren. Das nützt erfahrungsgemäß auch nichts. Das Wort Hysterie allein ist wohl noch häufiger umgebracht worden als selbst die Psychoanalyse und doch wird es sicher länger leben als wir zusammen. Die Bezeichnung Neurose behält ja auch insofern immer noch eine gewisse Bedeutung, als sich hier oft seelische und körperliche Störungen ziemlich unentwirrbar vermischen.

systems verweise ich auf die zusammenfassenden Darstellungen von v. BERGMANN und BILIGHEIMER, LANGLEY, L. R. MÜLLER, SCHILF, E. A. SPIEGEL, PH. STÖHR jun., CHR. KROETZ. Es sollen hier nur ganz kurz diejenigen Tatsachen und Meinungen ins Gedächtnis zurückgerufen werden, deren Erwähnung für diese Darstellung unerläßlich erscheint. Hervorgehoben sei zunächst die Erkenntnis von der *Ubiquität der vegetativen Innervation* [1]. Das autonome Nervensystem steht nicht nur den Funktionen der allein vegetativ innervierten Organe vor, sondern ist auch in einer noch nicht ausreichend zu kennzeichnenden Weise (Muskelstoffwechsel? Tonus?) an den Leistungen der Skeletmuskulatur beteiligt (ORBELI, BRÜCKE, SCHILF). Die quergestreifte Muskulatur ist somatisch *und* vegetativ innerviert. In einem wunderlichen Verhältnis zu dieser Ubiquität der vegetativen Innervation steht die Tatsache, daß nach Entfernung selbst ausgedehnter Teile des sympathischen und parasympathischen Nervensystems die Ausfallerscheinungen relativ geringfügig sind. An Katze, Hund, Affe ist von CANNON und seinen Mitarbeitern (zit. bei KROETZ) schließlich die sympathische Ganglienkette von den Ganglia stellata bis zu den Ganglien oberhalb des Beckenrandes entfernt worden. Dadurch wurde auch der cervicale Teil abgeschnitten (Passage der präganglionären Fasern des Halsteils durch die Ganglia stellata). Dennoch konnten zahlreiche dieser so weitgehend sympathektomierten Tiere noch monatelang weiterleben; darunter eine Katze, der noch außerdem eine Nebenniere entfernt und das Mark der anderen zerstört worden war, so daß (wie die spätere Sektion ergab) kein chromaffines Gewebe zurückgeblieben war. Man hat gemeint, auf Grund dieser Erfahrungen, die ja darlegen, daß zur Erhaltung des Lebens das autonome Nervensystem nicht notwendig sei, diesem auch die Bezeichnung „Lebensnerven" (L. R. MÜLLER) absprechen zu sollen (CANNON, E. SCHILF). Immerhin ist zu bedenken, daß diese weitgehend sympathektomierten Tiere doch nur unter den schützenden Bedingungen des Laboratoriums ihr Leben weiter fristen konnten, und daß ihre Lebensmöglichkeit unter den natürlichen Bedingungen der Außenwelt ganz erheblich gelitten hatte. Sie waren, vor allem infolge der Unfähigkeit, äußeren Gefahren und Schädigungen (Kälte, Wärme, Muskel und Herz beanspruchende Abwehrleistungen usw.) ausreichend Widerstand und Ausgleich zu leisten, unter normalen Bedingungen lebensunfähig. Zur primitivsten Lebensbemeisterung mindestens scheinen die „Lebensnerven" doch unerläßlich zu sein.

Bevor ich eingehe auf das Zusammenspiel autonomer nervöser Vorgänge und Wirkungen mit chemischen körpereigenen Reizstoffen soll noch kurz auf die Doppelinnervation vegetativ gesteuerter Organe hingewiesen werden. Diese Doppelinnervation, die möglicherweise nur wenige Ausnahmen kennt — (fehlende parasympathische Innervation der Schweißdrüsen?) [2] ist zugleich eine doppelsinnige, insofern als eine sympathisch bewirkte Funktion parasympathisch gehemmt wird und umgekehrt. Diesem anscheinenden Antagonismus gegenüber läßt sich jedoch darauf hinweisen, daß es sich bei mehr organismischer Betrachtungsweise „in Wahrheit um eine synergistische Innervation der *Gesamtfunktion*" handeln kann, wobei eben nur die *Teile* eines Organes antagonistisch (durch *denselben* Nerven) beeinflußt werden: z. B. *Vagus:* Kontraktion der Muskeln des Magenkörpers und Erschlaffung des Schließmuskels; *Sympathicus:* Kontraktion des Schließmuskels am Magenausgang und Erschlaffung der Muskulatur des Magenkörpers.

---

[1] Vgl. hierzu besonders auch G. TH. BRÜCKE: „Fortschritte in der Erkenntnis des vegetativen Nervensystems."

[2] Vgl. KROEZ: S. 1745; O. FOERSTER: Zbl. Neur. 50, 764; der nachgewiesen hat, daß es außer dem Sympathicus noch andere durch Pilocarpin erregbare parasympathische Schweißnerven gibt.

Die fruchtbare Konzeption einer Vagotonie bzw. Sympathicotonie (EPPINGER und HESS) im Sinne des elektiven Überwiegens eines dauernd gesteigerten Vagustonus über den Sympathicustonus und umgekehrt, läßt sich nach späteren Untersuchungen (v. BERGMANN und seiner Schule, E. FRANK, SCHILF, I. BAUER, R. SCHMIDT u. a.) nicht mehr ganz aufrecht erhalten. Es scheint so zu sein, daß keines der zur Prüfung hauptsächlich verwandten Pharmaca (Pilocarpin, Atropin-Adrenalin, Ergotamin) streng auswählend wirkt (LEWANDOWSKI, L. R. MÜLLER, E. FRANK, BILLIGHEIMER und G. v. BERGMANN usw.), so daß also auch ein experimenteller Erweis einer Vagotonie streng nicht zu erbringen ist. Überstarke pharmakologische Reaktionen am vegetativen Nervensystem sind häufig; sie sind aber weniger ein Beweis für eine sympathische oder parasympathische Übererregbarkeit als für eine Überempfindlichkeit des gesamten Rezeptivapparates, und somit „ein Stigma abnormer Organempfindlichkeit überhaupt" (E. FRANK). An die Stelle der EPPINGER-HESSschen Lehre einer Vagotonie-Sympathicotonie, deren einprägsame Wirkung gerade von ihrer zugespitzten Typisierung ausging, sowie von ihrem großen Aspekt auf Konstitutionsgruppen mit bestimmter Krankheitsbereitschaft, ist mehr und mehr die Überzeugung getreten, daß es reine Formen kaum gibt, sondern nur Mischformen: d. h. eine Stigmatisation im vegetativen Nervensystem überhaupt (G. v. BERGMANN). Von LESCHKE wird jedoch auch neuerdings gerade die klinische Brauchbarkeit der EPPINGER-HESSschen Vagotonielehre betont. Die Verschiebung des vegetativen Gleichgewichtes nach der parasympathischen Seite derart, daß alle parasympathisch wirkenden Reize zu abnorm gesteigerten Reaktionen führen, lasse sich in der klinischen Symptomatologie bei vielen Menschen finden; und diese zeigten auch das entsprechende pharmakodynamische Verhalten. Überempfindlichkeit gegen Morphin und Pilocarpin finde sich bei denselben Menschen, die zu vasomotorischen Störungen mit Gefäßkrämpfen neigten, leicht seekrank würden, an Asthma bronchiale litten, an Laryngospasmen, Supersekretion, Superacidität und Spasmus des Magens; die Extrasystolen zeigten bei dauernd langsamem Puls mit respiratorischer Arrythmie, spastische Obstipation, colica mucosa, leichtes Schwitzen usw. Freilich hebt auch LESCHKE hervor, daß die klinischen Erscheinungen wie die pharmako-dynamischen Reaktionen selbst bei ausgesprochenen Fällen nur einzelne Organe und Organsysteme beträfen, sich aber niemals im gesamten Sympathicus oder Vagus abspielten: etwa Fehlen jeder gesteigerten Erregbarkeit des Herzvagus bei spastischer Obstipation. JOS. WILDERS hat in einer Arbeit über das von ihm sog. „Ausgangswertgesetz" nachzuweisen versucht, worauf das Versagen der pharmakodynamischen Nachprüfungen an Vagotonikern und Sympathicotonikern beruhe. Auch von ihm konnten jedenfalls unter den größten Kautelen individuell konstante Reaktionen nicht regelmäßig erzielt werden. Er glaubt zu finden, daß die Differenz erklärt werden kann mit der Differenz der Ausgangswerte (etwa von Puls und Blutdruck) bei den einzelnen Versuchen. Der Ausfall einer vegetativen Reaktion ist in erster Linie abhängig von dem bereits bestehenden Erregungszustand der vegetativen Nerven, bzw. dem Tätigkeitsgrad der vegetativen Organe: je höher Erregungszustand bzw. Tätigkeitsgrad sind, desto geringer ist die fördernde, desto stärker die hemmende Wirkung. „Erreicht aber der Erregungszustand *höhere Grade,* dann kommt es infolge des Bestehens antagonistisch wirkender Systeme bei fördernden Mitteln, bei sehr geringen Erregungsgraden bei hemmenden Mitteln zu paradoxen Reaktionen." Wie schwierig es ist, sich dem Zwang zur gegensätzlichen Typisierung auf dem Gebiet vegetativer Funktionskomplexe zu entziehen, geht aus der bekannten Aufstellung von B- und T-Typen hervor, wie sie W. JAENSCH gerade aus der v. BERGMANNschen Schule im Anschluß an Arbeiten von E. R. JAENSCH eingehend dargelegt hat, ohne daß sich aber beide Typen mit den Begriffen vagotonisch oder sympathicotonisch in Einklang bringen ließen[1].

Die Unzulänglichkeiten einer pharmakologischen Diagnostik — aber auch der Erkenntnis vegetativer Korrelationen überhaupt — liegen zum guten Teil in der Schwierigkeit, ja Unmöglichkeit, zu entscheiden, ob jeweils fördernde oder antagonistisch hemmende Einflüsse wirksam sind. Dazu kommen eine Reihe von Untersuchungsergebnissen, die es wahrscheinlich machen, daß die Funktion autonom innervierter Organe nicht unmittelbar und allein auf einen *nervösen* Impuls schließen läßt, sondern daß gleiche Wirkung ausgehen kann von körpereigenen chemischen Stoffen oder auch Elektrolyten (Kationen, K', Ca'', H'). Es werden im Körper, besonders bei Leistungsaufwand der Organe, Stoffe gebildet (Hormone), die in spezifischer Zusammenarbeit mit den verschiedenen Anteilen des autonomen Nervensystems die sympathischen und parasympathischen Wirkungen hervorrufen. Die großen Gegenspieler im Sinne solcher inkretorischen Synergisten scheinen dabei zu sein das *Adrenalin* (CANNON) und das *Insulin* (?) (H. STAUB, ROSENBERG)[2]. Neuere Untersuchungen seit O. LOEWIS Entdeckung (1921) einer vagotropen und sympathicotropen Substanz im Herzen bei Reizung des Vagusstammes bzw. des Accelerans legen die Vermutung nahe, daß es außer den genannten inkretorischen Synergisten noch andere „sympathico"- bzw. „parasympathicomimetische" Stoffe gibt, nämlich solche, die bei Reizung vegetativer Nerven in den Erfolgsorganen selbst entstehen („Lokalhormone" E. TH. BRÜCKE). Durch die nervösen Impulse werden intracellulär wirksame Hormone erzeugt, die nunmehr erst jene Wirkungen hervorrufen, die früher etwa für eine unmittelbare Folge der Vagus- bzw. Acceleranswirkung am Herzen galten. Hierzu gesellen sich noch weitere Stoffwechselprodukte (Serumeiweiß, Eiweißabbauprodukte, Lipoide), die insbesondere die Adrenalinwirkung fördern oder hemmen oder die wie das Histamin einen fast parasympathicomimetischen Charakter besitzen (E. FRANK)[3]. Neben einer nervösen und humoralen Beeinflussung der Adrenalinsekretion ist in den letzten Jahren noch diejenige einer *ionalen* untersucht worden (TRENDELENBURG[4], S. G. ZONDEK u. a.), ohne daß hier schon ausreichend gesicherte und unbestrittene Befunde vorliegen.

Bereits EPPINGER und HESS vermuteten, daß die Tonisierung der Endapparate (und damit auch ihr Erregbarkeitsgrad) chemisch erfolge. Im Anschluß an Arbeiten von FRIEDRICH KRAUS, die darauf abzielen, das vegetative Nervensystem einzugliedern in das Gesamt eines vegetativen Systems überhaupt, rückt unter anderem auch E. FRANK von dem Begriff eines „Nervenendapparates" ab. Es handle sich vielmehr um einen Rezeptivapparat der Zelle, den er nach dem Vorschlag von KRAUS und ZONDEK als das *vegetative Betriebsstück der Zelle* bezeichnet[5].

Immer wieder erscheinen im Lauf der Jahre denkerische Bemühungen, die einigermaßen Sichtung und Überblick geben wollen über die hier kaum angedeutete Verwickeltheit vegetativen Geschehens, und die — Ungeklärtes hypothetisch überbrückend — die ursächlichen und zeitlichen Zusammenhänge, die morphologischen und funktionellen Eigentümlichkeiten vegetativer Organe und

---

[1] Eine *echte Vagotonie* (bei jedoch *auch* erhöhtem Sympathicotonus) tritt ein im Anschluß an die Decerebrierung (SHERRINGTON, MAGNUS und KLEE: zit. bei E. FRANK); ein überwiegend vagotonisches Verhalten zeigt das parkinsonistische Syndrom; ein überwiegend sympathicotonisches Erscheinungsbild lassen viele Fälle von Thyreotoxikose erkennen.
[2] Allerdings scheint dem *Adrenalin* eine ungleich höhere Bedeutung zuzukommen.
[3] Zusammenfassende Darstellung und Literatur bei KROETZ.
[4] TRENDELENBURG: Hormone, S. 1. Berlin 1930.
[5] „Wir vindizieren diesem komplizert gebauten Betriebsstück zwei Fangarme ... — einen adrenalinophilen (mit dem Sympathicus im Kontakt befindlichen) und einen cholinophilen (mit dem Parasympathicus korrespondierenden) — welche einem gemeinsamen ionenempfindlichen Grundstück aufsitzen" (E. FRANK).

Vorgänge bis hinauf zu seelischen Entsprechungen und charakterologischen Determinanten vereinfachend zusammenfassen: Vagotonie — vegetative Stigmatisation — Basedowide und tetanoide (B. u. T.) Typenschau — vegetatives System und „Tiefenperson" sind solche Entwürfe. Wiederholt ist auf die „mehrfache Sicherung" vegetativer Vorgänge hingewiesen worden[1], und im Verein damit auf deren *mehrfache zentrale Steuerung und Regulation*[2]. Die Befunde und ihre Deutung sind aber auch hier umstritten; dies gilt besonders von den sog. *Stoffwechselzentren* im Zwischenhirn und ihrem Einfluß. (Vgl. die Diskussion um diese Fragen in den Verhandlungen der Gesellschaft Deutscher Nervenärzte in Hamburg 1928: E. FRANK, E. P. PICK, I. P. KARPLUS, H. SPATZ, F. H. LEWY.) Auch hier zeigt sich — wenigstens physiologisch gesehen — die Neigung, den Begriff vegetatives Zentrum im Anschluß an W. R. HESSsche Gedankengänge aufzufassen im Sinne einer ganzheitlichen Betrachtung der vegetativen Abläufe. Zentrum bedeutet nicht die Stätte, deren Zerstörung oder Reizung von umschriebenen Ausfällen oder Leistungen begleitet sind, sondern Zentrum ist „ein potentieller Repräsentant der nach einem bestimmten Leistungsergebnis orientierten Funktionsordnung von Erfolgsorganen". Dieses besondere Steuerungsorgan: Zentrum „baut aus den von der Peripherie einlaufenden Afferenzen ein Erregungsgebilde auf, dessen wieder nach der Peripherie fließenden Entladungen die Erfolgsorgane zu einem geordneten Zusammenwirken veranlassen" (W. R. HESS[3]). In ähnlicher Weise spricht BRÜCKE davon, daß es sich nicht um *ein* vegetatives Zentrum handle, sondern um eine große Zahl, vielleicht nicht histologisch, sondern nur nach ihrer Funktion trennbarer vegetativer Koordinationszentren, gewissermaßen um die Repräsentation einer visceralen Eupraxie. Auf eine Erwähnung der aufgestellten vegetativen Zentren im Rückenmark, Medulla oblongata, Mittelhirn, Hypothalamus, Corpus striatum und Rinde und ihrer Funktionen muß hier verzichtet werden. Auch diese Zentren können auf chemischem Wege (Hormone, Stoffwechselprodukte) in ihrer Erregbarkeit beeinflußt werden. Eine wichtige Rolle aber spielt im Rahmen dieser Arbeit die Möglichkeit einer corticalen (L. R. MÜLLER u. a.) und psychischen, insbesondere affektiven Erregung vegetativer Zentralstätten im Zwischenhirn. Ihre enge Nachbarschaft (im Hypothalamus) zu zentralen Regulationsbezirken affektiven Geschehens und emotioneller Ausdrucksbewegungen legt von vornherein den Gedanken an eine Verkoppelung zu bestimmter Leistungsgemeinschaft nahe. Jedenfalls läßt uns eine Reihe von Tatsachen über die psychische Beeinflussung des vegetativen Systems — wovon im nächsten Abschnitt näher gesprochen werden soll — mit zureichender Begründung annehmen, daß der Hypothalamus der Übertragung psychischer und corticaler Erregungen dient.[4]

---

[1] „Demnach sind die Symptome einer generellen Sympathicuserregung und einer gesteigerten Adrenalinsekretion vollkommen identisch, und es ist zur Kontrolle, ob unter bestimmten Bedingungen eine allgemeine Sympathicuserregung oder nur eine Nebennierensekretion eintritt, oft nötig, Versuche an nebennierenlosen Tieren zu wiederholen, um den einen Faktor sicher ausschalten zu können. In der organischen Natur hängt der Erfolg eines biologischen Geschehens nur ganz selten von der Funktion eines einzigen Mechanismus ab, fast immer finden wir eine mehrfache Sicherung; dementsprechend ist auch die Nebenniere selbst von sympathischen Fasern sekretorisch innerviert, so daß bei jeder Steigerung des Sympathicustonus gleichzeitig eine vermehrte Adrenalinmenge ins Blut sezerniert wird, und die Symptome der Sympathicuserregung sehr oft sowohl auf die direkte Nervenerregung als auch auf eine Hyperadrenalinämie zu beziehen sind ...." E. TH. BRÜCKE: Mitt. Ges. dtsch. Naturforsch. 4, 927 (1927).

[2] „Auch wenn man nach KRAUS das vegetative nervöse und endokrine System zu einem einheitlichen vegetativen zusammenfaßt, so ist doch auch in diesem die nervöse Regulation das Übergeordnete" (LESCHKE).

[3] HESS, W. R.: Regulation des Blutkreislaufes. Leipzig 1930.

[4] SPIEGEL: Die Zentren des autonomen Nervensystems. Monographie 1928. — REICHART, M.: Hirnstamm und Psychiatrie. Mschr. Psychiatr. 68.

b) Einfluß seelischer Vorgänge auf vegetative Funktionen [1].

Gewisse körperliche Begleiterscheinungen seelischer Vorgänge sind seit jeher sprichwörtlich. Die mimischen Äußerungen: Röte vor Scham, Zorn, Blässe vor Angst, Sträuben der Haare, Schweißausbrüche, Tränen, graue Schlaffheit des Kummers und so fort, sind jedem geläufig und werden unmittelbar als Ausdruck bestimmter zugeordneter Affekte und Stimmungen verstanden. In diesem Zusammenhang wird in der Regel auf die JAMES-LANGEsche Theorie der Affekte verwiesen: Das was wir Gemütsbewegung nennen, ist sekundär, ist erst die Summe der Empfindungen, die wir von den körperlichen Vorgängen haben; diese körperlichen Vorgänge aber folgen *unmittelbar* der psychischen Erfassung des erregenden Vorganges. Das hieße: Die vegetativ bedingten Erscheinungen (Erröten, Herzklopfen, Tränen usw.) treten nicht, wie heute meistens angenommen wird im zeitlichen Anschluß an die Affekte auf, sondern die Gemütsbewegungen folgen den vegetativen Vorgängen zeitlich und ursächlich. SHERRINGTON [2] schaltete an einer Hündin operativ so gut wie alle Eingeweide vom Großhirneinfluß aus. Dennoch zeigte diese Hündin keine Änderung in ihren emotionellen Äußerungen: Zorn, Freude, Furcht usw.; nur die vom vegetativen System abhängigen Erscheinungen (Sträuben der Haare usw.) blieben aus. Damit muß die Auffassung von JAMES auch experimentell als widerlegt gelten [3].

In älteren experimentell-psychologischen Arbeiten (Literatur darüber bei H. W. v. WYSS [4], R. METZNER) wurden die körperlichen Begleiterscheinungen von Zuständen geringer-seelischer Erregung (sog. gefühlsindifferente Erregungen; Tätigkeitsformen [MARTIUS]) sowie von Affekten untersucht; insbesondere wandte man sich den Kreislaufvorgängen und der Atmung zu.

Man fand bei angestrengter Aufmerksamkeit bestimmte Kurven am Plethysmogramm (E. WEBER: Anstieg, kurze Senkung, erneuter Anstieg); der Blutdruck steigt, die Pulszahl nimmt im wesentlichen zu (LEHMANN). Die Atmung ist verflacht und beschleunigt. WEINBERG [5] untersuchte bei affektschwachen psychischen Reizen (Klingelzeichen, Zuruf von Worten) einen größeren Verband vegetativer Erscheinungen (Pupille, Atmung, Elektrokardiogramm, Plethysmogramm) in Reaktionsgleichzeitigkeit. Er fand ein regelmäßig gleichsinniges Überwiegen sympathisch bzw. parasympathisch gesteuerter Funktionen derart, daß „Erhöhung des Bewußtseinsniveaus begleitet wird von einer erhöhten Sympathicuswirkung und Erniedrigung desselben von einer vermehrten Parasympathicuswirkung" (sog. „psychophysiologischer Reflex"). Man wird bei diesen diskutierten Zusammenhängen zwischen Bewußtseinshelligkeit und vegetativem Verhalten daran denken, daß ja gerade für die Schlaf-Wachfunktionen von verschiedener Seite (EPPINGER, v. PAPP und SCHWARZ [6], besonders aber wiederholt von HESS) ein Intensitätswandel vor allem der sympathischen Innervation angenommen wird; möglicherweise aber auch ein Überwiegen parasympathischer Einflüsse am Gehirn (HESS). Es klingt hier schon deutlich die

---

[1] Vgl. hierzu HANSEN: Psychische Beeinflussung des vegetativen Nervensystems. — WYSS, H. W. v.: Der Ausdruck der Gemütsbewegungen. Nervenarzt 2 (1929). — Einfluß psychischer Vorgänge usw. Handbuch der normalen und pathologischen Physiologie, Bd. 16,2. Berlin 1931. — MONAKOW, P. v.: Über die zentrale Repräsentation vegetativer Funktionen. Schweiz. Arch. Neur. **32** (1933).
[2] SHERRINGTON: Zit. bei BRÜCKE: Mitt. Ges. dtsch. Naturforsch. **1928**, 923.
[3] *Nachtrag bei der Korrektur:* Eine Darstellung vorwiegend amerikanischer Ergebnisse über körperliche Befunde bei seelischen Störungen bringt CAMERON, D. EWEN in Objective and experimentel Psychiatry, New-York 1935. Für ihn ist freilich das „Seelische" im wesentlichen nur Epiphänomen körperlicher Vorgänge, besonders auch die Affekte.
[4] v. WYSS H. W.: Einfluß psychischer Vorgänge usw.
[5] WEINBERG: Z. Neur. **85**, 543; **86**, 375 (1923).
[6] EPPINGER, v. PAPP u. SCHWARZ: Über das „Asthma cardiale". 1924.

Konzeption einer grundsätzlichen Funktionsverteilung auf das sympathische und parasympathische System an, wie sie HESS[1] später gegeben hat. Das vegetative System arbeitet nach zwei Fronten: Entfaltung aktueller Energie, Entfaltung von Leistung: ergotropes Prinzip = Sympathicuswirkung; und demgegenüber Entlastung der Gewebe, Erhaltung der Leistungsmöglichkeit, Restitution: histotropes Prinzip = Parasympathicuswirkung. Eine sichere Entscheidung in bezug auf Wirkung und Folge zwischen Bewußtseinsniveau und vegetativen Vorgängen läßt sich aus den WEINBERGschen Untersuchungen nicht treffen. v. WYSS[2] meint im Anschluß an HESSsche Gedankengänge und im Gegensatz zu WEINBERG, daß der erhöhte Bewußtseinszustand *Folge* der Sympathicuserregung sei.

HANSEN weist gerade auch an diesem Beispiel mit Recht darauf hin, wie schwierig Fragen nach „Ursache und Wirkung innerhalb der Vitalvorgänge" zu beantworten seien. Größeres Interesse als den vegetativen Entsprechungen des Aufmerkens, des „Wachseins", gilt jedoch denjenigen der ausgesprochenen Gefühlstöne sowie der Affekte. Die Erscheinungen sind ja hier ungleich lebhafter und eindringlicher; sie legen von vornherein den Gedanken einer spezifischen Zuordnung sympathischer und parasympathischer Reaktionen zu bestimmten Gefühlsqualitäten noch näher. Wie später gezeigt werden soll, läßt sich jedoch eine solche Korrelation nur sehr bedingt annehmen [3].

Eine große Fülle von Untersuchungen gelten den affektiven Auswirkungen am *Kreislaufsystem*. Ursprüngliche Befunde (MENTZ, LEHMANN, BRAHN u. a.) schienen zwischen elementaren Gefühlstönen (Lust-Unlust) und bestimmten Pulsverläufen (Verlangsamung-Beschleunigung) kennzeichnende Beziehungen zu ergeben. MARTIUS hat schließlich nachgewiesen, daß gesetzmäßige Beziehungen solcher Art nicht bestehen. Zu dem gleichen Ergebnis kamen in bezug auf plethysmographische Feststellungen der Blutverschiebung DE JONG, KÜPPERS und BICKEL: Jede psychische Tätigkeit, gleichviel ob sie die Betonung der Lust-Unlust, Spannung oder Lösung tragen, sei begleitet von der gleichen plethysmographischen Kurve (kurz dauernde Volumzunahme, gefolgt von länger dauernder Volumsenkung) [4]. Die Frage, wieweit an der affektiv einsetzenden Blutverschiebung die Blutreservoire beteiligt sind (BARCROFT, CANNON, zit. bei W. H. v. WYSS), kann hier nur aufgeworfen werden. Beobachtungen über Verhalten des Hirnvolumens bei Lust- und Unlustgefühlen (BERGER, BICKEL, E. WEBER usw.) haben keine sicheren Ergebnisse gebracht.

Von großer Bedeutung sind Feststellungen über das Verhalten des *Blutdrucks*. Er ist für die Dauer seelischer Erregung, aber auch in einer gewissen Nachzeit erhöht (KNAUER, KNAUER und BILLIGHEIMER). Eine Blutdrucksenkung fand PAL bei Schmerzwirkung (tabische Krisen), aber auch bei Angst (Examen), Schreck wurde sie beobachtet, und zwar sowohl systolisch wie diastolisch (KNAUER und BILLIGHEIMER). Den Einfluß seelischer Erregungen auf den Blutdruck von Hypertonikern hat unter anderem FAHRENKAMP nachgewiesen. Läßt die seelische Spannung nach, so geht auch die Spannung der Gefäßwand zurück. Über einfache Verlangsamung und Beschleunigung der Herzaktion hinaus sind auch Herzunregelmäßigkeiten beobachtet worden: Extrasystolien (HANSEN); diese allerdings nur bei kreislaufinsuffizienten Patienten während der großen Visite, bei Vorbereitung zur Faradisation. HANSEN weist

---

[1] HESS: Klin. Wschr. **1925** I, 1353; **1930** I, 1009.
[2] WYSS, v.: Schw. Arch. Neur. **19**, 3 (1926).
[3] Hierzu und zum folgenden siehe auch: HANS ZWEIG: Das Leib-Seeleproblem und seine Auswirkung in der Medizin. Zbl. Neur. **61**, 1 (1932).
[4] Wegen der Streitfrage, ob die Erregung von Herz und Gefäßen gleichzeitig oder unabhängig voneinander erfolge, siehe auch A. WEINBERG: Psyche und unwillkürliches Nervensystem. Z. Neur. **86**, 375 (1923).

in diesem Zusammenhang auf die wichtigen Studien von E. H. HERING [1] hin. HERING fand, daß bei seinen Versuchstieren die Disposition zu Kammerflimmern und Herztod bei Narkose um so größer war, je aufgeregter die Hunde und Katzen vor der Chloroformnarkose waren.

Wichtige Ergebnisse brachten die Untersuchungen von PAWLOW und seiner Schule. Es gelang ihm, an Hunden die Magensekretion durch psychische Reize zu beeinflussen. Versiegen der Magensekretion fand BICKEL beim Hunde im Anblick einer Katze, CANNON schlagartigen Stillstand der Magenbewegung bei der Katze im Anblick eines Hundes. Ähnliches sahen v. BERGMANN und KABISCH. Auch beim Menschen wurden Hemmungen der Magensekretion beobachtet, bzw. Steigerung bei freudiger Stimmung während des Essens (SCHROTTENBACH; RÖMER und SOMMERFELD bei Kindern).

Über so mehr oder minder umschriebene Organbeeinflussungen hinaus kommt es aber im Verlauf von Affekten und Verstimmungen, auch zu Änderungen im Stoffwechsel. So fand CANNON eine Emotionsglykosurie bei sehr erregten Tieren, die nach Entfernung der Nebennieren (Wegfall der Adrenalinabscheidung) unterblieb (zit. nach HANSEN). Die Frage nach einer solchen Glykosurie ist beim Menschen allerdings sehr umstritten (KNAUER; dagegen v. NOORDEN und ISAAC). Vorübergehende Glykosurien bei lebhaft erregten Geisteskranken (Katatone, ängstlich Depressive) sind den Psychiatern jedenfalls ziemlich geläufige Erscheinungen [2]. Freilich liegen die Verhältnisse hier viel zu verwickelt, als daß derlei Befunde die These einer Emotionsglykosurie stützen könnten. Als Folgen affektiver Einflüsse wurden weiterhin Änderungen der Stoffwechselgröße, des Wasser- und des Mineralhaushaltes (Phosphaturie) beschrieben (GRAFE, DEUTSCH, HEILIG und HOFF u. a.).

Die Methodik experimenteller Erforschung psychophysischer Abhängigkeiten wurde dadurch bereichert, daß man systematisch *suggestive Beeinflussungen*, vor allem in der Hypnose, heranzog. HANSEN weist darauf hin, daß schon ERNST WEBER beschrieb (1910), wie allein durch die Suggestion: der Arm hebe sich, eine Blutverschiebung nach dem in der Einbildung bewegten Glied eintrat von gleicher Art, als wenn die Muskulatur dieses Armes wirklich angespannt und das Glied gehoben wurde. Gerade diese Erscheinungen, die als ,,sinngemäße Realisierung" von suggerierten Affekten, bzw. ,,in der Einbildung gegebenen Situationen" (HANSEN) und — suggestiv erlebten Eingriffen in das eigene Körpergeschehen gedeutet werden können, und in der Regel so gedeutet werden, sind für die Pathogenese der sog. Organneurosen wichtig geworden. Der Vorteil dieser Methode liegt darin, daß der Bewußtseinsumfang eingeengt und durch diese konzentrative Umschaltung der Körper in ungewöhnlicher Weise unter den dominierenden Einfluß einer bestimmten und beabsichtigten Gefühlslage kommt. Man darf so vielleicht erwarten, neben einer besonderen Lebhaftigkeit auch eine besonders reine Zuordnung vegetativer Äußerungen zu bestimmten Elementargefühlen anzutreffen, selbst wenn man die Schwierigkeit mit in Betracht zieht, die darin liegt, daß ja auch die ,,Hypnose" mit ihrer eigentümlichen Bewußtseinslage schon ,,für sich" nicht ohne Einfluß auf die vegetativen Vorgänge bleiben kann [3]. Aber dieser Hinweis läßt bereits erkennen, wie unmöglich es ist, an dem gegenseitigen Bedingungsspiel einer jeweiligen seelischen und körperlichen Gesamtsituation vorbeizusehen. Darauf wird im Rückblick über diesen Abschnitt näher eingegangen werden.

Hervorzuheben sind zunächst die Arbeiten, die sich mit dem Einfluß suggerierter Affekte auf die ,,Verdauungsfunktionen" befassen. HEYER fand, daß

---
[1] HERING: Münch. med. Wschr. 1916 I, 521.
[2] LAUDENHEIMER: Münch. med. Wschr. 1925 II, 1843. — LANGE, JOH.: BUMKES Handbuch der Geisteskrankheiten. Spez. Teil II.
[3] KIRSCHBERG, DEUTSCH und KAUF, LENK, HEYER.

die Magensekretion, die auf Suggestion von Nahrungsaufnahme einsetzte, durch affektive Einflüsse verschiedener Art gestört wurde, und zwar ohne spezifische Korrelation; nur schien die Einwirkung unlustbetonter Reize rascher zu erfolgen. Ähnliche Ergebnisse fand HEYER in bezug auf die Peristaltik des Magens.

PAWLOW hatte bereits an Tieren nachgewiesen, daß durch Vorzeigen von Speisen Magensaft abgesondert wurde, der quantitativ und qualitativ von der Art dieser Speisen abhing. Beim Menschen fand HEYER ebenfalls entsprechende spezifische Magensekretion auf vorgezeigte Speisen. Zu etwas anderen Ergebnissen kamen HEILIG und HOFF: Suggerierte Aufnahme von Lieblingsspeisen führte zu superazider Sekretion (bei Norm- und Subaziden), auch dann, wenn diese Lieblingsspeise etwa sehr fett war und also bei qualitätsspezifischer Wirkungsweise hätte hemmenden statt fördernden Einfluß haben müssen. Umgekehrt rief die Suggestion von Abscheu erregenden Speisen eine subazide Sekretion hervor, selbst wenn die Speise „normalerweise" die Säureproduktion hätte anregen müssen. Auch hier bestanden in beiden Versuchsreihen gleichsinnig fördernde oder hemmende Einflüsse auf die Peristaltik.

Die Ergebnisse HEYERs sind von HANSEN und DELHOUGNE bestätigt worden. Schon aus diesen einander scheinbar widerstreitenden Befunden geht hervor, wie vielschichtig im Einzelfall die Bedingungen sind, wie es hier zu einem Gegenspiel kommt zwischen gegebenen Affekten etwa und „normgemäßer" Wirkung von Speisen, d. h. Reizen der Umwelt. Es sei im Anschluß daran hingewiesen, auf weitere Untersuchungen von HEYER, die dartun, wie sehr bei allen solchen Erwägungen die individuelle Eindrucksfähigkeit zu beachten ist, besonders aber die augenblickliche seelische Eindrucksbereitschaft und das funktionelle Entgegenkommen einzelner Organsysteme. In der Hypnose beobachtete HEYER ein unterschiedliches Verhalten des Blutdruckes bei Kreislaufgesunden und bei Hypertonikern. Das Absinken des Blutdruckes erfolgte bei den Gesunden in einigen Minuten bis auf den Ausgangswert; bei Hypertonikern dagegen zog sich diese Rückbildung über 2 Stunden hin. Man kann gegenüber manchen tiefenpsychologischen und psychotherapeutischen Deutungsverstiegenheiten nicht genug auf die Anschauung von HANSEN verweisen, daß zwar das vegetative Nervensystem in der Lage sei, „die somatische Realisation der personalen psychischen Erlebniswelt zu vollziehen, unabhängig in gewissen Grenzen von der realen Struktur und den Reizen der Umwelt", daß aber diesen Äußerungen „in der Funktionsbreite und der Funktionsgewohnheit der Organe natürliche Grenzen gezogen sind". HANSEN weist dabei hin auf die Möglichkeit eines sog. psychogenen — auch experimentell in der Hypnose erzeugten — Fiebers. Aber in den positiven Fällen bestand eben noch eine Labilität der Wärmeregulation nach kaum abgelaufenen, organisch begründeten Temperatursteigerungen [1]. Für das Verständnis suggestiver — wie HANSEN meint — angeschauter und anschaulich erkannter, eingebildet (ideagen) wirksamer Realisationen im Körperlichen erscheint es wichtig, anzumerken, daß in diesen Fällen nicht einfach „Fieber" suggeriert wurde, sondern kurz zurückliegende Situationen, in denen Fieberanstiege stattgefunden hatten und erlebt worden waren (KOHNSTAMM und FRIEDMANN, LADECK, EICHELBERG).

Einzelne Ergebnisse experimentell hypnotischer Studien am Kreislaufsystem und an den Stoffwechselvorgängen sollen noch kurz Erwähnung finden. Anstiege und Abfälle der Schlagfolge unter suggerierten Affekten fand ASTRUCK. Anfängliche Senkung des Minutenvolumens, dann Steigerung über das Ausgangsniveau mit Pulsbeschleunigung stellten LAUBER und PANNHORST unter dem

---

[1] Auch HOFF meint, daß in solchen Fällen wohl stets irgendwo eine organische Bereitschaft zu Temperaturen (Herde in der Lunge, Tonsillen usw.) bestehen.

Einfluß suggerierter Freude fest. Dieselben Autoren fanden auch als vegetative Ausdruckswirklichkeit einer hypnotisch suggerierten Arbeitssituation deutliche Schwankungen im Minutenvolumen. Vorübergehende Blutdruckerhöhung bei suggerierten Affekten fanden KRONFELD, bei Suggestion von Bewegungen KLEMPERER.

Die *Wärmeregulation* wurde besonders von HANSEN und GESSLER studiert. Die Versuchsperson, liegend im warmen Zimmer, reagierte auf die Suggestion, sie läge im Schnee, sogleich mit einer Stoffwechselsteigerung (20—30%), so als läge sie wirklich im kalten Winter und kühle sich ab. Eine wirkliche Temperaturverminderung auf 10^0 C im Zimmer rief bei der Versuchsperson keine Verbrennungssteigerung hervor, wenn ihr suggeriert wurde, sie liege auf einer sonnehellen Sommerwiese oder im warmen Zimmer.

Funktionsverwirklichungen suggestiver Einflüsse auf den Wasserhaushalt fand MARX: Suggestion des Wassertrinkens (wie am VOLLHARDschen Wassertag) führt zu entsprechender Verdünnung des Blutes und Harnvermehrung; suggestiv eingebildeter Durst zu umgekehrtem Verhalten.

Noch umstritten sind Untersuchungen des Kohlehydrathaushaltes, worauf schon oben bei der Emotionsglykosurie hingewiesen wurde. Auch hier scheint — ähnlich wie beim sog. psychogenen Fieber — ohne organische Bereitschaften abnormer Art eine suggestive Beeinflussung des Zuckerstoffwechsels nicht möglich zu sein [1].

Eine Steigerung des O_2-Verbrauches bei Suggestiverlebnissen depressiven Inhaltes fand GRAFE (bis zu 25%); auch einen plötzlichen Gewichtssturz um 2 kg glaubt er nach starker Erschütterung und Sorge beobachtet zu haben (?)

Zu den besonders eindrucksvollen Suggestivwirkungen gehören hypnotisch hervorgerufene Erscheinungen an der Haut (Blasenbildungen, Verschwinden von Warzen, Blutungen) [2]. Es handelt sich ja hierbei um Symptome ungewöhnlicher Art, die auch nur bei anscheinend besonders vegetativ disponierten Persönlichkeiten hervorgerufen werden können, und deren Beziehungen zu den Erscheinungen der Stigmatisation bis in die letzte Zeit mit einiger Vorsicht diskutiert werden (SCHINDLER, HANSEN, KROETZ usw.).

c) Die Wirkungsweise seelischer Beeinflussung vegetativer Funktionen.

Der kurze Überblick über eine seelische Beeinflussung vegetativer Äußerungen im Experiment läßt, so unklar auch Einzelheiten der Wirkungswege und Wirkungsweise noch immer sind, doch eben die Möglichkeit einer solchen ursächlichen Verkettung als sicher annehmen; die alltägliche — nicht nur ärztliche — Erfahrung lehrt darüber hinaus, daß sie häufig ist. ,,Wie gegenüber vielen Reizen der Umwelt, erweist sich gerade das unwillkürliche Nervensystem auch gegenüber seelischen Einflüssen als sehr reaktionsbereit. Die notwendige Anpassung des Vegetativen an die Um- und Innenwelt bedingt einen steten Wechsel im Tonus und in der Erregbarkeit aller Teile des vegetativen Nervensystems und damit in der Anspruchsfähigkeit gegen Reize der verschiedensten Art" (E. P. PICK). Diese Umstimmung und dauernde Gewinnung eines neuen vegetativen Gleichgewichtes geschieht in beständiger Korrelation mit körpereigenen chemischen Stoffen. Ich erinnere an den oben gegebenen Hinweis auf die Arbeitsgemeinschaft des sympathico-adrenalen Systems und auf die Schwierigkeit, innerhalb solcher Wirkungszusammenhänge eine genaue Sonderung nach steuernden und gesteuerten Funktionen zu vollziehen. Wenn man sich vorstellt,

---

[1] Vgl. hierzu HANSEN und die Untersuchungen von GIGON, AIGNER und BRAUCH an Diabetikern.

[2] Vgl. hierzu I. H. SCHULTZ, W. SCHINDLER.

daß seelische Erregungen an einem repräsentativen Zentrum für vegetative Vorgänge etwa angreifen, und daß nun eine allgemeine Erregung des sympathischen Nervensystems stattfindet — so ist das eine vielleicht einleuchtende aber allzu vereinfachende Annahme. Ja, es ist nicht einmal immer zu entscheiden, ob es sich bei den sympathischen Symptomen nicht um Folgen einer starken Adrenalinausschüttung ins Blut handelt. (Als Testmöglichkeit wird auf die Beteiligung der Schweißdrüsensekretion hingewiesen, da diese nur durch direkten Nerveneinfluß, nicht durch Steigerung der Adrenalinkonzentration im Blut hervorgerufen werden kann.) Außerdem wird infolge der sympathischen Innervation der Nebennieren — durch ausgedehntere sympathische Erregung — auch die Adrenalinausschüttung erhöht werden [1]. Hinzu aber kommt, worauf bisher schon gelegentlich verwiesen wurde, der Umstand, daß auch das animale Nervensystem, der zentrale Apparat selbst auf verschiedene Weise beeinflußt wird. „Die durch das vegetative System vermittelten, erregbarkeitsändernden, umstimmenden Einflüsse, erstrecken sich nicht nur, wie wir früher annahmen, auf die peripheren Erfolgsorgane, sondern auch die höchst entwickelten Zentren unseres Nervensystems unterstehen den allgemeingültigen Organisationsgesetzen, zu denen auch die vegetative Innervation zu zählen ist" (E. TH. BRÜCKE). Wieweit schließlich eine solche Auffassung vom zentralen Nervensystem — bis zur Hirnrinde — als einem Erfolgsorgan vegetativer Nerveneinflüsse gedacht wird, geht aus der schon erwähnten Anschauung von W. R. HESS über die Schlaf-Wachregulation hervor. Von tiefliegenden umschriebenen Teilen des Gehirns (elektrische Reizung bei Katzen im Hirnstamm in der Gegend des 3. Ventrikels) kann eine so weitgehende Umstimmung des — vorwiegend ja seelischen — Gesamtverhaltens hervorgerufen werden, wie es der Schlaf darstellt, den W. R. HESS für einen parasympathischen Erfolgsakt hält.

Der Einfluß sympathischer Wirkungen auf das sensible System im Sinne einer Erregbarkeitsverminderung oder Steigerung für Schmerzreize wurde von PETTE sowie von FOERSTER, ALTENBURGER und KROLL nachgewiesen. Diese Ergebnisse sollen hier Erwähnung finden, nicht nur weil sie auch eine sympathicogene Umstimmung des animalen Nervensystems in seinem peripheren Abschnitt dartun, sondern weil sie gleichzeitig eine Deutungsmöglichkeit für den Mechanismus hysterischer Anästhesien und Hyperästhesien nahelegen. Eine gewisse experimentelle Bestätigung dieser Annahme fanden ALTENBURGER und KROLL bei chronaximetrischen Untersuchungen suggestiver Einflüsse auf die Änderung der Reizschwelle („besser fühlen!" „schlechter fühlen!"). Die adäquate Wirkung solcher Suggestionen war immer nur in solchen Hautgebieten nachzuweisen, deren Sympathicusversorgung intakt war, nicht aber bei Patienten mit Sympathicusläsionen.

Wenn auch die nervösen Substrate psychischer Tätigkeit [2] wie das ganze animale Nervensystem für bestimmte Einflüsse als ein „Erfolgsorgan" des vegetativen Nervensystems aufgefaßt werden können; und wenn man annehmen darf, daß auf diesem Wege auch gewisse Stimmungen und Verstimmungen entscheidend miterzeugt werden (klimatische Einflüsse; Verstimmung, Reizbarkeit bei Föhn [DE RUDDER]; Wirkung von Giften [Cocain: W. R. HESS]), so kann doch nicht bezweifelt werden, daß der eine Ablauf einer solchen Wirkungskette, nämlich der vom seelischen Einfluß zum vegetativen Erfolg unserer Erfahrung nach häufiger ist, und daß auch die Forschung für diese Ablaufsweise gesichertere Ergebnisse erbracht hat.

---

[1] Daß aber z. B. auch bei Reizung des Hypothalamus Blutdrucksteigerungen vorkommen, die nicht etwa durch Adrenalinausschüttung infolge Sympathicuswirkung hervorgerufen sind, haben KARPLUS und KREIDL nachgewiesen.

[2] Ein anatomischer Nachweis dafür ist bisher nicht erbracht.

Es fragt sich nun, wie beschaffen die seelischen Reize sein müssen, die einen solchen Einfluß gewinnen. A. WEINBERG meint, daß Reize, die „für die Versuchsperson eine psychische Bedeutung haben, eine Gleichgewichtsstörung im vegetativen System hervorrufen, wobei noch ein bestimmter „erhöhter Bewußtseinszustand" vorausgesetzt wird (s. oben S. 485). Das soll heißen: Seelische Erlebnisse, die einen etwas angehen und die außerdem eingebettet sind in einen Zustand besonderer Wachheit. Ich glaube, daß man auf einen solchen Zustand von Bewußtseinserhöhung als einer besonderen Voraussetzung wird verzichten können; soweit er unmittelbar an eine affektive Erregung gebunden ist, ist eben der Effekt der Motor und soweit eine solche Bindung an Gemütsbewegungen sich nicht nachweisen läßt, bleibt ernstlich zu erörtern — und wie mir scheint, kaum zu entscheiden —, ob das hohe Bewußtseinsniveau nicht bereits Folgeerscheinung einer vegetativen Beeinflussung cerebraler Apparate ist, im Sinne von W. R. HESS. Man muß sich nur freimachen von der Auffassung, als ob es „reine" seelische Funktionen wie Wahrnehmungen, Vorstellungen, Erinnerungen usw. gäbe und muß bedenken, wie untrennbar ihnen Gefühlstöne beigemischt sind. Wo solche Gefühlstöne stärker anklingen, da führen sie zu mehr oder minder deutlichen Auswirkungen im vegetativen Gebiet: Ja, diese körperlichen Begleitsymptome gehören mit hinein in die Begriffsbestimmung der Affekte. Die ausschlaggebende Rolle der emotionellen (thymogenen) Einflüsse im Gesamt seelischer Einwirkung auf vegetative Vorgänge wird heute nicht ernstlich bestritten, durchaus in Übereinstimmung mit der Wichtigkeit, die dem Hirnstamm gegenüber dem Cortex seit Jahren für viele psychischen Leistungen beigemessen wird (M. REICHARDT, KLEIST, FR. POLLACK u. a.).

d) Begriff des Organismus.

Es ist wiederholt darauf hingewiesen worden [1], wie sehr Organempfindungen aus dem Körper am Aufbau von Vitalgefühlen und Stimmungen mitbeteiligt sind. Auch darin zeigt sich eine Beziehung zwischen vegetativen Organen und „Gefühlssphäre". Ja man kann sich vorstellen, daß es so zu Verschmelzungskreisen zwischen verwandten Gefühlsqualitäten kommt, die zum Teil aus seelischen Erlebnissen stammen, zum Teil eben solche Stimmungsanteile sind, herrührend von Organempfindungen. Klingt *ein* bestimmter Gefühlston an, so mit ihm der ganze ursprünglich in sinnvollem Zusammenhang mit ihm stehende „Gefühls-*Kreis*" (R. MATTHAEI). Auf diese Weise ließe sich eine Erklärung dafür finden, daß ein Sinnesreiz — auswirkend über die Gefühlssphäre und solche Empfindungskreise — zu vegetativen Reaktionen führt an einem Organ, das mit dem auslösenden Reiz in keiner sonst erkennbaren oder „zweckvollen" Beziehung steht. Man erkennt, daß eine solche Betrachtungsweise vom Gestaltproblem her gewonnen wurde und ich führe sie an, um zu zeigen, wie unbefriedigend heute allenthalben eine isolierte Betrachtung von Leistungen und Organen erscheint. Es gilt dies für das Zusammenspiel vegetativer Vorgänge überhaupt; für die Verknüpfung vegetativer Funktionen verschiedener Organsysteme untereinander (enge Korrelation zwischen Zirkulationssystem, Temperaturregulierung, Verdauungsfunktionen, Sexualfunktionen: W. R. HESS); dann für die wechselweise Beeinflussung des animalen und vegetativen Nervensystems, bzw. psychischer und vegetativer Funktionen.

Das Gesamtverhalten des *Organismus* ist es, von dem es jeweils abhängt, in welcher Weise seelische Einflüsse etwa zur Auswirkung gelangen [2]. Daß die

---
[1] SCHELER, KURT SCHNEIDER, W. R. v. WYSS u. a. m.
[2] Vgl. hierzu auch I. D. ACHELIS: Der ärztliche Begriff des Organismus. „Ein Organismus ist nicht eine gleichsam nachträgliche Verknüpfung von Organen, sondern ein Ineinander von Funktionen, die in sehr verschiedener Weise durch Organe repräsentiert sind."

Forschung dabei herkommen wird von der isolierenden Untersuchung der Organsysteme, ja einzelner Organfunktionen, aber auch immer wieder zurückkommen muß zur experimentellen Ergründung solcher Einzelleistungen bedarf wohl keiner besonderen Begründung und wird, soweit ich sehe, ernstlich nicht bestritten.

e) Psychovegetative Korrelationen und Leib-Seele-Problem.

Über den körperlichen Organismus als eines lebendig wirkenden Ganzen hinaus weisen aber die seelische Beeinflußbarkeit vegetativer Funktionen und umgekehrt die Möglichkeit vegetativer Umstimmung des Gehirns mit ihren seelischen Begleiterscheinungen, insbesondere solchen emotioneller Art auf eine Ganzheit noch höherer Ordnung hin: auf die leib-seelische Einheit des Individuums nämlich oder wenigstens auf das Ganze seiner leib-seelischen Funktionen. Die Möglichkeiten, in denen metaphysischem bzw. rational psychologischem Denken die leib-seelischen Beziehungen erscheinen (Wechselwirkung oder Parallelismus in ihren verschiedenen Auffassungen), können hier nicht diskutiert werden[1]. O. SCHWARZ meint in temperamentvoller Weise, daß es ein Leib-Seele-,,Problem" nur in der Medizin gebe, weil eigentlich nur hier ,,der Fragestellung aus einer größeren Lebensdringlichkeit der Beantwortung" der nötige Affektgehalt erwachse. Eine solche Auffassung wird zwar kaum allgemeine Zustimmung finden, aber sie weist doch entschieden darauf hin, daß die medizinische Einstellung zum Leib-Seele-,,Problem" überwiegend praktisch gerichtet ist. Es ist ihr um die Korrelationen körperlich-seelischen Geschehens vor allem deshalb zu tun, weil in ihrem Bereich krankhafte Regulationsstörungen beobachtet werden, die zu therapeutischem Handeln zwingen. Von der Arbeitshypothese eines neutralen psychophysischen Parallelismus gehen auch neuere medizinische Betrachtungen über die körperlich-seelischen Beziehungen nicht ab[2]. Immerhin hat gerade die Beschäftigung mit den sog. psychoneurotischen Syndromen zur Annahme geführt, daß ein *Wirkungs*-Zusammenhang zwischen psychophysischen Korrelationen bestehen müsse. Es wird dabei besonders unterstrichen, wie häufig in diesem Wirkungszusammenhang das Seelische die Stellung des Bewirkenden einnimmt. Eine ,,Psychogenie" in diesem Sinn kann jedoch nie ein existenzielles Hervorgehen bedeuten, oder die Auslegung körperlicher Vorgänge als Epiphänomene des Seelischen. Die psychologische Bemühung um das Neuroseproblem hat sich mit der Annahme eines Wirkungszusammenhanges leib-seelischen Geschehens und mit der Diskussion um die Akzentverschiebung von der Somatogenese zur Psychogenese nicht zufriedengegeben. Auf eine Darstellung derjenigen Lehren medizinischer und philosophischer Autoren, die hier klärend und fördernd gewirkt haben (GOLDSTEIN, FR. KRAUS, V. BERGMANN, W. STERN, PALAGYI, KLAGES, SCHELER), kann verzichtet werden. Ich verweise auf die obengenannte skizzierende Zusammenfassung von HANS ZWEIG. Die Abtrennung des Körperlichen vom Seelischen wird verstanden als eine künstliche Scheidung des *einen* organisch Ganzen, eben des menschlichen Organismus, und diese Scheidung ist bedingt durch die verschiedene Weise, in der dieses organische Gesamtgeschehen von uns betrachtet wird (GOLDSTEIN) und betrachtet werden *muß*, da das Seelische objektiv nicht erfaßbar ist — oder doch nur teilweise — wie der Körper, sondern nur subjektiv erlebt wird.

---

[1] S. hierzu u. a. HANS ZWEIG: Zbl. Neur. **61**, 1 (1932). — JAKOBI u. WINKLER: Arch. f. Psychiatr. 1930. — SCHNEIDER, K.: Pathopsychologie im Grundriß. — WENZEL, A.: Das Leib-Seele-Problem, 1933 (ausführliche und kritische Darstellung!).

[2] S. etwa O. SCHWARZ: Philosophische Grenzfragen der Medizin. Leipzig: Georg Thieme 1930. S. 70: ,,Ob man zwei aufeinander abgestimmte oder gegenseitig sich bewirkende Substanzen denkt, oder nur zwei Aspekte derselben Substanz annimmt, oder nur von bestimmten Reaktionsbereitschaften spricht, festgehalten muß nur das Moment der Entsprechung werden."

Die Lebenseinheit des Seelischen und Körperlichen findet sich in besonderer Zuspitzung betont bei H. SCHELER, der die Grenze des Seelischen mit der des Lebendigen überhaupt zusammenfallen läßt. Eine gewisse Trennung seelischer Funktionen von einer Sphäre des Geistigen, in dem vitales Leben (Empfindungen, Gefühle) erst zu *Erlebnissen* wird, findet sich bei PALAGYI, REICHARDT. Von hier gehen deutliche Brücken zu Auffassungen etwa von O. SCHWARZ: Es gibt über die psychophysisch-neutrale Gegebenheitsweise unseres vitalen Lebens hinaus noch eine geistige Stellungnahme dazu, ein Erlebnis unseres vitalen Lebens [1].

Gegen „die unerträgliche Verquickung der Begriffe seelische Funktion und geistiger Gehalt seelischer Erlebnisse" in dem einen Wort „psychisch" wendet sich L. BINSWANGER. Gerade von der Pathologie her gesehen muß ein solcher Hinweis beachtlich erscheinen. Neben den allgemein-menschlichen psychophysisch normalen Abläufen und Betriebsstörungen steht, sie mitbestimmend und mitbestimmt durch sie die individuelle innere Lebensgeschichte eines Menschen, d. h. die unaufhörliche Kette seiner seelischen Erlebnisse und der geistige Zusammenhang ihrer Erlebnisgehalte. Der *kranke* Mensch hat *seine* Krankheit und nimmt in seiner Weise Stellung zu ihr. Wenn man von einer Banalisierung des *Leib-Seele*-Problems absieht, wie sie etwa O. SCHWARZ vornimmt (s. S. 492), dann läßt sich zusammenfassend folgendes sagen: Der Zusammenhang zwischen psychischen und körperlichen Vorgängen bleibt uns unbegreiflich, „selbst dann, wenn wir wüßten, was sich auf beiden Seiten entspricht. Dieses tatsächliche Wissen allein aber wäre Sache des Mediziners; alles weitere gehört in die Philosophie" (BUMKE). Der Mediziner rechnet mit der Tatsache psychophysischer Korrelationen (POLLNOW). Damit ist zugleich gesagt, daß wir von einer Psychogenie körperlicher Erscheinungen nur vergleichsweise reden können. Umschreibungen wie: psychische Inbetriebsetzung (HEYER); seelisch anregen, hervorrufen statt verursachen (SIEBECK); in Erscheinung treten lassen usw. sind zwar unverbindlicher aber dadurch nicht besser. Empirisch läßt sich dartun, daß an der Vermittlung zwischen der objektiv biologischen und der subjektiv psychologischen Situation (POLLNOW) das „vegetative System" die entscheidende Rolle spielt. Dabei ist die neuronale Steuerung nur der eine Vermittler zwischen den Erfolgsorganen; sie ist von den Einflüssen hormonaler und ionaler Art in der Auswirkung nicht zu trennen (v. BERGMANN). Es ist denkmöglich, daß sich der nervöse Einfluß vorwiegend auswirkt in einer Verschiebung des Elektrolytmilieus der Zelle.

Die Innigkeit der Zusammenhänge körperlicher und seelischer Abläufe und die Labilität sog. körperlicher „Ausdrucksvorgänge" seelischen Geschehens läßt sich am psychogalvanischen Reflexphänomen (VERAGUTH) erkennen. Umstritten ist die Frage, ob allein der Affekt das psychogalvanische Phänomen auslöst, indem durch vegetative Einflüsse eine Verminderung der Gewebspolarisation der Haut (GILDEMEISTER) zustande kommt (WITTKOWER und FECHNER). Die Frage erscheint müßig, da es seelisches Geschehen ohne wenigstens einen Hauch von Gemütsbeteiligung — jedenfalls normalerweise — nicht gibt [2].

---

[1] Um die bewußtseinstranszendentale Art dieser vitalen Vorgänge zu kennzeichnen, spricht SCHWARZ auch von einem „*Lebnis*" unserer selbst.

[2] POLLNOW meint gar: Wenn man den Begriff der Affektivität in einem weiten Sinne gebrauchen will, so ließe sich das Affektive mit dem Psychischen identifizieren. — Wenn etwa eine Versuchsperson von I. H. SCHULTZ nach langjährigem autogenem Training seinen Puls von 76 auf 44 oder auch auf 144 Schläge dressieren konnte, ohne Einschaltung von affektbetonten Erlebnissen, so wird das wohl richtig sein; aber es wird dieses Kunststück dennoch nicht ohne jede affektive Beteiligung vor sich gehen, so wenig wie bei dem bekannten vegetativen Virtuosen, der unter anderem die schönste Gänsehaut bekam, aber nur, wenn er sich sehr lebhaft in eine winterliche Situation versetzte.

Wenn man nun aber doch über die physiologische und klinische Empirie hinaus das Bedürfnis hat mit den Fragen einer dualistischen Kausalität, einer Wechselwirkung, eines psychophysischen Parallelismus (den anzunehmen BLEULER für einen „Unsinn" erklärt) sich auseinanderzusetzen, so kann in der Tat dem Arzt eine Denkmöglichkeit einleuchtend erscheinen, wie sie etwa v. BERGMANN vorzutragen nicht müde wird. Die organische, beseelt-leibliche Existenz Mensch stellt ein psychophysisches Gesamtgeschehen dar, daß uns als Vorgang in der Welt der Objekte erscheint, das aber zugleich untrennbar in sich enthält ein Geschehen in der Welt des Subjektes, weil „aus einer einzigen Welt zwei getrennte Welten künstlich durch unser Erkennen konstruiert werden, um zu forschender Erkenntnis kommen zu können" (v. BERGMANN)[1].

II. Die organneurotischen Betriebsstörungen.

1. Allgemeiner Teil.

a) Verursachung und Entstehung.

Im Mittelpunkt organneurotischer Reaktionen und Verläufe steht die *gestörte Funktion* von Organen oder Organsystemen, die vom vegetativen Nervensystem gelenkt werden. Wieweit die Annahme gerechtfertigt erscheint, daß es eine

---

[1] In einer Anmerkung sei hier wenigstens hingewiesen auf die Lehrmeinung des Philosophen NIKOLAI HARTMANN, die unter anderem auch von POLLNOW und von v. BERGMANN zitiert wird. Der Parallelismus zerreiße die Einheit des Menschen und setze eine konstruierte Zweiheit an ihre Stelle. Er übersieht, daß gerade die Einheit als Phänomen gegeben ist. Es herrscht eine beiderseitig unübersteigbare Problemscheide, eine Trennung der Problemgebiete und wissenschaftlichen Methoden, aber keine seiende Dualität .... „Niemand zweifelt, daß organisches Leben sich vom Physisch-Materiellen wesenhaft unterscheidet. Aber es besteht nicht unabhängig von diesem; es enthält es in sich, beruht auf ihm, ja die Gesetze des Physischen erstrecken sich tief in den Organismus hinein. Was nicht hindert, daß dieser über sie hinaus noch seine Eigengesetzlichkeit habe, die in jenen nicht aufgeht. Solche Eigengesetzlichkeit überformt dann die niedere, allgemein physische Gesetzlichkeit.

Ähnlich ist es mit dem Verhältnis des seelischen Seins zum organischen Leben. Das Seelische ist, wie die Bewußtseinsphänomene beweisen, dem Organischen durchaus unähnlich, es bildet offenbar über ihm eine eigene Seinsschicht. Aber es besteht überall, wo wir ihm begegnen, in Abhängigkeit von ihm, als getragenes Sein. Wenigstens kennen wir in der wirklichen Welt kein Seelenleben, das nicht vom Organismus getragen wäre. Wollte man hieraus schließen, daß es auch keine eigentümlichen Bestimmtheiten und Gesetze habe, die nicht in denen des Organischen aufgehen, so würde man wiederum das Phänomen verkennen und der ‚Erklärung von unten' verfallen. Die Psychologie hat es über jeden Zweifel erhoben, daß hier eine spezifisch-seelische Eigengesetzlichkeit waltet; wir kennen sie zwar noch wenig (die Psychologie ist ja eine junge Wissenschaft), aber alles, was wir von ihr erfassen, zeigt deutlich ihre Eigenart, Selbständigkeit, Unableitbarkeit. Das seelische Sein ist also zwar getragenes Sein, aber in seiner Eigenart ist es bei aller Abhängigkeit autonom..."
„Die Abhängigkeit der höheren Seinsschicht ist aber durchaus keine Beeinträchtigung ihrer Autonomie. Die niedere Schicht ist für sie nur tragender Boden, conditio sine qua non. Die besondere Gestaltung und Eigenart der höheren hat über ihr unbegrenzten Spielraum. Das Organische ist zwar getragen vom Materiellen, aber sein Formenreichtum und das Wunder der Lebendigkeit stammen nicht aus ihm her, sondern treten als ein Novum hinzu. Ebenso ist das Seelische über dem Organischen, das Geistige über dem Seelischen ein Novum. Dieses Novum, das mit jeder Schicht neu einsetzt, ist nichts anderes als die Selbständigkeit oder ‚Freiheit' der höheren Kategorien über den niederen. Es ist eine Freiheit, welche die Abhängigkeit auf ihr natürliches Maß einschränkt und so mit ihr in der Einheit eines durchgehenden kategorialen Schichtungsverhältnisses koexistiert. Man kann ihr Gesetz in Vereinigung mit dem vorigen so aussprechen: die niederen Kategorien sind zwar die ‚stärkeren', aber die höheren sind über ihnen dennoch ‚frei'.

Das Gesetz der Stärke und das der Freiheit bilden zusammen ein unlösliches, durchaus einheitliches Verhältnis; ja sie bilden im Grunde eine einzige kategoriale Dependenzgesetzlichkeit, welche das Schichtenreich der Welt von unten auf bis in seine Höhen beherrscht..."
Aus NICOLAI HARTMANN: Das Problem des geistigen Seins. Berlin-Leipzig 1933. S. 14, 15 und 16.

Grenze und Gegensätzlichkeit zwischen funktionellem Leiden und organischer Krankheit nicht gebe (v. BERGMANN), soll in einem späteren Abschnitt über den Verlauf dieser Betriebsstörungen dargelegt werden. Hier geht es zunächst um die pathogenetische Hauptfrage, wie und in welchem Ausmaß in diese Steuerung, bzw. gestörte Steuerung *seelisches* Geschehen eingreift. Denn es sollte füglich nur dann von ,,Organneurosen" gesprochen werden, wenn der seelische Anteil im Aufbau den Akzent erhält. Von vornherein muß ich jedoch — im Gegensatz zu KRONFELD u. a. — erklären, daß mir die ,,tiefenpsychologische Arbeit auf diesem Gebiet" vielleicht weiter getrieben, aber nicht gesicherter erscheint, ,,als man dies von der pathophysiologischen Forschungsseite sagen kann". Erkenntnis und Deutung gibt es hier wie da, aber im Psychologischen und Pathopsychologischen ist das Erkennen schwerer und das Deuten leichter. Einzelne Etappen auf dem Wege pathophysiologischer Forschung wurden bereits im ersten Teil erwähnt: Organminderwertigkeit, Vagotonie-Sympathicotonie; ,,Stigmatisation im — zunächst — vegetativen *Nerven*system", schließlich im ,,vegetativen System" schlechthin; vegetative Konstitutionstypen; Polygenie funktioneller Störungen; ,,Abbau" der Organneurosen.

In solchem *Abbau* (v. BERGMANN) gipfelt schließlich und anscheinend notwendig die zunehmende Vertiefung pathophysiologischer Erkenntnisse, und erweist so aufs neue, daß man zwar von der *Lebens*einheit des menschlichen Organismus durchdrungen sein kann, und dennoch sich genötigt sieht, klinisch die Leib-Seele-Schranke anzuerkennen, und sei es auch nur nach der Akzentverschiebung auf die körperlichen oder seelischen Anteile an der Störung von Organfunktionen. Über solche Erkennung scheinbar rein neurotischer Beschwerden als latenter und larvierter Krankheitsbilder, als ,,formes frustes" ist seit v. BERGMANNs Vorgang wiederholt berichtet worden. Ich erinnere nur an die neurotisch gedeuteten epiphrenalen Betriebsstörungen, wie sie v. HATTINGBERG als ,,Atemkorsett" beschrieb, während v. BERGMANN als organische Ursache eine Hernie des Oesophagus — mit einer Alteration der beiden nn. vagi — aufdeckte; weiter an die tabischen, saturninen und nicotinogenen Magenspasmen (CURSCHMANN u. a.), sowie an gewisse Magenbeschwerden, die HANSEN — unter Hinweis auf eine Arbeit von LANGENSKIÖLD — als Ausdruck einer Forme fruste der Tetanie beschrieben hat. Von hier zu den vegetativen Konstitutionstypen ist nur ein Schritt.

JOH. LANGE hat in einem Fall von ,,Hysterie" hingewiesen auf Kranke mit bestimmten somatischen Komplexen, die ,,bei den leisesten Anstößen zum Vorschein kommen", und bei denen man allenthalben an eine Störung in der Ca-Verwertung denken könne: ,,Echte Stigmatisierte" im Sinne SCHINDLERs, Menschen mit Neigung ,,zur multiplen Hautgangrän" mit ,,hysterischem Fieber" entfernteren Beziehungen zum exsudativen und zum Migränekreis, mit ,,starren Visionen" im Sinne des tetanoiden Typus von JAENSCH.

Es wurde schon erwähnt, daß die Lehre von EPPINGER und HESS über die Vagotonie auch deshalb so fruchtbar war, weil sie den großen Aspekt auf die Konstitutionstypen mit bestimmter vegetativ-nervöser Krankheitsbereitschaft lenkte. OTTOMAR ROSENBACH hatte 1879 zuerst über einen wahrscheinlich auf einer Neurose des Vagus beruhenden Symptomenkomplex mit Herz- und Magenbeschwerden sowie Luftmangel berichtet. Wie sehr die ,,Vagotonie" in ihrem klinischen Wert umstritten ist, wurde im ersten Teil dargelegt; ebenso die häufigen Versager im Nachweis des zugeordneten einseitigen pharmakodynamischen Verhaltens. Dennoch scheint weder darüber noch über die tatsächliche Häufigkeit oder Seltenheit solcher oder *bevorzugt* vagotonischer Symptomenkomplexe bei vagotonischer Labilität Einigkeit zu herrschen. DANIELOPOLU und CARRIOL[1]

---
[1] DANIELOPOLU u. CARRIOL: Arch. Mal. Cour **1923**, No 3.

haben eine Modifikation des Atropinversuches angegeben, die es erlauben soll, alle Mischungen von Vago- und Sympathicotonie oder -hypotonie festzustellen, einschließlich der Amphotonie. Bei aller Unzulänglichkeit empirischer Forschung scheint mir die Annahme doch begründet zu sein, daß bestimmten vegetativen Konstitutionen bestimmte seelische Verhaltensbereitschaften sowohl wie bestimmte Funktionseigenheiten und funktionelle Störungen von Organen zugeordnet sind. Möglicherweise ist ja auch die Fähigkeit, an verwandten Erscheinungen überwiegend das Gemeinsame oder unerbittlich das Trennende zu sehen und als entscheidend zu werten von so different vegetativer Konstitution mit abhängig. Der „Typus" einer Vagolabilität mit Überempfindlichkeit gegen Morphin und Pilocarpin läßt sich auch klinisch anscheinend eher erhärten als derjenige einer Sympathicolabilität mit Adrenalinüberempfindlichkeit. Ausdruck einer *vorzugsweisen Vagolabilität* sind (LESCHKE u. a.): vasomotorische Störungen mit kalten Händen und Füßen, oft mit venöser Stauung und Blaufärbung, vasculäre Hypotonie, Bradykardie, respiratorische Arrhythmie, Migräne, anginöse Beschwerden, Asthma bronchiale, Neigung zum Seekrankwerden, Laryngospasmus, Supersekretion, Superacidität plus Spasmus des Magens; vermehrte Peristaltik und Neigung zu Durchfällen; größerer Flüssigkeitsverbrauch; leichtere Neigung zum Fettansatz. Als Kennzeichen des *Sympathicolabilen* gelten: Tachykardie mit Neigung zur Blutdrucksteigerung, hoher steiler Anstieg und rascher Abfall der Adrenalinblutdruckkurve, kugelige Form des Herzens mit lebhafter Aktion, Extrasystolen, die durch Atropin nicht zu beeinflussen sind, Erregbarkeit der Vasomotoren mit leichtem Erblassen und Erröten, Glanzauge, Konvergenzschwäche (mit Neigung zu Akkommodationskrämpfen wie bei Vagotonikern) und ganz allgemein: fehlende Bereitschaft für die organneurotischen Störungen des Vagotonikers. Wenn also auch auf der einen Seite eine jeweilig individuell verschiedene Zusammenordnung etwa von: Bradykardie, Atemstörungen bis zum Asthma bronchiale, Hyperacidität, Neigung zu Durchfällen; auf der anderen von Tachykardie, Anacidität, Schweißausbrüchen, Tremor beobachtet wird, so ist doch wiederum nicht zu verkennen, wie wenig *eindeutig* sympathicolabil die basedowoiden Persönlichkeiten, oder — wie v. BERGMANN im Anschluß an I. BAUER sie nennt —, die konstitutionell Thyreotischen sind. Gerade auf sie aber treffen die obengenannten Merkmale einer sympathisch labilen Konstitution zu. Bei ihnen findet sich beispielsweise in der Regel ein Überwiegen des vagotonischen Verhaltens der Darminnervation mit vermehrter Peristaltik und Neigung zu Durchfällen, und weit seltener eine Gruppe mit sympathischer Hemmung der Magen- und Darminnervation bis zu atonischer Obstipation und Meteorismus. Gerade am Beispiel des Hyperthyreotischen wiesen schon PÖTZL, EPPINGER und HESS auf die Neigung zur Mischung, zur Aufspaltung vegetativer Labilität in den verschiedenen Innervationsgebieten hin; so wie klinisch doch recht häufig überwiegend *vago*labile Persönlichkeiten eine erhebliche Puls*beschleunigung* aufweisen. Wie schwierig im einzelnen die Zuweisung bestimmter Funktionsstörungen zu bestimmter oder überhaupt zu einer Labilität des vegetativen Nervensystems ist, geht etwa daraus hervor, daß der Pylorospasmus so lange dem Vagotoniker zugesprochen wurde, bis ihn KLEE als Sympathicusfunktion erkannte, und daß ständige Bradykardie bei sonst normalem Herzen nicht ohne weiteres auf vermehrten Vagustonus zurückzuführen ist, sondern daß hierbei der Ansprechbarkeit des Erfolgsganzen der entscheidende Einfluß zukommen kann (WENCKEBACH, zit. nach v. BERGMANN). Es wurde schon oben erwähnt, daß v. BERGMANN an die Stelle einer so polaren Typisierung: Vagotonie-Sympathicotonie eine Labilität im gesamten vegetativen Nervensystem setzte. Innerhalb der Gesundheitsbreite findet er Gruppen mit veränderter humoraler Struktur und einem entsprechend andersartigen, vegetativen Verhalten, die beide nicht akzidenteller Natur sind, sondern wesentliche Konstitutionsmerkmale. Für eine ganz große Gruppe solcher „vegetativ Stigmatisierten" gibt es eine Beziehung zu den Schilddrüsenhormonen. Darauf weist der biologische Test der REID-HUNT-Reaktion hin: Für die Maus erhöht sich die Dosis letalis von Acetonitril nach Vorbehandlung mit Schilddrüsenpräparaten (v. BERGMANN und GOLDNER, OEHME und PAAL usw.). Menschen solcher Art mit einem „Miniaturbasedow ohne Morbus", einem „Mikrobasedow", einer „thyreotischen Konstitution" (I. BAUER, v. BERGMANN) neigen zum Schwitzen, zu Dysmenorrhöe, zu Tachykardie und Temperaturerhöhung, zu Tenesmen der Gallenblase, zu Dyskinesien im Magen- und Darmtractus; sie zeigen Ulcusdisposition, sind meist schlank, leptosom, haben Glanzauge und etwas vergrößerte Schilddrüse, sind affektlabil, reizbar, hastig. Wenn v. BERGMANN neuerdings den Begriff der vegetativen Stigmatisation von der ursprünglich gemeinten Beschränkung auf das *vegetative Nervensystem* befreit und erweitert hat, auf eine Stigmatisation im *vegetativen System überhaupt*, so ist das die selbstverständliche Konsequenz aus den neueren physiologischen Ergebnissen, die an die Stelle des vegetativen Nervensystems wenigstens drei beständig ineinandergreifende Regulationssysteme setzen, ionale Umstimmungen, hormonale Einflüsse, nervöse Impulse. Auch der berühmte Fund von FRIEDRICH KRAUS aus dem Rudolfspital in Wien über die Degeneration des Vagus im Falle eines rein vagoneurotischen Kardiospasmus mit Oesophagusdilatation läßt sich, wie v. BERGMANN zeigt, sehr wohl als sekundäre Nervenschädigung durch Druck oder Zerrung deuten *infolge* von langjährigem Kardiospasmus mit Oesophagusdilatation.

Es gibt nach den klinischen Erfahrungen keinen anderen Weg als die Reaktionsbereitschaft der einzelnen Organe zu untersuchen und diese Reaktionsbereitschaft als Symptome der Labilität im *gesamten* vegetativen System zu verstehen. In den Gruppen der konstitutionell nervösen Menschen, der „Neuropathen", der „Neurosebereiten" spielt diese vegetative Stigmatisation als angeborene Labilität *typischer* Art trotz verschiedener Mischung der klinischen Erscheinungen die somatisch entscheidende Rolle. Es seien hier aus der Fülle der Literatur nur drei kennzeichnende Hinweise erwähnt. I. H. SCHULTZ nennt die konstitutionelle Nervosität, die „Neurosenbereitschaft" eine Diathese im Sinne von HIS. Sie sei „ein individuell angeborener, oftmals vererbter Zustand, der darin besteht, daß physiologische Reize eine abnorme Reaktion auslösen, und daß Lebensbedingungen, welche von der Mehrzahl der Gattung schadlos vertragen werden, krankhafte Zustände bewirken". LICHTWITZ meint, daß an der Neurose Menschen von besonderer somatischer und psychischer Konstitution erkranken. „Muskelschwache, schlaffe Haltung, hängende Gesichtszüge, weiche Beschaffenheit der Gewebe, lose Gelenke, Glanzauge, rascher Wechsel der Hautfarbe, Neigung zu mechanischer und spontaner Dermographie, derbe Arterien und Hautvenen, Neigung zu Schwitzen, Neigung zu Tränen sind die wesentlichen äußeren Kennzeichen der neurotischen Konstitution. Ermüdbarkeit, Neigung zu Frösteln und zu frieren, vermehrtes Schlafbedürfnis, aber unruhiger und durch wüste Träume gestörter Schlaf, dem unfrohes Erwachen folgt; Schreckhaftigkeit, taktile und sensorische Überempfindlichkeit..... sind die .....Merkmale der Neurosenbereitschaft. Alle diese Merkmale kann man unter der Rubrik reizbare Schwäche zusammenfassen." Gegenüber einer so mehr summarischen Darstellung ist — etwa von REICHARDT, von ZUCKER — versucht worden, bestimmte neuropathische Formen und Verlaufstypen herauszuheben. Bei einer charakteristischen Unterform der vegetativen Neurose jenseits des 35. Lebensjahres hat ZUCKER konstante Besonderheiten am Habitus, gleichartige objektive Störungen, und subjektiv ähnliche Beschwerden beobachtet: schlaffer Turgor, geringes Fettpolster, vorgealtertes Aussehen, Hyperacidität des Magens, vorzeitige Rigidität der Gefäße, geringe Schweißbildung, geringe Dermographie.

Die dispositionellen, konstitutionellen, ja familiär-hereditären Anteile am Aufbau neurotischer und insbesondere organneurotischer Reaktionen und Verläufe, wie sie hier erwähnt wurden, und wie sie auch sonst in der Literatur eine Rolle spielen — ich verweise nur auf die konstitutionellen und familiären Bereitschaften zur arteriellen Hyper- und Hypotonie, zur Migräne, zum Asthma, zu Sekretionsstörungen und Dyskinesien des Magen- und Darmtractus — werden heute wohl von fast allen Autoren anerkannt, selbst wenn sie von manchen, vorwiegend psychotherapeutisch eingestellten Autoren bagatellisiert werden. Für die Organneurosen mit ihren mehr minder isolierten funktionellen Betriebsstörungen liegt es nahe, in den Kreis der ererbten oder erworbenen Störungsbereitschaft eben dieses Organ oder Organsystem selbst miteinzuziehen. Die Lehre von einer *Organminderwertigkeit* (A. ADLER), schon früh gefaßt, hat neuerdings auch von klinischer und physiologischer Seite besondere Bestätigung gefunden [1].

Auf die Deutung von Organminderwertigkeit als besonderer Lebensform, wie dies ALFRED ADLER und seine Schule wollen, wird später einzugehen sein; hier soll der Begriff nur im somatisch funktionellen Sinn gemeint sein, als individuelle Beschaffenheit bestimmter Organe, die dazu führt, daß dieses Organ in der Funktion zurückbleibt, dadurch den notwendigen Anforderungen des Lebens nicht gewachsen ist und infolgedessen häufig bei normaler und erst recht bei übermäßiger Beanspruchung erkrankt [2]. Dieses „somatische Entgegenkommen" (S. FREUD) der Organe und dessen subjektives Erfühlen in den Mißempfindungen (PÖTZL, JAHRREISS u. a.) ist für die *Organbestimmung* oder sog. *Organwahl* bei den Organneurosen allem Anschein nach von erheblicher Bedeutung, und zwar nicht nur als konstitutionelle Disposition, sondern gerade auch als erworbene Organerkrankung geringen Grades (v. WEIZSÄCKER).

Neben einer besonderen Labilität von vegetativem Nervensystem und Erfolgsorgan, hat man schließlich auch geglaubt, eine erhöhte Ansprechbarkeit von endokrinen Drüsen- und Drüsensystemen annehmen zu können. Das jeweils unterstellte Organsystem werde dann Äußerungsort der Neurose (ALKAN).

Es wurde schon erwähnt, daß man die Organminderwertigkeit nicht nur somatisch verstanden wissen will, sondern auch als bestimmte *Erlebnisform* (A. ADLER); in dem psychoanalytischen Begriff des „somatischen Entgegenkommens" ist als notwendige Ergänzung mitgedacht ein seelischer Konflikt und sein symbolischer Ausdruck; und *Organwahl* bedeutet die — seelische — Determinierung eines Organs zur abnormen Funktion. Es eröffnet sich also von hier aus das Bereich des Psychischen und die Frage nach dem Anteil am Aufbau der sog. Organneurosen. Nirgends scheint dieser Anteil so deutlich zu sein wie hier, freilich auch nirgends so deutbar und zur Deutung verführend. Die gestörte Funktion wird verstanden als Ausdruck des Seelischen. Das kann generell nicht verwundern. Es wurde ja im ersten Teil dargelegt, wie untrennbar seelischen Abläufen emotiver Art vegetative Vorgänge zugeordnet sind, die als Erblassen und

---

[1] So E. FRANK „Abnorme Reaktionen und Reaktionsbereitschaften vegetativ innervierter Organe brauchen nicht zu beruhen — wie es die Definition der Neurosen erfordern würde — auf einer Dauererregung (Tonus) oder Übererregung nervöser Zentren: sondern überstarke Reaktionen auf das sympathicomimetische bzw. parasympathicomimetische Pharmakon erweisen eine Übererregbarkeit beider Fangarme oder des gesamten Rezeptivapparates, sind also ein Stigma von abnormer Organempfindlichkeit, nicht von nervöser Übererregbarkeit." Die isolierte erhöhte Reaktionsbereitschaft vom vegetativen System gelenkter Organe betonen auch J. BAUER, H. CURSCHMANN, v. BERGMANN, SIEBECK, v. WEIZSÄCKER, HANSEN u. a.

[2] Vgl. hierzu die Kontroverse zwischen E. KAHN und A. ADLER im Nervenarzt 1.

Erröten als Tränen und Zittern, als Pulsbeschleunigung und Leuchten der Augen sehr ausdrücklich in Erscheinung treten. Es besteht kein ernstliches Hindernis, auch hinter Funktionsstörungen des Herzens, der Atmung, des Darmes usw. nach ihrem allgemeinen oder besonderen Ausdruckswert zu fahnden. ,,Man kann", meint KEHRER, ,,diese Körperteile (sc. die inneren Organe) geradezu als die innere Front des gemütlichen Ausdrucksapparates ansprechen, dessen äußere das Spiel der Mienen und Gesten und die Lautsprache darstellen." Eine solche Betrachtungsweise kann sich nicht genügen lassen an der einfachen Annahme einer Ausdrucksbedeutung vegetativ gesteuerter Organfunktionen, sondern sie wird darauf abzielen, bestimmte, regelmäßige, ja gesetzmäßige Beziehungen zwischen beiden nachzuweisen, derart, daß die Neurose in ihrer somatischen Ausdrucksform ,,dem physiologischen Funktionsplan des Organismus folgt" (v. WYSS). So hat v. WEIZSÄCKER versucht, die ,,spezifische psychische Valenz" der Verdauungsfunktion im ganzen und in seinen Teilen darzustellen, indem er sich fragte, welche ,,psychischen Gebiete" mitsamt ihren neurotischen Fehlformen den einzelnen Organgebieten adäquat zugeordnet sind. Er stellt mit der gebotenen Vorsicht zunächst folgende Korrelationen auf: 1. Die Außensinne, willkürliche Muskulatur und Bewegungsapparat, gewisse Kopforganisationen tragen den Konflikt mit der Umwelt, sind Ausdrucksgebiet von traumatischem Konflikt, von Geltungs- und Tendenzneurosen. 2. Die anatomischen Übergangsgebiete von Innen- und Außensinnen, von willkürlicher und unwillkürlicher Muskulatur am anourogenitalen Pol mit ihren Funktionsentgleisungen: Aerophagie, Rumination, Brechneurose, Obstipation usw. entsprechen den neurotischen Erledigungen im Konflikt der Willkür mit der Autonomie der Organe, dem Kampf des Neurotikers mit sich selbst, der vernunftbestimmten mit der triebbestimmten Seite der Psyche. 3. Die rein autonomen Gebiete vom Oesophagus bis zum Mastdarm erscheinen v. WEIZSÄCKER als Ausdrucksgebiete der Person am wenigsten geklärt. Hier spiele sich wohl die neurotische Erledigung eines innersten Existenzkampfes ab, wie etwa in den hypochondrischen Syndromen, bis ,,an die Stelle des inneren Menschen schließlich die inneren Organe treten". 4. Im System der endokrinen Apparate sieht v. WEIZSÄCKER das Ausdrucksgebiet der sog. Temperamente.

Organwahl bedeutet demnach, daß ein bestimmter Konflikt auch ein bestimmtes Ausdrucksgebiet im Körperlichen wählt. So fragwürdig uns auch diese Beziehungen im einzelnen noch sind und bleiben werden, so führen doch auch sie zu der denkerischen Konsequenz und sind von ihr aus zu verstehen, daß an die Stelle des Begriffes einer psychogenen oder somatogenen Reaktion die Anschauung ,,einer letzten Identität der beiden Reihen tritt, welche nur durch die Betrachtungsform, nicht in der Sache selbst auseinanderfallen".

In verwandter Weise sucht v. WYSS im Anschluß an die HEsssche Lehre von der ergotropen Funktionsweise des Sympathicus, der histotropen des Parasympathicus — wie sie im ersten Teil skizziert wurde, die entsprechenden Funktionen als vorbestimmte Ausdrucksmittel elementarer Konflikte zu begreifen. Die sympathicogen gesteigerte Kreislauf- und Atmungstätigkeit im Angstanfall erhält so die Bedeutung von Ausdrucksmitteln des leidenschaftlichen Kampfes um die Selbstbehauptung. Parasympathische Erscheinungen wie Ohnmachten, vermehrte Darmperistaltik, Harndrang dagegen sind Ausdruck einer widerstandslosen Selbstaufgabe der Persönlichkeit. In der Tat handelt es sich in solchen und ähnlichen Funktionssteigerungen und Entgleisungen um Erscheinungen, die unmittelbar als Ausdruck heftiger Gemütsbewegungen und schwieriger seelischer Lagen erlebt und verstanden werden, und zwar so häufig, daß sie alltägliches Sprachgut geworden sind: Es preßt einem das Herz ab, es schlägt einem auf den Magen, es schnürt mir die Kehle zu, es läuft kalt über den Rücken, der Ekel würgt mich usw. Es läßt sich ohne schwierige Konstruktionen verstehen, daß ein ekelhaftes Erlebnis und schließlich nur mehr die lebhafte Erinnerung daran zum Erbrechen führen. Sowie man jedoch beginnt, an Stelle solcher unmittelbaren Ausdrucksbeziehungen Symbolbeziehungen zu setzen, gelangt man möglicherweise zu einer tieferen und zuweilen auch treffenden Einsicht in verwickelte Zusammenhänge, aber doch eben zu einer nur gleichnishaften Deutung, die plump und schief wird, sobald man sie aus ihrer schwebenden Sphäre löst. So mag sich etwa gelegentlich hinter einem Erbrechen als determinierendes Erlebnis die Schwierigkeit einer schlechten aber ,,nicht gebrochenen" Ehe verstecken. Oder hinter Kopfschmerzen steht die *Symbolfunktion* des Kopfes: das Selbst; sein Schmerz ist die symbolische Repräsentation des Leidens im Selbst oder am Selbst (KRONFELD). Die verschluckte Luft des Aerophagen steht für den Ärger, die Kränkungen, Niederlagen, die er ,,hinunterschluckt", und so fort. So kann eine Organsymbolik als bestimmend gedacht werden und gelegentlich bestimmend sein für die ,,Wahl" der neurotischen Betriebsstörung; nicht weniger als eine Organminderwertigkeit; oder auch ein zufälliges Zusammentreffen von seelischem Trauma mit organischer Erkrankung. So schwankt die Erkenntnis und das Ringen um sie zwischen der Feststellung unverbindlicher Gleichzeitigkeit und dem Postulat unentrinnbarer, vorgebildeter Gesetzmäßigkeit.

Eine besondere Bedeutung für die Organdetermination, ja für die Pathogenese der Organneurosen überhaupt, hat die Übersetzung der PAWLOWschen Lehre von den *bedingten Reflexen* ins Psychologische erlangt (HANSEN, PANNHORST; ADLERSBERG und PORGES, KÜPPERS, BUYTENDYK usw.). Die seelischen Ausdruckserscheinungen im vegetativen Bereich sind *unbedingte* Reflexe; dagegen sind die *bedingten* Reflexe nervöse Abläufe besonderer Art. PAWLOW meint, daß sie sich im Experiment als mechanisch bedingte Verbindungen zwischen inadäquatem Reiz und Reaktion darstellen lassen: Speichelsekretion bei Hunden auf akustische, optische Reize. Eine solche Dressur durch Erfahrung ist aber ohne psychische Beteiligung am ,,Reflexablauf" nicht zu verstehen. Unbedingter und bedingter Reflex gehören zu einer Situation zusammen und werden auch so aufgefaßt. Nur weil die gegebenen Reize als Signal verstanden werden, und nur, soweit sie diesen Charakter des Signals tragen, sind sie wirksam, und können körperliche Funktionen in Gang setzen. ,,So kann eine Gesamtlebenssituation je nach ihrer emotionalen Intensität und ihrer gleichzeitig — oft wohl nur zufällig — gegebenen Organverknüpfung zu einer Bindung führen, kraft deren künftighin eine jede Teilgegebenheit des Erlebnisinhaltes die Dignität eines Signalmerkmales für einen jeweils durch die Ausgangssituation bestimmten Organablauf bekommt (HANSEN). Auf solche Weise kann — genau wie in den Experimenten PAWLOWS — eine bestimmte Organfunktion von ihren üblichen biologischen Beziehungen wie abgelöst und verselbständigt erscheinen; und eine Loslösung und Dysfunktion kann schließlich allein durch die *Vorstellung* eines Erlebnisses und des bedingenden Signales ausgelöst werden. Wie fest und wie labil zugleich gewisse Organfunktionen durch die bedingten Reflexe der Erziehung und Gewohnheit geregelt sind, läßt sich etwa am Defäkationsvorgang zeigen. Das Wunder der endlich gelungenen Dressur am Kleinkind wird beim Erwachsenen selbstverständliche, in der Norm unerschütterliche, oft auf die Minute ,,automatisch" geregelte Leistung; und doch besteht noch immer häufig genug eine so labile Verbindung zwischen ,,Reiz und vegetativem Effekt", daß eine Änderung der gewohnten Umgebung, die neuen Eindrücke einer Reise schon genügen, um den gewohnten Ablauf durch neue Bedingungsreize zu stören.

Solche Signale stammen aber keineswegs nur von außen. Die Organfunktionen sind ja dauernd begleitet von mehr oder minder unterschwelligen

Empfindungen und Mißempfindungen vitaler Art, auf deren möglichen Wert als „Anzeichen für lebensfördernde und lebenshemmende Vorgänge innerhalb des Organismus" SCHELER nachdrücklich und im Gegensatz zu den peripheren und umschriebeneren „sinnlichen" Gefühlen hinweist. Wie sehr solche Mißempfindungen zu einer *dauernden* Quelle von seelischer Beunruhigung, immer vermehrter ängstlicher Zuwendung zu bestimmten Organfunktionen werden und damit endlich auch zu deren Dysfunktion führen können, erhellt schon aus der bekannten Erscheinung, die SCHELER so kennzeichnet, daß „alle vitalen Gefühle.. durch die Zuwendung der Aufmerksamkeit auf sie in ihrem normalen Ablauf zum mindesten gestört werden und sinnvoll und normal nur jenseits der Helligkeitssphären der Aufmerksamkeit fungieren" (s. auch JAHRREISS). Von hier aus erhellt auch der Wert des Lebensgefühles und „der Signale des veränderten Lebensgefühles" sowie der Affektspannungen in Lagen der Erwartung, Befürchtung, ängstlichen Erregung für das Zustandekommen von Organneurosen; zugleich aber auch die Tatsache, daß es entscheidend ist, wie jemand zu echten oder nur übertrieben lebhaft empfundenen Organbeschwerden oder schließlich auch zu objektiv registrierten Funktionsstörungen Stellung nimmt. Die Art dieser Stellungnahme, das Nichtbeachten, Entwerten oder Überwerten, das Bekämpfen und Fertigwerden, das Willkommenheißen und Aufbauschen vor sich und anderen, die ergebene Hinnahme lästiger Störungen oder die Hingabe an sie ist abhängig von der konstitutionell verschiedenen seelischen Widerstandskraft überhaupt, von der Beschaffenheit des augenblicklichen „vitalen Turgors", aber auch von der *Bedeutung*, die derlei subjektiven Mißempfindungen und Funktionsstörungen — offen oder maskiert — für die Existenz der Betroffenen zukommt. Auch hier greifen körperliche und seelische Funktionen sowie geistiger Gehalt eines individuellen Lebens kaum überschaubar ineinander, faktisch untrennbar, und in ihrer gegenseitigen Bindung und Abhängigkeit nur gewaltsamem Sondern und gelindem Deuten einigermaßen zugänglich. Jede Stellungnahme beschließt in sich die Frage nach der Bedeutung desjenigen, zu dem Stellung genommen wird; und diese Frage ist ohne Zweck- oder Zielfrage, ohne finale Betrachtungsweise nicht zu lösen. Gerade von der Konzeption der Organminderwertigkeit aus ist ja ADLER zur „Individualpsychologie" gekommen, zur Allerweiterung des finalen Gedankens in Neurose- und Persönlichkeitsgestaltung, zum Begriff des „Zweckstrebens" aus alles überschattendem Minderwertigkeitsgefühl und Geltungsstreben. Der hysterische Modus im engen Sinn einer — wenigstens zunächst — absichtsvollen seelischen Regie ist damit getroffen; und damit die Verwendung, Fixierung und der Ausbau auch organneurotischer Reaktionen.

Aus allem, was bisher angeführt wurde, erhellt die *Polygenie* (CURSCHMANN) der sog. Organneurosen: Sehr verschiedenartige Ursachen können die gleiche Funktionsstörung bewirken, und für deren Zustandekommen ist nicht *eine* Ursache verantwortlich zu machen, sondern ein vielschichtiges Bedingungsspiel körperlicher und seelischer Anteile. Es scheint so zu sein, daß der Anstoß oder auch die bewirkende Hauptursache an sehr verschiedener Stelle innerhalb der Kette von Erfolgsorganen bis zum seelischen Bereich liegen kann, und zwar jeweils verschieden selbst für die gleichen Störungen bei derselben Persönlichkeit, ohne daß dies am subjektiven Verhalten oder den objektiven Phänomenen zu erkennen wäre. Ob etwa ein Asthmaanfall psychisch ausgelöst ist (durch Signalerlebnis, unmittelbar thymogen durch Schreck, hysterisch-tendenziös usw.) oder durch bestimmte Allergene, oder durch Organüberempfindlichkeit bei normalen Reizen oder durch irgendeine Kombination von alle dem läßt sich fast nie mit genügender Sicherheit entscheiden, nicht einmal aus dem Erfolg oder Mißerfolg einer Behandlungsmethode. Da nun seelisches Geschehen nicht ohne affektive

Beteiligung, affektive Vorgänge nicht ohne vegetativen „Ausdruck" im Körperlichen ablaufen, so ist der Rang des Seelischen im Aufbau von „Neurosen" vegetativ gesteuerter Organe kaum zu überschätzen. Dabei ist jedoch an eine Schranke zu erinnern, die schon oben erwähnt wurde: daß nämlich dem somatischen Ausdruck psychischer Erlebnisse „in der Funktionsbreite und der Funktionsgewohnheit der Organe natürliche Grenzen gezogen sind" (HANSEN). Die konstitutionelle Labilität der vegetativen — nervösen, humoralen, ionalen — Steuerungen mag in engerer Beziehung zur konstitutionellen seelischen Labilität stehen, vielleicht sind es nur zwei Seiten *eines* funktionalen Geschehens; aber, psychische und vegetative Labilität sind im Ausmaß ihrer neurosebildenden Kraft von der Intaktheit oder Minderwertigkeit des Erfolgsorganes entscheidend abhängig.

Man muß sich von dem Vorurteil freimachen, daß organneurotische Reaktionen *nur* am *unversehrten* Organ geschehen — eher das Gegenteil ist der Fall — und daß funktionelle Betriebsstörungen am geschädigten Organ seelisch nicht ausgelöst sein könnten. Sie sind es eher häufig. Darauf wird im nächsten Abschnitt noch einzugehen sein.

Die folgende Tabelle bringt in schematischer Darstellung einen Überblick über die Vielschichtigkeit der organneurotischen Bedingungen.

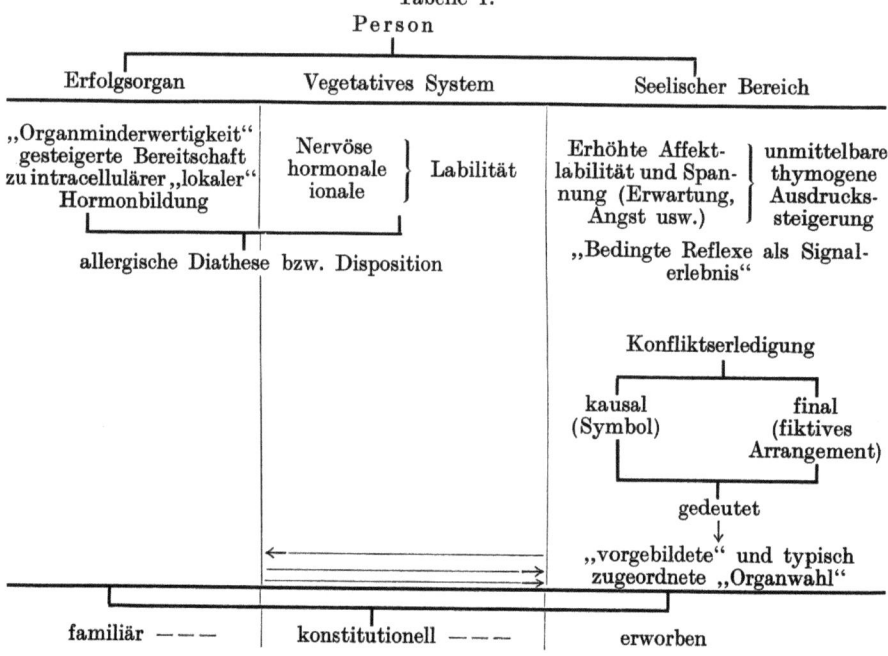

Tabelle 1.

b) Erkennen und Verlauf.

Wenn es auch — um mit STAEHELIN zu reden (zit. nach v. BERGMANN) — theoretisch gleichgültig ist, wo man den Ring der vielgliedrigen Kausalitätskette löst, wie sie soeben geschildert wurde, so ist doch praktisch und dem Einzelfall gegenüber die Wahl kaum willkürlich. Darin liegt die diagnostische Aufgabe beschlossen und zugleich ein Teil hoffnungsfreudiger Therapie. Wie man es auch nennen mag: Strukturanalyse, Schichtendiagnose, konzentrische Analyse — immer bedeutet es die gleiche Forderung, die Aufbaubedingungen einer Organneurose nicht nur festzustellen, sondern auch nach ihrem Wert abzustufen, und nach Möglichkeit zu ergründen, ob der Akzent auf dem Körperlichen oder dem Seelischen ruht.

Eine pharmakodynamische Prüfung, deren physiologischer und pathophysiologischer Wert selbst umstritten ist, wird hier nicht weit führen. Die funktio laesa ist ja gegeben, ihre körperliche Abhängigkeit selbstverständlich, und wo gröbere Organschäden ernstlich auszuschließen sind, wird die feinere Diagnostik vielleicht noch allergische Überempfindlichkeiten gegen bestimmte Antigene nachweisen können. Alles das überhebt den Arzt nicht einer eingehenden Persönlichkeitsanalyse, wozu die Lebensschilderung und nicht selten Lebensbeichte des Patienten gehört. Organneurotische Störungen unterliegen grundsätzlich den gleichen Erkenntniswegen wie die hysterischen Reaktionen im Gebiet der willkürlichen Muskulatur, der sensiblen und sensorischen Bereiche: nämlich dem ätiologischen und dem symptomatologischen (E. GUTTMANN). Die erste Methode zielt darauf ab, ,,die seelische Verursachung nachzuweisen und das seelische Festhalten verständlich zu machen", die zweite stützt sich auf ,,eine empirische Klassifizierung der Einzelsymptome als solcher, denen keine Organveränderung zugrunde liegt" (GUTTMANN). Die fortschreitende Diagnostik organischer Schäden hat bekanntlich zu einem ,,Abbau" gewisser hysterischer Reaktionen sowohl wie insbesondere der Organneurosen geführt (v. BERGMANN). Es wurden schon oben die ehemals als neurotisch gedeuteten Beschwerden einer Insuffizienz des Hiatus oesophageus und der Oesophagushernie erwähnt; die verschieden organisch bedingten Magenspasmen; die pseudoneurasthenische Achylie bei Anämie, die Magenneurose als forme fruste der Tetanie. Auch hierbei ist es sehr wohl möglich, daß gelegentlich von emotiven Einflüssen her eine Auslösung der Beschwerden, ihre Häufung oder längere Fixierung geschieht. Von nur psychisch erfaßbaren Abläufen her erscheint die Betriebsstörung eines Organes wesentlich auch als eine Ausdrucksform seelischer Funktionen und Erlebnisse, und umgekehrt von nur somatisch faßbaren Veränderungen her als eine wesentlich organisch bedingte Störung. v. BERGMANN rechnet die Organneurosen insgesamt zu den Cavetediagnosen, d. h. zu denjenigen, die nur mit Vorbehalt und innerer Unruhe gestellt werden und immer eine Mahnung zu sorgfältigster somatischer Diagnostik bleiben sollten. So verstanden, ist mit der Forderung nach Abbau der Organneurosen ,,keine Kluft gerissen zu ihren seelischen Ausdrucksanlässen; vielmehr ist nur die innige dynamische Beziehung jener beiden Pole speziell um ihren Ausdruckseffekt strenger betont" (HANSEN)[1]. Die Kenntnis der Organneurosen, vor allem aber die ,,somatisch" eingestellte Beschäftigung mit ihnen, hat wesentlich mit dazu geführt, den ,,fließenden Übergang von funktionell pathologischem Geschehen, zu morphologisch nachweisbarem aufgezeigt zu haben, im Morphologischen der Pathologie ein Dokument der gestörten Funktion zu sehen" (v. BERGMANN). Wenn man so konsequent die Funktion in den Mittelpunkt der Betrachtung rückt, ist es verständlich, wie gerade die leichten Krankheitsformen, die formes frustes, die ,,Mikrofälle" als Organneurosen erscheinen; wie sich krankhaft veränderte, stabil gewordene Reaktionslagen erhalten, und doch nur durch die veränderte Reaktion selbst nachweisbar sind; wie derlei leichte organische Beeinträchtigungen zunächst nur in psychischen Erscheinungen als den oft feinsten Indicatoren sich ankündigen:

---

[1] Grundsätzlich ist es hier wie bei den hysterischen Reaktionen. ,,Die Verfeinerung des diagnostischen Rüstzeuges kann uns nur darüber belehren, daß wir zu Unrecht Fälle der Gruppe der Rentenneurose eingereiht haben, die tatsächlich zu der der organischen Unfallfolgen gehören. Die Unterscheidung dieser Gruppen selbst ist aber damit ebensowenig angetastet, wie umgekehrt irgend etwas gegen den Begriff der organischen Unfallfolge gesagt wäre, wenn wir ..... in anderer Richtung dazu gelangten, einige von den Kranken, die wir früher als organisch Geschädigte angesehen haben, jetzt als Simulanten zu entlarven" (E. STRAUSS).

in Ermüdung, Gedächtnisschwäche, Zerstreutheit, Erregung (v. BERGMANN); und wie schließlich die Grenze und Gegensätzlichkeit zwischen funktionellem Leiden und organischer Krankheit auch nach der Seite des Verlaufes fällt, indem „ein echter Circulus vitiosus von Funktionsstörung zu organischer Erkrankung und von organischer Erkrankung zu Funktionsstörung besteht" (SIEBECK).

Diese Organschäden aus gestörter Funktion haben in der Literatur der psychophysischen Beziehungen und der Organneurosen eine beträchtliche Rolle gespielt (v. BERGMANN, DURIG, ALKAN usw.). Ihre Tatsache ist weder grundsätzlich noch für viele Einzelfunde mehr zu bestreiten. Es kann dabei sozusagen geradlinig zu greifbaren anatomischen Veränderungen kommen, oder — was wohl häufiger ist — bereits bestehende morphologische Schäden, die jedoch klinisch noch latent waren, werden nun auch klinisch zu Organkrankheiten.

Aus den beiden folgenden Tabellen (die ich der Monographie von ALKAN entnehme) lassen sich diese Beziehungen im einzelnen erkennen.

Tabelle 2. 1. Magen-Darmkanal.

	Wirkung der exzitativen psychogenen Neurose			Wirkung der depressiven psychogenen Neurose		
	funktionell	anatomisch		funktionell	anatomisch	
		direkt	sekundär		direkt	sekundär
Auf den Oesophagus	Oesophago-Cardiospasmus	Idiopathische Dilatation	Ulcus pept. oesophag.			
Corpus ventriculi				Atonie und Ptosis ventriculi	Gastritis ex atonia	
Antrum ventriculi	Antrotomie		Ulcus paraphyloric.			
Duodenum			Ulcus duodeni			
Jejunum und Ileum						
Appendix	Appendicitis, Spasmus		Seltene Formen von Appendicitis			
Colon	Spastische Obstipation	Spastischer Ileus	Rezidiv, Colitis	Atonische Obstipation		
Rectum						
Anus	Sphincter-Spasmus		Chronische Fissura ani			

Es läßt sich so etwa eine Reihe aufstellen von gelegentlichen psychisch mit bedingten Kontrakturen glatter Muskulatur, zu Dauerkontraktionen mit Anämisierung, besonders an Hohlorganen; mit regressiven neurobiotischen Veränderungen (Ulcus ventriculi, Colitis ulcerosa), weiter über einen Spasmus zu muskulärer Hypertrophie der oberhalb gelegenen Partien (Hypertrophie des linken Ventrikels bei essentieller Hypertonie); außerdem führen Spasmen oder Lähmungen an röhrenförmigen Organen zu Flüssigkeitsstauungen und damit zu krankhaften Schädigungen durch Gärungsvorgänge oder Konzentrationsänderungen (Stauungsoesophagitis ALKAN).

Obgleich solche anatomischen Schäden nach funktionellen Störungen nicht selten beobachtet werden, so kann man doch auch nicht sagen, daß sie den

Organneurosen häufig oder gar als Regel folgten. Mir scheint ein solcher Ausgang viel eher dazu angetan, nachträglich die Diagnose einer entscheidend thymogenen und erlebnisbestimmten Betriebsstörung anzuzweifeln. Besonders *isolierte* Organstörungen sind verdächtig auf eine überwiegend *nicht* seelische Verursachung (H. CURSCHMANN), selbst dann, wenn ein seelischer Zusammenhang noch so eindeutig ist und der Symbolcharakter der Funktionsstörung gewissermaßen auf der Hand liegt. Die Anschauung vegetativer Symptome als Ausdrucksformen des Seelischen ist zwar eine immer *auch* mögliche Betrachtungsweise; aber eben nur eine, und nicht immer wird gerade sie den wirklichen, d. h. wirkenden Zusammenhängen gerecht. Es ist eine gefährliche Einseitigkeit und fast ein geistiger Hochmut, wenn man hier dem Körper nicht geben will, was des Körpers ist.

Man darf auch nicht übersehen, daß gelegentlich echte Organerkrankungen „in seelische Regie" (HEYER) genommen werden, ja im Grunde ist dieses Verhältnis nur eine Zuspitzung der neurotischen „Organdetermination" durch dispositionelle Organbereitschaft (Organminderwertigkeit). Bei der Unsicherheit einer Diagnostik nach dem Verfahren der „Ausschließung", ist die strenge Forderung einer wirklich positiv gesicherten seelischen Herleitung organneurotischer Reaktionen (KRONFELD u. a.) zu begrüßen. Sie ist ja die obenerwähnte ätiologische Methode. Daß sie allein *ohne* subtile somatische Untersuchung, ohne den Kontrollweg über somatische Phänomene und ihre Bewertung zu gesicherten Ergebnissen führt, ist nach dem heutigen Stand unseres Wissens nicht anzunehmen.

Tabelle 3. 2. Kreislaufsystem.

	Wirkung der exzitativen psychogenen Neurose		
	funktionell	anatomisch	
		direkt	sekundär
Auf das Herz	Extrasystolen; Tachykardie	Hypertrophie gegen periphere Widerstände	Dasselbe, Dilatation
Auf die Aorta		Juvenile Atheromatose	
Auf die Arterien			
Auf die Arteriolen	Essentielle Hypertonie	Arteriosklerose, Retinitis angiospastica, Apoplexie, rote Granulaniere	
Auf die Capillaren		Raynand	Erythromelalgie
Auf die Venen			

Im vorhergehenden Abschnitt wurde schon darauf hingewiesen, wie sehr Entstehung und Verlauf der Organneurosen von der individuellen Stellungnahme zu körperlichen Mißempfindungen und Funktionsstörungen abhängig sind. Man kann versuchen, von typischen psychopathischen Verhaltungsweisen her (hypomanisch, depressiv, sensitiv, geltungssüchtig usw.) zu entsprechenden Reaktions- und Verlaufstypen der Organneurotiker zu kommen, und neben körperbaulichen Zuordnungen auch Zuordnungen zu vegetativen Organisationen zu ermitteln. Ansätze dazu finden sich in den Arbeiten von KRETSCHMER, ENKE, W. JAENSCH, I. H. SCHULTZ, KRONFELD, V. WEIZSÄCKER, HANSEN u. a. Die teilweise Symptomengemeinschaft mit den einfach konstitutionell Nervösen, den nervös Erschöpften (neurasthenische Reaktion), den „Hypochondern" wurde wiederholt beschrieben (BUMKE, KAHN, BRAUN, I. H. SCHULTZ, STERTZ, JAHRREISS). Allen ist die vegetative Stigmatisation gemeinsam; die größere isolierte oder multiple Organbereitschaft (somatisches Entgegenkommen) und Betriebsstörung zeichnet den Organneurotiker aus; die Fähigkeit, mit seinen

Beschwerden fertig zu werden, den konstitutionell Nervösen; die Bereitschaft zu Krankheitseinbildungen mit oder ohne funktionelle oder anatomische Organstörung den Hypochonder. Das unterschiedliche Verhalten liegt also hier vorwiegend in charakterologischen Eigenschaften, zum Teil wohl auch in bestimmten Schlüsselerlebnissen und seelischen Konflikten, die freilich wieder abhängen von dauernden oder vorübergehenden Reaktionsbereitschaften der Persönlichkeit.

Organneurotische Verläufe sind nicht nur „vielschichtig" verursacht, sondern oft auch vielgestaltig. Es wurde schon erwähnt, daß dabei eine überwiegende Zuordnung entweder zum parasympathischen oder zum sympathischen Funktionskreis nicht die Regel ist; aber — wie mir scheint — auch nicht gerade die Ausnahme. So kann jemand wechselnd an spastischer Obstipation, an gelegentlichen Krampfzuständen im Bereich der Atmung und an Migräne leiden, oder fast ausschließlich an Migräne und nur gelegentlich im Anschluß daran an erschwerter Atmung, Bradykardie, dann Obstipation. H. CURSCHMANN spricht von einem „Schauplatzwechsel" der neurotischen Reaktionen und verweist auf gelegentliche „organneurotische Museen". Heftige akute und sehr vielfältige funktionelle Betriebsstörungen beschreibt LOEWY als vegetative Anfälle. Ich habe mich von der seelischen Auslösung solcher Anfälle, die nicht häufig sind, nie recht überzeugen können; dagegen fand ich bei allen eine hypochondrisch-überbesorgte Einstellung, die freilich bei der unmittelbar erlebten Angst nicht wundernehmen kann. Wenn man bedenkt, daß eine besondere Form schwerer vegetativer Beeinträchtigung, nämlich die echte endogene Depression (*vitale Depression* K. SCHNEIDER; Melancholie) mit einer Fülle von vitalen Mißempfindungen wie Herzangst, Herzdruck, Beklemmung, Obstipation, Appetitlosigkeit, Kopfdruck gleichzeitig einhergehen kann mit tiefster Niedergeschlagenheit, Verzweiflung, seelischer und motorischer Hemmung, schließlich mit unbegründeten Selbstvorwürfen und wahnhaften Ideen depressiven Inhaltes (Versündigung, Verarmung), dann ist theoretisch unschwer einzusehen, wie oft leichte, beginnende Melancholien als Herz-, Darm-, Magenneurose verkannt werden; besonders dann, wenn der körperliche Anteil der vitalen Depression im subjektiven Erleben sowohl wie im klinischen Bild überwiegt und die gedrückte, lustlose Stimmung, die seelische Hemmung erst sorgfältig erfragt werden müssen (DREYFUS, BUMKE, JOH. LANGE).

c) Behandlung.

Die Vorträge und Diskussionen auf dem Psychotherapeutenkongreß 1927 in Nauheim geben ein gutes Bild vom Stand der Behandlung organneurotischer Störungen sowohl, wie von der Stellungnahme einzelner Autoren zu ihr. Nach dem, was bisher über den Aufbau, den Verlauf und die Erkennung dieser seelisch in Gang gesetzten, bedingten, festgehaltenen, verschlimmerten Betriebsstörungen gesagt wurde, ist leicht abzuleiten, daß eine solche Behandlung als die wirksamste erscheinen muß, der nicht nur eine exakte Analyse der organischen Komponenten vorausgegangen ist (KATSCH, HANSEN, SCHINDLER, I. H. SCHULTZ, HOMBURGER u. a.), sondern die sich auch *sowohl* den körperlichen, *wie* den seelischen Bedingungen handelnd zuwendet.

Die folgende Tabelle bringt einen *schematischen Überblick der Behandlungswege*:

Als das besondere, ja fast erstaunliche Ergebnis bei Durchblick der Literatur erscheint mir viel weniger die Tatsache, daß es noch immer *Nur*-Psychotherapeuten und *Nur*-Somatiker strengster Observanz gibt, sondern daß man sich auf psychotherapeutischer Seite weitgehend den alten, bis in die letzte Zeit als Charlatanerie und peinliche Drastik verpönten Methoden der reinen oder teilweisen suggestiven und hypnotischen Behandlung zugewandt hat. Der Erfolg blieb nicht aus, und ich halte es nicht für notwendig, ihn dadurch zu schmälern, daß man seinen — wie man etwas verschämt meint — selbstverständlich! *nur* symptomatischen, vorübergehenden Charakter betont. Daß auch jede psychisch wesentlich mitbedingte funktionelle Organstörung im Gesamt einer individuellen Person nicht ohne „Bedeutung" sein kann, daß sie zuweilen selbst Symbolcharakter und Tendenzwert besitzen mag, ist nicht ernstlich zu bestreiten; aber es bestehen sehr erheblich verschiedene Akzentuierungen, je nachdem eine solche Organneurose mehr unmittelbar seelischen *Funktionen* des Affektes zugeordnet ist oder tatsächlich auf den geistigen Bereich der inneren Lebensgeschichte und ihrer Dauerkonflikte zurückgeht. Alle Psychotherapie, die wesentlich Erziehung ist, mag und muß sich zuweilen solcher tief verwurzelten Organneurosen annehmen.

Bei ihren Trägern ist die neurotische Fehlleistung nicht selten nur *eine* Reaktionsweise ihrer „psychopathischen" Persönlichkeit. Daß auch hier die charakterologischen und affektiven Anlagen alle Psychotherapie jedenfalls in ihrem Erfolg begrenzen — aber auch in der Methode der Wahl begrenzen sollten, halte ich für gewiß.

Es ist kennzeichnend, daß gerade für diejenigen Wege seelischer Behandlung die Erfolgsaussichten

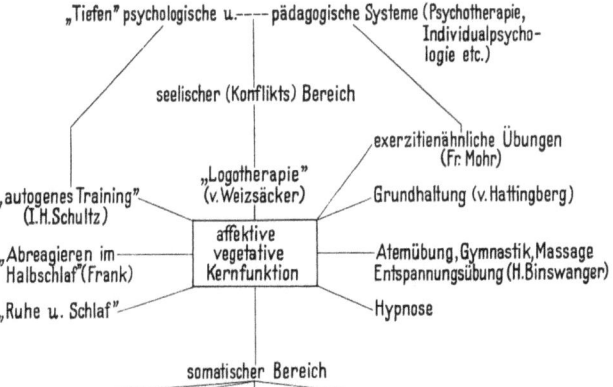

Tabelle 4. Behandlungswege.

günstig sind, die sich der „Entspannung" sowohl wie der aktiven „Bemeisterung" seelisch-körperlicher Vorgänge zuwenden. Das „autogene Training" von I. H. SCHULTZ ist hier an erster Stelle zu nennen. Die Patienten sollen — und können es nach I. H. SCHULTZ in ganz ungewöhnlichem Ausmaß — lernen, durch innere Konzentration sich zu entspannen. Sie lernen das durch systematisches rationelles Üben, auch gruppenweise. Körpermuskulatur, Herztätigkeit, Gefäßregulierung, Atmung, Vorgänge im Leib, im Kopf, werden ganz allmählich unter ärztlicher Kontrolle „erobert". Es geschieht dies in einem Zustand von Versenkung, oder doch jedenfalls von „Außenabkehr und Innenwendung". Der Schüler lernt es, diese Umschaltung in einem hypnosegleichen Zustand schließlich ohne jede Hilfe selbst herbeizuführen. Daß es sich dabei um ein so *rationelles* Vorgehen handelt, wie es I. H. SCHULTZ selbst anscheinend meint, und wie es v. HATTINGBERG bemängelt, möchte ich allerdings bezweifeln. So wie es im autogenen Training auf die seelische „Haltung" dem Körper gegenüber ankommt und damit also auf eine sehr erzieherische Beeinflussung, ja fast auf nichts weniger als auf die Gewinnung einer neuen Einstellung zu Ich und Umwelt, so hat v. HATTINGBERG *seine* psychotherapeutische Methode unter den Zentralbegriff der „Grundhaltung" gebracht. Die Methode geht durchaus vom Körperlichen aus, hat — wie das autogene Training — Beziehungen zum Yogha — und wurde angeregt durch die Erfahrung des „Atemkorsetts" (s. o.!) am „eigenen Leibe". Atemübungen, Gymnastik, Massage sind förderliche Teilübungen. „Grundhaltung ist eine natürliche und zugleich persönliche, seelisch-leibliche Einheit." Es fällt v. HATTINGBERG nicht leicht, zu sagen, was er damit meint: „Wie Geist Halt in der

Freiheit ist, so ist das Seelische wesentlich Haltung. Es ist freilich Unendliches darüber hinaus, in einem schöpferischen Urgrund und ewiges Werden, Liebe. Hier aber können Namen grundsätzlich nicht mehr sein als völlig leerer Schall. Was sich begrifflich fassen läßt, ist allein Haltung." Es ist, soweit ich es verstehe, „autogenes Training", nur mit einer größeren Betonung von persönlichkeitsgemäßer Selbstentfaltung und religiöser Bindung.

„Einfacher" sind die Methoden, in denen das Suggestive überwiegt, oder jedenfalls unmittelbarer in Erscheinung tritt: so das Abreagieren im Halbschlaf von FRANK. HANSEN weist mit Recht darauf hin, daß durch diese immer wiederholte Produktion neurotischer Symptome in einem psychischen Ausnahmezustand die beständig wirkenden Signalmerkmale, ähnlich wie in den PAWLOWschen Versuchen, ihrer Wirksamkeit beraubt werden, da die gleichzeitige Reizung durch *wesentliche* Merkmale der *Objekte* unterbunden ist. Über die einfachen Entspannungsübungen, Hypnose, braucht hier nichts weiter gesagt zu werden. Selbst Ruhe und Schlaf können, richtig eingeschaltet, Förderliches leisten, besonders bei den Neurosen des Kreislaufsystems (DURIG, ALKAN usw.). Es gibt u. a. Migräniker — selbst epileptisch Kranke, die ja beide ein pathogenetisches Teilstück für den Anfall gemeinsam haben — deren Attacken sich bei Entziehung des üblichen, und wie sich damit erweist, notwendigen Mittagsschlafes häufen.

Die Signalmerkmale verlieren ihre Wirksamkeit auch dann, wenn „der Symptombindung ihr organischer Angriffspunkt durch *Organtherapie* entzogen wird" (HANSEN). Im einzelnen kann hier nur auf die diätetischen, antiallergischen, pharmakologischen, aber auch klimatischen, balneologischen Möglichkeiten verwiesen werden. Wichtig scheinen mir noch zwei Hinweise zu sein. Einmal darauf, daß man die nicht organisch geschädigten Organe dadurch nicht funktionsbereiter und funktionstüchtiger macht, daß man sie „schont", zum anderen darauf, daß es gelegentlich „scheinbar" neurotische und zugleich scheinbar lebensbedrohliche Funktionsstörungen geben kann, denen aber eine lebensrettende Funktion innewohnt, die keine psychologische Analyse und keine Abstellung zulassen [1].

---

[1] ACHELIS, J. D.: Der ärztliche Begriff des Organismus S. 58 f. ... „Nehmen wir an, daß ein Herzkranker, der bei Bettruhe leidlich kompensiert ist, vor stärkere Anforderungen gestellt wird. Er leiste Muskelarbeit, die stärkere Durchblutung verlangt. Genau wie bei vielen Gesunden steigt die Herzfrequenz; es ist aber sehr bald der Punkt erreicht, wo die Frequenzsteigerung nicht mehr zur Vermehrung des Minutenvolumens, sondern zu seiner Verminderung führt. Die Blutversorgung der Peripherie wird durch die sinsetzende Regulation verschlechtert. Ähnlich liegt es bei der Atmung. Auch die Lungendurchlüftung wird schlechter, wenn eine gewisse Frequenz überschritten wird. Das Ergebnis der Regulation ist, da hier das Herz vor der Muskulatur funktionell versagt, zunächst eine Gehirnanämie, dann ein Kollaps — das Endergebnis meist eine Schädigung des Herzmuskels für längere Zeit. Ein solcher Kranker wäre sehr viel besser daran, wenn er nicht regulierte. Freilich wären auch dann seine Muskeln während der Arbeit nicht hinreichend durchblutet. Sie würden sich verhalten wie Muskeln, denen die Blutzufuhr abgeschnitten ist, sie würden in kürzester Zeit ermüden, und die gefährliche Anstrengung, die den Herzen schadet, würde einfach nicht ausgeführt werden können. Eine sehr wohltätige Ruhe würde sich von selbst einstellen. Das Gegenteil ist der Fall: die sympathische Erregung, die zur Erhöhung der Herzfrequenz führt, scheint sich dem ganzen Organismus mitzuteilen. Der Sympathicus ruft wohl meist Gesamterregungen hervor, und seine Wirkungen auf einzelne Organe sind häufig Laboratoriumsprodukte. Jedenfalls ist es eine unangenehme, oft wohl sogar schädliche Nebenerscheinung der erhöhten Herzfrequenz, daß der Kranke erregt und nervös ist. Er benimmt sich mit etwas unheimlicher Genauigkeit konträr zu dem, was man zur Heilung wünscht. Er soll ruhig liegen und ist zappelig, er soll sich nicht aufregen und gerät über jede Kleinigkeit in Wut, er soll schlafen und wälzt sich schlaflos im Bett. Sind diese Symptome erst einmal überwunden, ist der erste Schritt zur Heilung gemacht. Das Gesamtverhalten ist so verändert, daß es zu jenem verhängnisvollen Kollaps hindrängt, wenn nicht ein Arzt oder ein energischer eigener Wille eingreift. Meines Erachtens darf man diesen

2. Besonderer Teil.

Eine ausführliche klinische Darstellung, insbesondere eine eingehende spezielle Pathologie organneurotischer Betriebsstörungen, kann hier nicht gegeben werden. Das Gebiet erstreckt sich auf eine Reihe von Organsystemen, deren zureichende Kenntnis nicht nur internistische Vorbildung, sondern noch dermatologisches, gynäkologisches, urologisches .Fachwissen voraussetzt. Dem Psychiater und Neurologen ist es vor allem darum zu tun — und damit wird er sich auch in der Regel begnügen müssen, — grundsätzlich zum Aufbau der Organneurosen Stellung zu nehmen und dabei, sowie bei der Frage der Behandlung, besonders dem seelischen Anteil in der Kette der Bedingungen nachzugehen. Praktisch ist er auf die Mitarbeit der betreffenden Fachärzte angewiesen und diese auf seine Unterstützung. Für die Physiologie, insbesondere auch die Innervationsverhältnisse der einzelnen Organe- und Organsysteme muß ich auf die Darstellung der Anatomie und Physiologie des vegetativen Nervensystems verweisen.

a) Kreislaufsystem.

Herz und Gefäße sind den seelischen Erlebnissen, vor allem dem affektiven Geschehen besonders innig verbunden. Erröten und Erblassen, sowie Störungen im Rhythmus, der ,,Eurythmie" des Herzens sind objektive Zeichen, die jeder kennt; und die Empfindungen und Mißempfindungen bis zur qualvollen und gegenstandslosen *Angst*, die in der Herzgegend gefühlt werden, sind im eigenen Erleben vom Schmerz der Trennung, der ängstlichen Besorgtheit, dem Druck des Kummers oft schwer zu trennen.

Die *Angst* steht als subjektive Klage und faßbarer Ausdruck im Mittelpunkt vieler neurotischer Störungen, ja man hat sie gelegentlich überhaupt zu ihrem ,,Kernproblem" machen wollen (WEXBERG). Jedenfalls ist sie — in einigermaßen ausgeprägter Form — so sehr körperlich *und* psychisch und so innig in einem Wirkungskreis zusammengefügt, daß es nicht zu verwundern ist, wenn man mit guten Gründen für ihre Psycho- wie für ihre Somatogenese, oder auch für eine Sowohl- als — auch — Entstehungsweise plädiert hat. Die Angst als seelischer Ausdruck einer Libidostauung (nach sexueller Abstinenz, Coitus interruptus usw.) ist bekannt. Man hat sie aber auch pathophysiologisch als Folge von Hormonretention oder unabgebauten Stoffwechselprodukten infolge sexueller Abstinenz zu erklären versucht (REICH), infolge einer toxischen Wirkung auf den Vagus. Jedenfalls ist Angst ein seelisches Erlebnis und insoweit trifft SCHILDERS Auffassung zu, daß Angst erst dann Angst sei, wenn das Subjekt die eigentümlich gefärbten Unlustempfindungen infolge vegetativer Erregungen nicht bewältigen kann. L. BRAUN möchte die Angstempfindung überhaupt nur im Herzen entstehen lassen; die Schilderung der Kranken mit Anfällen von Angina pectoris legen diese Vermutung nahe. Auch scheint mir die gegenstandslose, oft jagende Angst mancher Psychotischen ohne greifbare Herzstörung und ohne die klinischen Erscheinungen einer Angina pectoris nicht dagegen zu sprechen, selbst wenn hier in anderer Weise von Zentralstätten des vegetativen Nervensystems her das Herz in Erregung versetzt würde. Bei der *Behandlung* von *Angstattacken* darf man nicht übersehen, daß es nicht nur seelische, sondern auch pharmakologische Mittel gibt. W. MISCH und MISCH-FRANKL empfehlen

---

Zustand nicht psychologisch auflösen, so sehr auch gewisse Ähnlichkeiten mit der Neurose auffallen. Würde es nämlich gelingen, diese Erregtheit, diesen ,,neurotischen" Zustand, ganz zu beseitigen — und dazu gehörte auch die ,,Beruhigung" des Herzens —, würde der Tod in akuter Kreislaufinsuffizienz eintreten. Denn abgesehen davon, daß er für die Heilung nicht günstig ist, ist dieser Zustand der einzige, in dem der Kranke noch existieren kann.

Acetylcholin (0,1 intramuskulär) oder Paeyl (4—6 Tabletten), da der Cholineffekt dem sympathicotonen Angsteffekt genau entgegengesetzt sei. Sie sahen schlagartige Beseitigung der Angst.

Unter den noch heute im ärztlichen Sprachgebrauch summarisch und unverbindlich sog. ,,Herzneurosen" spielen die *Rhythmusstörungen* eine beachtliche Rolle. Gerade die ,,Unregelmäßigkeiten des Herzschlages" aber haben seit WENCKEBACHs Untersuchungen (1914) dazu geführt, den verschwommenen Begriff der Herzneurose abzubauen. Für das Gebiet der Rhythmusstörungen ist er nach FR. KRAUS und NICOLAI als erledigt anzusehen. v. BERGMANN betont, daß sein Begriff der *Betriebsstörung* — wie er bisher auch hier wiederholt verwandt wurde — die Frage aufhebe, wieweit den Extrasystolen, dem Herzblock grob anatomische Veränderungen (Entzündung, Schwiele, Infarkt) zugrunde lägen oder nur unsichtbare biologische kolloidale Strukturänderungen, oder wieweit sich diese verbänden mit intramuralen und extrakardialen Störungen der Nervenfunktion, und wieweit außerdem neben anderen zentralen Einflüssen affektiv gesetzte Funktionsänderungen hineinspielten. ,,Das gleiche Phänomen am Herzen, etwa die Extrasystolie kann psychogene wie organische Grundlage haben; bei beiden ist im Betrieb Störung." Bei Affekten kann es selbst zu einer absoluten Arrhythmie kommen (KREHL, HANSEN). Es sei hier noch einmal auf die entscheidende Tatsache hingewiesen, daß es eine bestimmte Resistenzfestigkeit von Organen gegenüber seelischer Beeinflussung gibt, daß aber zum Bereich organneurotischer Reaktionen beispielsweise auch eine solche absolute Arrhythmie infolge seelischer Einflüsse auf ein *organisch schon geschädigtes* Herz gehört. Ein gelegentlich erwähntes Verhalten derart, daß primär psychisch bedingte Extrasystolen bei gesundem Herzmuskel als ruckartiges Gefühl in der Herzgegend empfunden wurden, während die auf Myokardschäden beruhenden Extrasystolen nicht zu Bewußtsein kamen, scheint kein ausreichendes differentialdiagnostisches Kriterium zu sein. Am Zustandekommen einer unregelmäßigen Herztätigkeit können beteiligt sein: intramurale Plexus- und Ganglienzellen, extrakardiale Hemmungs- und Erregungsnerven (Vagus, Accelerans), feinste physikalische, chemische Änderungen im Sinusknoten, im HISschen Muskelbündel, im ASCHOFF-TAVARA-Knoten, in der Herzmuskelfaser. Affektive Einflüsse (keineswegs nur solche sexueller Herkunft), vegetative Einwirkungen (neurolaner, hormonaler, ionaler Art)[1], Zustand des Herzens als des Erfolgsorgans sind auch hier vielschichtig zusammengefügt und häufig genug — wie es scheint — nur ungenau zu scheiden. Ob etwa die *respiratorische Arrhythmie* vom zentralen Tonus oder vom Erfolgsorgan abhängt, läßt sich am lebenden Menschen kaum ermitteln (v. BERGMANN). Zur ,,thyreotischen Konstitution" (Mikrobasedow) gehört wie zum Basedow die Tachykardiebereitschaft, die unter dem Einfluß von Affekt, Muskelarbeit, Adrenalin gleicherweise manifest werden kann (s. auch BANSI). Die Herabsetzung der Reizbarkeit durch Chinin, Chinidin ist bekannt; ebenso die Digitalis-,,Nebenwirkung" der Extrasystolen, des Herzblockes.

HERZ hat ein Zustandsbild beschrieben, das den Herzneurosen zugezählt zu werden pflegt und das er ,,Phrenokardie" genannt hat: Atemsperre, Herzklopfen, Herzstiche. Die Pathogenese ist, soweit ich sehe, noch nicht geklärt. Die seelische Verursachung aus erotischen Konflikten mag zuweilen einleuchtend erscheinen. Möglicherweise aber handelt es sich dabei um eine ähnlich mechanische Irritation der Nervi vagi, wie sie v. BERGMANN als epiphrenale Neurose bei der Oesophagushernie beschrieben hat.

---

[1] Auf die Ähnlichkeit zwischen Calcium- und Sympathicus-, Kalium- und Vaguswirkung hat S. G. ZONDEK hingewiesen.

Funktionsstörungen der Arteriolen. Die Gefäßstörungen haben nicht nur für den Internisten, sondern auch für den Nervenarzt zunehmend an Interesse gewonnen. Ich erinnere an Arbeiten von OTFRIED FOERSTER, von SPIELMEYER und seiner Schule, von K. NEUBÜRGER, ED. KRAPF. Besonders die Beziehungen der Hypertonie zu allgemeiner Gefäßlabilität, zu bestimmten Körperbauformen, zu seelischen Eigentümlichkeiten und klinischen Erscheinungen von häufig anfallsartigem Charakter (KRAPF) — Migräne, Epilepsie, angioneurotische Attacken — sind hier zu nennen. Die feinere Diagnostik des Blutdruckverhaltens durch das sympathicomimetische (?) Adrenalin (Adrenalin-Blutdruckkurven; DRESEL); die fortlaufenden Messungen (Blutdruckkurven!) nach FAHRENKAMP, die mikroskopische Beobachtung der Unruhe im Capillarsystem, die Schlafdruckmessungen mit dem Normergebnis einer Senkung (KATSCH), die Registrierung feinster Ausschläge unter seelischem Einfluß beim Lesen, Schreiben usw. durch FR. LANGE und die damit gesicherte Erkenntnis, daß der Blutdruck auch normalerweise Ausdruck des wechselnden Gefäßtonus ist, haben den Hypertonus immer mehr als *funktionelles* Verhalten erkennen lassen. Allen Hypertonien ist ein bestimmtes Funktionsverhalten gemeinsam (DURIG, V. BERGMANN; OTFRIED MÜLLER usw.). Durch tonische Verengerung des Gesamtquerschnitts der terminalen Strombahn, der Arteriolen, wird infolge des erhöhten Widerstandes auch der Blutdruck dynamisch-mechanisch erhöht. Den normalen Blutdruck regelt eine Vielzahl von Kräften: Vasoconstrictoren und Dilatatoren halten sich das Gleichgewicht; durch Depressor und Splanchnicus wird dafür gesorgt, daß abnorm hohe Drucke nicht auftreten können. Durch funktionelle Wirkung kann ein Hochdruck nur zustande kommen, wenn die Regulation gegen Druckerhöhung geschädigt ist, oder wenn die druckerhöhenden Reize die druckherabsetzenden Regulationen in ihrer Wirksamkeit überbieten (DURIG). Eine solche Regulationsstörung kann einsetzen „zentrogen, hämatogen, reflektorisch" (DURIG), denn für den Zustand der Arteriolen ist die Einstellung der Zentren, die von der Peripherie beeinflußt werden können und die ihrerseits wieder die Peripherie beeinflussen, von gleicher Bedeutung, wie das hormonale Verhalten, das ionale Milieu, die Serumstruktur (v. BERGMANN). Die Einstellung eines variablen Ruhetonus geschieht (wohl überwiegend) zentral, aber auch peripher (DURIG). K. DRESEL hat, unter der Annahme, daß es eine Selbstregulierung des Blutdruckes gebe nach Art der Temperatur- und Blutzuckereinstellung, ein subthalamisches Blutdruckzentrum (KARPLUS und KREIDL) und eine „striäre Hypertonie" angenommen. Auf eine Störung der zentralen Blutdruckregulation wird auch die Blutdrucksteigerung bei Schrumpfnierenerkrankung zurückgeführt, so gut wie bei essentieller Hypertonie (LESCHKE). Reizung des Vasoconstrictorenzentrums (etwa durch Kohlensäure, die im Experiment zur Hypertension führt: GOLLWITZER-MEIER 1929, zit. bei v. BERGMANN), abnorme Erhöhung seiner Erregbarkeit oder derjenigen der Umschalteganglienzelle, der Gefäßganglien oder der Synapsien an den Gefäßen, schließlich auch Erregbarkeitssteigerungen an den Erfolgorganen selbst, den Gefäßmuskeln können eine Hypertension mit verursachen (DURIG). Auch das Verhalten der Depressorfunktion in der Aorta ist wichtig, deren Zerstörung zu einem Dauerhochdruck führt (HERING). Reflektorisch kann eine Enge der harnabführenden Wege eine Hypertension zur Folge haben. „Der Dauerkatheter bei einem Prostatiker läßt alle diese Funktionsstörungen oft noch restlos zurückgehen" (v. BERGMANN). Aber auch innersekretorische Vorgänge (Pubertät, Involution) können einen blutdrucksteigernden Einfluß ausüben; nach septischen Infektionen bei schwerer Commotio cerebri sah man gelegentlich einen dauernden Hochdruck verschwinden. Man darf in diesem Zusammenhang daran erinnern, daß vereinzelt bei genuin epileptischen Kranken die Anfälle nach einem Schädeltrauma ausbleiben können. Nach neueren Untersuchungen von ED. KRAPF liegt es nicht so fern, zwischen beiden Ereignissen sogar engere Beziehungen zu vermuten, da eine abnorme Labilität der Blutdruckregulierung, vor allem die Hypertension am pathogenetischen Aufbau des epileptischen Anfalles häufiger als bisher angenommen wurde, beteiligt zu sein scheint.

Für die organneurotischen Störungen der Blutdruckregulierung sind nach den bisherigen fragmentarisch dargestellten Ergebnissen von besonderer Bedeutung die Frage der seelischen Wirkungsbreite auf das Gefäßsystem und die Frage nach den Grundlagen der essentiellen Hypertonie. Über den Einfluß seelischer Vorgänge auf den Blutdruck wurde schon im ersten Teil einiges erwähnt. Klinisch bedeutsam ist hier wie bei allen organneurotischen Störungen der Umstand, daß sich ein seelischer Einfluß auch da nicht ohne weiteres ausschließen läßt, wo nachweislich ein organischer Schaden vorliegt; und daß andererseits keine funktionelle Hypertonie *allein* durch seelische Einwirkungen besteht. Auch der gesunde Gefäßapparat ist Ausdruck für feinste seelische Regungen; aber niemals läßt er Reaktionen beobachten von solchem Ausmaß, wie sie durch Emotionen beim krankhaft erhöhten oder abnorm labilen Blutdruckverhalten üblich sind. An der Aufrechterhaltung oder Entstehung der Hypertension sind Änderungen im Stoffwechsel mitbeteiligt (VOLLHARD, FAHRENKAMP u. a.), wie sie auch unter Gemütsbewegungen beobachtet werden (FAHRENKAMP). Es wurde oben der Adrenalintest von DRESEL erwähnt; unter emotiven Vorgängen kommt es — möglicherweise auch zentral gesteuert — zu einer Ausschüttung von Adrenalin, das dann peripher angreift und zu Blutdrucksteigerungen führt. Wichtig sind Untersuchungen von FR. LANGE und von K. FELIX über eine blutdrucksenkende Substanz — durch Erweiterung der Arteriolen —, die sich vom Kallikrein wie von anderen, ähnlich auf den Depressor wirkenden Substanzen (Acetylcholin, Histamin) unterscheidet. Es handelt sich dabei um ein Guanidinderivat. Auffällig ist dessen häufiges Vorkommen sowohl bei essentieller Hypertonie (vermindert im Blut, vermehrte Ausscheidung im Harn) wie bei nephrogener (vermehrt im Blut, vermindert im Harn), während LANGE bei einer Gruppe alter Menschen mit erhöhtem Blutdruck die Verhältnisse ganz wie bei Blutdruckgesunden fand. Es wäre möglich, daß es sich bei den essentiellen Hypertonieformen um eine konstitutionelle Eigentümlichkeit handelt. Die Erblichkeit — man hat an einen dominanten Erbgang gedacht (FR. KAUFMANN) — scheint heute gesichert zu sein. Die familiären Anfälligkeiten auf dem Gebiet der Gefäßlabilität (Hypertonie, Apoplexie, Angina pectoris vasomotorica, Migräne, Gefäßstörungen an den Extremitäten usw.) drängen sich immer wieder auf. Daneben bestehen im Rahmen des konstitutionellen Hochdrucks häufig (R. SCHMIDT) Hyperglykämie, Glykosurie, Gicht, Diabetes, Adipositas, Polycythämie, pyknischer Habitus oder wenigstens deutlich pyknische „Einschläge". Die *Hypotonie* mit ihren Beziehungen zum leptosomen Typus, zu Tuberkulose, Carcinom, perniziöser Anämie usw. ist gewissermaßen der konstitutionell gegebene Gegenpol (F. W. STEIN, KLOTZ, WULFFTEN-PALTHE u. a.). Auch DRESEL hat die These einer striären Hypertonie verfochten und zum Teil mit der konstitutionellen Bedingtheit der Hypertonie, ihren Zusammenhängen mit dem Diabetes und zugleich mit der Wichtigkeit seelisch-emotioneller Einflüsse auf den Hochdruck begründet.

Es gibt eine latente Bereitschaft zum arteriellen Hypertonus, sie ist häufig ohne greifbare Symptome. Fortlaufende Blutdruckkurven (FAHRENKAMP), Funktionsprüfungen mit dem Nachströmungsversuch (FR. LANGE) können sie dennoch frühzeitig erhärten. Aber auch unter Einflüssen, die bei normalem

Ruhetonus der Gefäße mühelos ausgeglichen werden, wird eine solche latente Hypertonie offenkundig: durch ein heißes Bad, bei schwülem Wetter, durch Blutdruckerhöhung statt Senkung bei Hyperventilation usw. (v. BERGMANN). Auch die Gemütserregung ist ein solcher Test. LESCHKE fand im Kriege bei Frontkämpfern Blutdruckwerte von 180 mmHg für lange Zeit und er meint, daß bei *disponierten* Individuen eine derartige Blutdrucksteigerung auch weiterhin bestehen und zum Krankheitsbilde der genuinen Hypertonie führen kann. Aber sie kann eben auch für mehr oder minder lange Zeit wieder völlig zur Norm zurückkehren, wenn es gelingt, in geeigneter Weise den Patienten seelisch zu entspannen und abreagieren zu lassen. Dabei hilft schon viel, daß man ihn nicht unnütz anspannt; die iatrogene Schädigung spielt gerade bei den Hypertonikern ein bekannte Rolle (BUMKE). Man darf nicht vergessen, daß jede ärztliche Bemerkung, die ängstliche Vorstellungen weckt, sehr leicht zu einem neurotischen „Signalmerkmal" werden kann. Dem ersten heftigen Stoß auf den abnorm labilen Gefäßtonus, gleichviel ob er psychisch oder unmittelbar vegetativ ausgelöst wurde, kommt möglicherweise ein „sensibilisierender" Einfluß zu, der nie wieder ganz auszugleichen ist.

Es kann nicht wundernehmen, daß in der Therapie der Hypertonus-„Neurosen" die seelischen Entspannungsmethoden an der Spitze stehen. Sie wurden oben skizziert. Schon gut dosierte Ruhepausen schaffen Nützliches. Ohne diätetische und sonstige Lebensregelung, ohne medikamentöse Behandlung (mit Luminaletten, Luminal, Prominal, Doryl usw.) wird man auf die Dauer nicht auskommen. Es sei unter den vielen Beispielen in der Literatur wenigstens der Patient von OTFRIED MÜLLER erwähnt, dessen Blutdruck von 280 mm Hg allen somatischen Behandlungsversuchen trotzte, aber nach einer Aussprache über Verfehlungen in der Ehe auf 150 abfiel und noch nach Jahren 130 betrug. Die Herzhypertrophie war nicht ganz zurückgegangen. Immer ist zu bedenken, daß nicht nur seelischer Druck den Blutdruck steigert, sondern, daß auch der Blutdruckkranke psychisch in erhöhtem Maß labil ist (ED. KRAPF u. a.). Diese Labilität der gemütlichen Äußerungen, die gelegentliche Unfähigkeit, sie normal zu bremsen, läßt häufig schon nach der Schilderung eine Hypertension als Ursache vermuten.

Klinisch und pathologisch-anatomisch ist die Lehre genügend erhärtet, daß ein rein funktioneller Hochdruck Jahre hindurch bestehen kann, ohne zu organischen Schäden zu führen. In der Regel bleiben sie jedoch nicht aus. Der Blutdruck sinkt nicht mehr zur Norm zurück, Arteriosklerose und Herzhypertrophie werden nachweisbar. Die häufigste Ursache der kardiovaskulären Dekompensation ist die chronische Blutdruckerhöhung (v. BERGMANN).

Angina pectoris vasomotorica. Die Diagnose der Angina pectoris ist leicht, wenn sie mit typischen Anfällen einhergeht, sie ist im allgemeinen schwierig, sowie es um die Abgrenzung gegenüber „psychogenen", organneurotischen Störungen kommt, die sehr ähnliche Beschwerden aufweisen. „Noch heute gehen sicher eine Fülle von Menschen unter der Diagnose ‚Herzneurose', bei denen erst später, manchmal erst nach Jahrzehnten die Inkongruenz zwischen Sauerstoffnachfrage und -angebot des Herzens durch das Auftreten von Schmerzphänomenen deutlich wird" (v. BERGMANN).

Es wurde oben schon auf den von HERZ sog. Symptomenkomplex der „Phrenokardie" hingewiesen, und auf die unzureichende ursächliche Herleitung aus sexuellen Konflikten; ein Teil dieser Fälle gehört sicher in das Gebiet der Angina pectoris, ein anderer, wie mir scheint, zu dem Komplex der Oesophagushernie (v. BERGMANN, s. oben).

Unmittelbare Ursache der Anfälle sind Gefäßkrämpfe mit Blutdruckerhöhung, und zwar bei der Angina pectoris mit organischer Grundlage, der die *Angina pectoris vasomotorica* als eine besondere Form *ohne* anatomische Schädigung des Herzens oder seiner Kranzarterien gegenübergestellt wird.

Die konstitutionellen Beziehungen zur essentiellen Hypertonie wurden schon erwähnt. Wir für diese gilt auch die Wirksamkeit seelischer Erregungen und der therapeutische Einfluß der Entspannung. Bis zu einem gewissen Grad kann bei beiden vegetativen Betriebsstörungen vom Arzt eine seelische Prophylaxe ausgeübt werden. Daß daneben eine somatische Allgemeinbehandlung und eine medikamentöse Behandlung der Anfälle notwendig ist, braucht hier nicht mehr betont zu werden. Aber — es gibt durchaus Fälle von vasomotorischer Angina pectoris, denen gegenüber jede Organtherapie versagt, während die Psychotherapie Wunder wirkt. Von der Nützlichkeit oder der Zulänglichkeit einer symbolischen Deutung der Anfälle, deren Ausdrucksgewalt nicht zu übersehen ist, habe ich mich noch nicht recht überzeugen können.

Eine Diagnosetabelle, die einer Arbeit von EDENS[1] entnommen ist, läßt synoptisch die Schwierigkeiten der Beurteilung erkennen und zugleich ersehen, daß ohne erfahrene internistische Beratung dem Psychiater und Neurologen von jeder Behandlung eines Angina pectoris-Syndroms abzuraten ist. Als das sicherste differentialdiagnostische Kriterium bezeichnet EDENS: die Zeichen von Herzschwäche, sowie deren Besserung und die Besserung der Angina pectoris durch Strophantin - Enphyllin. Die günstige Wirkung des Strophantins spricht für Angina pectoris auf organischer Grundlage, gegen Angina pectoris vasomotorica. Da aber funktionelle und organische Störung ein Stück Ausdrucksgemeinschaft besitzen (v. WEIZSÄCKER), so spielen Gefäßkrämpfe bei der organischen Form eine Rolle, und die Gefäßspasmen der vasomotorischen Form können organische Veränderungen schaffen.

b) Funktionelle Störungen der Atmung.

Atemstörungen sind häufig, ihre Verursachung und Entstehungswege so „komplex" (MATTHES), daß selbst beim Asthma bronchiale die Synopsis und Synthese der Forschungsergebnisse im allgemeinen und die spezielle Analyse des Einzelfalles mehr eine Erkenntnis vorzutäuschen als wirklich zuzulassen scheinen. Im Anschluß an die sog. Kreislaufneurosen seien zunächst die primär cardial bedingten dyspnoischen Beschwerden kurz erwähnt. Durch Versagen des linken Herzens kommt es zur Stauung im kleinen Kreislauf; die Lunge wird „starrer", das Atmen mühsam und erschwert, die Ventilation der Alveolen schlechter, die Arterialisation des Blutes ungenügend; die erhöhte Kohlensäurespannung erregt das Atemzentrum, erzwingt eine forcierte Atmung, bedingt den großen Lufthunger, der nicht gestillt werden kann. So kommt es zur großen Atemnot des Asthma cardiale (SIEBECK). In den Entstehungskreis können auch — anfallsauslösend oder verlängernd — psychische Momente eingeschaltet sein, aber man muß sich hüten, die wesentlich organische Grundlage auch in ihren Anfängen zu übersehen und ins psychologisch Deutbare umzusetzen. Ich darf hier auf eine Bemerkung von KRONFELD verweisen, daß es breite Zonen gäbe, wo von einer ausdrucksmäßigen Bedeutung der Organstörungen keine Rede sein könne.

Die nervöse Hyperpnoe, die Tachypnoe und „Schauspieleratmung" (VORKASTNER) ist neuerdings als neurotische Atmungstetanie geschildert worden (ADLERSBERG und PORGES), in dem eine Wirkungsreihe vom Affekt über Hyperventilation, Alkalose — Verringerung der Ionisierung des Blutcalciums — Steigerung der tetanoiden Symptome angenommen wird. Man sieht sie nicht

---

[1] EDENS, ERNST: Über Angina pectoris vasomotorica. Münch. med. Wschr. **1932 II**, 1874 f.

Tabelle 5 nach E. EDENS.

Nr.		Angina pectoris vasomot.	Angina pectoris	Herzinfarkt
1	Vorkommen Anfall	Meist Frauen	Meist Männer	Meist Männer
2	Anfall	Teilerscheinung einer allgemeinen spastischen Vasoneurose	Auch ohne Zeichen einer allgemeinen Vasoneurose	Unabhängig vom Zustand des Gefäßnervensystems zur Zeit des Anfalles
3	Beginn des Anfalles	Mit peripherischen Gefäßstörungen	Mit Herzbeschwerden	Mit Herzbeschwerden
4	Auflösung des Anfalles	Kälte, Ermüdung, oft von Entzündungsherden	Anstrengung, Kälte, Erregung, Blähung	Oft in der Ruhe oder im Schlaf
5	Im Intervall	Meist vasomotorische Beschwerden	Ohne Beschwerden	Mit längere Zeit anginöse Beschwerden nach dem Anfall
6	Dauer des Anfalles	Minuten, Stunden	Minuten	Stunden, Tage
7	Haltung im Anfall	Unruhig, oft Erleichterung durch Bewegung	Vermeidung jeder Bewegung	Unruhig, zuweilen Umhergehen
8	Schmerz	Meist geringer als Beklemmung	Oft in der Mitte des Brustbeins	Oft im unteren Teil des Brustbeins, durch Nitrite und Xanthinpräparate nicht beeinflußt
9	Shockerscheinung	Fehlen	Fehlen	Vorhanden
10	Puls	Labil	Unverändert	Klein und oft auch beschleunigt
11	Blutdruck	Labil	Unverändert oder erhöht	Oft erniedrigt
12	Herztöne	Unverändert	Unverändert	Leise, zuweilen Galopprhythmus, perikardiales Reiben
13	Erbrechen	Fehlt	Fehlt	Oft
14	Dyspnoe	Fehlt	Fehlt	Oft vorhanden
15	Stauungserscheinung	Fehlen	(Fehlen)	Häufige Folge des Anfalles
16	Temperatur	Normal	Normal	Erhöht
17	Leukocytose	Fehlt	Fehlt	Vorhanden
18	Elektrokardiogramm	Normal	Oft verändert	Gewöhnlich charakteristisch verändert

selten in Verbindung mit ängstlich gefärbter psychotischer Erregung aber auch als hysterische Ausdruckssteigerung mit oder ohne Anfall. Atembehinderungen durch *Rhinitis nervosa* (KUTTNER) habe ich gelegentlich als *familiäre* Eigentümlichkeit beobachtet; psychische Auslösung ist dabei so wenig obligatorisch wie psychische „Symptomverarbeitung". Funktionsstörungen, Mißempfindungen müssen eine subjektive Bedeutung erlangen, ehe sie in seelische Regie genommen werden können.

Das *Asthma bronchiale* ist ein Paradigma für unser Wissen und Nichtwissen im Bereich der Organneurosen. Seine Pathogenese ist in den letzten Jahren emsig und von verschiedenen Einfallspforten her bearbeitet worden (STORM VAN LEUWEN; KÄMMERER, VEIL, HANSEN, I. H. SCHULTZ, KRONFELD, ESKUCHEN, KLEWITZ, POLLNOW, PETOW und WITTKOWER u. a.). Willkürlich kann der Atem nur eine kurze Spanne angehalten werden, dann greift der schützende Reflex ein, der über den Vagus zur Kontraktion der Bronchialmuskulatur führt. Im Tierversuch führt Vagusreizung zum Bronchialmuskelkrampf und vermehrter Schleimabsonderung. Infolge dieser Kontraktion erweitern sich sogar die muskelfreien Alveolen und das Zwerchfell tritt tiefer (THEOD. BEER, zit. nach LESCHKE). Zentrale, periphere oder reflektorische Vagusreizung mit Spasmen der Bronchialmuskeln als Ursache des Asthmas hat BIERMER 1870 angenommen. LESCHKE u. a. reihen Bronchialasthma unter die parasympathischen Neurosen ein. Bei chemischen Reizungen, besonders aber beim anaphylaktischen Shock kommt es zu den gleichen Erscheinungen wie bei experimenteller Vagusreizung im Tierversuch. Durch das artfremde Eiweiß tritt eine Änderung im kolloidalen Verhalten ein, und dadurch eine Reizung der myoneuralen Verbindungsstellen des Parasympathicus mit der glatten Muskulatur. Es kommt zum Asthma, zur Erschlaffung des Herzmuskeltonus, zu Blutdrucksenkung und vermehrter Fülle im Splanchnikusgebiet, besonders in der Leber. Hautjucken, Urticaria, Erbrechen, erhöhte Peristaltik mit Abgang von blutigem Schleim im Knochenmark werden beobachtet (LESCHKE). Das Bronchialasthma stellt also nur einen Teil aus dem Gesamtgeschehen des anaphylaktischen Shocks dar, und zwar denjenigen, der auf einer anfallsweisen „Neurose" des Lungenvagus beruht, und zu Bronchialmuskelkrampf mit Lungenblähung, vermehrter Sekretion zähen Schleimes durch die Bronchialschleimhaut führt, sowie zu deren Schwellung durch Erweiterung ihrer Blutgefäße. Beim Meerschweinchen ist der anaphylaktische Shock ein typischer Asthmaanfall, beim Menschen überwiegt die Kreislaufinsuffizienz (LESCHKE). Unter den pathogenetischen Bedingungen muß nach diesen Ergebnissen einer *lokalen* Überempfindlichkeit, konstitutionellen Organminderwertigkeit oder erworbenen Organschwäche eine wesentliche Rolle zukommen. Sie kann ihren Ort haben in der Bronchialschleimhaut, im Gebiet des Lungenvagus, in zentralen Innervationsstätten im Zwischenhirn, die Ursache sind für Veränderungen des Wasser- und Mineralstoffwechsels beim Asthma (VEIL); aber sie können auch beruhen auf einer örtlichen Konzentration des Antigens am Reaktionsort. LESCHKE weist z. B. darauf hin, daß Nahrungsmittelidiosynkrasie mehr zu Erbrechen, Durchfall, Urticaria führt; Pollen, Blütenstaub dagegen häufiger zu Bindehautkatarrh, Schnupfen, Asthma.

Von KRONFELD sind familiäre Inhärenz, regionale Verbreitung, Bindung an geologische Bodenstrukturen als Asyle des Nichtwissens bezeichnet worden; eine Trennung des allergischen Asthmas von psychogenen (HANSEN) hält er für einen Verlegenheitsausweg und bezieht sich auf KLEWITZ, der bei einer Impfung von 600 Fällen zu keiner sicheren Unterscheidung des psychogenen vom allergischen Asthma gelangen konnte. Immerhin hat KLEWITZ in 35% (von 423 Fällen) eine spezifische Heredität nachgewiesen! Die therapeutische Einstellung von KRONFELD, der unter Widerspruch von WITTKOWER u. a. die Psychotherapie der internistischen Somatotherapie für überlegen erklärte, aber gleichsam vermittelnd zur Unterstützung der „nicht restlos befriedigenden" Psychoanalyse die „alten Waffen" der Hypnose und Suggestion empfiehlt, kennzeichnet die theoretische wie die praktisch-therapeutische Sachlage genügend. Es gilt für alle Organneurosen, daß sie eine somatische Basis haben und daß die Psychotherapie nicht selten den körperlichen Behandlungsmethoden überlegen ist; *auch* da, wo den seelischen Einflüssen nur ein akzidenteller Charakter zukommt. Vielleicht hat dieses Verhalten seine Ursache darin, daß die seelische Einwirkung im Kettenreflex der Pathogenese an *jedem* Glied angreifen kann, bis hinunter zu den ionalen Verschiebungen, d. h. zu dem tiefsten physikalisch-chemischen Reaktionssystem des Organismus. I. H. SCHULTZ unterstreicht diese Tatsache mit Recht. Den einzelnen körperlichen Mitteln kommt eine so erschöpfende Wirkungsbreite und -tiefe nicht zu. *Wie* diese seelische Wirkung vor sich geht, ist letzten Endes nicht zu ermitteln. Wenn es auch manche Menschen im „autogenen Training" lernen mögen, durch reine konzentrative Vergegenwärtigung einer unwillkürlich ablaufenden Funktion so mit ihr umzugehen wie mit einer willkürlichen, so ist es mir doch unerfindlich, was dann etwa bei der Heilung von Warzen unter psychischer Behandlung vor sich geht, und beim Bronchialasthma verstehe ich es eigentlich nicht besser. Wenn SCHILDER meint, daß die Erklärung der Organneurose aus körperlichen Veränderungen zur Zeit unmöglich sei, und daß der psychologische Weg weiterführe, so habe ich den Eindruck, daß man sich einfach täuscht. Nicht über die Unzulänglichkeit des somatologischen Wissens und nicht über die universelle Wirkungsbreite und den häufigen Wirkungsvorgang aller psychotherapeutischen Methoden vor den somatischen; wohl aber über die tatsächliche Schlüssigkeit angenommener verständlicher Zusammenhänge zwischen Symptom und Ausdrucksbedeutung, sowie bestimmter kausaler Beziehungen, zwischen seelischer Funktion und organneurotischer Entgleisung. Daß man aus dem Erfolg allergischer Behandlung nicht auf rein allergisches Asthma schließen dürfe und aus dem Erfolg einer psychischen Behandlung nicht auf die überwiegend psychische Veranlassung, wird auch — wie mir scheint zutreffend — betont. Auch der epileptische Anfall wird gelegentlich emotiv ausgelöst, nicht so sehr selten sogar der erste, und ebenso kann eine echte melancholische Phase nach seelischem Trauma einsetzen. Die überwiegende Bedeutung der — konstitutionellen — aber wohl gerade hierbei auch dispositionellen Bereitschaft wird man dennoch nicht ernstlich bestreiten können. Die Meinung von HANSEN u. a., daß es allergische und nicht allergische Formen des Bronchialasthmas gebe, halte ich für sehr wahrscheinlich zutreffend, oder vielleicht besser ausgedrückt: es gibt kein Bronchialasthma ohne Organschwäche; aber die Manifestationsbereitschaft ist verschieden, auch in bezug auf das individualtypische Verhalten, und ebenso vorzugsweise die Resistenzschwäche gegenüber verschiedenen allergischen, klimatischen, psychischen Einflüssen. Daß *jeder* Asthmaanfall zuweilen auch psychisch ausgelöst werden kann, spricht — nach allem, was hier vorgetragen wurde — nicht gegen diese Auffassung.

Zur psychischen Behandlungsweise des Bronchialasthmas kann ich im übrigen auf den allgemeinen Teil verweisen. Gerade das Asthma soll in seiner ursächlichen Verankerung weit in die Konfliktssphäre der Persönlichkeit hineinragen, auch wenn man nicht gerade mit der Psychoanalyse als letzte Determinante die Angst vor der Ablösung von der Mutter und den entsprechenden Protest dagegen annimmt, aber die Domäne ist die Ruhebehandlung. Die hypnotische psychogymnastische Übungsbehandlung von LAUDENHEIMER sei hier besonders erwähnt, ebenso das autogene Training von I. H. SCHULTZ: „Im speziellen stellen wir den Asthmatiker darauf ein, den gesamten Nasenrachenraum bis zum Kehlkopf mit einem Kühleerlebnis unterempfindlich zu machen und eine entsprechende Schleimhautabschwellung zu begünstigen; Luftröhre, Bronchien und Lungenraum werden dagegen intensiv wärmend durchströmt." Internistische Kontrolle ist dabei notwendig und die Behandlung selbst bis zur geforderten und erfolgbringenden Meisterschaft des Patienten zeitraubend.

Somatische Behandlung mit den parasympathisch hemmenden sympathisch fördernden Mitteln (Adrenalin, Suprarenin [im Asthmolysin wirksam] Sympathol) ist bekannt. Eine neueste Übersicht über die Therapie bringt I. H. SCHULTZ[1] auf die hier besonders verwiesen sei. Die allergischen Behandlungsmethoden erfordern spezielle Kenntnisse (s. Arbeiten von STORM VAN LEUWEN, KÄMMERER, v. BERGMANN u. a.).

---

[1] SCHULTZ, I. H.: Fortschr. Neur. **1933**.

c) Neurosen des Verdauungssystems.

An den funktionellen Störungen im Bereich des Verdauungssystems vom Mund bis zum After hat sich die psychische Beeinflussung von Organfunktionen früh exakt und eindringlich nachweisen lassen (PAWLOW, HEYER, v. BERGMANN, KATSCH) aber es hat auch gerade in ihrem Bereich der Abbau der Organneurosen energisch eingesetzt und ist noch keineswegs abgeschlossen. Selbst an einem so wohlbekannten Symptomenkomplex wie dem Kardiospasmus wird durch v. BERGMANNs Untersuchungen über die Hiatushernie des Oesophagus gerüttelt. Zu diesen freien Hiatushernien rechnet v. BERGMANN auch diejenigen Fälle, bei denen im Röntgenbild ein Höhertreten der normalerweise subphrenisch gelegenen Anteile des Oesophagus bzw. der Kardia zu beobachten ist. Bei 10 von 17 Fällen von Kardiospasmus konnte nun nachgewiesen werden, daß ein abgeschnürter Anteil des Kontrastmittels säckchenförmig oberhalb des Hiatus zu liegen kam; dieser Abschnitt wurde für den Magenanteil gehalten.

Neben dem Krampf der Kardia sind im Bereich bis zum Magen eine Reihe von Betriebsstörungen zu nennen, über die ausführlicher u. a. H. CURSCHMANN berichtet hat. Die *Speichelstockung* (Xerostomie, Mundtrockenheit) spielt als unmittelbar thymogene Unterfunktion keine allzu seltene Rolle; man kann sie ja den Kontaktneurosen (G. v. STOCKERT) zurechnen, die nur deshalb so selten zum Arzt führt, weil sie — abgesehen von Berufsrednern, Schauspielern — zwar subjektiv unangenehm ist, objektiv meist aber unauffällig bleibt im Gegensatz etwa zum Stottern. Wie bei diesem und den Funktionssperrungen überhaupt, kommt es besonders leicht zur Verschlimmerung durch ängstliche Erwartung ihres Eintretens. *Aerophagie* (Luftschlucken), Rülpsen und Regurgitieren mit *Rumination* finden sich gelegentlich bei ein und demselben Menschen, manchmal sogar mit Erbrechen. In einem Falle meiner Beobachtung war eine Rumination so wie CURSCHMANN diese beschreibt — Beförderung von Speiseteilen in den Mund ohne Widerwillen, ohne Nausea, reflektorisch und ohne besondere Kenntnisnahme — das erste Anzeichen eines Ulcus duodeni. Es blieb auch nach operativer Heilung bestehen und gewann in der konfliktreichen Lage dieses Mannes — eines mittleren Beamten — den psychischen Wert einer Waffe gegen Ansprüche der Umwelt: Hindernis im Umgang mit dem Publikum. Auf ein familiäres Vorkommen der Rumination hat CURSCHMANN hingewiesen.

v. BERGMANN hebt hervor, wie in unzulässiger Weise funktionelle Störungen zu Krankheiten gestempelt wurden. Die *nervöse Dyspepsie* ist oft nur der Ausdruck eines Reizmagens und dieser wieder fast identisch mit einer Gastritis mit und ohne Ulcus (KATSCH). Supersekretionen und Superacidität sind zu einem großen Teil dem Ulcusleiden zugeordnet, die fraktionierte Aushebung hat den Klettertypus der Säurewerte als ein wichtiges Symptom des Ulcus duodeni erwiesen. Die REICHMANNsche *Krankheit* (Gastrosuccorrhoe), bei der ungeheure Saftströme ausgebrochen werden können, ist Ausdruck einer gestörten sekretorischen Funktion, meist bei einem Ulcus pylori (Ulcérés à crises tabiformes). WESTPHAL und KATSCH haben 1913 bei einer Schilderung des neurotischen Ulcus duodeni darauf hingewiesen, daß vegetative Begleiterscheinungen (Hyperperistaltik oder Pylorospasmus) sowohl wie vegetative Stigmen verschiedener Art vorhanden waren; das Krankheitssyndrom des Duodenalgeschwürs deuten sie als vegetativ-neurotisches Kranksein bei Ulcus duodeni. Die Lehre, daß eine primäre Gastritis zur Ulcusbildung führe (KONJETZNY) ist verlassen; dasselbe gilt von der Infarkttheorie. Dagegen zeigen neuere Arbeiten (BÜCHNER, SILBERMANN u. a., zit. bei MOSCOWICZ), daß ein hyperaktischer Magensaft die Magenwand schädigen kann, jedoch nur in der Zone der Pylorusdrüsen[1]. Auch die Darmwand ist ungeschützt. Histaminähnliche Substanzen sind dafür besonders angeschuldigt worden (KATSCH); die Hyperaktivierung des Magensaftes kann verschiedene Ursachen haben, neurogene sowohl wie allergische und psychische. Das gilt auch für die Sekretionskrisen der REICHMANNschen Krankheit. Vaguserregende Pharmaca, etwa Cholin, steigern die Sekretion und die Salzsäureabsonderung des Magens. Unter den nervösen Stigmen bei Ulcuskranken haben schon WESTPHAL und KATSCH basedowoide Zeichen angeführt; in der Tat ist es so, daß die Mehrzahl der konstitutionell Hyperthyreotischen hinsichtlich ihrer Magen-Darmfunktionen sich „paradoxerweise" (LESCHKE) wie Vagotoniker verhalten, neben einer kleinen Gruppe, deren Magen-Darmmotilität sympathisch gehemmt ist. Reizung des Sympathicus (splanchnici) führt im Experiment zur Kontraktion des Schließmuskels am Pylorus. Die Wirkung des Atropins am Magen hat durch die Untersuchungen von KLEE (periphere Reizungen nach hoher Rückenmarkdurchtrennung bei Katzen) zur Klärung geführt. Ist ein Sympathicustonus vorhanden, dann hemmt Atropin die Magenperistaltik und den Tonus. Auf diesen spasmolytischen Effekt gründet sich die v. BERGMANNsche Atropinbehandlung beim Ulcus, beim spastischen Sanduhrmagen und bei Tenesmen der Gallenwege (v. BERGMANN und BILLIGHEIMER, LESCHKE). Atropin führt, wie Adrenalin, zu einer Herabsetzung der Magensaftabsonderung und seines Gehaltes an Salzsäure und Pepsin. Die Abgrenzung der sog., psychisch mehr oder minder verursachten und zu beeinflussenden vegetativen Magenneurosen gegen das Ulcus ventriculi ist noch immer schwer. RUHMANN versucht eine schärfere Definition der Organminderwertigkeit von Magen und Darm zu geben, indem er eine angioneurotische Organdiathese annimmt, mit Neigung zu funktionell-nervösen Störungen im peripherstem Gefäßabschnitt entsprechend einer teilweisen vasoneurotischen Diathese (OTFRIED MÜLLER).

Besondere *charakterologische Eigentümlichkeiten* bei Männern mit leichten, psychotherapeutisch rasch kurierten Magenbeschwerden verschiedener Prägung hebt VOGEL hervor: Ausgeprägter Ordnungswille bis zur Pedanterie, Sparsamkeit bis zum Geiz bei ausgesprochen ordentlichem sozialen Verhalten. Im Anschluß an eine Erschütterung der Lebensordnung (Arbeitslosigkeit usw.) traten die — hypochondrisch umsorgten — Beschwerden auf. Die primitive Deutung einer Ausdruckssymbolik des Hinunterschluckens von Ärger und Verdruß für die Aerophagie wurde schon erwähnt, sie spielt angeblich auch eine Rolle beim Kardiospasmus und anderen neurotischen Störungen der Magenfunktionen; im Gegensatz etwa zu den hitzigen, explosiblen, aber rasch abreagierenden Hypertonikern. Auf das gallige Temperament und die funktionellen Tenesmen der Gallenwege (SCHINDLER) sei ebenfalls verwiesen. Untersuchungen wie die von VOGEL werden den wirklichen Zusammenhängen wohl am ehesten gerecht, da sie die unmittelbare, konstitutionell gegebene Abhängigkeit zwischen vegetativem Verhalten, Persönlichkeitsstruktur und neurotischen Reaktionen ahnen lassen. Die Ausführungen v. WEIZSÄCKERS zum Aufbau der Magen-Darmneurosen wurden schon früher dargelegt.

Es seien in diesem Zusammenhang auch nachdrücklich die Arbeiten von ROSENFELD erwähnt, der dem vegetativ körperlichen Unterbau die kausale Hauptrolle zuschreibt. Die Linie zu den Charakterologien von EWALD und neuerdings von E. BRAUN, aber auch zu den Ergebnissen KRETSCHMERs und seiner Schule kann hier nur angedeutet werden.

---

[1] H. HANKE meint nachweisen zu können, daß eine Disharmonie des vegetativen Systems nicht mittelbar über vasomotorische Reaktionen, sondern unmittelbar, peptisch, im Sinne der Überwertigkeit des Magensaftes, wie es BUCHNER besonders betont, zu erosiven Schädigungen der Magenschleimhaut führt.

Gegenüber dem Luftschlucken hat das *Erbrechen* gelegentlich eine nicht zu übersehende Ausdrucksbedeutung, nämlich Ekel und Abwehr. Aber die oft bedrohliche Gegenwart sehr eindeutiger Organkrankheiten darf darüber nicht vergessen werden (KLIMKE, SCHINDLER). Wieweit Enteroptose, Atonie des Magens und Darmes, zuweilen kombiniert mit Anacidität wirklich auf seelischem Wege zustande kommen, ist mir fraglich. Die gelegentlich geäußerten (SCHINDLER) Beziehungen zur Depression dürfen jedenfalls nicht anders verstanden werden denn als klinisch den seelischen Erscheinungen nebengeordnete Symptome: die gemeinsame Ursache ist doch wohl eine primär vegetative Störung. Daß man in der Tat durch hypnotische Beeinflussung ein Höher- und Tieferstehen des Magens vor dem Röntgenschirm beobachten kann (HEYER), beweist nichts für die Genese im Einzelfall.

Durchfälle infolge nervöser Hyperperistaltik bei häufig familiärer vegetativer Funktionsbereitschaft gegenüber Angst, Schreck oder überhaupt jedem akuten und heftigen Affekt sind bekannte Ausdrucksformen der „inneren Front" (KEHRER). Von fast allen Funktionsstörungen im Bereich der Bauchorgane werden sie am wenigsten hypochondrisch ausgedeutet. Möglicherweise bergen sich auch hinter diesem Verhalten — über die Gesamtorganisation der Tiefenperson hinweg — Beziehungen zu Charakter und Temperament der Betroffenen. Jedenfalls zeigen organneurotische Hypochonder mit der häufigen Neigung zu Pedanterien und egoistischen Einstellungen weit häufiger Neigung zu spastischer Obstipation.

Die *Colica mucosa* läßt in ihren klinischen Äußerungen sowohl wie im pathologischen Aufbau Beziehungen zum Asthma bronchiale erkennen, sowie zur Urticaria und dem eosinophilen Dickdarmkatarrh (SCHINDLER, v. BERGMANN u. a.). Sie ist keine Lokalkrankheit, sondern Ausdruck eines allergischen Reizzustandes.

Man hat beim Lesen der Literatur, auch der großen Monographien und der Übersichten (KATSCH, KANTOR, v. BERGMANN, FLEISCHER, KNUD FABER, SCHIFF, H. CURSCHMANN) den Eindruck, daß auf dem Gebiet der Magen-Darmstörungen die Rolle des psychogenen Moments mit großer Vorsicht diskutiert werde. Dem Goethewort, das in neuerer Zeit öfters angeführt wird, wonach das Außen das Innen und das Innen das Außen sei, mag nicht bestritten werden, daß es auch für den großen Aspekt auf den beseelten menschlichen Organismus zutrifft. Aber im Empirischen bleibt, selbst wenn man das Reich der berühmten Übergänge weit faßt, das Außen außen und das Innen innen, und zwar um so betonter, je mehr man — wohl wissend um das Sowohl-Als auch funktioneller Störungen — das diagnostische Können treibt.

Grundsätzlich ist zur psychischen *Behandlung* der Magen-Darmneurosen nichts anderes zu sagen als zu den Kreislauf- und Atemstörungen. Vor übertriebener psychotherapeutischer Aktivität, trotz gelegentlich guter Erfolge wird gewarnt (SCHINDLER, LEIBOWITZ, v. BERGMANN); unter den somatischen Methoden verwahrt sich v. BERGMANN gegen die „primitive Dermatologie der Schleimhautbehandlung" mit Berieselung durch Glaubersalzwasser und Höllensteinlösungen. Funktionell angepaßter sind die Entspannung der Muskelschichten durch Atropin, Belladonna, Papaverin. Gegen eine übertriebene Schondiät bei nicht organischen Schäden haben sich u. a. I. H. SCHULTZ ausgesprochen.

d) Urogenitalsystem.

Auch die Harnblase ist als „Fangnetz und Spiegel seelischer Konflikte" bezeichnet worden (STUTZIN und WARNER). Durch die neuropsychische „Mischung von Autonomie, Automatie und Willensregulierbarkeit, andererseits durch ihre seelische und somatische Einbeziehung in die Sexualsphäre" sei sie sogar besonders dazu geeignet. Immerhin ist wenigstens ihre Ausdrucksmöglichkeit beschränkt: *Polakisurie, Retention, Inkontinenz* und *Enuresis*. Jede dieser Formen kann Symptom einer organischen Erkrankung sein. Selbst hinter der sog. Enuresis nocturna können sich nächtliche epileptische Krampfanfälle verbergen und jede organische Miktionsstörung kann *als* Funktionstonsleistung von seelischen Einflüssen abhängig sein. Auch eine Blasenstörung bei multipler Sklerose läßt sich durch Hypnose und andere suggestive Einflüsse bessern. Daraus läßt sich weder ihre „seelische Verursachung" ableiten, noch läßt sich bestreiten, daß auch Funktionsleistungen bei einem organischen Pathos über das vegetative System seelischen Einwirkungen zugänglich sind.

Das Problem der *Enuresis* ist noch nicht gelöst. Komplizierte seelische Beziehungen, etwa zwischen Onanie und Enuresis als Schuldersatzhandlung (KLÄSI, zit. nach O. SCHWARZ) scheinen mir viel seltener zu sein als man häufig annimmt. Das gleiche gilt von einer individualpsychologischen, finalen Deutung des Symptoms. Eine Organminderwertigkeit darf man wohl mit Recht zumeist annehmen, worin sie liegt, ist unbekannt. Daß sie etwa nur die Blase, eine erhöhte Tonusbereitschaft des Detrusor, eine Sphincterschwäche betreffen müßte, ist nicht einzusehen. Mein Lehrer G. ASCHAFFENBURG pflegte in seinen Vorlesungen darauf hinzuweisen, daß man es nicht selten erleben könne, wie bei einem Enuretiker, kaum daß er abends uriniert habe, das Bett schon wieder „schwimmen" könne. Die Organschwäche könnte also auch im Harnbereitungssystem liegen und ähnlich einer REICHMANNschen Krankheit zu Sekretionskrisen führen. Die Enuresis hat keine einheitliche Genese. Psychische Stumpfheit kann am Aufbau ebenso beteiligt sein wie seelische Lebhaftigkeit. Bei solcher Persönlichkeitsprägung scheint mir den Miktionsträumen mit ihrer plastischen Deutlichkeit doch eine Bedeutung für die Enuresis zuzukommen. Das Verwunderliche ist ja zunächst die Tatsache, daß die kleinen Kinder relativ rasch lernen, ihre Blasenfunktion auf bestimmte regulierende Bedingungsreflexe einzustellen, nicht aber, daß sie es nicht lernen. Erziehungsfehler, Umweltschäden können zu Falschgewöhnungen führen, aber da, wo die Organminderwertigkeit oder ein ihr konstitutionell vielleicht zugeordnetes vegetativ nervöses *und* seelisches Verhalten oder eine dieser Bedingungen beeinflußbar sind, helfen drastische Mittel nicht selten überraschend. Sie setzen sich anscheinend mit ihrem Signalwert als eine Art „Schlafwache" durch. Von hier aus scheint mir die alte Anschuldigung der ungewöhnlichen Schlaftiefe für das Zustandekommen der Enuresis nicht ganz so unberechtigt zu sein, wie man zum Teil meint (O. SCHWARZ, FEER[1]). Die *neurotische Harnverhaltung* und die sog. *Reizblase* sind seltene Erscheinungen.

Unter Leistungsstörungen des *Genitalsystems* sei zunächst auf die männlichen Formen: Impotenz und gehäufte Pollutionen hingewiesen. Bei dem Rang, den die Genitalfunktionen im seelischen Haushalt einnehmen, kann es nicht verwundern, daß Leistungshemmungen und Fehlleistungen zu seelischen Konflikten führen und umgekehrt. Hier erweisen sich in jedem Fall psychophysische Persönlichkeit, Lebensgeschichte und neurotische Störung in jeweils neu zu ermittelnder Abhängigkeit. Es ist ja bekannt, wie von solcher Sphäre aus die Psychoanalyse entstanden ist und mit ihr die Ära der „tiefenpsychologischen" Forschungen und Erkenntnisse; ein Ausläufer ist die Lehre von der „Psychogenese" körperlicher Funktionsstörungen.

Die *weiblichen Genitalstörungen* sind entsprechend der anatomischen und physiologischen Organbeschaffenheit und in Übereinstimmung mit dem betonten

---

[1] Siehe hierzu die neuere Darstellung von CHRISTOFFEL, der die Enuresis nocturna als die häufigste motorische Schlafstörung (Schlafhandlung) bezeichnet und sie in die Nähe der Zustände von Schlafwandel rückt.

Zyklus der Vorgänge und dem „Generationsgeschäft" vielfältiger als die männlichen (A. MAYER, WALTHARD, HAHN, GRÄFENBERG, MEYER-RÜEGG, NOVAK und HARNIK, CIMBAL u. a.).

Frigidität, Dyspareunie, Vaginismus entsprechen etwa den männlichen Potenzstörungen. Ob es Frigidität als anlagebedingtes Persönlichkeitsmerkmal überhaupt gibt, wie oft sie angegeben oder verschwiegen wird, und wie oft sie tatsächlich neurotische Hemmung oder Waffe ist, läßt sich nach Literatur und psychiatrischen Erfahrungen kaum abschätzen.

Vaginismus ist wohl sicher eine wesentlich seltenere Situationsentgleisung als die männliche Impotenz.

Dagegen sind Störungen der *Menstruationsblutungen, Dysmenorrhoe* und *Fluor albus* häufiger. Es sind Erscheinungen, die gewissermaßen eine Stufe tiefer im Körperlichen liegen und der vitalen Person unmittelbarer verknüpft sind als der geistigen. Eine pathogenetische Strukturdiagnose der Gemütsbewegungen, des endokrinen Apparates, der vegetativen Abläufe, der Beschaffenheit des Erfolgsorganes, ist im einzelnen hier so schwierig wie bei allen Organneurosen. Ich verweise vor allem auf die Arbeiten von A. MAYER, die auch reichliche Kasuistik aus der „Sprechstunde" bringen.

Die Psychotherapie gestörter Genitalfunktionen zerschlägt oft den gordischen Knoten, ohne daß diese praktische auch eine erkenntnismäßige Lösung wäre.

e) Haut.

Psychovegetative Erscheinungen an der Haut sind alltäglich und werden im Erröten und Erblassen unmittelbar als seelischer Ausdruck „verstanden". Aber es gibt konstitutionelle Unterschiede in der Bereitschaft zu diesen Reaktionen, die regelmäßig in der Jugend leichter auftreten als im Alter. SACK weist darauf hin, wie häufiges Erröten eine Erweiterung der Gesichtscapillaren, ja eine Stase herbeiführen könne, bis es auf diesem trophisch gestörten Boden zu einer echten Acne rosacea mit Teleangiektasien und Gewebshypertrophien kommt.

Immerhin erhellt schon aus diesem Beispiel, daß es eine schiefe Auffassung wäre, die Acne rosacea etwa schlechthin als psychogene Dermatose anzusprechen. Man tut, soweit ich sehe, von vornherein gut, bei den nicht banalen Hauterkrankungen (Ekzem, Psoriasis usw.) seelische Bedingungen in ihrem Wirkungswert nicht zu überschätzen (BETTMANN), wenn auch im Einzelfall ein Ekzem etwa auf dem Boden eines seelisch ausgelösten Juckreizes mit folgendem Kratzen entstehen kann, oder zum Anlaß wird für reaktive Verstimmung und Besorgtheit, die nun ihrerseits über vegetative Einflüsse hinweg eine Besserung hintanhalten kann. Gerade der Nervenarzt sieht diesen Weg, bei dem eine Hauterkrankung oder eine umschriebene, entstellende Hautanomalie zu Minderwertigkeitsreaktionen führt, häufiger als den der seelischen Verursachung. Aber auch gemeinsame biologische Wurzeln bestehen zuweilen zwischen Psoriasisschüben etwa und melancholischen Phasen.

Hautjucken, Pruritus, *Urticaria* dagegen sind pathologische Erscheinungen an der Haut, bei denen sich emotive Einflüsse häufig und überzeugend nachweisen lassen. Dazu gesellen sich *Herpes*, QUINCKEsches Ödem, *Ergrauen* der Haare. Die allergische Genese dieser Störungen ist in gleicher Weise wie etwa beim Bronchialasthma, bei der Colila mucosa zu werten. Bei einer konstitutionellen oder dispositionellen Bereitschaft kann ein psychischer Shok, eine Konfliktsangst usw. Hautreaktionen hervorrufen; gelegentlich aber kann auch einmal ein solcher Shock eine „humorale Umwälzung erzeugen, eine Kolloidoklasie", die nun zur Hautreaktion führt (DRACOULIDÈS, JOLTRAIN, SACK). Für die *Urticaria*-Quaddelbildung ist die ursächlich notwendige Ausscheidung von Histaminsubstanzen nachgewiesen (DOERR, zit. bei SACK). Diese können allergisch, aber auch vom Sympathicus aus freigesetzt werden. Psychischer Reiz führt zur Quaddelbildung auf dem Weg sympathischer Erregung oder durch Auslösung allergischer Reaktion zu örtlicher Histaminausscheidung und zur Urticariaquaddel. Im einzelnen liegen die seelisch funktionellen Verhältnisse und die Beziehungen zur geistigen Persönlichkeit wie bei allen organneurotischen Reaktionen. BUNNEMANN meint sogar, analog etwa zu den Anschauungen v. WEIZSÄCKERS am Verdauungsapparat, daß man schon jetzt Hautkrankheiten unterscheiden könne, die auf sexuellen Konflikten beruhten, weiter solche, in denen sich eine Angst um die Existenz kundgibt, dann solche, die der Ausdruck eines grauenerregenden Erlebnisses sind usw.

Der psychotherapeutische Erfolg, nicht zuletzt durch Hypnose, ist zuweilen verblüffend. So wenn etwa bei einem Pruritus, der keinem der Mittel aus imponierend aufgereihten Töpfchen weichen wollte, nach kurzer Zeit Besserung der Beschwerden und damit ein Aufleben der ganzen Persönlichkeit einsetzt. Dasselbe gilt von quälenden Juckanfällen, bei denen sich gut erkennen läßt, wie zwischen Reiz und Beachtung ein circulus vitiosus besteht, wie aber auch Häufigkeit des Juckreizes und des Kratzens konstitutionell verschieden angelegt sind, wie sie durch nervöse Erschöpfung oder seelische Erregung in ihrer Intensität gesteigert werden und bei Wohlbefinden sich bessern, wie aber auch Falschgewöhnung oder Erziehung von Einfluß sein können.

Vielleicht erweist sich nirgends so eindringlich und überzeugend das Wirkungsausmaß des Seelischen auf körperliches Geschehen wie an den *spontanen Hautblutungen* (SCHINDLER, JACOBI) und an den wunderwirkenden „Besprechungen" oder Kochsalzinjektionen usw. bei *Warzen* (L. GRUMACH). Solche Vorgänge sind dazu angetan, den Unwissenden mit abergläubischen, ja mystischen Vorstellungen zu erfüllen, dem Wissenden aber führen sie vor Augen, daß er zwar Bruchstücke von Wirkungswegen kennt und hoffen darf, neue zu entdecken, daß er aber „das Wirkende" im lebendigen Leib-Seele-Organismus nur höchst unzulänglich in seine Bildersprache übersetzen kann.

Anhang.

Die sog. „Koordinationsneurosen".

1. Allgemeiner Teil.

Aus der Fülle neurotischer Reaktionen und Entwicklungen lassen sich diejenigen Betriebsstörungen, die einzelne Organe für sich zu betreffen oder von ihnen auszugehen scheinen, als Organneurosen bezeichnen und wenigstens begrifflich scharf von anderen Formen abgrenzen. Ihnen sind nach Ursache und Entstehung, aber auch im Erscheinungsbild unter allen seelisch *mit* hervorgerufenen und festgehaltenen körperlichen Störungen die sog. Koordinationsneurosen zunächst verwandt. Jedoch schon die Tatsache, daß sich diese Koordinationsneurosen an der quergestreiften, willkürlich beeinflußbaren Muskulatur abspielen, macht es notwendig, sie von den „Organneurosen" zu trennen. Man nennt sie häufig auch „*Beschäftigungsneurosen*", *koordinatorische* Beschäftigungsneurosen, oder *Beschäftigungskrämpfe,* um damit wesentliche Merkmale ihrer Entstehung und Erscheinung zu kennzeichnen. Allen Koordinationsneurosen ist gemeinsam und bestimmt ihren *Begriff,* daß es sich um Funktionsstörungen solcher Muskelgruppen handelt, die bei bestimmten Bewegungsabläufen („Beschäftigungen, Tätigkeiten") gemeinsam und in genauem Zusammenspiel in Tätigkeit treten. Diese Tätigkeiten wurden ursprünglich erlernt, um schließlich fast völlig automatisiert zu verlaufen. Lehrbeispiele solcher koordinatorischen Neurosen und zugleich die weitaus wichtigsten unter ihnen sind *Schreibkrampf* und *Stottern*.

Bei diesen Formen neurotischer Störungen ist der gleiche Streit der Meinungen um seelische oder organische Verursachung entbrannt wie bei den Organneurosen und es wiederholt sich hier bei zunehmender Kenntnis *auch* organisch bedingter Störungen erscheinungsbildlich gleicher Art ein ,,Abbau der Neurosen", wenigstens bis zu dem Grad, daß ein besonders körperliches Entgegenkommen konstitutioneller oder erworbener (dispositioneller) Art meistens und zurecht angenommen wird. Die seelischen Veranlassungen, Vergröberungen und Fixierungen koordinatorischer Neurosen erhalten insofern eine eigene Note, als die betreffenden Tätigkeiten sich vor den Augen und Ohren anderer abspielen. Das gilt vor allem für das Sprechen und seine Koordinationsneurose: das Stottern. So bezeichnet etwa J. S. GALANT das Stottern als eine *sozioaffektive Dysphasie,* wie denn überhaupt die Nomenklatur auf dem Gebiet der Stimmheilkunde etwas eigenwillige Wege geht. v. STOCKERT hat für das Stottern und eine Reihe anderer Neurosen den Begriff der *Kontaktneurose* geprägt, denn es handle sich dabei um eine Manifestation von Störungen (,,funktionelle Dysfunktionen") [!], ,,die gleichsam unter der Kontrolle eines Partners verlaufen". Aber wie man auch die seelischen Faktoren am Aufbau einschätzen und deuten mag, — psychoanalytisch oder individualpsychologisch, oder weniger konstruktiv als Erwartungsangst und störende Aufmerksamkeitszuwendung zu automatisierten Handlungen, oder als mehr minderbewußte Äußerungsformen jeweils verschiedener Lebenskonflikte und seelischer Haltungen,— so gibt es doch eine Reihe von Tatsachen, die mindestens ein körperliches Entgegenkommen allgemein neuropathischer Art, oder eine mehr umschriebene konstitutionelle oder dispositionelle Funktionsminderwertigkeit immer wahrscheinlicher machen. HION hat in einer Arbeit, die FRÖSCHELS anführt, gefunden, daß unter 295 Stotterern überwiegend häufig ,,einzige" Kinder seien, und glaubt dieses Ergebnis im Sinne der ADLERschen Individualpsychologie auswerten zu können. FRÖSCHELS fand demgegenüber unter 1813 Fällen 565 einzige Kinder und 514 mit einem Geschwister. SZONDI, der 100 Stotterer konstitutionsanalytisch untersuchte, hält das Stottern für eine erbbedingte, genuine Spracherkrankung aus dem dimer-recessiven Erbkreis: Epilepsie — Migräne — Stottern. Ein familiäres Auftreten, zuweilen in dominantem Erbgang, hat schon LENZ erwähnt; ob die gelegentliche Diskordanz bei E. Z. (SIEMENS) durch Umwelteinflüsse erklärt werden muß (v. VERSCHUER), scheint mir fraglich zu sein. SZONDI fand jedenfalls häufig Migräne und Epilepsie unter den Müttern von Stotterern und schreibt auch diesen selbst eine größere Neigung zu Epilepsie und Eklampsie zu als der Durchschnittsbevölkerung. In 20% der Fälle fand er extrem große oder kleine Schädelmaße; 71% zeigten Auffälligkeiten des Vasomotoriums einschließlich atypischer Capillarbilder, die auch schon bei den Eltern beobachtet wurden. Auf die häufige *Linkshändigkeit* in der Verwandtschaft von Stotterern und bei diesen selbst wiesen neuerdings wieder TRAVIS und JOHNSON hin, die meinen, daß auch zwischen dem Beginn des Stotterns und dem Wechsel von Linkshändigkeit zu Rechtshändigkeit ursächliche Beziehungen bestehen. KISTLER fand eine auffallende Häufigkeit von Linkshändern unter Stammlern, aber nicht unter Stottern. Es läßt sich auch nicht übersehen, daß eine Reihe von schwachsinnigen oder epileptischen Stotterern keine ,,Neurose" bekommen. CIAMPI führt diese Tatsache dafür an, daß das Stottern keine Angstneurose sei; nicht die Angst mache Stottern sondern das Stottern Angst; aber auch diese Angst fehle dann, wenn — bei Oligophrenen usw. — das Stottern nicht richtig beurteilt werde, oder doch jedenfalls Minderwertigkeitsgefühle fehlen. Es gibt aber auch hochbegabte Stotterer, deren Stottern sich nicht verschlimmert, weil ihnen ein gütiges Geschick nur sehr kümmerliche Mindergeltungsgefühle gab, mit denen sie jedenfalls fertig wurden, ehe es zur Kontaktneurose kam.

SEEMANN hat in ziemlich hohem Maße bei kindlichen, weniger bei erwachsenen Stotterern eine Erschwerung der Nasenatmung festgestellt (adenoide Wucherungen u. a. Ursachen). Er meint, daß es dadurch zu einer Behinderung der thorakalen Atmung und damit zu einer Verminderung der Alkalireserve im Blut komme, die nun ihrerseits die Funktion des *vegetativen Systems* ändere. O. WUTH erwähnt u. a., daß bei gewissen Formen des Stotterns eine höhere Alkalescenz des Speichels gefunden worden sei. Eine Störung im vegetativen System bis hinauf bis zu den Zentralstätten im Diencephalon wird in verschiedenen Abwandlungen als konstitutionelle oder dispositionelle Ursache oder Mitursache des Stotterns angesprochen. So meint etwa SEEMANN: Die psychischen Erregungen benutzen den Weg über die — in ihrer Funktion durch die Alkaliverminderung im Blut gestörten — vegetativen Zentren, die nun ihrerseits über das striopallidäre System jene Betriebsstörungen hervorrufen, die das Stottern bedingen. CIAMPI spricht von einer Anomalie der myostatischen Innervation. SOVAK meint, das Gleichgewicht des vegetativen Systems sei bei der Mehrzahl der Stotterer gestört; das Stottern selbst sei aber nicht einfach durch diese Störungen hervorgerufen, sondern vegetative Labilität und Stottern hätten ihre gemeinsame Ursache in einem cerebralen Schaden. v. STOCKERT drückt sich wieder etwas positiver aus, wenn er als somatische Grundlage der Kontaktneurosen eine Enthemmung des striopallidären Schaltapparates annimmt. Es müssen dies ja nicht gleich wie *er* meint, pathologisch-anatomische Veränderungen sein.

Sehr ähnlich lauten die pathogenetischen Vorstellungen über das Zustandekommen des *Schreibkrampfes*. Bei encephalitischem Parkinsonismus hat SITTIG, nach früheren Beobachtungen von LEMOS, LEVY, das Auftreten eines Schreibkrampfes beobachtet und zwar bemerkenswerterweise in einem Fall, bei dem extrapyramidale Störungen sonst kaum vorhanden waren. Die Krampfbewegungen vor allem in den beiden ersten Fingern und in der Hand setzten auch beim Essen, beim Anfassen von Papier und anderen Bewegungen ein, bei denen mit Daumen und Zeigefinger zugefaßt wurde. Einige weitere Beobachtungen von Schreibkrampf bei „Striatumläsionen" beschreibt E. ADLER. HALLERVORDEN bemängelt zurecht, daß man einen so komplexen Vorgang wie den Schreibkrampf wohl kaum mit *einer* Zentralstätte in Verbindung bringen könne und daß überdies gerade bei Encephalitikern das Striatum frei bleibe und vorwiegend die Substantia nigra geschädigt sei. Eine „extrapyramidale Grundlage" des Schreibkrampfes nimmt auch *Rost* an. Jedenfalls bestand in seinem Fall eine klassische Form dieser Neurose 5 Jahre lang ehe andere, vom Schreibakt unabhängige Erscheinungen einsetzten und zwar tetanieforme Spasmen der Finger und unwillkürliche Bewegungen von athetoidem Charakter; allmählich entwickelte sich eine dauernde tonische Flexion der Hand. Freilich läßt sich aus solchen sicher organisch verursachten „symptomatischen" Formen des Schreibkrampfes nur die Vermutung ableiten, daß auch dem essentiellen Schreibkrampf, oder wenigstens einer Gruppe davon und vielleicht noch anderen Koordinationsneurosen eine zentrale Leistungsschwäche ererbter, angeborener oder erworbener Art als *ein* unerläßlicher pathogenetischer Faktor zugrunde liegt. Ich möchte daran erinnern, daß die quergestreifte Muskulatur somatisch *und* vegetativ innerviert ist und möglicherweise auch an der Regulation des Muskeltonus beteiligt ist (ORBELI, BRÜCKE, SCHILF).

Angeborene „Tonusveränderungen" im Sinne der DUPRÉschen Paratonie als Voraussetzung dür das Entstehen des Schreibkrampfes betont neuerdings

CALLEWAERT; die vermehrte Neigung zu Muskelspannungen, Vorkommen von Mitbewegungen und die allgemeine neuropathische Konstitution lassen an eine Schädigung zentraler Steuerungen denken. Wenn man erwägt, daß die „Beschäftigungsneurosen" im Gegensatz zum Stottern überwiegend häufig erst im mittleren Lebensalter auftreten, so ließe sich vermuten, daß für diese Neurosen erworbene und periphere Schädigungen ursächlich doch eine größere Rolle spielen. Man kann aber gegen eine solche Auffassung mit guten Gründen mancherlei einwenden. Es wäre möglich, daß mit zunehmendem Alter und vielleicht frühzeitiger als man annehmen möchte, Dysfunktionen in den vegetativen Zentralstätten einsetzen, oder auch im extrapyramidalen System ohne daß ihnen nachweisbare pathologisch-anatomische Befunde zugrunde liegen, sondern vielleicht kolloidchemische oder andersartige Abänderungen. Vielleicht treten solche Änderungen abnorm frühzeitig dann auf, wenn ein frühkindliches Trauma schon eine erhöhte zentrale vegetative Labilität gesetzt hat. ROSANOFF hat kürzlich festgestellt, daß frühgeborene, untergewichtige Kinder leichter eine Hirnschädigung bei der Geburt erleiden und daß Knaben davon häufiger betroffen werden als Mädchen. Es ist aber bekannt, daß unter Stotterern und Kranken mit Schreibkrampf der männliche Anteil überwiegt. Für den Schreibkrampf ließe sich das aus äußeren Umständen erklären, für das Stottern wohl kaum. Wie hoch im übrigen eine, wenn auch nicht sicher faßbare, körperliche Grundlage, nämlich das „konstitutionelle oder dispositionelle Entgegenkommen", gerade für das Stottern veranschlagt wird, geht schon daraus hervor, daß eine solche Prädisposition selbst für das „induzierte" Nachahmungsstottern angenommen wird (WEISS und BARCZINSKI).

Man muß versuchen, der Ursachenkette jedes einzelnen Falles einer koordinatorischen Neurose nachzugehen; es wird sich dann nicht selten, und zwar bei den „Beschäftigungsneurosen" häufiger als beim Stottern zeigen, daß eine „echte Neurose" im Sinne einer seelischen Verursachung und Fixierung — wenn auch auf dem Boden einer besonderen Anlage — nur mit Zurückhaltung diagnostiziert werden kann, und daß zuweilen nachweisbar andere, organische Schäden die Hauptursache darstellen. So erwähnt etwa SITTIG in der obenangeführten Arbeit frühere Befunde von ANDRÉ THOMAS (Halsrippe bei Schreibkrampf); von BOURGIGNON und FAURE-BEAULIEU (partielle Neuritis des n. radialis infolge Arthritis deform. der Halswirbelsäule), von FR. KRAMER, der in einem Fall eine Atrophie des rechten Daumenballes nachwies. COSTEDOAT und AUJALEU analysierten 3 Fälle von Schreibkrampf, in denen neben einer angeborenen nervösen „Übererregbarkeit" und seelischen Störungen noch jeweils ein verschiedener Organschaden bestand (Osteophyten an Körpern der Halswirbel; RECKLINGHAUSENsche Krankheit; Scapulo- humerale Arthritis und Periarthritis). Gefäßerkrankungen, neuralgische Beschwerden als auslösende Bedingung sind häufig beschrieben worden, desgleichen eine unzweckmäßige Art des Schreibens selbst: Harte Federn, verkrampfte Haltung usw. Je mehr man bestrebt ist, organischen und jedenfalls außerseelischen Bedingungen nachzugehen, um so geringer wird die Zahl überwiegend seelisch verursachter „echter" Koordinationsneurosen sein. Es wiederholt sich hier die Erscheinung, die bei den Organneurosen ausführlicher beschrieben wurde, daß nämlich eine „neurotische Reaktion" am Beginn einer organischen Erkrankung des Nervensystems stehen kann und daß sie gleichwohl seelisch ausreichend determiniert zu sein scheint. So habe ich kürzlich eine Kranke mit schon recht fortgeschrittener multipler Sklerose gesehen, bei der vor Jahren — und zwar von Neurologen und Psychiatern — für lange Zeit ein Schreibkrampf diagnostiziert wurde. Allerdings hätten wohl schon damals die Klagen über Parästhesien in den Händen und vor allem die Tatsache, daß der Schreibkrampf auch links bestand — ohne daß die Kranke jemals Schreibmaschine geschrieben hatte — eher an einen zentralnervösen Prozeß denken lassen sollen. Daß andererseits zwischen organischer Erkrankung und ihrem Erlebnis mit aller störenden Beachtung, Beobachtung, Befürchtung ein geschlossener Kreis gegenseitiger Abhängigkeit und schädlicher Förderung besteht, ist bekannt genug.

Für die *Behandlung* gelten die gleichen Grundsätze, wie sie im Abschnitt über die Organneurosen ausführlicher dargestellt wurden. Kennzeichnend ist nur die Unerläßlichkeit einer „gymnastischen" Behandlung mit Ruhigstellung, motorischer Entspannungsübung und Neulernen von Sprechen, Schreiben und anderen berufsmäßigen Hantierungen. Aber Ähnliches strebt ja die Psychotherapie, besonders das autogene Training (I. H. SCHULTZ) auch für die Organe und Organsysteme an, die dem willkürlichen Einfluß in der Norm jedenfalls weitgehend entzogen sind.

2. Besonderer Teil.

a) Koordinatorische Beschäftigungsneurosen (Bewegungsneurosen).

Der *Schreibkrampf (Mogigraphie, Graphospasmus)* gilt noch immer mit Recht als Paradigma einer neurotischen Betriebsstörung, bei der ohne erkennbare organische Beeinträchtigung Muskelgruppen, die bei einer bestimmten, ursprünglich erlernten und allmählich automatisierten Leistung zusammenspielen, allmählich anfangen zu „krampfen". Bei den ganz reinen Formen bleibt auch dieser Krampf auf die eine Tätigkeit (Schreiben, Klavierspielen usw.) beschränkt. Die wissenschaftliche Kenntnis des Schreibkrampfes datiert seit CH. BELL (zit. bei CURSCHMANN). Männer sind häufiger befallen als Frauen und wenn wohl nicht zureichend bezweifelt werden kann, daß an dieser Verteilung die Tatsache schuld ist, daß mehr Männer als Frauen berufsmäßig schreiben und daß somit dem bestimmten Beruf *eine* auslösende Ursache zukommen wird, so wurde doch im allgemeinen Teil ausgeführt, daß dies möglicherweise nicht der einzige Grund ist für das ungleiche Befallensein der Geschlechter. Auch bei Kindern zeigt sich der Schreibkrampf gelegentlich und es wäre vielleicht lohnend, diesen Fällen auch mit Hilfe graphologischer Methoden nachzugehen. Bei Schriftuntersuchungen an Stotterern hat sich gezeigt (ROMÁN-GOLDZIEHER, SCHULMANN), daß enge Beziehungen zu verschiedenen Formen der Sprachstörungen, insbesondere zum Stottern bestehen. Es fanden sich Abwandlungen des Tempos, der Flüssigkeit des Ablaufes, schließlich weitgehende Störungen des Rhythmus. Bei Messung mit dem Graphodyn ergaben sich hohe Druckwerte. Es ließe sich denken, daß gelegentlich beiden Formen koordinatorischer Neurosen eine gemeinsame konstitutionelle oder dispositionelle Ursache zugrunde liegt und daß sie auf einer außergewöhnlichen Bereitschaft zur „Tonisierung" bestimmter Muskelgruppen beruht. Freilich trennt man von jeher unter den Erscheinungsformen des Schreibkrampfes von der eigentlich *spastischen,* die *paralytische* ab und kennt überdies noch eine *neuralgische* und eine *Tremor*-Form. Ich stimme CURSCHMANN zu, wenn er meint, daß sich gerade unter dem mit grobem Zittern der Hand- und Unterarmmuskeln verlaufenden Schreibkrampf hysterische Reaktionen oder organische Krankheiten, etwa eine multiple Sklerose, verbergen können. Mißempfindungen, ja schmerzhafte Gefühle in der betroffenen Muskulatur sind beim Schreibkrampf häufig und meist von einem Affekt des Mißmutes begleitet, der zu einem ungeduldigen Erzwingenwollen des Schreibaktes, aber noch häufiger zum verzagten Aufgeben führt oder zu gelegentlichen hypochondrischen Befürchtungen. Es soll aber auch eine rein neuralgische Form geben, wie CURSCHMANN meint sogar nicht selten, bei der es zwar zu

Parästhesien und Schmerzen komme, ohne daß jedoch eine Neuritis vorliegt; und bei der ein Krampf oder auch eine funktionelle Parese nicht eintritt. Lediglich der Schmerz, der beim Schreibakt einsetzt, verhindert das Schreiben. Aus eigener Erfahrung ist mir kein Fall dieser Art bekannt geworden. Gerade die Angaben in der Literatur, daß dieser neuralgische Typus häufiger Übergänge zum *hypotonisch-paralytischen* zeigen soll und umgekehrt lassen vermuten, daß sich bei beiden Formen gelegentlich doch organische Prozesse abspielen, auch wenn deren Diagnose aus den Erscheinungen nicht gesichert werden kann und neuropathische Stigmen sowie bekannte oder einleuchtend konstruierte seelische Gründe die Annahme einer „echten" Beschäftigungsneurose zu sichern scheinen. Der wirklich spastische Schreibkrampf stellt sich — wie auch die übrigen Formen in der Regel allmählich ein; das Tempo der Entwicklung hängt weitgehend ab von der Art, wie diese Störung erlebt und wie zu ihr Stellung genommen wird.

Es gibt auch rein neuropathische Unterbrechungen des Schreibaktes, Unsicherheiten, Verzerrungen des Schriftbildes, ohne daß es in derlei Fällen zu einem Krampf bestimmter Muskelgruppen kommt. Ich habe das bei allgemein neuropathischen Persönlichkeiten gesehen, bei denen schon eine harte Feder, die ungewohnte Dünne oder Dicke eines Halters, zu glattes oder auch zu rauhes Papier eine neurotische Schreibunsicherheit und die Neigung zu Unterbrechungen hervorrief. Die Überanstrengung besonders der Supinatoren durch fehlerhaftes Schreiben wird unter den pathogenetischen Faktoren immer wieder angegeben. Es kommt neben zunehmender Ermüdbarkeit zum Kleben am Federhalter und damit an Buchstaben, bis schließlich nach diesen Vorboten ein Krampfen der Beuger, besonders an den beiden ersten Fingern einsetzt, gelegentlich aber auch ein Streckkrampf des extensor indicis. Im weiteren Verlauf kann es zu einem Spreizen der Finger, ja einem krampfhaften Einschlagen des Daumens in die Hohlhand kommen; schließlich können alle am Schreibakt mitbeteiligten Muskeln des Armes bis zum Schultergürtel (Pro- und Supinatoren, Biceps, Triceps, Deltoideus) von diesem Krampf befallen sein. Die Störung führt gelegentlich zu einer „totalen peripheren Agraphie" (CURSCHMANN), d. h. zu einer völligen neurotischen Schreibunfähigkeit — während das Schreiben mit der Maschine selbst in derlei Zuständen noch ohne Mühe möglich sein kann. Es ist leicht einzusehen, daß in jedem Fall von Schreibkrampf seelische Einflüsse auftreten können, die das Leiden schon in seinen ersten Anfängen lebhaft zu steigern vermögen. Taktile Empfindungen und mit dem Schreibakt verknüpfte Gemeingefühle, aber auch die Einzelheiten der gesamten Bewegungsleistung, die alle sonst unter der Bewußtseinsschwelle ruhen, werden empfunden und registriert und unterbrechen damit den automatisierten Ablauf des Schreibaktes.

MOHNKOPF hat gezeigt, in welcher Weise eine solche Automatisierung von Handlungen, d. h. ein fast Unwillkürlichwerden ursprünglich willkürlich ausgeführter und erlernter Hantierungen vor sich geht. Die bewußten Antriebe fallen fort; bei Ausführung der Bewegung selbst tritt das kontrollierende Bewußtsein mehr und mehr zurück, dadurch wird eine größere Gleichzeitigkeit und Schnelligkeit von Bewegungen erreicht und außerdem die Fähigkeit, eine zweite Nebenleistung mit zu vollziehen. Jede Aufmerksamkeitszuwendung zur motorischen Form des Geschehens stört in einem und schließlich in allen diesen Gliedern den Bewegungsablauf. Unsicherheit, Erregung, Befürchtung, Erwartungsangst steigern das Übel mehr und mehr. Daß neben diesen mehr reaktiven seelischen Äußerungen auch seelische Konflikte einen Schreibkrampf verschlimmern oder auslösen können, ja daß sie dies entscheidend zu tun imstande sind, wurde wiederholt erwähnt. Auch kann der Schreibkrampf, wie jede andere Beschäftigungsneurose in echte und sicher nicht ganz zweckunbewußte hysterische Regie genommen werden. Die Differentialdiagnose gegenüber den sog. „Pseudo"-

formen bei hysterischen Zittern kann hier nicht immer leicht sein; das sichere Ausschließen einer doch organischen Ursache, oder Mit-Ursache ist jedoch nach meinen Erfahrungen schwieriger. Die *Behandlung* richtet sich nach der Pathogenese. Ruhe, Entspannungsübungen, Unterstützen des Schreibens durch allerlei Hilfen (breite, weiche Federn, möglichst Steilschrift, besondere Halter wie NUSSBAUMsches Bracelet, ZABLUDOWSKYs Federhalter) sind wohl notwendiges Requisit jeder Therapie. Die Berücksichtigung des — in der Regel ja neuropathischen — Allgemeinzustandes sowie der seelischen Wurzeln und schädlichen Einflüsse für den Schreibkrampf selbst, schließlich in manchen Fällen ernsthafte Psychopädagogik verstehen sich heute von allein. Die Prognose ist nicht gerade günstig; Besserungen lassen sich aber in den meisten Fällen erzielen.

Andere *Beschäftigungsneurosen* spielen praktisch eine weit seltenere Rolle. Die allgemeinen Voraussetzungen sind die gleichen wie beim Schreibkrampf, wenn auch jeweils andere, eben für die besondere Beschäftigung kennzeichnende Muskelgruppen befallen werden. So gibt es einen *Pianisten-* und einen *Geigerkrampf* (diesen vorwiegend linksseitig); einen *Telegraphistenkrampf* (CRONBACH); aber auch einen Krampf bei *Melkern*, bei *Falzern, Schneidern, Schustern* usw. Bei einem *Zigarrenwickler* sah ich eine „Beschäftigungsneurose" nach Schädeltrauma und zwar derart, daß die Fingerkuppen nicht mehr mit der früheren Kraft und Geschwindigkeit gegen die Hohlhand sich abwickeln konnten und sehr rasch unter Eintritt von Paraesthesien ermüdeten. Auch über Beschäftigungskrämpfe an den *Beinen* ist berichtet worden, so bei *Tänzerinnen*, Maschinennäherinnen, aber auch bei Soldaten. Hypertonische und hypotonische neurotische Funktionsstörungen im Bereich der *Lippen* wurden bei *Bläsern* beobachtet, in der *Zunge* bei Klarinettenbläsern (STRÜMPELL, STADLER zitiert bei OPPENHEIM, CURSCHMANN usw.). OPPENHEIM warnt vor einer Verwechslung all dieser seltenen Störungen mit echten *Arbeitslähmungen* (professionellen Paresen). Die Differentialdiagnose wird freilich nur da sicher möglich sein, wo neuritische oder andere Erscheinungen organischen Gepräges nachzuweisen sind.

b) Stottern.

Die funktionellen Störungen der Sprache sind im Laufe der letzten Jahre wiederholt und eingehend, z. T. monographisch dargestellt worden. Es hängt dies mit ihrer großen praktischen Bedeutung zusammen und damit einhergehend, mit der Tatsache, daß das Gebiet ein besonderes Maß spezialistischer Ausbildung und Erfahrung voraussetzt. Es hat sich allmählich eine eigene Disziplin entwickelt, die das gesamte Gebiet der Sprach- und Stimmheilkunde umfaßt. Von psychiatrisch-neurologischer Seite sind diesem Gebiet durch den Ausbau der Psychotherapie und neuerdings durch phonetische Untersuchungen (ZWIRNER) Anregungen zugeflossen. Hier kann nur auf das Stottern eingegangen werden, das als koordinatorische Störung schon von KUSSMAUL gedeutet wurde (reizbare Schwäche der sprachlichen Koordinationsapparate). Es darf nicht verwechselt werden mit dem *Stammeln*, das bestimmte Fehler der Aussprache umfaßt (Näseln, Lispeln, Stammeln bei einzelnen Lauten: T K usw.). Es handelt sich hier um Fehler der Aussprache, während das Stottern einen Fehler des Redeflusses darstellt, eine spastische Hemmung des Sprechens (H. GUTZMANN-NADOLECZNY). Das Stammeln stellt im wesentlichen eine Hemmung der sprachlichen Entwicklung dar mit allerlei Ersatzgewohnheiten und geringem oder fehlendem neurotischen Beiwerk, während für das Stottern ein mehr umgekehrtes Verhalten zutrifft. Allerdings hat schon GUTZMANN darauf hingewiesen, daß doch recht häufig auch das kindliche Stottern auf Eigentümlichkeiten der Sprechentwicklung mit zurückzuführen sei. Normalerweise tritt zwischen dem 3. und 4. Lebensjahr eine gewisse Sprachnot ein, ein

„physiologisches Stottern", das seine Ursache in dem Mißverhältnis zwischen sprachlichem Äußerungsbedürfnis und Sprechenkönnen, zwischen Gedanke und Wort hat. Ein übereiltes, hastiges Reden mit Stockungen, Verlegenheitslauten findet sich gelegentlich auch bei Erwachsenen von fahrigem Temperament und wird als *Poltern* bezeichnet. Auch dieses Poltern unterscheidet sich von der Sprachneurose Stottern dadurch, daß der charakteristische Hemmungszwang, „Dekoordinierung des Bewegungsablaufes" (v. STOCKERT) fehlt. Die Pathogenese und davon abhängend die Nomenklatur sind im Laufe der letzten Jahre häufig umstritten worden (FRÖSCHELS, HOEPFNER, NADOLECZNY u. a.). NADOLECZNY stellt verschiedene Bezeichnungen in seinem Referat 1931 zusammen: Intentionsneurose, Sprachzwangsneurose (TRÖMMER), Erwartungsneurose (ISSERLIN), Angstneurose (L. FRANK, HOMBURGER), Minderwertigkeitsneurose (SCRIPTURE), Kontaktneurose (v. STOCKERT), Striatumneurose (SCHILDER); dazu kommt der Ausdruck: sozioaffektive Dysphasie (I. S. GALANT). Eine besondere, von K. KLEIST und im Anschluß daran vor allem von NADOLESZNY bekämpfte Skala von Bezeichnungen stammt von HOEPFNER und ist vielfach übernommen worden. Sie schließt sich eng an seine Auffassung von der Psychogenie organsymptomatischer Sprachstörungen an: *Assoziative Aphasie* als rein psychogene Sprachstörung = Stottern. Im Gegensatz zu organischen Artikulationsstörungen („Sprachataxie"), bei denen das Bild der Gesichtsverzerrungen, der auffallenden Mitbewegungen, der Wortumgehung, aber auch der Angst des Stotterers fehle, liege beim Stottern die Ursache der spasmoiden Sprechbewegungen bzw. Hemmungen nur im Vorstellen. Zu der *„primär ataktischen"* Wiederholung von Silben und Lauten gesellt sich gewissermaßen ein Zuschuß an Sprechleistung, der unter den Formen der *„dynamisch-motorischen,* der *sensorisch-aphatischen* und der *abstraktiv-psychopathischen Rekonstruktionswillkür"* verlaufe. Es bildet sich seelisch ein Störungsbewußtsein aus, das über den Weg der Litteral-Verbalnegation und der abstraktiv-psychopathischen Funktionsnegation bis zur Lebensnegation sich entwickeln könne. Die Bedeutung des Willkürlichen („Assoziativen") für die Entstehung des Stotterns ist neben HOEPFNER besonders von FROESCHELS, aber auch von v. STOCKERT u. a. betont worden, während sich ältere Autoren, aber auch NADOLECZNY gegen die Allgültigkeit dieses Weges ausgesprochen haben. Soviel darf heute wohl als gesichert gelten, daß sich jedenfalls in sehr vielen Fällen (FRÖSCHELS meint — immer; NADOLECZNY fand es in $^2/_3$ von 300 Kranken) das Stottern aus dem Silben- und Lautwiederholen, oder auch aus dem Langziehen eines Lautes (FLATAU) entwickelt. Ein gewisses pathogenetisches Schema wird neben HOEPFNER insbesondere von FRÖSCHELS angegeben, der sogar die Zwangsläufigkeit dieser Stotterentwicklung betont: es kommt nach dem noch physiologischen Wiederholen von Lauten und Silben zum Pressen, dann zu Mitbewegungen, zum Zucken und Aufblähen der Nasenflügel, später zu einem raschen, manchmal sich jagenden Wechsel zwischen Pressen und Wiederholung, dann zur Lautfurcht, bis am Ende *„kaschiertes Stottern"* auftritt: Kurzes Verstummen, Erröten, starrer Blick, Nasenflügelatmen und dahinter eine deutliche innere, ängstlich gefärbte Erregung. Daß gleichwohl allem Stottern eine besondere Organbereitschaft, Organminderwertigkeit zugrunde liegt, wird heute wohl übereinstimmend angenommen. Es wurde schon erwähnt, daß dies auch für die Fälle des „induzierten" und des — von manchen Autoren davon noch abgetrennten — *Nachahmungsstotterns* gilt, die beide angeblich auch ohne Anamnese, allein aus der Art des Stotterns erkannt werden können. Auch die vermutete Art dieser Krankheitsbereitschaft wurde im allgemeinen Teil bereits abgehandelt. Es soll hier noch ausgeführt werden, daß Konstitutionsuntersuchungen auf Grund der KRETSCHMERschen Typenlehre kein sicheres Ergebnis brachten. Auch NADOLECZNY hat Cyclothyme und

Schizothyme in seinem Material gefunden; er hebt auch die Erblichkeit des Stotterns und gleichzeitig die Tatsache hervor, daß unter 1000 Fällen mehr als die doppelte Anzahl stotterfreier Geschwister vorhanden war: Ein Ergebnis, das gegen eine nennenswerte Bedeutung von Ansteckung und Nachahmung spricht. Daß sich im Lauf der Jahre, auch ohne ärztliche oder ohne nennenswerte — jedenfalls sachkundige — Behandlung das Stottern bis auf geringe Reste (initiale Mitbewegungen, einzelne Flickworte) oder nur noch gelegentlich, situativ bedingtes Deutlicherwerden verlieren kann, ist nicht allzu selten zu beobachten; auch das Zurücktreten beim Chorsprechen, beim Singen, bei heilpädagogischen Übungen — im Gegensatz zum Verhalten in häuslicher Umgebung — ist häufig beschrieben worden. Es hängt dies mit seelischen Einflüssen (Mühegeben, Gehenlassen, Verlieren von Ängstlichkeit) zusammen; beim Singen aber vielleicht auch damit, daß es sich hierbei um willkürlich erlernte und „bewußter" ausgeführte Bewegungen handelt als beim Sprechen (CIAMPI), so wie ja auch gelegentlich ein mehr schauspielerhaftes oder pathetisches Sprechen das Stottern fast verschwinden läßt. Mir scheinen gerade solche Beobachtungen, wie auch die Neigung zu Mitbewegungen ein Hinweis darauf zu sein, daß dem Stottern eine zentralnervöse — vielleicht extrapyramidale Anlageschwäche zugrunde liegt, unbeschadet aller Anerkennung seelischer Mitursachen bis zu tiefgehenden Lebenskonflikten.

Die *Behandlung* des Stotterns wird neben der Übungsbehandlung (HOEPFNER ist soweit ich sehe, allerdings ein Gegner aller Versuche dieser Art) genau wie bei den übrigen, mehr isoliert sich abspielenden Neurosen pädagogisch-psychotherapeutische Methoden anwenden und je nach den Umständen — etwa bei der sog. „*initialen Form des Stotterns*" (FRANK) im Verlauf echt neurasthenischer Reaktionen — auch allgemein roborierende Mittel verordnen müssen. Eine Erziehung in Stotterkursen wird von *Rothe* abgelehnt und statt dessen die Errichtung von Klassen für Sprachgestörte, womöglich bis zum Schulende gefordert. Eine Therapie, die die ganze Persönlichkeit erfasse, erziehe, neu einstelle, ist auch hier ein etwas hochgespannter Wunsch, der selten Wirklichkeit wird.

Literatur.

A. *Monographien und zusammenfassende Darstellungen.*

ADLER, ALFR.: Studie über Minderwertigkeit von Organen. München 1907 u. 1927. — ALKAN, LEOP.: Anatomische Organkrankheiten aus seelischer Ursache. Stuttgart 1930. — BAUER, J.: Die konstitutionelle Disposition zu inneren Krankheiten. Berlin 1924. — BERGER, H.: Über die körperlichen Äußerungen psychischer Zustände. Jena 1904. — BERGMANN, G. v.: Klinische funktionelle Pathologie des vegetativen Nervensystems. Handbuch der normalen und pathologischen Physiologie, Bd. 16, H. 1. Berlin 1930. — Funktionelle Pathologie, eine klinische Sammlung von Ergebnissen und Anschauungen einer Arbeitsrichtung. Berlin 1932. — BERGMANN, G. v. u. E. BILLIGHEIMER: Das vegetative Nervensystem und seine Störungen. Handbuch der inneren Medizin von G. v. BERGMANN u. R. STAEHELIN, Bd. 5, Teil II. Nervensystem 2. Berlin 1926. — BICKEL: Die wechselseitigen Beziehungen zwischen psychischem Geschehen und Blutkreislauf mit besonderer Berücksichtigung der Psychosen. Leipzig 1916. — BIEDL: Innere Sekretion. Berlin 1916. — BLEULER, E.: Affektivität, Suggestibilität, Paranoia, 2. Aufl. 1926. — BRAUN, E.: Psychogene Reaktion. BUMKES Handbuch der Geisteskrankheiten, Bd. 5, Spezieller Teil I. Berlin 1928. — Die vitale Person. Leipzig 1933. — BRAUN, L.: Herz und Psyche in ihren Wirkungen aufeinander. Leipzig u. Wien 1926. — BRÜCKE, G. TH.: Fortschritte in der Erkenntnis des vegetativen Nervensystems. Naturwiss. 1928. — BUMKE, O.: Die Störung des sympathischen Systems. Handbuch der Neurologie von LEWANDOWSKY, Bd. 1. 1910. — Die Revision der Neurosenfrage. Referat Kassel 1925. — Verh. Ges. dtsch. Nervenärzte. Münch. med. Wschr. **1925 II**, 1815 f. — Lehrbuch der Geisteskrankheiten, 3. Aufl., 1929. — Die Psychoanalyse (eine Kritik). Berlin 1931.

CANNON: Bodily changes in pain, hunger, fear and rage. New York u. London 1929. — CIMBAL: Die Bedeutung der endokrinen Vorgänge für Psychosen und Neurosen. Handbuch der inneren Sekretion von MAX HIRSCH, Bd. 3, Lief. 4. Leipzig 1928.

Das vegetative Nervensystem. Verh. Ges. dtsch. Nervenärzte Hamburg **1928**. — DRESEL: Erkrankungen des vegetativen Nervensystems. Spezielle Pathologie und Therapie innerer Krankheiten. Herausgeg. von KRAUS u. BRUGSCH, Bd. X, Teil 3, Nervenkrankheiten 3. 1924. — Die Neurosen des vegetativen Nervensystems. Vagotonie und Sympathicotonie. Erg. Med. **1921**. — DREYFUSS: Über nervöse Dyspepsie. Jena 1908. — DURIG, A.: Über Blutdruck und Blutdruckmessung. Wien. med. Wschr. **1932** I, 6—9, 82—85, 112—114. EPPINGER u. HESS: Die Vagotonie. Berlin 1910. — EPPINGER, v. POPP u. SCHWARZ: Das Asthma cardiale. Berlin 1924.
FABER, KNUD: Die Krankheiten des Magens und Darmes. Berlin 1924. — FAHRENKAMP: Die psychophysischen Wechselwirkungen bei den Hypertonieerkrankungen. Hippokrates-Verlag 1926. — FENDEL, HEINZ: Die vegetative Neurose als kausaler Faktor in der Genese körperlicher und seelischer Erkrankungen. Frankfurt 1927. — FLEISCHER, FR.: Die Magenneurosen. Ergebnisse der gesamten Medizin. Herausgeg. von TH. BRUGSCH Bd. 8, H. 1/2. Berlin u. Wien 1926. — FLEISCHHACKER, H.: Die trophischen Einflüsse des Nervensystems. Handbuch der normalen und pathologischen Physiologie, Bd. 10. 1927. — FRANK, LUDW.: Affektstörungen, Studien über ihre Ätiologie und Therapie. Berlin 1913. — FRÖHLICH, A.: Pharmakologie des vegetativen autonomen Nervensystems. Handbuch der normalen und pathologischen Physiologie Bd. 10. 1927.
GRODDECK: Psychische Bedingtheit und psychisch-analytische Behandlung organischer Leiden. Leipzig 1917. — GUTTMANN, E.: Organische Krankheitsbilder hysterischen Gepräges. Fortschr. Neur. 4 (1932).
HARTMANN, NIKOLAI: Das Problem des geistigen Seins. Berlin u. Leipzig 1933. — HESS, W. R.: Die Regulierung des Blutkreislaufes. Leipzig 1930. — Die Regulierung der Atmung, gleichzeitig ein Beitrag zur Physiologie des vegetativen Nervensystems. Leipzig 1931. — HEYER, G. R.: Das körperlich-seelische Zusammenwirken in den Lebensvorgängen. Grenzfrag. Nerv.- u. Seelenleb. **1925**, H. 121. — HOFFMANN, H. F.: Das Problem der Neurosen in moderner klinischer Beleuchtung. Ref. 57. Verslg südwestdtsch. Neur. u. Psychiater 1932. Z. Neur. **1932**, 141, 267. — HOLUB, ARTHUR: Die Lehre von der Organminderwertigkeit. Leipzig 1931.
JAENSCH, W.: Grundzüge einer Physiologie und Klinik der psychophysischen Persönlichkeit. Ein Beitrag zur funktionellen Diagnostik. Berlin 1926. — JAHRREISS, W.: Das hypochondrische Denken. Arch. f. Psychiatr. **92** (1930).
KÄMMERER, H.: Allergische Diathese und allergische Erkrankungen. München 1926. — KAHN, EUGEN: Psychopathische Persönlichkeiten. BUMKES Handbuch der Geisteskrankheiten, Bd. 5, Spez. Teil I. — KATSCH: Magenneurosen. Handbuch von MOHR-STAEHELIN, 2. Aufl., Bd. 3. 1926. — KAUFMANN, FR.: Pathologie des arteriellen Hochdrucks. Handbuch der normalen und pathologischen Physiologie, Bd. 7, H. 2. — KEHRER, F.: ,,Neurosen." Handwörterbuch der medizinischen Physiologie von BIRNBAUM. Leipzig 1930. — KLAGES, LUDWIG: Ausdrucksbewegung und Gestaltungskraft. Leipzig 1923. — KLEWITZ: Das Bronchialasthma. Dresden u. Leipzig: Theodor Steinkopff 1928. — KLOTZ, R.: Die organischen Grundlagen der Neurasthenie. Dresden u. Leipzig: Theodor Steinkopff 1929. — KRAUS, F.: Syszygiologie der Person. Leipzig 1916 u. 1923. — Allgemeine und spezielle Pathologie der Person-Tiefenperson. Leipzig 1926. — KREHL, L. v.: Krankheitsform und Persönlichkeit. Leipzig 1929. — KRETSCHMER, E.: Körperbau und Charakter. 5. u. 6. Aufl. Berlin 1926. — KROETZ, CHRISTIAN: Allgemeine Physiologie der autonomen nervösen Correlationen. Handbuch der normalen und pathologischen Physiologie, Bd. 16, Teil II. 1931. — KRONFELD, A.: Psychophysische Beziehungen bei den Organneurosen. Jkurse ärztl. Fortbildg **1932**, H. 5. — KÜPPERS, E.: Puls, Blutdruck, vasomotorische Störungen, Blutverteilung. BUMKES Handbuch der Geisteskrankheiten, Bd. 3. Berlin 1928.
LAIGNEL-LAVASTINE, DE: La méthode concentrique dans l'étude des psichonévroses. Leçons cliniques de la Pitié. Paris 1927. — LANGE, JOHANNES: Die endogenen und reaktiven Gemütserkrankungen etc. BUMKES Handbuch der Geisteskrankheiten, Bd. 6, Spez. Teil II. — LANGLEY: Das autonome Nervensystem, Teil I. Berlin 1922. — LESCHKE, E.: Erkrankungen des vegetativen Nervensystems. Handbuch der inneren Sekretion, Bd. 3, 1. Hälfte. Leipzig 1928 und ,,Nachtrag" 1931. — LEWY, F. H.: Die Lehre vom Tonus und der Bewegung. Berlin 1933. — LEYSER, EDG.: Das Neurosenproblem vom lebenswissenschaftlichen Standpunkt aus. Berlin 1927.
MACKENZIE, J.: Angina pectoris. London 1923. — MATTHAEI, R.: Das Gestaltproblem. München 1929. — MAYER, A.: Psychologisches aus der gynäkologischen Sprechstunde. Würzburg. Abh. **27**, H. 12. Leipzig 1932. — MOHR, FR.: Psychophysische Behandlungsmethoden. Leipzig 1925. — MONAKOW, P. v.: Über die zentrale Repräsentation vegetativer Funktionen. Schweiz. Arch. Psychiatr. **32** (1933). — MONAKOW, C. v. u. R. MOURGUE: Biologische Einführung in das Studium der Neurologie und Psychopathologie. Hippokrates-Verlag 1930. — MOSSO, A.: Kreislauf des Blutes. Leipzig 1881. — MÜLLER, L. R.: Die Lebensnerven. Berlin 1924. — Lebensnerven und Lebenstriebe, 3. Aufl. Berlin 1931. — MÜLLER, OTFRIED: Die Blutdruckkrankheit.

Oehme, Curt u. Herm. Paal: Die Reid-Hunt-Reaktion. Erg. inn. Med. **44**, 214 (1932). — Oswald: Psyche und vegetatives System. Berlin 1929.
Pawlow, J. P.: Die höchste Nerventätigkeit (das Verhalten) von Tieren. München 1926. — Pollnow, Hans: Das Leib-Seele-Problem und die psychophysischen Korrelationen. Brugsch-Lewys Biologie der Person, Bd. 2, S. 1001—1092. 1931. — Pophal: Das vegetative Nervensystem und seine klinische Bedeutung. Erg. inn. Med. **19**.
Redlich, E.: Referat über die Neurosenfrage. Verh. dtsch. Nervenärzte **1925**. — Romberg, v.: Lehrbuch der Krankheiten des Herzens. Stuttgart 1925. — Rosenfeld, M.: Die Beziehungen innersekretorischer Vorgänge zu psychopathologischen Phänomenen. Zbl. Neur. **57**, 1 (1930). — Rudder, M. de: Wetter und Jahreszeit als Krankheitsfaktoren. Berlin 1931.
Scheler, M.: Die Stellung des Menschen im Kosmos. Darmstadt 1928. — Schilder, P.: Organneurosen. Jkurse ärztl. Fortbildg **19** (1928, Mai). — Schindler, R.: Nervensystem und spontane Blutungen mit besonderer Berücksichtigung der hysterischen Ekchymosen und der Systematik der hämorrhagischen Diathesen. Abh. Neur. **1927**, H. 42. — Schneider, K.: Die abnormen seelischen Reaktionen. Leipzig u. Wien 1926. — Pathopsychologie im Grundriß. Handbuch für psychische Hygiene. Berlin 1931. — Schottky, Johannes: Innere Krankheiten und Psychiatrie. Fortschr. Neur. **5** (1933). — Schröder, P.: Stimmungen und Verstimmungen. Leipzig 1930. — Schultz, I. H.: Konstitutionelle Nervosität. Bumkes Handbuch der Geisteskrankheiten, Bd. 5, Spez. Teil I. 1928. — Die seelische Krankenbehandlung. Jena 1930. — Organneurosen als psychotherapeutisches Problem. Fortschr. Neur. **4** (1932). — Das autogene Training. (Konzentrative Selbstentspannung.) Leipzig 1932. — Schwarz, O.: Psychogenese und Psychotherapie körperlicher Symptome. Wien 1925. — Spiegel, E. A.: Autonomes Nervensystem. Handbuch der normalen und pathologischen Physiologie, Bd. 10. 1927. — Die Zentren des autonomen Nervensystems. Monographien Neur. u. Psych. **1928**, H. 54. — Stertz, G.: Die neurasthenische Reaktion. Bumkes Handbuch der Geisteskrankheiten, Bd. 5. Berlin 1928. — Storm van Leeuwen: Allergische Krankheiten. Berlin 1926. — Straus, Erw.: Geschehnis und Erlebnis. Berlin 1930. — Szondi, L.: Die Revision der Neurastheniefrage. Leipzig 1930.
Trendelenburg, P.: Die Hormone, T. 1. Berlin 1929.
Veraguth: Das psychogalvanische Reflexphänomen. Berlin 1909. — Vorkastner: Organneurosen. Handbuch der Neurologie, herausgeg. von Lewandowsky.
Weber: Der Einfluß psychischer Vorgänge auf den Körper. Berlin 1910. — Weizsäcker, V. v.: Die Neuroregulation. Verh. dtsch. Ges. inn. Med. Wiesbaden **1931**. — Wenkebach: Die unregelmäßige Herztätigkeit. Leipzig 1914. — Wenzel, A.: Das Leib-Seele-Problem. Leipzig: F. Meiner 1933. — Wyss, W. H. v.: Einfluß psychischer Vorgänge auf Atmung, Pulsfrequenz, Blutdruck und Blutverteilung. Handbuch der normalen und pathologischen Physiologie, Bd. 16, II, S. 2. — Körperlich-seelische Zusammenhänge in Gesundheit und Krankheit. Leipzig 1931.

B. Einzelarbeiten.

Achelis, J. D.: Der ärztliche Begriff des Organismus. Vorträge des Instituts der Geschichte der Medizin Leipzig, Bd. 3. 1930. — Adler: Beiträge zur Lehre von der organischen Grundlage der Psychoneurosen. Österr. Ärzteztg **9**, Nr 23 (1912). — Adler, A.: Über corticale und funktionelle nervöse Blasenstörungen. Dtsch. Z. Nervenheilk. **65**, H. 1/2 (1920). — Das organische Substrat der Psychoneurose. Vortrag, Bd. 6. — Die Individualpsychologie in der Neurosenlehre. Dtsch. med. Wschr. **1929 I**, 213. — Adlersberg u. Porges: Die neurotische Atmungstetanie. Wien. Arch. inn. Med. **8** (1924). — Altenburger, H. u. F. W. Kroll: Über die vegetative Beeinflussung des sog. Nervensystems. Pflügers Arch. **223** (1929). — Suggestive Beeinflussung der Sensibilität. Z. Neur. **124**, 538 (1930). — Allers, R.: Psychotherapie. Psychogenese und Psychotherapie körperlicher Symptome, herausgeg. von O. Schwarz. Wien 1925. — Aschner: Über einen noch nicht beschriebenen Reflex vom Auge auf Kreislauf und Atmung. Wien. klin. Wschr. **1908 II**. — Astruck, P.: Über psychische Beeinflussung des vegetativen Nervensystems in der Hypnose. Arch. f. Psychol. **45**, 266 (1923).
Bäumler: Über die Beeinflussung der Herztätigkeit in der Hypnose. Münch. med. Wschr. **1917 II**. — Bansi, H. W.: Kreislaufstudien beim Basedow und bei der Herzneurose. Z. klin. Med. **110**, 633—684 (1929). — Bauer, J.: Zur Funktionsprüfung des vegetativen Nervensystems. Dtsch. Arch. klin. Med. **107** (1912). — Die individuelle Konstitution als Grundlage nervöser Störungen. Psychogenese und Psychotherapie körperlicher Symptome, herausgeg. von O. Schwarz. Wien 1925. — Zur Kenntnis der Neurosen des Rectums. Med. Welt **1932**. — Beckmann, K.: Über Änderungen in der Atmungsregulation durch psychische und pharmakologische Einflüsse. Dtsch. Arch. klin. Med. **117** (1915). — Behrenroth, E.: Die sexuelle psychogene Herzneurose (Phrenokardie). Dtsch. med. Wschr. **1913 I**, 106. — Bergmann, G. v.: Die nervösen Erkrankungen des Magens. Verh. dtsch. Ges. inn. Med. **1924**. — Von chronischer Gastritis, Achylia gastrica und gastrogenen

Diarrhoen. Jkurse ärztl. Fortbildg **1926**. — Zum Abbau der „Organneurosen" als Folge interner Diagnostik. Dtsch. med. Wschr. **1927** Nr 49. — Die „vegetativ Stigmatisierten". Med. Klin. **1928,** 844. — Z. klin. Med. **108** (1928). — Psychophysische Vorgänge im Bereiche der Klinik. Dtsch. med. Wschr. **1930** II, 1684—1688. — BERGMANN, G. v. u. M. GOLDNER: Die vegetativ Stigmatisierten und die Reaktion nach REID-HUNT. Z. klin. Med. **108,** 100 (1928). — BETTMANN, S.: Zur Frage der psychogenen Hauterkrankungen. Nervenarzt **1,** 513—520 (1928). — BICKEL: Über die wechselseitigen Beziehungen zwischen den Vorgängen des Bewußtseins und der Innervation des Gefäßsystems. Med. Klin. **1915** I. — BIER: Höchstleistungen durch seelische Einflüsse und Daseinsnotwendigkeiten. Münch. med. Wschr. **1924** II. — BILLIGHEIMER: Über einen Antagonismus zwischen Pilocarpin und Adrenalin. Beitrag zur Innervation der Schweißdrüsen. Arch. f. exper. Path. **88** (1920). — Das Problem der Schweißdrüseninnervation und seine Bedeutung für die Klinik. Münch. med. Wschr. **1921** I. — BING, R.: Über lokale Muskelspasmen und Tics, nebst Bemerkungen zur Revision des Begriffes der Psychogenie. Schweiz. med. Wschr. **1925,** 933. — BINSWANGER, H.: Beobachtungen an entspannten und versenkten Personen. Nervenarzt **1929,** 193. — BINSWANGER, L.: Lebensfunktion und innere Lebensgeschichte. Mschr. Psychiatr. **68** (1928). — BINSWANGER, OTTO: Zur Pathogenese der Organneurosen. Dtsch. med. Wschr. **1928** II. — BLEULER, E.: Psychophysische Theorien in der Auffassung der Hysterie. Z. Neur. **141** (1932). — BLOCH, BRUNO: Über die Heilung der Warzen durch Suggestion. Klin. Wschr. **1927** II. — BLOEDORN, W. A.: Cardiacs neuroses. Ann. clin. Med. **4** (1925). — BOENHEIM, FELIX: Endokrin bedingte Neurosen. Arch. Verdgskrkh. **42,** H. 4 (1928). — BOGEN: Experimentelle Untersuchungen über psychische und assoziative Magensaftsekretion beim Menschen. Arch. ges. Psychol. **117** (1907). — BRAENKER, W.: Die Anatomie und Chirurgie des vegetativen Nervensystems. Verh. Ges. dtsch. Nervenärzte Hamburg **1929**. — BRAHN, M.: Experimentelle Beiträge zur Gefühlslehre. Philos. Stud. **18** (1903). — BRAUN, L.: Psychogene Störungen der Herztätigkeit. Psychogenese und Psychotherapie körperlicher Symptome. Herausgeg. von O. SCHWARZ. Wien **1925**. — Über Asthma bronchiale. Psychogenese und Psychotherapie körperlicher Symptome. Herausgeg. von O. SCHWARZ. Wien **1925**. — Die Psyche der Herzkranken. Z. Psychol. **1,** 106 (1928). — BRILL, E.: Zur Frage des vegetativen Systems bei Hautkranken. Dtsch. med. Wschr. **1932** II. — BRÜCKE, E. TH. VON: Einflüsse des vegetativen Nervensystems auf Vorgänge innerhalb des animalischen Systems. Erg. Physiol. **34,** 220 (1932). — BUMKE, O.: Der Arzt als Ursache seelischer Störungen. Dtsch. med. Wschr. **1925** I. — Ziele, Wege und Grenzen der Psychiatrischen Forschung. Handbuch der Geisteskrankheiten, Bd. 1, Allg. Teil 1. — BUNNEMANN: Über die Erklärbarkeit suggestiver Erscheinungen. Mschr. Psychiatr. **34,** 349. — Über die Organfiktion. Beiheft 1 zu den Annalen der Philosophie. Leipzig: Felix Meiner. — Über psychogene Dermatosen. Z. Neur. **78,** 115 (1922). — Neue Beiträge zur Frage der Psychogenese von Hautsymptomen. Z. Neur. **88,** 589 (1924). — Tatsachen dermatologischer Psychogenese und daraus sich ergebende Folgerungen. 2. allg. ärztl. Kongr. Psychother. **1927**. — BUYTENDIJK: Kritik der Reflextheorie auf Grund der Erforschung der Verhaltensweisen beim Tier. Verh. dtsch. Ges. inn. Med. **1931**.

CANNON, W. B.: The JAMES LANGE Theory of emotions: a critical examination etc. Amer. J. Psychol. **39** (1927). — Erg. Physiol. **27,** 380 (1928). — The autonomic nervous system. Lancet **1930** I; 1109. — CENI, CARLO: Psiche e vita organica. L'attivita psico-neuroendocrina. Milano Ist. edit. Sci. **1925**. — CHRISTOFFEL, H.: Einiges über Neurosen und Psychoneurosen, Physiogenese und Psychogenese. Praxis **1925,** Nr 30. — Zur Biologie der Enuresis. Z. Kinderpsychiatr. **1** (1934). — CIMBAL, W.: Dysmenorrhoe als Organneurose. Arch. Frauenkde u. Konstit.forsch. **12,** H. 3 (1926). — Die vegetativen Äquivalente der Depressionszustände. 18. Jverslg Ges. dtsch. Nervenärzte **1928**. — CRAMER, H. u. E. WITTKOWER: Über affektiv somatische Veränderungen. Klin. Wschr. **1930,** 1296. — CURSCHMANN, H.: Zur Frage der Organneurosen. Med. Klin. **1926** II. — Über nervöse Dyspepsien. Klin. Wschr. **1925** II. — Die somatische Symptomatologie der Organneurosen. Verh. Ges. dtsch. Nervenärzte **1928**.

DANIELOPOLU u. CARRIOL: Arch. Mal. Coeur **1923,** No 3. — DANISCH, F.: Innere Sekretion und vegetatives Nervensystem. Klin. Wschr. **1928** I. — DATTNER, B.: Über Pharmakotherapie der Neurosen. Dtsch. Z. Nervenheilk. **1925**. — Neue Wege der Neurosentherapie mit Ausblicken auf den zyklischen Formenkreis. Z. Neur. **104,** 256 (1926). — Ernährungsprobleme in der Neurologie und Psychiatrie. Z. Neur. **111** (1927). — Analysen zur Somatogenese der Neurosen. Klin. Wschr. **1929** I. — DAVID, E.: Über die Pathogenese von Angstzuständen, sowie über ihre Therapie. Psychiatr.-neurol. Wschr. **1926** I. — DENNING, H., K. FISCHER u. K. BERINGER: Psyche und vegetatives Nervensystem. Dtsch. Arch. klin. Med. **167,** 26 (1930). — DEUTSCH: Psychoanalyse und Organkrankheiten. Internat. Z. Psychoanal. **1922,** H. 3. — Experimentelle Studien zur Entstehung der Organneurose. Verh. Kongr. inn. Med. **1923**. — DEUTSCH, F. u. E. KAUF: Psychophysische Kreislaufstudien. Z. exper. Med. **32** (1923). — DIEDEN: Die Innervation der Schweißdrüsen. Dtsch. med. Wschr. **1918** II. — DRACONLIDES, N.: L'émotion considérée comme antigene on créant

un terrain propre a l'éclosion des Dermatoses (psychodermatoses). Bull. Soc. franç. Dermat. **39**, H. 8 (1932). — DREIKURS, RUDOLF: Das nervöse Symptom. Wien. med. Wschr. **1932** I.
EDENS, E.: Münch. med. Wschr. **1932** II. — EICHELBERG: Durch Hypnose erzeugtes ,,hysterisches" Fieber. Dtsch. Z. Nervenheilk. **1921**, 352. — ELLER, JOS. JORD.: Neurogenic and psychogenic disorders of the skin. Med. J. a. Rec. **129** (1929). — ENKE, W.: Die Affektivität der Konstitutionstypen im psychogalvanischen Versuch. Z. Neur. **138** (1932). — ESKUCHEN: Die Pathogenese des Asthma bronchiale. Klin. Wschr. **1926** I. — EXNER, ROB.: Grundumsatz und spezifisch-dynamische Wirkung bei Neurosen. Z. Neur. **121**, 308 (1929).

FAHRENKAMP, K.: Psychomotorische Beziehungen beim Herzkranken. Nervenarzt **2** (1929). — FELDBERG, W. u. E. SCHILF: Histamin und histaminähnliche Substanzen. Zbl. Neur. **52** (1929). — FELIX, K.: Chemie der stofflichen Kreislaufregulation. Klin. Wschr. **1933** I, 5. — FLANDIN, O. N.: Les réactions cutanées d'origine émotive. Ref. Zbl. Neur. **45**, 112. — FLATAU, G.: Angstneurosen und vasomotorische Störungen. Med. Klin. **1913** II. FOERSTER, O.: Diskussionsbemerkung. Zbl. Neur. **50**, 795. — FOERSTER, O. u. H. ALTENBURGER: Über die Beziehungen des vegetativen Nervensystems zur Sensibilität. Med. Klin. **1929** I, 519. — FOERSTER, O., H. ALTENBURGER u. F. W. KROLL: Über die Beziehungen des vegetativen Nervensystems zur Sensibilität. Z. Neur. **121** (1929). — FRANK, E.: Die parasympathische Innervation der quergestreiften Muskulatur und ihre klinische Bedeutung. Klin. Wschr. **1920** II. — Die Klinik und Pathologie des vegetativen Nervensystems. 18. Jverslg Ges. dtsch. Nervenärzte 1928. — FRIEDLÄNDER: Psychoneurose und Diabetes insipid. Ges. Nervenärzte 1910. Z. Org. **3**. Zbl. Neur. **2**, 344 f. — FRÖHLICH u. MEYER: Zur Frage der viszeralen Sensibilität. Klin. Wschr. **1922** II.

GESSLER, H. u. K. HANSEN: Über die suggestive Beeinflußbarkeit der Wärmeregulation in der Hypnose. Dtsch. Arch. klin. Med. **156** (1927). — GIGON, A., E. AIGNER u. W. BRAUCH: Über den Einfluß der Psyche auf körperliche Vorgänge. Schweiz. med. Wschr. **1926** II. — GLASER: Psychische Beeinflussung des Blutserumkalkspiegels. Klin. Wschr. **1924** I. — Die inneren Organe unter dem Einfluß des willkürlichen und unwillkürlichen Nervensystems. Dtsch. med. Wschr. **1925** I. — GOLDSCHEIDER, A.: Die Neurosenfrage. Dtsch. med. Wschr. **1927** II. — GOLDSTEIN, K.: Die Beziehungen der Psychoanalyse zur Biologie. Ber. 2. allg. ärztl. Kongr. Psychother. **1927**. — Das psychophysische Problem in seiner Bedeutung für ärztliches Handeln. Ther. Gegenw. **72** (1931). — Zum Problem der Angst. Allg. ärztl. Z. Psychother. **2**, 409. — GOLLWITZER-MEIER: Pflügers Arch. **222** (1929). — GRÄFENBERG, E.: Die Reichweite des psychogenen Faktors in der Frauenheilkunde. Allgem. ärztl. Z. Psychother. **2**, 665 f. (1929). — GRAFE u. MAYER: Z. Neur. **86** (1923). — GRAFE, E. u. L. MAYER: Über den Einfluß der Affekte auf den Gesamtstoffwechsel. Z. Neur. **1927**, 47. GRAFE u. TRAUMANN: Z. Neur. **62** (1920). — GRUENZWEIG, B.: Proteinkörpertherapie bei Störungen im vegetativen Nervensystem. Ref. Zbl. Neur. **50**, 775 (1928). — GRUMACH, L.: Über Suggestivbehandlung von Warzen. Münch. med. Wschr. **1931** II. — GUBERGRITZ, M.: Darmneurosen. Arch. Verdgskrkh. **44** (1928).

HAHN, B.: Die Psychogenese gynäkologisch-sexueller Symptome und deren psychotherapeutische Behandlung. Fortschr. Med. **44**, 676 (1926). — Innere Sekretion und Neurose. 2. allg. ärztl. Kongr. Psychother. **1927**. — HANKE, H.: Vegetativ peptische und toxische Gastritis im Experiment. Klin. Wschr. **1934** I, 1461. — HANSEN, K.: Die Organdetermination in den psychogenen Neurosen. Verh. dtsch. Ges. inn. Med. **1924**. — 1. allg. ärztl. Kongr. Psychother. Baden-Baden 1926. — Analyse, Indikation und Grenze der Psychotherapie beim Bronchialasthma. 2. allg. psychother. Kongr. 1927. — Zur Theorie der Symptombildung in der Neurose. Nervenarzt **1** (1928). — Psychische Beeinflussung des vegetativen Nervensystems. Naturwiss. 1928. — Magenbeschwerden als Ausdruck einer forme fruste der Tetanie. Nervenarzt **1** (1928). — Zur Frage der Psycho- oder Organogenese beim allergischen Bronchialasthma und den verwandten Krankheiten. Nervenarzt **3**, 513 (1930). — HANSEN, K. u. W. REISCH: Über humorale Herznervenwirkung. Z. Biol. **92** (1932). — HATTINGBERG, V.: Das Atemkorsett. Münch. med. Wschr. **1928** II. — HATTINGBERG, H. v.: Aufbau der Grundhaltung als Aufgabe wahrhafter ärztlicher Psychotherapie. Med. Welt **1932**, 1337. — HEIDEMANN, H.: Zwei Fälle abnormer Pigmentierung im Anschluß psychischer Affekte. Ugeskr. Laeg. (dän.) **1932**. — Ref. Zbl. Neur. **67**. — HERZ, M.: Die Herzneurosen. Ref. STULZ, Bd. 1, S. 282 f. — HERZBERG, A.: Der Erregungshemmungskonflikt in der Ätiologie der Neurosen. Allg. ärztl. Z. Psychother. **1**, 464 (1928). — HESS, L.: Bemerkungen zur Pathologie der Herzneurosen. Wien. med. Wschr. **1911** II. — Somatische und autonome Innervation. Wien. klin. Wschr. **1929** I. — HESS, W. R.: Über die Wechselbeziehungen zwischen psychischen und vegetativen Funktionen. Schweiz. Arch. Neur. **15/16** (1925). — Funktionsgesetze des vegetativen Nervensystems. Klin. Wschr. **1926** II, 1353. — Stammganglion. Reizversuche. — Ber. Physiol. **42**, 5, 6. Physiol. Tagg 1927, Frankfurt a. M. — Die Funktion des vegetativen Nervensystems. Klin. Wschr. **1930** II. — HEYER: Psychische Faktoren bei organischen Krankheiten. Münch. med. Wschr. **1922** II.

HEYER, G. R.: Magensekretion und Psyche. Verh. 31. Kongr. inn. Med. 1921. — Die Magensekretion beim Menschen unter besonderer Berücksichtigung der psychischen Analyse. Arch. Verdgskrkh. 27/29. — Psychische Einflüsse auf die Motilität von Magen und Darm. Zugleich ein Beitrag zur Gastroptosenfrage. Klin. Wschr. 1923 II. — Psychogene Funktionsstörungen des Verdauungstraktes. Psychogenese und Psychotherapie. Wien 1925. — HEYER, G. R. u. K. BÜGLER: Möglichkeiten und Grenzen der Psychotherapie bei Organneurosen. Kasuistische Mitteilungen etc. Dtsch. Z. Nervenheilk. 98, 123 (1927). — HIGIER, HENRYK: Allgemeine Neurosen, Psychoneurosen und Organneurosen in der modernen inneren Medizin und ihre rationelle Behandlung (poln.). 1929. Ref. Zbl. Neur. 54, 727. — HOCHE, ALFR.: Pathologie und Therapie der nervösen Angstzustände. Dtsch. Z. Nervenheilk. 41 (1911). — HOFF, HANS: Beitrag zur Beziehung funktioneller und organischer Symptome. Nervenarzt 5 (1932). — HOFF, H. u. P. WERNER: Über psychovegetative Schaltungen und ihre Beeinflussung. Klin. Wschr. 1928 I, 346. — HOFFMANN, HERM.: Über psychogene Beschwerden. Dtsch. med. Wschr. 1928 II. — Zbl. Neur. 53, H. 7. — HOMBURGER, A.: Die Gefahren der Überspannung des psychotherapeutischen Gedankens. Nervenarzt 1 (1928). — HUMMELSHEIM: Zur Diagnose und Therapie psychogener Augenstörungen. Arch. Augenheilk. 99, H. 1/2 (1923).

IBRAHIM, J.: Pathologische Beugungsreflexe als Grundlagen neurologischer Krankheitsbilder. Neur. Zbl. 30 (1911). — ISENSCHMIDT u. KREHL: Über den Einfluß des Gehirns auf die Wärmeregulation. Arch. f. exper. Path. 70 (1912).

JACOBI, E.: Psychogene Spontanblutungen der Haut. Arch. f. Psychiatr. 88, 631 (1924). — JACOBI, W. u. H. WINKLER: Arbeiten zur Ideengeschichte der Psychiatrie. I. Mitt. Zur Psychophysiologie der Gefühle. Arch. f. Psychiatr. 91, 162—170 (1930). — JAMIN: Die Zwerchfellneurosen. Münch. med. Wschr. 1919 II. — JANNUSCHKE, H.: Neurasthenie, Angst und Kreislaufapparat. (Klinisch-pharmakologische Studien.) Wien. med. Wschr. 1929 II. — JOLTRAIN, ED.: L'émotion, facteur de déséquilibre humoral et de dermatoses. Bull. Soc. franç. Dermat. 39, 8 (1932). — JONG, DE: Die Hauptgesetze einiger wichtiger körperlicher Erscheinungen beim psychischen Geschehen usw. Z. Neur. 69 (1921).

KAHN, EUGEN: Bemerkungen zur Frage der Organminderwertigkeit. Nervenarzt 1, H. 1 (1928). — KANTOR, J. L.: Neurogenic and psychogenic disorders of the alimentary canal. J. nerv. Dis. 70 (1929). — KARPLUS, J. P. u. KREIDL: Beziehungen der Hypothalamuszentren zu Blutdruck und innerer Sekretion. Pflügers Arch. 215, 667 (1927). — KATSCH, G.: Über Pathogenese und Erscheinungsform der Magenneurosen. Klin. Wschr. 1926 I. — Die Klinik der Magenneurosen. Verh. Ges. Verdgskrkh. 1927. — Zur Pathologie der bedingten Reflexe. Wien. klin. Wschr. 1930 I. — KATSCH u. WESTPHAL: Das neurotische Ulcus. Mitt. Grenzgeb. Med. u. Chir. 26, H. 3 (1913). — KATZ, D. u. R.: Psychologische Untersuchungen über Hunger und Appetit. Arch. ges. Psychol. 65, 269 f. — KISS, JOS.: Über den psychogenen und neurogenen Fluor. Zbl. Gynäk. 1932, 1640 f. — KLEMPERER, E.: Blutdruck und Pulsuntersuchung bei Gesunden. 24. Kongr. inn. Med. 1907. — KLIMKE, WILH.: Über psychogenes und habituelles Erbrechen. Dtsch. med. Wschr. 1932 II. — KLOTZ, R.: Die Atonie der Kapillaren als Organ-Grundlage von Neurasthenie und Neurosen. Z. Kreislaufforsch. 153. — Über Insuffizienz von Hypophyse und Adrenalsystem, ein Beitrag zur Entstehung von Neurasthenie und Neurosen. Endokrinol. 4 (1929). — KNAUER, A. u. E. BILLIGHEIMER: Über organische und funktionelle Störungen des vegetativen Nervensystems. Z. Neur. 50, 199 (1919). — KOGERER, H. Über die theoretischen Grundlagen der Neurosenbehandlung. Wien. klin. Wschr. 1926 I. — KRAPF, ED.: Über die epileptiformen Anfälle bei ALZHEIMERscher und die Anfälle bei PICKscher Krankheit. Arch. f. Psychiatr. 93, 3 (1931). — Über Spätepilepsie. Arch. f. Psychiatr. 97, H. 3 (1932). — Über cerebrale Störungen bei Hypertonikern. 5. Tagg Kreislaufforsch. 1932. — Seelenstörungen der Blutdruckkranken. Habil.schrift 1933. — KRAUS: Vegetatives System und Individualität. Med. Klin. 1922 II. — KRAUS, F.: Über das Neuroseproblem. Klin. Wschr. 1927 I. — Anatomische und physiologische Studien über vegetative Regulationen. Z. klin. Med. 121 (1932). — KRAUS u. ZONDEK: Klin. Wschr. 1922 II, 1753. — KREHL: Über funktionelle Erkrankungen. Ther. Gegenw. 1902. — Über nervöse Herzerkrankungen und den Begriff der Herzschwäche. Münch. med. Wschr. 1906 II. — KRETSCHMER, M. u. R. KRÜGER: Über die Beeinflussung des Serumkalkgehaltes in der Hypnose. Klin. Wschr. 1927 I. — KROLL, FR. W.: Über das Vorkommen von übertragbaren schlaferregenden Stoffen im Hirn schlafender Tiere. Z. Neur. 146 (1933). — KRONFELD, A.: Über Psychotherapie gestörter Organfunktionen usw. Ber. 4. allg. ärztl. Kongr. Psychother. Leipzig 1929. — KÜPPERS, E.: Kritisches zur Lehre von den bedingten Reflexen. Dtsch. Z. Nervenheilk. 111, 215. — KUTTNER, A.: Rhinitis serosa, eine Neurose der Nase in Parallele zu den Neurosen des Verdauungstraktes. Arch. Verdgskrkh. 37, 128 f. (1926). — KUTTNER, H. P.: Versuch einer Strukturanalyse des nervösen Magens. Arch. Verdgskrkh. 27 (1926). — KUTTNER, L.: Zur Differentialdiagnose der Magenneurose und ihre Beziehungen zur Therapie. Ther. Gegenw. 53, 4 (1912). — KYLIN, ESKIL: Moderne Gesichtspunkte in der Neurosenfrage. Sv. Läkartidn. 22, 9 (1925). Ref. Zbl. Neur. 42, 315 (1926).

LAIGNEL-LAVASTINE, M.: Die konzentrische Methode in der Diagnostik der Psychoneurosen. Nervenarzt 1, 520—528 (1928). — LANGE, FRITZ: Dtsch. med. Wschr. 1932 I. — Der stoffliche Anteil an der Regulation des Kreislaufes, seine Bedeutung für die Hypertonie. Klin. Wschr. 12, Nr 5 (1933). — LANGE, JOH.: Ein Fall von Hysterie. Wiss. Sitzg dtsch. F.Anst. Psychiatr. Zbl. Neur. 47 (1927). — LAUBER, HEINR. u. R. PANNHORST: Über psychische Beeinflussung des Herzminutenvolumens. Z. klin. Med. 1930. — LAUDENHEIMER: Psychotherapie des Bronchialasthmas. Ther. Gegenw. 1926, H. 8. — LEHMANN, G.: Über einen möglichen humoralen Wirkungsmechanismus bei Reizung sympathischer Nerven zu den Muskeln. Z. Biol. 92 (1932). — LEIBOWITZ, O.: Ulcus ventriculi und Psychotherapie. Nervenarzt 2 (1929). — LENK, E.: Blutdruck und Hypnose. Dtsch. med. Wschr. 1920 I. — LESCHKE, E.: Die Ergebnisse und Fehlerquellen der bisherigen Untersuchungen über die Begleiterscheinungen seelischer Vorgänge. Arch. ges. Psychol. 3 (1914). — LEWANDOWSKY: Z. Neur. 14 (1913). — LEWY, F. H.: Die Bedeutung der Nervenzentren für die Magenneurose. Verh. Ges. Verdgskrkh. 1927. — LEYSER, E.: Herzkrankheiten und Psychosen. Mschr. Psychiatr. 25, Beih. (1924). — LICHTWITZ, L.: Allgemeine Übersicht über Visceralneurosen. Klin. Wschr. 1929 II. — LILIENSTEIN, S.: Psychoneurosen bei Herzkrankungen (Kardiothymie). 2. allg. psychother. Kongr. 1927. — LÖWI, O.: Über humorale Übertragbarkeit der Herznervenwirkungen. Pflügers Arch. 198 (1921). — LOEWY, P.: Der vegetative Anfall. Mschr. Psychiatr. 52 (1922).

MARANON, G.: Contribution à l'étude de l'action émotive de l'adrénaline. Rev. franç. Endocrin. 2 (1924). — MARCINOWSKI: Die Bedeutung der Weltanschauungsprobleme in der Heilkunst. Z. Psychother. 1929 I, H. 3. — MARTIN, P. u. FL. GRAF: Über die Wirkung schmerzhafter Eingriffe auf den Blutdruck bei Gesunden, bei Nervösen und bei Hypertonikern. Münch. med. Wschr. 1926 I. — MARX, HELLM.: Diurese durch bedingten Reflex. Klin. Wschr. 1931 I, 64 f. — Psychosom. Wechselwirkungen. Klin. Wschr. 1933 I, 689 f. — MATTHES, M.: Die Pathogenese und die Erscheinungsform der Herzneurosen. Klin. Wschr. 1926 I, 393. — Über das Asthma bronchiale. Wien. med. Wschr. 1929 I. — MAUTHNER, O.: Über einige psychogene bzw. psychogen-organische Symptome im Bereich des Kehlkopfes und Rachens, der Nase und des Gehörorgans. Mschr. Ohrenheilk. 62 (1928). — MAYER, A.: Über psychogene Entstehung gynäkologischer Symptome. 1. allg. ärztl. Kongr. Psychother. Baden-Baden 1926. — Psychogene Störungen der weiblichen Sexualfunktion Psychogenese. und Psychotherapie körperlicher Symptome, herausgeg. von O. SCHWARZ, Wien 1925. — MENTZ, P.: Die Wirkung akustischer Sinnesreize auf Puls und Atmung. Philos. Stud. 11 (1893). — MEYER-RUEGG: Die psychisch bedingten Leiden im weiblichen Genitale. Schweiz. med. Wschr. 1925 II. — MISCH, W. Medikamentöse Behandlung der neurotischen Angstzustände. Dtsch. med. Wschr. 1932 II. — MISCH, W. u. K. MISCH-FRANKL: Die vegetative Genese der neurotischen Angst und ihre medikamentöse Beseitigung. Nervenarzt 5 (1932). — MOHR: Über die Behandlung der Organneurosen. Ther. Gegenw. 1922, H. 11. — MOLHANT: Essai de pathogénie et de traitement biologiques des troubles nerveux, dits contionels. Régulation psichique et regulation biologique etc. etc. Bull. Acad. Méd. Belg. 8, 119—176 (1928). — MONAKOW, v.: Biologie und Psychiatrie. Schweiz. Arch. Neur. 4, 13 (1919). — MOOS, ERW.: Psychische Einflüsse auf das Blutgefäßsystem. 2. allg. ärztl. Kongr. Psychother. Nauheim 1927. — MORAWITZ, P.: Zur Ätiologie und Therapie der angioneurotischen Ödeme (QUINCKE). Fortschr. Ther. 2, H. 17 (1926). — MOSKOWITZ, L.: Über die Entstehung der Magengeschwürkrankheit (Gastropathie). Klin. Wschr. 1930 I, 385.

NEUBÜRGER, KARL: Verh.ber. 5. Tagg Kreislaufforsch. 1932. — NEUTRA, W.: Zur Entstehung der Neurosen. Vorl. Mitt. Wien. med. Wschr. 1926 I. — NIESSL V. MAYENDORF: Zur Neurosenfrage. Allg. Z. Psychiatr. 83 (1926). — NOVAK, J. u. M. HARNIK: Die psychogene Entstehung der Menstrualkolik und deren Behandlung. Z. Geburtsh. 96, 239 f. (1929).

PANNHORST, R.: Beitrag zur Klinik der bedingten Reflexe. Nervenarzt 5 (1932). — PAWLOW: Die bedingten Reflexe bei Zerstörung verschiedener Bezirke der Großhirnhemisphären beim Hund. Verh. Ges. russ. Ärzte 1907. — Die äußere Arbeit der Verdauungsdrüsen. NAGELS Handbuch der Physiologie, Bd. 2. — PENDE, R.: Rapporti patogenetici e confini clinici fra nervosi e malattie organiche. Rinasc. med. 4, 551, 574 f. (1927). — PETTE, H.: Über gewisse Formen durch konstitutionelle Abartigkeit gekennzeichnete Neurasthenie. Dtsch. Z. Nervenheilk. 97, 200 (1927). — Das Problem der wechselseitigen Beziehungen zwischen Sympathicus und Sensibilität. Dtsch. Z. Nervenheilk. 100 (1927). — Die Hyperventilation als Methode zur Objektivierung vegetativer Phänomene. Vortr. 55. Wandersvslg südwestdtsch. Neurol. u. Psychiater 1930. — PICK, E. D.: Dtsch. Z. Nervenheilk. 106 (1928). — PICK, P.: Pharmakologie des vegetativen Nervensystems. Dtsch. Z. Nervenheilk. 106 (1928). — PILCZ, A.: Erkrankungen des Zentralnervensystems und Verdauungstrakt. Wien. med. Wschr. 1929 I, 53. — PÖTZL, O.: Über einige Wechselwirkungen hysteriformer und organisch cerebellarer Mechanismen. Jb. Psychiatr. 3 (1917). — PÖTZL, EPPINGER u. HESS: Wien. klin. Wschr. 1910 II, 1831. — POLLACK, FR.: Die Stellung des vegetativen Nervensystems im psychocerebralen Bauplan. Z. Neur. 137

(1931). — POLLNOW, H., H. PETOW u. E. WITTKOWER: Beiträge zur Klinik des Asthma bronchiale und verwandter Zustände. 4 Teile zur Psychotherapie des Asthma bronchiale. Z. klin. Med. 110, 701—721 (1929). — POTOTSKY, C.: Psychogenese und Psychotherapie von Organsymptomen beim Kinde. Psychogenese und Psychotherapie körperlicher Symptome. Wien 1925.
RAIMANN, E.: Fortschritte der Neurosenlehre. Wien. med. Wschr. 1927 II. — REICHARDT, M.: Hirnstamm und Psychiatrie. Mschr. Psychiatr. 68 (1928). — Über die sog. Neurosen. Dtsch. med. Wschr. 1930 I. — Klin. Wschr. 1930 II. — Die psychogenen Reaktionen, einschl. der sog. Entschädigungsneurosen. Arch. f. Psychiatr. 98. — ROSENBACH, OTTOMAR: Dtsch. med. Wschr. 1879 I. — ROSENFELD, M.: Die vegetative Neurose in ihren Beziehungen zu psychischen Störungen. Mschr. Psychiatr. 60 (1925). — ROST, G. A.: Hautkrankheiten. Fachbücher für Ärzte. Herausgeg. von Schriftleitung der Klin. Wschr. Berlin: Julius Springer 1926. — RUDORICI, A. et A. KREIDLER: Le déséquilibre végétatif dans les névroses. Revue neur. 33, 1123 (1926). — RUHMANN, WALTHER: Angioneurotische Organdiathese von Magen und Darm. Med. Welt 1932.
SACK, W.: Allergische Reaktionen als neurotisches Symptom. 56. Verslg südwestdtsch. Neur. u. Psychiater 1932. Zbl. Neur. 65, 443. — SACK, W. TH.: Die Haut als Ausdrucksorgan. Arch. f. Dermat. 1926. — Zur Kasuistik und Problematik psychogener Dermatosen. Nervenarzt 2 (1929). — SAENGER, M.: Über die psychische Komponente unter den Asthmaursachen. Berl. klin. Wschr. 1912 I. — SCHIFF, ARTHUR: Über Magenneurosen. Karlsbad. ärztl. Vortr. 8, 347 (1927). — SCHILDER, P.: Psychogene Parästhesien. Dtsch. Z. Nervenheilk. 64 (1919). — Das Leib-Seelenproblem vom Standpunkt der Philosophie und naturwissenschaftlichen Psychologie. Psychogenese und Psychotherapie körperlicher Symptome. Herausgeg. von O. SCHWARZ. Wien 1925. — Der gegenwärtige Stand der Neurosenlehre. Klin. Wschr. 1927 I. — The somatic basis of the neurosis. J. nerv. Dis. 70 (1929). — SCHINDLER, R.: Die Psychoneurosen des Verdauungstraktes. Ber. allg. 2. ärztl. Kongr. Psychother. Bad Nauheim 1927. — Die Behandlung der Psychoneurosen des Verdauungstraktes. Arch. Verdgskrkh. 44 (1928). — SCHMIDT, R.: Tonusproblem und Vagotonie. Z. klin. Med. 86 (1918). — SCHNEIDER: Über die Entstehung und Behandlung des Asthma bronchiale. Zbl. inn. Med. 1925. — SCHNEIDER, ALB.: Zur Differentialdiagnose organischer und nervöser Angina pectoris. Med. Welt 1932. — SCHOLZ, WILH.: Über Herzneurose. Wien. klin. Wschr. 1928 I, 951. — SCHULTZ, I. H.: Stigmatisierung und Organneurose. Dtsch. med. Wschr. 1927, II 1584 — Psychologie und Psychotherapie bei Herzschwäche. Med. Welt 4, Nr 37. — Erlebnis, Haltung, Organneurose. Vortr. 18. Jverslg Ges. dtsch. Nervenärzte Hamburg 1928. — Psychogramm und Charakterologie. Vortr. Kongreßber. 3. Kongr. Psychother. Leipzig 1928. — Psychologische Bemerkungen zur Therapie der Angina pectoris. Dtsch. med. Wschr. 1930 I. — Die Grundtypen des psychologischen Aufbaues sog. Organneurosen. Vortr. Ges. inn. Med. Berlin 1931. Ref. Klin. Wschr. 1931 I, 91. — SCHULTZ u. REICHMANN: Zur Psychopathologie des Asthma bronchiale. Dtsch. med. Wschr. 1923 I, 33. — SCHULTZ-HENCKE, HARALD: Zur Diskussion der Organneurosen. Nervenarzt 1, 661 (1928). — SCHUR, H.: Über nervöse Störungen der Magenfunktion. Z. ärztl. Fortbildg 1926, 69. — Nervöse Störungen der Ernährung und Verdauung (zugleich ein Beitrag zur Theorie der Organneurosen). Wien. med. Wschr. 1927 I. — SCHWARZ, O.: Psychogene Störungen der männlichen Sexualfunktion (psychogene Impotenz). Psychogenese und Psychotherapie etc. Wien 1925. — Das Problem des Organismus. Psychogenese und Psychotherapie körperlicher Symptome. Wien 1925. — Über psychogene Nierenschmerzen. Allg. Z. ärztl. Psychother. 1, 28 (1928). — Medizinische Anthropologie. Eine wissenschaftstheoretische Grundlegung der Medizin. Leipzig 1929. — Das Leib-Seele-Problem in der Medizin. Vortr. Inst. Gesdh.Med. Leipzig 3 (1930). — SHERVINGTON, C. S.: Experiments on the value of vascular and visceral factors on the genesis of emotion. Proc. roy. Soc. Lond. 66 (1900). — SIEBECK: Über kardiale Dyspnoe. Klin. Wschr. 1929 II, 2121. — Die psychophysischen Beziehungen der Organfunktion und ihre therapeutische Beeinflussung. Z. ärztl. Fortbildg 1933, H. 8. SPEER, ERNST: Die reaktive Seelenstörung. Grundsätzliche Bemerkungen zur Neurosenfrage. Dtsch. med. Wschr. 1929 II. — STECKEL: Zur Psychologie der Schmerzphänomene, insbesondere des Kopfschmerzes. Fortschr. Sex.wiss. 2 (1926). — STEIN, F. W.: Hypotonia nervosa, ein konstitutionelles Krankheitsbild. Med. Klin. 1929 I. — STERN: Zur Frage der psychogenen Dermatosen. Z. Neur. 79 (1922). — STOCKERT, F. G. v.: Zur Sprache der Neurotiker. Wien. med. Wschr. 76 (1926). — Stottern, ein Beitrag zur Frage der neurotischen Organwahl. Wien. med. Wschr. 78, 972 f. (1928). — Klinik und Ätiologie der Kontaktneurosen. Klin. Wschr. 1929 I. — STRANDBERG, J.: Psyche und Hautkrankheiten. Psychogenese und Psychotherapie körperlicher Symptome. herausgeg. von O. SCHWARZ. Wien 1925. — STRANSKY, ERW.: Einige Gesichtspunkte zur Neurosenlehre. Wien. med. Wschr. 1926 I, 111 f. — STUTZIN, J. J.: Uroneurosen. Med. Klin. 23 (1927). — STUTZIN, J. u. H. WARNER: Die Harnblase als Ausdrucksgebiet für neuropsychische Vorgänge. Med. Klin. 1928 II, 1467. — SZYMANSKI, J. S.: Wandlungen der Seelenauffassung im Laufe der Zeiten. Arch. f. Psychiatr. 94 (1931).

TARCHANOFF, J. R.: Über willkürliche Acceleration der Herzschläge. Pflügers Arch. **35** (1885). — TUCZEK, KARL: Kathartische Analyse und Heilung einer Magenneurose. Nervenarzt **1**, 600 (1928).
VEIL, EBERHARD: Herzneurose und organische Herzinsuffizienz. Karlsbad. ärztl. Vortr. **9** (1928). — VOGEL, P.: Über neurotische Magen- und Darmbeschwerden. Z. Neur. **141** (1932). — VOGT, C.: Einige Ergebnisse unserer Neurosenforschung. Naturwiss. **9**, H. 18 (1921).
WALTHARD: Psychoneurose und Gynäkologie. Mschr. Geburtsh. **36**, Erg.-H. (1912). — WEINBERG, A.: Psyche und unwillkürliches Nervensystem. Z. Neur. **85/86** (1923). — WEIZSÄCKER, V. v. Über neurotischen Aufbau bei inneren Krankheiten. Vortrag. Ref. Zbl. Neur. **41**, 688. — Der neurotische Aufbau bei den Magen- und Darmerkrankungen. Dtsch. med. Wschr. **1926** II. Ges. Dtsch. Nervenärzte Kassel 1925. — WENCKEBACH: Experimentelle Studien zur Entstehung der Organneurosen. Kongreßber. dtsch. Ges. inn. Med. **1933**. — WEXBERG, E.: Die Angst als Kernproblem der Neurose. Dtsch. Z. Nervenheilk. **88** (1926). — WILDER, JOS.: Das „Ausgangswertgesetz" usw. Z. Neur. **137** (1931). — Zur Pharmakotherapie und -diagnostik der vegetativ nervösen Erkrankungen. Vortrag. Ref. Zbl. Neur. **57**, 437. — WIMMER, A. (Kopenhagen): Über „dyskrine" Familien. Diskussionsbem. Zbl. Neur. **50**, 771. — WITTKOWER, E. u. OTTILIE FECHNER: Über affektiv somatische Veränderungen. V. Mitt. Der psychogalvanische Reflex. Z. Neur. **1931**, 676. — WOLLENBERG, R.: Der heutige Stand der Lehre von den Neurosen. Dtsch. med. Wschr. **52**, 2061 (1926). — WULFFTEN-PALTHE, P. M. v.: Leiodystonie. Geneesk. Tijdschr. Nederl.-Indië **72** (1932). Ref. Zbl. Neur. **67**, H. 3/4. — WYSS, W. H. v.: Vegetative Reaktionen bei psychischen Vorgängen. Schweiz. Arch. Neur. **19** (1926). — Der Ausdruck der Gemütsbewegungen. Nervenarzt **2**, 534 (1929).
ZAPPERT, J.: Über Gewohnheitsneurosen. Fortschr. Med. **45** (1927). — ZONDECK, S. G.: Untersuchungen über das Wesen der Vagus- und Sympathikuswirkung. Dtsch. med. Wschr. **50** (1921). — Biochem. Z. **132**, 362 (1922). — Klin. Wschr. **1923** I, 382. — Arch. f. exper. Path. **143** (1929). — ZUCKER: Über eine charakteristische Unterform der vegetativen Neurose. Dtsch. Z. Nervenheilk. **101** (1928).

Anhang: Die sog. Koordinationsneurosen.

I. Monographien und Referate.

CURSCHMANN, H.: Koordinatorische Neurosen. Handbuch der inneren Medizin, herausgeg. von V. BERGMANN u. STAEHELIN, Bd. 5, 2. Aufl. 1926.
FLATAU, TH. S.: Die Krankheiten der Sing- und Sprechstimme. Handbuch der Hals- usw. Heilkunde, Bd. 5. 1929. — Stottern. Tagg dtsch. Ges. Sprach- und Stimmheilkunde. Leipzig 1928. — FRÖSCHELS, E.: Lehrbuch der Sprachheilkunde, 2. Aufl., 1925.
GUTZMANN, H.: Die Fachliteratur über Stimm- und Sprachstörungen und über die Phonetik von 1919—1925. Internat. Zbl. Ohrenheilk. **25** (1926). — Die Fachliteratur über Stimm- und Sprachstörungen und über die Phonetik von 1925—1928. Internat. Zbl. Ohrenheilk. **30** (1929). — GUTZMANN, H.-NADOLECZNY: Die funktionellen Störungen der Stimme und Sprache. Handbuch der inneren Medizin, herausgeg. von BERGMANN u. STAEHELIN, 2. Aufl., Bd. 5, 2. 1926.
HOEPFNER, TH.: Grundriß der psychogenen Störungen der Sprache. Psychogenese und Psychotherapie körperlicher Symptome. herausgeg. von O. SCHWARZ. Wien 1925.
NADOLESCZNY: Physiologie der Stimme und Sprache. DENKER u. KAHLES Handbuch der Hals-Nasen-Ohrenheilkunde, Bd. 1, S. 621. 1925. — Kurzes Lehrbuch der Sprach- und Stimmheilkunde mit besonderer Berücksichtigung des Kindesalters. Leipzig 1926. — Sprach- und Stimmheilkunde. Fortschr. Neur. **1931**, 56 f. — Sprachstörungen. Handbuch der Hals- usw. Heilkunde, Bd. 5. Berlin 1929.
OPPENHEIM, H. u. M. NONNE: Die Beschäftigungskrämpfe. Lehrbuch der Nervenkrankheiten, 7. Aufl., Bd. 2, S. 1980. 1923.
ZWIRNER, EBERHARD: Die Phonetik in ihrer Beziehung zur Neurologie und Psychiatrie. Fortschr. Neur. **1930**, 363 f.

II. Einzelarbeiten.

ADLER, EMIL: Über einige Fälle von Schreibkrampf bei Striatumläsion. Nervenarzt **5**, 295 (1932).
BINSWANGER, L.: Zum Problem von Sprache und Denken. Schweiz. Arch. Neur. **18** (1926).
CALLEWAERT, H.: La crampe des écrivains. Influence de techniques professionnelles défectueuses. J. de Neur. **30**, 814 (1930). — CIAMPI, LANFRANCO: Neue ätiopathogenetische und therapeutische Auffassung des Stotterns. Bol. Inst. psiquicatr. Fac. Ci. méd. Rosario **4**, 1—26 (1932). Ref. Zbl. Neur. **68**, 509. — COSTEDOAT et AUJALEU: La crampe des écrivains.

Paris méd. **1932** II. Ref. Zbl. Neur. **66**, 837 (1933). — CRONBACH: Telegraphenkrampf. Arch. f. Psychiatr. **37**, 243.

FRANK, D. B.: Intentionales Stottern und Klarheit des Bewußtseins. Z. Neur. **123** (1929). — FRÖSCHELS, E.: Zur Frage der Geschwisterzahl von Stotterern. Wien. klin. Wschr. **1933** II, 1291. — Symptomatologie des Stotterns. Mschr. Ohrenheilk. **68**, 814 (1934). — FRÖSCHELS, E. u. I. MOSES: Über die Konstitution assoziativ-aphatischer (stotternder) Kinder. Wien. med. Wschr. **1926** II, 873.

GALANT, JOH. SUSM.: Über die sozialen Mechanismen der sozioaffektiven Dysphasie (Stottern). Schweiz. med. Wschr. **1933** II, 714. — GUTZMANN-NADOLECZNY: Übungsbuch für Stotternde. Osterwieck 1926.

HOEPFNER, TH.: Stottern und assoziative Aphasie. Z. Neur. **94** (1924).

ISSERLIN, M.: Psychologisch-phonetische Untersuchungen. I. Mitt. Allg. Z. Psychiatr. **75** (1919). — Psychologisch-phonetische Untersuchungen. II. Mitt. Z. Neur. **94** (1924). — Die pathologische Physiologie der Sprache, I. Teil. Erg. Physiol. **29** (1929).

KISTLER, K.: Linkshändigkeit und Sprachstörungen. Schweiz. med. Wschr. **1930** I, 2. — KRAMER, FRANZ: Z. Elektrol. u. Röntgenkde **10**, 104 (1908).

MOHNKOPF, WILHELM: Zur Automatisierung willkürlicher Bewegungen, zugleich ein Beitrag zur Lehre von der Enge des Bewußtseins. Z. Psychol. **1933**, 130.

ROSANOFF, ARON, J. CHRISTINE V. JNMAN-KANE: Relation of premature birth underweight condition at birth to mental deficiency. Amer. J. Psychiatr. **13**, 829 (1934). — ROST, BRONISLAW: Der Schreibkrampf auf extrapyramidaler Grundlage. Neur. polska **16/17**, 265—270. Ref. Zbl. Neur. **75**, 377 (1935). — ROTHE: Die Umerziehung. Halle 1929. — ROTHE, KARL C.: Das Entwicklungsstottern als sprachneurotischer Prozeß. Z. pädagog. Psychol. **30**, 566 (1929).

SCHULMANN, A.: Schriftuntersuchungen an Stotterern. Verh. internat. Ges. Logopädie **38—39** (1935). — SEEMANN, M.: Über somatische Befunde bei Stotterern. Mschr. Ohrenheilk. **68**, 895 (1934). — SITTIG, OTTO: Über Schreibkrampf bei Encephalitis epidemica. Klin. Wschr. **1929** I, 794. — SOVAK, M.: Sympathikusreflex der Stotterer. Čas. lék. česk. **1933**, 164. Ref. Zbl. Neur. **69**, 612. — STEIN, LEOPOLD: Zur Symptomwahl bei der assoziativen Aphasie. Wien. med. Wschr. **1931** II, 1596. — Die Behandlung der assoziativen Aphasie. Mschr. Ohrenheilk. **68**, 920 (1934). — STERN, HUGO: Die Notwendigkeit einer einheitlichen Nomenklatur für die Physiologie, Pathologie und Pädagogik der Stimme. Berlin-Wien 1928. — STOCKERT, F. G. v.: Klinik, Ätiologie und Therapie des Stotterns. Dtsch. Z. Nervenheilk. **98**, 284 (1927). — Stottern, ein Beitrag zur neurotischen Organwahl. Wien. med. Wschr. **1928** II. — Klinik und Ätiologie der Kontaktneurosen. Klin. Wschr. **1929** I, 76. — Die Psychogenese des Stotterns. Mschr. Ohrenheilk. **68** (1934). — SZONDI, L.: Konstitutionsanalyse von 100 Stotterern. Wien. med. Wschr. **1932** II. — Konstitutionsanalyse psychisch abnormer Kinder. Halle 1933.

TRAVIS, LEE EDWARD and WENDELL JOHNSON: Stuttering and the concept of handedness. Psychologic Rev. **41**, 534 (1934). — TRÖMNER, E.: Das Stottern — die Sprachzwangsneurose. 2. Tagg dtsch. Ges. Sprach- u. Stimmenheilk. Leipzig 1929.

WEISS, D. u. L. BARCZINSKI: Zur Erkennung des Nachahmungsstotterns. Arch. f. Psychiatr. **95** (1931). — WUTH, OTTO: Chemie der Psychosen. Fortschr. Neur. **5** (1933).

Namenverzeichnis.

Die *kursiv* gedruckten Ziffern beziehen sich auf die Literatur.

Abbott, W. *424.*
Abrami 235, *245.*
Achard 395, 399, *406.*
Achelis, J. D., 491, 508, *533.*
Acton 357, *408.*
Acuna 362, *408.*
Adam 322.
Addison 350.
Adie 37, *84,* 90, 113, 122, 123, 129, 136, *140, 242.*
Adler 127, 377, 442, *533.*
— A. *471,* 498, 501, *531, 533.*
— E. *525, 539.*
Adlersberg 157, 500, 514, *533.*
Adrian 324.
Adson, Alfred W. 280, 318, 319, 328, 344, 366, *401, 405, 408, 409, 420.*
Affleck 252, 266.
Agnello 181, *242.*
Aiello, G. 328, *405, 408.*
Aiginger, J. *471.*
Aigner 489, *535.*
Airy 177, *242.*
Aja, Sáinz de 372, *419.*
Ajmar, Fr., *421.*
Aka 254.
Akobdszanjanz, G. 323, *409.*
Alajouanine 180, 326.
Albers 255.
Albrecht, K. 306, 460.
— Th. *471.*
Alda 235, *242.*
Alessandri, Roberto 261, 371, *401.*
Alexander 82, *84,* 460.
Aljavdin, A. *409.*
Alkan, L. 498, 504, 508, 531.
Allan, W. 168, 189, 217, *242,* 266, 274, 280, 361, *409.*
Allen, Edgar V. 46, 47, 48, 63, 76, *84, 85,* 246, 249, *401, 420.*
Allende 51, *84.*
Allers, R. *471, 533.*
Alquier 344, 348.
Altenburger, H. 48, *84,* 490, *533, 535.*
Alurralde, Mariano 259, *401.*
Alvarez, E. *419.*
Alzheimer 40, 84.
Amabilino, R. *401.*
Amat, Marin 182, 235, *244.*
Amyot, R. 395, *424.*
Anastazy *403.*
Anderson 13, *84,* 182, *242,* 248.

André, Y. 286, 314, *420, 422.*
Andrews 334, *414.*
Andriezen 51, *84.*
Angelesco 248.
Anitschkoff 326.
Anselmino, K. 312, *421.*
Antona, L. de *402, 405.*
Antonelli 176, 209, *242.*
Antoni 456, *471.*
Apert 40, *84,* 226, 237, *242.*
Apostol *245.*
Appelbaum, S. J. 256, *401.*
Arady, K. v. 318, 321, 322, 325, 326, 351, 353, *409.*
Arazzi 295.
Archambault 330, 331, 334, *414, 423.*
Aretaeus 33, *84,* 88.
Armani, L. 351, 363, *409.*
Armas *421.*
Arnaud 267, *404, 420.*
Arndt 351, *471.*
Arning 252.
Aronstam 314.
Artom, M. 313, *409.*
Asai, J. 374, *416.*
Aschaffenburg, G. 196, 521.
Aschenheim, E. *164.*
Aschner *533.*
Assmann, H. 202, *242,* 260, 267, 269, 274, 385, *400, 401, 424.*
Astruck, P. 488, *533.*
Atkin 259.
Atzler, E. *471.*
Aubrun, W. *423.*
Auerbach 199, 202, *242,* 287, 293, 294.
Aujaleu 526, *539.*
Auld 76, *84,* 390.
Avezzu 287, 292, 293.
Awguschewitsch, P. *414.*
Awtokratow, P. M. 452, 467, *471.*
Ayala 394.
Aydillo 138, *140.*
Aymès 256, 312, *420.*
Ayres 326.

Babinski 197, *242,* 393.
Babonneix 200, *242.*
Bachenheimer, M. *164.*
Back, E. *471.*
Backmann 331.
Baelz 451.

Bäumler 33, *84, 533.*
Baguette *404.*
Bailey, H. 109, *140,* 312, 382, *401.*
— Percival *417.*
Bajpayee, A. *401.*
Balaban, N. *409,* 451, *471.*
Balbi, E. *406.*
Balfour 199.
Balint 76, *84.*
Ball, Erna 312, 315, 316, 328, 379.
— E. F. 219, 235, *242.*
Baller 364.
Ballerini 304, 373, *408.*
Ballet 111, 118, 122, *140,* 185, *242,* 299, 315.
Balló, B. *422.*
Balogh 118, *140.*
Balyeat 167, 220, 223, 234, *242.*
Bansi, H. W. 510, *533.*
Baralt 177, *242.*
Barbara 129, 134.
Barbash 47, *84.*
Barber, H. W. *421.*
— L. F. *401.*
Barbier *420.*
Barborka 236, *242, 244.*
Barbot 312, 326.
Barcroft 486.
Barczinski, L., 526, *540.*
Barenne, Dusser de 383.
Barker 261, 282.
Barkman, Ake 336, 344, 345, 356, *409.*
Barlow 252, 261.
Barmwater, Knud 259, *401.*
Barnhoorn 80, *85.*
Barraquer 336.
Barrel 334.
Barrows 368.
Barsony, Th. *421.*
Barthélemy, R. 313, 314, 328, *409, 411.*
Baruk, H. 283, 323, *405, 411.*
Basch, G. 354, *414, 421, 423.*
— M. *414, 421.*
Basombrio, G. 313, 353, 354, 414.
Basset, A. *416.*
Bassi 339.
Bassoe 93, 110, *140.*
Basta 351.
Bastedo 224, *242.*
Batman 248.

Bau 352, *409*.
Bauer 109, 111, 117, 118, 312, *471*.
— J. 112, 134, 369, *471*, *482*, 496, 497, 498, *531*, *533*.
Baugh 8, *84*.
Bayet 306, 307.
Baylac 46, *84*.
Bazan, F. *424*.
Bazin 284.
Beader 261.
Beard, G. M. 455, 456, *471*.
Beau, Henri 278, *404*.
Beauchant 369, 381.
Beauchesne, H. *422*.
Beaulien 526.
Beauvieux *245*.
Becher, E. 435, *471*.
Bechterew 66, *84*.
Beck, A. 247, 248, 255, 266, 280, 381, *401*.
Becker, S. *424*.
Beckmann, K. 254, *533*.
Bedarida, N. *405*.
Beecher 219, *242*.
Beer, Th. 331, 332, 334, 349, 516.
Beevor 20, *84*.
Begg 252.
Behague 63, *84*.
Behmak *212*.
Behrend 164.
Behrenroth, E. *533*.
Bejarano, J. 246, 351, *401*, *409*.
Bejlin, J. 283, 284, *405*.
Bell, Ch. 527.
Bellavitis 65, *84*.
Bellinger 47.
Ben, F. *414*.
Bénard 347.
Benatt, A. *420*.
Benda 287, 290, 293, 295, 380.
Bender 253, 256.
Benedek, L. 138, *140*, 273, *401*.
Benjamin, E. *471*.
Bennett, T. J. 249, 267, *401*.
Benoist 298.
Benson 256.
Berencsoy 221, *242*.
Berg, H. J. van den 222, 224, 234, *242*.
— W. *242*.
Berger, H. 174, 203, 204, *242*, 304, 305, 340, 341, 486, *531*.
Bergmann, G. v. 456, 457, *471*, *481*, *482*, 487, *492*, *493*, *494*, *495*, *496*, *497*, 502, 503, 504, 510, 511, 513, 517, 518, 519, 520, *531*, *533*.
Bergson 326, 330.
Beringer, K. *534*.
Berlit, B. *471*.
Bernard, Claude 203, 249.

Bernard, L. *401*.
Bernhardt 89, 90, 91, 92, 94, 96, 97, 101, 105, 108, 109, 110, 111, 112, 113, 116, 117, 118, 119, 120, 121, 122, 123, 124, 126, 138, 139, *141*, 185, 193, *242*, 251, 256, 288, 299.
Bernheim 164.
Bernheimer 182, 24?.
Bernstein, E. 335, *414*.
Bernuth, F. v. *421*.
Bero, Bes de 4, *84*.
Bertaccini, G. *409*.
Bertellotti 351.
Bertin, E. 313, *409*.
Bertolani 48, *84*.
Bertrand, J. *421*.
Bervoets 266.
Besançon *405*, *421*.
Bettmann, S. 306, 310, 329, 386, 388, 522, *405*, *416*, *534*.
Beumer 164.
Beutter 395.
Beyer 177, *242*.
Beyermann 94, 106, 107, 116, 117, 118, *140*.
Biancalani, A. *408*.
Bibrowicz, W. 454, *474*.
Bickel 486, *531*, *534*.
Biedl 204, *242*, *531*.
Bielschowsky 51, *84*.
Bienvenue, A. 278, *403*.
Bier 129, *141*, *534*.
Biermer 516.
Biernacki *471*.
Bieulac 30, *84*.
Bikeles, G. 287, *406*.
Billigheimer, E. 221, *242*, *449*, *450*, 459, 462, 463, *471*, *473*, *481*, *482*, 486, 519, *531*, *534*, *536*.
Bing, R. 167, *242*, 287, *406*, *534*.
Bingel 49, *84*.
Binswanger, H. *534*.
— L. *534*, *539*.
— O. 4, 10, 41, 61, *84*, 196, 446, *471*, *493*, *534*.
Bircher 370.
Birk 154.
Birnbaum, K. 439, 440, 450, 467, *471*.
Biro 63, *84*.
Bisgaard 48, 55, *84*, *86*.
Bitot 330, 338.
Bittorf 374.
Bize, P. R. *423*.
Bjering 247.
Blaauw 256.
Blamontier 205, 223, 236, *245*, 377, 384, 399, *419*.
Bland 256, 259, 262.
Blaschko 329.
Blatt, O. 351, *409*.

Blaustein, N. 369, 376, 378, *416*.
Pleuler, E. 51, *84*, *471*, 494, *531*, *534*.
Blitzstein 172, *242*.
Bloch, Br. 270, 279, 329, *400*, *534*.
— E. *401*.
Bloedorn, W. A. *534*.
Blomfield 247.
Blum, K. 273, *471*.
Blumreich 66.
Boadmann 276, *414*.
Boas, E. 110, 122, *140*, *405*.
Bode, H. G. *421*.
— O. 309, 315, *414*, *423*.
Boe, Hilmar 366, *423*.
Boeck 286.
Bönheim, C. E. 331, 338, *414*, *471*.
Boenheim, F. *534*.
Boerner 367, 372.
Boettiger 285.
Bogaert, Ludo van 127, *140*, 176, 239, *243*, 261, 270, 330, 377, 381, *401*, *402*, *414*, *417*, *424*.
Bogart, A. *416*.
Bogdanovic 366.
Bogen *534*.
Boggon, R. H. 280, *401*.
Bohn *422*.
Bohns 167.
Bohumiczky, E. 398, *416*.
Bojovitsch 83, *84*.
Boks 394, 395.
Bolten, G. C. 193, 223, *242*, 299, 302, 303, 306, 307, 311, 350, 369, 372, 383, 392, *408*, *416*.
Bombarda 326.
Bombi, G. 273, *401*.
Bond 5, 40, 45, 67, 83, *86*, 223, *242*.
Bonhoeffer, K. 40, *84*, 102, 113, 114, 115, 119, *140*, 438, 440, 441, 442, 446, 451, 452, 464, 465, *471*.
Bonn 241, *242*.
Bonnaire 74, *84*.
Bonnal 241.
Bonnet, H. *421*.
— L. M. *408*.
Bonnier 44, *84*, 200, *242*.
Booth 270.
Boothby 47, *84*.
Bootli, J. A. *403*.
Borak, J. 255, 270, 277, 278, 304, 305, *401*, *405*, *408*, *416*.
Borchardt, L. *471*.
Bordoni 193.
Boretius 248.
Borghesan, E. 256, *401*.
Bornstein 182, *242*.

Borovsky, M. 269, 332, *401*, *414*.
Borries, G. 369, *416*.
Bory, L. 328, *409*, *414*.
Bosanyi 259.
Bose, du 280, *402*.
Bossert 30, *84*.
Bost, Cr. 330, 331, *414*.
Bostock 138, *140*.
Bostroem 446.
Bouchard 181, 217, 218.
Bouchaud 242.
Bouché 242.
Boucher, R. *424*.
Bourgignon 332, 526.
Bourneville 29, 74, *84*, 189.
Boutelier 318, 328, *404*, *411*.
Bouttier 29, 35, *84*, 321.
Bouveyron 226, 237, 242, 330, 334, 335.
Bovis, de 280.
Bowen 293.
Bowman 16, 47, *84*.
Boyce 54, *84*.
Boyden 236.
Bracchi 287, 290.
Brack 222.
Braeucker, W. 240, 242, 277, 279, 280, *401*, *416*, *424*, *534*.
Brahn, M. 486, *534*.
Brailowsky 121, *140*.
Brain, Russell 29, 47, 65, 77, 80, *84*, *85*.
Bramann 273.
Brams 172, *242*.
Bramwell 39, *84*, 312, 364.
Brandenburg 299, *406*.
Brandess, Theo *401*.
Brasch 183, *242*, 248.
Bratz 40, *84*, 162.
Brauch, W. 489, *535*.
Braun, E. 460, 462, 467, 468, 471, 505, 519, *531*.
— L. 471, 509, *531*, *534*.
Bravais 20, 31, *84*.
Bregmann, L. E. 365, *402*, *409*.
Bregs, P. *402*.
Breitmann, M. 365, *422*.
Brengues 261.
Breslauer 269.
Brickner 225, *245*.
Bridge 54, 77, *84*.
Briese, M. 347, 348, *412*.
Brill, E. *534*.
Brissaud 200, 261, 329, 340, 347, 350, 355.
Broadbent 25, 32, *84*.
Brock 105, 107, 123, *140*, 278, *421*.
Brocq 363.
Brodnitz 273, *403*.
Brodskij, L. *412*.
Bromberg 100, 123, *140*.
Bronson 306, 311.
Brooke, Ch. 276, 350, *402*.

Brosse 377, *417*.
Broustet, P. *422*.
Brown, George E. *401*, *402*, *406*, *409*, *420*, *421*.
— Grafton *416*.
— Graham 14, 29, 39, 65, *84*, 129, 223, 234, *213*, 289, *401*, *402*, *405*, *406*.
— H. 246, 258, 267, 274, 280, 287, 318, 319, 320, 328, 344, 366, 398, *409*.
— T. R. 85, *243*.
Browne *84*.
Brown-Séquart 39, *84*, *129*.
Bruch *140*, *406*.
Bruchanski 451, *471*.
Brücke, G. Th. 481, 483, 484, 490, 525, *531*, *534*.
Brückner, St. *423*.
Brühl 46, *84*, *86*.
Brünauer, R. 312, 313, 316, 320, 322, 325, 329, 337, 344, 345, 347, 348, 349, 350, 351, 356, 358, 359, 360, 361, 362, 363, 364, 365, 366, *410*.
Brüning, F. 280, 299, 306, 333, 365, 366, *400*, *406*.
Brünniche 248.
Brugsch, Th. *407*, 457, 461, 462.
Bruhns 318.
Brunet, R. *421*.
Brunner 204.
Bruns 273, 329.
Brunschweiler, H. 313, 315, *409*.
Brusset, J. 353, 354, 359, *413*.
Brussilowski, L. 451, *471*.
Bruusgaard, E. *409*.
Buchanan, A. 172, 189, 217, *242*.
Buchwald 358.
Budina, R. 334, 335, *414*.
Büchler, P. 270, *402*, *409*.
Büchner 518, 519.
Bügler, K. *473*, *536*.
Bürger, H. 297, 480.
Buendia, B. 377, *418*.
Bulle, E. 307, 408.
Bulloch 368.
Bumbacesca 91, 119, *141*.
Bumke, O. 133, 438, 440, 441, 446, 451, 455, 462, 468, 469, *471*, 477, 478, 480, 493, 505, 506, 513, *531*, *534*.
Bungenberg de Jong, W. J. H. *416*, *420*, 486, *536*.
Bunnemann 523, *534*.
Burchard 380.
Bureau, Y. 353, 354, *411*.
Burnier 264, 278, 318, 320, 321, 328, *403*, *410*.
Burns 314.
Burr 30.

Bury 293, 328, *409*.
Buscaino 52, 65, *84*.
Buschke, A. 325, 360, *409*.
Busy 261.
Buytendijk 500, *534*.
Buzzard 13, *84*.
Bywater, H. 261, *402*.

Cabannes 339, 340.
Cachera, René *421*.
Caesar *243*.
Cagiati 343.
Cailliau 314, *412*.
Calhoun, F. P. 256, 291, *402*, *406*.
Callenberg, J. *416*.
Callewaert, H. 526, *539*.
Calman 261, 266, 385.
Calmeil 29, *84*.
Calmette 248, 332, 340.
Calvé, Le 369, 396, 399.
Campbell, D. 55, *84*, *140*, *423*.
Cameron 435.
Canale, P. *416*.
Caneo 47, *84*.
Cannon, W. B. 481, 483, 486, 487, *531*, *534*.
Cantalamessa 183, 185, *243*.
Capecchi, E. *416*.
Capone *402*.
Capparoni 218, *242*.
Caraman, Z. 325, 353, *412*.
Cardenal, M. Ch. 325, *413*.
Cardi 257, 266, 346.
Carle 350, *422*.
Carlill 138, *140*.
Carnevalis *424*.
Caro *409*.
Carol, W. *409*.
Carp, L. 256, *402*.
Carpenter 49, *84*.
Carré 88.
Carriol 495, *534*.
Carsaman 349.
Carteaud, A. *410*, *414*.
Casaubon, A. *416*, *419*.
Casazza, R. 408.
Časovnikov, R. *416*, *424*.
Casper, A. 324, *413*.
Cassirer, R. 246, 255, 266, 277, 281, 282, 283, 286, 287, 288, 289, 292, 293, 294, 295, 296, 297, 299, 312, 314, 322, 324, 330, 331, 336, 337, 341, 352, 355, 360, 379, 382, *400*, *406*, *407*, *471*.
Castana 246.
— V. *402*.
Castellino 257, 266, 284, 346, 392.
Casters 176, *243*.
Catalano 34, *84*.
Cattaneo, Donato 271, *402*.
Cavagnes 306.

Cavazzani 287, 290, 294.
Cave 89, 90, 91, 93, 96, 97, 98, 99, 100, 101, 104, 105, 106, 107, 108, 109, 111, 114, 115, 116, 118, 119, 122, 123, 124, 125, 138, *140*.
Cazacou 395.
Cederberg 287, *421*.
Celasco, Juan 350, *409*.
Celice, J. 314, *410*.
Celsus *84*.
Ceni, C. 55, *84*, *534*.
Cerkes, A. 325, *409*.
Černi, L. 334, 336, 337, 363, *414*.
Cernjavskaja, D. *400*.
Cerutti, P. *424*.
Cervais *403*.
Cervenka, J. 392, *416*.
Cestan 4, *84*.
Chabbert 181, 182, 183, *243*.
Chajes 306, 309.
Challier 259.
Challiol, V. *416*.
Charcot 20, 70, *84*, 176, 177, 178, 180, 181, 182, 186, 187, 192, 196, 197, 208, 217, 218, 237, *243*.
Chardonneau 293, *408*.
Charles 201, 225, *243*.
Charrin 226.
Charvát, J. 399, *416*.
Chasanow, M. *414*, 423.
Chauffard *402*.
Chauvet 350.
Chavany 341, *415*.
Chevalier 293, *407*.
Chevang 341.
Chiari 348.
Chiray 224, 236, *243*.
Chiavuttini 261.
Chirée 66, *84*.
Chomereau, B. *414*.
Chorosko 37, *84*, *85*.
Christiani 293.
Christiansen 175, 177, 178, 180, 187, 189, 190, 192, 193, 194, 196, 218, 228, 236, *243*.
Christoffel, H. 521, *534*.
Church 168, 228, *243*.
Chvostek 142, 145, 261, 311.
Ciampi, L. 524, 525, 531, *539*.
Cid, J. M. 394, *416*.
Cimbal, W. 462, 463, *471*, 522, *531*, *534*.
Claparède 129.
Clark 66, *84*, 179, *213*.
— Pierce 20, 24, 28, 34, 45, 51, 66, 81, 83, *81*.
Clarke 14, *84*, *407*.
Claude, H. 8, 46, 52, *84*, *86*, 248, 258, 279, 283, 393, *402*, *405*.

Cobbs 4, 45, 46, 47, 53, 54, 55, 56, 59, 76, *84*, *85*, *86*, *87*, *243*.
Coca 390.
Cockayne 312.
Cohen 116, 138, *140*, 262, 270, 279, 302, 306, 377, 381.
Cohn, Toby 276, 282.
Coke 390.
— F. 222, 235, *243*.
Cole, J. *424*.
Collet 37, *86*.
Collier 11, 20, 33, 38, *84*, 266, 290, 293, 328.
Collins 138, *140*, 299, 300, 315, 335, 367, 376, 377.
Collip 47.
Colman 21, *84*.
Colson 252, 259.
Comby, Jules 167, *405*.
Comel, M. *420*, *422*.
Consiglio 226, 237, *243*.
Cookson 30, *84*.
Cooper, Astley 53, *84*, 372, 383.
Cordiviola, L. *422*.
Cords, R. *414*.
Cornil, M. 234, *243*, 267, 277, 305, *401*, *406*, *407*, *420*, *424*.
Cornu 175, 193, 195, 200, *243*.
Corregro 364.
Costa, Mendes da 387.
Costedoat *539*.
Coulaud 347.
Couput 323, 324, *409*.
Courrèges, de 278, 314, *402*, *410*.
Court 308.
Courtades 371.
Courtois, A. *422*.
Courtsio 314.
Covisa, J. S. 314, 351, *409*.
Craig, Mc, K. 267, *420*, *422*.
Cramer, A. H. 30, *84*, *471*, *534*.
Creak 140.
Créhange, J. L. *413*.
Cremieux 224, 245.
Crichlow, R. S. 277, *402*.
Crichton 14, *84*.
Crinis, de 8, 46, *84*.
Crocher 321.
Crocq, J. 281, 282, 283, *405*.
Croftan 218, 220, *243*.
Cronbach 529, *540*.
Cronheim 237, *244*.
Crosti, A. 315, *409*.
Crouzon 4, 34, *84*.
Crowder 390.
Cullen 477.
Culver 256, 278.
Čumakov, N. *409*.
Cuneo 55, *84*.
Cunningham, W. F. 259, 267, *402*.

Curschmann, H. 66, 84, 92, 100, 112, 120, 135, *140*, 142, 148, 166, 167, 168, 171, 172, 173, 174, 183, 192, 198, 204, 217, 220, 222, 223, 226, 227, 230, 237, 239, 241, 242, *243*, 257, 290, 293, 296, 297, 298, 299, 300, 301, 302, 303, 305, 306, 316, 324, 331, 332, 338, 355, 361, 366, 369, 372, 399, *400*, *407*, *409*, *424*, 461, *471*, 480, 495, 498, 501, 505, 506, 518, 520, 527, 529, *534*, *539*.
Curtis 223, *243*, *421*.
Curtius, F. 386, 387, *416*, *472*.
Cushing 202, 256, 277.
Cushny 80, *84*.
Czerny, W. *410*.

Dahmen, O. 329, *402*, *405*.
Daiber, G. *472*.
Dalma 46, *84*.
Dana 340.
Dandry 84.
Dandy 49, 53, 82, *84*, 240, *243*.
Daneri, M. 364, *413*.
Danielopolu 495, *534*.
Daniels 90, 102, 109, 111, 122, 123, 124, 138, *140*.
Danilewskaya, E. 326, *409*.
Danisch, F. *534*.
Dannhauser 65, *84*.
Dardani, Remo *414*.
Dardignac 248.
Darling 80.
Dattner, B. 223, 235, *243*, *472*, *534*.
Daunic 264, *402*.
Dávalos, M. *402*.
Davanzo 221, *243*.
Davenport 41, 61, 62, *84*.
David, E. *534*.
— H. 200, *242*, 363, *410*, *411*.
Davis, L. 255, 299, *402*, *407*, *410*.
Davson of Penn, Lord 201, 223, *243*.
Debove 394.
Debray 318, 335.
Debré, R. 172, *243*.
Debrez 243.
Decastello, V. 315.
Dechaume, J. *244*, 267, *404*.
Declause 247.
Dederding, D. 380, *416*.
Defrance 247, 248.
Dehio 248, 266, 287, 290, 294, 295, 298, 307.
Dejeane 239, *243*.
Déjérine 62, *84*, 189, 217, *243*, 299, 301, 303, 339.
Delafontaine *140*.

Namenverzeichnis.

Delarne *411*.
Delas 328, *413*.
Delasiauve 65, *84*.
Delbecke, R. 261, 270, *401*.
Delcroix *410*.
Delhaye, A. 395, *416*.
Delherm 278, 315, 323, 324, *404, 409*.
Delhougne 488.
Delille *402*.
Delmas 66, *84*.
Delorme 239, *243*.
Demel, R. 280, 281, *400, 402*.
Denney, H. 357, *409*.
Denning, H. *534*.
Denyer 111, *140*.
Depisch 350.
Dercum 80, *84*, 116, 117, 118, *140*.
Deroto 353.
Desaux, A. 383, *425*.
Desbonnets *403*.
Determann 174, 177, 178, *243*.
Deutsch, E. 487, *416, 534*.
— F. *534*.
Devoto, A. 318, 319, 354, *409, 416*.
Deyl 200, *243*.
Diamond 224, *243*.
Dickerson 240, *243*.
Dickinson, W. 326, 395, *418, 425*.
Dide 34, *84*, 262.
Didier 254, 306.
Didsbury 199, *243*.
Dieck 296.
Dieden *534*.
Diehl 368.
Dielmann 46, *84*.
Diethelm 370, 374, 381, 383.
Diller 382.
Dinkelacker 367, 368, 377, 381, 383, 399.
Dinkler 307, 308, 309, 310, 344, 346, 347, 348, 355.
Diss *409*.
Dittrich, O. *406, 416, 424*.
Divry 80, *84*.
Dixon 248.
Dociades, L. *472*.
Döbel 361.
Döllken 206, 239, *243*.
Doerr, R. 390, 523, *416*.
Dominguez 252.
Donath 363.
Doran 62, *84*.
Dorst, St. F. *424*.
Douady, D. 323, *411*.
Doutrelepont 306, 307, 308, 310.
Dove 266.
Dowling, G. B. *409*.
Dowman 33, *85*.
Doyle 90, 102, 109, 111, 122, 123, 124, 138, *140*.
Dracoulidès, N. 522, *534*.

Dreikurs, R. *472*, 535.
Dresel, K. *472*, 511, *532*.
Dreyfuss 283, *406, 417*, 506, *532*.
Driak, F. *424*.
Drought 80, 87, 121, *141*.
Druitt 260.
Drysdale, H. H. *416*.
Duane 243.
Dubois-Reymond 173, 196, 202, 203, 204, 212, 216, *243, 407*.
Dubreuilh, W. 357, *409*.
Ducocher 262.
Dünger 293.
Duerdoth 248, *402*.
Dufke, Fr. 372, *416*.
Dufour 209, *243*, 248, 318, 328.
Duke, W. W. *416*.
Dukemann 261.
Dumas, A. 293, *407, 420*.
Dumitresco 176, 185, 244.
Duncan, Glen 47, *84*.
Dunlaß, H. 369, *416*.
Dunsmure 39, *84*.
Dupérié, R. 247, *402*.
Dupré 350.
Durante, L. 280, *402*.
Durham, R. 354, *409*.
Durig, A. 504, 508, 511, *532*.
Durupt, A. *421, 423*.
Dutaillis 180.
Dutil 20, *84*.
Duval 241, *243*.
Duvoir, L. *422*.
Dwight 187.

Ebbecke, U. 288, *416, 472*.
Eberhard 340.
Ebert 255.
Ebstein 322.
Echeverria 29.
Economo 114, 127, 129, *140, 437*.
Eddowes 321.
Edeiken, L. 323, *409*.
Edel, K. 66, *84*, 111, 112, 121, *140, 422*.
Edens, E. *400*, 514, *535*.
Edgeworth 76, *84*.
Edinger 199, *243*.
Egger 299, 301, 303, 312.
Eggleston 47, *86*.
Eguchi, H. 326, *409*.
Ehlers, H. 181, *243*.
Ehrenclou, A. 336, *415*.
Ehrenwall 377.
Ehrmann, F. S. 312, 313, 316, 320, 322, 325, 326, 329, 337, 344, 345, 347, 348, 349, 350, 351, 356, 358, 359, 360, 361, 362, 363, 364, 365, 366, *409, 410*.
Eibrink, G. A. H. 333, 340, *415*.

Eichelberg 488, *535*.
Eichhorst 252.
Eicken 288.
Eiselt *416*.
Eisner 390.
Elias, H. 283, *406*.
Ellenbrock 330.
Eller, Jos. Jord. 535.
Elliotson 66, *84*.
Ellis, R. W. B. *416, 424*.
Elman 53, *84*.
Elsberg 53, 55, 59, *84*, 86.
Elsner 291, 294.
Ely 243.
Emminghaus 337.
Enderle *424*.
Enke, W. *472*, 505, *535*.
Enrico, C. 347, 351, *410*.
Ensor 368, 388.
Entres, J. L. *472*.
Eppinger, H. 218, *472*, 482, 483, 485, 495, 496, *532, 537*.
Epstein, St. 193, 344, 363, *422*.
Erben 462.
Erdmann 222.
Erichton 367.
Eriksson, J. *402*.
Erkes 364.
Erlanger, B. *164*.
Ermakov 120, *140*.
Esau *423*.
Escat 187, 231, *243*.
Escherich 143, 152, 153, 155, *164*.
Eschweiler 371.
Eskuchen 390, 398, 399, 515, *535*.
Eslevič 116, 117, 118, *140*.
Esquirol 4, 15, 74, *84*.
Estländer 248.
Etienne 283, 395.
Ettinger 385.
Eulenburg 173, 200, 203, *243*, 288, 290, 295, 318, 325.
Eusière 66, *84*.
Evans, E. *416*.
Everke 48, *84*.
Ewald 434, 437, 519.
Exner, R. 435, 469, *471*, 535.
Eyrich 470.
Ezickson, W. J. *416*.

Faber, H. *424*.
— Knud *423*, 520, *532*.
Fabre 167, 172, *243*.
Fackenheim 76, *84*.
Façon, E. 110, *140*, 335, *415*.
Fagge 25, *84*.
Fahrenkamp, K. 241, *472*, 486, 511, 512, *532, 535*.
Fajngold, L. 3.9, *410*.
Falta, W. 353, 392, *472*.
Faure 526.
Favier 328.

Favory, A. 326, 350, *113*.
Fay, Temple 49, 50, 54, 82, *84, 86,* 280, *402.*
Fechner, O. 493, *539.*
Fecht *243.*
Fedorow 315, 319.
Feer, E. W. 149, 155, 297, 369, 377, 521, *407, 416.*
Feiling, A. 280, *402.*
Feinberg, N. *472.*
Feldberg, W. 269, 270, 271, *535.*
Felix, K. 512, *535.*
Fellner *401.*
Fendel, H. *532.*
Fényes, J. 319, 322, *410.*
Féré 4, 9, 15, 20, 29, 30, 61, 66, *85,* 121, 174, 175, 176, 177, 178, 179, 189, 190, 192, 193, 209, 212, 380.
Féréol 375.
Fernandez, S. *402.*
Fernell 199.
Fernet 353, 354, *411.*
Ferranini 293.
Fessler, A. 325, *410, 422.*
Feudel, H. *472.*
Fiehrer, A. 350, *422.*
Filia 65, *85.*
Filiol 320, *410.*
Fillié *410.*
Fincher 33, *85.*
Finckh 62, 63, *85.*
Finder *416.*
Finger 288.
Finkelnburg, R. 447, *472.*
Finkelstein 150, 156, 311, *408.*
Finlay 326.
Firth 35, *85.*
Fischer, B. 51, 55, *85,* 89, 90, 100, 102, 110, 111, 120, *140,* 212, 248, 251.
— E. 118.
— F. 88, 111.
— J. *140.*
— K. *534.*
— O. 335.
Fischl, R. *410.*
Fisher 201, *243.*
Flach, Auguste 132.
Flandin, Ch. 235, 371, 399, *400, 402.*
— O. N. *535.*
Flarer, F. 353, *406, 410, 422.*
Flatau, G. 166, 167, 168, 169, 171, 173, 174, 175, 176, 177, 178, 179, 180, 181, 186, 187, 188, 189, 190, 192, 193, 194, 195, 197, 198, 200, 202, 209, 217, 218, 230, 235, 241, *243, 472,* 530, *535.*
— Th. S. *539.*
Fleischer, Fr. 520, *532.*
Fleischhacker, H. *532.*
Flesch 53, *85.*

Fletcher 323, 362.
Fliederbaum *416.*
Flint, Gordon 423.
Florentin 370, *420.*
Florian 395.
Flothow, P. G. *400.*
Fodor 224, *243.*
Foerster, O. 11, 24, 35, 49, 54, 55, 59, 64, *85,* 206, *243,* 273, 357, *400,* 481, 490, 511, *535.*
Förster, E. 447, 469, *411.*
Fog 54, *85.*
Follet 395.
Follmann, J. *422.*
Fontaine, R. 348, 365, *403, 411, 420.*
Ford 30, *85.*
Fordyce, A. 321, 340, *415.*
Forel, O. L. 313, 315, *409.*
Forestier *245.*
Fornara 313.
Fornero, A. 271, *402.*
Forni 193.
Forsberg 374.
Forster, F. E. 299, 365, *406, 472.*
Foshay 47, *85.*
Fossier *407.*
Foster *85.*
Fouché 123, *140.*
Fournier, J. C. 183, 226, *244,* 370, 381, *418, 424.*
Fox, Taylor 80, *85,* 255.
Franckel *411.*
Fränkel 237, *243.*
Frank 47, *85.*
— D. B. *540.*
— E. 482, 483, 484, 498, 508, *535.*
— L. 530, 531, *532.*
— Ph. *424.*
Franke 364.
Frankel *421.*
Frankhauser 80, *85.*
Frankl-Hochwarth, von 142, 148, 153, 227, 299, 305, 330, 450, 509.
Franz 226.
Freemann 390.
Frei, Magda 164.
Frémy 314.
French 394.
Frenkel 283, 379, *420, 421.*
Frenkl, *417.*
Freud, S. 42, 97, 198, 452, 498.
Freudenberg, E. 76, *85,* 142, 151, 152, 156, 157, 158, 163, 164, *164.*
Freudenthal 375.
Freund, E. 122, *140,* 238, *410,* 445.
Frey, E. K. 279, 307, *408, 420.*
Frick, F. 328, *402, 410.*
Fried 48, *85.*
Friedel 247.

Friedemann 256, 435.
Friedenwald, J. 264, *402.*
Friedheim 325.
Friedländer 224, 235, *243, 535.*
Friedmann, M. 37, *85,* 88, 136, 160, 161, 264, 299, 335, 361, *435,* 446, 447, 452, 467, *472,* 488.
Frink 40, *85.*
Frisch, Felix 46, 47, 48, *85,* 105, *140.*
Fritz 388.
Fritzsche, G. 352, *410.*
Frocassi 113, *140.*
Frödeberg 91, 95, 100, 101, 111, 117, *140.*
Fröhlich, A. 206, *532, 535.*
Fröschels, E. 524, 530, *539, 540.*
Fromhold 331.
Fromm, N. K. 330, 331, 334, *414, 423.*
Frunkin 93, 97, 107, 110, 114, 116, 118, 120, 123, *140.*
Fry 47, *84.*
Fuchs 80, *85, 243,* 256, 377, 462.
— A. 182, 209, *243,* 256.
Fürstenheim 324, *413.*
Fuerstner 374, 393.
Fuhs, H. 386, *417.*
Fulton, John F. 61, *85,* 109, *140,* 251, 280, 382, *402, 417.*
Furbush 61, *86.*
Fuss 324, 351.

Gadaud *418.*
Gadrat, J. *410, 417, 422.*
Gaensslen 222, 223, *243,* 371, 384.
Gänssler 384.
Gärtner 78, *85.*
Gagel, O. 266, *420.*
Gaillard 248.
Gaisböck 221, *243.*
Galant, J. S. 524, 530, *540.*
Galen 4, 31, 88, 199.
Galenko, W. 284, *406.*
Galezowski 176, 177, 180, 197, *243.*
Gallavardin, L. *402.*
Gallois, J. *420.*
Gamble 48, 76, *85.*
Gamper 127.
Gans, O. 344, *400, 407.*
Garcin 119, *140.*
Gardère 336.
Garner, V. *408.*
Garnier, M. 396, *417.*
Garra, A. 381, *424.*
Garrigues 248, 251, 256.
Garrod 74.
Gasne 282.
Gaspardi 248.

Gaspero, di 46, *85*.
Gaté, J. *410*.
Gatellier, J. *423*.
Gauch, S. 278, 314, 364, *402*, *410*.
Gaucher 306.
Gaupp, R. 439, 458, 464, 465, 466, 468, *472*.
Gauthron *416*.
Gay, P. J. *424*.
Gazia, H. *410*.
Gebbing, M. *472*.
Geist 331.
Gelb, A. 459, *472*.
Gélineau 88, 89, 93, 94, 102, 112, 119, 120, 131, 135, *140*, 161.
Gennes, I.. de *402*.
Georges 248, 252, 258, 266, 267, 269, *402*, *403*, *423*.
Georgi 46, *85*.
Gerbis, H. 247, 273, 304, *403*.
Gerhardt 290.
Gerhartz 377.
Gerlach, F. 399, *417*.
Germain, St. de 348.
Germes 252.
Gernez, L. *403*.
Gerrard 287.
Gerson *243*, 350.
Gerstmann 99.
Gersung 335.
Gesell 340, 342, 343, *415*.
Gessler, H. 489, *535*.
Gewin 247.
Geyelin 52, 76, *85*.
Ghelfi 259.
Gibert 259.
Gibney 321.
Giebler 185, 186, *243*.
Gierlich 435, 457, 461, 462, *472*.
Giesen 123, *140*.
Gigon, A. 489, *535*.
Gilbert 261.
Gildemeister 493.
Gillespie 119, *140*.
Gillies, H. *423*.
Gilmoor 322.
Giovanni 266.
Girons, St. 284.
Giroux, R. 279, *403*.
Gjessing, H. Chr. *424*.
Glasberg 363.
Glaser *535*.
Glasser 329, 353, *410*.
Glen, R. *405*.
Glénard, Roger *420*.
Glorieux 393.
Gnesda 393.
Goebell 273.
Göring, D. 355.
Gött 30, *85*, 142, 147, 158, 290.
Goette 290.
Goldbladt 204.
Goldbloom 76, *85*.

Goldflam 89, 107, 108, 119, 121, 122, 124, *140*.
Goldmann 157, *164*.
Goldner, M. 497, 534.
Goldscheider, A. 336, 433, 438, 458, 462, *472*, *535*.
Goldschlag, F. 394, 395, 396, *417*.
Goldschmidt 322, 346, 347.
Goldsmith, W. *410*.
Goldstein, K. 349, 447, 459, *472*, 480, 492, *535*.
Goldzieher 527.
Golla 80, *85*.
Gollwitzer *164*, 511, *535*.
Golomb, J. 359, *410*.
Golsmid 314.
Gómez, F. 369, *417*.
Gonzalez-Aquilar, J. *400*.
Goodheart 350.
Gordinier 382.
Gordon, A. *417*.
— H. 18, *85*, 172, 226, *243*, 347, 348, *410*.
Gotch 54.
Gottesmann, J. *410*.
Gougerot, H. 264, 278, 318, 319, 320, 328, *403*, *410*, *422*.
Gouin, J. 278, *403*.
Govin 220, 234.
Gowers 4, 5, 9, 10, 11, 12, 14, 15, 16, 17, 20, 21, 23, 25, 27, 36, 38, 44, 61, 62, 63, 65, 67, 70, 76, *85*, 88, 93, 119, 120, 121, 138, 167, 174, 192, 217, 238, 239, 241, *243*, 261, 334.
Gozzano 100, 101, *140*.
Grabs 339.
Graçoski *406*.
Gradle 193, *243*.
Gräfenberg, E. 522, *535*.
Graf, Fl. *537*.
Grafe, E. 339, *472*, 487, 489, *535*.
Graham, Douglas 276, *403*.
Grant, R. T. 157, *164*, *417*.
Grasset 169, *243*, 323, 326, 328, 356.
Graves 83, *85*, 286, 287, 290, 293, *407*.
Gray, A. M. H. *422*.
Grazia, de 266.
Greiwe 266.
Grenet, H. 258, 266, 267, 269, *403*.
Grenier 286, 290.
Greving, R. *472*.
Grimes, E. 166, *243*.
Grimm *417*.
Griveaud 328, *410*.
Grjasev, F. *407*.
Groddeck *534*.
Grödel, Fr. 314, 318, *410*.
Groer, v. 151.

Groot jr., J. de 378, *417*.
Gros, A. 273, *403*.
Gross 137, 306, 369, 375, 377, 378.
Gruber, G. B. 275, 294, 346, *400*.
Grün 89, 106, 120, 121, 139, *140*.
Grünfeld 321, 325, 349, 361.
Grünstein 176, 177, *243*.
Grünzweig, B. *535*.
Grütz, O. 329, *415*.
Grugent 273.
Gruhle 4, *85*, 136, *140*.
Grumach, L. 523, *535*.
Gruszecka, A. 102, 113, 118, 140, 261, *403*.
Gstrein 288, 290, 291, 292, 293, *403*.
Guarini, C. 323, *422*.
Gubergritz, M. *535*.
Gubler 186, *243*.
Günther 119, *140*.
Guillain, G. 119, *140*, 314, 326, 350, *410*, *423*.
Guillaumin, Ch. O. 383, *405*, *414*, *423*, *424*.
Gutfreund 306.
Guth 322.
Guttmann, E. 40, 48, 49, 54, 64, *84*, *85*, 235, 305, 462, *472*, 480, 503, *532*,
Gutzmann, H. 529, *539*, *540*.
György 150, 155, 156, 157, *164*.

Haase, W. 408.
Hachez, E. 386, *417*.
Hadlich 205, *243*.
Haelst, A. van *410*.
Haenel 119, 121, 330.
Haeseler 457.
Haguenau, Y. 235, *245*, *416*.
Hahn, B. 522, *535*.
— H. 462, *472*.
— J. 218, 220, 226, 227, 238, *243*, 303, 381, *400*, *408*.
Haig 218, 220, *243*, 261.
Hajos, W. *417*.
Halban, v. 230, *243*.
Halbertsma, Tj. *422*.
Haldin *410*.
Hall, M. 80, *85*, 192, 202, 203.
Hallé, J. *422*.
Hallervorden 525.
Hallopeau 329.
Halpert 257.
Halstedt 371, 376.
Hamburger 167, 172, *243*.
Hamilton 48, *85*, 288, 294, 295.
Hammer 276, 351, 363.
Hammerschlag 460.
Hammond 74, *85*, 203.
Handford 318.
Handwerk 380.

Hanke, H. 519, *535*.
Hanse, M. *472*.
Hansen, K. *472*, 480, 485, 486, 487, 488, 489, 495, 498, 500, 502, 503, 505, 506, 508, 510, 515, 516, 517, *535*.
Hardy 250, 328.
Hare, Francis 56, 74, *85*, 204, 236, *243, 407*.
Harlay 348.
Harnik, M. 522, *537*.
Harrington 378.
Harris 32, *85*, 110, 138, *140*, 238, *243*.
Hartenberg 29, 46, 65, *85*, 199, *243*.
Hartmann 166, 199, 217, 241, *243*, 285, 296, 312, 325, 326, 354, 358.
— N. 494, 532.
Hartsock 224, 236, *243*.
Hartung 226, 237, *243*.
Harvier, P. 362, *410*.
Hascovec 299.
Hase 307.
Haskovec 351.
Hastreiter 248.
Hatousek 361.
Hatry 322, 351, *410*.
Hattendorff 334, 335.
Hattingberg, v. 495, 507, *535*.
Hauptmann, A. 436, 439, 447, 468, *472*.
Haushalter 312.
Hausman *86*.
Hawke, E. K. 385, *419*.
Hay, K. 284, *406*.
Heberer 83, *85*.
Hebra 364.
Heidemann, H. *535*.
Heidenhain 389.
Heilbronner 37, *85*.
Heilig 487, 488.
Heiligenthal 335.
Heimann, V. 293, 322, 351, 369, 385, 392, 398, *410*, *418*.
Heine, J. *400, 420*.
Heinemann 332.
Heinisman, J. 363, *410*.
Heinz, R. 469, *472*.
Heissen 302, *408*.
Heitz, J. 463. 417.
Hektoen 325, 346, 347.
Held 55, *85*.
Heller, J. 254, 312, 318, 321, 325, 329, 344, 361, 364, 365, 388, *400, 407*.
— Th. *472*.
Hellpach, W. 443, 450, 451, 454, 456, 462, 465, *472*.
Hellwig 239, *243*.
Helmholtz 77, *85*.
Helsmoortel 330.
Hendriksen 54, *85*.

Henke, H. 475, *538*.
Henneberg 94, 111, 112, 120.
Hennecaut 248.
Henning 73, *85*, 394.
Henoch 287, 293, 374.
Henry 247, 260.
Henschen 171, 199, *243*.
Héraux, A. *404*.
Hercog, Paul *422*.
Herczeg 363.
Hering, E. H. 486, 487, 511.
Hermann, R. 113, *140, 403, 420, 424*.
Herpin 4, 7, 10, 73, 77, *85*.
Herringham 321.
Herschmann 128, *140*.
Hertoghe 226, *243*, 283, 284, 395, 399.
Herxheimer 285, 296, 318, 344, 355, 356, 358, 361.
Herz, M. 262, 278, 302, 306, 375, 510, *535*.
Herzberg, A. *535*.
— W. R. 128, 130, 134, 218, 354, *472*, 449, 482, 483, 484, 485, 490, 491, 495, 496, *532, 535, 537*.
Hetény 224, *243*.
Heuk 262, 263.
Heusner 316.
Heuyer, G. 393, *400, 424*.
Hever *140*.
Heverogh *140*, 187, 189, *243*.
Heyer, G. R. 449, 469, 487, 488, 493, 505, 518, 520, *473, 532, 535, 536*.
Heyerdahl 167, 217, *243*.
Heymann 163, 373.
Heymanowitsch *243*.
Higgins 241.
Higier, H. 365, *400, 536*.
Hill 53, *85*, 204, *243*.
Hillemand, P. 287, *407, 414*.
Hiller 335.
Hillmann, H. J. 325, 353, *400*.
Hilpert 112, 120, 121, 138, *140*, 177, *243*.
Himmelweit, F. *472*.
Hincky *410*.
Hines jr., E. A. *424*.
Hintner 306, 307, 308, 310.
Hion 524.
Hirose 293.
Hirsch 83, *85*, 127, 279, 330, 334.
— A. 164, 279.
Hirschberg, N. *473*.
Hirschfeld, R. 246, *400, 407*.
His, W. 369, *473*, 497.
Hlaváček, Vl. 388, *417, 424*.
Hnatek 248, 251.
Hoche, A. O. *404*, 440, 444, 449, 450, *473, 536*.

Hochenegg 246, 261, 266.
Hochsinger 30, *85*, 159, 160.
Hodge 201, *243*.
Höflmeyer 332, 333.
Hönighaus, L. *420*.
Hoepfner, Th. 530, 531, *539, 540*.
Hoesslin, R. v. 248, 253, 263, 278, 462, *473*.
Hoff, H. 89, 105, 107, 109, 111, 112, 114, 115, 118, 121, 123, 124, 134, *140, 473*, 487, 488, *536*.
Hoffa 329, 355, 365.
Hofferbert, A. *473*.
Hoffmann, H. 145, 282, 285, 330, 331, 334, 341, 342, 344, 350, 351, 353, 361, *410, 536*.
— H. F. 478, *532*.
Hofmann, E. 386, 387, *417*.
Hoke, E. 370, *417*.
Holland 257.
d'Hollander 37, *84*.
Holm 248, 251.
Holmes, Oliver Wendell 33, 35, 38, *85*, *87*, 220.
Holschaw, F. 270, *403*.
Holst 203, 248, 256.
Holström 47, *85*.
Holub, A. *532*.
Homburger, A. *473*, 506, 530, *536*.
Homen 380.
Hope 394.
Hopkins 357, *409*.
Hoppe 325, 356.
Hopphan, E. *424*.
Horinchi 288, 293, *407*.
Horn, P. 442, 447, 449, 451, 462, 463, *473*.
Hornowski 293, 294, 295, 347, 348.
Horoshko 76, *85*.
Horowitz, A. 323, 353, *412*, *423*.
Horrax 43, *85*.
Horsch, K. *421*.
Horsley 49, 54, *85*.
Hortolomei 244.
Hoshina, K. 287, *421*.
Hoyen 248.
Hryniewiecki, St. 383, *417*.
Hubert 314, 318.
Huchard 218.
Hudelo 357, *410*.
Hudovernig 181, 183, *243*.
Hübner 248, 331, 332.
Hürlimann 323, 379.
Hürthle 203.
Huet 363.
Hufschmidt 320, 353, *410*.
Huguenin, R. 396, *417*.
Huldschinsky *164*.
Hummelsheim *536*.
Huntzinger 224, 234, 236, *244*.

Namenverzeichnis.

Hurmuzache, Cl. *406*.
Hurst, F. 227, *243*, 390.
Husler, J. 141 f., *165*.
Hustin 242.
Hutchinson 254, 259, 260, 314, 329.
Hval 292, 293, *407*.

Ibrahim, J. 149, 150, *165*, *536*.
Imperiale, C. 274, *403*.
Inclan, José Luis *400*.
Innran, J. Chr. V. *540*.
Ipsen, Johs *400*.
Isaac, P. 248, 252, 258, 266, 267, 269, *402*, *403*, 487.
Isanos, M. 347, 348, *412*.
Ischlondsky, N. E. *473*.
Isenschmidt, R. 445, *473*, *536*.
Ishida, Iwao 287, *421*.
Isola, D. 313, 352, *411*.
Isovesco 261.
Isserlin, M. 451, *473*, 530, *540*.
Iterson, van 371.
Ivanoff, S. 374, *417*.
Iwai 261, *403*.
Iwamura 144.
Iwanow *473*.

Jaceoud 203, *243*.
Jack 242.
Jackson, Hughlings 4, 5, 10, 13, 14, 16, 20, 22, 25, 31, 35, 38, 39, 41, 56, 58, 59, 77, 78, *85*, 182, 193, *243*.
Jacob 273, 313, 318, 325, 328, 353, 354, 395, *404*, *411*.
Jacobi, E. *473*, 523, *536*.
— W. 46, *85*, 308, *400*, *531*.
Jacquelin, A. *421*.
Jacquet 200, *243*, 335.
Jadassohn 338, 349.
Jaensch, E. R. *473*, 482.
— W. 435, 482, 495, 505, *532*.
Jaffé, K. *411*.
Jahn, D. *473*.
Jahrreiss, W. 195, *243*, 467, *473*, 477, 498, 501, 505, *532*.
Jakob 318, 325, 328, 353, 354.
Jakobi 492.
Jakobsohn 110, 111, 122, 126, *140*.
James 326, 485.
Jamhanzi 29, *85*.
Jamieson 377.
Jamin *536*.
Jancsó *417*.
Jandova 374.
Janet 40, *85*.
Janichewski 363, *411*.
Janota 138, *140*.
Janowski, W. *472*.
Jansen 333, 340, *415*.
Jansion *406*.

Januschke, H. 435, *473*, *536*.
Janzen 88, 91, 110, 116, 118, 122, 126, *140*.
Jaques 348.
Jaroschy, W. 395, *417*, *424*.
Jasiénski, J. *420*.
Jaso, E. *406*.
Jeanselme 320, 321, 349, *411*.
Jedlicka, V. 347, 348, 350, *411*.
Jelgersma 51, *85*.
Jeliffe 93, 107, 111, *140*, 272, 279, *421*.
Jelsma, F. *405*.
Jendrassik 101, 330, 334, 338.
Jenkin 76, *85*.
Jenny, Ed. 386, *417*.
Jirasek *407*.
Joachim 185, *243*.
Job 54, 77, *84*, *85*.
Jörgensen 165.
Johannsen 286, 357, *409*.
Johanson 250.
John 47, *85*.
Johnson, W. 80, *85*, 247, 397, *418*, *424*, 524, *540*.
Jolly 118, 120, 177, 209, *243*, 339.
Joltrain, E. 235, 369, *417*, *421*, *424*, 522, *536*.
Jones 51, 52, *86*, 299.
Jonnesco 83, *85*, 239, *243*.
Joppich 347.
Jordan, A. 313, 320, *411*.
Josat 4, *85*.
Josefowitsch 314, 326.
Joseph 307, 367, 370, 381, 385, 386.
Jossmann *415*.
Jourdanet 200, *243*.
Jourdens 285.
Juliusburger, O. *473*.
Jung, A. 363, *418*, *422*.
Juster 312, 363, *411*, *412*, *421*.
Justin, L. *405*, *421*.

Kabisch 487.
Källmark, F. *417*.
Kämmerer, H. 202, 207, 217, 220, 235, 238, *243*, 374, 384, 389, 390, 391, 515, 517, *417*, *532*.
Kaglin, E. *473*.
Kahane 276, *400*.
Kahler 89, 102, 107, 109, 112, 116, 117, 118, 119, 120, 134, *140*, 349.
Kahn, E. 450, 452, *473*, 498, 505, *532*, *536*.
— W. 323, 324, 354, *408*, *409*.
Kaku, T. 298, *421*.
Kalischer 325, 358.
Kambayashi 354.
Kammann 106, 114, 115, *140*.
Kamp 380.

Kanavel, A. B. 299, *402*, *407*.
Kane *540*.
Kanko, Yoshitomo 348, *422*.
Kanno, E. 325, 351, *411*.
Kantor, J. L. 520, *536*.
Kaplinski 89, 126, *140*.
Kaposi 306, 307, 312, 318, 329, 364.
Kappis *407*.
Karger 76, *85*.
Karplus, J. P. 181, 186, 193, *243*, 304, *400*, 436, 449, 484, 490, 511, *536*.
Karrer *164*.
Kartje 282, 283.
Kashida 145.
Kast 201, *243*.
Katsch, G. 506, 511, 518, 519, 520, *532*, *536*.
Katz, D. R. *536*.
Kauf, K. E. 487, *534*.
Kaufmann, Fr. 512, *532*.
Kaunitz, J. 275, *400*.
Keefe 370.
Kehrer, F. 112, 393, 435, 459, 460, 461, 462, 463, *473*, 477, 478, 479, 520, *532*.
Keilmann, Klaus *411*.
Keith 54, 77, *85*, *86*.
Keller, H. 94, 131, *140*, 209, *243*, 326, *473*.
Kelling 224, *244*.
Kellog 223, *243*.
Kelly, S. 287, 294, *407*.
Kennedy, Foster 14, 39, 45, 49, *85*, 107, 112, 113, *140*, 202, 223, *244*, 381, 383, *417*.
Kernohan, J. W. 267, *420*, *422*.
Kerpolla 205, 235, *243*.
Kerr, W. 277, *403*.
Kestenbaum 128.
Kiaer, Sven *403*.
Kick 308.
Kierkegaard, S. 450, *473*.
Kiess 351.
Kimber 81, *85*.
Kindberg 199.
Kirschberg 487.
Kirschenberg, E. 331, 339, *415*.
Kiss, J. *536*.
Kisthinios, N. 279, *403*.
Kistler, K. *540*.
Kitaigorodskaja, O. *415*.
Kiuzhi 354.
Kläsi 521.
Klages, L. 492, *532*.
Klappenbach, W. 254, *403*.
Klauder *407*.
Klausner 237, *244*.
Klee 483, 519.
Klein *415*.
Kleine 120, 122, 137, *140*.
Kleist, K. 437, 491, 530.

Klemperer, E. 489, *536*.
Klewitz 515, 516, *532*.
Klimke, W. 520, *536*.
Klinger 354.
Klingmann, W. O. 330, 331, 361, *411*.
Klingmüller, V. 364, *406*.
Klinkart 369.
Klotz, R. 435, *473*, 512, *532, 536*.
Kluge *140*.
Knapp 36, *85*, 183, 191, *244*, 335.
Knauer, A. 449, 450, 459, 462, 463, *473*, 486, 487, *536*.
Kneidel 62, *85*.
Knjažanskij *415*.
Knowledge *85*.
Koch, J. L. A. *403*, *473*.
Kocher 82, *85*, 202, *244*.
Köbner 386.
Kölle 362.
Köllner, H. 459, *473*.
Koelsch 273, *400*.
Koenig, Paul 374, 377, *417*.
Königstein 291, 293, 354.
Körner 332.
Köster 254.
Kogerer, H. 51, *85*, *536*.
Kogoj, Fr. 319, 344, 345, 351, *411*.
Kohnstamm, O. 435, 467, *472*, 488.
Kolb 326.
Kolisch 247, 266.
Kollarits, J. 181, *244*, *473*.
Kolle 241, *244*.
Kollewije 118, *140*.
Kolodan 280.
Kolodny, A. *403*.
Konjetzny 518.
Kopczynski 314, 340.
Kopf, H. 270, 279, *403*.
Koplik 150.
Kopp 307.
Koppius 287.
Korn 330.
Kornfeld 261, 266, 349.
Korns, H. M. *424*.
Koshewnikow, A. M. 37, *85*, 340, *415*.
Kosmadis, W. 319, *400*.
Kowalewsky, P. J. 166, 190, 193, 200, *244*, *473*.
Kracht 331, 332.
Kraeger, F. 292, *407*.
Krämer 177, *244*.
Kräpelin, E. 196, 449, *473*.
Kraetzer, A. 247, *403*.
Krafft-Ebing, v. 190, 193, 196, 197, 200, 244, *473*.
Kramer, F. 526, 540.
Kramsztyk 220, 226, *244*.
Krapf, E. 511, 512, 513, *536*.
Krasnowa, P. *411*.
Kraus, A. *411*, 436, *536*.

Kraus, E. J. 344, 345, 346, 347, 348, 355, *403*, *411*, 436, 462, *536*.
— F. 119, 135, *140*, 270, 314, *407*, 436, 462, *473*, *483*, 484, 492, 497, 510, *532*, *536*.
Krause, W. M. 113.
Krebs, E. 312, 325, 326, 354, *411*.
Kreeger 312.
Krehl, L. v. *474*, 510, *532*, *536*.
Kreibich 253, 307, 308, 309, 310, 374, 396.
Kreidl 436, 449, 490, 511, *536*.
Kreindler, A. 107, 127, 283, 335, *406*, *415*, *538*.
Kren 312, 320, 321, 322, 324, 325, 347, 350, 351.
Kretschmer, E. 45, *85*, *444*, 456, 461, *474*, 505, 519, *532*, *536*.
— M. *536*.
Kretz, J. 399, *424*.
Krieger 349.
Krijnen, J. *417*.
Krisch 179, *244*.
Krisowski 259.
Kroemer 325.
Kroetz, Chr. *474*, 481, *483*, 489, *532*.
Krogh 270.
Kroll, F. W. 490, *533*, *535*, *536*.
— M. 319, 337, *400*.
Krompecher 344, 355.
Kroner 259.
Kronfeld, A. 452, *474*, 489, 495, 500, 505, 514, 515, 516, *532*, *536*.
Krotoska, M. *415*.
Krueger, R. 331, 334, *536*.
Kruglow, A. *407*.
Krumbholz 37, *85*.
Krysztalowicz 344.
Kubo, H. *419*.
Kuczska, W. *411*.
Külbs, F. 451, 469, *474*.
Kümmel jr., H. 259, 280, *400*, 460.
Künkel, F. *474*.
Küppers, E. 437, 449, *474*, 486, 500, *532*, *536*.
Kuerbitz 372.
Kugler, E. *474*.
Kujaschansky 340.
Kulkow, R. *415*.
Kulkow, A. 46, *85*, 340, *415*.
Kulm 375.
Kummer 351.
Kunos *243*.
Kunstmann 287, 294, 299, *407*.
Kuntz 248.
Kunz, M. *474*.
Kupferberg 237.

Kuré, Ken 270, 348, 364, *422*.
Kurzrok 225, *245*.
Kussmaul 53, *85*, 529.
Kuttner, A. 515, *536*.
— H. P. *536*.
— L. *536*.
Kylin, E. *536*.
Kyriaco *140*.
Kyrle, J. *400*.

Labarraque 170, *244*.
Lacasseyne, J. *404*.
Ladalle 330.
Ladeck 488.
Laederich, L. *422*.
Laennec *411*.
Laewen, A. 299, *407*.
Lährs 248.
Ladalle 330.
Lafon 254, 351.
Lafora 51, *85*, 121, 138, *140*.
Lagade, J. *421*.
Lagarde 284.
Laignel, L. 267, 281, 288, 351, 369, 399, *400*, *407*, *417*, *421*, *532*, *537*.
Laing 224, *244*.
Lamacq 198, *244*, 339.
Lamoc *140*.
Lamotte 349, *414*.
Landau, A. *403*, *420*.
Lande 330, 338.
Landgraf 287.
Landis, E. 257, 271, *404*, *406*.
Landry 37, *85*, 381.
Landwehr 377.
Langdon 29, 65, *85*, 339.
Lange, C. de 183, 232, *244*.
— Fr. *537*.
— Joh. 455, *473*, *474*, 480, 485, 487, 495, 506, 511, 512, *532*, *537*.
Langenskiöld 495.
Langeron *403*.
Langley 481, *532*.
Langmead 361.
Lannois, Maurice 286, 287, 289, 290, 294, 295, 394.
Lanzenberg 329, 353, *410*.
Lapersonne 176, *244*.
Lapinsky, M. N. 277, *403*.
Laqueur 276, 277, 299, *400*.
Larsen, Erik 341, *423*.
Lartigue *403*.
Lasegue 193, 217, 222, *244*.
Lassila, W. *403*.
Latham 203, *244*.
Lauber, H. 331, 332, *415*, 488, *537*.
Laubry 377, *417*.
Laudat 221.
Laudenheimer *140*, 220, 226, 237, *244*, 487, 517, *537*.
Laudon 375.
Laurenti 248.

Laurentier 264, *402*.
Laval, F. *417*.
Lavallée 291.
Lavastine, M. 267, 281, 288, 351, 369, 399, *407*, *417*, *421*, *532*, *537*.
Lawson, R. S. 280, *403*.
Layani, F. 281, 282, 283, 284, 285, 286, 298, *406*, *421*.
Lechelle, P. 119, *140*, 322, *411*.
Leclerc 176, *244*, 314.
Lecoulant 328, *413*.
Lederer 149, *165*.
Ledoux, E. *406*.
Leeuwen, Storm van 223, 235, *245*, 368, 369, 370, 383, 390, 391, *419*, 515, 517.
Legrain 313, 353.
Lehmann, G. 485, 486, *537*.
— W. 280, 306, *400*.
Lehmkuhl 37, *85*.
Lehner, E. 222, 227, *244*, *417*.
Lehrnbecher, A. 264, *403*.
Leibbrand, W. *473*.
Leibovici, R. *421*.
Leibowitz, O. 520, *537*.
Leidler, R. 460, *474*.
Leiner 351, *411*.
Leischner 235, *244*.
Lelong 313.
Lemon, W. S. *416*, 525.
Lenk, E. 278, 487, *537*.
Lennon, W. *424*.
Lennox 4, 45, 46, 47, 48, 54, 55, 56, 76, *85*, *87*.
Lenoir 74, *85*, 306, 308.
Lenstrup, E. 340, 342, *415*.
Lenz 524.
Leopold *417*.
Lepinay 320, *422*.
Lereboullet, P. 284, 313, 351, 362, *406*, *411*.
Leredde 346, 347, 348, 363.
Léri, A. 230, 313, 314, 328, 331, 334, 339, 395, *411*, *415*, *417*.
Leriche, R. 49, *85*, 258, 279, 280, 299, 348, 363, 365, *400*, *403*, *407*, *411*, *420*, *422*.
Lermoyez 34, *87*, 240.
Lerner, M. L. 256, *401*.
Leroy 28, *85*.
Leschke, E. 436, 462, *474*, 482, 484, 496, 511, 513, 516, 519, *532*, *537*.
Leskowski 334.
Lesné 310, 369, *417*.
Leube 349.
Leubuscher, P. 454, *474*.
Leuret 65, *85*.
Leven *424*.
Levi, A. *244*.
Lévi, L. 44, 46, *85*, 112, 200, 225, 226, 227, 237, *244*, 290.

Levin 90, 97, 102, 107, 109, 110, 111, 117, 123, 126, 136, *140*.
Levinsohn *242*.
Lévy, Gabrielle *411*.
— Georges *411*, *412*.
— Leopold, M. 30, *86*, 264, 270, 284, 287, 314, 315, 330, 353, 369, *417*, *421*, 525.
Levy, S. *405*.
Lewandowski 240, *244*, 482, *537*.
Lewellys 261.
Lewen 224, 241.
Lewin 287, 290, 293, 295, 312, 315, 318, 321, 329, 342, 344, 354, 361, 364, 365, 370.
Lewinsohn 183.
Lewis, Thomas 269, 270, 271, 280, 295, 296, *404*, *406*, *421*.
Lewontin 310.
Lewy, F. H. 120, *140*, 304, 484, *532*, *537*.
Ley 127, *140*, 226, *244*, *417*.
Leyser, E. 55, *85*, *406*, *474*, *532*, *537*.
Shermitte, J. 88, 90, 108, 110, 113, 114, 119, 124, 131, 133, 138, *140*, 314, 315, 347, 352, *411*, *414*.
Lichtwitz, L. 119, 350, 362, *410*, 497, *537*.
Lichty 221.
Lieben 372, *417*.
Liebner, E. 313, *411*.
Lilienstein, S. *537*.
Lind 48, 50, *85*.
Lindber, K. *417*.
Lindemann 369.
Lindenmeyer 238, *244*.
Lindner 383.
Linossier, A. 313, 314, 328, *411*.
Linser 388.
Lippmann, A. 235, *244*, 255, *474*.
Lisi, de 91, *140*.
Lisser 259.
List, C. F. *415*.
Little 306, 349.
Liveing 166, 169, 171, 175, 176, 177, 189, 192, 193, 198, 200, 217, *244*.
Livieratos, S. G. *422*.
Livinston, W. K. *404*.
Locock 77, *85*.
Loeb, L. 330, 332, 338, 339, *417*.
Löblowitz 308.
Loeft, van der 80, *85*.
Löhe 310, *421*.
Loeper 221, *244*.
Loessl, J. 273, *404*.

Löwenberg, R. D. 46, *85*, *411*, *415*.
Löwenfeld, L. 88, 93, 94, 112, 132, 138, *140*, 193, 195, *244*, 452, *474*.
Loewenheim 370.
Löwenstein, K. *140*, *474*.
Löwenthal 202.
Löwi, O. 483, *537*.
Loewy, P. 97, *140*, 335, 460, *474*, 506, *537*.
Logan 59, *86*.
Long 37, *85*.
Longcope, W. 314, 347, 348, 352, 353, *411*.
Lopez 97, 112, *140*.
Lorenz 29, *85*, 199.
Lorenzo, R. *411*.
Lortat 273, 313, 318, 325, 328, 353, 354, 395, *404*, *411*.
Losetschnikow 322.
Loubiere, M. *404*.
Louste 312, 314, 363, *411*, *412*, *418*.
Love, W. S. jr. 264, *402*.
Lovén, K. 374, 379, *424*.
Lovett 374.
Lovner 65, *85*.
Loyal 299, *402*, *407*.
Lubbers 222, 234, 235, *244*.
Lublinski 375.
Lucas 30, *85*.
Lucretius *85*.
Ludwig 389.
Lührs 225, 237, *244*.
Luithlen 312, 316, 344, 360.
Luksch 127.
Lundborg 34, *85*, 350.
Lunedei *418*.
Luntz 335.
Lusignan, H. *424*.
Lusitanus, Zacutus 312.
Lust 116, *140*.
Lustig 255.
Lutz, W. 354, 378, *400*.
Lutzenberger 182, *244*.
Luzzato 287, 350.
Lyle 266.
Lyon, G. 236.

Mabille 394.
MacCallum, W. 344, 348, *412*.
MacDonald, J. 53, *86*, 377, *418*.
MacGregor 341.
MacKay, W. 47, *244*, 340, 341, 342, 363, 379, *412*, *418*, *422*, *424*.
Mackenzie, J. 532.
MacLeod, J. 47, *86*, *418*.
Macpherson 262.
McBridge 261.
M'Call 248.
McClure 224, 234, 236, *244*.

McCrudden, Fr. H. *413, 419.*
McDonnell 77, *86.*
McDougall, W. 28, *86, 474.*
McGuire 397, *418, 424.*
McIlvaine, James *418.*
McKendrick 33, *86.*
McKennan 48, *86.*
McNamara 120, *140.*
McQuarrie 77, *86.*
Macera, J. M. *408.*
Machol 293.
Machton 324.
Mader 247.
Maes 8, *86.*
Magnus, G. *400,* 483.
Maire, Roger 359, *412, 423.*
Makarow 109, 133, *140.*
Malchers 258.
Malossi, C. *412.*
Mamerto *408.*
Mamou, H. 326, 351, *413, 422.*
Mangelsdorf 172, *244.*
Mankowsky, B. 107, 113, 114, 115, *140,* 315, 318, 340, *412, 415.*
Mann, L. 457, 461, *474.*
Mannheimer 372.
Mannini 34, *86.*
Manthey, P. 335, *415.*
Mantle 256.
Manz 180, *244.*
Marañon, G. 282, 284, *406, 421, 537.*
Marburg, O. 62, *86, 244,* 278, 304, 305, 330, 331, 332, 335, 363, *400.*
Marchand 29, 48, 65, *86,* 87, 248, 252, 262.
Marcinowski *537.*
Marcozzi *418.*
Marcus, Henri 259, 261, 268, 269, *404.*
— Herbert *404.*
— M. *412.*
Margolin, G. S. 261, *404.*
Margolis 221, *244.*
Marie, Pierre 65, 80, *86,* 349.
Marina 182, *244.*
Marinesco, G. 104, 107, 110, 115, 127, 129, *140,* 326, 335, 349, *406, 415.*
Mariotti, E. *418.*
Markow, G. 119, *140,* 326, *409.*
Marmon 350.
Marotte 315.
Marquézy, R. 326, *404.*
Martin, P. 35, *86,* 299, *537.*
Martinet 272, 283.
Martinez, Z. V. *401.*
Martinico, G. 370, *418.*
Martius, F. 435, *474,* 485.
Marx, H. 489, *537.*
Maškileisson, W. L. N. 352, 353, 386, *412, 418.*
Maso, P. dal 271, *402.*
Massaglia 55, *86.*

Massalongo 186, *244.*
Massee 116, *141.*
Masslow 146, *165.*
Matas 370.
Mathes, P. *474.*
Mathez, A. 284, *406.*
— J. A. *406.*
Mathieu, P. 167, 232, *244,* 350, 370, 372, *422.*
Matras, A. *412, 422.*
Matsui, S. 347, 348, 351, *412.*
Matthaei, R. 491, *532.*
Matthes, M. *537.*
Matusis, J. 398, *418.*
Matzdorff 102, *140.*
Mauriac, P. *404,* 422.
Mauthner, O. 180, *244,* 460, *474, 537.*
Maxwell, L. A. I. *418.*
May, E. 283, 284, 287, 292, 294, 373, 386, 392, *406, 407, 418, 421.*
Mayer, A. *474,* 522, *532, 537.*
— J. *410.*
— L. *415, 472, 535.*
Mayerhofer 457, 461, *474.*
Mayesima 299, *407.*
Mayo, W. I. 280, 366, *420, 422.*
Mayr, J. *400.*
Meier *164,* 511, *535.*
Meige, H. 175, 178, *244,* 393, 394, *424.*
Meisal, Nin 271, 403.
Melkersson, E. 382, *418.*
Melli, G. 396, *418.*
Memmesheimer 394, *418.*
Menagh, F. R. 370, *418.*
Mendel, E. 120, 167, 173, 182, 198, 204, 217, 239, *244,* 330, 338, 350, 368, 380, 388.
Mendel, F. 182.
— K. 168, *244,* 335, *407, 474.*
Menninger 66.
Mentz, P. 486, *537.*
Meschede, H. 280, *404.*
Messing, Z. 279, *404.*
Mészáros, K. 319, *412.*
Mettler 388.
Metzner, R. 485.
Meyer 522, *535, 537.*
— A. *420.*
— F. 37, 46, 55, *86,* 206, 257, 273, 318, 323, 328, 335, 377, *403, 407.*
— Jean *403.*
— M. *474.*
— S. *474.*
Mezzatesta, F. *415.*
Mgebrov, M. *412.*
Mibelli 222.
Michaelis, O. 326, 328, 362, *412, 422.*
Michail, D. *418.*
Michelet 312, *412.*

Miget *140.*
Miklós *417.*
Milbradt, W. *422.*
Milian, G. 315, 323, 352, 353, *412, 424.*
Milizyn 76, *86.*
Millard 362.
Miller, H. 387.
— T. 16, 47, 76, *86,* 102, 223, 235, *244,* 387, *418.*
Millet, R. *418.*
Mills 14, 33, *86,* 291.
Milroy, W. F. 394, 397, *418.*
Milton 367, 374, 384.
Mindlin, S. 288, *400.*
Mingazzini 129, 134, 180, 183, 192, 195, 196, *244,* 261.
Minor, L. *244,* 252, 341, *474.*
Minot 223, 224, 236, *244.*
Minza 113.
Mirallié 339.
Mirenghi, N. U. *404, 420.*
Misch, W. 390, *418,* 450, *474,* 509, *537.*
Missriegler 96, 138, *140.*
Mitchell 105, *141,* 249, 286, 287, 290, 291, 293, 294, 298.
Miverghi 270.
Mixter 49, *86.*
Moebius, P. J. 166, 167, 169, 171, 173, 176, 177, 180, 181, 186, 192, 197, 200, 206, 208, 217, 218, 230, 238, *244,* 263, 270, 303, 330, 338, 455, 456, *474.*
Moehlig, R. 205, *244,* 350, *412.*
Möllendorf 173, 203, 204, *244.*
Moellenhoff 118, *140.*
Moersch, F. 195, *244.*
Mohnkopf, W. 529, *540.*
Mohr, Fr. *407, 532, 537.*
Molhaut *537.*
Moll 291.
Mollaret, P. 119, *140, 423.*
Moloney 219, *244.*
Monahan, J. J. *404.*
Monakow, C. v. *532, 537.*
— P. v. 479, 485, *532, 537.*
Monbrun 180.
Mondio, E. *404.*
Monier 278, 312, 326, *404, 412.*
Moniz, E. 372, 395, 396, *418.*
Monro 246, 247, 248, 253, 256, 259, 260.
Monroe 253.
Montesano 315.
Montgomery 254, 256, 278, 340, 341.
Moon 52.
Moormeister 307.
Moos, Erw. *537.*
Morat, P. *417.*
Morawiecka, J. 322, 349, *412.*
Morawitz, P. 369, *418, 537.*

Moreau 62, 86, 119, *140*, 189, 227, *245*.
Morel 291, 323, 324, *409*.
Morenas *244*.
Morgan 256, 259, 287, 293, 298.
Morgenstern 150.
Moriarty 76, 77, *86*.
Morichau 369, 381.
Morison 15.
Moro 146, 151, 155.
Morris 276, 378.
Morrow 318.
Morse 30.
Morselli 61, *86*, 315.
Morton, B. William *418*.
— J. 138, *140*, 271, *404*.
Mosenthin 351.
Moses, J. *540*.
Mosler 364.
Mosso, A. 183, 226, 244, *418*, *424*, *433*, *532*.
Moszkowicz, L. 366, *415*, 518, *537*.
Motschutkowsky 146.
Mott 51, *86*.
Motte, de La 66, *86*.
Moulonguet, P. *422*.
Mounstein 266.
Mourgue, R. 479, *532*.
Mourson 248.
Moxon 25, *86*.
Mucha, V. 246, 247, 268, 269, 272, 276, 311, *408*, *420*.
Muck, O. 205, *244*.
Mühlpfordt, H. *418*.
Mühsam 322.
Müller, A. 33, 47, *86*, 199, *244*.
— E. F. *474*.
— F. C. *474*.
— H. 386, *418*.
— L. R. 202, 206, 212, *244*, 303, 319, 333, 334, 338, 342, 353, 377, 381, 462, 469, *474*, 481, 482, 484, *532*.
— O. 235, *244*, 251, 258, 302, 307, 310, 319, 334, *400*, 511, 513, 519, *532*.
Münch, W. 370, *418*.
Münzer 91, 108, 109, 110, 113, 115, 119, 123, 124, 136, *140*.
Muncford, P. B. 253, 293, 299, *404*, *407*.
Munson 50, *86*.
Muratoff 339.
Murray *712*.
Muskens 4, 8, 9, 20, 23, 27, 30, 34, 44, 59, 62, 63, 66, *86*.
Musso 183, 226, *244*, 370, 381, *418*, *424*, *433*, *532*.
Myers, B. 138, *140*, *424*.
Myerson 63. *86*.

Nachman 65, *86*.
Nadoleczny 529, 530, *539*, *540*.
Naegeli 312, 313, 350, 353, 354, 384, *400*, *41?*.
Nageotte *422*.
Napp, V. *418*.
Nardelli, L. *406*.
Nast 222, 234, *244*.
Natousek 322.
Naudaschew 261.
Naunyn 315, 350.
Navarro 51, *84*.
Negro 101.
Neisser 119, *140*.
Nekam 273.
Nemlicher, L. J. 331, 334, *415*.
Nerrlinger *86*.
Netter 221, 226, 235, *245*.
Neuberger 310.
Neubürger, K. *474*, 511, *537*.
Neuda 369, 376, 378, 381.
Neumann, A. 185, *244*, 321, 364, 370, *418*.
Neumark 322.
Neustaedter 331.
Neutra, W. *537*.
Nevermann 118, *140*.
Newmark 111.
Nicati 175, *244*.
Nicolai 510.
Nicolas, J. 113, 138, *140*, *404*.
Nieden 293.
Niekau 253, 258, 289, *407*.
Nielsen, J. M. *86*, 195, *244*, 287, 318, *407*.
Nielson 47, *86*, *407*.
Niessl v. Mayendorf *537*.
Ninde 45, *86*.
Ninhei-Sai 261.
Nissl 266.
Noak 92, 110, 111, 112, 119.
Nobl 363.
Nobécourt 248, 283, 286, 287, *404*, *407*.
Nösske 277.
Noïca, D. 334, *415*, *418*.
Nörstrom 199, *244*.
Nonne, M. 230, *244*, 394, 438, 442, 452, 457, 461, 465, 466, *474*, *539*.
Noorden, v. 352, 361, 487.
Norvig 48, *86*.
Nothhafft, v. 312, 344, 346, 347, 348, 349, 356, 361, 362.
Nothmann 336.
Nothnagel 39, 44, 81, *86*, 212, 282, 299, 350.
Notkin 40, *86*.
Nouhuys, F. van *425*.
Novak, J. 522, *537*.
Novoa, Santos R. 407, *425*.
Nussbaum 529.

Obanio 16, *86*.
Obregia, J. 282, 283, *406*, *415*.

Obständer, E. *423*.
Ochsenhandler 76, *86*.
Odermath 206, *244*.
Oddy, H. *425*.
Oeconomakis 285.
Oehlecker 273.
Oehme, K. 389, *418*, 497, *533*.
Ohm, J. 459, *474*.
O'Leary, P. A. 318, 319, 328, 344, 366, *409*, *412*.
Oliaro, Tomaso 381, *425*.
Oliver, E. L. *412*.
Olkon, D. M. 371, *418*.
Olmsted 59, *86*.
Oppel, W. A. 281, *404*.
Oppenheim, H. 39, 40, *86*, 97, 120, 121, 136, 137, 162, 168, 169, 187, 188, 189, 192, 197, 198, 204, 217, 218, 239, 241, *244*, 255, 256, 275, 296, 301, 306, 316, 330, 331, 332, 333, 334, 335, 337, 358, 359, 360, 361, 364, 380, 461, *474*, 529, *539*.
— M. *412*.
Oppenheimer 370.
Orbelli 481, 525.
Orbinson 335.
Orlof, P. 318, 321, 325, *412*.
Orlowski 37, *86*.
Ormerod 182, 299, 374.
Ormond 179.
Ormsby 255, 366.
Orr 51, *86*.
Orsos, E. *405*.
Osborne 279.
Osler 260, 261, 318, 368, 383.
Osman 396.
Osnato 46, 47, 48, *86*.
Ossokin 76.
Ostertag 212, 232, 233, *244*.
Ostrowski, St. 359, *412*.
Oswald *533*.
Otte. H. *421*.

Paal, H. 497, *533*.
Paderstein 183, 186, *244*.
Padilla 290, 294, *407*.
Pässler, H. 204, *244*, 445, *474*.
Packard 377.
Pagès 332, 340.
Paget 286, 290.
Pagniez 4, 45, 55, *86*, 222, 224, 234, *244*, 398.
Pahl *475*.
Paisseau, G. *412*.
Pákozdy 185, *244*.
Palagyi 492, 493.
Pal, J. 205, 206, 210, 211, 213, 231, *244*, *475*.
Pallasse 267, 404.
Pallet 180.
Palmieri 350.
Palthe, P. M. v. 512, *539*.

Pancoast 49, *86*.
Pancrazio, F. 404.
Pandelesco 176, 185, *244*.
Panegrossi 314, 350.
Pannhorst, R. 488, 500, *537*.
Panofsky 374, *418*.
Panse, F. *475*.
Paparcone 334.
Papastratigakis 113, *140*.
Papp, v. 485.
Pappenheim 46, *86*.
Paraf 235, *245*.
Paralt 177.
Pardee 226, 237.
Parhon, C. J. 51, *86*, 226, *244*, 325, 347, 348, 349, 353, 392, 395, *412*.
Parisot 267, 277, *401*, *406*, *407*, *420*.
Parrisius 257, 258, 259, 263, 281, *407*.
Parry 187, 202.
Parvulesco, N. *418*.
Pasini, A. *422*.
Paskind 91, 97, 100, 106, 110, 112, 120, 123, 124, *140*.
Pasteur 256, 369, 373, 377, 384, 385, 392, 398, 399, *414*, *418*, *419*.
Paton, T. *409*.
Patrick, H. 30, *86*, *412*.
Patry *86*.
Patrzek 315.
Patterson 46, *87*.
Paulian 201, *244*.
Pauliny 271, *404*.
Paunesco *140*.
Pautrier, L. M. 319, 320, 353, 354, 359, 362, *412*, *422*.
Pawlow, J. P. 449, *475*, 487, 488, 500, 518, *533*, *537*.
Pawlowski 315.
Payenneville *412*.
Peake, Pemberton 203, *244*.
Péhu 282.
Pelizäeus 322, 326.
Pellissier, L. 249, *401*.
Peloquin *418*.
Pende, R. 284, 392, *537*.
Pendleton 76, *85*.
Penfield 44, 49, 52, 64, 83, *85*, *86*.
Penning, C. P. *425*.
Penta 104, 106, 114, 138, *140*.
Pepa, A. *416*.
Pepper, O. *418*.
Per, M. 315, *412*.
Pereira, A. *418*.
Peritz, G. 199, 221, *244*, 305, 366, *412*, *475*.
Pernet, J. 318, *412*.
Péron 395.
Perrier 113, *140*.
Pérrin 261, 320, 323, 353, *410*, *412*.
Personali 287, 293.

Perutz, A. *422*.
Pesopoulos *418*, *425*.
Pessler 173.
Pest 172.
Petelin, S. 315, 353, 355, *412*.
Petermann 77, *86*.
Petersen, W. F. *474*.
Peterson 47, *86*, 228, *243*.
Petges, G. 313, 328, 351, *412*, *413*, *422*.
Petit 180, 248.
Petov *243*.
Petow, H. 515, *538*.
Petráček, E. *425*.
Petrillo, L. *415*.
Petruschky, J. *475*.
Pette, H. 127, 437, 490, *537*.
Pettow 224, 235.
Petz 193.
Peyre 90, 110, 119, 124, *110*, 325, *413*.
Peyri, J. *413*.
Pezzali 47, *86*, 288.
Pezzi 187, *244*.
Pfab, B. *404*.
Pfaff 221.
Pfanner 108, 109, 112, 116, *140*.
Pfaundler, M. *475*.
Pfeiffer, B. 46, 55, *86*, 446, *475*.
Pfister 89, 105, 266.
Phillips, W. 188, 193, *244*, 368, 369, 390, 391, 398, *418*.
Philippson 364.
Phleps 255, 256, 257, 259.
Phocas 248.
Piazza 264, 341.
Pichaud *245*.
Pichler 179, *244*.
Pick, A. *475*.
— E. D. *408*, 446, 484, *537*.
— P. 484, *537*.
— W. 29, 65, *86*, 178, *244*, 299, 301, 307, 336, 358, *423*, 446.
Piéchaud, F. *404*.
Pierini, L. *406*, *425*.
Piéron 65, *86*.
Pike 53, 59, *84*, *86*.
Pilcz, A. 63, *86*, *537*.
Pilotti 51, *86*.
Pinard, Marcel 350, *422*.
Pineles 151, *406*.
Pinkus 329.
Pirquet, v. 144.
Pison *244*.
Pissling 339.
Pitres 33, *86*, 266.
Plavec 201, *244*.
Pletzer 380.
Podeano *140*.
Pötzl, O. 11, 46, *86*, 128, 130, 131, 132, *140*, 480, 496, 498, *537*.
Pogorelsky *408*.

Pohl, R. 325, *410*, *422*.
Polano, M. K. *425*.
Policard 258.
Poll *140*.
Pollack, Fr. 491, *537*.
Pollak, E. *244*, 269, 331, 333, 340, *404*.
— F. *404*, *415*, *537*.
Polland, R. *401*.
Pollnow, H. 493, 494, 515, *533*, *538*.
Pollock 61, *86*, 236, *244*.
Pollosson 37, *86*.
Pongs *475*.
Popea 47, *86*.
Popescu 221, *244*.
Pophal *533*.
Popova, N. 120, *140*, 334, *415*.
Popovicin 221, *244*.
Popp, v. *532*.
Poppelreuter, W. 447, *475*.
Popper 12.
Porges 157, 500, 514, *533*.
Porot 294, 295.
Portal 4, *86*.
Posey 181, *245*.
Pospelow 261, 293, 310, 315.
Post, W. E. 221, *245*.
Poster 46.
Potain 291, 328.
Pototzky, C. *475*, *538*.
Potpeschnigg 152.
Poulton, E. P. 249, 267, *401*.
Poumeau *402*.
Poussepp, L. 201, 313, *413*.
Powell 248.
Prakken, J. R. *413*, *422*.
Prange 92, 100, 112, 120, 135, *140*.
Pratz 51.
Prentis 288.
Prestora 260.
Pribram 270.
Price 273.
Prichard 31, *86*.
Prieto, J. 351, *409*.
Princi 293, *407*.
Prior 51, 52, *86*.
Prout 20, 28, 34, 51, 81, *84*, *86*.
Prussak, S. *409*.
Prussakowa, S. 352, *409*.
Prynton 395.
Puach 293, *408*.
Puech *408*.
Pulawski 380, 399.
Pulay 354.
Purkinje 129.
Putnam 39, *86*, 221, *244*, 299, 303.

Queroy 37, *85*.
Quincke 201, 202, *244*, 366, 367, 368, 369, 370, 371, 373, 374, 375, 377, 378, 379, 380, 382, 384.

Rabot 34, *86*, 349, 357, *410*.
Rachford 245.
Racine *412*.
Rackemann 390.
Rad, v. *245*, 381.
Radimska 374.
Radoničič, K. 287, 291, *406*, *407*.
Radot, V. 119, *140*, 180, 193, 203, 204, 205, 217, 218, 221, 222, 223, 225, 227, 228, 234, 235, 236, *245*, 369, 373, 377, 384, 385, 392, 398, 399, *414*, *418*, *419*.
Raecke 41, *86*, 446, *475*.
Raeschke *418*.
Raimann, E. *475*, *538*.
Rajka, E. 222, 227, *244*, *406*, *419*.
Rake, G. 325, 346, 348, *413*.
Ramazotti, V. *413*.
Ramirez 234, *245*, 390.
Ramond 395.
Ramskill 77, *86*.
Randak 278.
Rapin 367, 368, 377, 381, 394, 395.
Rappoport, B. J. 287, 331, 334, *407*, *415*.
Rasmussen 346.
Ratner, F. 107, 109, 112, 114, 115, 116, 120, 122, 123, *140*, 335, *415*.
Ratshford 221.
Raullet 209, *245*.
Raulston 223, 235, *244*.
Rauzier 169, *243*.
Ravault, P. P. *402*.
Raven 368.
Raymond 192, 315, 324, 326, 329, 331, 335, 348, 349.
Raynaud 246, 247, 248, 251, 253, 256, 259, 265.
Rebattu 48, *86*.
Redlich, Emil 33, 46, 55, 66, *86*, 87, 88, 91, 92, 93, 94, 95, 97, 98, 100, 101, 102, 106, 107, 108, 109, 110, 111, 112, 113, 114, 115, 116, 117, 118, 119, 120, 121, 122, 123, 124, 125, 126, 127, 128, 129, 132, 133, 134, 135, 136, *140*, 153, 191, 192, *245*, 446, 477, 478, *533*.
Reese 245.
Regelsberger 462, *475*.
Reich, W. 65, *86*, 452, 509, 535.
Reichardt, M. *245*, 437, 444, 446, 468, *475*, 491, 493, 497, *538*.
Reiche 238, *245*, 248.
Reichmann *538*.
Reiner 204, *242*, 324, 351, 354.

Reiss 247, 331, 332.
Remak 393.
Rémond 221, 236, *245*.
Renaut 306.
Rendu 248.
Rennedy, Roger *422*.
Renshaw 254, 306.
Rentz 179, *244*.
Renzo, di 48.
Retezeanu, C. J. 301, *421*.
Revington 189.
Reynolds *86*.
— Russell 4, 15, 22, 25, 34, 35, 62, *86*.
Rham 256.
Rheindorf, G. 418, *425*.
Ribbière 226.
Ribot 41.
Richards, jr. 220, *242*, 395, *418*, *425*.
Richet fils, Ch. 76, *87*, *420*.
Richter, A. 245.
— H. 245.
— C. P. 107, *140*, 186, 238.
Riecke 386, *418*.
Rieder, W. 258, 268, 269, 271, 280, *404*.
Riehl 306, 374.
Rietschel, H. 150, *165*, 259.
Rietti 394, 396, 399.
Riley 166, 225, 226, *245*.
Rille 321.
Rimé 315, 352, *412*, *414*, *423*.
Rimpler 181, *245*.
Rinkel 167, 220, 234, *242*, *245*.
Rio, del 182, *245*.
Ritti 262.
Riva 256, 259.
Rives, J. *413*.
Rivière 167, 232, *245*.
Rizatti 91, 113, 114, 115.
Roasenda 303.
Roberts, St. R. *245*, *407*, *413*.
Robinson, J. 47, *86*, 273, *403*.
Robiolis 175, *244*.
Rocaz, Ch. 297, *407*.
Roch *421*.
Roche, J. 351, *406*, *408*, *413*, *421*.
Rodiet 29, *86*.
Roederer, J. 320, 324, *413*, *415*, *422*.
Römer 487.
Röper, E. *475*.
Roesch 350.
Röthler 309, 311.
Roger, H. *140*, 178, 224, *245*, 256, 314, 315, 420.
Rogers, J. B. 77, *86*, *405*.
Rohrer 177, *245*.
Rojtmann, R. 398, *418*.
Rolandi 112, *141*.
Rolland 33, *86*.
Rolleston 251, 390.
Román 527.
Romano 181.

Romberg, v. 200, *245*, 330, 338, *533*.
Rominger, E. *475*.
Ronzini, M. *404*.
Roques *140*, 256, 259.
Rosanoff, A. 526, *540*.
Rose 192, 199, *245*.
Rosenbach, O. 199, *245*, 459, 495, *538*.
Rosenberg 371, 483.
Rosenfeld, H. 241, 310, 322, *421*, 519.
— M. *475*, 519, *533*, *538*.
Rosengart 292.
Rosenstein 206, 231.
Rosenthal, C. 90, 94, 96, 100, 102, 104, 105, 106, 107, 111, 112, 113, 115, 116, 118, 119, 123, 124, 130, *141*, 239, 337, 361, 369, 382, *418*.
Rosett 54, *86*.
Ross 293.
Rossbach 172, 350.
Rossolimo 185, *245*.
Rost, Br. *540*.
— G. A. 291, *538*.
Rothe, K. C. 531, *540*.
Rothfeld, J. 90, 97, 100, 104, 105, 107, 109, 116, 122, 123, 131, 137, *141*, 281, 282, *406*.
Rothlin 221, *245*.
Rothmann, H. *475*.
— St. 59, *86*, *245*, 311, 330, 353, *413*.
Rothmund 326.
Rotnes, P. *413*.
Rotschild, H. de 226, 264, 270, 283, 284.
Rottmann 183, 208.
Rouques 361.
Roussel, F. J. 383, 404, 418.
Routier, D. *420*.
Roux 167, 232, 241, *243*, *244*, 347, 351.
Rouzaud 221, 236, *245*.
Rove 220, 234, *245*.
Rowe, A. W. *413*, *419*.
Rows 5, 40, 45, 66, 83, *86*.
Roxburgh, A. 320, *413*.
Royle, N. D. 280, *404*.
Rubaltelli, E. *425*.
Rubaschow, S. 340, *404*.
Rubaszew, S. *404*.
Rud, Einar 257, 258, 263, 271, 279, *404*.
Rudder, M. de 490, *533*.
Rudeau 245.
Rudorici, A. *538*.
Rudzki 293, 294, 295.
Ruegg 522, *537*.
Rülf 247, 262.
Ruhemann, Ernst 267, 385, *419*.
Ruhmann, W. 519, *538*.

Rumpel 374.
Runge, W. 273, 458, 459, *476*.
Rupert 224, *245*.
Russell 4, 25, 44, 76, *86*.
Russi, F. 351, *413*.
Ryle 44, *86*.

Sabrazès 340.
Sachs 46, *86*, 266, 287, 294, 295, 299, 331.
— F. *165*, 287.
Sack, W. 522, 523, *538*.
— W. Th. *401*, *408*, *538*.
Sänger, M. 217, *245*, 459, *538*.
Sager 107, 127.
Sahli 209.
Sai 261.
Saint Girons, Fr. *406*.
Sainton, P. J. 108, *141*, 247, 288, 294, 295, 326, 350, 351, *407*, *413*, *422*.
Saishiro *403*.
Saito 299, *407*.
Sajitz 237, *245*.
Salin 261.
Salkan, D. 318, 355, *413*.
Salle, La *414*, *423*.
Salles 384.
Salmon 117, 129, 134, *141*, 339.
Salus 119, 332.
Samada 306.
Samaja, R. *421*.
Samuel 330, 338.
Sandiford 47, *84*.
Sands 80, *86*.
Sannicandro, G. 270, 279, *354*, 364, *404*, *406*, *413*.
Santos, Novoa 378.
Sarbó, v. 62, *86*, 193.
Sargent 64, *86*.
Sattler 349.
Saundby *245*, 299.
Savill 292, 302, 328.
Sawasaki 48, *86*.
Scala, G. 355, *413*.
Scarpa, A. *422*, *425*.
Schaffer 30, *85*, 193.
Schäffer, H. 142, 248, 326, 361, *402*, *419*.
Schalabutoff 276.
Schalit, A. 374, *419*.
Schapiro, B. *475*.
Scharnke 457, *475*.
Schaxel, J. 446, *471*.
Scheer 164, *165*.
Scheiber 256.
Scheler, M. 491, 492, 493, 501, *533*.
Schelven, van 238, *245*.
Schenk 287.
Scherber *412*.
Schieck 341, 342.
Schiff, A. 520, *538*.
— E. 53, *86*, 150.

Schilder, P. 89, 99, 110, 111, 115, 116, 117, 138, *141*, 191, *471*, *475*, 479, 509, 530, *533*, *538*.
Schilf, E. 270, 271, 481, 482, 525, *535*.
Schindler, R. *475*, 489, 495, 506, 513, 519, 520, 523, *533*, *538*.
Schirmacher 287, 289, 290, 298, *407*.
Schlapp 31, *86*.
Schlesinger, H. 143, 235, *245*, 292, 293, 315, 332, 334, 335, 339, 367, 368, 372, 373, 374, 377, 378, 379, 380, 381, 383, 385, 386, 393, *407*, *419*.
Schmelinski 292.
Schmidt 54, *85*.
— A. 172. 181, *245*, 325.
— K. E. 183, *245*.
— R. 293, 299, 300, *475*, 482, 512, *538*.
Schmidt-Weyland 269.
Schmiergeld 37, 52, *84*, *86*.
Schmitz, A. H. *475*.
Schneider, A. 467, *538*.
— K. *164*, 467, *475*, 491, 492, 506, *533*, *538*.
Schob 178, *245*.
Schoch, A. 386, *419*.
Schönberg 255.
Schöne, F. 192, *245*.
Schöngut, E. 362, *413*, *422*.
Schönhof 278, 363, 366.
Schönlein 374.
Scholl 352.
— K. *410*.
Scholtz 350, 361.
Scholz, W. 364, *538*.
Schorer, G. 377, 378, *419*.
Schott 262.
Schottin 200, *245*.
Schottky, J. *533*.
Schottmüller 237, *245*.
Schou 52, 76, *86*.
Schreiber 276, 277, 286.
Schreus, H. *419*.
Schröder, P. *475*, *533*.
Schrottenbach 487.
Schubiger 324, 356, *419*.
Schüller 202, *245*.
Schütz 282, 290.
Schulmann, A. 370, 527, *540*.
Schulte 341.
Schultz, J. H. 322, 372, *419*, 462, *475*, 479, 480, 489, 497, 505, 506, 507, 515, 516, 517, 527, *538*.
Schultz-Heucke, Harald *475*, *538*.
Schultze, F. 177, 189, 193, 194, 200, 227, 236, *245*, 299, 314, *475*.
Schultzer, Poul 383, *419*.

Schulz 248, 306, 346, 347, 350.
Schupfer 30, *86*.
Schur, H. *538*.
Schuster, J. 188, *245*.
— P. *475*.
Schwab, O. 127, 447, *475*.
Schwartz 76, *86*, *245*, 290, 291.
Schwarz, E. *425*, *532*.
— O. 485, 492, 493, 521, *533*, *538*.
— P. 291, 351, *413*, *532*.
Schwarzkopf, A. *420*.
Schweinitz 185, *245*.
Schwerdt 362.
Scimone 219, *245*.
Scolari, E. F. 318, 328, *413*, *422*.
Scott, W. M. 271, 347, *404*.
Scripture 530.
Seale, E. *413*.
Sedan 210, *245*, 256, *420*.
Sedillot 201, *245*.
Sée 283, *406*.
Seelig 334.
Seemann, M. 525, *540*.
Séglas 74, *86*.
Segura 364.
Seidelmann 248, 273.
Seishiro 261.
Seitz, L. *475*.
Sellei, Josef 316, 326, 356, 362, 398, *413*, *419*, *422*, *423*, *425*.
Sels 127, *140*.
Selter, P. 297, *421*.
Selye, H. *413*, *423*.
Semerau *475*.
Seminario, C. 364, *413*.
Semon 97, 112.
Sempan *140*.
Senator 290, 314.
Sepp 207, *245*, 382.
Sequeira, J. 351, *419*.
Serejski 90, 93, 97, 107, 110, 114, 115, 116, 118, 120, 123, *141*.
Serio 287.
Sevane, C. *418*.
Seyler 325, 356.
Sézary, A. 273, 318, 326, 328, 350, *413*, *422*.
Sgalitzer, M. 278, 304, 305, 363, *400*.
Shanahan 30, *86*.
Shaw, M. 262, 294, 295, 331, 415, *423*.
Sherrill 76, *86*.
Sherrington, C. S. 55, 483, 485, *538*.
Shinazono 293.
Shinkle, C. E. *404*.
Shionoya 186, *245*.
Shoemaker 276.
Shoji, Y. *423*.
Sibley, W. K. *401*.

Sicard 34, *86*, 175, 186, 193, 235, 240, *245*, 331, 335, 363.
Siebek 493, 498, 504, 514, *538*.
Siebelt 451, *475*.
Sieben, H. 306, *425*.
Siebert 116, *141*, 335.
Siebley 308.
Siegrist 178, 209, *245*.
Siemens, H. W. 283, 312, 368, 386, 387, 394, *401*, *419*, *423*.
Siemianowski, M. *475*.
Sieshiro, Iwai 261, 271.
Sieveking 73, *86*, 193.
Sikle 193.
Sikora 370.
Silbermann 100, 518.
Silberstein 279.
Silley 276.
Simon, A. 169, 247, *405*, *419*.
Simons, E. *245*, 257, 303, 336, *419*.
Simpson 261, 280, *405*.
Simson, T. *475*.
Singer 89, 119, 122, 135, 288, 289, 290, 291, 292, 293, 347, 349, 361.
Sinkler 299, 303, 306.
Sioli, F. 51, *87*, *475*.
Sirota, L. 353, 362, *413*.
Sittig, O. 11, 12, *86*, 176, *245*, 525, 526, *540*.
Sjögren 47, *86*.
Skaletz, H. 388, *425*.
Sklarz 306, 309, 310, 311.
Skvorcov 120, *140*.
Sladen 282.
Slatmann, A. F. 372, 373, *419*.
Slaughter, W. H. 248, 340, *405*.
Slesinger, E. G. *401*.
Sloane, P. *423*.
Slobodnik, M. 372, *419*.
Smirnitsbuj, J. *415*.
Smith, A. E. 368, *419*, 421.
— Jens. Chr. 217, *245*, 254, 293, *408*.
Smolensky, A. *473*.
Soecknick *164*.
Söderberger 334.
Sohier 278, 314, 364, *410*.
Solis 262, 270, 279, 302, 306, 377, 381.
Solomon 91, 98, 106, 107, *141*.
Somalo, Marcos *419*.
Somer 95, 102, 119, *141*.
Sommer, R. 470, *475*.
Sommerfeld 487.
Sorsby, A. 331, *415*, *422*.
Souques 133, 182, 227, *245*, 282, 332, 334.
Sourdel, M. 420.
Southard 30, 50, 61, *85*, *86*, *87*.
Southey 260.

Sovak, M. 525, *540*.
Spangler 76, *86*.
Spatz, H. 484.
Speer, E. *538*.
Sperling, O. 109, 119, 210, 122, 123, *141*, *475*.
Spiegel, E. A. *419*, *475*, 481, 484, *533*.
Spiegler 314.
Spieler 259.
Spielmeyer 51, *86*, 213, 232, 287, *408*, 511.
Spiller 36, 37, 40, *87*, 113, *141*, 181, *245*, 287, 291, 294.
Spillmann, L. 312, 314, 329, *413*, 414.
Spiro *418*, *425*.
Spitzer 201, *245*.
Spitzy, H. *419*.
Spota 259.
Spratling 9, 26, 44, 61, 62, *87*.
Spurling, R. G. *405*.
Spuzic 235, *245*.
Stadler 529.
Staedtler 287.
Staehelin 369, 377, 378, *407*, 502.
Staemmler 267, 339, 374, *405*, *418*.
Stahl 299.
Stalker 298, *408*.
Stallmann 40, *87*.
Stantien, E. *424*.
Starr 385.
Staub, H. 483.
Steckel, W. 83, *87*, 220, 371, *538*.
Steffens 40, *87*.
Stein, F. W. 218, 220, 226, 238, *243*, *475*, 512, *538*.
— L. *540*.
Steiner, G. K. 298, 362, 369, *413*, *423*, *475*.
Steinitz, H. 324, *413*.
Stelwagon, A. *419*.
Stelzner, H. 464, *476*.
Stembo 324.
Stengel 89, 105, 107, 111, 112, 114, 118, 121, 123, 124, 134, *140*.
Stephens, G. 257, *405*.
Stepp 155.
Sterling, Wl. 36, *87*, 204, 221, 226, *245*, 331, 352, 390, *413*, *419*.
Stern, A. 182, *538*.
— G. 48, *84*, 370, 375, *419*, *538*.
— H. *540*.
— W. 492.
Sternberg, H. 270, 282, 326, *418*.
Sternthal 321, 322, 325, 326, 356.
Sterting 382.

Stertz, G. 36, *87*, 437, 440, 446, 448, 454, 460, 461, 466, 468, *476*, 505, *533*.
Steven 326, 348.
Stevens 225, 237, *245*.
Stewart 35, 53, *87*, 273, 319.
Stief, A. 330, 336, *415*, *423*.
Stiefler, Georges 112, 113, 114, 115, 118, 119, 122, 126, *141*, 238, *245*, 330, 331, 334, 335, 338, 357, 363, 369, *415*, *423*, *476*.
Stieglitz 361.
Stier, E. 37, *87*, 162, 330, 331, 338, 341, 342, 343, 444, *476*.
Stierlin, E. 451, *476*.
Stillé 292.
Stiller, B. 220, *476*.
Stilling 330, 331, 340, 341.
Stocker 392.
Stockert, F. G. v. 113, *140*, 392, 518, 524, 525, 530, *538*, *540*.
Stockmann 199.
Stöckl, E. 351, *413*.
Stöhr, Ph. jr. 206, 212, *245*, 481.
Stöltzner 259.
Stöwsand, W. *476*.
Stokes, J. *408*.
Stolkind, E. 261, 315, *420*, *423*.
Stolpertus 367.
Stolz, Ch. *419*.
Stookey 55, *84*.
Stopford 273, *405*.
Storm van Leeuwen, W. 223, 235, *245*, *419*, 515, *533*.
Stoye, W. *413*.
Stradin, P. 263, 264, *405*.
Sträussler 101.
Strandberg, J. 285, 354, 364, *421*, *538*.
Stransky, E. 89, 105, 107, 110, 111, 118, 120, 123, 132, 138, *141*, *538*.
Strasburger 238, *245*.
Straus, E. 305, *408*, 503, *533*.
Strauss 77, *84*, 90, 92, 93, 94, 95, 100, 102, 109, 112, 113, 114, 115, 117, 124, 129, 132, *141*, 246, 261, 266.
Strempel, R. 386, 387, *416*.
Strohmeyer 241, *245*.
Strom, A. 352, *413*.
Stroomann 238, 242, *245*.
Strouse 384.
Strukow, A. 347, 348, 352, *413*.
Struebing 367, 368, 377, 381, 384.
Strümpell 202, 222, *245*, 350, 529.
Strunz, F. 351, *413*.
Stubenrauch 306.

Stüber 62, *87.*
Stühmer 386, 388.
Studnička, B. 325, 351, 361, 363, *414.*
Stukovsky 237, *245.*
Sturge 289.
Stursberg 257.
Stutzin, J. J. 520, *538.*
Sucher, A. 398, *419.*
Surat, W. 334, *415.*
Susini, M. 394, 399, *119.*
Susman, E. 52, *86,* 183, *245,* *417.*
Sutova, T. 366, *414.*
Swieten, van 15.
Symonds 113, 114, 124, *141,* 217.
Syz 53, *87.*
Szarka, V. *405.*
Szatmary 118, *141.*
Szondi, L. 194, *245,* 435, *476,* 524, *533, 540.*
Szymanski, J. S. *538.*

Tachau 284.
Taft 51, *87.*
Takats, G. de 280, *405.*
Talbot 47, 77, *87.*
Talley 375.
Tamburri, T. *401.*
Tandler, J. *476.*
Tanka, D. 330, *415.*
Tarchanoff, J. R. *539.*
Tardieues, A. *414.*
Targowla 46, 262.
Tarp 371.
Taubert 293.
Tedesco 261.
Tedeschi 322.
Teed 200.
Teglbjoerg 76, *86.*
Telford 273, *405.*
Tenner 53, *85.*
Tercero, M. *406.*
Terplan 267.
Terrien *245,* 341, *415.*
Tertius *407.*
Teske 314.
Tesone, P. *419.*
Thalmann 350.
Thaysen 205, *245.*
Thibièrge 306, 314, 322, 325, 354, 356, *414.*
Thiébaut 312, 325, 326, 354.
Thiele, R. 89, 90, 91, 92, 94, 96, 97, 101, 105, 107, 108, 109, 110, 111, 112, 113, 115, 116, 117, 118, 119, 120, 121, 122, 123, 124, 126, 138, 139, *141, 476.*
Thiemich 152, 158, 160.
Thiriol 312, 351, 359.
Thom 30, 46, 50, 63, 76, *87.*
Thomas, A. 526.

Thomas, E. 174, 179, 200, 221, 231, *245,* 283, 284, 286, 346, 347, 348, 363, *406, 419, 420.*
— W. A. *245,* 283.
Thomsen 186, 201, *245.*
Thomson 201, 237, *245.*
Thorspecken, O. *165.*
Thoyer 119, *140.*
Thrash 116, *141.*
Thurzó, E. de 46, *87,* 138, *140, 405.*
— J. *405.*
Tilanus 341.
Tillgren 47, *86.*
Timme 226, 237, *245.*
Tinel, J. 83, *87,* 248, 258, 279, *402.*
Tissot 166, 199, 230, *245,* 283, 379, *420.*
Tobias, Norman *415.*
Tobiesen 394.
Todd 20, 31, *87.*
Toen 313.
Tönnes, W. *405.*
Tönnies 247.
Török, L. 222, *244,* 383, 384, 390, 405, 406, 419.
Toheverria *87.*
Tokarski, K. 271, 272, *405.*
Tolosa, Colomer E. 261, 275, 276, 319, *405, 414.*
Tommasi, L. 314, 322, 329, *414.*
Toomy 283.
Torrvella, M. *406.*
Tóth 271, *404.*
Touchard 344, 346, 351.
Toulouse 29, 48, 65, 76, *87.*
Touraine *423.*
Tourette, Gilles de La 238.
Touton 306.
Towaine *414.*
Traband 331.
Trambusti, B. *405.*
Traumann 374, *535.*
Trautmann, E. 239, *245, 476.*
Travis, L. E. 524, *540.*
Trémolières, F. 347, 352, 370, 411, *414.*
Treumann 374, *535.*
Trendelenburg, P. 483, *533.*
Trepte, G. *415.*
Trescher 47, *86.*
Treu 331.
Trevisanello 55, *87.*
Triboulet 224, 236, *243.*
Trincas, M. 280, *405.*
Trömner, E. 94, 129, 135, *141,* 183, 208, *245,* 331, *415,* 530, *540.*
Trombert 301, 303.
Trousseau 5, 21, 25, 36, *87,* 217, 231, *245.*
Truffi G. 308, 309, 311, *423.*
Tscherback 341.

Tsellios, P. A. *422.*
Tsiminakis 53, *87,* 89, 110, 114, 115, 116, 121, 123, *141.*
Tsuchida 350.
Tsuji 287, 292, *408.*
Tucker 48, *87.*
Tuček, K. *539.*
Turettini 369, *419.*
Turnbull 370.
Turner, Aldren 4, 20, 30, 40, 51, 61, 62, 63, 66, 74, 76, *87.*
Turpin 145.
Tylor 80.
Tzank 239, *245.*

Uffenheimer 148, 157.
Uhlenhuth 326, 347, 362.
Ullmann 314, 323, 381, 389.
Ullmo, A. 319, 359, *412.*
Ullrich, O. *405.*
Ulrich, M. 78, *87,* 173, 176, 177, 181, 189, 192, 197, 217, 218, 227, 228, *245,* 247, *405.*
Unna 346.
Unverricht 34, *87.*
Urbach 120, *141.*
Urbantschitsch 248.
Urechia 91, 119, *141,* 230, *245,* 282, 301, *406, 421.*
Usse 252, 262.
Uyematsu 54, 55, 59, *87.*

Vadasz 100, 101, 123, 138, 139, *141.*
Vaillard 266.
Valensi 330.
Valkenburg, van 12, *87.*
Vallentin 386.
Vallery, P. 119, *140,* 180, 193, 203, 205, *245,* 349, 369, 373, 377, 384, 385, 392, 398, 399, *414, 418, 419.*
Vallette, A. 352, *414.*
Valobra 307, 369, 375, 394, 396.
Vassilevskij, M. *424.*
Vaughan, W. 223, 234, *245,* 385, *419.*
Vazquez, R. *415.*
Vedel 293, *408.*
Veil, E. 341, *415,* 515, 516, *539.*
Velde, van der 348.
Ventura, J. R. *405.*
Veraguth 16, *87,* 493, *533.*
Véran, P. 288, 294, 295, *407.*
Vercellino, L. *421.*
Verdelli 248, 256.
Verhogen 315,

Verneuil 248.
Vernieuwe *425*.
Verotti, Italo 315, *414*.
Verschuer, v. 524.
Verworn, M. 433, *476*.
Vicol, A. 47, *86*, 334, *415*.
Vidal 235, 318, 328, 364.
Viehweger 351.
Viéla, A. *417*.
Vietti 239, *245*.
Vigano, E. 363, *414*.
Vignal, E. 405, *414*.
Vigne, P. *410*.
Vigoureux 394.
Villaret, M. 261, 284, *405*, *406*, *421*.
Villaverde 88, 100, 111, 116, 123, 138, *141*.
Vinard, J. 278, 312, 326, *404, 424*.
Vincent, Cl. 284, 393, *421*.
Vinning 44, *87*.
Viole, P. L. *403, 417*.
Virchow 330, 338.
Vivado, A. 340, *415*.
Vliet, van 394.
Voelcker, F. 371, *425*.
Vogel, P. *476*, 519, *539*.
Vogelsang 183, *245*.
Vogl, A. *425*.
Vogt, C. 30, *87, 476, 539*.
Vohwinkel, K. H. 320, 329, 337, *414*.
Voisin 192.
Volhard 206, 272, 335, 512.
Voljfsohn, N. *415*.
Volland 52, *87*.
Vollmer, H. 48, 76, 77, *87, 412*.
Voncken *405*.
Voringer 362.
Vorkastner 514, *533*.
Voss 175.
Vossius 326.
Voto, de 362.
Vul, J. 318, *414*.
Vulpian 256, 286.

Wadson, A. *422*.
Wadsworth 185.
Wagenmann 256.
Wagner 83, *87*, 100, 101, 107, 114, 115, 116, 124, 139, *141*, 329, 331, 369.
Wakefield, E. G. *424*.
Waldorp, C. 313, 353, 354, *414*.
Walinski, F. 435, *476*.
Walker 390.
Wallis 46, *87*.
Walter 46, *85, 410*.
Walthard 522, *539*.
Walther 47, *87, 420*.
Wandel 248.
Ward 46, *87*.
Warfield, L. M. 398, 399, *420, 425*.

Warner, H. 520, *538*.
Warren 256, 385.
Wartenberg, R. 49, *87*, 331, 332, 335, *415*.
Wason 367.
— J. M. *420*.
Wasservogel 335.
Watermann 39, *86*.
Watkins, R. M. 398, *420*.
Watson 50, *87*.
Watts, J. W. 266, *420*.
Weber *533*.
— E. 203, *215*, 247, 288, 449, 458, 459, *476*, 485, *486*, 487, *533*.
— F. Parkes 292, 294, 297, 312, 315, 328, 384, 385, 394, 397, 399, *406, 408, 414, 420, 421, 423, 425, 533*.
— L. W. *476*.
Wedrow, N. 271, 279, *405*.
Wedroy 270.
Weech 120, 126, *141*.
Weed 50, *87*.
Weeks 47, 62, 76, *84, 87*.
Wegner 180, *245*.
Weidner 76, *87*.
Weil 372.
Weiler, K. *476*.
Weill, Jean 331, *415, 423*.
Weimann 51, *87*.
Weinberg, A. A. 330, 334, 449, *476*, 485, 486, *539*.
Weir 105, *141*, 286, 287, 290, 291, 293, 294, 298.
Weiss, D. *245*, 246, 250, 251, 256, 257, 265, 306, 319, 370, *420*, 526, *540*.
Weissenbach, R. J. 283, 314, 354, *405, 414, 423*.
Weissmann 221, 226, 235, *245*.
Weitz 223.
Weizsäcker, V. v. 444, *476*, 498, 499, 505, 514, 519, 523, *533, 539*.
Welti, Max *425*.
Wenckebach 496, 510, *533, 539*.
Wenderowič 96, 102, 112, 113, *141*.
Wennberg *414*.
Wenzel, A. 492, *533*.
Werner, P. 109, 326, *473, 536*.
Wernstedt 165.
Werther 351, 363, *408*.
West 329.
Westphal 51, 66, *87*, 88, 89, 95, 102, 111, 120, 124, *141*, 173, 183, 224, *245*, 256, 315, 322, 347, 348, 519, *536*.
Wexberg, E. *476*, 509, *539*.
White 314.
Whitehouse 362.
Whiting 375, 388.

Whytt 230.
Wickenthal, K. *476*.
Widal 221, 222, 235, *245*, 390.
Widowitz 385.
Wiechowsky 203, *245*.
Wieg *476*.
Wiener 179, *245*, 287, 294, 295, 299.
Wiersma 45, *87*.
Wiesel 330, 332, 338, 339.
Wieting 276.
Wigley, M. 314, *414*.
Wiggleswoorth 50, *87*, 266.
Wildbrandt 217, *245*, 459, *538*.
Wilder, Josef 47, 77, *87*, 100, 112, 119, 136, *141*, 435, *476*, 482, *539*.
Wildermuth 63, *87*.
Wilhelm 371, 386, 388.
Wilks 77, *87*.
Will 372, *412*.
Willan 374.
Williams, Duckworth 77, *87*.
Williamson 332, 334.
Willrich 350.
Wills 383.
Wilmaers 119, *141*.
Wilson 1, 89, 90, 91, 95, 97, 98, 100, 101, 102, 103, 104, 105, 107, 113, 119, 120, 121, 122, 123, 129, 133, 136, *141*, 224, *245*.
Wimmer, A. 36, *87*, 109, 119, 120, 122, 123, *141, 539*.
Winchell *420*.
Windscheid 302, 447, *476*.
Winfield 362.
Winkelman 50, *84*.
Winkler, H. 492, *536*.
Winter 48, 83, *87*.
Wirz, Fr. *420*.
Wise *420*.
Wittels 83, *87*.
Wittkower, E. *476*, 493, 515, 516, *534, 538, 539*.
Witzel 239, *245*.
Wohlfahrt 91, 92, 94, 97, 107, 109, 110, 111, 114, 115, 118, 120, 124, *141*.
Wohlwill, F. 183, *401, 476*.
Wolf, Benita 151, 352.
— M. *414*.
Wolff, E. 273, 390.
— H. G. 331, *415*.
— J. 54, *87*, 335, 336.
Wollenberg, R. 452, 459, 460, 464, 465, *476, 539*.
Wolters 344, 347, 348.
Woodcock 39, *87*.
Woodnut 293.
Worcester 51, *87*.
Woringer, Fr. 359, *409, 412*.
Worster 80, *87*, 121, *141*.
Wright 47, *85*.
Wulfften 512, *539*.

Wuth, O. 46, *87*, 213, 435, 525, *540*.
Wwedensky 266.
Wyss, W. H. v. 449, *476*, 485, 486, 491, 499, *533*, *539*.

Yamagata, K. 348, *422*, *423*.
Yarian 383.

Zabludowsky 529.
Zade 459.
Zadek 292, 293, 323, 351, *408*.
Zador 89, 93, 109, 118, 120, 121, *141*.

Zambacco 356.
Zander 46, *86*.
Zappert *165*, 192.
Zande, F. van der *409*.
Zappert, J. *539*.
Zaroshy 395.
Zass, R. *424*.
Zeebi, P. *418*.
Zeek, P. 397, *424*.
Zehrer, H. 96, 102, 107, 109, 118, 119, 122, *141*, *414*.
Zeller, O. *405*, *408*.
Zengerle 306.
Zeydner 223, *245*.
Zha 273.

Ziehen 121, 162, 181, 185, 186, 342, 343.
Ziegenweidt 331, 332, 334.
Ziegler, K. *141*, *476*.
Zieler 306, 307.
Zierl 269, 296, *408*.
Zimmern, A. *421*.
Zondek, S. G. 129, *141*, 353, 483, 510, *536*, *539*.
Zoon, J. 363, 425.
Zorn 353, 354, *410*, *411*, *412*.
Zucker, K. 393, *476*, 497, *539*.
Zuntz 66, *87*.
Zuppa, A. 363, *414*.
Zweig, H. *476*, 486, 492.
Zwirner, E. 529, *539*.

Sachverzeichnis.

Abbau der Organneurosen 495, 503, 518, 524.
ABDERHALDENsche Reaktion 119.
Abducenslähmung 182.
Absenzen, gehäufte 160.
Acetylcholin, Angstaffekt 510.
Achylia gastrica und RAYNAUDsche Krankheit 264.
Achylie, pseudoneurasthenische 503.
Acne rosacea 522.
Adrenalinausschüttung und sympathische Symptome 490, 512.
Aerophagie, Ausdruckssymbolik 518 f.
Affekte, 488.
— Arrhythmie 510.
— Intensität der 96.
— Tonusanfälle 95.
— Verdauungsfunktion 487.
Affekt-epileptische Zustände 162.
Affektinkontinenz, organische 466.
Affektive Erregung:
— Bewußtseinserhöhung 491.
— Zwischenhirn 484.
Affektiver Tonusverlust 101.
Affektkrämpfe, respiratorische 162.
Affektstoß und Regulationsstörung 450.
Aggression, affektiver Tonusverlust 96.
Aggressionstrieb 97.
Akroasphyxia atrophica 281 f.
— chronica, Diagnose 284.
— — endokrines System, Dysfunktion 284.
— — Erblichkeit 283.
— — Nebenniereninsuffizienz 284.
— — Polyneuritis 285.
— — Schilddrüsentätigkeit, Störungen der 284.
— — Sensibilitätsstörungen 281.
— — Sklerodermie 329.
— — Symptomatologie 282.
— — Syringomyelie 285.
— hypertrophica 281.
Akrocyanose 281 f.
Akrodermatitis chronica atrophicans 285.
— — — Erythromelie 296.

Akrodynie 297.
Akromegalie, Akroasphyxia chronica 285.
— Akroparästhesien 305.
— Erythromelalgie 297.
— Hemihypertrophie 342.
Akroparästhesien 299 f.
— Anämie, perniziöse 305.
— Anklopferkrankheit 304.
— Capillaruntersuchung 302.
— Heredität 302.
— Neuropathie 301.
— Neurosen, professionelle 304.
— Ödem, QUINCKEsches 373, 385.
— Pathologie 301 f.
— Sklerodermie 321.
— Sklerose, multiple 305.
— Tabes 305.
— Tetanie 305.
Alkalireserve im Blut 435.
— und Stottern 525.
Alkoholismus, pseudoneurasthenische Syndrome 429.
Alopecia congenita 387.
ALZHEIMERsche Krankheit 52.
Amylnitrit 239.
Anacidität 520.
Anämie, perniziöse 305.
Anfall, reaktiver 94.
Anfälle, subcorticale 100.
— vegetative 506.
Angina pectoris 514, 515.
— — vasomotorica 513 f.
Angiokeratoma Mibelli 312.
Angioneurosen, gewerbliche 273.
Angiospastische Theorie 213.
Angst und Coitus 452.
— und neurotische Störung 509.
— Regulationsstörung 450.
— und Stottern 524.
Angstattacken, Behandlung von 509 f.
Anklopferkrankheit 304.
Anlage, psychopathische 465.
Antrieb und innere Sekretion 437.
— vitaler, Assimilationsstörung 464.
Antriebsschwäche und vegetative Regulationsstörung 438.
Aphasie, assoziative 530.

Apnoë 146.
Äquivalent des Tonusverlustes 99.
Äquivalente, epileptische s. Epilepsie.
Arbeitslähmung 430.
Arbeitslähmungen, Beschäftigungsneurose 529.
Arrhythmie, absolute 510.
— respiratorische 462, 510.
Arsenintoxikation, chronische 312.
Arterien, passagere Kontraktionszustände 256.
Arteriolen, Funktionsstörungen der 511.
Arteriosklerose 439, 446.
— pseudoneurasthenische Syndrome 429.
Arthritis 296.
Arthrogryposis 155.
Asphyxie, lokale 251, 264, 286.
— symmetrische 286.
Assimilation 429, 430.
— kumulative 432.
— und Schlaf 464.
— Stoffwechselausgleich 431.
Astasie 94.
Asthenopie 459.
Asthma bronchiale 514, 515 f.
— — Heredität des 516.
— — Vagusreizung 516.
— cardiale 514.
Ataxie, vasomotorische 262.
Atemkorsett 495.
Atmung, funktionelle Störungen der 514 f.
Atmungstetanie 157.
— neurotische 514.
Atonie 520.
Atropinbehandlung, Ulcus 519.
Atropinversuch und Vago- und Sympathicotonie 496.
Augenzittern der Bergleute 459.
Aura, epileptische s. Epilepsie.
Auraerscheinungen, nichtepileptische 91, 100, 169.
Ausdruck und Symptom 505, 517.
Ausdrucksvorgänge, körperliche 493.
Ausgangswertgesetz 98, 482.
Autointoxikation, gastrointestinale 356.

Handbuch der Neurologie XVII. 36

Sachverzeichnis.

Basedowoid 435.
BASEDOWsche Krankheit:
— Schreck 435.
— Sklerodermie 314.
— Syndrom, vitales 438.
— Tachykardiebereitschaft 510.
Begutachtung, neurasthenische Reaktion 443f.
Belastungen, affektive und Emotionsstöße 450.
Beriberi, Symptome, erythromelalgieähnliche 293.
Beruf, neurasthenische Reaktion 454.
Beschäftigungsneurosen 523, 526f., 529.
Betrachtungsweise, finale 501.
Betriebsstück, vegetatives der Zelle 483.
Bewegungsneurosen 527f.
Bewußtsein, Pyknolepsie 136.
Bewußtseinsniveau, Erhöhung 485.
Bewußtseinsstörungen siehe Epilepsie.
Bewußtseinszustand, erhöhter und Reize 491.
Bicarbonat-Tetanie 157.
Biogenbildung, Funktionssubstrat 432.
Biogene, Aufbau und Zerfall der 431.
Biotonus 430.
Blasenstörung, Hypnose 521.
Blitzkrämpfe 37.
Blutdruck, Absinken 488.
— und seelische Erregung 486.
Blutdruckkurven 511.
Blutdrucksenkende Substanz, Untersuchungen 512.
Blutkalk 110.
Blutzuckerkurve, alimentäre, Schwankungen der 435.
Bradykardie 496.
Bronchitis fibrinosa 377.
Brombehandlung 121.
Bronchialasthma, Organschwäche 517.
Bronchitis fibrinosa mit Asthma 377.
— spastisch asthmatische 150.
Bronchotetanie 149.
Brüste, intermittierende Anschwellung der 376.
Bulbärparalyse, progressiva 314.
Bulbusdruckversuch (ASCHNER) 462.
Bullosis mechanica dystrophica mutilans 387.

Capillarmikroskop 288.
Capillaruntersuchung 302, 319.
CHEYNE-STOKESsche Atmung, Einschlafen 137.
Chorea, Hemiatrophie 331.
— QUINCKEsches Ödem 371f.
— Sklerodermie 314.
Chronaxiemessung 145.
Chûte 94.
CHVOSTEKsches Phänomen 142, 153.
Coitus interruptus und Angst 452.
Colica mucosa 520.
Coupieren von Anfällen 33, 80f., 100.
Crises solaires 377.

Dämmerzustände 194.
— epileptische s. Epilepsie.
Dauerdefekte nach Migräneanfällen 179.
Degeneratio genito-sclerodermica 352.
Depression, endogene 506.
Depressionen, neurasthenische 467f.
Depressionszustände 194.
Depressive Reaktion, Inhalt 448.
Dermatose, psychogene 522.
Dermographismus 462.
Diathese, angioneurotische exsudative 385.
— nervöse 426.
Dissimilation, Phase der 429f.
— Steigerung der 431.
— verstärkte 432.
Dissimilationsprodukte und Stoffwechselkreislauf 438.
Dissoziationszustände 104, 105.
Doigt mort 251.
Doppelinnervation 481.
Drüsen, endokrine 116.
Duodenalstenose 241.
DUPUYTRENsche Kontraktur 322.
Durchfälle und „innere Front" 520.
Dysgrypnien 105.
Dysmenorrhöe 522.
Dyspareunie 522.
Dyspepsie, nervöse 518.
Dysphasie, sozioaffektive 524.
Dysphrenia hemicrania 196.
Dystrophia musculorum progressiva 261, 315.

Einschlafsucht 135.
Einschleifung von Fehlfunktionen 444.
Eklampsie, Epilepsie 66.
— tetanoide 147.

Ekzem 522.
Elastofibrose 346.
Elektrolyte 483.
Emotion, Erschöpfung 451.
— vegetatives System 449.
— s. auch Affekt und Ausdruck.
Emotionsglykosurie 487.
Encephalitis lethargica, Hemiatrophie 331.
— — Sklerodermie, diffuse 315.
— vegetativa 297.
Encephalitisformen, abortive Narkolepsie 113, 114.
Endarteriitis obliterans 274.
Endogene Nervosität 467.
Endokrine Erkrankung und Funktionsverschiebung 434.
— Störungen 224, 270, 279, 284, 293.
Entartung, nervöse 455.
Enteroptose 520.
Enuresis 521.
Epidermolysis bullosa, flüchtiges Ödem 386.
— — hereditaria 371.
Epilamptische Anfälle 162.
Epilepsia minor s. Epilepsie. petit mal.
Epilepsie, Absinth 53.
— Acidose 48 f., 54, 57, 77.
— Äquivalente, psychische 22, 40.
— Ätiologie 43, 61, 71.
— Affect-Epilepsie 40.
— akinetische 38.
— Alkalose 48, 54.
— Alkoholismus 52.
— allergische Erscheinungen 76.
— Altersverteilung 61, 71.
— ALZHEIMERsche Krankheit 52.
— Ammonshornsklerose 51.
— Anämie 52.
— — cerebrale 60.
— Anfälle 1, 2, 3, 6, 7, 14. 18 f., 21, 32, 34, 35, 39, 47, 49, 55, 67 f.
— Anfall, Behandlung des 80.
— — Bewegungs-Typen 23 f.
— — cataplectischer 43.
— — Corneal-Reflex 25.
— — Coupieren 33.
— — Cyanose 18, 26.
— — Dauer 18.
— — Defäkation 25.
— — Einnässen 18, 25.
— — Erblassen, anfängliches 25, 26.
— — Erection 25.
— — generalisierter 7, 18, 58, 71.
— — Häufigkeit 71.

Epilepsie, Anfall, Hypertension 512.
— — Jahres-Kurve 65.
— — klonische Phase 18, 23 f.
— — Mechanismus 58.
— — nächtliche 25, 68.
— — negative Symptome 60.
— — Periodizität der 71.
— — psychasthenischer 40.
— — Pupillen 18, 25.
— — Reflexe 25.
— — Samenerguß 18, 25.
— — Schaum vor dem Munde 24.
— — Schrei 18, 22.
— — Serien 27.
— — Speichelfluß 25.
— — Tageszeiten 29.
— — Theorie, angiospastische 213.
— — Theorien, physiologische 59.
— — tonische Phase 18.
— — vasovagaler 42 f.
— — visceraler 3.
— — voll entwickelter 7.
— — Weinen 25.
— — Zeitfaktor 25.
— Anfall-Bereitschaft 58.
— anfallsfreie Zeit 71.
— Angstneurose 42 f.
— Anorexie 9.
— Anstaltsbehandlung 76.
— Antiepileptica, Geschichte der 73.
— arc de cercle 69.
— Arteria carotis, Druck auf 53.
— Arteriosklerose 52.
— Asphyxie 52.
— Atemstillstand 72.
— Atmung 35.
— Atmungs-Krampf 3.
— Atrophie, Hirnwindungen 50.
— — lobäre 50.
— attitudes passionelles 69.
— Augenmigräne 179.
— Aura 3, 7, 9 f., 17, 19, 55 f., 61, 69.
— — akustische 17.
— — Angst 14 f.
— — Bewegungs-Empfindungen 12.
— — complexe 12, 17.
— — Entzückung 15.
— — epigastrische 12.
— — Farbensehen 16.
— — Gelächter 15.
— — Geschmack 15.
— — Häufigkeit der verschiedenen Arten 10, 15.
— — olfactorische 16.
— — optische 16.
— — Parästhesien 10, 11.

Epilepsie, Aura, psychische 13.
— — Schmerz 11.
— — Sinnesgebiete 15.
— — uncinata 13, 31, 42.
— — Depersonalisations-Typus 14.
— — — abortiver Typus 14.
— — — Erinnerungen, panoramaartige 14.
— Automatismen, präconvulsive 9.
— BABINSKIsches Zeichen 20, 69.
— Begleiterscheinungen 52.
— Behandlung 73 f.
— — Alkohol 81.
— — Amylnitrit 81.
— — Arsen 79.
— — Arznei 77 f.
— — Belladonna 80.
— — Borax 80.
— — Brom 54, 77 f.
— — Bromacne, Schwefelsalbe 79.
— — chirurgische 81 f.
— — Chloral 81.
— — Chloroform 81.
— — Crotalin 76.
— — Dauer 78.
— — Dialacetin 80.
— — Digitalis 80.
— — Eisen 80.
— — Exstirpation des Ganglion cervicale 83.
— — Gardenal 79.
— — Gélineau's dragées 79.
— — Ingwer 81.
— — Kalk 80.
— — Liquordrainage 82.
— — Lumbalpunktion 81.
— — Luminal 54, 79, 81.
— — Magnesiumsulfat 82.
— — Milchinjektion 76.
— — Nitroglycerin 80.
— — Paraldehyd 81.
— — Peptoninjektion 76.
— — Petit mal 79.
— — Proteininjektion 76.
— — psychotherapeutische 83.
— — Sauerstoff-Einatmung 81.
— — Scopolamin 81.
— — Status 81, 17.
— — Strophantus 80.
— — Strychnin 80.
— — Sympathektomie, periarterielle 83.
— — symptomatische 80.
— — Traubenzuckerinjektionen 82.
— — Trepanation 82.
— — Vaccine 76.
— — Zinkoxyd 80.
— Berufswahl 75 f.

Epilepsie, Bevölkerungsschichten, Beteiligung der 61.
— Bewegungen, koordinierte 24.
— Bewegungs-Störungen, postencephalitische 3.
— Bewegungstypen 23.
— Bewußtlosigkeit 7, 12, 18 f., 23, 33 f., 38, 42, 60, 69.
— Bleivergiftung 52.
— Blitzkrämpfe 37.
— Blut 45 f.
— — Cholesterin 47.
— — Fibrin 46.
— — Serum-Eiweiß 46.
— Blut-Gerinnungszeit 46.
— Blutkörperchensenkung 46.
— Blutliquorschranke 51, 53.
— Blutregulation, Kerne, bulbäre der 59.
— Blutviscosität 46.
— Blutzucker 47.
— BROADBENTS Gesetz 32.
— Bromvergiftung 79.
— BROWN-SÉQUARDS Epilepsie 39.
— cerebrale Kinderlähmung 82.
— Charakter, epileptischer 41, 45.
— chirurgische Befunde 49.
— Corpora amylacea 51.
— Coupieren der Anfälle 33, 80 f.
— Creatinin 46.
— Dämmerzustände, postepileptische 21.
— Definition 4.
— — ätiologische 5.
— — physiologische (H. JACKSON) 5.
— Dehydration des Gehirns 54.
— „Déjà vu"-Typus der Aura 14.
— Diät 77.
— — fleischlose 76.
— — Hunger- 54, 76.
— — ketogene 54.
— — salzfreie 76.
— Diagnose 67 f.
— Druck, intrakranieller 53.
— Eheverbot 73.
— Eiweiß-Stoffwechsel 46.
— Ekchymosen 21.
— Eklampsie 66.
— Embolie 52.
— Encephalitis 52.
— Encephalographie 49.
— Endarteriitis 52.
— Endokrinologie 51.
— Enthirnungsstarre 23, 35.
— Entladung 5, 59.
— Eosinophilie 46.

Epilepsie, ependymale Granulationen 50.
— Epilepsia larvata 22.
— — maior 27.
— — partialis continua 36.
— — procursiva 21.
— Epileptikerserum 48.
— epileptogene Felder 55.
— Epistaxis 9, 65.
— eugenische Bestrebungen 73.
— Exhibition 21.
— experimentelle 52 f.
— extrapyramidale 36.
— Facies epileptica 44.
— Familiengeschichte 43.
— Ferment, antiproteolytisches 46.
— Fett-Stoffwechsel 47.
— Fieber 26, 43 f.
— Folgezustände 7, 20f., 191.
— forensische Frage 22.
— Friedmannsche Krankheit 161.
— Gähnen 43.
— Ganglien, periventrikuläre 51.
— Geburtstrauma 73.
— Gefäßkrampf 57.
— Gefäßsymptome 25.
— Gehirngewicht 50.
— Gehirnoberfläche 49.
— Gelegenheitsursachen 75.
— geographische Verteilung 61.
— genuine 1.
— — angioneurotisches Ödem 383.
— — galvanische Zuckungswerte 144.
— Geschichte der 4.
— Geschlechter, Beteiligung der 61.
— geschlechtliche Funktionen, Einfluß 65.
— Goldsolreaktion (C. Lange) 46.
— Grand mal 7, 58.
— Grundumsatz 47.
— Halluzinationen des Geruchs und Geschmacks 14.
— Harnstoff 46.
— Heilung durch fieberhafte Erkrankung 74.
— Heißhunger 9.
— Hemianopsie 17.
— Hemiatrophie 331.
— Hemicranischer Anfall 212.
— Hemmung 60.
— herdförmige Veränderungen 50.
— heredofamiliäre Erkrankung 1.
— Herzblock 52.
— Herzkrankheiten 52.

Epilepsie, Hinstürzen 7, 37.
— Hirnabsceß 52.
— Hirnblutung 52.
— Hirndruck 82.
— Hirnfunktionen, Schemata 18.
— Hirngeschwülste 52.
— Hirnschwellung 52, 54, 82.
— Hirntrauma 52f.
— Histopathologie 51.
— Hitze, Einfluß der 65.
— Hydrocephalus 52.
— Hygiene, allgemeine 74f.
— Hyperventilation 54.
— hypoglykämische Anfälle 47.
— Hypophyse 48, 52.
— Hysterie 22, 33.
— hysterische Anfälle 69f., 57.
— Hystero-Epilepsie 40.
— idiopathische 1, 33, 70.
— Immunität 74.
— infantile 29.
— Infektionskrankheiten 52.
— Insulinhypoglykämie 54.
— Interferometrie 46.
— Intervalle 27.
— intracorticale Reaktionen 60.
— ischämische Veränderung 51.
— Jackson-Anfälle, Coupieren der 80.
— Jacksonsche 11, 23f., 31f., 57, 59, 64, 68.
— Jahreszeiten, Einfluß der 65.
— Kalcium 47.
— Keimdrüsen 48.
— Kinderkrämpfe 71.
— Kinderlähmung, cerebrale 33, 82.
— Klassifikation 4f.
— Kleinhirnanfälle 34.
— Kleptomanie 21.
— klimakterische 30.
— klinische Typen 26f.
— Kohlehydrate 47.
— Konflikte, unbewußte 66.
— koordinierte 36.
— Kopfschmerz 13, 20.
— kosmische Einflüsse 64.
— Krampfschwelle 53.
— Krankheitseinheit 2.
— kryptogenetische 71, 74.
— Kurzschlußtheorie 61.
— Lähmung, motorische 33.
— — postepileptische 20.
— Lebensgefahr 72.
— Leukocytose 46.
— Leukopenie 46.
— Liquor cerebrospinalis 46, 48f.
— — — Gesamteiweiß 46.
— Liquordruck 46.

Epilepsie, Liquorstauung 52, 56.
— Liquor-Zellgehalt 46.
— Luftdruck, Einfluß 65.
— Makropsie 16.
— makroskopische Veränderungen 50.
— Mastix-Reaktion 46.
— Menièresche Anfälle 69.
— Meningitiden 52.
— Menopause 66.
— menstruelle 27, 29, 35, 65.
— Migräne 43, 189f.
— Mikropsie 16.
— Mittelhirn 58.
— Mittelhirnreflex 35.
— Monoepilepsie 36.
— Morbus sacer 4.
— motorische Zentren, Erregung 59.
— Muskelkrämpfe 7.
— Myalgie 20.
— myoclonische 8, 33f., 51, 59, 68.
— Myoclonus-Epilepsie (Unverricht) 34.
— „myriad spells" 37.
— Nachtwandeln 21.
— Namengebung 4.
— Narkolepsie 43, 120, 136.
— Nebennieren 48, 52.
— Nebenschilddrüse 47.
— Neuralgien, paroxysmale 38.
— Ödem, supracorticales 56, 82.
— Ohnmachtsanfälle 69.
— Pacchionische Granulationen 50.
— Palaeothalamus 42.
— Paragraphie 18.
— Paraphasie 18, 21.
— Pathogenese 55f.
— — endokrine Veränderungen 55.
— — humoraler Faktor 56.
— — mechanischer Faktor 56.
— — neuraler Faktor 55.
— — p_H-Quotient 57.
— — vasculärer Faktor 56.
— pathologische Anatomie 49f.
— — Physiologie 45f.
— Periode, 24 Stunden 78.
— Periodizität 27.
— periventrikuläre 41f.
— Petit-mal, Behandlung 79, 80.
— — Häufigkeit 27.
— Petit-mal-Anfälle 6, 7, 19, 21, 22, 35, 37, 44, 57, 59, 64, 68, 71.
— p_H 48, 49.
— Picksche Krankheit 52.
— Plexus chorioideus 51.

Epilepsie, Prodrome 8 f.
— Prognose 37, 71.
— Pronation, epileptische 20.
— Prophylaxe 73 f.
— Protein-Überempfindlichkeit 46.
— Pseudoangina 42.
— Pseudosklerose 52.
— Psychoanalyse 42, 66, 83.
— Psychogenese 66, 67, 83.
— Psychotherapie 83.
— Puls 26, 35.
— PURKINJE-Zellen 51.
— Pyknolepsie 28, 37, 71.
— Rassen, Beteiligung der 61.
— Reflexe 20.
— Reflex-Epilepsie 38 f., 57.
— Reizbarkeit 9.
— retinal-arterieller Krampf 25.
— Rinden-Reizung, experimentelle 59.
— Rotation 35.
— Säurebasen-Gleichgewicht 48, 54.
— ,,Salaam" tics 37.
— Sauerstoffspannung in den Geweben 54.
— Schilddrüsen 47, 52.
— Schlaf 20, 65.
— Schwangerschaft 48, 66, 74.
— Schwindelanfälle 19.
— — MENIÈRE 69.
— Schwitzen, anfallsweises 35.
— senile 30.
— Sensibilitätsstörungen, objektive 8.
— sensitive 192.
— sensorische 68.
— Sklerodermie 314.
— Sklerose, diffuse 52.
— — multiple 52.
— — tuberöse 52.
— Späteklampsie 153 f., 158.
— Spontanheilung 72.
— Sport bei 75.
— Sprachstörung 192.
— Status, Behandlung des 81.
— — epilepticus 20, 28, 72, 79.
— — Tod im 28.
— Sterblichkeit 72.
— Stigmata 44.
— Stirnhirnsymptome 58.
— Stottern 524.
— striäre 35.
— subcorticale 36.
— Sympathektomie, periarterielle 56, 83.
— Symptomatologie 6 f., 22 f., 128 f.
— — abgesehen von den Anfällen 44 f.
— Syphilis 52.

Epilepsie, System, sympathisches 51.
— Tetanie 47, 153 f., 158.
— Theorie der Entstehung 60.
— — der Erregung 59.
— Thrombose 52.
— Thymus 52.
— Tic 3.
— tonische Phase 23, 34 f., 68.
— Toxine, endogene 55.
— Trauma 63 f.
— traumatische, Behandlung chirurgische 82.
— Traumzustände 9, 13 f.
— Tuberkulose 52.
— Typus, kombinierter 27.
— — nächtlicher 29, 65.
— — Tages- 9, 65.
— Unruhe 8.
— Urin 19.
— Vaguskerne 42.
— Varianten, akustikomotorische 39.
— — epileptische 31 f., 71.
— — sensorische 38 f.
— — vegetative 41.
— Vasomotoren-Reflex 55.
— Ventrikel, dritter 42 f.
— — vierter 42, 44.
— Ventrikelerweiterung 50.
— Vererbung 57 f., 62, 71, 73 f.
— Verstimmungszustände 41.
— Verwachsungen, intermeningeale 50.
— Verwirrungszustände, vorübergehende 68.
— Wandertrieb 20, 21 f.
— Wassermannsche Reaktion 46.
— Wasserstoffionenkonzentration 48.
— Wasserstoffwechsel 82.
— Zelleinschlüsse 51.
— Zellen, chromophile 52.
— Zentralwindung, vordere 58.
— Zentren, vegetative 41.
— Zuckerspiegel 47.
— Zuckungen 19.
— Zungenbiß 18, 83.
Epileptoid, neuropathisches beim Kind 162.
EPPINGER-HESSsche Lehre 482.
Erbrechen 520.
ERBsches Phänomen 143.
Ergotamin 239.
Ergotismus 275.
Ergotropes Prinzip 486.
Ergrauen der Haare 522.
Erholung 430.
Erlebnis, Reaktion 448.
Erlebnisform, Organminderwertigkeit 498.
Ermüdung 90, 431.

Ermüdungsgifte, Stoffwechselkreislauf 438.
Erregbarkeit, latente 141.
— manifeste 141.
Erschöpfung 429 f., 433.
— BASEDOWsche Krankheit 435.
— Emotion 451.
— psychische, neurasthenische Reaktion 440.
— Sinnestäuschung 459.
Erwachen, verzögertes psychomotorisches 105.
Erweckbarkeit 93.
Erythema exsudativum multiforme 296.
— indurativum 284.
— multiforme 397.
— nodosum 397.
Erythrocyanose 284.
Erythrodermie 296.
Erythrödem, synonymisches 297.
Erythromelalgie 286 f.
— Ätiologie 287.
— Akrosphyxia chronica 298.
— Akromegalie 297.
— Arthritis der kleinen Gelenke 296.
— berufliche Überanstrengungen 287.
— Blutbild 292.
— capillarmikroskopische Untersuchungen 288.
— Diagnose 296 f.
— Diathese, neuropathische 293.
— endokrine Störungen 293.
— Erysipel 296.
— Gangrän 291.
— Gefäßkrankung 294.
— Gliosis spinalis 293.
— Knochenatrophie 291.
— Metatarsalgien 296.
— Myelitis 293.
— Ödem, entzündliches 296.
— — QUINCKEsches 292, 385.
— Paralyse 293.
— pathologische Anatomie und Pathogenese 294 f.
— Phlegmone 296.
— Plattfuß, entzündlicher 296.
— Polycythämie 292.
— Polyneuritis 285, 293.
— Prognose 298.
— Psychosen 293.
— RAYNAUDsche Krankheit 291.
— Röte 288.
— Schmerz 288.
— Schwellungen 288.
— Sklerodaktylie 328.
— Sklerodermie 292.

Erythromelalgie, Störungen, trophische 290.
— Symptomatologie 288.
— Tabes dorsalis 293.
— Tarsalgien 296.
— Therapie 298.
— thermische Schädlichkeiten 287.
— Tumor, extramedullärer 293.
— Zentralnervensystem, organische Affektion 293.
Erythromelie, Akrodermatitis chronica atrophicans 296.
Erythroprosopalgie-BING 287.
Eunuchoidismus 438.
Exogene Reaktionsformen 428 f.
Exophthalmus, rezidivierender 377.
Exsudativer Prozeß (Gehirn) 202, 207.
Extrapyramidales System Dysfunktion 526.
Extrasystolie 510.
Extremitätenlähmung, periodische 137.

Facialislähmung 183, 185, 315, 331.
— rezidivierende, Arthritismus 369.
Facialisphänomen 142, 153.
Fasciculäre Zuckungen 179.
FEERsche Krankheit 297.
Fettsucht 107 f.
Fieber 174, 185.
— psychogenes 488.
— vegetatives System 445.
Flimmerskotom 176, 177.
Fluor albus 522.
Fremdneurosen 479.
FRIEDMANNsche Krankheit 160 f.
Frigidität 522.
Funktion, gestörte, organneurotische Reaktion 494.
Funktionelle Erkrankungen und Neurose 478.
Funktionsablauf, vegetativer 437.
Funktionssubstrat 434 f.
Funktionsunregelmäßigkeiten vago-sympathicotonische 458.

Gähnanfall 91.
Ganglienkette 481.
Gangrän, Abgrenzung von postinfektiöser und kachektischer 274.
— Ergotismus 275.
— Erythromelalgie 291.
— Formen des Vorkommens 252.

Gangrän, multiple, neurotische 310.
— postinfektiöse 274.
— RAYNAUDsche 249, 252.
— symmetrische, Beriberi 273.
— Zehen und Füße 276.
Gastritis 518.
Gastrointestinale Störungen 356, 390.
Gastrosuccorrhoe 518.
Geburtshelferhandstellung 143, 148.
Gefäßerkrankungen 230, 259, 270, 294.
Gefäßkrampf (Gehirn), Lokalisation 208.
— Migräneanfall 205 f.
— Vertebralissystem 210.
Gefäßkrisen, Lehre von den 205.
Geigerkrampf 529.
Gefühls-Kreis 491.
Gefühlssphäre und vegetative Organe 491.
Gefühlsstörung 178.
Gelegenheitskrämpfe 147, 154, 159.
Gelenkergüsse 379.
GÉLINEAUsche Krankheit 88.
GÉLINEAUsches Syndrom 135.
Gelolepsie 137.
Geloplegie 137.
Gemütsbewegung 485.
Genußmittel, übermäßiger Gebrauch 445.
Gereiztheit 465.
Gesichtsfeldeinengung, Ermüdung 459.
Gesundheitsgewissen 467.
Gleichgewicht, vegetatives 489.
Gleichgewichtsstörungen 187, 188.
Gliosis spinalis, Erythromelalgie 293.
— — Hautgangrän, multiple, neurotische 310.
Glossy skin 357.
Glottiskrampf 145.
Grand mal s. Epilepsie.
Grippeanfälle, neurasthenisches Syndrom 445.
Grundhaltung, YOGHA 507.
Guanidinderivat 512.
Guanidin-Tetanie 157.

Hämoklasische Krise 221, 222.
Halsrippe und Raynaudsymptome 262, 273.
Halssympathicus 173, 215.
Harnverhaltung, neurotische 521.
Hautblutungen, spontane 523.

Hautgangrän, multiple, neurotische 306 f.
Hautgangrän, multiple neurotische:
— Behandlung 311.
— Diagnose 311.
— Gesamtverlauf 308.
— Hysterie 310.
— Neuritiden, periphere 310.
— Ödem, flüchtiges 386.
— — QUINCKEsches 373.
— Tabes 310.
— Vasomotorensystemstörung 309.
— Verschorfung 309.
Hautreflexe, neurasthenische Reaktion 461.
HEADsche Zone 329.
Hemianopsie 176, 178, 179.
Hemiatrophia cruciata 335.
Hemiatrophia faciei progressiva:
— Ätiologie 331 f.
— Alopecie 333.
— Augenmuskellähmung 331.
— Chorea 333.
— Echinococcus 339.
— Encephalitis 331.
— Epilepsie 331.
— Facialislähmung 331.
— Haare 333.
— Herpes 333.
— Kaumuskelkrämpfe 334.
— Lues 339.
— MARCUS-GUNNsches Phänomen 331.
— mesencephale Läsion 339.
— neuropathische Belastung 331.
— Paralyse 339.
— pathologisch-anatomische Befunde 338.
— Poliomyelitis 331.
— Pupille-Lichtstarre 334.
— Sklerose, multiple 339.
— Sympathicusaffektion 334.
— Syringomyelie 339.
— Tabes 339.
— Torticollis 331.
— Trauma 331.
— Trigeminusaffektion 334.
— Tumor (Dura) 339.
— Zungenmuskeln 331.
Hemiatrophia totalis einer Körperhälfte 335.
Hemicrania cerebellaris 188.
— continua 169.
— facioplegica 185.
— sympathico-paralytica 203.
— sympathicotonica 203.
Hemihypertrophia cruciata 340.
— faciei 340.
— totalis 341.
Hemihypertrophie, Akromegalie 342.

Hemihypertrophie, Syringomyelie 342.
— Zunge 342.
Hemiparästhesie 178.
Hemiparese 179.
Hemiplegie 179, 184.
— chronisch-neuropathische Ödeme 393.
— Kombination mit Erythromelalgie 293.
Hemmung, innervatorische und Tonusverlust 131.
— kataleptische 94.
Heredodegeneration 338.
Herpes 333, 522.
— zoster gangraenosus 310.
Herzangst 467.
Herz, Erkrankung mit Erythromelalgie-Symptomen 294.
Herzinfarkt 515.
Herzkranke, Cyanose 296.
Herzneurosen 510.
Herztetanie 150.
Hinken, intermittierendes 275, 297.
Hirngeschwulst 230.
Hirnnervenlähmungen, Sitz der 208.
Hirnrinde, sensible, Überempfindlichkeit der 435.
Hirnschlaf und Körperschlaf 104, 127.
Hirnstamm und psychische Leistungen 491.
Hirntraumen, Folgezustände nach 439, 446.
Hirntumor, Einleitungsphase 439.
— pseudoneurasthenische Syndrome 429.
Histotropes Prinzip 486.
Hörfähigkeit, Ermüdungssymptome der 460.
Homme momie 326.
Hormonale Frühjahrskrise 156.
Hormone 483.
Hydrocephalus, Migräne, symptomatische 230.
Hydrops abdominalis intermittens 378.
— hypostrophos tendovaginarum 378.
Hygiene, körperlich-seelische, neurasthenische Reaktion 470.
Hyperakusis 460.
Hyperidrosis palmaris 387.
Hyperpnoë, nervöse 514.
Hyperthyreotische, konstitutionell, und Magen-Darmfunktion 519.
Hypertonie, Gefäßlabilität 511.
— genuine 512, 513.

Hypertonie, striäre 511, 512.
Hypertonus-Neurosen, Therapie der 513.
Hyperventilation, Schlafanfall 93.
Hyperventilationstetanie 157.
Hypnolepsie 135.
Hypnose, psychophysische Abhängigkeiten 487.
Hypochonder, Obstipation 520.
— vegetative Stigmatisation 505.
Hypochondrische Reaktion 427, 469.
Hypochondrisches Denken und Mißempfindung 467.
Hypogenitale Hand 284.
Hypoglykämie, spontane 137.
Hypophyse, Insuffizienz 284.
— nervöse Erscheinungen 435.
Hypotonie und leptosomer Typus 512.
Hysterie, Komplex, somatischer 495.
— Reflexverstärkung, willkürliche 461.
Hysterische Anfälle 69f.
— Erscheinungen und organische 479.
— Prägung, organisch bedingter cerebraler Leistungsausfälle 480.
— Reaktion 427, 468.
— Überlagerung der neurasthenischen Reaktion 470.

Impotenz 521.
Indican im Urin 435.
Individualpsychologie (ADLERsche) 524.
Infektionskrankheiten, Folgezustände nach 446.
— Neurasthenie 428.
Infektionsprodrom, Syndrom, vitales 445.
Initialkrämpfe 147, 154, 159.
Inkontinenz 521.
Innere Organe und Sklerodermie 325.
Innervation, vegetative Ubiquität 480.
Intoxikation, infektiöse und nervöse Symptome 445.
Iritis, rezidivierende, Hydrops intermittens 381.
Isolierungsphänomene 479.

JACKSON-Epilepsie s. unter Epilepsie.
JAMES-LANGEsche Theorie der Affekte 485.
Jatrogene Schädigung 513.

Kachexie 325.
Kalkablagerungen 354.
Kallikrein 279.
Kardiospasmus, Ausdruckssymbolik 519.
— Hiatushernie des Oesophagus 518.
— vagoneurotischer 497.
Kardiovasculäre Störungen, Erschöpfungsneurasthenie 462.
Kardiovasculärer Symptomenkomplex, Schreckneurose 463.
Katalepsie, Tonusverlust, affektiver 138.
Kataleptische Starre 94.
Katarakt 326.
Katatonie 262.
Kenotoxine 430.
Kernneurosen 479.
Klimakterium 438.
Körperschlaf 127.
— Hirnschlaf 104.
Körperschlafanfälle 133.
Kohlehydrathaushalt und suggestiver Einfluß 489.
Kolloidoklasie 522.
Konfliktstopographie 479.
Konstitution 111, 134, 426.
— thyreotische 497, 510.
Konstitutionell Nervöse, neurasthenische Reaktion 453.
Konstitutioneller Hochdruck 512.
Konstitutionstypen, vegetative 495.
Kontaktneurose, striopallidärer Schaltapparat 525.
Kontaktneurosen 518, 524.
Kontrastreaktionen 466.
Konzentrationsunfähigkeit 464.
Koordinationsneurosen 523f.
Koordinationsstörungen der einzelnen Schlafkomponenten 130.
Kopfschmerz 169, 170, 177, 181, 460.
Krämpfe, allgemeine 147.
— psychasthenische 162.
— tonisch-klonische 179.
Krampfkrankheiten, intermediäre 141.
Krankheitsbilder, latente 495.
Krankheitseinheiten 427.
Kreislaufsystem 509f.
— affektive Auswirkungen am 486.
Kriegsbeschädigung 139.
Kriegsschädigungen, psychische 450.
Kurzschlußtheorie 61.
Kyphoskoliose 324.

Labilität, konstitutionelle der vegetativen Steuerungen 502.
— vasomotorische 262.
Lachen und Schlaf 104.
Lachschlag 94, 136.
Lähmung, cerebrale Kinder- 33.
— paroxysmale 183.
Laryngospasmus 145.
Lebensgeschichte, innere 493.
— — und Organneurose 507.
Lebensnerven 481.
Leib-Seele-Problem 477.
— und psychovegetative Korrelationen 492 f.
Lepra 273.
Lichtempfindlichkeit, galvanische 459.
Lichtreflexbewegung 459.
Lidflattern 459.
Linkshändigkeit und Stottern 524.
Lipodystrophia progressiva 336.
Lipodystrophischer Typus 352.
Lipomatose 264.
Liquorzirkulationsstörung, SPITZERs Theorie 201.
Lokalhormone 483.
Lues 119, 249, 259, 274, 313.
Luftschlucken 518.
Luminal 238, 242.

Magentetanie 157.
Maschinennäherinnen, Krampf bei 529.
MASSLOWsches Respirationssymptom 147.
Melker, Krampf bei 529.
Melorheostose 395.
MENIÈREsches Syndrom, vasomotorische Störung 380.
Meningitis serosa und neurasthenische Reaktion 448.
Menstruationsblutungen 522.
Migräne, Ätiologie der 217 f.
— Alkalireserve 221.
— Alkohol 242.
— allergische 219, 222, 234.
— Alter 167.
— anatomische Schädigungen bei 232.
— Anfallsformen 166.
— angiospastische Theorie der 202, 217.
— — Syndrome 204.
— Anlage zur 217, 228.
— Appetitlosigkeit 172.
— assoziierte 178.
— Augenmigräne 175 f., 209.
— — und homonyme Hemianopsie 209.
— Aurasymptome 169.

Migräne, Basen-Säure-Gleichgewicht 221.
— Bauchmigräne 172.
— Bauchoperation 241.
— Behandlung, Acetylcholin 239.
— — Alttuberkulin 235.
— — Brom 237.
— — Brom-Papaverin-Luminal 238.
— — Chinin 239.
— — Crotolin 235.
— — Duodenalsonden 236.
— — Eigenblut- 235.
— — Fußbäder 241.
— — Histamin 235.
— — im Anfall 241.
— — Kalk- 237.
— — Luminal 238, 242.
— — Milchinjektionen 235.
— — Moloid 239.
— — Morphin 242.
— — Nahrungszusammensetzung 223, 235.
— — Nitroglycerin 239.
— — Nitrokörper 239.
— — Ovariumpräparate 237.
— — Papaverin 238.
— — Papaverininjektion, intravenöse 241.
— — Paracodin 241.
— — Pepton- 235.
— — Pferdeserum 235.
— — roborierende Kuren 239.
— — Schilddrüsen- 237.
— — Typhusvaccine- 235.
— Beruf 168.
— Brechreiz 171.
— Brustmigräne 174.
— Dämmerzustände 194.
— Darmsymptome 174.
— Dauerdefekte bei 232.
— Depressionszustände 194.
— Desensibilisierung, allgemeine 234.
— Diät 223, 235, 236.
— Differentialdiagnose 231 f.
— dissoziierte 178.
— Duodenalstenose 241.
— endokrine Störungen 224.
— Epilepsie 43, 189 f.
— Erbrechen 171.
— Ernährungsstörungen, ischämische 212.
— exsudativer Prozeß (Gehirn) 202, 207.
— For. interventricular. Monroi 201.
— Gefäßerkrankungen 230.
— Gefäßnerven 206.
— Gersondiät 236.
— Gesichtskrampf 175.
— gichtige Anlage 218.
— hämoklasische Krise 221 f.

Migräne, Häufigkeit der 166, 176.
— Halssympathicus-Läsion 215.
— Halssympathicusoperation 240.
— Halssympathicussymptome 173, 204.
— Harnsäureretention 220.
— Harnsymptome 174.
— Hemicrania sympathicotonica 203.
— hereditäre Beziehungen zwischen Epilepsie und Migräne 189.
— Herzbeschwerden 173.
— Hinterhauptschmerz 171.
— Hirnnervenlähmungen 208.
— Hirnnerven-Reizsymptome 174.
— Hydrocephalus, angioneurotischer 201.
— Hypertonie 205.
— Hypophyse 226.
— Hypophysentheorie 200.
— hysterische Reaktionen bei 197.
— interparoxismale Symptome bei 198.
— JACKSON-Anfälle, sensible 192.
— Kältereiz als auslösender Faktor 205, 227.
— Kalkstoffwechsel 221.
— Kindermigräne 167.
— Kleinhirnsymptome 188.
— Kompresse 241.
— Konstitutionstypus und 220.
— Kopfschmerz 169 f., 177, 181.
— Kopfschmerzpulver 241.
— Kopftrauma 228.
— Leberfunktionsstörung 201.
— Liquorzirkulationsstörung 201.
— Luftveränderung 227, 242.
— Lumbalpunktion 202, 242.
— Magenerscheinungen 172.
— Magenptose 241.
— Massage 241.
— myalgische Theorie der 199.
— Naseoperation 241.
— Nebenschilddrüse 226.
— Nervensystem, vegetatives 218.
— operative Eingriffe 239.
— ophthalmoplegische 180 f.
— — Facialislähmung 183, 185.
— — Fieber 185.
— — Häufigkeit 181.
— ovarielle 225, 237.

Sachverzeichnis.

Migräne, Oxalämie 221.
— Pathogenese der 199 f.
— Pentosurie 221.
— Periodizität 168.
— Petit-mal-Anfälle 190.
— pontomesencephale Form der 187.
— Prognose 232.
— Prophylaxe 242.
— psychische Erscheinungen im Anfall 173.
— — Störungen bei 194 f.
— Pupillenerweiterung 173, 204.
— QUINCKEsches Ödem 371, 382, 390.
— reflektorische 226.
— Reflextheorie 199.
— Schilddrüse 226.
— Schwellungen 173.
— Schwindelanfälle 187.
— Sehstörungen 176, 209, 212.
— Sinus-caroticus-Reflex 204.
— Sondenversuch (MUCK) 205.
— Sprachstörung 178, 192.
— Status hemicranicus 168, 233.
— Stoffwechselvorgänge 220.
— Stottern 524.
— Stuhlregelung 236.
— Sympathektomie 240.
— Sympathicussymptome, allgemeine 173.
— symptomatische 167, 229f.
— — Bleivergiftung 231.
— — Hirngeschwulst 230.
— — Hirnlues 230.
— — Malaria 230.
— — Nierenkrankheit 230.
— — Oculomotoriusgeschwulst 230.
— — Otosklerose 231.
— — Paralyse 230.
— — Pathogenese 214.
— — Sklerose, multiple 230.
— — Tabes 230.
— Therapie der 233 f.
— Tonsillotomie 241.
— Trigeminusneuralgie 231.
— Vagotonie 219.
— Verdauungsstörungen 223.
— Vererbung bei 217.
— Vestibularisapparat 188.
— Wetterwechsel 227.
— zentrale Theorien 200.
Migräneäquivalente 172, 173, 177, 187, 195.
Migräneanfall, auslösende Ursachen 221 f., 227 f.
— Dauer 169.
— Ende 175.
— Eosinophilie 223.
— Fieber 174.
— Folgezustände 192.

Migräneanfall, Gefäßkrampf 206.
— — im Vertebralissystem 210.
— Gefäßkrampf-Lokalisation im Gehirn 208.
— Gefäßkrisen (PAL) 205.
— gewöhnlicher 169 f.
— Pathomechanismus 199.
— psychische Erregung 227.
Migränesymptome, Lokalisation der 211.
Migränoepilepsie 190.
Migraine ophthalmique 175.
Mikrobasedow 497.
— Tachykardiebereitschaft 510.
Mikrofälle 503.
MIKULICZsche Krankheit, Ödem 376.
MILROYsche Krankheit 394.
Mißempfindungen und Depression 506.
— somatisches Entgegenkommen der Organe 498.
Morbus WESTPHAL-GÉLINEAU 88.
Morphinismus 438.
Mors subita infantum 146.
Mundtrockenheit 518.
Muskelerregbarkeit, mechanische 461.
Muskelwogen 461.
Myalgische Theorie 199.
Myoclonusepilepsie siehe Epilepsie.

Nachahmungsstottern 530.
Nachtdienst, übermäßiger 455.
Narkolepsie 87f.
— ABDERHALDENsche Reaktion 119.
— Adynamic 94.
— ätiologische Faktoren 111.
— Alkohol und Anfall 93.
— Allergie 120.
— Arteriosklerose 120.
— atypische Zustände der 102.
— Aufwecken 93.
— Aura 91.
— Blutbefund 108, 109.
— Blutkalk 110.
— Blutzucker 110.
— Capillarbild 109.
— Dissoziationserscheinungen 104.
— Drüsen, endokrine 116.
— Einschlafanfälle 94.
— Encephalitis 113.
— Encephalogramm 110.
— Epilepsie 120, 136.
— familiäre 112, 113.
— Fettsucht 107f.

Narkolepsie, forensische Bedeutung 139.
— FRIEDMANNsche Krankheit 161.
— Genitaldrüsen 117f.
— Grundumsatz 107f.
— Habitus 110.
— Häufigkeit der 124.
— Heredität 111.
— Hyperventilation 93.
— Hypogenitalismus 118.
— Hypophyse 116.
— Hysterie 137.
— kataleptische Starre 94.
— Keimdrüsen 117.
— Konstitution 111, 134.
— Kopftrauma 139.
— Kriegsbeschädigung 139.
— Liquor 110.
— Lokalisation der 127.
— Lues 119.
— Lymphocytose 107f.
— Menstruation 118.
— Nachtschlaf 106.
— Nasenbluten 120.
— neurologischer Befund bei 107.
— Pathogenese 128f.
— Polycythämie 119.
— posttraumatische Gruppe 119.
— psychisches Bild 110.
— Pubertät 124.
— RAYNAUDsche Krankheit 109.
— Reizerscheinungen, motorische 91.
— Röntgenbefund 110.
— Schädeltraumen 119.
— Schlaf, narkoleptischer und Ruhe 89.
— Schlafäquivalente 131.
— Schlafanfall siehe auch Schlaf und Schlafanfälle.
— Schlafstörung und Schlafumkehr 106.
— Schlafzentrum 129.
— Senkungsgeschwindigkeit 110.
— Spasmophilie 161.
— Stoffwechsel 110.
— symptomatische 133.
— Therapie 138, 139.
— Thyreoidea 117.
— Tonusverlust siehe Tonusverlust.
— Tuber cinereum 129.
— Vagotonie 109.
— vegetatives System 107, 109f.
Nervenendapparat 483.
Nervensystem, animales, sympathicogene Umstimmung 490.
— organische Erkrankungen 310.

Nervenverletzungen, Folgeerscheinungen von 273.
— Hautgangrän 310.
— und vasomotorische Störungen 273.
Nervöse Depression (BUMKE) 452.
— Regulationsstörung der Organfunktion 457.
Nervosität, Begriff 426.
— konstitutionelle 426f., 440f.
— und ländliche Bevölkerung 456.
Nervus acusticus, Ausfallserscheinungen des 185.
— facialis, Reizsymptome des 175.
— hypoglossus, Ausfallserscheinungen des 185.
— oculomotorius, Geschwülste des 186.
— supraorbitalis, Druckempfindlichkeit des 171.
— trigeminus, Ausfallserscheinungen 183.
— trochlearis, Lähmung 182.
Neuralgiforme Schmerzen 460.
Neuralgischer Typus, Schreibkrampf 528.
Neurasthenie, Begriff der 426.
— exogene Entstehung der 426.
Neurasthenische Depression 452.
— Melancholie (FRIEDMANN) 452.
— Reaktion 427f.
— — Ätiologie 440f., 445.
— — Begriff der 428.
— — Höhensonnenbestrahlung bei 469.
— — hydrotherapeutische Maßnahmen 469.
— — und körperliche Krankheit 444.
— — körperliche Symptome 458.
— — Lebensalter 453.
— — Nebenniere 435.
— — Prognose 466.
— — psychische Symptome 463.
— — Randsymptome 456.
— — Reizflucht 433.
— — Schlafmittel 469.
— — Therapie 468f.
— — vitales Syndrom 453.
Neuritis optica, vasomotorische Störung 380.
Neuronschwelle, Erniedrigung der 432.
Neurose, Begriff der 477.
— vegetative 497.
Neurosenbereitschaft 497.
Neurosen, Gruppierung 479.

Nicotin, Mißbrauch von 451.
Nicotin-Gebrauchseinschränkung 469.
Nicotintremor 461.
Nystagmoid, neurasthenisches 457f.
Nystagmus der Grubenarbeiter 459.

Oculomotoriuslähmung 180, 183.
Ödem, Begriff 389.
— akutes umschriebenes s. Ödem, QUINCKEsches.
— angioneurotisches s. Ödem, QUINCKEsches.
— chronisch-neuropatisches 393.
— entzündliches 296.
— QUINCKEsches 310, 328, 366f.
— — Akroparästhesien 373, 385.
— — Allergene 369, 390.
— — Anaphylaxie 390.
— — Anurie 376.
— — Aphasie, komplette motorische 381.
— — Arzneimittel 369.
— — Asthma 390.
— — Augenlider 374.
— — Basedow 373.
— — Behandlung, desensibilisierende 398.
— — — Eigenserum- 399.
— — — Organpräparate 398.
— — — Peptonlösung 399.
— — Blutaustritt 374.
— — cerebrale Symptome 381.
— — Chorea 371, 372.
— — Diagnose 392f.
— — Diarrhöen, profuse 378.
— — Diathese, gichtische 369.
— — — neuropathische 371.
— — Ekzem 390.
— — Eosinophilie 384.
— — Epiglottis 376.
— — Erbrechen 377.
— — Erschöpfungszustände, körperliche 371.
— — Erythromelalgie 292.
— — Facialislähmung 382.
— — Fieber 383.
— — Gelenkergüsse 379.
— — Glottis 388.
— — Gravidität 372.
— — Hämoglobinurie, paroxysmale 381.
— — Harnentleerung 381.
— — Hautblutungen 374.
— — Hebephrenie 372.
— — Hemiplegie, passagere 381.

Ödem, QUINCKEsches, Heredität 368.
— — Heufieber 390.
— — HORNERsches Syndrom 374.
— — Hysterie 393.
— — Idiosynkrasie 390.
— — Kaumuskulatur 374.
— — Kieferklemme 379.
— — Klimakterium 372.
— — Lähmung, periodische 382.
— — Larynx 377.
— — Lunge 377.
— — Magen-Darm-Erscheinungen 377.
— — Malaria 370.
— — Melancholie 372.
— — Meningitis serosa 381.
— — Menstruation 372.
— — Migräne 371, 382, 390.
— — Muskeln 373.
— — Nahrungsmittelallergene 369.
— — Nervenkrankheiten, organische 372.
— — Neuralgien 370, 379.
— — Neurosen 371.
— — Oculomotoriuslähmung, rezidivierende 371, 382.
— — Opticusaffektion 380.
— — Organneurosen 522.
— — Paralyse, myasthenische 382.
— — Pathogenese 389f.
— — Prognose 388.
— — Proteinintoxikation 390.
— — Puerperium 372.
— — RAYNAUDsche Krankheit 373, 385.
— — Schleimhäute 376.
— — Sehnenscheidenanschwellung 378.
— — Serumkrankheit 390.
— — Sklerodermie 373.
— — der Speicheldrüsen 375.
— — Symptomatologie 373f.
— — Tabes dorsalis 372.
— — Tachykardie 381.
— — Tetanie 372.
— — Therapie 397f.
— — Trauma 371.
— — Trophoedème Meige 372.
— — Tumor, Rückenmark 372.
— — Urticaria 384, 390.
— — Ventrikel, dritter 382.
— — Spasmophilie 151.
— — stabiles, flüchtiges Ödem 397.
Oedème blanc, Hysterie 393.
— bleu, Hysterie 393.
— ségmentaire 394.

Sachverzeichnis.

Oesophagushernie 495, 503, 513.
Onanie und emotionelle Schädigung 452.
Organdetermination 505.
Organdiathese, angioneurotische 519.
Organe, somatisches Entgegenkommen der 498.
— vegetative Gefühlssphäre 491.
Organempfindungen 491.
Organerkrankung, larvierte 456.
Organfunktionen, vegetativ gesteuerter, Ausdrucksbedeutung 499.
Organismus, Begriff des 477, 491f.
Organminderwertigkeit 498, 505.
— Enuresis 521.
Organneurosen 426, 477f.
— Abbau der 495.
— Aufbau der 495.
— Behandlung der 506f.
— Krankheitsformen, leichte 503.
Organneurotische Betriebsstörungen 494f.
Organsymbolik 500.
Organwahl und Konflikt 499.
— und Organneurosen 498.
Orgasmolepsie 137.
Orthostatisch-epileptoider Symptomkomplex 161.
Osteomalacie, Tetanie, idiopathische 155.
Osteomalacischer Typus der genito-sklerodermatischen Degeneration 352.
Otosklerose 231.
Ovarium, Störungen 284.
Oxalämie 221.

Pacylbehandlung bei Angstattacken 510.
Padutin 279.
Paralyse, progressive, Erythromelalgie 293.
— Pseudoneurasthenische Erscheinung 293, 446.
Paranoide Reaktion 448.
Parasympathicuswirkung und Bewußtseinsniveau 485.
— histotropes Prinzip 486.
Parkinsonismus, encephalitischer Schreibkrampf 525.
Partialkonstitutionen 426.
Pavor nocturnus 103, 105.
Periarteriitis nodosa, multiple neurotische Hautgangrän 310.
Periodik und Funktion des vegetativen Nervensystems 130.

Peroneusphänomen 143, 153.
Person, vitale 435, 436f., 477.
— — Zwischen-Mittelhirn 437.
Petit-mal s. Epilepsie.
Pfötchenhand 148.
Phosphat-Tetanie 157.
Phrenokardie 510, 513.
Pianistenkrampf 529.
PINK-Disease 297.
Pollakisurie 521.
Pollutionen, gehäufte 521.
Poltern und Stottern 530.
Polygenie der Organneurosen 501.
Polyneuritiden, neurasthenische 461.
Polyneuritis 273, 285, 293, 457.
Postinfektiöse Schwächezustände 439.
— — und neurasthenische Reaktion 453.
PROLsches Phänomen 143.
Pruritus 522f.
Pseudohalluzinationen auf akustischem Gebiet 460.
— Erschöpfung 459.
Pseudolipom 376.
Pseudoneurasthenische Erscheinungen 428, 439f., 446f.
Pseudoschlafzustände 104.
Psoriasis 522.
Psychasthenie 427.
Psychische Leistung und Hirnstamm 491.
Psychogene Entwicklungen 467f.
— Reaktionen, Definition 448.
— — und hysterische Reaktionsformen 449.
— — neurasthenische Reaktion 467, 468.
Psychogenese, körperlicher Störungen 477.
Psychoneurosen 478.
Psychopathie 196.
Psychopathische Belastung und Krieg 442.
— Persönlichkeiten 427.
— — und neurotische Fehlleistung 507.
Psychophysische Korrelationen 493.
Psychose, symptomatische 429.
Psychosen, symptomatische Folgezustände nach 446.
Psychotherapeutische Methoden, Wirkungsvorgang 517.
Psychotherapie, Angina pectoris vasomotorica 514.
— Anlage 507.
— Asthma 516.
— und neurasthenische Reaktion 469.

Psychovegetative Erscheinungen der Haut 522.
Ptosis 458.
Pupillenerweiterung, neurasthenische Reaktion 459.
Purpura toxica 374.
Pyknolepsie 88, 136.
— Epilepsie 28, 37, 71.

QUINCKEsches Ödem s. Ödem.
QUINQUAUDsches Phänomen 461.

Rachitikerzähne 151.
Rachitis und Tetanie 156.
Randneurosen 479.
RAYNAUDsche Krankheit 246f.
— — Ätiologie 246f.
— — Arteriosklerose, diffuse 259.
— — Arthritis urica 260.
— — Basedow 264.
— — Behandlung, chirurgische 279.
— — — elektrische 276.
— — — Heißluft 276.
— — — Massage 276.
— — — medikamentöse 278.
— — — physikalische 276.
— — — Stauung 277.
— — — Strahlen- 277.
— — Blutdruck 256.
— — Calcinosis interstitialis 264.
— — capillar-mikroskopische Beobachtungen 257.
— — Dementia paralytica 261.
— — Demenz, senile 262.
— — Dermatomyositis 261.
— — Diät 276.
— — Diagnose 272f.
— — Dystrophia musculorum progressiva 261.
— — endokrine Störungen 270.
— — Ganglien, sympathische 267.
— — Gangrän 249, 252.
— — s. auch Gangrän.
— — Gefäßerkrankung 259, 270.
— — Gliosis 261.
— — Hämoglobinurie, paroxysmale 260.
— — Halsrippe 262, 273.
— — Hemiplegie 261.
— — hereditäre Disposition 247.
— — Herzerkrankung 259.
— — Hydrocephalus 261.
— — Infektionskrankheiten 248.
— — Kälteschäden 275.

RAYNAUDsche Krankheit, Katatonie 262.
— — Knochen-Veränderung 255.
— — Labyrinthstörungen 256.
— — Lues 249, 259, 274.
— — Magengeschwür 264.
— — Malaria 248.
— — Manie, akute 262.
— — Melancholie 262.
— — Meningitis, luische 261.
— — Nägel 254.
— — Narkolepsie 109.
— — Nerven, periphere, Erkrankungen der 261f., 270.
— — Ödeme 264, 373, 385.
— — Pachymeningitis cervicalis hypertrophica 261.
— — Panaritien 254.
— — Paralysis agitans 261.
— — Pathogenese 268f.
— — pathologische Anatomie 266f.
— — plethysmographische Untersuchungen 257.
— — Poliomyelitis anterior chronica 261.
— — Polyneuritis 273.
— — Pseudobulbärparalyse 261.
— — psychische Erregungen 248.
— — Radiculitis chronica 261.
— — Schrumpfniere 259.
— — Schweißsekretion 255.
— — Sehstörungen 256.
— — Sensibilitätsstörungen, objektive 255.
— — sklerodermatische Veränderungen 254.
— — Sklerose, multiple 261.
— — Speicheldrüsen-Anschwellung 264.
— — Symptomatologie 249f.
— — Tabes 261.
— — Teleangiektasien 264.
— — Tetanie 261.
— — Tränendrüsenanschwellung 264.
— — Traumen 248.
— — trophische Störung 252.
— — Tuberkulose 249.
— — Tumor medullae spinalis 261.
— — vasomotorische Störungen 250.
— — Verlauf 264f.
— — Zentralnervensystem-Erkrankung 262, 270.

Reaktion, neurasthenische s. neurasthenische Reaktion.
RECKLINGHAUSENsche Krankheit 387.
Reflex, bedingter 432, 500.
— neurasthenische Reaktion 461.
— psychophysiologischer 485.
— seelische Ausdruckserscheinungen 500.
— Tonusanfälle 100.
Reflex-Abschwächung 462.
Reflexempfindlichkeit, galvanische 459.
Reflexphänomen, psychogalvanisches (VERAGUTH) 493.
Reflextheorie 199.
Regulationsinstanz des vegetativen Systems 436.
Regulationsschwäche, endogene 441.
Regulationsschwankungen, vegetative Funktionsstörungen innerer Organe 462.
Regulationsstörung, vegetative 457f.
Regurgitieren 518.
REID-HUNT-Reaktion 497.
Reizbare Schwäche 432f., 457.
Reizbarkeit der lebendigen Zelle 431.
— neurasthenische 432.
— übergroße 426, 428.
Reizblase 521.
Reizempfänglichkeit, Störungen der 465.
Reizerscheinungen, motorische 91.
Reizsamkeit, neurasthenische, Folgen 465.
Reizsymptome, Hirnnerven 174.
Reservekräfte 430.
Retention 521.
Rêverie 104.
Reversibilität, Einschlaf- und Tonusanfälle 100.
— und Schlaf 92.
Rheobase 145.
Rhinitis nervosa 515.
Rhythmusstörungen 510.
Ringskotome, flüchtige 459.
Rückbildungsalter und neurasthenische Schädigung 454.
Rührseligkeit und Neurasthenie 465.
Rumination 518.

Sauerstoffmangel der Gewebe 435.
Schauspieleratmung 514.
Schichtneurosen 479.
Schichtstar 151.
Schilddrüse und nervöse Erscheinungen 435.

Schilddrüsentätigkeit, Störungen 284.
Schlaf, Aufbau-Phase 429.
— Hirnschlaf 104.
— Körperschlaf 104.
— Lachen und 104.
— narkoleptischer 89.
— normaler 90.
— Tonusumstellung und 431.
— Überarbeitung 441.
Schlafanfälle 87, 89, 90, 106, 129.
— Calcium 93.
— Coupieren der 90, 100.
— Dauer 93, 101.
— Häufigkeit 93, 101.
— ohne Schlaf 103.
— ohne Tonusverlust 123.
— Provozieren 93.
Schlafbedürfnis 89.
Schlafenzug und Genußmittel 445.
— neurasthenische Reaktion 455.
— psychische Schädigung 451.
Schlafhunger 464.
Schlafkoordination 133.
Schlafsteuerungszentrum, Funktionsanomalien 132.
— Lokalisation des 127, 128.
Schlafstörung, Behebung der 469.
— neurasthenische Reaktion 463f.
— vegetative Regulationsstörung 438.
Schlafsucht 106, 134.
Schlaftrunkenheit 104.
Schlaf-Wachfunktion 485.
— Störungen der 458.
— vegetative Gesamtumstellung 438.
Schlaf-Wachregulation 490.
Schlafzentrum 127, 437.
Schlafzustand, sexuelle Erregung 104.
Schmerz, Einfluß sympathischer Wirkungen 490.
— neurasthenische Reaktion 460.
— vegetatives Nervensystem 436.
Schneider, Krampf bei 529.
Schnupfen, vasomotorischer 376.
Schreck, Erkrankung und 435.
— RAYNAUDsche Krankheit 248.
— Vasomotorium und 449f.
— vitale Person und 439.
Schreckneurosen 463.
Schreibkrampf 524f., 527f.
Schreibunsicherheit, neurotische 528.

Schützengrabenerfrierungen 328.
Schuster, Krampf bei 529.
Schwäche der Leistung 432.
— und neurasthenische Reaktion 428.
— reizbare 432 f.
— — und vegetative Regulationsstörung 438.
Schwächezustände, hyperästhetisch-emotionelle 428, 446.
— postinfektiöse, konstitutionelle Nervosität 455.
Schwindel 187, 188, 460.
Selbststeuerung des Stoffwechsels 430.
Sella turcica, Röntgenbefunde 116 f.
Shock, anaphylaktischer, und experimentelle Vagusreizung 516.
Signalmerkmal, neurotisches 513.
Sinnestäuschungen, optische und Erschöpfungszustand 459.
Sklerodermatische Maske 317.
Sklerodermie 312 f.
— Achylie 325.
— ADDISONsche Krankheit 350.
— Ainhum 357.
— Akroasphyxia chronica 329.
— Akrocyanose 329.
— Akrodermatitis 358.
— Akromikrie 323.
— Akroparästhesien 321.
— Albuminurie 326.
— Alopecia areata 320 f.
— Anämie, perniziöse 315.
— Anatomie, pathologische 344 f.
— Arsen im Urin 326.
— Arsenintoxikation, chronische 312.
— Artikulationsstörungen 325.
— Augenmuskelstörungen 322.
— bandförmige, Naeviszeichnung 329.
— Basedowsche Krankheit 314, 349.
— Behandlung, elektrischer Strom 363.
— — Massage 364.
— — Quarzlichtbestrahlung 363.
— — Röntgenreizbestrahlung der Thymus 363.
— — Sympathektomie, periarterielle 365.
— — Thyrheoidin 361.

Sklerodermie, Blutuntersuchungen 325.
— Blutzuckerwerte 354.
— Brustdrüsen-Atrophie 347.
— Bulbärparalyse 314.
— Calcinosis 350.
— capillaroskopische Untersuchungen 319.
— Cholesterinämie 354.
— Chorea 314.
— circumscripte 356.
— Diagnose 357 f.
— Dermatomyositis 361.
— Digestionsapparat-Störungen 325.
— Drüsen, endokrine 347.
— DUPUYTRENsche Kontraktur 322.
— Dystrophia musculorum progressiva 261, 315.
— en bandes 329.
— en plaques 329.
— Encephalitis 315.
— Epilepsie 314.
— Erkältung 313.
— Facialislähmung 315.
— Fascien 322.
— Fermentationsstörungen 356.
— Fiebersteigerungen 325.
— Gefäßerkrankung 355.
— Gelenke 324.
— Gelenkrheumatismus, chronischer 360.
— Geschwürsbildung 321.
— Glanzhaut 357.
— Glykosurie 326.
— Haarwachstums-Störung 321.
— Hautatrophien, idiopathische 358.
— Hemiatrophia faciei 336.
— Heredität 312.
— Herpes zoster 315.
— Herzerkrankungen 324.
— Hirnwindungen, Sklerosierung von 348.
— Hoden, atrophische 347.
— Hypophyse 347, 351.
— Infantilismus 351.
— Infektionskrankheit 313.
— innere Organe, Erkrankung 347.
— Insuffizienz, pluriglanduläre 351 f.
— Iontophorese 363.
— Kalkablagerungen 323, 354.
— Kataraktentwicklung 350.
— Kehlkopfmuskeln 322.
— Keimdrüsenstörungen 351.
— Knochenaffektionen 323.
— LANGERsche Spaltlinien 329.
— Lepra 357.
— Lymphocytose 325.

Sklerodermie, Mesenchymveranlagung 356.
— Morbus Addissonii 358.
— MORVANsche Krankheit 357.
— Motilitätsstörungen 322.
— Mundhöhle 324.
— Myasthenia gravis pseudoparalytica 315.
— Myélite cavitaire 348.
— Myelitis 314.
— Myokymie 322.
— Mysklerosen 322.
— Myxödem 358.
— Nägelveränderungen 321.
— Nebennieren 347, 350.
— Neurose, funktionelle 314.
— Ödem, QUINCKEsches 328, 358, 373.
— Oesophagus 325.
— Osteosklerosis disseminata 323.
— Ovarium-Fibrose 347.
— Parästhesien 321.
— Paralysis agitans 314, 350.
— Parathyreoidea 347.
— Pathogenese 349.
— Pankreasfermente 356.
— Pigmentation-Veränderungen 318, 319 f.
— Polymyositis subacuta 360.
— Polyneuritis diptherica 314.
— Progeria 351.
— Prognose 344.
— Purinstoffwechsel 354.
— Respirationsstörungen 325.
— Rückenmarkssklerose 348.
— Schilddrüse 326, 347, 349.
— Schleimhäute 324.
— Schweißsekretion 318.
— Schwerhörigkeit 322.
— Sehnenscheiden 322.
— Sensibilitätsstörungen 321.
— Sklerema neonatorum 359.
— Sklerodaktylie 326, 327 f.
— Sklerosierung von Hirnwindungen 348.
— Spinalganglien 348.
— Stadium atrophicum 317.
— — indurativum 317.
— — oedematosum 316.
— STILLsche Krankheit 324.
— Struma 326.
— Sympathicus 348.
— Symptomatologie 316 f.
— Syphilis 313.
— Syringomyelie 315, 357.
— Tabes 314.
— Teleangiektasien 318.
— Temperatur 319.
— Tetanie 350.
— Therapie 361 f.
— Thymusdrüse 351.
— Trauma 314.
— Trophödem 358.

Sklerodermie, Tuberkulose 313.
— Tumor cerebri 314.
— Urticaria 318.
— vitiligoähnliche Erscheinungen 320.
— Zahnfleischatrophie 321.
— Zentralnervensystem-Veränderungen 348.
— Zungenmuskel-Veränderungen 322.
Skleroedema adultorum 360.
Sklerose der Bauchganglien 267.
— multiple, Akroparästhesien 305.
— — Schreibkrampf 526.
Skotom 176, 209.
Somnosie 93.
Somnambulismus und Körperschlaf 103.
Späteklampsie 152 f.
— Epilepsie 153 f.
— KÖZ-Werte 153.
— Übererregbarkeitsphänomene 154.
Spasmophilie, Spätspasmophilie 152 f.
— tetanoide 141 f.
— — Prophylaxe und Therapie 163.
— — s. auch Tetanie, infantile und manifeste infantile.
— im weiteren Sinne 159 f.
— — Absenzen, gehäufte 160.
— — affekt-epileptische Zustände 162.
— — epilamptische Anfälle 162.
— — Epileptoid, psychopathisches beim Kind 162.
— — Friedmannsche Krankheit 161.
— — Krämpfe, psychasthenische 162.
— — Narkolepsie 161.
— — Symptomenkomplex, orthostatisch-epileptoider 161.
— — Wegbleiben junger Kinder 162.
Späteunuchoidismus 352.
Speichelstockung 518.
Spina bifida, Trophödem 395.
Spontangangrän 274.
Sprachstörung 178, 192, 524.
Stammeln 529.
Starre, kataleptische 94.
Status eclampticus s. Spasmophilie 147.
— epilepticus s. Epilepsie.
— hemicranicus s. Migräne.

Stigmatisierte, echte 495.
— vegetative 426, 458, 482, 484, 489, 505.
— — Begriff 457.
— — Schilddrüsenhormone 497.
Stimmritzenkrampf 145.
Stimmung und innere Sekretion 437.
— des Neurasthenischen 465.
Stimmungsgifte 445.
Stoffwechsel, innere Selbststeuerung 430.
Stoffwechselausgleich, Assimilation 431.
Stoffwechselzentren 484.
Stottern 524 f., 527.
— Behandlung 531.
— echte Neurose 526.
— extrapyramidale Anlageschwäche 531.
— induziertes 530.
— Organminderwertigkeit 530.
— physiologisches 530.
— und Stammeln 529.
Sturzanfälle, narkoleptische 94.
Suggestion und Magensekretion 488.
Suggestive Beeinflussungen und psychophysische Abhängigkeiten 487.
Symbolcharakter der Funktionsstörung 505.
Symbolfunktion 500.
Sympathektomie 279, 299.
Sympathicolabilität, Typus einer 496.
Sympathicotonie, Begriff der 263, 492.
Sympathicus 481.
Sympathicusläsionen und Suggestionen 490.
Sympathicuswirkung und Bewußtseinsniveau 485.
— ergotropes Prinzip 486.
Synkope, lokale 251, 264.
Syringomyelie, Akroasphyxia chronica 285.
— Hemihypertrophie 342.
— Ödeme, neurotische 392.
— Raynaudsche Krankheit 272.
System, vegetatives, Nekrose 311.

Tabes 230, 293, 305, 310, 314.
Tachypnoë 514.
Tänzerinnen, Krampf bei 529.
Teleangiostenose 346.
Telegraphistenkrampf 529.
Temperament, galliges 519.
Tetanie, akzidentelle 156.
— angeborene 155.

Tetanie, Atmungs- 157.
— beim Erwachsenen 154.
— Bicarbonat- 157.
— Epilepsie 47, 153, 158.
— Forme fruste der 495, 503.
— Guanidin- 157.
— Hyperventilations- 157.
— infantile, Apnoë 146.
— — Begriff 141.
— — Bronchotetanie 149.
— — Chronaxiemessung 145.
— — Chvosteksches Phänomen 142.
— — Erbsches Phänomen 143.
— — Facialisphänomen 142.
— — Geburtshelferhandstellung 143, 148.
— — Gelegenheitskrämpfe 147.
— — Herztetanie 150.
— — KÖZ-Werte 144 f.
— — Krämpfe, allgemeine 147.
— — Latenzzustand 142 f.
— — manifeste 145 f.
— — Mors subita infantum 146.
— — Ödeme 151.
— — Peroneusphänomen 143.
— — Pfötchenhand 148.
— — Prolsches Phänomen 143.
— — Prüfung der elektrischen Übererregbarkeit 143.
— — Schichtstar 151.
— — Schlesingersches Zeichen 143.
— — Schultzesche Variante des Facialphänomens 142.
— — Status eclampticus 147.
— — Stimmritzenkrampf 145.
— — trophische Störungen 141.
— — Trousseausches Phänomen 143, 148, 153.
— — Übererregbarkeit, elektrische 143.
— — — thermische 145.
— jahreszeitliche Verteilung der Tetaniefälle 155.
— latente, älterer Kinder 154.
— — Differentialdiagnose 159.
— Magen- 157.
— Ödem, Quinckesches 386.
— Parästhesien 141.
— parathyreoprive 157.
— persistente 151.
— Phosphat- 157.
— Prognose 157, 158.
— puerile 142, 152.

Sachverzeichnis.

Tetanie, Rachitis 156.
— Verlauf 151f.
— s. auch Spasmophilie, Späteklampsie.
Tetaniegesicht 148.
Tetaniezähne 151.
Thalamus, Affekt 98.
Thrombangitis obliterans 297.
Thyreoidismus 435.
Thyreotische, konstitutionell 496.
Thyreotoxikosen und nervöse Erscheinungen 435.
Tiefenperson 437, 484.
Tonusumstellung und Schlaf 431.
Tonusveränderungen, angeborene, Schreibkrampf 525.
Tonusverlust, abortiver 99.
— affektiver, Aggression 96.
— — Calciumschwankung 101.
— — Definition 131.
— — Lokalisation 128.
— — Narkolepsie 94.
— — ohne Schlafanfälle 123.
— — Ursache 97, 98.
— nichtaffektiver, spontaner, Anfälle 102.
— paradoxer 132.
— partieller 99.
Tonusverlust-Anfall, Affekte 95.
— Coupieren 100.
— Dauer 101.
— Häufigkeit 101.
— Reversibilität 100.
— Schlafanfall 92, 102.
Tonusverlust-Äquivalente 99.
Tonusverschiebungen im vegetativen System 430.
Training, autogenes 507.
— — Bronchialasthma 517.
Trauma 314, 331.
Tremor, neurasthenischer 461.
Triebe und Antrieb 465.
Trophoedème chronique héréditaire 394f.
Trophödem 394f.
Typenaufstellung (W. JAENSCH) 482.
Typus hemifacioscapulohumero-thoracicus 335.

Überarbeitung, geistige und Schlaf 441.
Überempfindlichkeit, krankhafte 431f., 438, 458.
— der Sinnesorgane 460.
Übererregbarkeit des Vestibularisapparats 460.
Übermüdung 429f.
— und Erschöpfung 441.
Übermüdungsschlaf, corticaler 89.
Ulcérés à crises tabiformes 518.
Ulcus duodeni 518.
— pylori 518.
Umstellung, Affektursache 98.
Urin, spastischer 174.
Urobilinogen im Urin 435.
Urogenitalsystem 510f.
Urticaria, emotive Einflüsse 522.
— Hautgangrän, multiple, neurotische 320.
— QUINCKEsches Ödem 373, 384, 390.
— Sklerodermie 318.

Vaginismus 522.
Vagotonie 482, 484, 496.
— Konstitutionstypen 495.
Vagotoniker, Schlafsuchtneigung 134.
Vagotonisches Verhalten der Vasomotoren und Narkolepsie 135.
Vagus, Doppelinnervation 481.
Vagusreizung, Bronchialmuskelkrampf 516.
Variante, SCHULTZEsche des Facialisphänomens 142.
Vasomotorium und körperlich-seelische Erschöpfung 457.
Vegetativ-nervöse Regulationsstörung 457f.
Vegetative Funktionen, Beeinflussung, seelische 489f.
— — Einfluß seelischer Vorgänge 485.
Vegetatives Nervensystem und Schmerzen 436.
— System, Begriff 436.

Vegetatives System, biologische und psychologische Situation 493.
— — und Erschöpfung 438.
— — Funktionen des Organismus 430.
Verdauungsfunktionen, Affekteinfluß, suggerierter 487.
Verdauungssystem, Neurosen 518f.
Verstimmung 465, 490.
— vegetative Regulationsstörung 438.
Vertäubung 460.
Vitale Person, Schreck 439.
— — Störungen der gesamten vitalen Person 463.
Vitales Syndrom 437f., 453.
Vitalgefühle, Aufbau von 491.

Wachanfälle 102, 104f., 133.
Wachen, Tätigkeit 429.
Wachzentrum 130.
Wärmeregulation und Suggestion 489.
Wärmereiz, Migräne 227.
Warzen 523.
Wasserhaushalt und suggestiver Einfluß 489.
Wegbleiben, spasmophiles 162.

Xerostomie 518.

Yogha 507.

Zentren, vegetative 484.
Zittern, Erblichkeit des 461.
— myoneurasthenisches 461.
Zivilisation, neurasthenische Reaktion 433, 455.
Zwischenhirn, affektive Erregung 484.
— regulative Funktionen 449.
Zwischenhirnsyndrom, STERTZsches 438.
Zwischen-Mittelhirn, Regulationsinstanz 436.
— Regulationsstörungen 439.
— vitale Person 437.

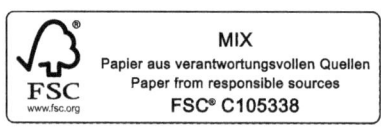

If you have any concerns about our products,
you can contact us on
ProductSafety@springernature.com

In case Publisher is established outside the EU,
the EU authorized representative is:
**Springer Nature Customer Service Center GmbH
Europaplatz 3, 69115 Heidelberg, Germany**

Printed by Libri Plureos GmbH
in Hamburg, Germany